Targeted & Controlled Drug Delivery

Novel Carrier Systems

Targeted & Controlled Drug Delivery

Novel Carrier Systems

S.P. Vyas
M.Pharm., Ph.D.
Post doc. (University of London, UK)
Professor (Pharm. Biotechnology), Deptt. of Pharmaceutical Sciences
Dean, Faculty of Technology
Dr. H. S. Gour University, Sagar (M.P.)

R.K. Khar
M.Pharm., D.B.M., Ph.D. (Sofia)
Professor & Head, Department of Pharmaceutics
Hamdard University, New Delhi

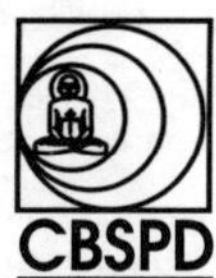

CBSPD

CBS Publishers & Distributors Pvt Ltd

New Delhi • Bengaluru • Chennai • Kochi • Kolkata • Lucknow • Mumbai
Gujarat • Hyderabad • Jharkhand • Nagpur • Patna • Pune • Uttarakhand

Targeted & Controlled
Drug Delivery
Novel Carrier Systems

ISBN-13: 978-81-239-0799-4

First Edition: 2002

Reprint: 2004, 2006, 2007, 2008, 2010, 2011, 2012, 2013, 2016, 2019, 2024, **2026**

Published by **Satish Kumar** Jain and Produced by **Varun Jain** for
CBS Publishers & Distributors Pvt Ltd
4819/XI Prahlad Street, 24 Ansari Road, Daryaganj, New Delhi 110 002, India.
Ph: 011-23289259, 23266861, 23266867 Fax: 011-23243014 Website: www.cbspd.com
e-mail: delhi@cbspd.com; cbspubs@airtelmail.in.

Corporate Office: 204 FIE, Industrial Area, Patparganj, Delhi 110 092, India
Ph: 011-4934 4934 Fax: 011-4934 4935 e-mail: publishing@cbspd.com; publicity@cbspd.com

Branches

- **Bengaluru:** Seema House 2975, 17th Cross, KR Road, Banasankari 2nd Stage, Bengaluru 560 070, Karnataka, India
  Ph: +91-80-26771678/79 Fax: +91-80-26771680 e-mail: bangalore@cbspd.com
- **Chennai:** 18/8B, Subbaraya Street, Shenoy Nagar, Chennai 600 030, Tamil Nadu, India
  Ph: +91-044-42032115, 044-26681266 e-mail: chennai@cbspd.com
- **Kochi:** 42/1325, 1326, Power House Road, Opp KSEB, Power House, Ernakulum Kochi 682 018, Kerala, India
  Ph: +91-484-4059061-65,67 Fax: +91-484-4059065 e-mail: kochi@cbspd.com
- **Kolkata:** 147, Hind Ceramics Compound, 1st Floor, Nilgunj Road, Belghoria, Kolkata-700056, West Bengal, India
  Ph: +033-25633055, 033-25633056 e-mail: kolkata@cbspd.com
- **Lucknow:** Basement, Khushnuma Complex, 7 Meerabai Marg (Behind Jawahar Bhawan), Lucknow-226001, UP, India
  Ph: +0522-4000032 e-mail: tiwari.lucknow@cbspd.com
- **Mumbai:** PWD Shed, Gala no 25/26, Ramchandra Bhatt Marg, Next to JJ Hospital Gate no. 2, Opp. Union Bank of India, Noorbaug, Mumbai-400009, Maharashtra, India
  Ph: 022-66661880/89 e-mail: mumbai@cbspd.com

Representatives

• Gujarat • Hyderabad • Jharkhand • Nagpur • Patna • Pune • Uttarakhand

For trade terms please contact customercare@cbspd.com
For general enquiries please contact info@cbspd.com

Printed at Glorious Printers, Jhilmil Industrial Area, Delhi, India

Preface

The present book "Targeted and Controlled Drug Delivery (Novel Carrier Systems)" is a concise and systematic presentation of concepts, and carrier(s), which could be used for controlled and targeted drug delivery at various levels of precision. Obviously, its first and foremost emphasis is on the significance of cell and molecular biology. The science of targeted drug delivery is burgeoning with new information and explosive out growth of technology and methodologies in this area. However, update of the recent developments and content remains to be central aim. It was resultant of long ranged sightness of Paul Ehrlich, who in early 20th century imaginated this "magic bullet" concept. Where a carrier system was proposed to simply carry the drug to its site of action and releasing it selectively while non-target sites should absolutely be exempted from drug effect. He coined the term "Magic bullet" for this event of selective drug delivery.

In the realm of targeted drug delivery, the parallel developments in allied sciences has casted a distinctive and formidable influence. Advances in recombinant technology and protein engineering offer possibilities of customized molecular design of protein/peptide drugs. Such advances not only help in elucidating drug biovagaries behaviour or cellular uptake or role of receptor and ligands but they would also assist greatly in engineering miniaturized molecular drug delivery devices. In such systems, molecule will contain in built navigation devices, homing component (ligand) and ferrying units (to negotiate or promote cellular fusion or uptake) in addition to potent pharmacodynamically effective group(s). Chemical modification(s) can be incorporated to improve in vivo stability and site selectivity. The synthetic analogues particularly retrospecific soft prodrugs are unique example of such advancements. Targeted controlled drug delivery in principle attempts to maximize therapeutic effect while curtail down contraindicative manifestation discernibly by delivering drug to or bringing it to the site (in therapeutically appropriate concentration) where it is needed.

The algorithm of drug carrier systems designed, developed and being epitomized and emergence of various concepts have honed and redefined the science of targeted drug delivery. The progress has animated the ephemeral dream by making it a practicable reality. The targeted drug delivery as a concept offers a rational method, to treat various diseases including, cancer, AIDS, infectious diseases, enzyme deficiencies, genetic disorders, etc.

The most effective central paradigm are receptor ligand interaction and mediated intracellular launch of carrier(s) for cytosolic intracellular drug delivery and they have provided new impetus to the concept. Targeted drug delivery functionally plunges upon an appropriate carrier system.

Carriers serve to negotiate specialized delivery functions through an ability intrinsic or acquired through incorporated instructions. Alternatively, extracorporeal administration form loci of localized reserves based on microspheres or nanoparticles from intelligent polymeric systems. Bioinspired and stimulant sensitive carriers provide means for drug release pulsation and modulation. The vast and variegated knowledge helps in engineering various purpose defined site specific customized carrier(s) including liposomes, niosomes, bioconjugates, chemical drug delivery systems, resealed erythrocytes, nanoparticles, microspheres, etc.

An overview on essentials of targeted drug delivery covering receptor ligand role in cellular uptake, phagocytosis, bioligands, differential expression of receptors, biochemistry of disease site, biobehaviour of carriers and other bioevents, which are critical in defining the ultimate destination of a carrier unit in body is a necessary prelude for proper understanding of strategy based drug targeting. Section I of the book is consisted of chapters on introduction to parenteral drug delivery, essentials of targeted drug delivery, chemical drug delivery systems and bioconjugate based systems for targeted drug delivery. Section II is comprised of colloidal carriers detailed in chapters on liposomes, niosomes, nanoparticles, microspheres, resealed erythrocytes, submicron emulsions, multiple emulsions and magnetically modulated drug delivery. Section III deals with applied targeted controlled drug delivery and it is consisted of chapters on drug delivery to brain, delivery to tumour and bone marrow targeting.

The book possesses and backs some more than 1500 references, 372 schematics and 103 tables. The chapters are structured in such a way that basic concepts, methodologies, applications and future perspectives give systemic understanding of subject where schematics explain the concepts for better retrieve. Furthermore, exhaustive update of subject is tabulated which provides a concise reference resource. The topics deal with carrier composites, which are most intensively studied and established. Thus it serves both as a text book as well as reference resource.

We wish to express our sincere gratitude to many research workers, whose findings we abridged and blended together to present a balanced and content rich overview of the subject. The text opens up deep details of processes of preparation, which could be of high benefit to industrial pharmacists. Contents are useful source of course material to post graduate students, research scholars and institutional scientists.

We are thankful to Mr. Vaibhav Sihorkar, Mr. Vivek Mishra, Ms. Preeti Venugopalan, Mr. Paramjit Singh, Mr. Sanyog Jain, Mr. Prabakaran D., Mr. Rajendra Pratap Singh, Mr. Amit Rawat and Mr. Praveen Dubey for their continual help in keying the manuscript, proof reading and skilful drawing of figures. We thank our families for their sincere support, patience and sparing us of responsibilities. We thankfully acknowledge various sources for basic ideas, landmark contributions and contents. The expert assistance and quality publication of this book by Mr. Satish Jain and Mr. Vinod Jain of CBS Publishers, New Delhi are sincerely acknowledged. We welcome suggestions from students, teachers and researchers, which will help improving the volume in future.

S. P. Vyas
R. K. Khar

Contents

Expanded Contents

SECTION I
General Considerations & Biochemical Concepts

SECTION II
Carrier Concepts in Drug Delivery

9. Nanoparticles 331-386

SECTION III
Site-Specific Drug Delivery

SECTION I

GENERAL CONSIDERATIONS AND BIOCHEMICAL CONCEPTS

CHAPTER 1

Introduction to Parenteral Drug Delivery

- Introduction
- Liposomes
- Niosomes
- Nanoparticles and microspheres
- Solid lipid nanoparticles
- Hydrogel nanoparticles
- Microparticles
- Long circulating microparticulates
- Specialized emulsions
- Multiple emulsions
- Emulsome™
- Long circulatory emulsions
- Resealed erythrocytes
- Supramolecular biovectors
- Lipoproteins
- Cyclodextrins
- Prodrugs
- Polymeric micelles
- Aquasomes
- Dendrimer
- Implant systems
- Systems for non-invasive systemic administration
- Conclusion
- References

Parenteral drug delivery seeks to optimize therapeutic index by providing immediate drug to the systemic pool in required quantity to treat emergency clinical episode(s) such as cardiac attack(s), respiratory arrests or to administer drugs which are extensively sampled and extracted or metabolized before reaching the systemic circulation. It is an ultimate requirement in the management of acute cases. Moreover, in the cases where colloidal carrier(s) are required to remain in vascular compartment or to be transported to a site in the body, the parenteral administration is inevitable. It is obvious, that the systems should possess optimal size and characteristics so as to negotiate desirable pharmacodynamic effects in a well defined manner. The body possesses a simile with typical water supplying system where blood rushes to traverse entire body through vascular conduits and may serve to carry drug(s)-containing carrier to the various locus of the body.

The parenteral drug delivery is mainly meant for drug concentration maintenance in systemic pool or other site of action(s). The release pattern from such systems may be, to sustain the pharmacodynamic effect or to target the drug at the site of its action. Moreover, some specialized autoregulatory circulating bioreactor like systems could also be customized for parenteral drug delivery. The delivery systems are drug carrier or conjugate system or may be prodrugs or chemical drug delivery systems. The target-oriented systems are generally programmed to release the contents at target bystander or intratarget locus or molecular levels. The drug is delivered in an explosive burst fashion or following a controlled or regulated release pattern. In the latter case drug release regulation could be monitored through bioresponsive behaviour of the system or it may be modulated from some external level using appropriate physical means, i.e. pH variation, magnetic field application or photo irradiation, etc.

The carrier systems are invariably ought to be colloidal stable dispersions of particulate or cellular materials. Classification of various parenterally administered colloidal carrier systems are schematically depicted in Figure 1-1. The parenteral drug delivery is affected through various routes of administration, which have a little in common other than the fact that invariably each route needs a hypodermal needle to inject the drug or delivery system in to the body. The drug delivery systems customized for parenteral administration in practice avoid or by pass a number of physiological and anatomical barriers. This entails for imposition of more rigorous constraints on compositions and preparation methodologies used. The most important routes for parenteral drug administration include intravenous and intramuscular, while subcutaneous being most preferred for vaccine(s) administration. Intravenous administration specially offers some distinctive advantages such as rapidity of action and direct administration of drug that allows physicians for dose titration at individual patient level. It results in much more predictable route related drug response and many drugs due to their biosusceptibility can not be administered through other route(s). Furthermore, delivery of drug can be monitored for release rate modulation, modification or termination. The preparations in real sense and terms should be free of any microbial load. It could preferably be achieved by using terminal sterilization. The latter in practice is attempted using autoclaving, however in the case of formulations based on thermosensitive and thermolabile materials terminal gamma rays irradiation or millipore filtration may with equal effects be adopted. In situations, where terminal sterilization does not work; it is advised that formulation using prefiltered materials be prepared in a fully aseptic environment. Furthermore, the solution or suspension must be compatible with the blood in regard to pH and tonicity. The preparation(s) with different pH should however ensure that on administration drug or carrier precipitation or peptization would not occur. The *in vivo* behaviour

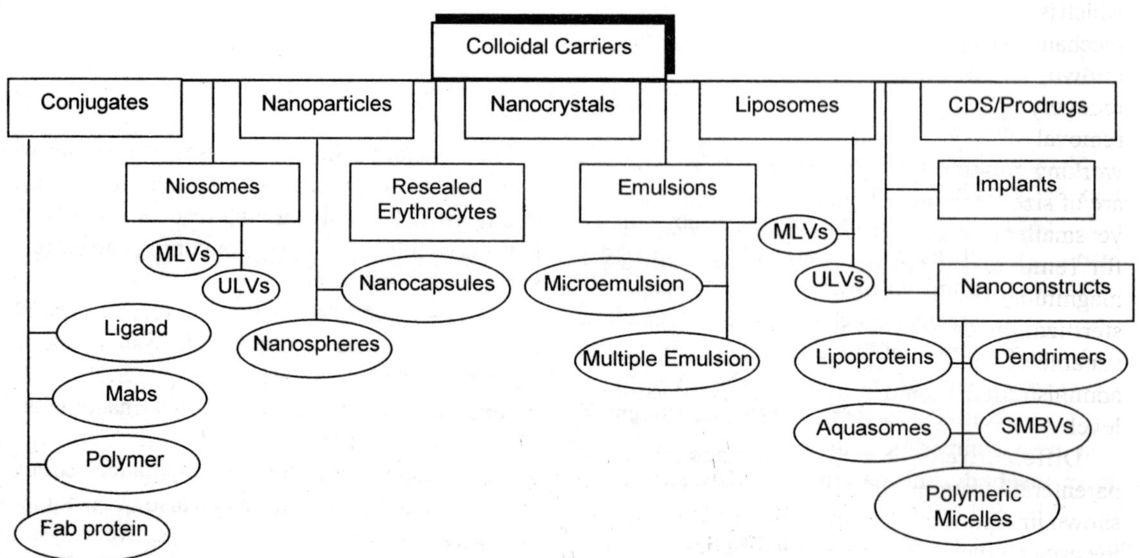

Fig. 1-1. Classification of Parenterally Administered Colloidal Carrier Systems

and instability of carrier composite may drastically affect over all disposition kinetics of drug in an unpredictable manner.

The parenteral drug delivery systems (PDDS) need to meet the basic requirements of parenteral products, i.e. sterility, apyrogenicity, reproducibility in performance, safety and efficacy. Methods of sterilization used are often the same, i.e. dry heat, moist heat, radiation and chemical means. However, every component of drug delivery device is ought to be sincerely scrutinized for effect of sterilization process on stability of the component and resultant effect on the formulation. It should also be considered, whether substitution of component would alleviate the problem or not. Similarly, a new possible option should be rigorously screened for its implications on the finished product. It appears that most of the colloidal dispersions are highly susceptible to heat and suffer peptization or aggregation. Therefore, ionization radiation in proper dose, which ensures absolute killing of microbial bioburden and also consoles and accounts for susceptibility of biotechnological drugs, should be used. The irradiation sterilization, however provides opportunity for graded approach, which could titre the precise dose of radiation optimum for complete killing of microorganisms. Furthermore, added to the existing problems, is the issue of bacterial 'death', which is defined as ceasing to exist. However, survival mechanisms devised by bacteria and viruses are now known, which raise an alarm in regard to their recovery of functionality. Nevertheless, complete removal of bioburden via aseptic filtration may offer working solution to the problem. Most of bacteria are of size larger than 1 μm but spherical forms are yet smaller in size. Therefore, the size range selected for removal should be at least three orders of magnitude, i.e. from 50 nm to 50 μm. Thus light sterilization or aseptic processing are seemingly suitable options. The products meant for parenteral administration should claim full sterility assurance level.

Different release mechanisms and biofate of parenterally administered systems are schematically shown in Figure 1-2. On intravenous administration the drug delivery systems traverse and span vascular compartment through pulmonary, systemic and tissue circulation. Oxygenated blood is pumped by left side of the heart through the aorta to body tissues. The deoxygenated blood from tissues is collected through veins and post vena cava in to the right part of the heart. It is then pumped through pulmonary vein to lungs for oxygenation. The circulation thus indicated the possible course of colloidal carrier(s) if they are not allowed to extravasate. The particles, which are sufficiently small to pass the pulmonary capillaries return to heart and circulated to tissues. Particles larger in size which escape pulmonary filter, are mechanically deposited in the capillaries or captured mainly by macrophages. The inflamed centres with excessive infiltrated macrophages thus become sites selectively traceable. Discontinuous basement membrane gives rise to small pores into endothelium. These are referred to as fenestrae with diameter from 30 nm to 100 nm. The particles smaller then 100 nm size escape circulation and taken up by hepatocytes. The capillaries of these organs are lined with active macrophages called Kupffer cells thus majority of particles escaping circulation for sequestration and retention by liver accumulate in Kupffer cells. The actively capturing system of liver is termed as reticuloendothelial system. Therefore, it is appreciated that to reach extravascular compartment the carrier must avoid opsonization and should be small enough in size. Furthermore, to be actively targetable it should be customized for site specificity using appropriate ligands. The release of drug may follow various patterns. The bystander explosive release is well exemplified by target sensitive immunoliposomes. The system typically based on conventional lipid with a derivatized lipid component; i.e. phosphatidylethylamine lined site specific immunoglobulin (PE-IgG). This conjugate participates in film structuring. On reaching the target under preferential affinity for target the PE-IgG mesogens laterally a partition leaving the vesicle leaky thus dumping the contents in the vicinity of target.

Cytosolic sustained drug release is based on strategy where a carrier construct enters a cellular target via receptor mediated endocytosis and categorically changes the pH of endosome. Due to change in pH the carrier loaded endosome does not fuse with lysosome thus remains as a cargo and

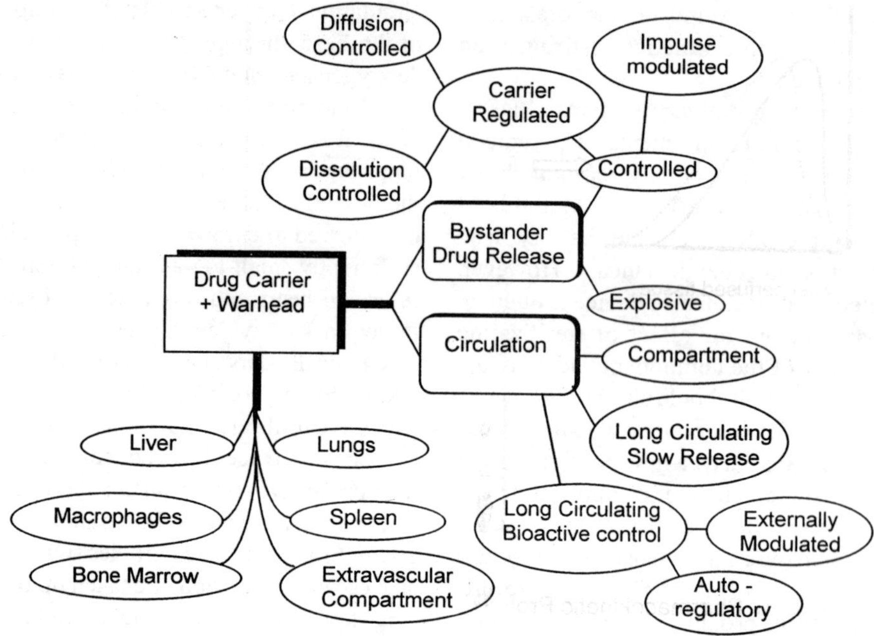

Fig. 1-2. Release Profile(s) and Biofate of Intravenously Administered System

releases drug contents slowly in to the cytosol(s). While another class of drug colloidal carrier(s) exploits or manipulates pH of endo-lysosomes and carrier unit leaks intact in to the cytosol. Thus it serves to constitute a cytosolic intracellular cargo for drug, which releases the contents in a controlled manner.

The targeted drug delivery to extracellular compartment is only possible following extravasation of carrier, and also the system should be engineered properly to span entire body, avoiding RES uptake to reach the site successfully, where it is retained due to receptor-ligand interaction. The circulating carrier could be arrested by site-specific ligands for ECM or cellular receptors.

Similarly, on intramuscular administration preferably in to deltoid, triceps, pectoral, and vastus lateralis muscles, the systemic availability depends on drug perfusion or diffusion in to the blood vascular system. Thus degree of site perfusion, nature of blood capillaries and volume of administered dose may affect drug diffusion (Fig. 1-3). Other than these, drug related paramter(s) might equivocally affect systemic availability of drug(s). The biofate of intramuscularly administered systems is schematically shown in Figure 1-4.

In order to construct and modify the pharmacokinetic behaviour and to maximize the therapeutic indices of drug(s) there have been intense renewed interests in the development of drug delivery systems. The therapeutic system engineered for the purpose provides manipulative modifications in therapeutic index vis-à-vis duration of activity. As it is known for controlled and novel drug delivery, they have various alternative route(s) of administration. The field of drug delivery and targeting has been revolutionized with the advent of a plethora of carrier systems that can be used either parenterally, topically, orally or by implantation. However, parenteral drug delivery remains the leading area of research, which led to the development of sophisticated systems that allow drug targeting and the sustained or controlled release of parenteral medicines. Figure 1-5 is showing possible release patterns obtained from parenterally administered systems. Intravenous and intraarterial administration particularly exploit blood as vehicle for transportation of carrier to the site(s). The colloidal

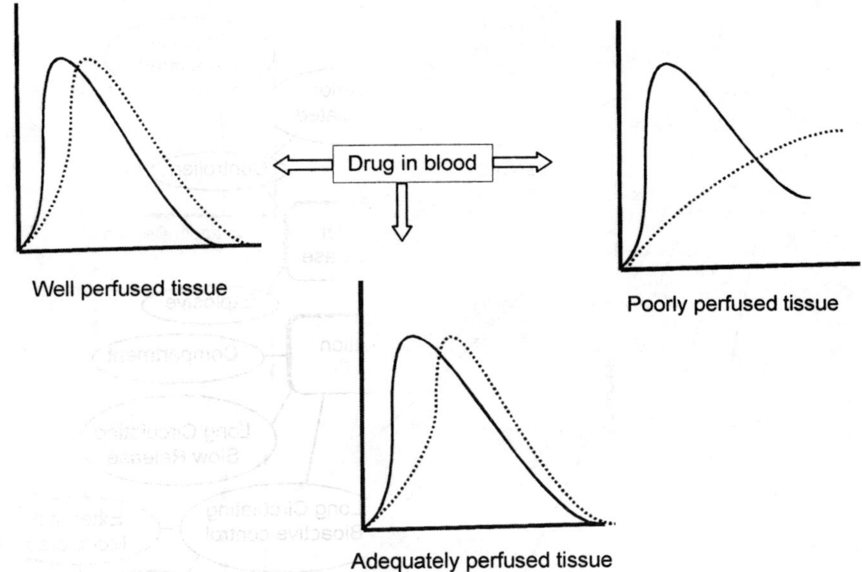

Fig. 1-3. Pharmacokinetic Profiles of drugs in Tissues of Varying Perfusion

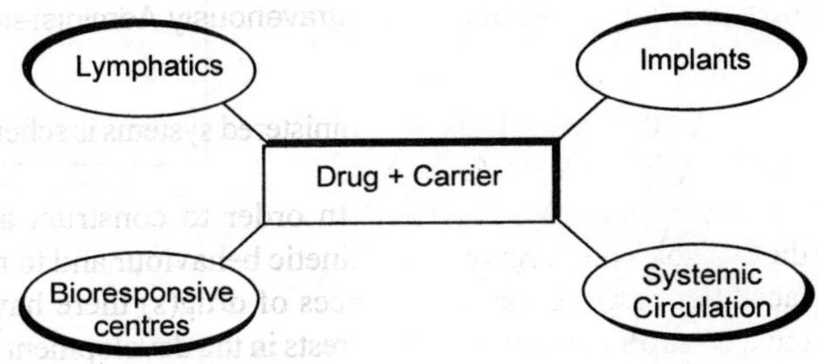

Fig. 1-4. Biofate of Intramuscularly Administered System

carrier may remain in vascular compartment as long circulating unit for controlled and prolonged drug release. The major carrier systems employed for drug delivery and site-specific drug targeting is tabulated (Table 1-1).

LIPOSOMES

Basically, liposomes are resultant of self-assembly of phospholipid molecules in an aqueous environment. The amphiphilic phospholipid molecules form a closed bilayer sphere in an attempt to shield their hydrophobic groups from the aqueous environment while still maintaining contact with the aqueous phase via the hydrophilic head group. The resulting closed spheres may encapsulate aqueous soluble drugs within the central aqueous compartment or lipid soluble drugs within the bilayer membrane. Alternatively, lipid soluble drugs may be complexed with cyclodextrins and subsequently encapsulated within the liposome aqueous compartment. The encapsulation within/or association of drugs with liposomes may alter drug pharmacokinetics, which may be exploited to achieve targeted therapies. Thus alteration of the liposome surfaces, and their further modifications are some of the requisites of optimized liposomal drug targeting.

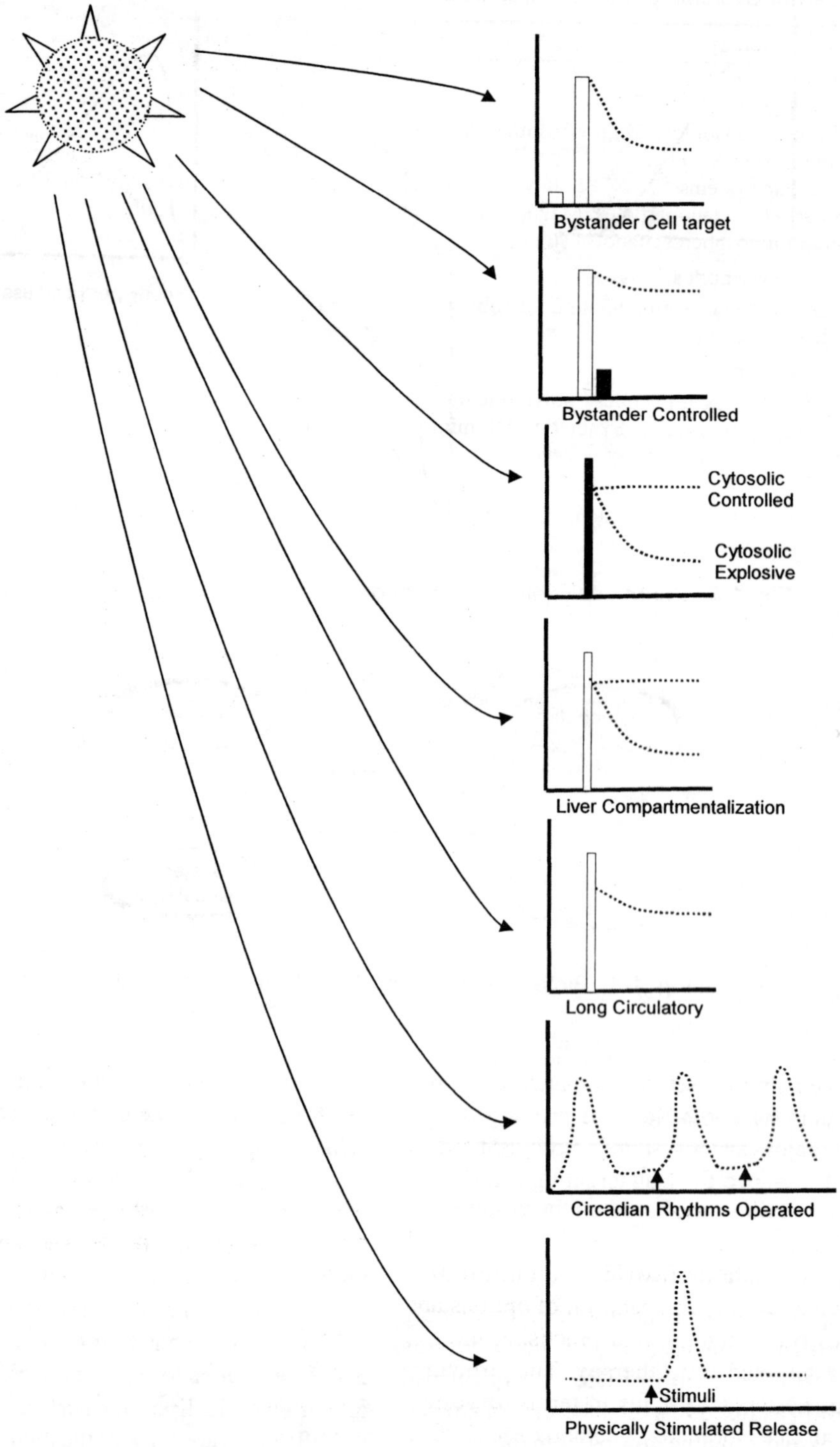

Bystander Cell target

Bystander Controlled

Cytosolic Controlled

Cytosolic Explosive

Liver Compartmentalization

Long Circulatory

Circadian Rhythms Operated

Stimuli

Physically Stimulated Release

Fig. 1-5. Schematic Showing Various Release Pattern(s) of Parenteral Drug Delivery Systems

Table 1-1. Carrier Systems Used For Targeted Drug Delivery

Drug delivery technology	Possible applications
Colloidal carriers Vesicular systems Liposomes; Niosomes; Pharmacosomes; Virosomes; Immunoliposomes Microparticulate systems Microparticles; Nanoparticles; Magnetic microspheres; Albumin microspheres; nanocapsules	Passive tumour targeting; Vaccine adjuvants, Passive targeting to lung endothelium in gene delivery, Targeting to regional lymph nodes, Targeting to cell surface ligands in various organs/areas of pathology, Sustained release depot at point of injection
Cellular carrier Resealed erythrocytes; serum albumin; antibodies; platelets; leukocytes	Passive targeting to liver tropics, enzyme replacement therapy and lysosomal storage diseases, as red cell substitute
Supramolecular delivery systems Micelles; reverse; mixed micelles; polymeric micelles; Liquid crystals; Lipoproteins; Synthetic LDL mimicking particles (supramolecule biovector system)	Passive targeting
Specialized emulsion system Multiple emulsions, microemulsions, lipid emulsions	Tumour targeting, Lipophilic drug administration vehicles, Targeting to cell surface antigens
Polymer based systems Signal sensitive; Mucoadhesive; Biodegradable; Bioerodible; Soluble synthetic polymeric carriers; Polymer (Poly-L-lysine)-drug conjugate	Localised depot systems for the treatment of infections and cancers, Sustained drug release systemic therapies
Bioconjugates including immunoconjugates Mabs; Immunological Fab fragments; antibody-enzyme complex & bispecific Abs; Immunotoxins, rCD4 conjugates	Site specific delivery
Prodrugs Prodrugs, ADEPT, VDEPT, GDEPT	Organ targeting, absorption enhancement, taste masking
Implant system	Controlled delivery of bioactives
Needle free injections	Decreased pain on injection, Increased bioavailability of intradermal vaccines
Others Aquasomes, Cochleates, Cyclodextrins	Lipophilic drug solubilization for parenteral use
Macromolecular carriers Glycoproteins; neo glycoproteins and Artificial Viral Envelope (AVE)	For antigen and DNA delivery
Lectins and polysaccharides	For targeted drug delivery

Vaious classes of liposome based on the vesicle type are shown in Figure 1-6.

The liposome and niosome technologies especially have provided a spectrum of options and opportunities for designing and practising the site specific and targeted drug therapy. The structural versatility of vesicular systems in terms of vesicle size, shape, surface morphology, composition, surface charge and bilayer fluidity; the ability to incorporate a wide range of drugs; or to carry cell-specific ligands could be exploited for clinical and therapeutic benefits.

Liposomes in Intracellular Infections

The intracellular pathogenic tropics are difficult biolocuses to treat due to drug or carrier related reasons. However, liposomes demonstrated appreciable potential and promises to overcome these

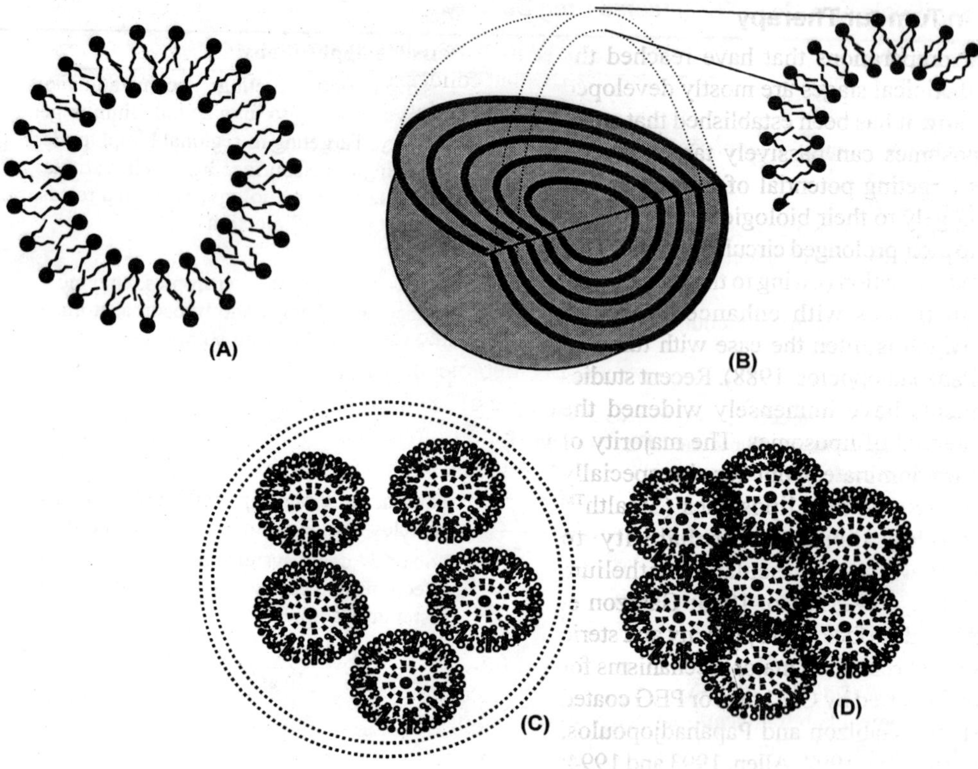

Fig. 1-6. Liposomes (A) Unilamellar Vesicle, (B) Multilamellar Vesicle, (C) Vesicle within Vesicle and (D) Multivesicular Liposomes

impediments and to make therapy possible. Liposome mediated treatment of fungal, viral, bacterial and protozoal infections takes the advantage of the natural targeting of liposomes to the RES-predominant organs and their "lysosomotropism" and "parasitotropism" (Vyas, 2001). The ability of liposomes to be taken up by macrophages and to concentrate in the liver and spleen undoubtedly makes them ideal for the treatment of diseases of the liver and spleen, such as leishmaniasis.

In the immunocompromised patients, the incidence of systemic fungal infections are more. Although parenteral amphotericin B (Amp B) displays an array of toxic and side effects, it is still the drug of choice in the majority of invasive fungal infections. The therapeutic index of Amp B has been improved by its incorporation in lipid carriers, which decrease Amp B toxicity (Hiemenz and Walsh, 1996; Wasan and Lopez-Berestein, 1998). Several lipid formulations of Amp B have been approved and are available commercially. These include AmBisome™ (Nexstar, Boulder, CO, USA), Abelect™ (The Liposome Company, Princeton, NJ, USA), Fungizone® (Bristol Myers-Squibb, Woerden, The Netherlands) and Amphotec™ (Sequus Pharmaceuticals, Merlo, CA, USA).

Similarly, targeting to lung has become a possible proposition by using O-stearoyl amylopectin and polyoxyethylene or monosialoganglioside coated liposomes. The encapsulation of the anti-tubercular agent rifampicin or isoniazid in liposomes, modulates the toxicity and improves the efficacy of these drugs. To summarise, liposomes by passively targeting the liver and spleen and also by actively targeting the lung have been shown to improve the efficacy and modulate the toxicity of certain anti-infectives.

Liposomes in Tumour Therapy

The liposomal preparations that have reached the preclinical and clinical stages are mostly developed for cancer therapy. It has been established that small and stable liposomes can passively target several tumours. This targeting potential of liposomes can be attributed largely to their biological stability and subsequently to their prolonged circulation time. This enables their extravasation (owing to their small size, 50-150 nm) in tissues with enhanced vascular permeability, which is often the case with tumours (Gabijon and Papahadjopoulos, 1988). Recent studies and developments have immensely widened the therapeutic potential of liposomes. The majority of the strategies predominately opt for the specially engineered long-circulatory liposomes (Stealth™ liposomes) having increased probability to extravasate to the tumour vascular endothelium (Woodle and Lasic, 1992; Allen, 1994; Gabizon et al., 1997). Increased surface hydrophilicity and steric hindrance, however remain as major mechanisms for long circulation imparted by GM1 and/or PEG coated liposomal systems (Gabizon and Papahadjopoulos, 1992; Woodle and Lasic, 1992; Allen, 1993 and 1994; Allen et al., 1998). The hydrophilicity contributed by various glycolipids and hydrophilic polymers is supposed to be the primordial for stealth behaviour of the liposomes. The alternative approaches include assimilation of transmembrane ion gradients to achieve effective drug retention, appending targeting ligands to enhance selectivity for disease sites/cells and fusogenic/internalizing components that augment intracellular delivery of liposomal contents.

Sterically stabilized liposomes particularly may be beneficial for passive targeting to macrophages. Although their macrophage uptake is less than the conventional liposomes, still half of the injected dose ultimately reaches phagocytic cells (probably due to protracted loss of PEG coating). In addition to liver and spleen macrophages, it even reaches deep tissue macrophages that is a practically inaccessible site. Small conventional liposomes and sterically stabilized liposmes can also be targeted to lymph nodes following subcutaneous administration. Lymph drainage from these injection sites, translocates liposomes to lymph nodes where they can exterminate metastases. Liposomes are also explored as potential gene and antigen carrying vehicles. Presently, the studies are largely devoted to plain cationic liposomes that condense DNA and deliver it non-specifically to various cells.

Two liposomal formulations namely, Doxil and DaunoXome, have been granted FDA approval and are marketed in USA, Europe, Japan and certain parts of Asia for the treatment of AIDS related Kaposi's sarcoma (Working et al., 1994; Forssen and Ross, 1994). DaunoXome was observed to be therapeutically more effective than conventional therapies, with reduced drug toxicity. Similarly, the use of Doxil in Kaposi's sarcoma has shown a high response rate in comparison to standard treatments.

The first and foremost requirement of gene manipulation is successful ferrying of target gene into the cells. This requires sophisticated strategies, which could smuggle this gene safe in to the target-organ/cells. A number of methods are available for transferring genes into cells and these include physical (e.g., electroporation, microinjection, particle bombardment), chemical (DEAE-dextran, polybrene-dimethyl sulphoxide, calcium phosphate precipitation, liposomes, poly-lysine conjugates) and biological (e.g., virus). The vehicles utilized for gene delivery can be viral (e.g., adenovirus, retrovirus and adeno-associated virus) and non-viral (e.g., liposomes and lipid-based systems, polymers and peptides) (Storm and Crommelin, 1998). Amongst the non-viral vector systems explored for gene delivery are liposomes and lipid complexes; especially engineered liposomes such as pH sensitive liposomes, cationic liposomes, fusogenic liposomes, genosomes, lipoplex, and lipopolyplex (Ledley, 1995).

Lipid gene complexes and delivery systems are the focus of several specialized high-technology companies. A number of their products are commercially available and a still larger number are in advanced phases of clinical trials. Some of the engineered liposomal and non-liposomal versions like pH sensitive cationic and anionic liposomes, pH sensitive immunoliposomes, fusogenic liposomes, genosomes (DNA-liposomes/lipid complexes), Lipofectin™ (lipid-DNA complex) have been investigated as the major gene vectors.

The role of liposomes has firmly been established as immunoadjuvants (enhancers of the immunological response), potentiating both cell mediated and humoral immunity. Liposomal immunoadjuvants release antigen slowly on intramuscular injection and they by themselves passively accumulate within regional lymph nodes. Strategies that enhance the targeting of liposomes to regional lymph nodes, for example the use of phosphatidylserine liposomes, may thus improve adjuvanticity (Oussoren and Storm, 1998). Liposomal vaccines can be made by associating microbes, soluble antigens, cytokines or deoxyribonucleic acid (DNA) with liposomes (Gregoriadis et al., 1996; Gregoriadis et al., 1997), the latter stimulating an immune response on expression of the antigenic protein (Gregoriadis, 1997). Liposomes bearing antigens are subsequently encapsulated within alginate lysine microcapsules (Cohen et al., 1991), and reportedly control antigen release and improve the antibody response. Liposomal vaccines may also be stored dried at refrigeration temperatures for up to 12 months and still retain their adjuvanticity (Kim and Jeong, 1995).

Other Liposome Applications

Another interesting liposome-based multivesicular formulation has recently been reported. This sustained release formulation, being developed by Depotech, has a particle size of 1-5 μm and is formed from phospholipids, cholesterol and the oil tripalmitolein. The system effectively controls the release of insulin-like growth factor I and is morphologically similar to the multivesicular niosome formulation. A similar formulation developed by Depotech for the intrathecal sustained release of cytarabine, Depocyt, has been recommended by the United States Food and Drug Administration's oncologic drugs advisory committee for accelerated approval, in the treatment of lymphomatous meningitis.

It can safely be said that liposomes are the most widely studied modern drug delivery system, meant for sophisticated drug delivery. They are leading carrier units to be clinically adopted as parenteral drug delivery system.

NIOSOMES

The success achieved with liposomal systems stimulated the search for other cost effective and stable vesicle forming amphiphiles. Non-ionic surfactants were among the first alternative materials studied. A large number of surfactants have since been found to self assemble into closed bilayer vesicles and most important of them are spans (sorbitan esters) and polyalkyl ether.

Non-ionic surfactant vesicles (niosomes or NSVs) are widely investigated as alternative vesicles and they are reported to mimic liposomes in several respects (Baillie et al., 1985). Niosomes are generated from the self-assembly of hydrated amphiphilic surfactant monomers. Various nonionic surfactants belonging to different chemical classes have been found to be useful alternatives to phospholipids in assembling vesicular carriers. The terminology does suggest that distinctions exist between niosomes and liposomes. They may differ in their chemical composition, but have similar physical properties. However, niosomes may also be prepared with ionic amphiphiles like negatively charged dicetylphosphate (DCP) or positively charged stearylamine (SA) in order to achieve a stable vesicular suspension.

Nonionic surfactants form a variety of aggregates from micelles to large vesicles, which can be used as drug delivery vehicles. This includes among others, drug carriers in oncology, for delivery of antiparasitic agents, cosmetic formulations, topical vehicles and as potential diagnostic devices (Florence, 1993; Yoshioka and Florence, 1994; Uchegbu and Vyas, 1998). Anticancer niosomes, if suitably designed, can accumulate within tumours like liposomes. Unlike non-stealth liposomes, 800 nm doxorubicin niosomes, possessing a triglycerol or 200 nm doxorubicin niosomes possessing a muramic acid surface are not taken up significantly by the liver; this behaviour suggests for their promising use as drug delivery carriers to organ(s) or sites other than liver and spleen.

Like liposomes, the uptake by the liver and spleen makes niosomes ideal for targeting diseases of these organs (Ahl et al., 1997). One such condition is leishmaniasis. Studies (Baillie et al., 1986; Hunter et al., 1988) suggest that niosomal formulations of sodium stibogluconate improve parasite suppression in the liver (Carter et al., 1988), spleen and bone marrow (Williams et al., 1995). Niosomes could serve as intramuscular cargo and depots for short acting peptide drugs, which are cleared fast from the circulation (Arunothayanun, et al., 1999).

Niosomes when tested as vaccine adjuvants were proven to be promising. These systems are potent stimulators of the cellular and humoral immune response (Brewer and Alexander, 1992; Hassan et al., 1996). The formulation of antigens as a niosome in water-in-oil emulsion further increases the activity of antigens (Yoshioka et al., 1995). The controlled release property of the emulsion formulation is probably responsible for enhancing the immunological response.

The understanding of amphiphilic assemblage, molecular topology, dimensional intricacies and possibility of molecular modelling have led to a variety of vesicles. Vesicles for use in drug delivery include those from amphiphilic carbohydrate and amino acid based polymers (Uchegbu et al., 1998a; Uchegbu et al., 1998b) and also from aged red blood cells (Grimaldi et al., 1997). The aged red blood cells were interestingly found to increase intracellular drug delivery to virus infected cells. Non-ionic surfactants and other amphiphiles may be used to prepare a number of different drug carriers with varied surface characteristics. This should provide the basis for the development of drug delivery vesicles with different biodistribution profiles for parenteral administration.

NANOPARTICLES AND MICROSPHERES

Nanoparticles and microspheres are first and foremost representative frontiers of colloidal drug delivery systems. They differ from liposomes and niosomes in that they are prepared from polymers and do not have an aqueous core but a solid polymer matrix. Microspheres and nanoparticles are usually prepared by the controlled precipitation of polymers solubilized in one of the phases of an emulsion. Precipitation of the polymer out of the solvent takes place on solvent evaporation, leaving particles of the polymer suspended in the residual solvent. Drug loading in both the cases may occur simultaneously with particle formation. The surfactants in the aqueous phase may be used to ensure particle size control. Microspheres may also be prepared by chemical cross-linking of soluble polymers and nanoparticles or by the polymerization of a monomer in a good solvent for the monomer but a poor solvent for the polymer or by high-pressure homogenization of a polymerized system. The loading of water soluble drugs into the hydrophobic polymer particle matrix is still difficult but may be enhanced by the salting out of the active ingredient using soluble inorganic salts, the formation of lipophilic ion pairs of soluble amine drugs with monoalkyl phosphate esters, or by exploiting the ionic attraction between basic amine drugs and the carboxylic groups of polylactic acid co-glycolic acid. Thus, these nanosized colloidal composites are capable of carrying a high drug load and of controlling the drug release in a predictable manner.

Most of the early investigations in the area of solid particulate drug delivery used non-biodegradable polymers such as polystyrene. However, recent studies have quite reasonably focused on the development of biodegradable or at least bioerodible particles. Polylactic acid, polyglycolic acid, poly ß-hydroxybutyrate and fibrin are biodegradable polymers used to make drug delivery particles, while the alkyl cyanoacrylates are bioerodible polymers. These solid nanoparticles and microspheres may be used to prepare sustained release parenteral formulations or to achieve drug targeting. Nanoparticles are defined as particulate dispersions having a size range between 30 and 500 nm while microspheres are defined as particulate dispersions having a particle size bigger than 0.5 μm. It is the sub-micron size of this delivery system, which makes them more efficient in certain drug therapy applications, such as in intracellular localization of therapeutic agents. These systems, in addition to sustained drug delivery have been investigated for various therapeutic applications.

Because of their small size, nanoparticles may be injected intravenously and used to target drugs to particular organs. The particles, after intravenous injection and non-polymer coated colloidal particulates, are cleared from the circulation by the liver and spleen. Therefore, to facilitate drug targeting in tumour tissue, avoidance of reticuloendothelial system is a priori (Illum and Davis, 1983; Verdun et al., 1990). The stealth character may be incorporated using polyoxyethylene block polymers. This may be achieved using block polyoxyethylene copolymers (Illum and Davis, 1984; Bazile et al., 1993; Verrecchia et al., 1995; Gref et al., 1994). The polymeric coat offers steric hindrance to opsonin or may promote adsorption of deopsonin to avoid macrophagic sequestration. Stealth nanoparticles may also be prepared by coating them with soluble polyoxyethylene (Leroux et al., 1996) or by using dialkyl polyoxyethylenes and phospholipids (Hodoshima et al., 1997). The hydrophobic portions of these amphiphilic molecules, in the latter case, comprise the core of matrix. Stealth nanoparticles increase the tumour accumulation and tumouricidal activity of anticancer drugs in mice. The accumulation of non-stealth doxorubicin nanoparticles within the Kupffer cells of the liver may be used to target hepatic neoplasm indirectly. The differential uptake of nanoparticles, i.e. by liver Kupffer cells but not by neoplasm cells could be exploited for bystander supplementation of drug(s) for the treatment of liver cancer.

In certain biomedical applications it is desirable and imperative that following i.v. administration, the colloidal particles should evade rapid recognition and uptake by the RES and subsequently achieve prolonged systemic circulation. These applications include a prolonged systemic drug delivery, use as an imaging agent or for site-specific localization of nanoparticles to organs other than the liver and spleen. This objective can be achieved by preparing nanoparticles from derivatized polymers or by surfacial modification of the preformed nanoparticles. Nanoparticles can be prepared with derivatized polymers, which orient their hydrophilic segment towards the aqueous bulk while hydrophobic segment(s) are shielded. Thus, the resultant surface has a hydrophilic characteristics and in effect evades recognition by RES (Gref et al., 1995). The alternative approach is surfacial modification of the preformed nanoparticles with different block co-polymers (Polaxamers™/ Pluronics™) or polyethylene glycols, which produce several fold higher systemic circulation time compared to unmodified nanoparticles (Torchilin and Trubetskoy, 1995).

Nanoparticles in Chemotherapy

The most promising application of nanoparticles is their use as carriers for antitumour agents (Couvreur et al., 1990; Kreuter, 1991). The tumours have enhanced endocytic activity and leaky vasculature, and this promotes accumulation of intravenously administered nanoparticles. The drug targeting to tumour tissues can be further facilitated and optimized by the "stealth" behaviour imparted by polyoxyethylene, which further effectively promotes extravasation. Stealth character can be imparted by coating plain nanoparticles with soluble polyoxyethylene, or by using dialykyl polyoxyethylene and phospholipids. PEGylated polystyrene nanoparticle and PEO grafted nanoparticle are shown in Figure 1-7 and 1-8, respectively.

Avoidance of Multidrug Resistance

The chemotherapeutic agents have limited success primarily due to the occurrence of multi-drug resistance (Endicott and Ling, 1989). It is often associated with the over-expression of a cell membrane glycoprotein of 170 kDa molecular weight (Kartner et al., 1985). The glycoprotein acts as an efflux pump and rejects positively charged amphipathic drugs from the cells as shown for bacterial transport proteins. Nanoparticles loaded drugs displayed better results in a number of chemotherapy refractory cancers both in animal and clinical models (Kubiak et al., 1989; Cuvier et al., 1992). As the particulate systems are localized in the lysosomes, it protects the loaded drug from the action of the P-glycoprotein, and also avoids immediate contact with P-glycoprotein transporter located at the plasma membrane.

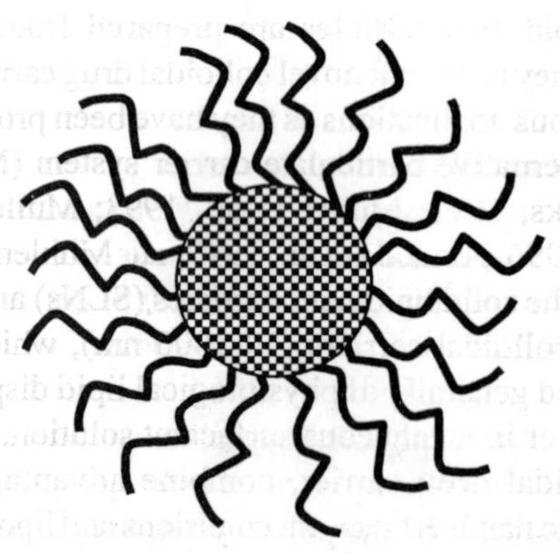

Fig. 1-7. PEGylated Polystyrene Nanoparticles

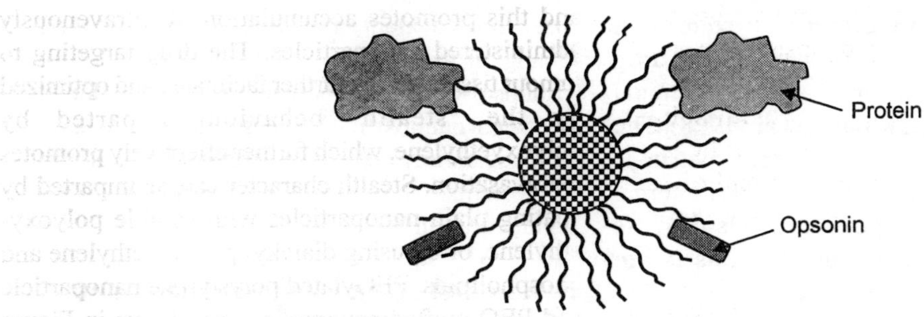

Fig. 1-8. PEO Grafted Polystyrene Nanoparticles with Opsonin Repelling Hydrophilic Surface

Adjuvant Effect for Vaccines

The nanoparticles with matrix entrapped or surface adsorbed antigen(s) have demonstrated an abstractive adjuvant effect following subcutaneous administration. This adjuvant effect can be attributed to the sustained release of the entrapped antigen or due to the improved uptake and subsequent processing of the nanoparticle bound antigen. Polymethylmethacrylate nanoparticles containing the influenza antigen induced significant antibody response in mice and offered protection against a mouse-adapted influenza virus challenge to a greater extent than the antigen alone or an alum preparation of the antigen (Kreuter, 1991). These workers also observed that the adjuvant effect increases with a decrease in particle size and an increase in hydrophobicity of the nanoparticles.

SOLID LIPID NANOPARTICLES

Solid lipid nanoparticles are prepared from solid lipids. They represent novel colloidal drug carrier for intravenous applications as they have been proposed as an alternative particulate carrier system (Muller and Lucks, 1991; Muller et al., 1993; Muller and Lucks, 1996; Almeida et al., 1997; zur Muhlen et al., 1998). The solid lipid nanoparticles (SLNs) are sub-micron colloidal carriers (50-1000 nm), which are composed generally of physiological lipid dispersed in water or in an aqueous surfactant solution. SLNs as colloidal drug carrier, combine advantages of polymeric nanoparticles, fat emulsions and liposomes and are simultaneously capable of avoiding some of their disadvantages. To overcome the disadvantages associated with the liquid state of the oil droplets, the liquid lipid was replaced by a solid lipid, which eventually transformed into solid lipid nanoparticles (Muller et al., 1993, Muller and Lucks, 1996).

Speiser, 1990 conducted the basic work in the area of solid lipid particles a decade back. The lipid nanopellets were prepared by first melting the lipid and it was then dispersed in a hot aqueous surfactant solution by stirring or ultrasonic treatment. Microemulsion technique was used for the preparation of solid lipid nanoparticles. The hot microemulsion containing the lipid was poured in to cold water leading to solidification of nanoparticles (Gasco, 1993). SLNs can also be produced by another diverse homogenization method at higher pressure for either melted or solid lipid (Muller et al., 1993 and 1995).

The SLNs offer some advantages compared to conventional particulate carriers (Muller et al., 1993; Muller et al., 1995; zur Muhlen et al., 1998) :

- Their small size and relatively narrow size distribution permits site-specific drug delivery.
- Controlled and sustained release of active drug can be achieved.
- The incorporated drug is protected from the onslaughts of biochemical degradation.
- Can be sterilized by autoclaving or gamma irradiation.
- Can be lyophilized and spray dried.
- Do not generate any toxic metabolites.
- Relatively cheap and stable.
- Ease of industrial scale production by hot dispersion technique.
- Surface modification can be easily performed.

SLN is a better alternative carrier system than conventional O/W emulsion if a prolonged drug release or a protection of drug against chemical degradation is desired (zur Muhlen et al., 1998). The drug incorporated into the solid lipid matrix is naturally better protected than in the oily internal phase of emulsion and liposomes. Also, SLNs facilitate prolonged drug release but this is not feasible with conventional emulsions.

In comparison to polymeric nanoparticles, the SLNs possess lower cytotoxicity. Due to the absence of solvents in the production process and a relatively low cost for the excipients required, its large-scale production is a viable proposition. They can be prepared by employing the simple process of high-pressure homogenization. As compared to liposomes, the SLNs protect the drug more effectively against chemical degradation since water has little or negligible access to the inner core of lipid particles.

HYDROGEL NANOPARTICLES

The self-assemblage and self-aggregation of natural polymer amphiphiles such as hydrophobized polysaccharides (like cholesteroyl pullulan, cholesteroyl mannan and cholesteroyl dextran) in water produces hydrogel nanoparticles (Akiyoshi and Sunamoto, 1992; Ohki et al., 1994; Akiyoshi et al., 1995, Nishikawa et al., 1996). The cholesterol bearing polysaccharides (CHP) self-aggregates to form monodisperse and stable hydrogel nanoparticles. In these nanoparticles, domains of the associated cholesterol groups of cholesteroyl polysaccharides offer non-covalent cross-linking points (Fig. 1-9). Changing the degree of substitution of cholesterol groups of CHP can modulate the size and density of hydrogel nanoparticles. These nanoparticles could be made bioinspired with customized delivery profile of proteins. They are safe version for parenteral administration.

Nano-crystals and Nano-suspensions

Recent investigations in drug delivery research are directed with defined emphasis on drug solubility problems and their redressal. Typical problems associated with poorly soluble drugs are low bioavailability and erratic absorption (oral administration) and problems of preparing parenteral dosage forms.

NanoCrystals™ (NanoSystems, Elan) and nano-suspensions are two recently introduced aspects to the drug delivery research. The basic concept is to convert micronized drug powders (i.e., microparticles) to drug nanoparticles. NanoCrystals™ are produced by dispersing the drug powder in a surfactant solution and the resultant suspension is subjected to a pearl milling process that can last from hours up to several days. To produce Nano-suspension (SkyePharm PLC; Drug Delivery Service, GmbH, Germany) the drug powder is dispersed in an aqueous surfactant solution by high speed stirring. The obtained macro-suspension is passed through a high-speed homogenizer that generates nano-suspension of the poorly water-soluble drug. Nanocrystals so obtained have

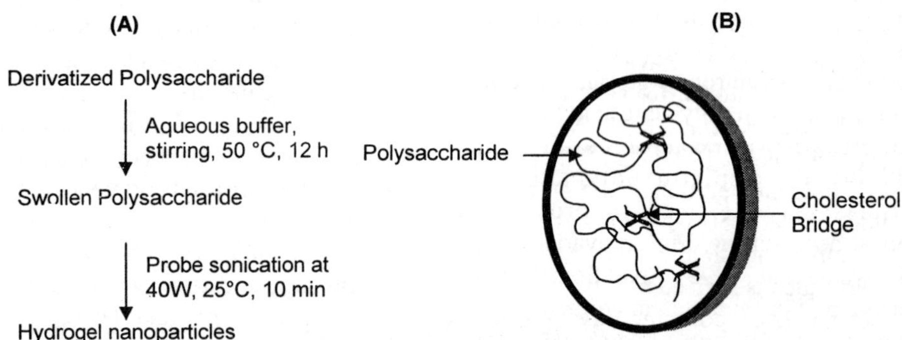

Fig. 1-9. Schematic of (A) Hydrogel Nanoparticles Prepared Using Cholesteroyl Polysaccharides, and (B) Structure of Hydrogel Nanoparticle

exceptionally high interfacial energy and thus on addition of phospholipid(s), amphiphiles tend to accumulate at solid/liquid interface and stabilize the nanocrystals thermodynamically to remain in suspension. Muller and co-workers, 2001 have discussed mucoadhesive nano-suspensions for surface-modified drug nanoparticles for site-specific delivery to brain.

MICROPARTICLES

Microparticles are generally injected either intraperitoneally, intramuscularly, subcutaneously or directly to the target organ and because of their large size (10-160 μm), they are used to provide a sustained release depot of the drug. Drug is gradually released on erosion or by diffusion from the particles. The rate of release may be increased by decreasing polymer molecular weight (Moritera et al., 1991; Mehta et al., 1994) and particle size (Sanchez and Alonso, 1995)and also by controlling the nature of the polymer/copolymer (Ruiz and Benoit, 1991).

Microparticulates for their distinctive chemo-embolism and chemotherapeutic effects were evaluated in experimental tumours, however their large particle size limits administration of these formulations by certain routes, thus ultimately limiting their potential. Hence, anti-tumour microparticles are either administered intraarterially in to blood supplying arteries straight or directly into the organ (Codde et al., 1993), or into body cavities such as the peritoneum (Ike et al., 1991). Doxorubicin ion exchange resin based microparticles have been found superior to the free drug when administered via the hepatic artery. Similarly, improved tumoricidal activity is seen in animals after intraperitoneal administration of mitozantrone chitosan (Jameela et al., 1996) or doxorubicin polylactic acid (Ike et al., 1991) microparticles when compared with the free drug and 100 μm cisplatin polylactic acid microparticles may be used to provide an intraperitoneal depot of the drug in ovarian cancer patients (Sugiyama et al., 1998). Apart from the intra-arterial and intraperitoneal routes, microparticles may also be injected directly into tumours. The direct injection of microparticles into solid tumours improvises the tumoricidal activity of the drugs 5-fluorouracil (Menei et al., 1996) and doxorubicin (Willmott and Cummings, 1987). Microparticles create an engineered minienvironment to the encapsulated bio active/protein or enzyme thus via effective immobilization may serve as artificial centre and substitute of body organs or tissues.

Biodegradable polylactic acid and polylactic acid co-glycolic acid microspheres are well appreciated immune adjuvant they provide a depot formulation of the antigen at the site of administration (Lima and Junior, 1999). The antigen is thus continually fed to the antigen presenting cells. Ovalbumin polylactic acid (Alpar et al., 1996) and polylactic acid/polyglycolic acid (O'Hagan et al., 1991) microparticles enhance the immune response to ovalbumin when compared with free ovalbumin on parenteral administration. Additionally, intramuscular injection of spermine-chondroitin sulphate microparticles enhances the virus specific immune response to rotavirus (Moser et al., 1996).

Depot formulations of short acting peptides have been successfully developed using microparticles technology. Such peptides include leuprorelin acetate (Okada and Toguchi, 1995) and triptoreline (Ruiz and Benoit, 1991), both luteinizing hormone releasing hormone agonists. Leuprorelin polylactic acid co-glycolic acid microspheres may be used as monthly and three monthly dosage forms in the treatment of advanced prostate cancer, endometriosis and other hormone responsive conditions (Okada and Toguchi, 1995). These microspheres effectively halt the progression of prostate cancer or endometriosis in patients and are currently marketed as Prostap SR.

Other peptides formulated as sustained release microparticles include the angiotensin receptor antagonist L-158809 for the treatment of hypertension (Lacasse et al., 1997), thyrotropin releasing hormone for central nervous system stimulation (Heya et al., 1994), salmon calcitonin (Mehta et al., 1994) for the treatment of hypercalcemia and postmenopausal osteoporosis and the immunosuppressant drug cyclosporin A. Detailed applications, method of preparation, etc. are discussed in the chapter on microspheres.

LONG CIRCULATING MICROPARTICULATES

The ultimate aim of drug therapy has been to deliver drug in requisite quantity exclusively to its therapeutic site or ensue a prolonged and controlled therapeutic effect. In either of cases, the carrier should remain long-circulatory in order to materialize and provide for site/carrier interaction followed by its eventual retention and accumulation at the site of action. In addition, it may remain in circulation while empirically releasing the contents slowly over protracted period of time. The needs entail for diversification of natural course of colloidal carrier biodisposition, i.e., passive accumulation. As it is discussed at places in this book, the role of opsonins and dysopsonins, where former after coating carrier(s) facilitate their opsonic removal by reticuloendothelial system (RES) predominant organs or macrophages, while latter following coating of carriers provide for their protection from such bio-sequestration and resultant early removal from systemic circulation.

The design of such system is largely based on collective knowledge gathered from various research disciplines including nature of RES, opsonization, dysopsonization and particle characteristics, surface hydrophilicity or hydrophobicity and surface modification strategies. Most of the strategies are based on the principle of RES uptake avoidance, which could be effectively executed by coating these particles with some known dysopsonins or behaviourally similar synthetic molecules. This not only imparts hydrophilicity to the surface but also contributes a distinctive steric barrier. Polyoxyethylene polymers of different molecular weights on coating (applying various methods) could render colloidal carriers to be long circulatory for sustained drug release or for targeted drug delivery. The application of stealth colloidal carriers has been extensively discussed in this book.

SPECIALIZED EMULSIONS

Emulsions are dispersions of one liquid inside a second liquid, where liquids being immiscible. Such dispersions (oil in water or water in oil) are stabilized by emulsifiers, which coat the droplets and prevent droplet coalescence by either reducing interfacial tension or creating a physical repulsion between droplets. Emulsions are usually used as a means of administering aqueous insoluble drugs by dissolution of the drugs within the oil phase or to prevent drug hydrolysis or drug uptake by infusion sets. It is recommended that emulsions destined for the intravenous (i.v.) route should have a submicron droplet size, although emulsions with a droplet size of 10mm have been used parenterally. Emulsions may also be used as drug targeting systems. Emulsion formulations, with a droplet size of 100 to 200nm, usually result in high drug liver uptake on i.v. injection. Emulsified drugs may be diverted from the liver on i.v. injection by incorporating polyoxyethylene surfactants as emulsifiers. Diversion from the liver prolongs the half life of the drug, allowing passive targeting to the lung, kidney and areas of inflammation. Active targeting may be achieved by conjugating antibodies to the distal ends of the polyoxyethylene chain emulsifiers, provided the emulsion droplets have a submicron droplet size. Emulsions may also be used to reduce drug toxicity. Use of a water in oil emulsion of amphotericin deoxycholate, as opposed to a solution, reduces the incidence and severity of renal impairment and chills in patients while still maintains the antifungal efficacy of the drug.

Recently, specialized emulsion systems like multiple emulsions (W/O/W or O/W/O), micro-emulsions and lipid emulsions have been investigated intensively as parenteral modes of drug delivery carriers, and effective adjuvant system in vaccine formulations.

MULTIPLE EMULSIONS

Multiple emulsions are complex type of emulsions and are a relatively new development in the field of emulsion technology. In the multiple emulsions the dispersed phase contains smaller droplets that have the same composition as the external phase. Since this involves double emulsification, these systems are also referred to as double emulsion. The multiple emulsions are also called "Liquid Membrane Systems" as the liquid film that separates the liquid phases and acts as a thin semipermeable film through which solute must diffuse in order to traverse from one phase to another. This liquid membrane may be hydrophilic or hydrophobic. The multiple emulsions can be either oil-in-water-in-oil (O/W/O) or water-in-oil-in-water (W/O/W) emulsion system.

Multiple emulsion systems have immense potential as a drug carrier since their vesicular structure with innermost phase is similar to that of liposomal vesicles and the selective permeability characteristic of liquid membranes. These properties have amplified the practical utility of multiple emulsions, especially as drug delivery systems. An O/W/O multiple emulsion may appear to be more beneficial dosage form since the extra partitioning step with drug initially in the internal oil phase is expected to be the rate-limiting step that may define the drug release characteristics.

Multiple emulsions have been exploited in various diverse applications like pharmaceutics, cosmetics, food and separation techniques. Their potential pharmaceutical applications include uses as red blood cell substitutes; treatment of drug overdosing; immobilization of enzymes; masking the taste of drugs; enhancement of gastrointestinal absorption; and as carriers for sustained release, lymphatic uptake and transdermal drug delivery. In addition to these applications, W/O/W emulsions have been used as intermediates for the preparation of microspheres.

EMULSOME™

Emulsome™ represents lipid based drug delivery systems with wide range of therapeutic applications especially for parenteral delivery of drugs, which are poorly water-soluble. Since lipophilic drugs have limited water solubility they may require an excessive quantity of surface active agents or co-solvents which often leads to undesirable toxic side effects. Emulsome particles are basically consisted of microscopic lipid assembly with apolar core (Fig. 1-10), which contains water insoluble drugs in the solution form without requiring any surface active agent or co-solvent. These fat cored lipid particles are dispersed in an aqueous phase. These systems are often prepared by melt expression or emulsion solvent diffusive extraction as discussed for preparation of nanoparticles. However, in place of emulgents an excessive quantity of phospholipids is used for their stabilization. The latter not only stabilizes the entire dispersion but excessive phospholipids assemble to form the lipid bilayered membrane similar to liposomes. In other words this system combines characteristics of lipid spheres and liposomes, i.e. characteristically with apolar core and liposomal crown (Surface). These systems can very

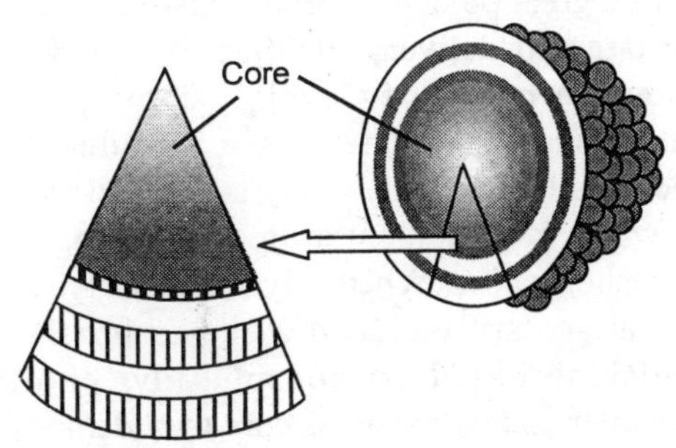

Fig. 1-10. An Insight into Emulsome™ Stucture

safely be used for parenteral administration of drug, adjuvant for vaccines, carrier containers for targeted drug delivery to liver, brain or RES rich organs. The active targeting has also been described to be a possible potentiality of this system by Pharmos, the adventer of the system.

LONG CIRCULATORY EMULSIONS

Emulsions and particularly O/W types, on parenteral administration are rapidly cleared from blood circulation, without negotiating much significant therapeutic benefits. They get accumulated in macrophages of liver and spleen and thus these organs tend to be major obstacles for delivering drug(s) to cells other than those in the RES. Therefore, to overcome such problems, various long circulating systems have been developed using various dysopsonic strategies.

Lipid emulsions stabilized using phospholipids are attractive and promising carrier system for systemic delivery of lipophilic drugs. O/W emulsions cross sectionally reveal to be consisted of an oil core surrounded by emulsifier(s) on the surface. Such emulsions are similar to liposomes when their ultimate surfaces are compared. The major differences between O/W emulsions and liposomes are that emulsions have monolayer of phosphatidyl choline on the surface and inside core is oil while on the other hand liposomes contain an outer bilayer of amphiphilic molecules such as phosphatidyl choline with a large aqueous compartment encapsulated within (Fig. 1-11). The lipid core microemulsions provide great potential and promises for controlled and targeted delivery of lipophilic drug(s). The system(s) could be developed for parenteral administration. They are biodegradable, biocompatible and physically stable and capable of carrying a large amount of lipophilic drugs in their hydrophobic core. When poly ethylene glycol (PEG) derivatives are included as co-emulsifier in to emulsions based on phosphatidyl choline as emulsifier and castor oil as core they demonstrate a typical stealthing character. The system resulted in a discernible effect on RES uptake which is almost avoided, while plasma profile suggests for their long circulation. The quantitative PEG co-emulsifier effect or blood circulation was observed to be incremental, however attained desirable level. Further the ability of PEG derivatives in prolonging the circulation time was recorded to be related to the chain length of PEG chain.

RESEALED ERYTHROCYTES

The membrane of erythrocytes can be transiently lysed or broken to yield higher permeability using osmotic variation, or by applying electric current for nanosecond(s) in the form of pulse. During this hyperpermeation membranolyzed phase, exogeneous substances could be encapsulated within the RBCs by bringing them in equilibrium with endogenous components and subsequently reanealing the RBCs by restoration of tonicity and incubating them at 37°C for resealing. The drug carrying capability of RBCs has been realized, which subsequently became a

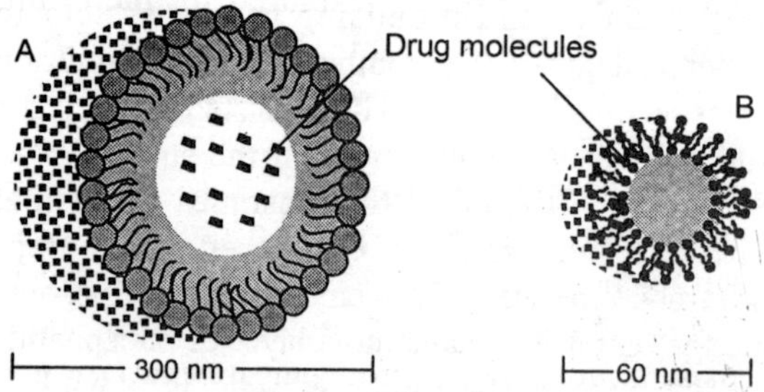

Fig. 1-11. Comparative Presentation of Lipid Emulsion Droplet (A) and Liposome (B)

central paradigm and established resealed erythrocytes as promising drug carrier. The erythrocytes lose their haemoglobin content at large when they are processed in laboratory for transient permeation applying various methods including osmolysis, electrical breakdown/electroencapsulation, endocytosis or other means and modes of perturbation. The haemoglobin loss in a way provides intracellular space for drug(s) to be incorporated. In fact during transient permeation phase there establishes an equilibrium between intra and extracellular contents especially the drug component. Furthermore, the permeable erythrocytes membrane can be resealed on restoration of temperature and tonicity of media. Thus, the drug bearing erythrocytes with minor variations in its membrane structure could be used as drug carrier for controlled or targeted drug delivery.

These carriers are specifically useful for lysosomal storage diseases. The RBCs being blood cellular components can be used safely as biological carriers. They could be absolutely autologous by source, thus exclude chances of immunological consequences and other contraindicative episodes. The methods essentially used for drug loading are classically free of organic solvent requirement hence residual solvent related problems are not encountered. Being non-immunogenic in nature they can be used as long circulatory drug/biological cargo. These carriers can selectively carry the contents to RES predominant organ in the body. Classically, the biological half life of resealed erythrocytes is 60-120 days depending on the method chosen for drug loading. The clearance reportedly follows a biphasic pattern. The contents of erythrocytes are released following phagocytosis or diffusion though the membrane or via some specific transport system. Membranolytic or membranotropic agents distinctively affect the integrity of the membrane and even they may translate them into various shapes including discocytes, achinocytes I, II and III.

Erythrocyte biocarriers as stated earlier can be used for treatment of lysosomal storage diseases, treatment of Gaucher's disease, liver tumour, parasitic diseases of liver and iron deposits of liver. The delivery of drug using these carriers to organs other than RES rich has been documented with the help of magnoresponsive erythrocytes under the guidance of external magnetic field. The studies are continuous, new horizons are emerging, clinical trials are testifying the therapeutic utility, yet they are required to circumvent and address various issues before they could become therapeutic carriers for clinical practices. The methodology relating to drug encapsulation, characterization and various biomedical approaches are discussed in this book.

Another version of biological carriers which seems fascinating is magnetizable monocytes. As reported they selectively sequester and phagocytose magnetic drug nanoparticles or nanocarriers, thus become drug loaded biocarriers responsive to external magnetic field. Obviously, their course of circulation and accumulation could be directed with the help of a magnetic field of an appropriate strength. Thus the carrier can be actively recruited at the site which is in need of drug and monocytes biofunctions. This strategy seems therapeutically rewarding with double targeting potentiality, i.e. the pharmacodynamic effect of carried contents and carrier therapeutically (biological activity, i.e. phagocytosis).

SUPRAMOLECULAR BIOVECTORS

Supramolecular biovectors (SMBVs) represent a classically customized drug delivery system which is colloidal in nature and able to mimic and negotiate the behaviour of endogeneous carriers, i.e. apoproteins and chylomicrons. Since, they can be deviced with differential core/crown characteristics they can encapsulate both hydrophilic and lipophilic drugs. Furthermore, the assemblage is principally a surface related phenomenon, it rarely requires sophisticated chemical methodologies. Thus they assemble under the command of interface as per the nature of assembling molecules, and define and decide the architecture of these units. The supramolecular systems are typically host-guest type and self-assembling type. Host-guest supramolecular systems are often combined at 1:1 molar ratio of host and guest. It is perceived to be a spatial accommodation of guest within the host component. It is reported that macrocyclic compounds possess an intramolecular cavity of classical molecular dimensions. These compounds are cyclodextrins, cyclophens, and crown ethers. They form inclusion type of complexes. Depending on the nature of the cavity they form complexes of hydrophilic/ hydrophobic drug molecules.

Self assembling on the other hand is resulted from spontaneous organization of specifically designed molecular components, which in effect form a thermodynamically stable system. The phenomenon of self organization proceeds involving design of system capable of spontaneously generating supramolecular entities, which are inclined to orient in a well defined way. Molecular crystals are self organizing structures while co-crystals could be referred to as self assembling structures. c-Defensin proteins represent a self assembling biosystem, which preferably assemble to form transmembrane channels into the membrane of virus and bacteria and lead to efflux of their cellular contents. Probably, so is the nature of staphyloccocal α-haemolysin and its various genetically and chemically modified variations like haemolysin or α,α- haemolysin which via the process of self assembly form the pores and invade the host system. It is interesting to note that the assemblage of biocomponent is modulated by bio-vagaries of vicinity and responds typically in an off and on manner or fashion. Furthermore, the crown of these systems and even the nature of the core may be customized via chemical modification of principal components. Accordingly, core composition may be designed. The second generation assemblage may be typically under the influence of vander Waal's forces, hydrogen bonding, hydrophobic interactions, charge transfer interactions or more so under dipole and ion-ion interactions. The lipoproteins and their mimics have been extensively explored for their clinical applications. These are cholesteryl esters or diglycerides surrounded by a monolayer of phospholipids with embedded one or more specific biodegradable, site specific, nanoscopic colloidal carrier capable of carrying a quantum of drug sufficient to negotiate pharmacodynamic effects. In regard to stability they are appreciably stable in plasma, while their hydrophobic internal core greatly resists the leaching of entrapped components. The studies suggest that applying the conjugation chemistry and exploring physicochemical character of a dipathic molecule, the similar architecture structures could be constructed which may carry hydrophilic drugs with equivalent level of success. The lipoprotein drug carrier redefines the biological fate of entrapped drug by selectively delivering it to the cellular compartments, which possess receptor ports for apoproteins. Furthermore, the chemical modification of apoprotein may redirect these carrier systems to the receptors other than lipoproteins under the navigation of appended ligands. There are variety of variations which could possibly adopted in drug carriers for the therapeutic purposes including drug targeting and/or controlled release. Liquid crystals, pharmacosomes, virosomes, proteosomes, etc. may carry structural analogy to these systems. Recently, the most important self-assembling systems reported include, microtubules and microcapillaries based on polymerizable lecithin, diacetylenic fatty acid chains or others. They have been reported as therapeutically useful drug carrying components for delivery of drugs to periodontal caries, vaginal cavity after their fragmentation serve as nanoconstructs for vaccine and bioactives delivery.

Orientation, Organization and Function

Spheres, discs, cylinders and columns are the characteristic structural features of both synthetic and supramolecular system. Spheres organize to form rings, discs forms columns, and rings and discs form cylinders and hexagonal superstructures (Fig. 1-12). In these molecular architecture systems the function is mainly based on the mode and order of molecular organization. The basic examples, range from life science dealing with proteosomes, to material science dealing with photoconductive discotic liquid crystalline mesophases.

Proteosomes and Multienzyme Complexes

When two or more enzymes catalyze two or more steps in a metabolic cascade, they generally form noncovalently associated multienzyme complex (Zubey, 1988). The organized complex permits a better catalytic turnover than the non-associated enzymes. Hence, proteosomes could be defined as high molecular weight multi-subunit enzyme complexes (approx. 700 kDa) with at least three distinct proteolytic activities (trypsin like, chymotrypsin like and peptidyl-glutamyl-peptide hydrolyzing type) (Arrigo et al., 1988). The catalytic activity of the proteosome particle is specifically due to the assembly pattern of enzymes and the working is highlighted accordingly.

Chylomicrons

After ingestion of fatty diet/fat, triglyceride lipids are first digested within the intestinal lumen, the digestion

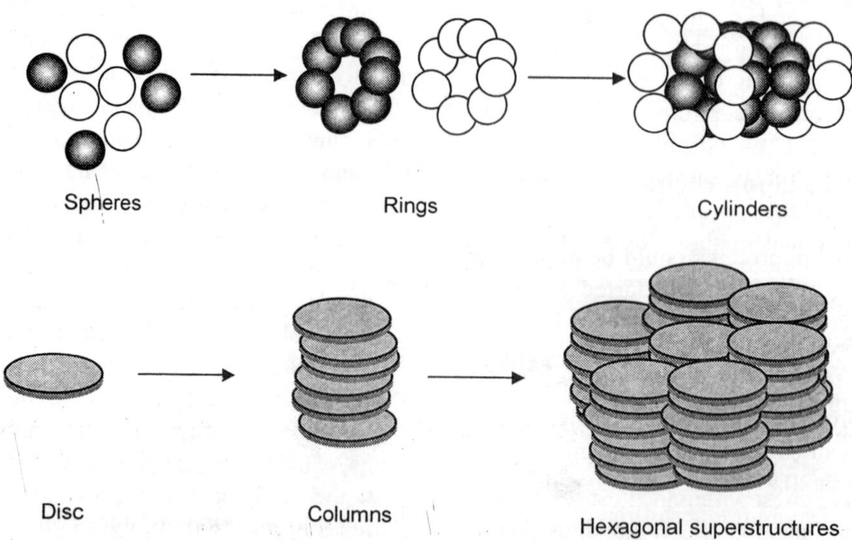

Fig. 1-12. Orientation Organization and Function of Supramolecular Systems

products are then absorbed by the enterocytes through chylomicrons. The specific lipoproteins (chylomicrons) are formed and secreted into the intestinal lymphatics for transport of fats (Tso and Balin, 1986). Their size ranges from 80-100 nm and density is less than 0.950 g/ml. These are translocated and secreted into lymph and subsequently enter blood circulation via thoracic duct. During circulation, the triglyceride component of the particles is rapidly hydrolyzed by lipoprotein lipase present on the surface of epithelial cells (Fielding and Havel, 1977; Bengtson and Olivercrona, 1988). This leads to the formation of chylomicron remnants, which are relatively enriched in cholesterol and apoprotein E (Lakshman et al., 1981; Borenztan et al., 1988). These remnants are rapidly cleared from the circulation by the liver. Readgreve, 1970 demonstrated that in rats 80% of the administered dose accumulates in liver after 4 minutes of injection of radiolabeled chylomicrons remnants. DeGroot and associates, 1981 reported that the parenchymatous cells are the main site for uptake of chylomicrons in liver. It involves a receptor mediated mechanism but specific receptor proteins for binding are yet to be identified. Thus these could be used for delivery of drug to parenchyma cells of liver following i.v. administration.

LIPOPROTEINS

Lipoproteins represent the major endogenous carriers that can be used for drug targeting. The major phenomenon related to their applicability in targeting is their extravasation for cellular interaction. The structure of lipoprotein is schematically shown in Figure 1-13.

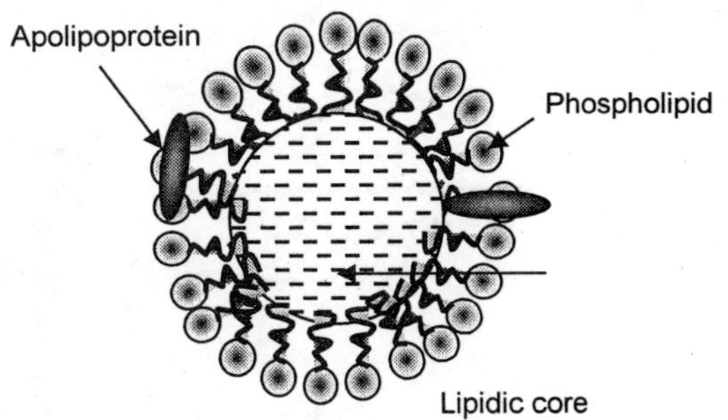

Fig. 1-13. Schematic Representation of the Structure of Lipoprotein

Extravasation of Lipoproteins for Cellular Interaction

Extravasation of lipoproteins could be appreciated when the lipoproteins are transported across the capillary wall into interstitial fluid that is in contact with the parenchymal cells of intact organ. Capillary endothelium offers the major barrier against extravasation process. The primary barrier limiting the permeability of capillary endothelium is that the most permeable capillaries are open sinusoids of liver and spleen which contain fenestration of about 100 Å diameter and permit easy penetrability to all classes of lipoproteins except chylomicron (Renkin, 1979). Thus, the concentration of a particular lipoproteins at sinusoidal surface of hepatocytes is similar to that in plasma. Many other organs like small intestine, endocrine glands, kidney may also contain the sinusoids. Since the aperture size is adequately smaller than 500 Å, it restricts the entry of most of the molecules.

All the major organs of body such as skeletal muscles, skin, adipose tissues, etc. are non fenestered and hence do not allow extensive passage of lipoproteins (Renkin, 1979). Hence lymph is one of the major sites for accumulation of lipoproteins. Further, the passage of lipoproteins across the central nervous system is limited due to the presence of tight junction endothelium (Renkin, 1979) leading to negligible to nil detection of VLDL and LDL levels in cerebrospinal fluid (CSF) (Pitas, et al., 1987). Interestingly HDL levels are detected in CSF containing apoprotein A-I and E (Roheim et al., 1979). However, the evidences reflect that apoprotin A-I might have reached CSF from plasma.

CYCLODEXTRINS

Cyclodextrins are water-soluble cyclic carbohydrate compounds with a hydrophobic cavity due to the specific orientation of the glucosidic substituents. Figure 1-14 schematically illustrates the amphiphilic β-cyclodextrin. These compounds form inclusion complexes with hydrophobic guest molecules, endowing such molecules with aqueous solubility. Only the modified cyclodextrins, such as hydroxypropyl β-cyclodextrin and sulphobutyl β-

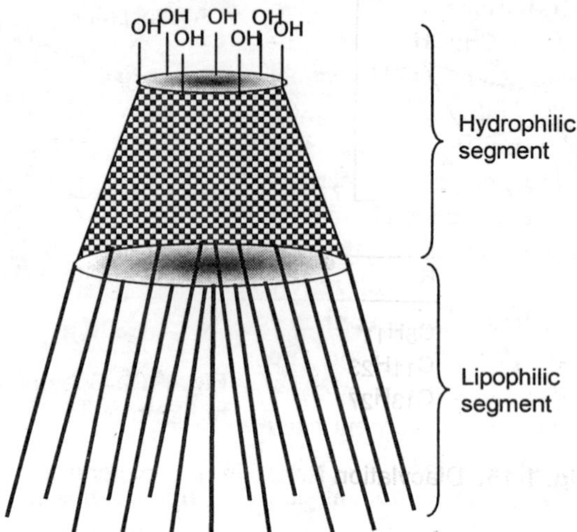

Fig. 1-14. Schematic Illustration of Amphiphilic β-cyclodextrin

cyclodextrin are regarded as parenteral molecular carriers. They have been used for solubilization of drugs, to stabilize and protect labile molecules and to therapeutically separate the incompatible components of a solution.

Cyclodextrins are used parenterally chiefly as pharmaceutical solubilizing agents. However, complexation with cyclodextrins also affects the pharmacokinetics and pharmacodynamics of certain drugs. It appears that the administration of cyclodextrin inclusion complexes does not alter the area under the plasma level time curve (AUC) when compared with the administration of drugs in suitable co-solvent formulations. However, when compared with an aqueous suspension of an insoluble drug, e.g. nimodipine, the relative increase in solubility afforded by the cyclodextrin inclusion complex does result in an increase in the drug AUC. Pharmacodynamically, the use of inclusion complexes reduces the sleep induction time of propofol compared with administration as an oil in water emulsion. This indicates a qualitative or quantitative difference in the handling of the drug *in vivo* when administered as a cyclodextrin inclusion complex compared with administration of an emulsion. Lipophilic drugs are believed to be rapidly released from cyclodextrin inclusion complexes on i.v. administration and complexation appears to enable the drug to enter the tissues in a larger amount and in an unaggregated state. Cyclodextrin inclusion complexes encapsulated within liposomes reduce drug urinary clearance.

An interesting study that proposes supramolecular customized assemblage of derivatized cyclodextrin in the form of nanospheres, which could serve as unique carrier system for drug(s) for their parenteral administration.

The diacylation of β-cyclodextrin (β-CD) imparts amphiphile character to β-CD, which on hydration assembles as spheres (Fig. 1-15). The diameter of spontaneously formed nanospheres has been measured to be 200-345 nm. The nanospheres have been proposed as promising biodegradable carrier for drug parenteral administration, as they are by intrinsic character of carrier itself, long circulating in nature.

PRODRUGS

The use of prodrugs in cancer chemotherapy for specific targeting of relatively toxic compounds to pathological areas is enjoying renewed research activity. Two of the technologies being evaluated at present are antibody directed enzyme prodrug therapy (ADEPT) and the use of polymeric prodrugs (or polymer drug conjugates as they are more commonly known). An algorithm of various prodrugs as chemical drug delivery systems is available. The concept classically deals with chemical modification

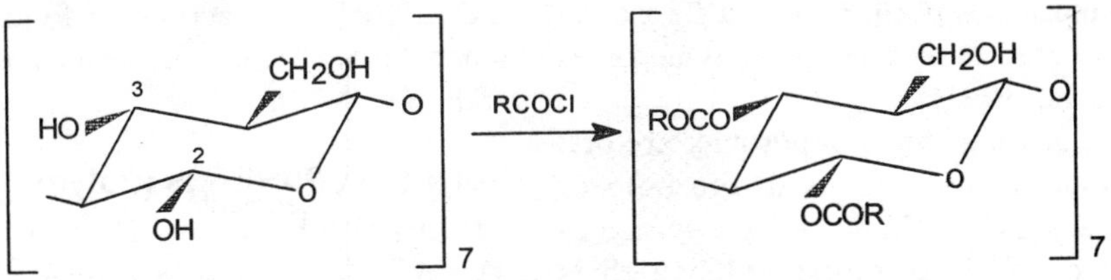

R	Compound
C_5H_{11}	β-CD-C_6
$C_{11}H_{23}$	β-CD-C_{12}
$C_{13}H_{27}$	β-CD-C_{14}

Fig. 1-15. Diacylation Reaction of β-cyclodextrin

of the drugs, which following parenteral administration undergo suitable changes (metabolize) yielding active principles at the site or body compartment exempting other body parts from unnecessary exposure to drugs. These systems could be designed specifically for body organs exploiting biochemistry and physiology of that organ. The organs, which could be targeted or delivered with active drugs, contain the enzyme responsible for metabolism of prodrug. The distribution of these enzymes is interestingly definite and specific. The various organs which have been delivered with the drug using this concept include, eye, kidney, liver, lungs, brain, lymphatics, etc. Further extensions of this technology include retrometabolic drug delivery or soft drugs. This is principally based on a lead compound which via inactive metabolite formation eventually generate an active drug thus it involves metabolism and activation processes. These systems are so designed that prodrug and generated metabolites both are soft to the biological system being isoelectronic or isosteric with drug metabolic analogues, they possess better pharmacodynamic activity and site specificity. Various systems based on this principle are discussed in chapter on chemical drug delivery.

Antibody Directed Enzyme Prodrug Therapy (ADEPT)

Several innovative strategies have been developed for the cell specific delivery of cytotoxic and antiviral agents and one such promising approach is the prodrug activation by antibody-enzyme conjugates. These antibody-coupled enzymes can be specifically targeted to the cells that express antigenic determinant (Senter et al. 1990). However, one of the major problems encountered with immuno-conjugates is the internalization of antibody. This problem can be duly addressed by ADEPT (antibody directed enzyme prodrug therapy). The generation of active derivatives in the proximity of the target cells leads to higher cellular and lower systemic concentration of the active drug. A Mab-β-glucuronidase conjugate as an activator of the prodrug epirubicin for the specific treatment of tumour has been reported (Hasima et al., 1992).

Another remarkable strategy for selective and specific chemotherapeutics is enzymosomes. Enzymosomes are basically liposomal constructs engineered to present a mini bioenvironment. In this strategy the enzymes are covalently immobilized or coupled to the surface of liposomes. Thus, following simultaneous administration of non-toxic prodrug and the immobilized enzyme, the former is transformed to a potent antitumour agent in the close proximity of tumour cell lines. The specificity of enzyme reaction limits the prodrug activation at the tumour site, through prior enzyme targeting by using liposomes, or via enzyme expressing gene delivery into the tumour cells (VDEPT). Figure 1-16 schematically presents the concept of targeted delivery of antitumour prodrug activating enzymes with immunoliposomes (ADEPT based liposomal system) also referred to as immuno-enzymosomes (Vingerhoeds et al., 1993).

The enzyme bearing immunoliposomes are first targeted to tumour cell lines with the help of appropriate Mabs. After binding of the immuno-enzymes, a prodrug is administered, which is activated by cell bound immunoenzymes in the vicinity of the tumour cells. Vingerboeds and co-workers in 1993 reported the coupling of the enzyme β-glucouronidase that activates prodrug epirubicin-glucouronide by converting it in to epirubicin. It was observed that pretreatments with enzymosomes (bearing no specific antitumour antibodies) or immunoliposomes (bearing no enzymes) were ineffective, but pre-incubation with immunozymes (enzymosomes) augmented the antitumour activity of the prodrug.

The choice of enzymes for ADEPT/VDEPT and the range of tumour antigen-targets is large, which increases the flexibility of these seemingly complex strategy in tumour chemotherapy and gene therapy. A wide spectrum of antigen specific targets is available that provides ample opportunities of targeting a range of tumours with Mab-enzyme conjugates (ADEPT). A number of antigen markers are also available that may be exploited for selective expression of prodrug activating enzymes coded by genes in GDEPT.

Sherwood, 1996 reported various enzyme-prodrug systems and proposed carboxypeptidase G2 enzyme and a nitrogen mustard prodrug based enzymosomes for clinical trials. Herpes simplex virus-thymidine kinase (HSV-tk) has been a leading candidate for VDEPT (virus directed EPT). Recently,

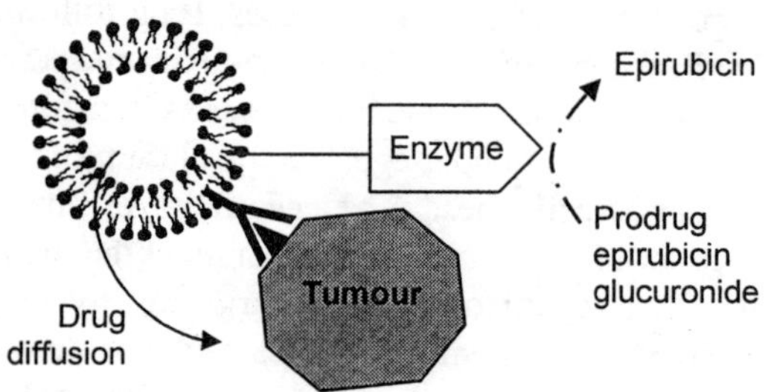

Fig. 1-16. Antibody Directed Enzyme Prodrug Therapy (ADEPT)

the ADEPT approach using folic acid in place of monoclonal antibody has been recommended (Reddy and Low, 1998).

Polymeric Prodrugs (Polymer Drug Conjugates)

The use of polymeric prodrugs, as pharmacodynamically active handles was first proposed nearly 25 years ago (Ringsdorf, 1975). It involves the use of an active substance and possibly a targeting moiety, both linked via spacers to a water-soluble polymeric backbone. From this basic blueprint number of polymer drug conjugates for cancer chemotherapy have been synthesized with cleavable drug polymer linkers. The various soluble polymeric prodrugs synthesized include prodrugs of daunorubicin (Hurwitz et al., 1980), doxorubicin (Seymour et al., 1994a), cisplatin (Maeda et al., 1993) and 5-fluorouracil (Nichifor et al., 1997). Polymer drug conjugates accumulate selectively within tumour tissue, leaking through the disorganized vasculature in a similar manner to that for liposomes. Clearance from tumour tissue is delayed due to the poor lymphatic drainage in the tumour surrounding. Tumour accumulation of polymer drug conjugates have eventually generate the enhanced permeation and retention effects (Matsumara and Maeda, 1986). Following i.v. administration the conjugate is taken up by tumour cells releasing active drug intracellularly (Duncan, 1992). It is not clear whether passive tumour targeting of polymer drug conjugates is influenced by the nature of the polymer backbone. However, passive tumour targeting is increased with an increase in polymer molecular weight (Pimm et al., 1996). The polymeric systems explored are largely prepared using non-biodegradable materials. Obviously, biodegradable polymers will be more acceptable, although care must be taken to ensure that biodegradation does not hamper the accumulation of conjugates in tumour tissue.

Passive tumour targeting with polymer drug conjugates could improve the tumoricidal activity of anticancer agents. Distribution to potential sites of toxicity, such as the distribution of doxorubicin to heart tissue (Yeung et al., 1991), is also decreased in the case of polymer drug conjugates. Doxorubicin polymer conjugates significantly increase the maximum tolerated dose of doxorubicin by selectively delivering the drug exclusively to site, which is situated away from potential toxicity (Vasey et al., 1996).

The polymer conjugates bearing galactose target hepatocytes and antibodies specific for an ovarian carcinoma cell line bind to ovarian carcinoma cells and target the site actively. Unfortunately, galactose-bearing polymer drug conjugates do not target hepatic carcinomas to any significant extent and preferentially locate in the normal liver tissue of mice and patients. This is due to the galactose receptor that is not sufficiently upregulated in neoplastic tissue. It is possible that liver targeting strategy may thus find a home in the treatment of non-neoplastic diseases. In summary, some interesting polymer systems with special therapeutic potentials are discussed in this book.

Biotin-avidin Conjugates

Biotinylated carriers or drugs on parenteral administration could be exquisitely be used for selective targeting of drugs. One of the most promising methods of tumour targeting is to make use of natural strong binding of avidin or streptividin to small molecule biotin (Longman et al., 1995a) (Fig. 1-17). Biotinylated molecules can be targeted in complex mixtures by using appropriate avidin or streptividin conjugates. If the biotinylated component has affinity for binding to a particular antigen or receptor of tumour, then the same can be located by the use of an avidin/streptividin conjugate containing a detecting molecule. A series of avidin or streptividin-biotin interactions can be built upon each other, utilizing the multivalent nature of each tetrameric avidin/streptividin molecule. The concept could be exploited with drug carriers as well. Liposomes with biotin modified lipids can be easily prepared and used to attach a variety of avidin/streptividin linked targeting proteins/ligands (Longman et al., 1995b). Non-specific protein based binding ligands (for example, avidin, streptividin, protein A or protein G) can be attached to liposomes through covalent conjugation methods. Moreover, the site directed targeting ligands, an antibody or biotinylated antibody, can subsequently be conjugated to the liposomes non-covalently using some non-

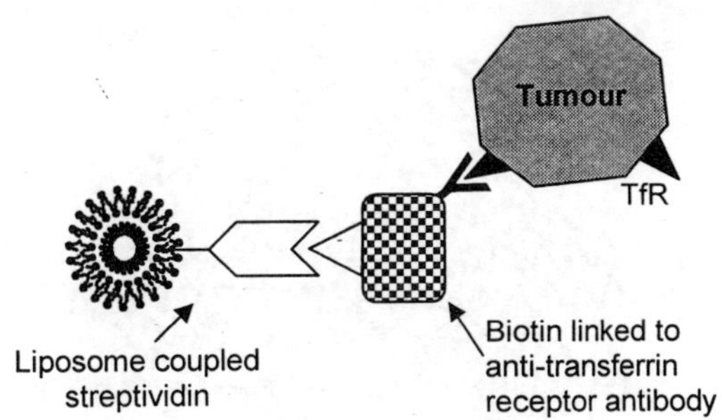

Fig. 1-17. Biotin-avidin/streptividin Conjugated Carriers, Where Avidin/streptividin Links the Delivery Systems and Biotinylated Targeting Ligand

specific binding ligands. This however restricts the use of only anti-target immunoglobulin molecules as site-directing ligands.

POLYMERIC MICELLES

Polymeric micelles are essentially based on amphiphilic block copolymers such as the Pluronics (polyoxyethylene polyoxypropylene block copolymers) self-assemble into polymeric micelles (Figure 1-18). Hydrophobic drugs may be solubilized within the core of the micelle (Kabanov et al., 1992; Batrakova et al., 1996) or, alternatively, conjugated to the micelle-forming polymer (Yokayama et al., 1990). Although micelles are rather dynamic systems, which continuously exchange units between the micelle structure and the free units in solution (Florence and Attwood, 1998), polyoxyethylene polyaspartic acid micelles are sufficiently stable in the blood and effectively alter the pharmacokinetics of solubilized drug (Kataoka et al., 1993). They thus circulate for prolonged periods and are capable of selectively delivering more drug to tumour tissue as compared to administration of the drug in solution (Kwon et al., 1993; Kwon et al., 1994). Pluronic micelles solubilizing epirubicin and doxorubicin increase the tumoricidal activity of these anticancer drugs (Batrakova et al., 1996) and polyoxyethylene polyaspartic acid micelle-forming block copolymers bearing covalently attached doxorubicin at the polyaspartic acid end reduce the toxicity of doxorubicin *in vivo* (Yokayama et al., 1990). Various intelligent polymeric systems have been developed which sensibly respond to the variation in biomilieu,

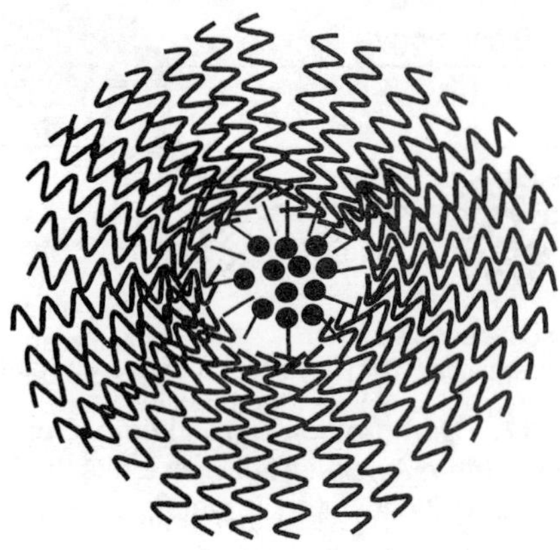

Fig, 1-18. Polymeric Micelle

i.e. variation in pH or temperature and accordingly termed as pH or temperature sensitive polymeric micellar system(s). Polymeric micelles bearing targeting ligands may also be used as drug targeting components. Pluronic micelles solubilizing the neuroleptic drug haloperidol may be targeted to the brain when conjugated to brain specific antibodies.

AQUASOMES

Aquasomes are three layered self-assembling compositions with ceramic carbon nanocrystalline particulate core coated with glassy cellobiose or alternatively degradable calcium phosphate nanocrystalline particle core coated with glassy pyridoxal-5 phosphate. Subsequently, drug/enzyme is non-covalently bound to the outer coating. In general these complex multicomponent particulate delivery systems are assemblies of simple polymers, complex lipid mixtures or ceramic materials with diameter ranging between 30 to 500 nm. As these are solid or glassy particles dispersed in an aqueous environment, they exhibit the physical properties of colloids and their mechanism of action is controlled by their surface chemistry. Aquasomes deliver their contents through a combination of specific targeting, molecular shielding and a slow and sustained release processes. Their large size and inherently active surfaces enable them to be loaded with substantial amounts of agents through non-covalent processes (Meijer et al., 1992). Moreover, owing to their size and relative structure stability, they avoid clearance by reticuloendothelial system or degradation by other environmental challenges.

Aquasome technology represents a platform system for preserving the conformational integrity and biochemical stability of bio-actives. It opens new vistas for vaccines, synthetic blood, drug delivery and gene therapy (Table 1-2).

Among various applications of aquasomes antigen delivery especially represents an illusive approach. A hydrophilic polyhydroxyloligomeric film of the disaccharide, cellobiose adsorbed on the carbon ceramic surface provides suitable conditions for efficient antigen delivery. Aquasomes are capable of eliciting a conformationally correct antibody mediated immunological reaction due to their potential of delivering the antigen in their native conformational state. Besides antigen, aquasomes have also been exploited for delivery of active insulin and haemoglobin (Kossovsky and Millett, 1991).

Aquasomes have also been envisioned for successful gene therapy. Figure 1-19 illustrates the attractive delivery system loaded with genetic material (Kossovsky, 1995). Studies revealed that aquasomes protect and maintain the structural integrity of the gene segment. A five-layered composition comprised of the ceramic nanocrystalline core, the polyoxyloligomeric film coating, the non-covalently bound layer of therapeutic gene segment, an additional carbohydrate film and a targeting layer of confomationally conserved viral membrane proteins, have been proposed for gene therapy. The aquasome vehicle would afford all of the potential advantages of viral vectors and simultaneous overwhelming the risk of irrelevant gene integration. Aquasomes are considered to be a rival of successful delivery vehicles like liposomes and also compete with modified adenovirus delivery vehicles and genetically engineered vaccines, however the simplicity of the chemistry provides an additional benefit for rapid development. Nevertheless, much more is to be explored before they can be adopted for clinical practices.

DENDRIMER

The term "Dendrimer" (Greek: dendron means tree and meros is part) graphically describes the chemical architecture of this new class of molecule. Dendrimers

Table 1-2. Applications of Aquasome-Based Molecular Delivery Technology

Use	Protein/Surface macromolecule	Rationale	Comment
Vaccines	Antigenic envelope proteins including EBV and HIV	To be effective, protective antibodies, the objective of vaccine therapy, must be triggered by conformationally specific target molecules.	Appears to be effective for a wide variety of antigens. Protective immunity not assessed. Long term toxicity not assessed.
Blood Substitutes	Haemoglobin	Co-operativity of haemoglobin is conformationally sensitive.	*In vitro* properties are similar to whole blood. *In vivo* properties including safety and toxicity not fully characterized.
Pharmaceuticals	Active drug such as insulin	Drug activity is conformationally specific.	Bioactivity of drugs preserved. Long term toxicity not characterized.
Gene therapy	Genetic Material	Targeted intracellular delivery.	Binding and release demonstrated. Targeting not currently reliable. Incorporates drug delivery and antigen delivery properties.
Enzymes	Polypeptide such as the enzyme, DNase	Activity fluctuates with molecular conformation.	Bioactivity of enzymes preserved. Long term toxicity not characterized.

*Adopted from Kossovsky, 1996

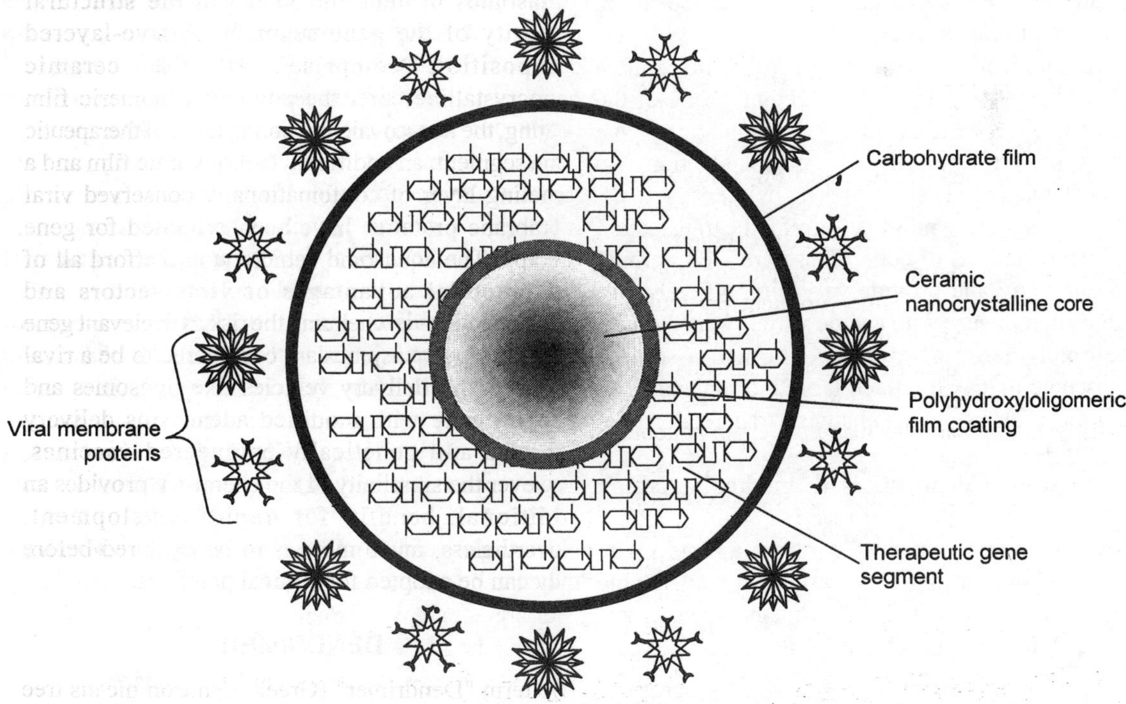

Fig. 1-19. Aquasomes for Gene Therapy

appear to be inert, non-immunogenic and non cytotoxic. These are highly branched three dimensional macromolecules with highly controlled structures with all bonds emanating from a central core. Generally, during dendrimer formation molecules emanate from a core and like a tree they more and more ramify with each subsequent branching unit referred to as generation. Dendrimer construction is fundamentally divided into two methods, the divergent method, where one branching unit after another is successively attached to the core molecule, hence the multiplication of the number of peripheral groups is dependent on the branching multiplicity. Secondly, convergent method, which involves the opposite course. The skeleton is built stepwise starting from the end group towards the inside and is finally treated with a core molecule to produce the dendrimer.

Basically, in the divergent method as the layers build outward from the core molecule the fractal or dendritic, nature of the growing structure emerges; large regions resemble the small Ys formed by triplets of monomers. The internal structure acquires a star like appearance and the final products as appear are called "Starburst Dendrimers".

The application of dendrimers in pharmaceutical and medical chemistry is fast becoming one of the most attractive areas. A variety of applications have been explored especially in gene transfection and medical imaging vis-à-vis as drug delivery systems. Dendrimers provide new platform for the transfection and manipulations of cells. These are well defined and non-toxic and provide very high efficiency of transfection *in vitro* with a wide variety of cell types. These polymeric moieties also furnish a soluble nanoscopic matrix to attach targeting molecules or other materials useful in enhancing transfection (Wu et al., 1994).

The use of dendrimers in medical imaging exploits the multiplicity of reactive chain ends and allows a large number of contrast agents to be introduced onto a single molecule in a controllable manner, thereby enhancing the imaging sensitivity. The dendimer based contrast agents utilize the well-defined structure and monodispersity of dendrimers. Raduchel, 1998 described the use of dendrimers in magnetic resonance imaging (MRI). The dendrimer, based MRI contrast agents (Fig. 1-20) provide greatly enhanced images of the heart, blood vessels and a variety of other organs (Fig. 1-21).

Being well-defined structure, compact globular shape, size, monodispersity and controllable surface functionalities dendrimers offer excellent candidature for drug delivery. Dendimers can be utilized as potential drug carriers in two ways, firstly drug molecules can be physically entrapped within the dendritic structure and secondly drug molecules can be covalently linked onto the dendrimer surface or other functionalities to produce dendrimer-drug conjugates. However, application of dendrimers as drug carriers should mainly focus on improving the design of the dendritic framework in terms of bio-compatibility and bio-distribution as most of the developed systems are unable to fulfil these requirements.

IMPLANT SYSTEMS

The intramuscular, subdermal, intracranial or other organospecific depots are largely based on implants which either limit high drug concentrations to the immediate area surrounding the pathology (Garvin et al., 1994; Fujita et al., 1997; Labhasetwar et al., 1994) or to provide sustained drug release for systemic therapy (Moo-Young et al., 1998; Lesser et al., 1996; Suhonen et al., 1995). Clinically, implant systems are recommended in situations where chronic therapy is indicated, such as hormone replacement therapy and chemical castration in the treatment of prostate cancer. Parenteral implants could be highly viscous liquids or semisolid formulations, both of which may be injected with a needle (Bernatchez et al., 1993). Alternatively, implants may be in the form of tiny rods impregnated with drug substances or a liquid, which gel following administration (Chandrashekar and Udupa, 1996; Haglund et al., 1996; Jeong et al., 1997). *In situ* forming gels either gel on diffusion of polymer solubilizing solvent from the injection site, leaving the polymer in contact with an aqueous environment *in vivo* or gel on cooling after being injected at an elevated temperature. *In situ* forming gels may be used to prepare sustained release formulations of oligonucleotides (Joshi et al., 1998) and non-steroidal anti-inflammatory agents

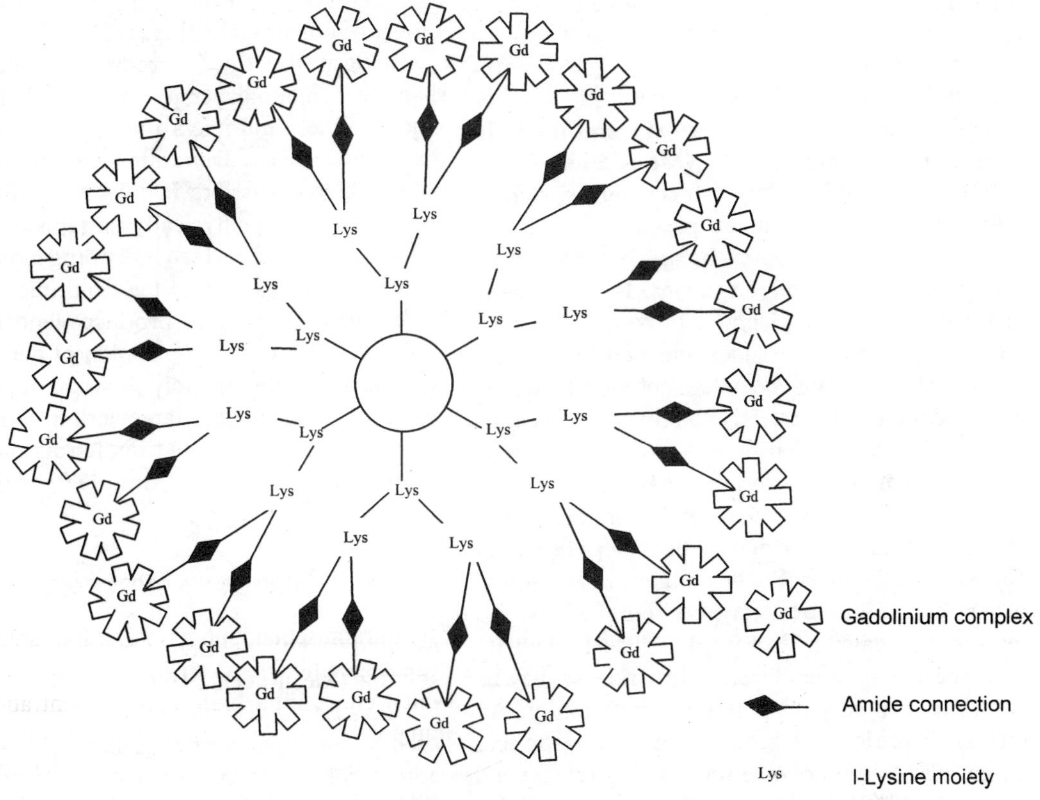

Fig. 1-20. A Dendrimer with 24 Complexed Gadolinium Ions Used as an MRI Contrast Agent

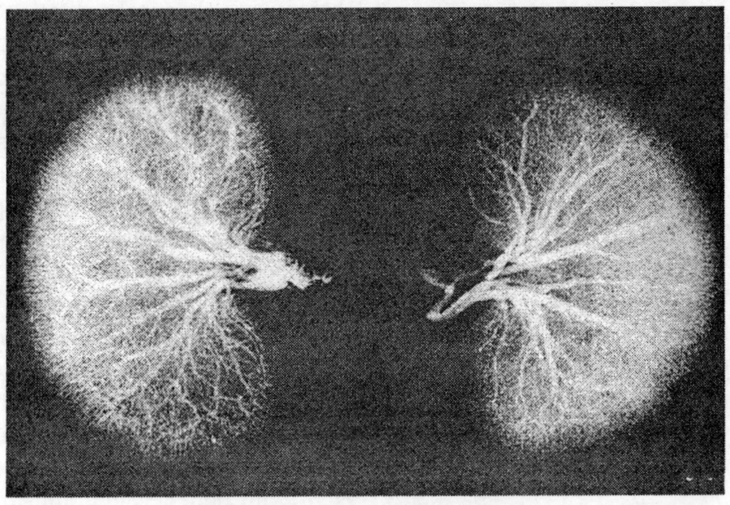

Fig. 1-21. MRI Image of Kidney

(Chandrashekar and Udupa, 1996). Implants intended for parenteral administration are prepared from a variety of polymeric materials including polysaccharides (Chen et al., 1995), polylactic acid co-glycolic acid (Kunou et al., 1995), and the non-biodegradable methacrylates (Moo-Young et al., 1998). Various principles or mechanisms such as diffusion, dissolution, vapour pressure (Fig. 1-22), osmosis (Fig. 1-23), ion-exchange, etc. have been exploited for implantable systems. Biodegradable materials, such as polylactic acid co-glycolic acid, are preferred as this excludes the need for surgical removal of the implant after treatment ends. However, non-biodegradable materials do provide therapeutic levels of drug for up to one year *in vivo*. Solid implants typically exhibit biphasic release kinetics, with an initial burst of drug followed by a slower release. The initial burst is usually due to the release of drug deposited on the surface of the implant although zero order release kinetics may be achieved by, for example, coating the implant with a drug impermeable material. Overall drug release may be controlled by varying polymer composition. An increase in the level of lactic acid in a polylactic acid co-glycolic acid copolymer retards drug release and an increase in the polymer molecular weight also retards drug release and prolongs drug effects *in vivo* (Meyer et al., 1995).

Drug release could be biophysically modulated using stimuli, to which a system responds, such as electrical stimuli in polyelectrolyte systems. The conventional pulsatile delivery systems such as the electrically triggered release of insulin from polydimethylaminopropylacrylamide gels (Kagatani et al., 1997). Solid implants avoid the peak levels associated with the administration of the drug in solution (Mestiri et al., 1995), thus limiting the toxic effects associated with the free drug. Implants are used for the delivery of anticancer agents as they are able to confine potentially toxic anticancer drugs to tumour sites and also allow sustained drug release. A viscous gelatin solution or galactoxyloglucan gel of mitomycin C administered intraperitoneally prolongs peritoneal and plasma clearance (Suisha et al., 1998). Tumoricidal activity of mitomycin C against a peritoneal ascites model was thus increased with use of the gelatin formulation in mice due to the presence of a depot of the gel in the peritoneum. Additionally, the intraperitoneal use of a 5-fluorouracil poly(ortho ester) implant improves the tumoricidal activity of

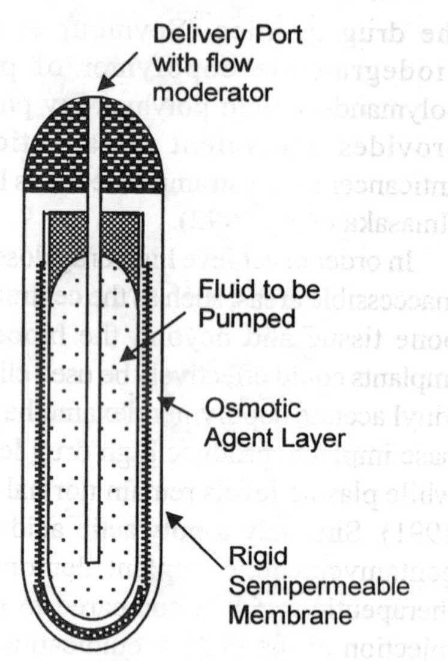

Fig. 1-23. Alzet® Implantable Osmotic Pump

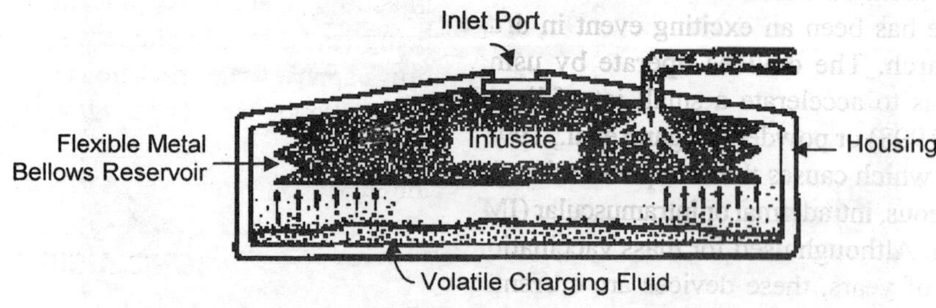

Fig. 1-22. Schematic Representation of a Vapour-Pressure Driven Pump (Rohde et al., 1988)

the drug in mice (Seymour et al., 1994b). A biodegradable copolymer of polylactic acid polymandelic acid polyhydroxy phenyl acetic acid provides equivalent therapeutic levels of the anticancer drug estramustine for as long as 10 weeks (Imasaka et al., 1992).

In order to achieve high drug doses in traditionally inaccessible areas, such as the central nervous system, bone tissue and beyond the blood-retinal barrier implants could effectively be used clinically. Ethylene vinyl acetate copolymer dexamethasone intracranial base implants produce high drug levels in the brain while plasma levels remain normal (Reinhard et al., 1991). Similarly a polylactic acid co-glycolic acid gentamycin bone implant demonstrated superior therapeutic regimen compared to an intramuscular injection of the drug at eradicating bone infections in a canine model. Additionally, polylactic acid co-glycolic acid scleral implants containing gancyclovir for the treatment of cytomegalovirus infection could maintain effective therapeutic levels of the drug in the vitreous humour and retina/choroid for over a period of three to five months.

It is concluded that implant systems, although have the obvious drawback of requiring administration through mini-surgical procedures, offer a means of achieving high drug concentrations in areas that are usually inaccessible to peripherally or vascularly administered drug. In addition, the high drug levels are maintained in sustained manner in these areas.

SYSTEMS FOR NON-INVASIVE SYSTEMIC ADMINISTRATION

The invention and successful demonstration of injection free parenteral administration of bioactives using a device has been an exciting event in drug delivery research. The devices operate by using compressed gas to accelerate a small jet of liquid (Rogge et al., 1998) or powder (Degano et al., 1998) at high speed, which causes the skin penetration for their subcutaneous, intradermal or intramuscular (IM) administration. Although used for mass vaccination for a number of years, these devices are currently being promoted as devices for the self-administration of parenteral drugs. Non-invasive parenteral administration should allow the painless injection of liquids and solids and also remove the risk of needle pricking associated injury to health care professionals. Some reports indicate an increased level of bruising (Verrips et al., 1998) and general discomfort (Prybylski et al., 1994) with jet injectors while others report a decreased level of general discomfort with the newer jet injectors (Domino et al., 1997; Bennett et al., 1998).

Intraject, Biojector and Medijector systems, while solids may be administered using Powderject's technology (Degano et al., 1998; Partsch et al., 1997). Fortunately, needle-free devices appear not to affect drug disposition when administered subcutaneously to patients and drug responses also remain largely unaffected when administration takes place by this route (Houdijk et al., 1997; Gerbert et al., 1996). However, a reduced bioavailability was observed after needle free (Biojector) i.m. injection of interferon β-1α when compared with i.m. administration with a needle. It appears that jet injectors are unable to administer the dose into the i.m. compartment efficiently and hence larger doses are required for effective i.m. injection with these devices (Domino et al., 1998). Reports are also available that indicate that the intracavernous administration of drugs for penile dysfunction may be affected by the use of jet injectors (Seyam et al., 1997). Powderject technology is currently being evaluated and used to develop intradermal DNA vaccines (Vanderzaden et al., 1998). A vaccine development collaboration agreement was recently signed by Glaxo Wellcome and Powderject to exploit this technology (Fox, 1998). The needle-less powder delivery device could administer the antigen and elicits cytotoxic T-cell responses with much lower doses of DNA than required by conventional needle injections. Needle-free injection devices currently being tested for the painless self-administration of drugs appear to be efficacious for subcutaneous and intradermal use. These devices also offer the possibility of improving patient responses to intradermally administered vaccines.

CONCLUSION

The past decade witnessed a real explosion in the number of technologies developed and available to control drug biodistribution. These **have been** exploited through particulate, soluble and implantable drug delivery systems. Passively targeted systems accumulate in the desired area of the anatomy or pathology due to the intrinsic properties of the materials/systems while actively targeted systems with targeting ligands or targeting antibodies could direct the carrier and contents to specific body sites. Drug carrier systems and technologies based on them such as those discussed above may be used to extend the patent life of the drugs but more importantly to control drug delivery on parenteral administration. Some of the newer systems, such as liposomal doxorubicin, may soon be licensed for new pathological indications. Additionally, the coming years may see some new formulation/drug delivery initiatives, such as the polymer drug conjugates and possibly the ADEPT systems as commercial products.

REFERENCES

Ahl P. L., Bhatia S. K., Meers P., Roberts P., Stevens R. and Dause R. (1997) *Biochim. Biophys. Acta* **1329**, 370.

Akiyoshi K. and Sunamoto S. (1992) *J. Surfactants Sci. Ser.* **44**, 289.

Akiyoshi K., Nishikawa T., Shichibe S. and Sunamoto J. (1995) *Chem. Lett.* 707.

Allen T. M. (1993) *Adv. Drug Del. Rev.* **13**, 285.

Allen T. M. (1994) *Trends Pharm. Sci.* **15**, 215.

Allen T. M., Hansen C. B. and Stuart D. D. (1998) In: Medical Applications of Liposomes, Lasic D. D. and Papahadjopoulos D. (Eds.), Elsevier, Oxford, 297.

Almeida A. J., Runge S. and Muller R. H. (1997) *Int. J. Pharm.* **149**, 255.

Alpar H. O., Ozsoy Y., Bowen J., Eyles J. E., Conway B. R. and Williamson E. D. (1996) *Proc. Int. Symp. Control. Rel. Bioact. Mater.* **23**, 861.

Arigo A.P., Tanaka K., Goldberg A.L. and Welch W.J. (1988) *Nature* **331**, 192.

Arunothayanun P., Turton J. A., Uchegbu I. F. and Florence A. T. (1999) *J. Pharm. Sci.* **88**, 34.

Baillie A. J., Coombs G. H., Dolan T. F. and Laurie J. (1986) *J. Pharm. Pharmacol.* **38**, 502.

Baillie A. J., Florence A. T., Hume L. R., Murihead G. T. and Rogerson A. (1985) *J. Pharm. Pharmacol.* **37**, 863.

Batrakova E. V., Dorodnych T. Y., Klinskii E. Y., Kliushnenkova E. N., Shemchukova O. B. and Goncharova O. N. (1996) *Br. J. Cancer* **74,** 1545.

Bazile D., Prud-Homme C., Bassoullet M. T., Malard M., Spenlehauer G. and Veillard M. (1993) *J. Pharm. Sci.* **84**, 493.

Bengtson G. and Olivercrona T. (1988) *Eur. J. Biochem.* **106**, 549.

Bennett J., Nichols F., Rosenblum M. and Condry J. (1998) *J. Oral Maxillofac. Surg.* **56**, 1249.

Bernatchez S. F., Merkli A., Tabatabay C., Gurny R., Zhao Q. H. and Anderson J. M. (1993) *J. Biomed. Mater. Res.* **27**, 677.

Borenztan J., Getz G.S. and Kotlar T.J. (1988) *J. Lipid Res.* **29**, 1087.

Brewer J. M. and Alexander J. (1992) *Immunology* **75**, 570.

Carter K. C., Baillie A. J., Alexander J. and Dolan T. F. (1988) J. Pharm. Pharmacol. **40**, 370.

Chandrashekar G. and Udupa N. (1996) *J. Pharm. Pharmacol.* **48**, 669.

Chen J., Jo S. and Park K. (1995) *Carbohydrate Polym.* **28**, 69.

Codde J. P., Lumsden A. J., Napoli S., Burton M. A. and Gray B. N. (1993) *Anticancer Res.* **13**, 539.

Cohen S., Bernstein H., Hewes C., Chow M. and Langer R. (1991) *Proc. Natl. Acad. Sci. USA* **88**, 10440.

Couvreur P., Roblot-Treupl L., Poupon M. F., Brasseur F. and Puisieux F. (1990) *Adv. Drug Del. Rev.* **5**, 209.

Cuvier C., Roblot-Treupel L., Millot J. M., Lizard G., Chevillard S., Manfait M., Couvreur P. and Poupon M. F. (1992) *Biochem. Pharmacol.* **44**, 509.

Degano P., Sarphie D. F. and Bangham C. R. M. (1998) *Vaccine* **16**, 394.

Domino E. F., Zsigmond E. K., Kovacs V., Fekete G. and Stetson P. (1997) *Int. J. Clin. Pharmacol. Ther.* **35**, 527.

Domino E. F., Zsigmond E. K., Kovacs V., Olajos B. and Fekete G. (1998) *Int. J. Clin. Pharmacol. Ther.* **36**, 458.

Duncan R. (1992) *Anti-cancer Drugs* **3**, 175.

Endicott J. A. and Ling V. (1989) *Ann. Rev. Biochem.* **58**, 137.

Fielding C.J. and Havel, R.J (1977) *Arch. Pathol. Lab. Med.* **101**, 225.

Florence A. T. (1993) In: Liposome Technology, Gregoriadis G. (Ed.), Vol. II, 2nd Ed., CRC Press, Boca Raton, FL, 157.

Florence A. T. and Attwood D. (1998) Physicochemical Principles of Pharmacy, 3rd Ed., Macmillan Press, Hampshire, 1.

Forssen E. A. and Ross M. E. (1994) *J. Liposome Res.* **4**, 481.

Fox S. (1998) *Genetic Engineer News* **18**, 24.

Fujita T., Tamura T., Yamada H., Yamamoto A. and Muranishi S. (1997) *J. Drug. Target.* **4**, 289.

Gabizon A. and Papahadjopoulos D. (1988) *Proc. Natl. Acad. Sci. USA* **85**, 6949.

Gabizon A. and Papahadjopoulos D. (1992) *Biochim. Biophys. Acta* **1103**, 94.

Gabizon A., Goron D., Horowitz A. T., Tzemach D., Lossos A. and Siegal T. (1997) *Adv. Drug Del. Rev.* **24**, 337.

Garvin K. L., Miyano J. A., Robinson D., Giger D., Novak J. and Radio S. (1994) *J. Bone Joint Surg. Am. Vol.* **76**, 1500.

Gasco M. R. (1993) *European Patent Application* 9 111 3152.2.

Gerbert J., Burns S. and Liedtke L. A. (1996) *J. Am. Podiatric. Med. Assoc.* **86**, 195.

Gref R., Domb A., Quellec P., Blunk T., Muller R. H., Verbavatz J. M. and Langer R. (1995) *Adv. Drug Del. Rev.* **16**, 215.

Gref R., Minamitake Y., Peracchia M. T., Trubetskoy V., Torchilin V. and Langer R. (1994) *Science* **263**, 1600.

Gregoriadis G. (1997) *Pharm. Res.* **15**, 661.

Gregoriadis G., Gursel I., Gursel M. and McCormack B. (1996) *J. Control. Rel.* **41**, 49.

Gregoriadis G., Leathwood P. D. and Ryman B. E. (1971) *FEBS Lett.* **14**, 95.

Gregoriadis G., Saffie R. and Da Souza J. B. (1997) *FEBS Lett.* **402**, 107.

Grimaldi S., Lisi A., Pozzi D. and Santoro N. (1997) *Res. Virol.* **148**, 177.

Haglund B. O., Josi R. and Himmelstein K. J. (1996) *J. Control. Rel.* **41**, 229.

Hasima H. J., Boven M., Vanmuijen M., Dejong J., vander Vijgh W. J. F. and Pinedo H. M. (1992) *Br. J. Cancer* **66**, 474.

Hassan Y., Brewer J. M., Alexander J. and Jennings R. (1996) *Vaccine* **14**, 1581.

Heya T., Mikura Y., Nagai A., Miura Y., Futo T. and Tomida Y. (1994) *J. Pharm. Sci.* **83**, 798.

Hiemenz J. W. and Walsh T. J. (1996) *Clin. Infect. Dis.* **22**, S113.

Hillery A. M., Toth I., Shaw A. J. and Florence A. T. (1996) *J. Control. Rel.* **41**, 271.

Hodoshima N., Udagawa C., Ando T., Fukuyasu H., Watanabe H. and Nakabayashi S. (1997) *Int. J. Pharm.* **146**, 81.

Houdijk E., Herdes E. and DelemarreVandeWaal H. A. (1997) *Acta Paediatrica* **86**, 1301.

Hunter C. A., Dolan T. F., Coombs G. H. and Baillie A. J. (1988) J. Pharm. Pharmacol. **40**, 161.

Hurwitz E., Wilchek M. and Pitha J. (1980) *J. Appl. Biochem.* **2**, 25.

Ike O., Shimizu Y., Ikada Y., Watanabe S., Natsume T. and Wada R. (1991) *Biomaterials* **12**, 757.

Illum L. and Davis S. S. (1983) J. Pharm. Sci. **72**, 1086.

Illum L. and Davis S. S. (1984) *FEBS Lett.* **167**, 79.

Imasaka K., Yoshida M., Fukuzaki H., Asano M., Kumakura M. and Mashimo T. (1992) *Int. J. Pharm.* **81**, 31.

Jameela S. R., Latha P. G., Subramoniam A. and Jayakrishnan A. (1996) *J. Pharm. Pharmacol.* **48**, 685.

Jeong B., Bae Y. H., Lee D. S. and Kim S. W. (1997) *Nature* **388**, 860.

Joshi R., Arora V., Desjardins J. P., Robinson D., Himmelstein K. J. and Iversen P. L. (1998) *Pharm. Res.* **15**, 1189.

Kabanov A. V., Batrakova E. V., Melik-Nubarov N. S., Fedoseev N. A., Dorodnich Y. and Alakhov V. Y. (1992) *J. Control. Rel.* **22**, 141.

Kagatani S., Shinoda T., Konno Y., Fukui M., Ohmura T. and Osada Y. (1997) *J. Pharm. Sci.* **86**, 1273.

Kartner N., Evernden-Porelle D., Bradley G. and Ling V. (1985) *Nature* **316**, 820.

Kataoka K., Kwon G. S., Yokoyama M., Okano T. and Sakurai Y. (1993) *J. Control. Rel.* **24**, 119.

Kim C. K. and Jeong E. J. (1995) *Int. J. Pharm.* **115**, 193.

Kossovsky N. (1995) Artificial Self-Assembling Systems for Gene Transfer, Presentation at the Cambridge Healthtech Institute Conference, Boston, MA.

Kossovsky N. and Millett D. (1991) *Mat. Res. Soc. Bull.* **9**, 78.

Kreuter J. (1991) *J. Control. Rel.* **16**, 169.

Kubiak C., Manil L., Clausse B. and Couvreur P. (1989) *Biomaterials* **10**, 553.

Kunou N., Ogura Y., Hashizoe M., Honda Y., Hyon S. H. and Ikada Y. (1995) *J. Control. Rel.* **37**, 143.

Kwon G. S., Yokoyama M., Okano T., Sakurai Y. and Kataoka K. (1993) *Pharm. Res.* **10**, 970.

Kwon G., Suwa S., Yokoyama M., Okano T., Sakurai Y. and Kataoka K. (1994) *J. Control. Rel.* **29**, 17.

Labhasetwar V., Underwood T., Gallagher M., Murphy G., Langberg J. and Levy R. J. (1994) *J. Pharm. Sci.* **83**, 156.

Lacasse F. X., Hildgen P., Perodin J., Escher E., Phillips N. C. and McMullen J. N. (1997) *Pharm. Res.* **14**, 887.

Lakshman M.R., Muesing R.A. and LaRose J.C. (1981) *J. Biol. Chem.* **265**, 3037.

Ledley F. D. (1995) *Human Gene Therapy* **6**, 1129.

Leroux J. C., Allemann E., DeJaeghere F., Doelker E. and Gurny R. (1996) *J Control Rel* **39**, 339.

Lesser G. J., Grossman S. A., Leong K. W., Lo H. N. and Eller S. (1996) *Pain* **65**, 265.

Lima K. M. and Junior J. M. R. (1999) *Braz. J. Med. Biol. Res.* **32**, 171.

Longman S. A., Cullis P. R. and Bally M. B. (1995a) *Drug Delivery* **2**, 156.

Longman S. A., Cullis P. R., Choi L., de Jong G. and Bally M. B. (1995b) *Cancer Chemother. Pharmacol.* **36**, 91.

Maeda M., Takasuka N., Suga T., Uehara N. and Hoshi A. (1993) *Anti-Cancer Drugs* **4**, 167.

Matsumara Y. and Maeda H. (1986) *Cancer Res.* **46**, 6387.

Mehta R. C., Jeyanthi R., Calis S., Thanoo B. C., Burton K. W. and Deluca P. P. (1994) *J. Control. Rel.* **29**, 375.

Meijer D. K. F., Jansen R. W. and Molema G. (1992) *Antiviral Research* **18**, 215.

Menei P., BoisdronCelle M., Croue A., Guy G. and Benoit J. P. (1996) *Neurosurgery* **39**, 117.

Mestiri M., Benoit J. P., Hernigou P., Devissaguet J. P. and Puisieux F. (1995) *J. Control. Rel.* **33**, 107.

Meyer J., Whitcomb L., Treuheit M. and Collins D. (1995) *J. Control. Rel.* **35**, 67.

Moo-Young A. J., Kuzuma P., Quandt H., Shlegel P. N., Bardin C. W. and Frick J. (1998) *Proc. Int. Symp. Control. Rel. Bioact. Mater.* **25**, 64.

Moritera T., Ogura Y., Honda Y., Wada R., Hyon S. H. and Ikada Y. (1991) *Investig. Ophthalmol. Vis. Sci.* **32,** 1785.

Moser C. A., Speaker T. J., Berlin J. A. and Offit P. A. (1996) *Vaccine* **14**, 1235.

Muller R. H. and Lucks J. S. (1991) *German Patent Application* P41 31 562.6.

Muller R. H. and Lucks J. S. (1996) *European Patent* 0605 497 B1.

Muller R. H., Jacobes C. and Kayser O. (2001) *Adv. Drug Del. Rev.* **47**, 3.

Muller R. H., Mehnert W., Lucks J. S., Schwarz C., zur Muhlen A., Weyhers H., Freitas C. and Ruhl D. (1995) *Eur. J. Pharm. Biopharm.* **41**, 62.

Muller R. H., Schwarz C., Mehnert W. and Lucks J. S. (1993) *Proc. Int. Symp. Control. Rel. Bioact. Mater.* **20**, 480.

Nichifor M., Schacht E. H. and Seymour L. W. (1997) *J Control Rel* **48**, 165.

Nishikawa T., Akiyoshi K. and Sunamoto J. (1996) *J. Am. Chem. Soc.* **118**, 6110.

O'Hagan D. T., Rahman D., McGee J. P., Jeffery H., Davies M. C. and Williams P. (1991) *Immunology* **73**, 239.

Ohki A., Naka K., Ito O. and Maeda S. (1994) *Chem. Lett.* 1065.

Okada H. and Toguchi H. (1995) *Crit. Rev. Therapeut. Drug. Carr. Sys.* **12**, 1.

Oussoren C. and Storm G. (1998) *Int. J. Pharm.* **162**, 39.

Partsch C. J., vonBuren E., Kuhn B., Sippell W. G. and Brinkmann G. (1997) *Eur. J. Pediatr.* **156**, 893.

Pimm M. V., Perkins A. C., Strohalm J., Ulbrich K. and Duncan R. (1996) *J. Drug. Target.* **3**, 375.

Pitas R.E., Boyles J.K., Lee, S.H., Hui D. and Weisgraber K.H. (1987) *J. Biol. Chem.* **262**, 14352.

Prybylski D., Santana S., Englender S. and Smith M. (1994) *Am. J. Epidemiol.* **139**, S71.

Raduchel B. (1998) *Polym. Mater. Sci. Eng.* **79**, 516.

Reddy J. A. and Low P. S. (1998) *Crit. Rev. Ther. Drug Carrier Syst.* **15**, 587.

Reinhard C. S., Radomsky M. L., Saltzman W. M., Hilton J. and Brem H. (1991) *J. Control. Rel.* **16**, 331.

Renkin E.M. (1979) *Acta Physiol. Scand.* **463**, 81.

Ringsdorf H. (1975) *J. Polym. Sci. Polym. Symp.* **51**, 135.

Rohde T. D., Buchwald H. and Blackshear P. J. (1988) In: Drug Delivery Devices, Tyle P. (Ed.), Marcel Dekker Inc., New York, 235.

Roheim P.S., Carey M., Forte T. and Vega, L. (1979) *Proc. Natl. Acad. Sci. USA* **76**, 4646.

Rogge M. C., Charenkavanich S., DiBiase M., Jones W., Knox S. J. and Alam J. J. (1998) *Drug. Delivery* **5**, 275.

Ruiz J. M. and Benoit J. P. (1991) *J. Control. Rel.* **16**, 177.

Sanchez A. and Alonso M. J. (1995) *Eur. J. Pharm. Biopharm.* **41**, 31.

Senter P. D. (1990) *FASEB J.* **4**, 188.

Seyam R. M., Begin L. R., Tu L. M., Dion S. B., Merlin S. L. and Brock G. B. (1997) *Urology* **50**, 994.

Seymour L. W., Duncan R., Duffy J., Ng S. Y. and Heller J. (1994a) *J. Control. Rel.* **31**, 201.

Seymour L. W., Ulbrich K., Steyger P. S., Brereton M., Subr V. and Strohalm J. (1994b) *Br. J. Cancer* **70**, 636.

Sherwood R. F. (1996) *Adv. Drug Del. Rev.* **22**, 269.

Speiser P. (1990) *European Patent* EP 0167 825.

Storm G. and Crommelin J. A. (1998) *Pharm. Science Tech.Today* **1**, 19.

Sugiyama T., Kumagai S., Nishida T., Ushijima K., Matsuo T. and Yakushiji M. (1998) *Anticancer Res.* **18**, 2837.

Suhonen S. P., Allonen H. O. and Lähteenmäki P. (1995) *Am. J. Obstet. Gynecol.* **172**, 562.

Suisha F., Kawasaki N., Miyazaki S., Shirakawa M., Yamatoya K. and Sasaki M. (1998) *Int. J. Pharm.* **172**, 27.

Torchillin V. P. and Trubetskoy V. S. (1995) *Adv. Drug Del. Rev.* **16**, 141.

Tso P. and Balin J.A. (1986) *Am. J. Physiol.* **250**, G715.

Uchegbu I. F. and Vyas S. P. (1998)

Uchegbu I. F., Schätzlein A. G., Tetley L., Brown M., Siddique S. and Jack V. (1998a) *Proc. Int. Symp. Control. Rel. Bioact. Mater.* **25**, 186.

Uchegbu I. F., Schätzlein A. G., Tetley L., Gray A. I., Sludden J., Siddique S. and Mosha E. (1998b) *J. Pharm. Pharmacol.* **50**, 453.

Vanderzanden L., Bray M., Fuller D., Roberts T., Custer D. and Spik K. (1998) *Virology* **246**, 134.

Vasey P. A., Duncan R., Twelves C., Kaye S. B., Strolin-Benedetti M. and Cassidy J. (1996) *Proceedings of the 9th NCI-EORTC Symposium on New Drugs in Cancer Therapy*, Amsterdam, 338.

Verdun C., Brasseur F., Vranckx H., Couvreur P. and Roland M. (1990) *Cancer Chemother. Pharmacol.* **26**, 13.

Verrecchia T., Spenlehauer G., Bazile D. V., Murrybrelier A., Archimbaud Y. and Veillard M. (1995) *J. Control. Rel.* **36**, 49.

Verrips G. H., Hirasing R. A., Fekkes M., Vogels T., VerlooveVanhorick S. P. and DelemarreVandeWaal H. A. (1998) *Acta Paediatrica* **87**, 154.

Vingerhoeds M. H., Hasima H. J., van Muijen M., vande Rijh, Cromellin D. J. A. and Storm G. (1993) *FEBS Lett.* **336**, 485.

Vyas S. P. (2001) In: Advances in Liposomal Therapeutics, Vyas S. P. and Dixit V. K. (Eds.), CBS Publishers, New Delhi, 230.

Wasan M. W. and Lopaz-Berestein G. (1998) In: Medical Applications of Liposomes, Lasic D. D. and Papahadjopoulos D. (Eds.), Elsevier, Oxford, 165.

Williams D. M., Carter K. C. and Baillie A. J. (1995) *J. Drug Target.* **3**, 1.

Willmott N. and Cummings J. (1987) *Biochem. Pharmacol.* **36**, 521.

Woodle M. C. and Lasic D. D. (1992) *Biochim. Biophys. Acta* **1113**, 171.

Working P. K., Newman M. S. and Huang S. K. (1994) *J. Liposome Res.* **4**, 667.

Wu C., Brechbiel M. W., Kozak R. W. and Gansow O. A. (1994) *Bioorg. and Med. Chem. Lett.* **4**, 449.

Yeung T. K., Hopewell J. W., Simmonds R. H., Seymour L. W., Duncan R. and Bellini O. (1991) *Cancer Chemother. Pharmacol.* **29**, 105.

Yokayama M., Miyauchi M., Yamada N., Okano T., Kataoka K. and Inoue S. (1990) *J. Control. Rel.* **11**, 269.

Yoshioka T. and Florence A. T. (1994) *Int. J. Pharm.* **105**, 1.

Yoshioka T., Skalko N., Gursel M., Gregoriadis G. and Florence A. T. (1995) *J. Drug Target.* **2**, 533.

Zubey P. (1988) Biochemistry, McMillan, London,1.

zur Muhlen A., Schwarz C. and Mehnert W. (1998) *Eur. J. Pharm. Biopharm.* **45**, 149.

CHAPTER 2

Molecular Basis of Targeted Drug Delivery

- The concepts of targeting
- Cellular biochemistry and molecular events in drug targeting
- Cell surface biochemistry and molecular targets
- Cell surface receptor expressed for immuno-regulatory molecules
- Future perspectives
- References

Most of the drugs introduced to clinical medicine exert their effects by interactive interference with cell and cell membrane related structure and functions through concentration dependent reversible interactions at specific receptor site(s). Obviously, to obtain a desirable therapeutic response, the correct amount of drug should be transported and delivered to the site of action with subsequent control of drug input rate. The distribution of other tissues therefore seems unnecessary, wasteful and a potential cause of toxicity. The developments of over past decades indicate explicit progress in the area of controlled and targeted drug delivery. It comes to be much more relevant in present context. What Juliano said "The practitioners of drug delivery research find themselves in difficult, however, interesting situation of being at a nexus between an ever growing stream of information about drugs and biological system, and ever expanding plethora of demands for more sophisticated therapeutic systems". It is apparent that most of diseases treated by cytotoxic agents not only demand for controlled drug delivery but also the pattern of delivery is directed to be specific, precise and defined at quantitative levels. The cell related biological regular events occurring in high order of specificity and precision offers basis for quantitative targeted drug delivery. There involved a number of essential bioligands for physiologic cell need and biosignaling. These operate through bioports referred to as receptors. The ligand-receptor interactions are highly stereospecific. Thus ligands or receptors could be exploited for site/cell specific drug delivery quantitatively in a well defined manner. Let us discuss and define various facets of essentials of drug targeting. One ever sought after yet unattained goal in clinical medicine remains to be the successful development of site-specific drug delivery systems. The practical realization of the concept shall be a great breakthrough in medical sciences. The precision programmed and site specificity of the system was poised as a "magic bullet" by Paul Ehrlich. It not only will ensure of site specificity, however will mitigate toxicity of drug(s) to non-target site(s) as a result of well controlled and attenuated drug level.

Selective drug delivery or targeting seeks to improve upon the benefit/risk ratio associated with drugs. Ideally, a drug intended for clinical use should have a high therapeutic index, which is a ratio of drug efficacy (therapeutic effect) and the drug toxicity (side effects). Many drugs, particularly chemo-therapeutic agents have narrow therapeutic window (low therapeutic indices) and their clinical use is limited and compromized by dose limiting toxic side effects. Approaches are being adopted either to control the distribution of drug by incorporating it in a carrier system or by altering the structure of the drug at the molecular level, or by controlling the input of the drug into the bioenvironment to ensure a programmed and desirable biodistribution. Rapid applications of the recent developments in molecular genetics are enabling both, the diagnosis of disease and understanding pathogenesis to the clock work precision, while advents on designing of novel drugs and delivery systems offer opportunities for radical cure of diagnosed diseases.

The efforts to improve drug effectiveness in therapeutics have been assisted by parallel developments in molecular and cell biology. On one hand, hybridoma and recombinant DNA technology have come strongly, and on the other, a number of cell membrane receptors and their interactions with respective ligands have been investigated and reported for many cell related biological functions. Such developments supported the successful developments of target oriented drug delivery systems.

The drug delivery technology has certainly infused new interests in seemingly traditional old drugs by providing trem new life specifically through their therapeutic targets. It is appreciated that, target oriented drug administration with improvements in therapeutic efficacy, reduction in side effects and optimized dosing regimen, shall be the leading trends in the area of therapeutics. Various aspects of the target oriented site specific delivery at cellular, molecular or sub-molecular level are discussed in this chapter.

THE CONCEPTS OF TARGETING

The concept of designing specified delivery system to achieve selective drug targeting has been originated from the perception of Paul Ehrlich, who proposed drug delivery to be as a 'magic bullet'. It was the very first report published on targeting (Paul Ehrlich, 1902) describing targeted drug delivery as an event where, a drug-carrier complex/conjugate, delivers drug(s) exclusively to the preselected target cells in a specific manner. Bangham's observation on phospholipid hexagonal liquid crystals, that they are permselective to the ions in a manner similar to biomembrane, led to discovery of artificial vesicular system based on phospholipid amphiphiles (Bangham, 1965). Gregoriadis, 1981 described drug targeting using novel drug delivery systems as 'old drugs in new cloths'.

Targeted therapy, as Ehrlich, 1902 proposed remains an unachieved goal yet, however the idea stimulated a long series of experiments that propounded the philosophy of targeting of drugs and genes and attracted present generation of researchers towards the problems and prospects associated with the concept. It is pertinent to discuss the concept and components, which are utilized in the targeting of drug(s). A number of essential aspects which should be considered for the designing of drug delivery systems to achieve this goal include target, carrier, ligand(s) and physically modulated components. Targeted drug delivery implies for selective and effective localization of pharmacologically active moiety at preidentified (preselected) target(s) in therapeutic concentration, while restricting its access to non-target normal cellular linings, thus minimizing toxic effects and maximizing therapeutic index (Gregoriadis and Florence, 1993).

Rationale of Drug Targeting

The site specific targeted drug delivery negotiates an exclusive delivery to specific pre-identified compartments with maximum intrinsic activity of drugs and concomitantly reduced access of drug to irrelevant non-target cells. The targeted delivery to previously in-accessible domains, e.g., intracellular sites, virus, bacteria and parasites offers distinctive therapeutic benefits. The controlled rate and mode of drug delivery to pharmacological receptor and specific binding with target cells; as well as bioenvironmental protection of the drug *en route* to the site of action are specific features of targeting. Invariably, every event stated contributes to higher drug concentration at the site of action and resultant lower concentration at non-target tissue where toxicity might crop-up. The high drug concentration at the target site is a result of the relative cellular uptake of the drug vehicle, liberation of drug and efflux of free drug from the target site.

Targeting is signified if the target compartment is distinguished from the other compartments, where toxicity may occur, and also if the active drug could be placed predominantly in the proximity of target site. The restricted distribution of the parent drug to the non-target site(s) with effective accessibility to the target site(s) could maximize the benefits of targeted drug delivery (Fig. 2-1).

Carriers

Carrier is one of the most important entities essentially required for successful transportation of the loaded drug(s) (Fig. 2-2). They are drug vectors, which sequester, transport and retain drug *en route*, while elute or deliver it within or in the vicinity of target. Carriers can do so either through an inherent characteristics or acquired (through structural modification), to interact selectively with biological targets, or otherwise they are engineered to release the drug in the proximity of target cell lines demanding optimal pharmacological action (therapeutic index). Delivery systems developed and exploited in the last decennia for ligand directed receptor mediated targeting are mainly focuses on liposomes and microparticulates, bioconjugates (drug-antibody conjugate, drug-polymer conjugates, drug-immunotoxin conjugates), fusogenic proteins and peptides and certain polymeric and macromolecular delivery systems.

An ideal drug carrier engineered as a targetable device should have the following features:

- It must be able to cross anatomical barriers and in case of tumour chemotherapy tumour vasculature.
- It must be recognized specifically and selectively by the target cells and must maintain the avidity and specificity of the surface ligands
- The linkage of the drug and the directing unit (ligand) should be stable in plasma, interstitial and other biofluids.
- Carrier should be non-toxic, non-immunogenic and biodegradable particulate or macromolecule and after recognition, and inter-

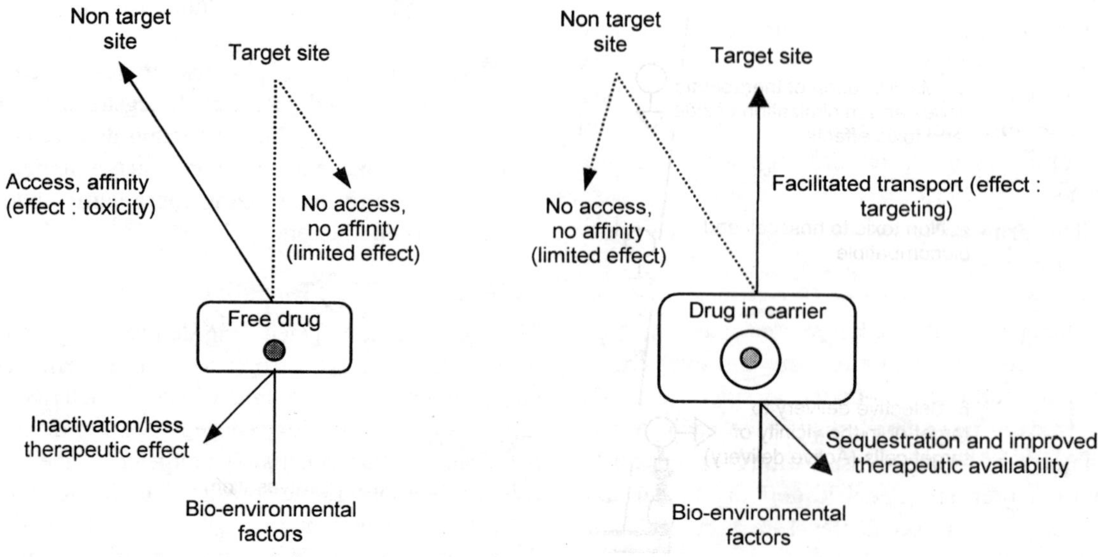

Fig. 2-1. Principle and Rationale of Drug Targeting

nalization, the carrier system should release the drug moiety inside the target organs, tissues or cells.

- The biomodules used for carrier navigation and site recognition should not be ubiquitous otherwise it may cross over the sites, defeating the concept of targeting.

The distinctive and defined intrinsic passivity of carrier at large decides its ultimate biodistribution. However, to promote its selective and intended association with any fixed cells, which are anatomically accessible to the carrier; the carrier must be able to recognize the cell(s) target; should bind to them and if necessary, penetrate into their interior. Similarly, tailoring the structural components of carrier systems (to take advantage of or tackling bioenvironmental properties) has led to the development of carrier systems of diversified nature and ultimately action specific. Some surface modifications of the carrier systems with particular ligands like sugars or monoclonal antibodies (Mabs) could impart a specific targeting potential to the carrier. Hence, in essence to deliver drug selectively to a target we should have versatile putative carriers and site-specific ligands.

Several carriers appended as pilot molecules to selectively deliver the drug to the intended cell lines have been reported (Table 2-1). Based on the nature of their origin they are categorized as endogenous (low density lipoprotein, high-density lipoprotein, chylomicrons, serum albumin, erythrocytes) and exogenous (microparticulates, soluble polymeric and biodegradable polymeric drug carriers). A variety of site specific and target oriented drug delivery systems have been developed and evaluated for their relative potentials.

Microparticulates have been investigated intensively during the last decade to explore and exploit intrinsic targeting potential of the plain or surface manipulated carriers. Advent of nanotechnology has infused new dimensions into the target oriented drug delivery through self-assembling supramolecules based nanostructures.

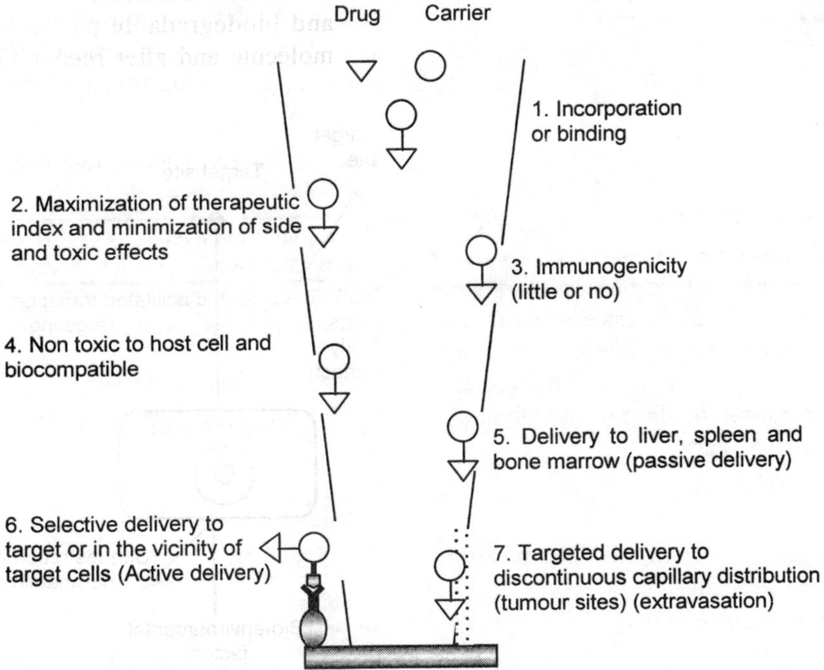

Fig. 2-2. Schematic Illustration of Requirement of Drug Carriers

Table 2-1. Carrier Systems Used for Targeted Drug Delivery*

1. Colloidal carriers
a) Vesicular systems
Liposomes; Niosomes; Pharmacosomes; Virosomes; Immunoliposomes
b) Microparticulate systems
Microparticles; Nanoparticles; Magnetic microspheres; Albumin microspheres; nanocapsules

2. Cellular carriers
Resealed erythrocytes; serum albumin; antibodies; platelets; leukocytes

3. Supramolecular delivery systems
Micelles; reverse micelles; mixed micelles; polymeric micelles; Liquid crystals; Lipoproteins (chylomicron; VLDL; LDL)
Synthetic LDL mimicking particles (supramolecule biovector system)

4. Polymer based systems
Signal sensitive; Muco-adhesive; Biodegradable; Bioerodible; Soluble synthetic polymeric carriers

5. Macromolecular carriers
a) Proteins, glycoproteins; neo glycoproteins and artificial viral envelopes (AVE)
b) Glycosylated water soluble polymers (poly-L-lysine)
c) Mabs; Immunological Fab fragments; antibody-enzyme complex & bispecific Abs
d) Toxins, immunotoxin & rCD4 toxin conjugates
e) Lectins (Con A) & polysaccharides

*Adopted from Vyas and Dixit, 1998

Levels of Drug Targeting

Targeted drug delivery may be achieved by using carrier systems, where reliance is placed on exploiting both, intrinsic pathway(s) that these carriers follow, and the bioprotection that they can offer to drugs during transit through the body. The various approaches of vectoring the drug to the target site can be broadly classified as:

- Passive targeting
- Inverse targeting
- Active targeting (Ligand mediated targeting and Physical targeting)
- Dual targeting
- Double targeting
- Combination targeting

Passive Targeting

Systems that target the systemic circulation are generally characterized as "passive" delivery systems (i.e. targeting occurs because of the body's natural response to the physicochemical characteristics of the drug or drug-carrier system. It is a sort of passive process that utilizes the natural course of (attributed to inherent characteristics) biodistribution of the carrier system, through which, it eventually accumulate in the organ compartment(s) of body. The ability of some colloids to be taken up by the RES especially in liver and spleen has made them as ideal vectors for passive hepatic targeting of drugs to these compartments. Passive capture of colloidal carriers by macrophages offers therapeutic opportunities for the delivery of anti-infectives for disease conditions that involve macrophage cells of the reticulo-endothelial system (RES) e.g., leishmaniasis, brucellosis and candidiasis (Table 2-2). Delivery into lysosomal compartment can also be affected for the treatment of certain lysosomal storage diseases, macrophage neoplasms and macrophage activation (Gregoriadis, 1981).

This category of targetable devices includes drug bearing bilayer vesicular systems as well cellular carriers of micron or submicron size range. The passive targetability of microparticulate drug carriers is due to the recognition of these exogenous

Table 2-2. Passive Hepatic Targeting for Macrophage Associated Diseases

Macrophage associated infected cell lines	Drugs proposed for encapsulation
Intracellular parasites	
Leishmaniasis; brucellosis; candidiasis	Antimalarial and anti-infective
Intracellular fungal infections	
Histoplasmosis; systemic mycoses	Antifungal (Amphotericin B)
Neoplasms	
Histiocytes medullar reticulosis; monocyte & hairy cell lukemia; Hodgkin's disease	Cytotoxic drugs
Viral infected diseases	Anti-viral drugs
Hepatitis	
Enzyme storage diseases	
Gaucher's disease, mucoliposes type II & III	Glucocerebroside and other enzymes

particulates either in the intact or in the opsonized form, by the phagocytic cells of the RES and this sensing behaviour is exploited to target MPS associated diseased cell lines (Table 2-2).

A major disadvantage of microparticulate carriers is that they cannot pass the endothelial cell lines, as a result extravasation is generally poor. Although some investigations claim that slow transcellular (vesicular) transport of liposomes and microspheres is possible through endothelia. The practical applications of microparticulate carriers are largely restricted to intravascular targets. Attempts have been made for targeting them to intravesicular non-RES cell lines and to increase circulation half life by exploiting strategies that involve modification of size, surface charge, composition, surface rigidity and surface hydrophilicity. These long circulatory modules, can then be relied as carrier base. However, to endow them with target specificity some site directing ligands could be appended on their surface site specific ligands can be immobilized with optimal targeting efficiency. Recent literature exhaustively deals with the pilot molecules (ligands) appended microparticles and liposomal systems.

Inverse Targeting

It is essentially based on successful attempts to circumvent and avoid passive uptake of colloidal carriers by reticuloendothelial system (RES). This effectively leads to the reversion of biodistribution trend of the carrier and hence the process is referred to as inverse targeting (Lazo and Hacker, 1986). One strategy applied to achieve inverse targeting is to suppress the function of RES by a pre-injection of a large amount of blank colloidal carriers or macromolecules like dextran sulphate (Illum et al., 1982; Illum et al., 1986; Tomlinson and Burger, 1987; Illum et al., 1989). This approach leads to RES blockade and as a consequence impairment of host defense system. Alternative strategies include modification of the size, surface charge, composition, surface rigidity and hydrophilicity of carriers for desirable biofate.

Recently available literature suggests modification of the surface by imparting distinctive hydrophilicity to the carrier particles, as an effective mode of targeting of drug(s) to non-RES organs. Davis and Hansrani, 1985 reported that phospholipid microspheres emulsified with Polaxamer 338 showed the lowest RES uptake in mouse peritoneal macrophages *in vitro*.

Illum and Davis, 1987 reported that Poloxamine 908, is another hydrophilic nonionic surfactant, which diverts normal RES uptake of coated emulsion and coated nanoparticles (polystyrene microsphere) to inflammatory sites in rabbits. Recently, Lee and co-workers, 1995 suggested inverse targeting of drugs to the sites other than RES rich organs by coating the lipid microemulsion (LM) with polaxamer 308. It has been suggested that surface hydrophilicity may reduce or even eliminate the adhesion of opsonin materials/HDL on to the surface of LM, which is believed to be an essential step in the process of phagocytosis responsible for ultimate uptake of LM by RES system.

Active Targeting

Conceptually, active targeting exploits modification or manipulation of drug carriers to redefine its biofate. The natural distribution pattern of the drug carrier composites is enhanced using chemical, biological and physical means, so that it approaches and identified by particular biosites. The facilitation of the binding of the drug-carrier to target cells through the use of ligands or engineered homing devices to increase receptor mediated (or in some cases receptor independent but epitope based) localization of the drug and target specific delivery of drug(s) is referred to as active targeting.

This targeting approach can further be classified it into three different levels of targeting: first order targeting (organ compartmentalization), second order targeting (cellular targeting) and third order targeting (intracellular targeting).

First Order Targeting

It refers to restricted distribution of the drug-carrier system to the capillary bed of a predetermined target site, organ or tissue. Compartmental targeting in lymphatics, peritoneal cavity, plural cavity, cerebral ventricles, lungs, joints, eyes, etc., represents first order targeting (It could also be categorized as a level of passive targeting).

The ability of liposomes to extravasate and penetrate into diseased states other than MPS is directly related to their size. Large liposomes (10 µ or above) are rapidly removed via mechanical filtration of lungs and from this size range down upto 150 nm are removed by tissue macrophages originated in the liver and spleen, which are the natural target for these vesicles (Fig. 2-3). In order to achieve significant levels in other tissues, liposomes of smaller size (≤100 nm) with a homogeneous distribution have been devel-oped. They could penetrate into either normal tissue having sinusoidal or fenestrated epithelium or otherwise into diseased tissue having altered capillary permeability. This has in turn increased the chances of achieving targeting *in vivo* to non-MPS cell linings.

Second Order Targeting

The selective delivery of drugs to a specific cell type such as tumour cells and not to the normal cells is referred as second order drug targeting. The selective drug delivery to the Kupffer cells in the liver exemplifies this approach.

Third Order Targeting

The third order targeting is defined as drug delivery specifically to the intracellular site of target cells. An example of third order targeting is the receptor based ligand-mediated entry of a drug complex into a cell by endocytosis, lysosomal degradation of carrier followed by release of drug intracellularly or gene delivery to nucleolus.

Ligand Mediated Targeting

Targeting components, which have been studied and exploited are pilot molecules themselves (bioconjugates) or anchored as ligands on some delivery vehicle (drug-carrier system). All the carrier systems, explored so far, in general, are colloidal in nature. They can be specifically functionalized using various biologically relevant molecular ligands including antibodies, polypeptides, oligosaccharides (carbohydrates), viral proteins and fusogenic residues. The ligands afford specific avidity to drug carrier. The engineered carrier constructs selectively deliver the drug to the cell or group of cells generally referred to as target. The cascade of events involved in ligand negotiated specific drug delivery is termed as ligand driven receptor mediated targeting.

Ligand mediated active targeting could be achieved using specific uptake mechanisms such as

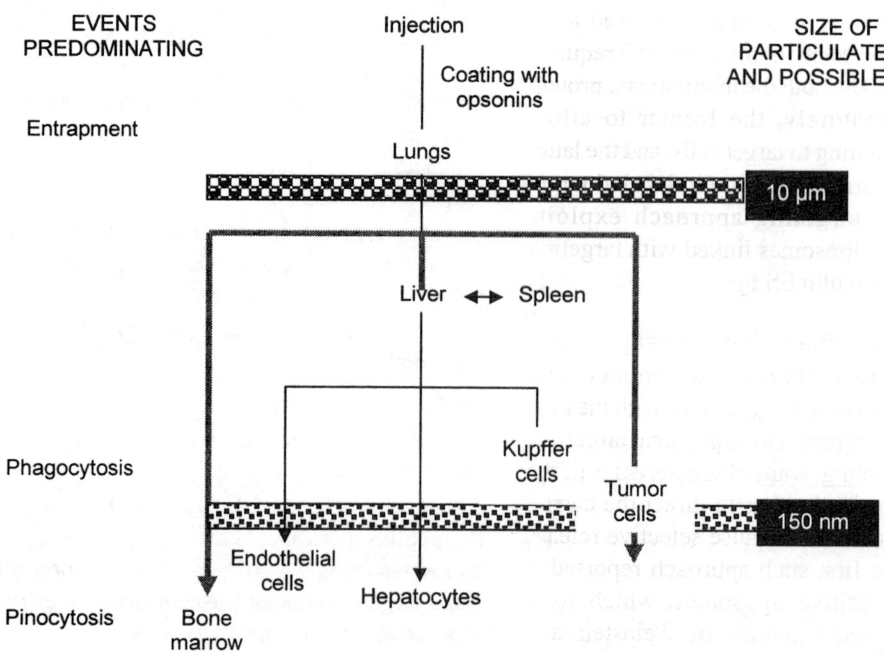

Fig. 2-3. Fate of Colloidal Carriers

receptor dependent uptake of natural low density lipoproteins (LDL) particles and synthetic lipid microemulsions of partially reconstituted LDL particles coated with the apoproteins. The apoprotein coat serves as a ligand for the LDL receptors expressed in the body. The ability of an immunoglobulin coated carrier to promote its accelerated interception by the liver and spleen, possibly via pathways involving Fc or C3B receptor mediated uptake, is one of the approaches that exemplifies and signifies active targeting. Recently, Balley and co-workers, 1997 described active targeting of the protein-coated liposomes using different targeting approaches: a two-step targeting approach and a direct approach. The study was based upon the specificity of biotin binding to avidin or streptividin. Biotinylated molecules can be targeted in complex mixtures by using the appropriate avidin or streptividin conjugates with carrier system. In the two step targeting approach, the first step prelabels target cells with biotinylated antibodies specific for a ligand on the target cell. At a predetermined time that was sufficient to allow for plasma elimination of free antibody, streptividin conjugated liposomes specific for biotin on the antibody prelabelled cells were administered. The active targeting is referred to as two step targeting approach for the fact that it requires the administration of the both the intermediate protein and liposomes separately, the former to allow accumulation and binding to target cells, and the latter to bind with the intermediate protein labeled target cells. The direct targeting approach exploits specificity by using liposomes linked with targeting ligands via a biotin-avidin bridge.

Physical Targeting (Triggered Release)

The selective drug delivery programmed and monitored at the external level (*ex vivo*) with the help of physical means is referred to as physical targeting. In this mode of targeting, some characteristics of the bioenvironment are used either to direct the carrier to a particular location or to cause selective release of its contents. The first such approach reported is the temperature sensitive liposomes, which were developed and applied to tumour by Weinstein and co-workers, 1979. The release of drug from temperature sensitive liposomes in the vicinity of a tumour (temperature status higher or equal to the phase transition temperature of constitutive lipids) is brought about by serum components mostly the lipoproteins, which at phase transition induce release of the entrapped drug.

It has been suggested that weakly anionic drugs, e.g. methotrexate, be released from liposomes preferentially at low pH regions of tumours. Yatwin and coworkers, 1980 have reported pH sensitive liposomes for selective release of contents at low pH. This approach was further modified with antitumour antibody anchored as a site directing ligand with pH sensitive components of the liposomes (pH sensitive immunoliposomes). The approach was found exceptional for tumour targeting as well as cytosolic delivery of entrapped drugs or genetic materials (Fig. 2- 4). In another approach, the application of external magnetic field has been suggested for localization of magno-responsive liposomes and microspheres within a preselected capillary bed.

Dual Targeting

This classical approach of the drug targeting employs carrier molecules, which have their own intrinsic antiviral effect thus synergies the antiviral effect of the loaded active drug. Based on this approach, drug conjugates can be prepared with fortified activity

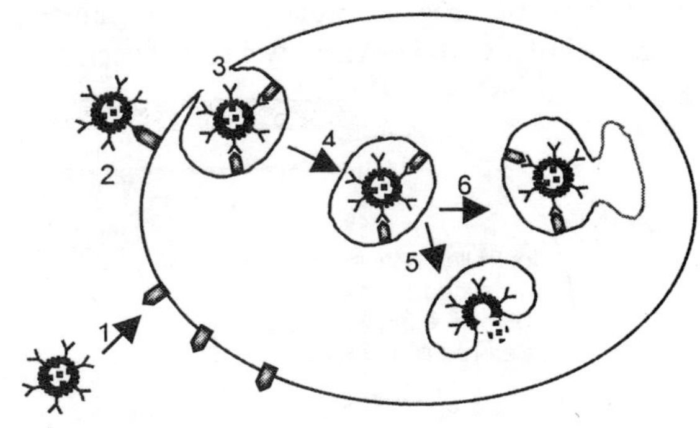

Fig. 2-4. pH Sensitive Cytosolic Delivery of Contents. 1. pH sensitive immunoliposomes bind with receptors via its Mabs component. 2, 3 and 4 indicates receptor-mediated internalization. 5 indicates cytosolic drug release at endosomal pH (4.5) and 6 indicates the fate of the system without the pH sensitive components.

profile against the viral replication (Jansen et al., 1991). A major advantage is that the virus replication process can be attacked at multiple points, excluding the possibilities of resistant viral strain development.

Double Targeting

For a new future trend, drug targeting may be combined with another methodology, other than passive and active targeting for drug delivery systems. The combination is made between spatial control and temporal control of drug delivery. This combination is represented in Figure 2-5.

The temporal control of drug delivery has been developed in terms of control drug release prior to the development of drug targeting. If spatial targeting is combined with temporal control release results in an improved therapeutic index by the following two effects. First, if drug release or activation is occurred locally at therapeutic sites, selectivity is increased by multiplication of the spatial selectivity with the local release/activation. Second, the improvement in the therapeutic index by a combination of a spatially selective delivery and a preferable release pattern for a drug, such as zero order release for a longer time period of the drugs. As shown in Figure 2-5 when these two methodologies are combined, it may be called "Double targeting".

In order to achieve a double targeting effect, site specificity of the drug, by virtue of targeting moiety, a high specificity module (mainly a photosensitizer)

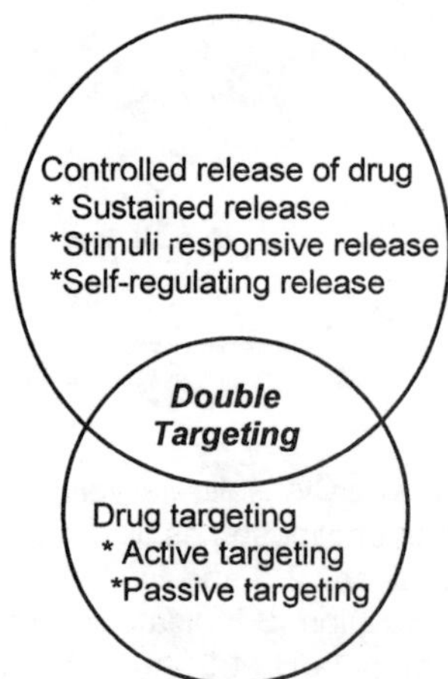

Fig. 2-5. The Concept of Double Targeting

is linked to antibodies. Mew and co-workers in a series of studies (1983, 1985) on such double targeting systems reported haematoporphyrin (Hp)-anti-M-1 antibody conjugates for the suppression of tumour following incandescent light exposure. Further, Hp-monoclonal antibody conjugates against a leukemia-associated antigen was shown to have selective phototoxicity. Conjugates of monoclonal antibody and photosensitizers were prepared using a spacer arm in order to circumvent direct coupling of drug and antibody molecules (Oseroff et al., 1986).

Similar double targeting systems were reported using different combinations of photosensitizer and antibody specific either to a particular antigen or to cell lines expressing cell specific receptors.

Combination Targeting

Petit and Gombtz, 1998 have suggested the term combination targeting for the site-specific delivery of proteins and peptides. These targeting systems are equipped with carriers, polymers and homing devices of molecular specificity that could provide a direct approach to target site. Modification of proteins and peptides with natural polymers, such as polysacc-harides, or synthetic polymers, such as poly(ethylene glycol), may alter their physical characteristics and favour targeting the specific compartments, organs or their tissues within the vasculature. Further vectorization of these modified proteins and peptides into vesicular or microparticulate carriers may take advantage of the intrinsic or inherited (through homing devices) properties of carrier to achieve a site specific active targeting of encapsulated contents. Some of the strategies are depicted in Figure 2- 6.

Problems Associated with targeted delivery systems

Several problems have been identified which require alterations in targeting strategies particularly, *in vivo*. These include:

- Rapid clearance of targeted systems specially antibody targeted carriers
- Immune reactions against intravenous administered carrier systems
- Target tissue heterogeneity
- Problems of insufficient localization of targeted systems into tumour cells

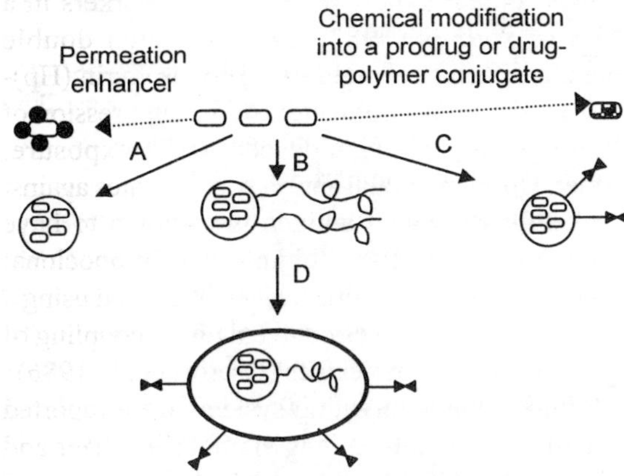

Fig. 2-6. Approaches used in Combination Targeting. Targeting can be achieved via physical (permeation enhancing), chemical (prodrug approach) or carrier encapsulation. Combination targeting using carrier approach can be signified when only carrier encapsulation (A) is accompanied by long circulatory attribute (B), ligand component (C) and/or long circulatory carrier with anchored ligand (D).

- Down regulation and sloughing of surface epitopes
- Diffusion and redistribution of released drug leading to no-specific accumulation

CELLULAR BIOCHEMISTRY AND MOLECULAR EVENTS IN DRUG TARGETING

Ligand mediated active targeting has emerged as a novel paradigm in targeting either at vascular compartment (first order) or cellular (second order) or intracellular (third order) levels (reviewed in Vyas et al., 2001 and Vyas and Sihorkar, 2000). Most of the carrier systems or bioconjugates explored so far, in general, can be utilized as a cargo-unit for the site-specific presentation and delivery of various bioactives using biorelevant ligands including antibodies, polypeptides, oligosaccharides (carbohydrates), viral proteins, fusogenic residues and molecules of endogenous origin. Various ligand-receptor systems are described which are investigated to date for targeted or cellular drug delivery. These include blood carbohydrate (lectin) receptors, Fc receptors, complement receptors, interleukin receptors, lipoprotein receptors, transferrin receptors, scavenger receptors, receptors/epitopes expressed on tumour cells and cell adhesion receptors. The role of receptors as molecular target has opened new opportunities for the cellular or intracellular targeting of drug(s) using carrier systems appended with targeting handles (ligands).

Several specific and non-specific cellular mechanisms have also been explored to facilitate the internalization and uptake of endogenous and exogenous ligands or ligand-carrier composites. Most of them exploit cell surface receptors (transmembrane proteins) or cell surface epitopes (determinants) that help mediate trafficking of ligands with the help of receptor mediated bioevents, mainly receptor mediated endocytosis (RME). Although not completely novel, area of receptor mediated endo- and trans-cytosis has recently gained a renewed interest due to the rapid progress and liaison in the fields of cellular and molecular biology and delivery systems. Ligand-mediated events are either currently exploited for targeted therapy of drugs or genes, or may appear as potential targets for future cellular targeting strategies. Cellular biochemistry and molecular events have dominated the research in the field of drug trafficking and subsequent biological disposition of drugs and delivery systems. Cell surface biochemistry and molecular portals have realized as delivery modules and are exploited for site specific and controlled drug delivery. Cell surface markers such as antigenic determinants or specific sequence of receptor sub units that serve as ligands are exploited and form basis of biochemical and molecular biology assisted delivery units. Receptor mediated cellular events have got major attention in the field of drug/gene delivery during last few years. The events mediated through the endogenous ligands/epitopes could be exploited for the designing of site specific and target oriented delivery systems.

CELL SURFACE BIOCHEMISTRY AND MOLECULAR TARGETS

Molecular targets for cellular targeting

Target could be described as a cell or group of cells in minority, identified to be in the need of treatment.

Some distinctive cellular elements present on the surface of the target cell(s), are considered to be pivotal in designing of carriers for targeting. Cell surface antigens, exploited in generating cell specific and non cross-selective antibodies; cell surface receptors, which recognize and internalize the macromolecular ligands and associated carrier; and cellular oncogenes or oncogenic viruses, serve as molecular targets. Molecular targets represent the most specific form of proteins and peptide drug targeting. In one sense, many protein and peptide drugs are themselves target orientated receptor-specific ligands. For example, insulin and steroidal drugs are sequestered and uptaken by specific cell receptors to affect their intracellular disposition. However, there are examples in which the function of a protein or peptide drug(s) enhanced when they are targeted to a specific site of action. Molecular targets provide a means for "active" drug delivery; i.e., the site to which the drug is ultimately delivered depends on the molecular specificity of the targeting agent rather than the physical characteristics of the drug or the drug delivery system (Table 2-3). Cell surface receptors are excellent ports which, may be effectively used in selective targeting of drugs,

Table 2-3. Target Organs or Compartments Exploited for Ligand Mediated Targeting

Macrophages and other phagocytic cells including Kupffer satellite cells, tissue macrophages, microglial cells of brain, langerhans cells of skin and blood macrophage or monocytes of MPS;
Non-phagocytic cells of RES including the liver endothelial cells (endocytic in nature) and vascular endothelial compartments
Lymphocytes and antigen presenting cells;
Accessible anatomical compartments, i.e. peritoneal cavity, cerebral ventricles, plural cavity, lungs, lymphatics and gastric mucosal cell lines;
Tumour cells with integrins mediating the expression of oncogenic proliferation
Vasoactive and angiogenic peptides expressed by malignant cells
Oncogenes or tumour suppressor genes
Cells *in vitro* for genome grafting or manipulation of DNA (genetic materials); and
Fibrin/site of clot formation

oligonucleotides or even genes by making use of their specific affinity ligands.

The appropriate targets either expressing a receptor or otherwise an epitope for carrier mediate interactions include macrophages, tumour cells or specific tissues or compartments.

In addition to their natural ligands, a number of other proteins and peptides can bind to the extra-cellular domain of receptors, including anti-receptor antibodies, and synthetic agonists and antagonists. These receptors binding proteins and peptides may overcome potential limitations of natural ligands for receptor-mediated drug delivery. Several receptors have been shown to regulate endogenous ligands or their functions with endocytic uptake as an initial step. These endogenous ligands include serum proteins (asialo-glycoprotein receptor) and serum lipids (LDL receptor). On the other hand, some ligands down regulate a number of receptors expressed on the cell surface (insulin and EGF receptor). Targeting receptors with their natural ligands have several limitations:

- First, the endogenously produced ligands may compete with exogenously delivered ligands for receptor binding. This limitation has been addressed by using anti-receptor antibody, which can preferably bind receptors in the absence or presence of ligands. Thus drug targeting via an anti-receptor antibody may circumvent competition between the drug carrier bearing suitable exogenously supplied ligands and the endogenous ligands for the target receptor.
- Second, exogenously delivered ligands mainly a hormone or growth factor may elicit an undesirable biological and immunological response. For example, systemic delivery of insulin as a ligand in non-diabetics can cause hypoglycemia. To address this problem, a proteolytic fragment of insulin, which retains high affinity for receptor binding yet possesses minimal effect on glucose homeostasis, has been shown to transcytosed across the blood-brain barrier.
- Third, certain ligands can bind multiple receptor types or isoforms which, are differentially expressed in various cells or

tissues. Isoform specific agonists and antagonists provide a means to differentiate between different receptors. Receptor antagonists block the binding of their natural ligand and thereby prevent receptor activation. For example, a series of both peptide and non-peptide antagonists for angiotensin II receptors have been developed. Drug delivery via receptor antagonists may offer the advantage of improved selectivity for receptor isoforms.

Receptor as Delivery Ports

Cell surface receptors are complex trans membrane proteins, which mediate highly specific interactions between cells and their extracellular milieu (cargo). Receptors however, are cellular markers and play an integral role in the regulation of cellular functions including, growth differentiation, metabolism, secretion, contraction and migration (Fig. 2-7). The two most common functions for receptors are to mediate the trafficking of their specific ligands and to transduce and regulate transmembrane signaling. Since receptors are differentially expressed in various cell types and tissues, they provide a basis for targeted drug delivery (Feener and King, 1998). Biochemical and physiological properties of receptors vary depending on both receptor type and cellular background (Fig. 2-8). It is likely that some receptor systems may be more suitable than others for receptor-mediated drug delivery. Receptors, therefore could be appreciated as the sensors expressed on target cells (or its intracellular domains) by which cells detect endogenous ligands/macromolecules. Receptors have highly specialized recognition sites with rigid structural requirements for binding signaling ligand. Receptors are primarily embedded in a cellular or subcellular membrane extending further as glycosylation (carbohydrate) pendent chains on the extracellular side. In the classical sense, an endogenous signaling molecule/ligand binds to its specific receptor (ligand binding under affinity and specificity) resulting in to the activation of receptors and a transmembrane signal reaches to the cellular

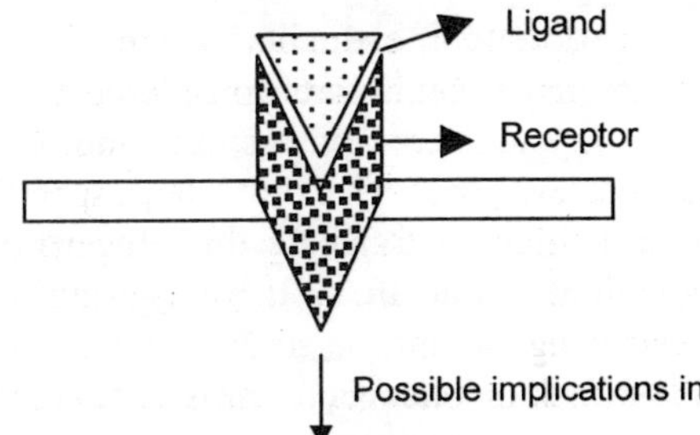

Fig. 2-7. Role of Ligand-Receptor Interaction in Various Fields

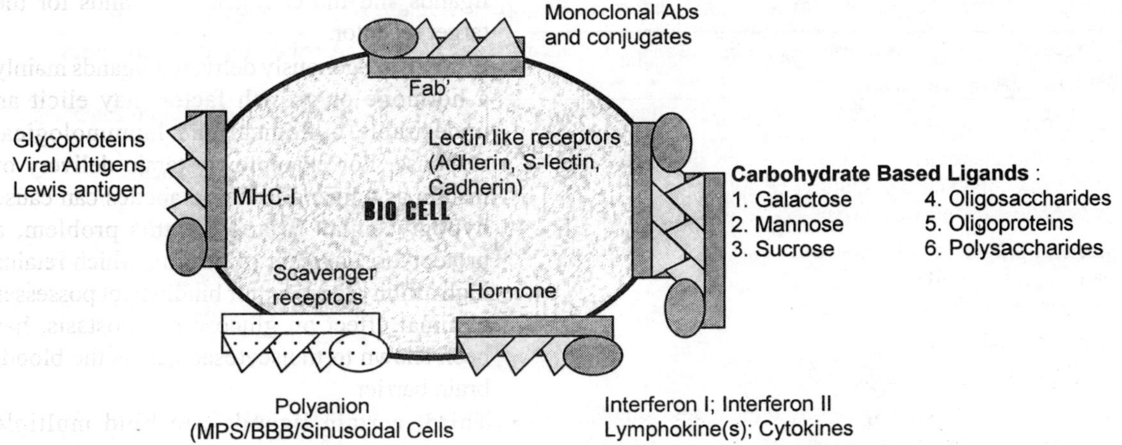

Fig. 2-8. Distribution and Classification of Various Receptors Expressed on the Biocell

interiors to negotiate the desired response at intracellular signal reception point. Exogenous ligands could be engineered with specific avidity towards the receptor(s) expressed on the target cell(s) and this approach could translate the concept of cellular as well as intracellular targeting into an adaptable practicing therapeutic strategy. Receptors are often identified and characterized according to their ligand binding properties. The regulation of receptor expression and ligand binding allows cells to modulate the hormonal and metabolic factors to dynamically interact with the surrounding to initiate a desirable and selective effect.

Specific and saturable ligand binding is a hallmark of receptors. These receptors are distributed (Fig. 2-8) as traffics between the plasma membrane and various intracellular compartments, such as endocytic vesicles and the Golgi apparatus. Certain types of receptors contain an intrinsic tyrosine kinase activity, which plays an essential role in their signaling while other receptors initiate their post-receptor signaling by coupling to cytosolic enzymes. Areas of potential importance to receptor mediated drug delivery include various receptor functions and cellular events like endocytosis, transcytosis, ligand-receptor complex, disposition and receptor regulation.

Ligands as Delivery and Targeting Tools

Ligands are carrier associated surface group(s), which can selectively direct the carrier to the pre-specified site(s) housing appropriate receptor units to serve as 'homing device' to the carrier/drug. The carrier systems interaction serve to assist presentation of ligands to their respective receptors localized on the cellular surface. Various ligands (Table 2-4) exploited for selective drug targeting include antibodies, polypeptides, oligo-saccharides, viral proteins, endogenous hormones and fusogenic residues etc. The ligands confer recognition and specificity upon carrier/vector and endow them with ability to approach the respective target selectively and deliver the drug. A ligand is neither, a shield, nor a motor, thus needs prolonged carrier/system circulation in-order to ensure target site accessibility for receptor-ligand recognition and interaction. Carrier target recognition is a prerequisite for ligand mediated targeting and provides a basis for using cell specific (receptor specific) ligands, attached to the carrier surface as a means of promoting recognition and conferring specificity. Ligands are often covalently anchored or non-covalently associated with the surface of the carrier in such a way that carrier tends to approach the specific cells, those expressing surface receptor, with a ligand specific affinity. Different ligands have been investigated so far in the pursuit to provide optimal targeting. The endogenous or exogenous ligands can be conjugated with either the drug or drug bearing delivery systems using various non-covalent and covalent techniques.

Table 2-4. Types of Ligands that are Internalized via Receptor-Mediated Endocytosis

Endogenous ligands	Immunological ligands	Glycoconjugate	Antibodies(Ab)/ conjugates
Transferrin	Recombinant CD molecules	Lectins	Polyclonal (heat aggregated) Ab
Folate	CD4/rCD4-toxin conjugate	Glycolipids	Monoclonal Ab (Mabs) specific to Fc/Fab'/ Complement
Lipoprotein	Major histo-compatibility complex (MHC)-peptide	Asialo-glycoproteins	Anti-idiotype or anti-anti-idiotype Ab against tumor epitopes
Epidermal growth factor	Interleukins	Neoglycoprotein	Haptens
Nerve growth factor	Interferons	Glyocosides	Bispecific Ab and Ab-enzyme conjugates
Insulin	ECM ligands, including RGD and YISGR	Viroproteins	Fab' or $F(ab)_2$ fragments
α-fetoprotein	Synthetic sLe^x Or sLe^A analogues	Polysaccharides	Single chain Fv protein (scFv)
Macroglobulin	Recombinant gp 120, gp41	Lipopolysaccharides	Immuno-toxins and chimeric toxins

LIGAND DRIVEN RECEPTOR MEDIATED DRUG DELIVERY

Design and development of potential carriers for cell specific delivery of therapeutics are immensely dependent on the selectivity of the carrier to the cellular receptors distributed variably at intracellular sites and on the surface of cellular systems. Other crucial factors include the anatomical and pathological barriers that have to be circumvented, *en route* before recognition site(s) are arrived. Intracellular mesogenic constraints as well as physiologic constraints are also encountered following receptor recognition. Similarly, cellular internalization is equivocally critical for intracellular routing, degradation and release of carrier contents.

Cellular Machinery that Drive Receptor Mediated Bioevents

Endocytosis

Endocytosis (phagocytosis and pinocytosis) has been defined as the internalization of plasma membrane with concomitant engulfment of extracellular cargo/ fluid. The process serves to selectively retrieve and assimilate various macromolecules from extracellular fluid for a variety of cellular functions. It is the main cellular activity involved in the internalization of the extracellular cargo and their vesicular coat proteins, which are subsequently processed via different pathways to appropriate intracellular targets. Phagocytosis is the engulfment of the endogenous and exogenous particulate materials, such as bacteria, erythrocytes, latex beads, colloidal particles and immunoglobulin molecules. It is performed by the phagocytic cells of the RES including the Kupffer cells of the hepatic sinusoids, the tissue fixed macrophages (histocytes) and the blood macrophages or monocytes. The process involves sequential steps of "recognition" (mediated by coating of blood components, mainly by opsonin and high density lipoproteins), "adhesion" (attachment of the particle to the macrophage cells of the RES) and "digestion" (whereby the particles are transferred to phagosome, phago-lysosome and finally to digestive vacuoles). Multiple attachment of particle associated ligands with membrane receptors is an essential stimulus for phagocytic capture of particles (Zippering).

On the other hand, pinocytosis is the uptake of small solutes and small droplets of extracellular fluid, the process is also known as 'cell drinking'. It is similar in many aspects to phagocytosis. It too involves the formation of intracellular vesicles from the plasma membrane, like 'phagosome'. These 'pinosomes' can carry extracellular materials for digestion to the lysosome. It occurs through nearly all nucleated cells.

Receptor Mediated Endocytosis (RME)

Based on the kinetics and other biochemical characteristics three internalization mechanisms have been proposed:

- Fluid phase pinocytosis;
- Adsorptive, receptor mediated pinocytosis, and
- Adsorptive, non-receptor mediated pinocytosis

As already noted, pinosomes only capture liquid and the solute(s), present in the extracellular fluid surrounding a cell (fluid phase pinocytosis). However, differential endocytic uptake is a prominent feature. This is possible by adsorptive pinocytosis, in which a solute binds to an external phase of the plasma membrane and drawn into the cell interior forming pinosome with solute concentration higher than that in the ambient liquid. This process can be highly efficient and could facilitate higher uptake rate as compared to substrate captured through fluid phase. Further, adsorptive pinocytosis can be categorized as: substrate-specific (receptor mediated) and non-specific. In the former, the cell surface recognizes and internalizes a liquid of narrowly defined structural composition, whereas in the latter substrate specificity is much broader, and vague.

Free drug and targeted drug carrier composites enter cells by different mechanisms. Free drug enters the cell interior via transmembrane diffusive transport or adsorptive (non-specific) pinocytosis, while cellular uptake of drug-carrier composites is mostly restricted to receptor mediated endocytosis. Figure 2-9 demonstrate transmission electron micrograph of receptor mediated endocytosis of liposomes.

When transported by diffusion, the drug will reach the cytoplasm of the cell, whereas all pinocytic processes are lysosomotropic. However, the rate and specificity of uptake by adsorptive pinocytosis is considerably slower compared to specific uptake by receptor mediated bioevents. Substrate specific adsorptive pinocytosis has been described for proteins, glycoproteins, lipoproteins and for a range of growth receptors. It has been realized that the fluid phase and receptor mediated pinocytosis are not separate cellular events, but they are different facets of the same event. Non-specific adsorption pinocytosis is responsible for the uptake of many non-glycosylated proteins particularly following cellular damage or protein denaturation.

Exogenous particulate material is also taken up by adsorptive non-receptor mediated endocytosis. Receptor mediated endocytosis (RME) is a well described system operating for cellular uptake of many endogenous and exogenous ligands. Specialized receptor proteins have been identified that operate for nutrients (LDL-cholesterol, Tf-iron), growth factors (EGF, insulin), viruses (influenza), toxins (diphtheria), glycoproteins (galactose terminating or mannose terminating glycoconjugates) and negatively charged macromolecular ligands.

Clathrin coated Receptor Mediated Endocytosis

The receptor molecules are heterogenous in structure but contain a common hydrophilic extracellular domain (ligand-binding domain) which contains glycosylation site. After binding of ligand to receptor (or sometimes independently) at the cell surface and clustering in the coated pits, internalization of the receptor ligand complex occurs via a clathrin coated vesicular intermediate (clathrin dependent pathways) which enters into cytosol. Sometimes the receptors along with their bound ligand are internalized without the coating of the clathrin protein (clathrin independent pathways) (Fig. 2-10).

Vesicular coat proteins mediate intracellular sorting of the cargo. These coat proteins serve several functions. They may concentrate cargo and their carriers (receptors) into nascent vesicles. They also form a scaffold upon which nascent vesicles may form. Finally, they serve to transport and target vesicles from the donor compartment to their appropriate destinations. Clathrin mediated endocytosis from the plasma membrane was among

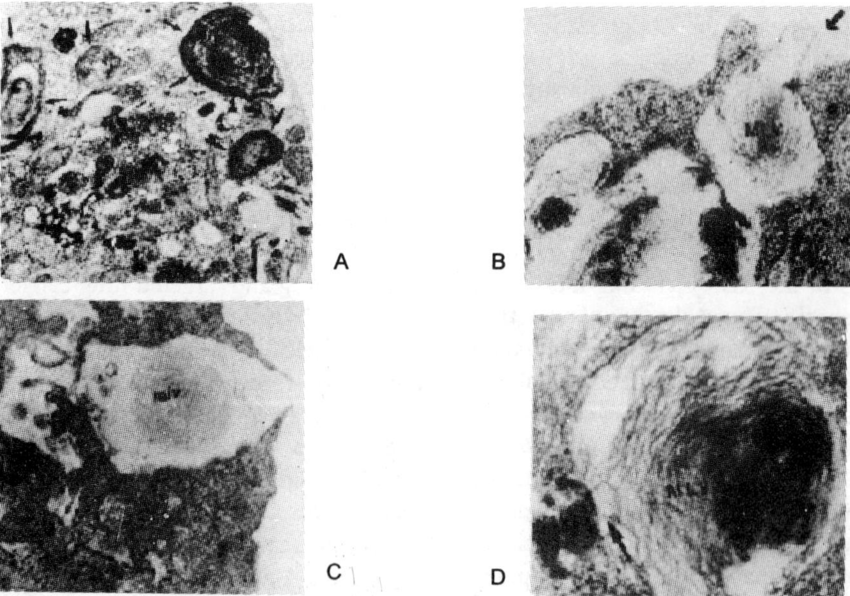

Fig. 2-9. Transmission Electron Microscopy Observation of Various Phases of Receptor Mediated Uptake of Liposome (A-D)

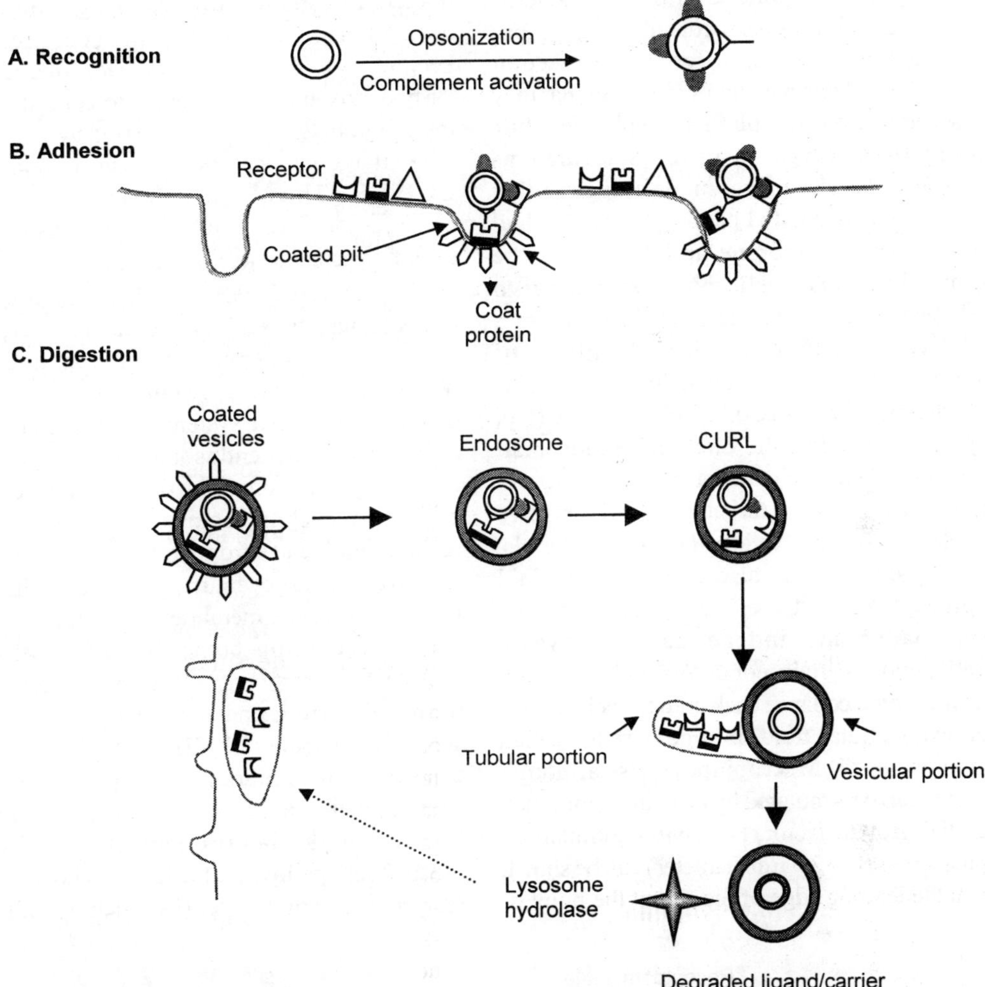

Fig. 2-10. Receptor Mediated Endocytic Uptake of Ligand. Role of *CURL* (Clathrin or Non-Clathrin Mediated Pathway) and Lysosomal Apparatus in the Release of the System in the Vicinity of Target

one of the first vesicular coat proteins identified at the electron microscopy level. Accordingly, it is one of the most characterized vesicular coats with respect to its biochemical compositions and role in protein sorting along the endocytic pathway (clustering of receptors in clathrin coated pits). Concentration of ligand-receptor complexes in these coated pits is mainly responsible for the rapid disposition of receptors, because any protein in coated pit, as it pinches off is internalized. Plasma membrane receptors that are responsible for the uptake of a variety of ligands including transferrin, alpha$_2$M, asialoglycoprotein, growth factors, diphtheria toxin, and immunoglobulins are internalized via a clathrin-mediated mechanism.

Clathrin Independent Endocytosis

Given the diversity of the incoming carrier composites and the need to process them in accordance with the hypothesis that coat proteins mediate vesicular transport and protein sorting, some clathrin independent endocytic pathways are explored recently. In contrast to RME appears to be independent of cellular cytoskeletal. Uptake through non-clathrin coated pit and macropinocytic pathway appears to involve components of the cytoskeleton (Fig. 2-11). Caveolae are also coated invaginations of plasma membranes but differ in the receptor disposition from clathrin coated vesicles in that they do not separate from the plasma membrane while unloading their cargo, a process termed as "potocytosis". An alternative model suggests that similar to clathrin-mediated pathway, caveolae bud from the plasma membrane and fuse with the endosome. The most well characterized cargo molecule undergoing potocytosis is folate. From a drug delivery standpoint, the advantage of potocytosis pathways over clathrin-coated RME pathways lies in the absence of the pH lowering step, thereby circumventing the classical endosomal/ lysosomal pathway. The concept may prove useful for the receptor mediated targeting of pH sensitive macromolecules or transfection of genetic materials. Additional processes can also contribute to fluid phase pinocytosis, but are independent of both clathrin coated and independent pathways. Classically, under certain conditions cultured cells from ruffles, which collapse back onto the cell surface and trap extracellular fluid in large vesicles called "macropinosomes". Macropinocytosis, although constitutive, can be simulated by growth factors such as epithelial growth factor. Following stimulation, macropinosomes (0.5-2.5 μm diameter) can be shown to form at the leading edge of the cell at the point of maximum membrane ruffling. In a recent development, early endosomal coat proteins have been identified and characterized. Interestingly, the early endosomal coat appears to consist of some of the subunits found in Golgi-associated, non-clathrin vesicular coat proteins known as coatomers or COPIES. Thus, the cell may use different combinations of existing coat proteins to regulated specific vesicular trafficking pathways.

In polarized cells, such as epithelial cells (enterocytes), the endocytic system is also polarized. The mode of its operation is more complex than non-polarized cells. Studies confirmed the presence of distinct endosomal systems in epithelial cells, the apical recycling endosome, and the basolateral recycling endosome. In these polarized cells, a common recycling compartment (CRC) exists that receives molecules from both apical and basolateral membranes, and eventually exocytose the contents to the appropriate membrane recycling components (apical recycling compartment or basolateral recycling compartment). Otherwise, direct exocytosis of apical sorting endosome (ASE) or basolateral sorting endosome (BLSE) takes place to apical or basolateral membranes, respectively. Endocytosis from either the basolateral or apical plasma membrane involves both clathrin-dependent and clathrin-independent pathways. Lasic, 1998 however, linked the generation of vesicles (by pinching off from lipid

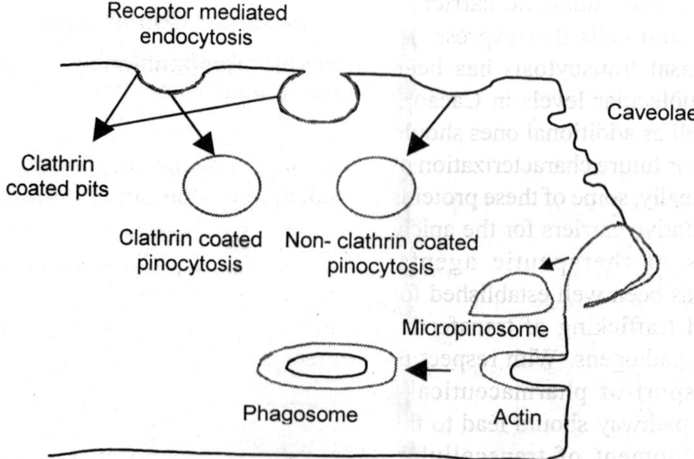

Fig. 2-11. Clathrin Independent Endocytosis either involving other Vesicular Coat Proteins (Caveolae) or Pinching-off of Macropinosomes.

tubules, exocytosis and endocytosis) and readsorption (fusion with plasma membrane) to the excess energy levels associated with various proteins and their conformational changes involved. It has been speculated that this excess energy can be conserved in the biological cells, where the fusion of the vesicles is constantly occurring. The excess energy, e, associated with each vesicle is around 10-50 kT, which corresponds approximately to the energy provided by the hydrolysis of several adenosine triphosphate (ATP) molecules (~15 kT per reaction). This analysis points to the possibility that some of the energy in the cell can be stored in the curvature of various vesicles and may become bioavailable upon vesicle fusion with the membrane, in a process that could be referred to as receptor independent energy driven endocytosis.

Ligand Mediated Transcytosis

Transcytosis is the process by which intracellular ligand or extracellular cargo internalized at one plasma membrane domain of a polarized cell is transported via vesicular intermediates to the contralateral plasma membranes. Much of the characterization of transcytotic pathway has come from the studies on transcytosis in the basolateral to apical direction. Accordingly, the polymeric immunoglobulin receptor (pIgR), a protein specialized for basal to apical transcytosis that recycles at the apical membrane as part of its transcytotic sojourn, has been used apparently as an apical endocytic carrier to introduce vector DNA into cells that express the pIgR. The apical to basal transcytosis has been however identified at molecular levels in Cacao 2 cells. This protein as well as additional ones should provide powerful tools for future characterization of transcytosis pathway. Ideally, some of these proteins may represent better putative carriers for the apical to basal transcytosis of therapeutic agents. Transcytosis pathway has been well established for the protein sorting and trafficking of transferrin, polymeric Ig, and viral pathogens. With respect to the delivery and transport of pharmaceuticals, characterization of this pathway should lead to the advances in the development of transcellular, transepithelial and transendothelial delivery systems.

Transcytosis is the principle mechanism involved in the receptor-mediated uptake of ligand(s). Ligand transcytosis suggests that exclusive localization of particulate does not occur necessarily within sinusoidal cells, but the particulate ligands may also end up in hepatocytes (in case, if hepatocyte is not capable to endocytose initially). VanBarkel et al. 1985 explored that colloidal gold particles coated with either lactosylated serum albumin or mannan are taken up initially by liver macrophages and endothelial cells, however subsequent redistribution to hepatocytes confirms ligand transcytosis to be operative *in vivo*. These cellular uptake characteristics constitute central dogma for ligand-receptor mediated drug targeting.

Recent studies in the area of cellular biology have reported specific proteins, named TAPs (transcytosis-associated proteins), that are particularly found on transcytotic vesicles and are believed to be required for fusion with the target membrane. Other methods to stimulate transcytosis involve the use of Brefeldin A (BFA), a fungal metabolite which has profound effects on the structure and function of the Golgi apparatus. In different studies, an increase in the number of apical transferrin receptors was recorded with either a concomitant decrease or unaffected basolateral Tf receptors. Brefeldin, by selectively modulating coat proteins influences the sorting process and may alter the transport pathway in a receptor mediated delivery system.

Intracellular Processing and Disposition of Drug-Carrier Composites

Receptor Recognition and Ligand-Receptor Interactions

Receptor recognition is a prerequisite for the ligand mediated targeting. The concept involves cell specific recognition of the carrier, internalization or binding of the drug conjugate, intracellular release and cellular retention of the active drug. These recognition sites could in principle serve for binding and/or endocytosis of receptor conjugated carriers for the intracellular delivery of drugs and genetic materials. Although such receptors often provide help for internalization followed by intracellular transport to degradative compartments, the relative rates of these processes in various cell types can be markedly different. In some cases only external binding occurs. In the latter case, local release of drug from carrier in the micro-bioenvironment of the cell membrane should then provide for a diffusive driving force for uptake by target cells. Both receptor and its density and affinity to a given substrate as well as the presence of competing endogenous ligands determine the extent of carrier receptor occupation and as a result the extraction of the carrier drug complex by the target tissue(s).

Ligand-receptor interaction at the cellular level leads to the consequences of site specific delivery through uptake of carried contents. Various ligands have been identified and used as novel navigators for selective delivery of drug(s). A drug conjugated to a ligand (neo-ligand) must obviously be constructed to preserve functional integrity of the active species following release from the ligand, whether the ligand is a small molecule or a macromolecule such as protein. However, the drug delivery strategies are based upon the ligand immobilized on a drug carrier and receptor interaction. In addition to being regulated by ligand, a number of other factors and agents, can modulate receptor-mediated endocytosis. Regulation of receptor mediated endocytosis was found to be influenced by protein kinase C (PKC). Internalization of both the insulin and transferrin receptors was increased following the activation of PKC by phorbol esters. The protein kinase and tyrosine kinase domains are investigated to play a main biological role as a ligand binding molecule providing strong evidences that protein phosphorylation can regulate receptor mediated endocytosis and intracellular trafficking.

Receptors lacking intrinsic protein kinase activity (as in the case of epidermal growth factor and insulin receptor) may also become associated with an active kinase following ligand-receptor interaction. The ability of selected receptors to initiate a cascade of protein phosphorylation as well as other second messenger signals upon ligand association suggests that careful engineering is a priori in the designing of ligand-drug chimera or ligand-carrier constructs bearing suitable bioactive agents.

Intracellular Processing of Receptor-Ligand Complex

Intracellular transport and processing after receptor mediated endocytosis and transcytosis vary markedly between different receptor-ligand systems and different cell types, and decides the fate of the drug-carrier composites into specific intracellular destinations. Subsequent to ligand-receptor dissociation, recycling of receptor to the plasma membrane and transportation of ligand to the lysosomal compartment is the most widely executed pathway. In this case, the ligands dissociate from their receptors in acidic environment of the endosome and eventually end up in lysosome, while the receptors are recycled via transport vesicles back to the cell surface for re use. This enables the target cell to endocytose the extracellular ligand at linear rates for hours. The time required for spanning the pathway from plasma membrane to endosomal compartment and receptor recycling to plasma membrane is on an average is 10-15 min for each round of endocytic cycle.

Receptors such as the ASGP, Tf, and LDL are able to negotiate several hundred rounds of endocytic pathway during a single receptor lifetime. On the other hand, ligand and receptors can show varied behaviour after RME other than the recycling of receptors. Other receptor-ligand complexes follow pathways other than the endosomal compartment. In some cases both the receptor and the ligand are degraded in lysosomes. In some cases both are transported through the cell, and the ligand is released by exocytosis at different surface loci of the cell from where it originated-a process called transcytosis. Receptors can follow one of at least 4 pathways from the endosomal compartment (Fig. 2-12). Receptors can return to the same plasma membrane domain, which they come from, leaving the ligand to be transported for lysosomal degradation or they can travel to lysosomes and with ligand bound to them, share the fate of the ligand (lysosomal disposition). Another pathway recycles them back along with the ligand to the site from where the receptor is being originated. A major pathway however is the transport to a different domain of the plasma membrane (transcytosis). The intracellular processing of ligands can also vary among different cell types. For example, insulin endocytosed by the insulin receptor is rapidly degraded in most cell types but is not sufficiently degraded by endothelial cells. The processing variations of different ligand-receptor complexes thus depend upon both the receptor and the cell type and ultimately influence the fate of internalized ligand(s).

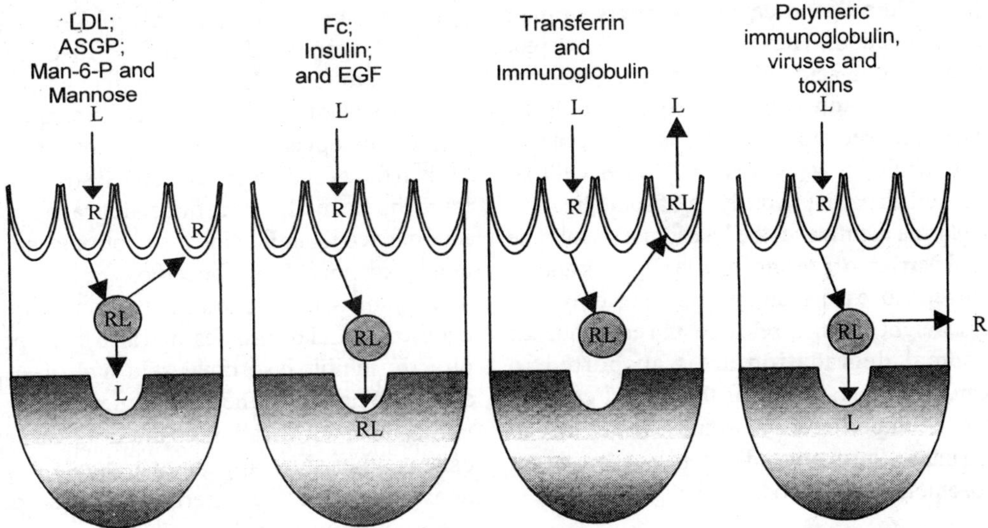

Fig. 2-12. Pathways of Receptor Internalizing and Recycling. Subsequent to Entry into Acidic Endosomes, Ligand and Receptors are Sorted and Trafficked Independently, Which may Result into Degradation, Recycling or Transcytosis of either Molecule. L=Ligand, R=Receptor.

Delivery of Drug-Carrier Composites to Acidic Endosomal and Lysosomal Compartments

Ideally, targeted drug carrier composites should be efficiently delivered to target cells, rapidly internalized, delivered to endocytic compartments and lysosomes and the free drug may diffuse in to the cytosol. For many receptors (e.g., LDL, ASGP, TfR) the internalization process is negotiated constitutively (without ligand-receptor binding) while in some cases formation of a ligand-receptor complex is mandatory for further cellular events (EGF receptors, insulin). The internalization is the key step in receptor mediated trafficking of the contents into the cellular compartments. If the target receptor is a molecule that is not internalized, or if its internalization is not induced by the ligand, the targeted drug composites is likely to have low targetability. Allen, 1997 demonstrated the impact of this concept in their studies with folic acid targeted liposomes appended with both internalizing and non-internalizing epitopes.

Followed by receptor mediated internalization, the ligand-receptor complex route to an acidic compartment through a maturation and fusion mechanism, after internalization. This prelysosomal sorting compartment is referred to as (compartment of uncoupling of receptor and ligand, CURL) endosome, or receptosome. The endosomal compartment is a complex structure of tubules and vesicles. The vesicles fuse with interconnected tubular elements called the trans Golgi, or with the components of CURL. The mechanisms by which endocytic substances are transported from early to late endosomes and finally to lysosomes are vague because the sub-cellular fate of targeting ligand is an intrinsic property of each ligand-targeted system. Some ligands are internalized, then subsequently transferred into endocytic vacuoles, then into fine anastomosed tubulo-vesicular structures, and then into lysosomes. Other proceeds directly from endocytic vacuoles to lysosomes. Two models have been postulated. The 'vesicle shunt model' assumes that early and late endosomes are pre-existing compartments that communicate through vesicle-mediate transport, while the 'maturation model' assumes that early endosomes mature gradually into late endosomes.

Numerous functions relevant to endocytic uptake of ligands and drug delivery occur in the endosomal and lysosomal compartment (pH 6-6.6 for endocytic vesicles, 5-6 for late endosomes, and 4-5 for lysosomal apparatus) and drive the intracellular disposition of the ligand coupled carriers to their respective destinations. These include ligand-receptor dissociation (due to acidic nature of the endosomal system), sorting and transport of internalized molecules and receptors to lysosome, plasma membrane, or Golgi apparatus or to other cellular targets as well as partial hydrolysis of some ligands. Like the plasma membrane, the lysosomal membrane is a natural barrier to macromolecular ligands and/or ligand appended carrier composites and only low molecular weight products released as a consequence of lysosomal degradation are transported to cytoplasm. The degradation of the ligand coupled drug-carrier composites in lysosomes is a key step in designing intracellular targeted system and constitutes the 'lysosomotropic' approach to drug targeting.

Delivery of Drug-Carrier Composites to Cytosolic Compartments

There have been various attempts to target the drug carrier composites directly to cytoplasm scavenging the endosomal and lysosomal compartments or facilitating their disposition from endosomes to cytosol. Different endosomolytic agents (choloroquine) or lysosomal membrane active pH-responding amphipathic helices based on fragments of the influenza virus haemagglutinin are used to promote translocation of immunotoxins or polymer-DNA complexes from endosomes to cytosol. Studies on virus fusion are consistent with pH-dependent events occurring within a subset of endosomes, which have an appropriate pH value. Instead of showing pH induced sorting (receptor-ligand dissociation), the virus coat proteins undergo a conformational change at pH 6.2, exposing its fusogenic components resulting in to the penetration of nucleocapsid into the cytosol ("microinjection") and forms the basis of various delivery strategies of viral origin. Another way of vesicle disruption can be achieved by exposing the cells simultaneously to adenovirus and an immunotoxin. Adenovirus escapes into the cytosol by disrupting the membrane of the endocytic vesicles, and as a consequence, the contents of the vesicles are released into the cytosol.

As mentioned elsewhere, the first step in the intracellular processing of ligand appended carriers is their sequestration and uptake into an endosome, which has an intravesicular pH of 5 - 5.5. If carrier can be engineered to become fusogenic upon exposure to this pH, then they may be able to fuse with the wall of the endosome releasing their contents into the cytoplasm of the cell before they become broken down and degraded in the lysosome. Attempt have been made to reduce degradation of the internalized ligands using lysomotropic amines such as ammonium chloride or carboxylic ionophores like monensin, which neutralize the acidic pH in late endosomes and lysosomes, and also by leupeptin that directly inhibit lysosomal acid hydrolases. These agents do not affect the rate of internalization or the intracellular localization of the drug-carrier composites rather they appear to reduce strongly the degradation of the internalized ligands in the endosomal apparatus.

Similar approaches for targeting the cytosol with pH sensitive ligands have been appreciated. Several studies using pH sensitive ligands that uncouple from receptors in the acidified endosomal environment have demonstrated that high concentrations of monensin (3-50 μM) block the delivery of the ligand to lysosomes. Such an effect was not observed for other ligands that do not dissociate from their receptors at the mildly acidic pH in the endosomes. Finbloom hypothesized that pH-sensitive ligands require dissociation from their receptors at acidic pH for the intracellular routing to lysosomes, whereas pH-insensitive ligands that do not uncouple from bound receptors in endosomes at pH 4-5 are shuttled to lysosomes even if pH gradients are disrupted by monensin and amines. pH sensitive immunoliposomes have been developed to release their contents in response to an acid triggering machinery within endosomal system following receptor-mediated endocytosis (RME). They undergo transient destabilization at a mildly acidic pH as found in the endosomes thus they could selectively deliver the contents to cellular components.

Receptor Mediated Gene Expressions using Conjugated Ligands

The preferred routes for the internalization of the DNA-ligand or DNA-lipid particles (or, otherwise receptor mediated targeting through virus bearing exogenous DNA) have not been clearly elucidated however, several ligand-receptor combinations have been exploited for the efficient internalization of the DNA particles (Fig. 2-13).

The delivery of exogenous DNA or DNA particles to a target tissue by viruses (retrovirus and adenoviruses) is dependent on several mechanisms ultimately leading to achieve cell-mediated internalization, trafficking and expression of the viral DNA. The mechanisms include:

- Endocytosis into an enveloped vesicle;
- Escape from cytoplasmic compartments by fusogenic mechanisms;
- Dissociation of the viral core and nuclear translocation of DNA, and
- Expression of specific genes included in virus.

On the other hand, DNA particles targeted by receptor mediated gene transfer are generally trafficked to degradative pathways and ultimately directed to lysosomes. However, a proportion of endocytosed ligand can escape lysosomal degradation in normal situations (diacytosis) that either recycles back to the membrane with the receptor bound or accompany the receptor to the Golgi apparatus thus leaking the contents of the lysosome into non-degradative compartment of the cell. It is possible that the association of ligand attached poly-L-lysine or PLL with the DNA permits the DNA particle to escape the endosomal and/or lysosomal degradative pathways. This could be achieved either by promoting a higher diacytic rate or simply by reducing the degradation of the DNA particle while normal diacytosis occurs, simultaneously adding to a more specific binding with receptor bearing cells.

After internalization, the DNA particles are transported to the nucleus and the genes are expressed. Gene transfer via receptor mediated endocytosis can be augmented by the use of pharmacological agents that disrupt the endocytic trafficking of DNA particle. Chloroquine has been used to increase expression of transgene delivered via transferrin receptor. Chloroquine acts by increasing the pH inside the lysosomes and therefore inhibits the activity of hydrolytic enzymes. However, chloroquine and other lysosomotropic agents, like monensin, may interfere with efficient transfection by inhibiting the recycling of receptor to the cell membrane from pre-endosomal vesicles.

Cellular Events for Vesicle Trafficking along Target Cell Cytoskeleton

Many recent advances in targeted drug delivery emphasize on regulation of the endogenous membrane trafficking machinery in order to facilitate

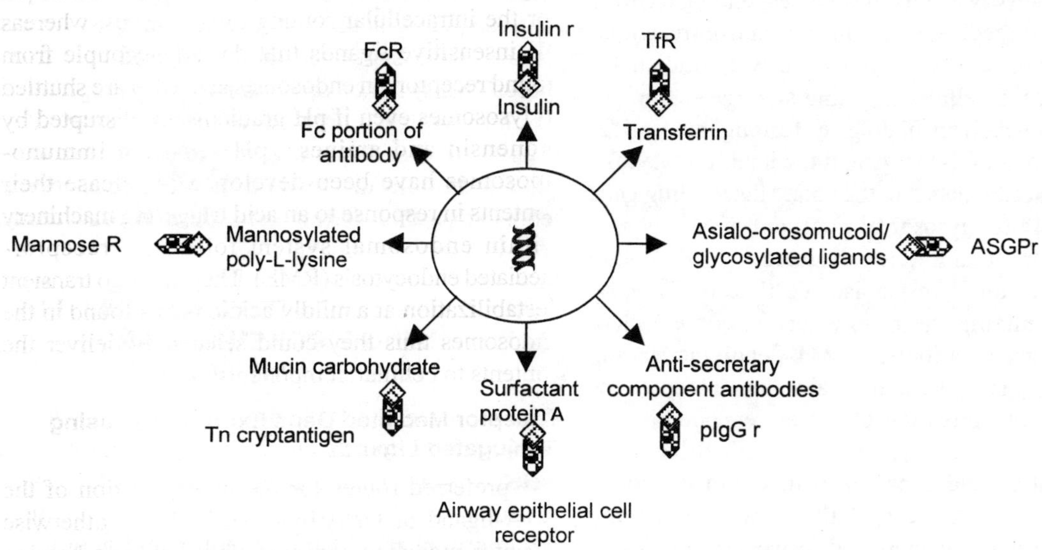

Fig. 2-13. Various Ligands used either as Conjugates or Sensing Molecules Anchored on Delivery Systems, Act as Vectors for Efficient Gene Expression or Gene Manipulation

uptake of polar drugs via receptor mediated endocytosis into target tissues.

A complete understanding of the cellular events involved in the movement of the surface-bound and extracellular components by endocytosis/transcytosis, and subsequent sorting of the internalized complex is essential. However, further regulation of sorting events (trafficking) within the endocytic pathway govern the intracellular destination and ultimate fate of the drug or drug-carrier conjugates. Recent investigations propose a role of the vesicular motor proteins (kinesin, cytoplasmic dynein and myosin) in numerous membrane trafficking events including endocytosis and transcytosis. Unlike coat proteins on the surface of the vesicles that determine the destination of the transport, motor proteins are responsible for the movement of the vesicles along cytoskeletons such as microtubules and microfilaments. Kinesin and cytoplasmic dynein are responsible for the movement of membrane vesicles along cellular microtubules (MTs) to and from cellular membrane compartments. On the contrary, certain members of the myosin family appear to drive and carry membrane vesicles along actin microfilaments (MFs) to and from membrane compartments.

Changes in the MT array and MT-based vesicle transport have been linked to corresponding changes in receptor-mediated endocytosis and intracellular sorting events. These events are well studied for ASGPr based cellular targeting strategies. A major limitation in delivery of drugs/genes/oligonucleotides by ASGP ligands is that ASGR mediated endocytosis results in accumulation of the bound ligand-drug/gene complex in the lysosomal pool and its subsequent degradation. Studies were conducted with DNA-ASG complex to improve persistence time of DNA by hepatectomizing the rats, where major effect of hepatectomy contributes to MT-depolymerization. This finding suggests that a major impediment to the stability and expression of protein encoded by the DNA is the efficient cytoplasmic dynein driven MT-dependent vesicle transport of ligand to lysosomal apparatus. The same hypothesis was tested and confirmed by Chowdhury and co-workers, 1993 who reported efficient transfection of foreign DNA complexed to ASGP-polylysine carrier in colchicine treated rat livers. The stability/persistence of DNA-carrier complex was increased from 48 h to several weeks. These findings illustrate the importance of understanding the individual membrane trafficking events in the target tissue, in order to regulate the intracellular destination of a drug (or drug-carrier) complex internalized by receptor mediated bioevents. In this particular case, it was important to down-regulate MT-based vesicle movement to the hepatocyte interior. In cases where movement to lysosomes is prerequisite for the specific delivery, MT-based vesicle transport could be a viable target for upregulation of traffic and presentation to lysosomal apparatus. Delivery devices appended with pH sensitive ligands appear to involve a microtubule based vesicle movement as a desired event for the intracellular trafficking as they require the acidic pH of the lysosomal pool for the triggered release of the encapsulated contents.

Future strategies in ligand mediated delivery of drug to a particular target tissue will involve the precise mechanisms for alterations of vesicle transport regulated and driven by the microtubule based motor proteins along the cytoskeletal MT-network. Although myosins have only recently been identified as vesicle motors (MFs), the identification of the steps in membrane trafficking facilitated by myosin will also facilitate a parallel approach with its corresponding actin-based vesicle motors. Recent studies have suggested that MT-based and actin-based (MFs) motor proteins may work together to facilitate vesicle movement, as recently reviewed by Langford. Consequently, the relevance of these vesicle motors in the field of receptor mediated endocytosis and, sorting in the desired target tissue, will be a major challenge.

RECEPTOR MEDIATED DRUG DELIVERY USING BIOCHEMICAL AND MOLECULAR LIGANDS

The approach of cellular drug targeting using ligand appended carriers is intimately dependent upon the selectivity and the distribution of the receptor bearing cellular targets in the body, followed by their recognition and ligand-receptor interaction, for intracellular routing of the drug-carrier complex. Various receptors for macromolecular ligands with the specificity for the cell type indicated are listed (Table 2-5). These blood cell specific receptors may serve as point port to cellular entry and constitute the fundamental principle of cellular drug targeting.

Blood cell receptors are comprised of a diverse range of cell surface lectins, immunoregulatory molecules and several macromolecular ligand-recognizing receptors. Similarly, under remodeled physiologic and biochemical situations the tumour cell surface associated determinants such as tumour cell surface receptors and antigenic determinants are being exploited for targeted drug therapy.

- Carbohydrate specific receptors: lectins and lymphocyte homing receptors;
- Cell surface receptors expressed on regulatory molecules: Fc receptors and complement receptors and their various sub types;
- Receptors for endogenous ligands/ macromolecules: scavenger, transferrin, folate and lipoprotein receptors

Carbohydrate Specific (Lectin) Receptors

Endogenous lectins are found on many normal and malignant cells, and are involved in various biological functions, acting as specific receptors and/or mediating endocytosis of specific glyco-conjugates. Glyco-conjugates (glycoprotein, glycolipid and glycosphingolipids) are regular components of the plasma membrane of the mammalian cells. The existence of membrane lectins, as 'carbohydrate specific receptors' present in the cell membrane (which recognize carbohydrate epitopes present as membrane glyco-sphingolipids and glycoproteins) suggests their clear role in cellular adhesion and recognition process. Therefore, glyco-conjugates specially recognized by membrane lectins may be used as carriers of metabolite inhibitors, toxic drugs, biological response modifiers and genetic materials. Alternatively, the membrane oligo-saccharide may constitute potential recognition sites for carbohydrate-mediated interaction between the cells (mammalian/microbial) and drug carriers bearing suitable site directing molecules (exogenous lectin ligands). Lectin receptors expressed on the various blood cells like macrophages, monocytes, endothelial cells, hepatocytes and lymphocytes are efficient in recognizing the complex oligosaccharide epitopes. The latter are also present on the cell surface or could be exogenous glyco-conjugate ligands mimics of endogenous carbohydrate epitopes. Some of the

Table 2-5. Cell Specific Receptors Expressed by various Cell Types in Bio-Environment

Cell types/ expression	Receptor(s)
Monocytes	Mannose 6-phosphate - t(n)GP, β-glucan
Hepatocytes	Galactose -t(n)GP (high-density), HDL, LDL, EGF, IgA, transferrin
Enterocytes	Maternal IgG, dimeric IgG, transcobalamin II
Macrophages	Mannose-6-phosphate- t(n)GP, galactose–t(n)GP, Man- Glc NAc -t(n)GP, fucosyl terminated glyco-conjugates
Kupffer cells	Mannose -t(n)GP, galactose-particles, polymeric negative charged proteins, complement factors, fucose, LDL, fucosyl based glyco-conjugates
T4 and other cells of immune system	Galactose -t(n)GP (low-density), interleukin, transferrin, CD4, complement
Fibroblasts	Mannose-6-phosphate-t(n)GP, transferrin, transcobalamin II, LDL, EGF
Endothelial cells	
i. Liver	Monomeric negatively charged proteins, Man-GlcNAc--t(n)GP, Fc receptors
ii. Blood brain	Transferrin, insulin
iii. Lung, diaphragm, heart	Albumin
Mammary acinar cells	Growth factor
Renal tubular cells	Low molecular weight proteins (cationic)
Tumor cells	Transferrin, folate, EGF receptor, fucose, TNF receptor, cell-adhesion components
Leukocytes	Integrin, selectin, cell adhesion molecules (CAM)

t(n) GP= Terminated (neo)-glycoprotein; HDL= High density lipoprotein, LDL= Low-density lipoprotein; EGF= epidermal growth factor; TNF= tumor necrosis factor; IgG= Immunoglobulin G; GlcNAc= N-acetyl- glucosamine

widely investigated lectins include galactose specific receptors (ASGPR, Asialo-glycoprotein receptor/ N-acetyl galactosamine (GlcNAc receptor); mannose receptors (Mannose terminating GPR/ N-acetyl glucosamine GlucNAc R); phosphomannosyl receptor (Man-6-P receptor); fucosyl and mannosyl-fucosyl receptor (MFR) and glucan receptor.

Membrane lectins usually recognize specific complex oligosaccharides with a high affinity and avidity while simple sugars with low avidity. For instance, the asialoglycoprotein receptor (ASGPR) binds N-acetyl lactosamine Galb4GlcNAcb-R type oligosaccharides or glycopeptide and the glycoproteins bearing such oligosaccharides. Biantennary branched oligosaccharide chains seem to have a preference for binding to lymphocytes, whereas tri- and tetra-antennary branches display a higher binding affinity for hepatic recognition system. Various kinds of extracellular ligands, such as hormones, growth factors, antibodies, viruses and toxins are taken up into cells by lectin-receptor mediated endocytosis. Human mononuclear phagocytes express a cell surface lectin receptor that specifically recognizes glycoconjugates bearing terminal galactose, mannose, mannose 6 phosphate (Man6P), fucose and GIcNAc residues. Receptor expression changes according to macrophage type and down regulation occurs upon activation of macrophages. In monocyte derived macrophages of human origin mannose receptor and mannose 6-phosphate receptor, both are expressed that bind the ligands followed by their receptor-mediated internalization. Human B and T lymphoblastoid cells also express mannose, glucose, GlcNAc, GalNAc, xylose and β-lactose specific lectins. Some of these receptors have been recorded to bind IgE. Lectins receptors with their ligands and specific expression sites are listed (Table 2-6).

Asialo-glycoprotein Receptor

The asialo-glycoprotein receptor was originally discovered during studies on the metabolism of serum glycoproteins. Upon removal of the terminal sialic acid residues from their N-linked oligosaccharides, they were rapidly cleared from the circulation and degraded in liver cells. It was discovered that terminal galactose residues in ASGPs are recognized by a receptor whose binding site is specific for D-galactose/N-acetyl D-galactosamine (GalNAc) and related galactose terminating- glycoproteins and galactoside-based ligands. Alternatively, The ASGPR has also been termed as 'mammalian hepatic lectin' or 'galactose specific receptor' or 'galaptins' and is completely characterized hepatocyte specific receptor.

Among monosachharides, N-acetyl-D-galactosamine is a better ligand than D-galactose. Consequently abundant physiological ligands exist, viz., asialo-fetuin, asialo-transferrin, asialo-ceruloplasmin, asialo-lactoferrin, asialo-orosomucoid, lac-BSA (a neo-glycoprotein), α_2-macroglobulin and hepatoglobulin, which traffic the carrier for ligand mediated targeting of cytotoxics and bioactives to hepatocytes and to hepatoma cell lines (HepG2) where the ASGPR are preferentially expressed. In addition, the construction of artificial ligands to the ASGP-receptor (Galactose-BSA and Galactose-cytochrome c) has been demonstrated which bind with high affinity to receptor on plasma membrane and become internalized and trafficked to lysosomal degradation with near physiological kinetics.

It is evident that different liver cells express specific galactose receptors and interact with different however specific ligand class. Hepatocytes avidly take up molecular and small sized particulate ligands (upto 8 nm) via ASGP receptors whereas endothelial cells take up small and intermediate sized galactose terminating ligands (Fig. 2-14). There exists a clear difference in the liver homing of the small or molecular ligands as compared against large, particulate and cellular ligands, although the initial recognition always involves terminal galactosyl groups. Van Berkel and co-workers, 1985 have reported that tris-galactoside terminated cholesterol (tris-gal-chol) liposomes or tris-gal-chol LDL are taken up preferentially by Kupffer cells but the smaller sized tris-gal-chol HDL were cleared by the hepatocytes. It is therefore conceivable to assume that ligand mediated uptake is size dependent.

Increased hepatic uptake of galactosylated liposomes does not necessarily mean that such liposomes end up as hepatocytes targeted. It was found in repeated experiments, using three different galactosylated liposomal formulations that such

Table 2-6. Membrane Lectins that Mediate Endocytic Trafficking Events

Lectin receptor	Ligand(s)	Cellular expression	Cell event
Asialoglycoprotein receptor/GlcNAc receptor	asialo-fetuin, asialo-transferrin, asialo-ceruloplasmin, asialo-lactoferrin, asialo-orosomucoid, lac-BSA, α2-macro-globulin and hepatoglobulin	Hepatocytes	Endocytosis
ASGP receptor	Oxidized LDL-terminated ligands	Hepatocytes	Endocytosis
Galactose particle receptor	Gal-particle (Tris-gal-chol)	Macrophage (kupffer cellss)	Endocytosis
Mannose/GluNAc receptor	agalacto-orosomucoid, ovalbumin, β-glucuronidase, mannan	Monocyte derived sinusoids/mature macrophages	Endocytosis
Phosphomannosyl receptor			
1. Cation independent (Insulin like growth factor-II)	Man-6-P (phosphorylated mannose ligands)	Freshly isolated monocytes	Endocytosis
2. Cation dependent	Man-6-P (phosphorylated mannose ligands)	Freshly isolated monocytes	Lysosomal enzyme trafficking
Mannosyl-fucosyl receptor		Macrophages, Hepatic endothelium	Endocytosis, secretion of glycoproteins
Fucosyl receptor	L-fucosyl glyco-conjugates, Gal-BSA, fucosylamine-conjugates	Rat kupffer cells, murine leukemia cell L1210	Endocytosis, over expression
β-Glucan	β-3 D-Glucan on heat killed yeast, zymogen glucan particles	Peritoneal macrophages, human monocytes	Endocytosis
Lymphocyte homing receptor	Vascular addresins	Lymphocytes	Recirculation to lymphoids

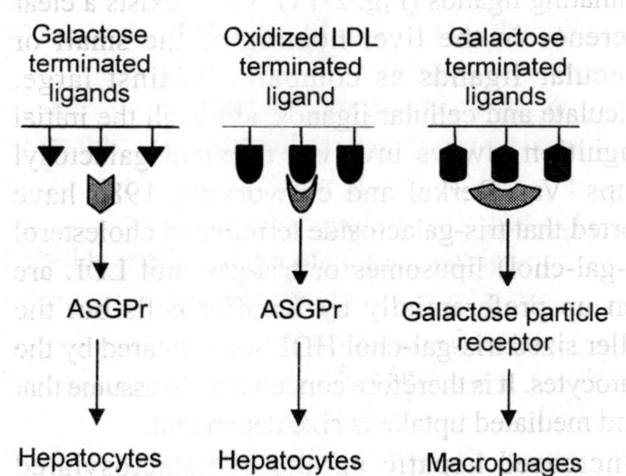

Fig. 2-14. Scheme Showing Affinity of Different Ligands Towards Asialo-glycoprotein Receptors and their Different Biological Fate

liposomes are selectively removed form circulation by Kupffer cells, probably their uptake is mediated via a galactose particle receptor. Macrophages (Kupffer cells) capture and accumulate particulate ligands of all types, but are ineffective in uptake of molecular ligands and known to express "galactose particulate receptors". Nevertheless, the composition of liposomes and nature of the appended ligands also determine the parenchymal (galactose specific receptor) or non-parenchymal receptor (galactose particle receptor) mediated uptake. The existence of galactose particle receptor on the plasma membrane of Kupffer cells raises interesting questions as regards to various factors that regulate the vectorial transfer of galactosylated liposomes to the hepatocytes. Spanjer and co-workers, 1985 reported that the bulk phospholipid composition of liposomes as well as the degree of oligosaccharide chain branching constitutes the determining factor in intrahepatic distribution of liposomes. ASGPr specific ligand lactosylceramide having disaccharide chain (as against tetrasaccharide chain of ASGP) was investigated for hepatocyte specific disposition after being immobilized on the surface of liposomes. However, a comparatively slower rate of uptake occurred. Nevertheless, down-regulation of the receptor in the diseased state has been an area that requires elaborate studies.

The studies indicative of roles of phospholipid compositions of the ligand appended targeting to different ASGP receptors are abound in the literature. Liposomes containing dimyristoyl-phosphatidyl choline as the major phospholipid constituent seemed to be preferentially taken up by the hepatocyte when lactosylceramide was used as ligand, whereas the Kupffer cells were the preferred site for sphingomyelin. They have also reported that liposomes having a triantenary galactose structure are preferentially taken up by the Kupffer cells. This effect has been attributed to a clustered arrangement of receptors on the Kupffer cells facilitating multiple bindings of receptor to particulate ligand. This does not however explicitly explain the reasons behind different fate of different galactosylated ligands.

The ASGP receptor serves as a convenient delivery port, since both natural ligands such as asialofetuin as well as synthetic galactose conjugates specific to ASGP are readily available. Two agents, toxic to hepatocytes or hepatic malignant cells, methotrexate and acetaminophen, have been rendered non-toxic by the subsequent addition of specific antidote coupled to asialo-fetuin, a ligand which binds to the ASGP receptor. The methotrexate and acetaminophen along with asialo-fetuin-antidote conjugates (folinic acid or N-acetylcysteine, respectively) were able to selectively deliver and rescue ASGP-receptor-bearing cells (but not the receptor negative cells). A similar approach was earlier utilized to deliver specific antimicrobial (antiviral) therapy to hepatocytes infected with *Ectromelia virus*. The antiviral agents, arabinoside and trifluorothymidine were complexed to asialo-fetuin and selectively delivered to hepatic parenchymal cells where they inhibited viral DNA replication. Receptor-mediated targeting of asialo-glycoproteins to highly specific receptors on parenchymal liver cells (hepatocytes) can be used to introduce new gene expression. Targeted delivery of DNA to liver cells via ASGP receptors was accomplished using a protein conjugate consisting of a cell targeting component composed of an ASGP ligand (asialo-orosomucoid) covalently bound to a DNA-binding component, a polymeric moiety, containing multiple positive charges (poly-L-lysine). Galactosylated poly-L-lysine and galactosylated ficoll are mimics of the neo-glycoproteins exploited to mediate hepatocyte targeting via ASGPR. Introduction of the particular plasmid DNA induces hepatocytes to synthesize proteins that are coded by the introduced genes. In addition, these systems are exhaustively studied for the delivery and targeting of anti-sense oligo-nucleotides to suppress endogenous gene expression.

Mannose, Mannosyl-Fucosyl (MF) Receptors

Specific cell surface receptors for mannose or N-acetyl galactosyl mannose-terminated-(neo)ligands including the lysosomal hydrolases are expressed on sinusoidal cells (especially endothelial cells) and Kupffer cells of the liver. Hepatocytes may present a cytosolic binding protein for mannose/N-acetyl glucosamine, but specific cell surface receptors (hepatic mannose receptor) are expressed excessively on endothelial cells and to a limited extent on cell membrane of Kupffer cells of the liver.

Mannose receptors are also found on alveolar and peritoneal macrophages, cultured circulating mono-neuclear cells and bone marrow cells. However, in the clearance of endogenous glycoproteins and exogenous glyco-conjugate ligands these cells may play a minor role, the great majority being cleared by hepatic mannose receptor. $\alpha\rightarrow(1,6)$ linked oligo-saccharides are better precursors than $\alpha\rightarrow(1,4)$ or $\alpha\rightarrow(1,2)$ linked residues as evident from *in vitro* macrophage binding studies. The mannose- or N-acetylglucosamine (GlucNAc)-terminated glyco-proteins as diverse as Rnase B (a naturally occuring mannose terminated GP), RnaseA (a nonglycosylated analogue with covalently attached-terminal mannose residues), agalacto-orosomucoid, ovalbumin, β-glucuronidase, mannan (a mannose terminated proteoglycan from yeast cell walls), or man/bovine serum albumin (a mannose-terminating neo-glycoprotein) have been discovered specific to the mannose/GlcNAc receptor in the liver. Expression of mannose receptors is frequent on monocyte derived mature macrophages, whereas mannose-6-phosphate (Man-6-P) recognizing lectin, also known as phosphomannosyl receptor is expressed on freshly isolated human monocytes. Two Man-6-P receptors are expressed on macrophages: a cation-independent (CI) receptor of 270 kDa also known as 'insulin like growth factor (IGF-II) receptor' and a low molecular weight cation dependent (CD) man-6-phosphate receptor essentially involved in lysosomal enzyme (lysosomal hydrolases) trafficking by fibroblasts.

Glycosylated polymers mainly poly-L-lysine has been investigated to possess carrier potential for drugs, oligonucleotides and genes to a number of well defined cell types through their interactions with membrane lectin receptors. Poly-L-lysine can be easily substituted with biological response modifier such as MDP, and with sugar derivatives such as mannoside or 6-phosphomannosides (Man-6-P) for targeting of biological response modifier to the macrophages or monocytes.

Coupling of mannose residues to the liposomal surface enhances their systemic clearance. Further, most of the liposomes disappearing from the circulation subsequently accumulate in the liver. The selective accumulation in liver remains however significantly inhibited by prior injection of mannan, indicating mannose receptor participation in the internalization of the liposome associated ligand. In experiments, where mice liver was previously perfused with mannosylated liposomes, the non-parenchymal cells were found to be seven times more efficient than the parenchymal cells in selective sequestration of mannosylated liposomes. Liposomes appended with amino-phenylmannoside are transported into the mouse brain across the blood brain barrier. This has been attributed to the presence of mannose-specific receptor located on the blood brain barrier. The rapid uptake of liposomes appended with mannose-terminating ligands by macrophages suggests them to be an ideal carrier system for macrophage targeting. Dumont and associates, 1990 observed that lipopolysaccharide (LPS) entrapped in mannosylated liposomes showed a reduced toxicity in animals hypersensitive to free LPS. They also observed that LPS targeted to tissue macrophages via mannosylated liposomes induced regression of experimental solid tumours in mice, and proved to be very effective against metastases in lung. However, it was noted that the level of mannose receptors expressed in the activated macrophages is very low (down-regulation of receptor). These findings should be conducive in designing appropriate ligand directed carriers to interact with carbohydrate receptors.

Mannosyl-fucosyl receptors (MFR) expressed on the mature macrophages and hepatic endothelium, bind mannose/fucose residues of the endogenous glycoprotein expressed on the surface of some bacteria and yeast. Evidences however, suggest that fucosylated asialo-transferrin (fucose $\alpha \rightarrow 1,3 \rightarrow$N-acetyl glucosamine adjacent to galactose) is cleared rapidly from the liver cells. Neither mannan nor derivatives of orosomucoid (that are cleared by binding receptors for galactose, N-acetyl glucosamine or mannose) could inhibit the clearance of fucosylated asialo-transferrin. Fucoidin, $\alpha \rightarrow (1,3)$ linked fucose was inhibitory for the receptor-mediated uptake, suggesting a L-fucose recognizing lectin receptor present on the liver cells especially on lymphocytes and mononuclear phagocytes (a separate entity from mannose/man-6-P receptor). Lectin receptors for sulfated polysaccharides are also present on lymphocytes, macrophages, polymorphonuclear leukocytes, mast cells and fibroblasts. Many more lectin binding proteins still to be explored could form molecular targets for the future cellular targeting strategies.

Human monocytes and peritoneal macrophages express a β-glucan recognizable lectin receptor. The glucan-binding site has been identified as a part of CR3 receptor. It mimics particulate activation of the alternative complement pathway. Membrane complement receptor type 3 (CR3) has lectin like properties and serves as a receptor for zymosan (with β-glucan as a component of the surface glycoprotein) along with its natural ligand, C3bi. Based upon these evidences, β-3D glucan from heat killed yeast and zymosan glucan particles have been appreciated as ligands for receptor mediated targeting to β-glucan receptors of the macrophage system. This receptor is also important in phagocytosis of bacterial and yeast surface determinants because glucan along-with mannose/fucose are components of surface glycocalyx of some bacteria and especially of yeast, and could form the basis of the targeted therapy.

Lymphocyte Homing Receptors

Lymphocytes undergo constant recirculation between the blood, lymph, lymphoid organs, and tissue spaces. Extravasation of lymphocytes in particular and leukocytes in general requires interaction between cell adhesion molecules (CAM) on the vascular endothelium and receptors for these CAMs on the circulating cells. The differential migration of lymphocyte subsets into different tissues is called 'trafficking' or 'homing'. In general naive (unprimed) B and T lymphocytes tend to home to various secondary lymphoid organs, such as the spleen, lymph node, or peyer's patches. These secondary lymphoid organs trap antigen or antigenic ligands and provide specialized microenvironments to support differentiation of antigen activated lymphocytes into effector and memory cells. Recirculating naive lymphocytes have cell surface receptors that recognize particular vascular addressin on the vascular endothelium of different secondary lymphoid tissues. Because these receptors direct the circulation of various populations of lymphocytes to particular lymphoid tissues, they are referred to as 'homing receptors'.

Lymphocyte homing receptors belong to a class of proteinaceous lectins, which include the serum mannose binding protein and mannose receptor on various tissue macrophages. These are lectin like receptors present on the cell membrane of various lymphocyte subsets, functionally indispensable to the recirculation of lymphocytes from the blood to lymphoid organs. The homing receptors on lymphocytes, which interact with tissue specific adhesion molecules on high endothelial venules (on CAM) direct recirculation of lymphocytes in a tissue specific fashion. Determinants specifically recognized by these lectins consist of mannose, fucose and fructose groups with their negative charged moieties. The negative charged moieties are generally based on the sulfate and phosphate groups like mannose-6-phosphate, fucose-4-sulfate, fructose-1-phosphate, fucoidin and phosphomannan. Recent evidences suggest the phosphorylated oligosacharides rather than sulfated oligosaccharides as the natural ligands for the lymphocyte homing receptors. Homing receptor lectins (mainly mannose) on lymphocytes is the probably only member that undergoes phagocytosis and mediates the extravasation and extracellular release of drugs.

CELL SURFACE RECEPTOR EXPRESSED FOR IMMUNOREGULATORY MOLECULES

Carbohydrates, often expressed as gangliosides, can act as cell surface receptors for regulatory molecules, e.g., interferons, thyroid-stimulating hormone, and for immunoregulatory molecules. The latter including factors mediating help and/or suppression of immune system, e.g., opsonins (Fc and complement), MHC class I & II glycoproteins, CD glycoproteins, interleukins, interferons, LFA and macrophage/monocyte colony stimulating factors (MCSF).

Fc Receptors

Immunoglobulins clustered on the surface of the target cell expose their tail regions (Fc) to be recognized by the Fc receptors (FcR) present on the surface of the macrophages and neutrophiles. Largely by means of such Fc receptors (Table 2-7) the phagocytic cells of mononuclear phagocytic system negotiate tumour cell killing with the help of ligand-associated anti-receptor or chimeric antibodies developed against the tumour cell surface antigenic determinants.

Antibodies as Biochemical Drug Carriers

Immunoglobulin developed against a surface determinant after immobilization on particulate or colloidal delivery systems could be targeted to the cells bearing Fc receptors via their Fc region or to the target antigen on the cell surface through Fab' region followed by internalization and release of the encapsulated bioactives. Mabs are now available for all the Fc receptors. Immunoglobulin fragments Fab' and $F(ab')_2$ or chimeras IgG developed against surface antigens or antigenic determinants are well

Table 2-7. Fc Receptors with their Preferential Binding Domains

Receptor type	Preferential binding	Mabs cloning
FcR1	IgG1 and IgG3	Cloned (32.2)
FcR2	IgG molecule/ligand complex	Cloned (IV-3)
FcR_{10}	-	Cloned (3G8, L23, VEP18)

known strategies to negotiate Fc receptor mediated drug/gene therapy. Mabs are now available for all the Fc receptors. Instead of using complete IgG portion, immunologically active fragments [$F(ab)_2$ and Fab'] have been used for improved access to the receptor bearing cells.

Recent developments in liposome technology possibly explore therapeutic applications involving site specific delivery of Mabs. Anti-target monoclonal antibody anchored on liposomes (immunoliposomes) with specific avidity directed to carbohydrate containing antigens have been investigated to deliver the drugs like Idoxuridine and Acyclovir in the treatment of Herpes Simplex Virus (HSV) infected cell lines. Instead of using complete IgG portion, immunologically active fragments [$F(ab)_2$ and Fab'] have been used and reported for improved targetability to the receptor bearing cells.

Antibody-associated liposomes containing antisense oligomer provide dual specificity: the antibody mediated selection of the particular cell lines along with the selectivity of the chosen mRNA sequence which is complementary to the liposome delivered oligomer. Khaw and co-workers, 1995 have also reported a novel adjunctive approach to seal the membrane lesions associated with acute myocardial infarction, using antimyosin Mabs directed, immunoliposomes. Here, an antigen on intracellular cytoskeletal myosin in hypoxic embryonic cardiocytes, is used as an anchoring site, and a specific antibody on immunoliposomes as a sensing ligand to *'plug and seal'* the membrane lesions. The study indicated that selective cell membrane sealing can prevent cell death in hypoxic cardiocytes, and this concept holds exploitable promises in different immunological consequences.

Recent developments related to sterically stabilized liposomes (SSL), renewed interest in systemic application of immunoliposomes due to their low RES uptake and long circulation half-life. This is as a result of their hydrophilic, opsonin repelling and sterically stabilized surface. The categories of these systems include liposomes that incorporate GM1 gangliosides or that coated with PEG polymers (protein pegylation), i.e., polymer grafted immunoliposomes, or polymer grafted micro-particulates. The development of new technologies for an efficient attachment of Mabs at the surface of PEG containing liposomes permits the resulting sterically stabilized immunoliposomes not only to exhibit greater recognition and target binding characteristics but also allows them to remain longer in circulation relative to classical immunoliposomes. Sterically stabilized liposome (SSL) mediated targeting of anticancer drug doxorubicin has been reported in the treatment of murine solid tumours, human solid tumour xenografts and human haematological cancers. The surface immobilized Mabs directed to tumour associated antigens for immuno-specific binding produce better therapeutic effect and reduce the level of non-specific binding to non-target cells.

Complement Receptors

Microbial polysaccharides could be used as ligands to activate the complement pathway (Alternative) or, otherwise the Fc region of the Ig molecule [or Fab'/$(Fab')_2$] as a signaling ligand to activate the complement pathway (Classic). In both the cases the complement component (C3) fragments C3b and C3bi are deposited on the target surface/ligand. C3b components of the complement make the target surface recognizable by both neutrophils and macrophages. Complement opsonized ligands could be readily phagocytosed by both monocytes and macrophages. Phagocytosis is mediated through binding of the signaling ligands to the specific complement receptor (CR) on the macrophage surface. Mabs specific for the CR are available and have been used till now mainly for receptor quantitation and to check the phagocytic avidity of the different CRs. (Table 2-8).

It has been recorded however, that SE (sheep erythrocytes) coated with C3b (EC3b) and C3bi

(EC3bi) could only be phagocytosed by the members of the MPS, if the uptake is additionally supported by another receptor or some additional binding site in the receptor protein itself. Infact, phagocytosis by complement coated system has been shown to be promoted by fibronectin serum amyloid P, interaction with FcR and/or glucan or mannan receptors.

The involvement of complement system in destabilization as well as in plasma clearance of liposomes is widely recognized. Kinsky, 1972 for the first time used antigen-carrying liposomes as models of the cell membrane to study the complement-induced damage of cells. The role of properly designed carriers has also been explored to induce alternative pathway of complement activation. Irrespective of the fact that whether classical or alternative pathway is operational in the destabilization of the carrier composites, complement factor C3b is commonly adsorbed to the carrier surface in both the cases. Once adsorbed it serves as an efficient opsonin to trigger rapid binding of the liposomes or similar carriers to C3b receptors on macrophages, followed by receptor mediated intracellular trafficking of contents. Some controversy exists about the relative contribution of the classical versus the alternative pathway. Czop and Austen, 1985 advocated for the predominant involvement of the alternative pathway, whereas Liu and co-workers, 1995 hold that the classical pathway is mainly responsible. As far as the classical pathway is involved, the occurrence of natural antibodies against lipid constructs in the serum is likely to be decisive. On the other hand, activation of the classical pathway has also been shown to occur without the involvement of antibodies. Liposomal charge, either positive or negative, is said to be important, although negatively charged lipids inhibit antibody-specific complement activation, whereas the alternative complement activation is said to be substantiated. Moreover, Liu and colleagues, 1995 emphasized the species dependence of complement-mediated liposomal clearance.

Table 2-8. Complement Receptors with their Preferential Binding Domains

Receptor type	Preferential binding	Mabs cloning
CR1	C3b	Cloned (CRbR, 44D)
CR3	C3bi	Cloned (Mo1, OKM1, D12)
CR4	C3b	Cloned (S-HCL-3, KiM1)

While ganglioside GM1 substantially increases circulation time in mice, it has opposite effects in rats. This is probably mediated via complement activation that is supposed to be induced by naturally occurring anti-GM1 antibodies in rat serum. Harashima and co-workers, 1994 focused attention on the importance of size of the particulate in complement activation. Complement dependent uptake by the liver in a perfused liver system increases with liposomal size, while opsonin-independent uptake is found to be size independent.

Interleukin Receptors

Interleukins and interferons constitute a family of potent lymphokines/cytokines that activate cells of the immune system. Recently, it has been demonstrated that at least two classes of receptor for IL-2 exist with markedly different affinity for ligand. All known biological actions of IL-2 have been correlated with occupancy of high affinity binding sites; the function of low-affinity sites however remains unknown. The designing of different target oriented delivery systems is based on the regulation of IL-2 receptor expression and their clearance from the surface of the target or activated cells. Various other IL receptors are present on blood cells involved in ligand endocytosis. These interleukin receptors including IL-5, IL-7 and IL-12 were characterized for their lymphopoietic activities and could become handle for future research and in field of ligand mediated targeting to desired receptor units (Table 2-9).

Despite its pleiotropic properties, immunotherapy with the respective cytokine ligands is restricted because these cytokines are rapidly cleared from the circulation and require high doses at which they induce toxic side effects. There have been various attempts to solve the problems associated with the delivery of cytokines to their desired receptor ports. Recombinant cytokines are developed to circumvent unfavorable effects associated with endogenous IL-2. Sato and co-workers, 1993 investigated biological

Table 2-9. Immuno-Bioligand Based Delivery Systems and Activity Profile

Target cell/ site	Delivery system	Activity
YAC-1 tumour cells/Meth A fibrosarcoma	Recombinant IL-2 immunocomplexed with Mabs against rIL-2	Induction of killer cells for anti-tumour activity
Murine CTLL-2 T cell line / human mitogen activated PBLs	Interleukin-2 chemically coupled to liposomes	Receptor mediated immunotherapy
Human tumour xenograft/ Severe combined immunodeficiency (SCID) mouse	IL-2 loaded poly(lactic acid) microspheres	Suppression of implanted tumour
IL-2 receptor bearing T cells (*in vitro*)	IL-2 in sterically stabilized liposomes	Anti-tumour activity in mice
Metastatic liver tumour	IL-2 in galactose containing liposomes	Enhancement of anti-tumour activity of lymphocytes
Hepatic sinusoidal lymphocytes/ hepatic metastasis in C3H/Me mice	IL-2 in galactose containing liposomes (Gal-lip-Il-2)	Activation of hepatic sinusoidal lympho-cytes and local anti-tumour activity in liver
IL-6 transgenic mice	Alginate-poly(L)lysine-alginate membrane microencapsulating SK2 hybridoma cells	Suppression of IgG1 plasmacytosis in the IL-6 transgenic mice
Liver sites in BALB/c mice	Recombinant human interferon-pullulan conjugates	Enhancement of IFN-induced enzyme (2-5A) activity

*Adopted from Vyas et al., 2001 with modifications

properties of an immune complex of recombinant interleukin-2 (rIL-2) and a monoclonal antibody against rIL-2 in mice for induction of killer cells and for antitumour activity. The results demonstrated that immune complex exerted a higher killer cell activity against YAC-1 cells and significant antitumour activity in a dose-dependent manner in Meth-A fibrosarcoma mice than rIL-2 or soluble IL-2 alone. In another development, polymer-conjugated cytokines (hybrid-cytokines), for instance PEG-modified interleukin-2 and PEG-modified interleukin-6 were shown to increase selectivity but could not curtail the unfavourable functions. However, the receptor mediated targeting using drug delivery systems has emerged as a novel concept in cytokine delivery. Targeted drug delivery using a variety of delivery systems including liposomes, microspheres, microcapsules, supramolecular biovectors, ceramics, and chimeric proteins, stabilizes the cytokines and expresses only the selective functions from other unfavorable functions *in vivo*. To further control pharmacokinetics and pharmaco-dynamics *in vivo*, drug delivery systems using hybrid cytokines are devised with increased stability and selectivity.

In an attempt to enhance the therapeutic efficacy of interleukin-2 (IL-2), recombinant IL-2 was encapsulated either in conventional or in long circulatory extravasating liposomes (sterically stabilized liposomes, SSL-IL-2). The latter bind selectively to IL-2 receptor bearing T-cells *in vitro*, indicating that the domain of the cytokine molecule involved in binding to the receptor is exposed to the outer liposomal membrane. The study demonstrated an improved immunomodulatory and antitumour activity of SSL-IL-2 in mice, suggesting the targetability of the system as compared against soluble IL-2. Furthermore, human recombinant interleukin-2 has been chemically coupled to the external surface of liposomes containing methotrexate as a candidate immunosuppressive agent. The system specifically directs the immunoliposomes to the activated T-cells expressing high affinity IL-2 receptor. The IL-2 bearing immunoliposomes presented a new class of cell-specific systems whose entry into the cytoplasm is controlled by cell surface receptor and associated cellular events. In order to further increase the targetability of the liposome encapsulate IL-2, a galactose receptor specific ligand was appended to facilitate the selective uptake by liver parenchymal cells bearing galactose-specific receptors. These Gal-Lip-IL-2 liposomes were administered to C3H/He mice and *in vitro* antitumour activity of hepatic sinusoidal lymphocytes and *in vivo* hepatic metastases measurements were made. The results confirmed earlier reports of Okuno and co-workers, 1998 in which they demonstrated maximum accumulation and the highest localized effects on the antitumour activity of the lymphocytes. The system with enhanced IL-2 presentation activated the hepatic sinusoidal lymphocytes and increased the local antitumour activity in the liver. Human recombinant interleukin were also used as ligand associated to supramolecular biovectors (SMBV). SMBVs are lipoprotein carriers appended with polymerized polysaccharide coat to mimic endogenous lipoprotein. The association of IL-2 with SMBVs modifies its *in vitro* proliferative activity and restores the activity of impaired IL-2.

Interferons

Some endogenous antiviral protein ligands like interferons (α and β) play an important regulatory role in the antiviral effect, bind to their specific receptors. On the other hand, γ-interferon activates neutrophils and may participate in the immune responses or may lead to macrophage activation. Even γ-interferon enhances expression of cellular receptors for other regulatory molecules like tumour necrosis factor. Incubation of several human tumour cell lines with human interferon-γ (IFN-γ) increased the specific binding of subsequently added ^{125}I-labeled recombinant human tumour necrosis factor (TNF). Interferon has been investigated mainly for their controlled delivery rather than site-specific delivery. However, some reports of the active targeting are documented where the conjugated recognition ligand like asialofetuin (specific for galactose specific receptors of hepatocytes), mono-clonal antibody (against glioma associated antigen), and pullulan (non-specific affinity towards hepatic receptors) enhanced the receptor specificity and avidity of the interferon.

MHC and CD Glycoproteins

Molema and Meijer, 1994 suggested that the interaction of specific MHC/peptide complexes with T cell receptor on the cell surface of CD4+ T cells is the key event in the T cell activation with the effective mediation of antigen presenting cells (APC). MHC-I is expressed on all nucleated cells whereas the expression of MHC-II occurs only on antigen presenting cells. The closed proximity of class-II MHC and polyanionic binding sites may indicate that CD4 receptor recognizes an endogenous anionic polysaccharide associated with the MHC carrier. In fact, class II MHC molecules carry a sulfated glycosaminoglycan that is essential for antigen presentation. Lymphocyte cell surface molecules such as CD2 (LAF2), CD22, CD4 and CD45 bind poly-anionic polysaccharides such as hyaluronic acid, sialic acid, dextran sulfate and heparin through their specific receptors. However, these anionic binding sites are different from those demonstrated by the families of selectins and integrins on lymphocytes. These immunoregulatory molecules could become as possible endogenous handles for either the possible exploitation of various receptor ports for the drug/gene targeting or for the effective presentation of the immunomodulators to the immune system.

Annemiek and co-workers, 1999 reported a well characterized liposomal carrier system in order to present MHC classsII/peptide complexes in a multivalent way to the immune system. This is the first report showing that MHC class/peptide liposomes can serve as 'artificial antigen presenting cells' for activation of CD4+ T cell hybridoma. As compared to soluble MHC classII/peptide complexes, the multivalency of liposomal complexes may be of an important advantage in immunotherapeutic applications rather than in drug targeting.

Receptors for Endogenous Proteins and Macromolecules

Lipoprotein Receptors (LpR)

Lipoprotein receptors (LpR) are instrumental for the transport of cholesterol and other lipids with their subsequent distribution and processing in the intracellular compartments (Table 2-10). Structurally, the lipoproteins consist of an apolar core, composed of triglycerides and/or cholesteroyl esters, surrounded by a polar monolayer of phospholipids and cholesterol. These complex structures accommodate several receptor-specific apo-lipoproteins (apo-LP).

A number of these apo-lipoproteins, e.g., apoB and apoE, have been demonstrated to function as ligands for receptor-mediated removal of the lipoprotein from blood.

Lipid and fatty acids are emptied in to the lymph from g.i.t. in the form of chylomicrons, and converted into chylomicron remnants by a lipoprotein lipase located on the surface of the vascular endothelial cells. Chylomicron remnants and a particular type of VLDL (very low-density lipoprotein), β-VLDL, are rapidly taken up by remnant receptors expressed on parenchymal liver cells and further processed via intermediate-density lipoprotein to low-density lipoprotein (LDL). LDL (low-density lipoprotein) is cleared mainly via specific LDL receptors (apo B and apoE), to a large extent by the liver, but peripheral tissues also participate substantially. High density lipoprotein (HDL) is secreted into circulation by the liver and intestine where HDL receptor, identified as ScR class B type 1 molecule, recognize and navigate the transfer of cholesterol from HDL to liver and non-placental steroidogenic tissues. As HDL and/or apoAI (the major apoLP of HDL) present various binding sites on different cell types and mediate the so-called reverse cholesterol transport, they are useful handles that can be manipulated accordingly to influence the cellular destination of the carrier systems. HDL particulate receptor has been shown to bind liposomes containing anionic phospholipids.

Recently, Rensen et al., 1997 have shown that particle size is a determinant of the intracellular fate of the apoE-containing particulate systems and their relative affinity towards LDLr or hepatic remnant receptor. In the study affinity towards the LDL receptors was demonstrated to be a function of particle size as 50 nm triglyceride emulsion particles displayed a much higher affinity towards the LDLr than 150 nm particles. The latter in turn had a stronger affinity towards the so-called remnant receptors. Similarly, small liposomes are being presented to these receptors after their binding with selective apo-E, the role of remnant receptor(s) and the LDLr seems critical in the intracellular delivery of these carriers. However, the research in recent years has presented convincing evidence that apo-LP is involved as complementary opsonin in the hepatocyte-mediated clearance of neutral liposomes from the blood. On the other hand, negatively charged (PS) liposomes, although adsorb significant amounts of apo-LP, are not cleared via apo-LP dependent mechanism, rather their disposition is mediated via complement activation and C3b opsonization.

Being endogenous in nature, lipoproteins or their apo-lipoproteins are non-immmunogenic ligands and escape recognition by RES system. However, they may also be exploited to target non-lipoproteins receptors following chemical modification of the their apo-lipoproteins. This is due to the fact that typical apo-LP apo-B is very firmly associated with the LDL particle and not readily susceptible for transfer or change. Apo-B has, however, been isolated and coupled to liposomes as LDLr specific ligand. Lundberg and co-workers, 1993 incorporated apo-B into phospholipid:cholesterol (2:1) liposomes and demonstrated specific (LDL-inhibitable) receptor-mediated interaction leading to uptake by CV-1 cells *in vitro*.

Acetylated-LDL as a ligand could be exploited to target endothelial liver cells exploring scavenger receptors expressed by these cells for polyanionic ligands. Lactosylation of LDL (tris-GAl-Chol-LDL) and HDL (tris-GAl-Chol-HDL) could be used as a means to target antivirals, antiparasites and immunomodulators to Kupffer cells and parenchymal liver cells (hepatocytes) respectively with galactose specific receptors (galaptins) expressed on these cells. LDL receptors are also involved in the efficient and transient gene expression. Wilson et al., 1992 introduced a plasmid containing cDNA for the human LDL receptor in LDL-receptor deficient rabbits in a model for familial hyper-cholesterolemia. The workers analyzed the exogenous LDL receptor mRNA level at different time intervals and found phenomenal transient gene expression and transcriptional activity.

Table 2-10. Major Lipoproteins and Preferred Ligands with Associated apo-LP

Receptor type	Ligands	Major apo-lipoprotein
Chylomicron	Chylo-micron	AL, AIV, B-48, CI, CII, CIII, E
VLDL	VLDL	B-100, CI, CII, CIII, E
LDL	LDL	B-100
HDL	HDL	AI, AII, E

Castignolles et al., 1994 developed synthetic mimics of natural endogenous particles (mainly LDL) and named them as "Supramolecular Biovector (SMBV)". These synthetic mimics incorporate bio-components as one of the construction element. SMBVs are lipoprotein-based carriers appended with polymerized polysaccharide with exterior coat layer of endogenous low-density lipoproteins (LDL). Vyas and co-workers, 1997 reviewed the composition and structure of these synthetic mimics of LDL and their possible role for site-specific drug delivery.

Jaitely and Vyas, 1999 characterized supra-molecular autovectoring systems for the targeted delivery of diclofenac diethylammonium to liver cellular tropics and the uptake was found mediated by the Kupffer cells of the liver. The supramolecular assemblages were consisted of the liquid crystalline phase surface stabilized with phosphatidylcholine. The targeting/autovectoring potential of supramolecular assemblages might be attributed to the fact that the system is comparable to the transporting form of cholesterol (liquid crystalline phase) in the body. Moreover, due to the nanometric size range and surface characteristics it could adsorb the apo-protein fragments present in the serum and could mimic endogenous lipoprotein to dictate the eventual course to the lipoprotein receptors expressed mainly on liver cells. Some of the biomedical applications in site-specificity of endogenous lipoproteins appropriately modified to achieve targetability are listed in Table 2-11.

Scavenger Receptors (ScR)

Scavenger cell receptors were discovered in 1979, during attempts to learn how cholesterol from low-density lipoproteins accumulates in macrophages in atherosclerosis plaques of patients with familial hyper-cholesterolaemia, who lack LDL receptors. In a series of studies thereafter, different macrophage scavenger receptors have been studied and explored using cDNA cloning and sequencing techniques (Table 2-12).

Scavenger receptors, which are expressed exclusively on endothelial liver cells and macrophages, mediate the uptake of a variety of polyanionic proteins/ligands or macromolecular complexes. These high binding sites are conserved on macrophages. They are capable of recognizing a number of structurally diverse polyanionic ligands such as modified protein (FITC coupled bovine serum albumin, acetylated or oxidized LDL), polysaccharides (Fucoidin dextran sulphate), polynucleotides (Polyinosinic and poly-guanylic acids) phospholipids (Phosphatidylserine), polyvinyl sulphate and bacterial lipopolysaccharide. Kupffer cells also express a specific receptor that recognizes both the particular terminal sugar and the negative charge present on the polyanionic glyco-conjugates. Similarly, receptors for monomeric negatively charged proteins are also expressed on liver endothelial cells.

The broad ligand specificity of scavenger receptors for polyanionic compounds makes them attractive candidates for mediating the bonding and intracellular uptake of negatively charged particulate systems especially PS liposomes. The liver is found to capture macromolecules having strong anionic charges, such as succinylated proteins and dextran sulfate, via scavenger receptor after intravenous injection in mice. It has been suggested that large succinylated and maleylated proteins should be useful as a carrier for the intracellular delivery of drugs specifically into the liver endothelial cells (Takakura and Hashida, 1996).

Macrophages are known to sequester and uptake chemically modified LDLs, such as acetylated LDL (acetyl-LDL) and oxidized LDL (Ox-LDL), via the macrophage scavenger receptors, leading to foam cell formation and massive intracellular accumulation of cholesteroyl esters. Chemically modified LDL (acetylated LDL) competes with liposomes for 60% of the binding sites on mouse peritoneal macrophages. However, experiments in cell culture systems with Cos cells transfected with type I and type II scavenger receptors from class A showed that these receptors were not able to bind and internalize PS containing liposomes. Only recently, it is reported that scavenger receptors from class B, which are members of the CD36 superfamily of selectins, are able to specifically bind liposomes containing anionic phospholipids. Furthermore, it has been shown that class B scavenger receptor functions as a receptor for HDL. The so-called oxidized low-density lipoprotein receptor, that has not been fully characterized, is shown to bind anionic ligands. Recently, Jinnouchi and co-workers,

1998 reported that glycoaldehyde-modifed LDL transforms macrophages into foam cells via macrophage scavenger receptors. These results were indicative of the fact that protein modified advanced glycation end products (AGE-LDL), if available *in situ*, are taken up by macrophage scavenger receptors and may take part to foam cell formation in early atherosclerosis lesions. They hold promise to be a targeting strategy of the future.

Transferrin Receptors (TfR)

Transferrin (Tf) is a major mammalian serum glycoprotein, transporting iron from sites of absorption and storage to tissue cells. Tf cell surface receptors present on all the growing cells render these cells as target modules selectively approachable through transferrins as carrier molecule. A diverse range of cell types including hepatocytes, fibroblasts, and blood brain endothelial cell lines and T4 cells express the transferrin receptors (TfR). TfR are present on actively dividing cell types implicating a role in growth and differentiation of a variety of cells. During activation, T-cells internalize and recycle their TfR. A successful gene delivery was demonstrated using a carbohydrate linked Tf-poly-L-lysine conjugate for efficient gene introduction in eukaryotic cells expressing the Tf receptors. Transferrin-poly-L-lysine and transferrin-protamine on complexation with plasma DNA demonstrate efficient binding and subsequent endocytosis by haematopoitic cells, leading to the expression of the transferred genes. Transferrin may be widely applied

Table 2-11. Biomedical Applications in Site-Specificity of Endogenous Lipoproteins appropriately Modified to Achieve Targetability

Modification	Method	Receptor(S) involved	Recognizing cell
Lactosylation of LDL (Tris-gal-chol-LDL)	Incubation of LDL with D-galactosyl-D-glucose) and sodium cyanoborohydrate)	Galactose particle receptor	Kupffer cells
Lactosylation of HDL (Tris-gal-chol-HDL)	Incubation of HDL with D-galactosyl-D-glucose and sodium cyanoborohydrate	Asialoglycoprotein (galactose-specific) receptor	Liver parenchymal cells
Acetylation of LDL	Incubation of LDL with acetic anhydride to modify glycine residue of apoprotein	Scavenger receptor (ScA, B and C)	Liver endothelial cells
Glycoaldehyde-modifed LDL	Incubation of LDL with glycoaldehyde in the presence of 0.5 mM EDTA	Scavenger receptor	Kupffer cells
Oxidized LDL (Ox-LDL)	Incubation of LDL with PBS and supplemented with 5 μM $CuSO_4$ for 24h (37 °C) and dialysing against PBS without cupric ion for 24 h (4 °C)	Scavenger receptor (ScA and B); Ox-LDLr	Kupffer cells
Lactosylated reconstituted HDL (LacNeoHDL)	Mixing of egg yolk PC and cholesteryl oleate with lactosylated HDL apo-lipoprotein	Galactose-specific receptor	Liver parenchymal cells

*Adopted from Vyas et al., 2001 with modifications

Table 2-12. Scavenger Receptors with Preferred Ligands

Receptor type	Ligands	Special cell type	Remarks
ScR-A	Acetyl-LDL, Ox-LDL, polyanionic ligands	Macrophages	Type-I and II, cloned
ScR-B	Acetyl-LDL, Ox-LDL, HDL, LDL, anionic lipids	Macrophages	CD36, super family, cloned
ScR-C	Acetyl-LDL, wide variety of polyanionic ligands	Drosophyla sp.	Cloned
Ox-LDLR	Ox-LDL, anionic lipids	Mammalian	95kDa membrane protein

*Adopted from Vyas and Sihorkar, 2000

as a carrier in the active targeting of anticancer agents, proteins and genes to primarily proliferating malignant cells that over-express transferrin receptors. However, most of the successful results obtained with the *in vitro* and *in vivo* application of this system are limited. This is probably due to competition of the administered system with endogenous transferrin, or due to the ubiquitous distribution of transferrin receptor and anatomical barriers. A recent review explores the possibilities of expression of TfR on proliferating cells, thus making these cells susceptible for intracellular delivery of antivirally active drugs/antisense oligomers (Table 2-13).

Folate Receptors

The vitamin folic acid (FA) enters cells through a carrier protein, termed as the reduced folate carrier, or via receptor mediated endocytosis facilitated by the folate receptor (FR). Because folate-drug conjugates could not serve as substrates of the former, they penetrate cells exclusively via FR-mediated endocytosis. The receptor for folate, also known as the folate-binding protein, is a glycosyl-phosphatidylinositol (GPI)-anchored membrane protein with an average molecular weight of 38 kDa. It mediates the cellular uptake of folate and the related coenzymes via receptor mediated endocytosis occurring at uncoated membrane regions termed as caveolae. Ligand binding to folate receptors stimulates their endocytic uptake by a clathrin-independent pathway (potocytosis) that has been exploited to negotiate a non-specific uptake of macromolecules and particulate drug delivery systems. In the potocytosis model of folate internalization, folate is proposed to bind receptor clustered around caveolae, i.e., specialized regions of the cell membrane enriched in cholesterol and other GPI anchored proteins. These caveolae then invaginate, forming a membrane-linked or cabled compartment within the cytoplasm. An integral proton gradient is then proposed to facilitate the release of the bound folate, allowing its movements across the caveolae membrane by an integral membrane anion carrier. In contrast, some reports suggest that FR exhibits no accumulation tendency in caveolae unless they are cross-linked with bivalent antibodies and also suggested the main involvement of coated pits rather than caveolae. Three receptor subtypes, α, β and γ, have been identified in humans. The γ-subtype is a rarely expressed secreted form, whereas the most common subtypes, α and β are membrane bound and have a high affinity for folic acid. Folic acid retains its receptor-binding activity upon conjugation to a macromolecule via its γ-carboxyl group. Therefore, folate derivatization can equivalently used to deliver foreign molecules into folate-receptor bearing cells.

Reddy and Low, 1998 have revised and summarized the folate receptor-mediated targeting approaches for the delivery of protein complex, low-

Table 2-13. Studies with Transferrin as an Endogenous Targeting Ligand

Target cell/ site	Delivery system	Activity (investigated)
Tumour cell (Hela, KB and colone); (Lovo, HL60, Hep2); H-mesothelioma tumour cell	Tf-methotrexate, Tf-adriamycin conjugate; Tf-polycation (poly-L-lysine/protamine) conjugate	Receptor mediated targeting to tumour cells
Rat brain cells	Maleimide grafted and Mabs (OX26) conjugated liposomes	Selective brain targeting
TfR^{+ive} human cancer cells	Biotinylated Tf-DNA conjugate	Gene delivery to human cancer cells
Murine melanoma cells	Avidin-polylysine conjugate complexed to biotinylated transferrin and DNA	Anti-HIV antisense delivery to brain
Murine OX-26	Fv antibody (Murine OX-26) streptividin fusion protein	Receptor mediated tumour targeting
Bladder cancer cell line (MGH-U1)	Tf-adriamycin conjugate	Receptor mediated targeting to bladder cancer cell lines

*Adopted from Vyas and Sihorkar, 2000

molecular weight chemotherapeutic agents, radioimaging agents, MRI contrast agents, genes, anti-sense oligonucleotides, ribozymes and immunotherapeutic agents. Proteins, drugs and imaging agents were effectively delivered to the folate receptor bearing cells by derivatization of endogenous folate with the therapeutically active modules (Table 2-14).

Tumour/viral cell Surface Biochemistry and Ligand Mediated Targeting Strategies

The drug-targeting concept was thought to be redefined as it has been severely invalidated in case of some pathological manifestations. For example, if endocytosis is required for cellular delivery, virus/tumour infected cells may be much less active in endocytosis due to the depletion of energy-rich metabolites or decreased expression of cell surface receptors. Success would seem to demand for some tumour cell associated receptors that are not found or expressed at extremely lower density level on the non-tumour cells. The molecular targets on the cells surface membrane of malignant cells may conveniently be divided in to following categories and could be targeted using the counter ligand or specially designed antibodies:

- Altered expression of cell adhesion molecules and their ligands
- Altered expression of certain receptors otherwise expressed by all eukaryotic cells, like insulin receptors and MHC class-I associated compound receptors.
- Exquisite expression of receptors during certain stages of cellular differentiation, like transferrin receptor (TfR), folate receptors, apo-lipoprotein receptor, c-kit receptors, hemopexin receptor and MHC class-II associated compound receptors.
- Altered expression of certain growth factors (epidermal growth factor receptor, EGFr) and certain vasoactive and angiogenic peptides.
- Expression of tumour vasculature epitopes, either of the endothelial cells or of the basement membrane supporting the endothelial cells or tumour stroma components (30.5 kDa antigen; CD19, CD34; endosialin; endoglin; F19 cell surface glyco-protein; fibronectin; fibrin; myosin and histone).
- Expression of surface determinants on malignant cells, like Ia antigens and tumour associated antigens (TAA).

Cell adhesion molecules are glycoproteins expressed on the cell membrane are involved in homotypic and heterotypic cell interactions through their respective receptors. Since cell-cell interactions are crucial in patho-physiological events, adhesion molecules play important roles in processes like wound healing, tumour metastasis, lymphocyte homing and granulocyte extravasation and expression of leukocyte receptors for ligands. These include members of cadherins and immunoglobulin super family (CAM), selectins and integrins (Fig. 2-15) and

Table 2-14. Studies using Folate as an Endogenous Targeting Ligand

Target cell/ site	Delivery system	Activity (investigated/ proposed)
KB and HeLa cells	Folate-PEG-PE (Doxorubicin)	Tumour targeting expressing FR
KB cell lines	Folic acid-Penicillin V-amidase (FA-enzyme conjugate)	Folate-targeted enzyme prodrug therapy
Tumour cell lines	Folic acid-single chain Fv conjugate	Folate-mediated immunotherpay (lysis of tumour cells by CTL in vitro)
CHO cells lacking folate receptor	Folic acid-PEG-PE (poly-L-lysine-DNA complex)	Folate-mediated non-viral gene therapy
HeLa cells	Folic acid-Cys^{287} (Pseudomonas exotoxin) conjugate	Efficient intracellular delivery and cytotoxicity of folate-linked toxins
Folate receptor expressing cancer cells (KB, HeLa, LoVo, SKOV3, SW620)	Folic acid-maytansinoid (DM1) conjugate	Selective killing of cancer cells expressing FR and non-toxic to normal cells lacking FR

Compiled and processed from a review by Reddy and Low, 1998

membrane associated proteoglycans. These cell adhesion moleculaes are exploited for tumour targeting and some of their applications are tabulated (Table 2-15)

Altered/Over Expression of Cell Specific Receptors

It is pertinent with the ligand-receptor mediated targeting approaches to discuss about the receptors either over-expressed or down regulated in the malignant target sites. Depending upon the over-expression (folate, transferrin, fucose and lipoprotein) or down regulation (ASGPr, mannose receptor), effective cellular targeting approaches could be engineered (Table 2-16). Folate receptors are over-expressed in several human tumours including ovarian carcinomas and epithelial cancers and hence been used as a targeting ligand and proposed to be superior over anti-target/anti-receptor monoclonal antibodies. Conjugates to FA linked to virtually any molecule or molecular complex of diameter <150 nm bind to the receptor possessing high binding affinity and enter the cell via receptor-mediated potocytosis. Since the same FA conjugates could not bind to FR negative cells even though they express the reduced folate carrier, the FA conjugates display significant selectivity for tumour cell *in vivo*. Liposomes conjugated to FA were also tested for targeting to neoplastic diseases. Unfortunately, poly(ethylene glycol) coating interfered with receptor recognition when the folate was directly linked to a PEG-linked phospholipid head group. To circumvent this

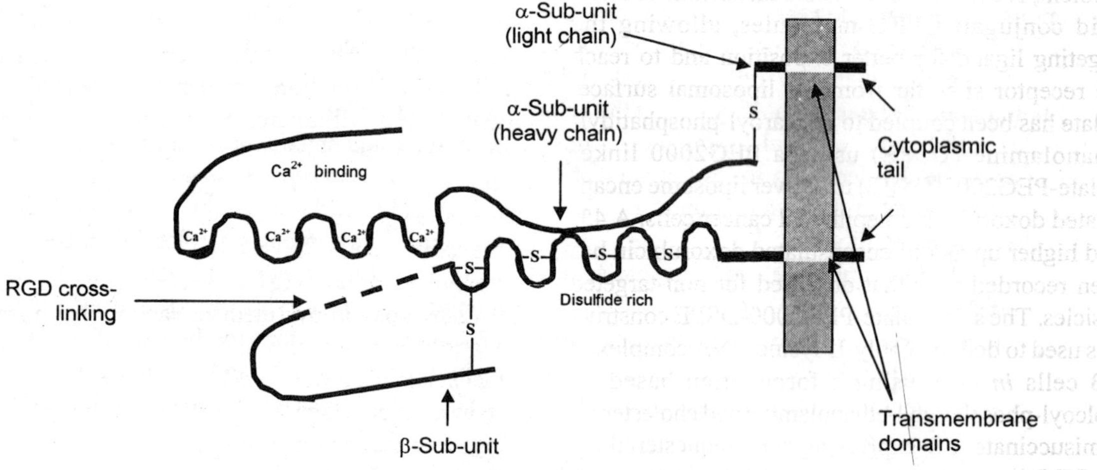

Fig. 2-15. A Typical Integrin Receptor

Table 2-15. Some Targeting Strategies using Endogenous Peptidic Segments of Cellular Adhesion Molecules (CAMs)

Receptor	Target cell/site	Ligand
Integrin αvβ3 (votronectin)	Tumour cell	Antibodies to αvβ3 (LM 609)
Integrin α5β1 (fibronectin)	Tumour cell lines	Synthetic peptide RGD (arginine-glycine-aspartic acid)
Integrin (laminine)	Tumour cell lines	Synthetic peptide YIGSR (tyrosine-isoleucine-glycine-serine-arginine)
Selectin	B16-BL6 murine melanoma cells	Sialyl Lexis X
E-Selectin	Inflammation induced mice	Sialyl Lexis X- Carboxymethyl pullulan conjugates

Table 2-16 Delivery Strategies Adopted to Target the Tumour Cells Using Over-Expressed Receptors as Molecular Ports

Target Receptors	Expression	Delivery strategies
Upregulation		
Folate	Ovarian carcinomas and epithelial cancers	Folic acid-Cys[287] (Pseudomonas exotoxin) conjugate, Folic acid-maytansinoid (DM1) conjugate
Fucose	Leukemia	N-(2-hydroxypropyl)methacrylamide co-polymer conjugates bearing N-linked fucosylamine and daunomycin.
Transferrin	T-cell leukemia, hematopoietic/ cancer cells	Tf-methotrexate, Tf-adriamycin conjugate; Tf-polycation (poly-L-lysine/protamine) conjugate, Biotinylated Tf-DNA conjugate
lipoprotein	Certain tumours	Porphyrin loaded lipoprotein (Photodynamic therapy)
Downregulation		
Asialoglycoprotein (ASGP)	Cirrhotic or tumour bearing livers	-
Mannose	Certain tumours	-

*Adopted from Vyas et al., 2001

problem, FA was attached to the distal ends of a few lipid conjugated PEG-molecules, allowing the targeting ligand for better exposition and to reach the receptor sites far from the liposomal surface. Folate has been coupled to distearoyl-phosphatidyl-ethanolamine (DSPE) using a PEG2000 linker (folate-PEG2000-DSPE) to deliver liposome encapsulated doxorubicin to epithelial cancer cells. A 45-fold higher uptake of encapsulated doxorubicin has been recorded over that observed for non-targeted vesicles. The same folate-PEG2000-DSPE construct was used to deliver a poly-L-lysine DNA complex to KB cells *in vitro* using a formulation based on dioleoyl-phosphatidyl-ethanolamine and cholesteroyl hemisuccinate. FR-expressing cells sequestered the FA-PEG-liposomes, however problems in regard to low unloading efficiency of entrapped drug after RME were encountered. A useful alternative as suggested by Reddy and Low, 1998 is to either incorporate a fusogenic peptide or to include in the liposomal formulation a lipid that acquires fusogenic properties only after entry into target cells. Although the fusogenic peptide can either be entrapped free within the FA-PEG-liposomes or covalently ligated to the liposomal surface, the former protocol is preferred, since it avoids induction of immune response against the fusogenic peptides.

An interesting observation of the receptor up-or down-regulation in normal and malignant cells could be seen in the case of lectin membrane receptors. It has been observed that asialo-glycoprotein receptor on the cell surface is depleted in normal hepatocytes of cirrhotic or tumour bearing livers, possibly due to a cellular redistribution and hence lower level of targeting was anticipated in patients with liver malignancies. On the other hand, the presence of fucose specific receptors capable of recognizing endogenous fucose-terminated ligands was reported on the surface of murine leukemia L1210. These over-expressed receptors were targeted by using polymers of N-(2-hydroxypropyl) methacrylamide bearing the alkylating agent sacrolysin, and additionally linked N-fucosylamine. It was demonstrated that conjugates containing fucosylamine were more cytotoxic than fucose free material against L1210 leukemia cells. Similarly, N-(2-hydroxypropyl)methacrylamide co-polymer conjugates bearing N-linked fucosylamine as well as the anthracycline daunomycin were targeted to leukemia cell lines. The latter was conjugated via a lysosomally degradable tetrapeptide (Gly-Phe-Leu-Gly) to the skeleton of the ligand-appended polymer. An 8-fold increased cytotoxic effect was recorded against L1210 cells cultured *in vitro* as compared to control, fucosylamine free conjugates. However, the same ligand conjugates showed no differential cytotoxic activity as compared against fucose free control to CCRF leukemia cells *in vitro*. It clearly indicates that the over expression of fucose binding lectins on the surface of certain tumour cell (L1210), mediate the targeting of these cells with fucose terminated ligands. Some types of tumour cells also express affinity receptors for LDL uptake, which may serve as means for ligand driven targeting of cytotoxic/bioactives to these cell lines. The number of receptors on normal cells is regulated by metabolic factors that are a function of intracellular amount of cholesterol and the rate of intracellular cholesterol synthesis. However, tumour cells lack many of the regulatory bioevents present in the normal cells, and in some tumour cells the regulation of the LDL-receptor is lost too. Such tumour cells express high number of LDL receptors under conditions where receptors in normal tissues are down-regulated. Not only cytotoxic drugs, but also photosensitizers porphyrins that incorporate well into lipoprotein carriers, may be delivered to tumour cells in this manner (reviewed by Bijsterbosch and van Berkel, 1990). In the so called photodynamic therapy, the tumour is localized with the help of porphyrin loaded lipoprotein using receptor mediated bioevents. This porphyrin-loaded tumour is subsequently exposed to irradiation or visible light. The porphyrin released at the target site act as photosensitizer and converts light energy to chemical energy, which results in severe biological damage of the target tissue (Fig. 2-16). However, solid tumours are poorly perfused and therefore not readily accessible for LDL, and this was the reason that these workers proposed drug-loaded or porphyrin-loaded LDL carriers for the eradication of the residual tumour cells.

Expression of Vasoactive and Angiogenic Epitopes on Tumour Vascular Endothelium

Tumour endothelial cells are a suitable target for targeted drug delivery and immunotherapy as they are accessible through the blood. The epitopes present on the tumour endothelial vasculature in the form of angiogenic peptides and adhesion molecules that interpaly between cells, soluble factors and extracellular matrix components could be exploited to negotiate targeting. At least 20 angiogenic peptides have been found on tumour vasculature that influence the endothelial cells directly (e.g., EGF and VEGF) or indirectly by inducing host cells to produce endothelial cell growth factors (e.g., TNF and TGF).

The epidermal growth factor receptor (EGFr) is over-expressed in a variety of human cancers and is reportedly involved in transduction of cell growth signals. Attempt has been made to target tumour cell lines using anti-EGF receptor antibodies. Fab fragment of anti-EGF receptorn antibody (B4G7) is conjugated with poly-L-lysine to form an affinity complex with DNA. The system was found excellent in *in vivo* targeted delivery of therapeutic genes to EGF-receptor hyperproducing tumour cells.

Rosenberg et al., 1987, targeted liposomes using a sandwich technique to the cultured rat pheochromocytoma and human melanoma cells expressing nerve growth factor receptors (NGFr). In their study these investigators incubated cells with biotinylated NGF and treated them with liposome-coupled streptavidin. Vascular endothelial growth factor receptor (VEGFR) antisense has shown to block expression of VEGFR and thereby suppresses the transforming phenotype of human carcinoma cell lines, KB cells. However, the delivery of VEGFR anti-sense oligonucleotides (ODNs) within liposomes that are further conjugated to folate via polyethylene glycol has recorded nine times higher uptake of ODNs than the uptake resulted in the case of plain liposomes and 16 times higher than soluble or non-encapsulated ODNs.

Endoglin, an essential component of the tumour growth factor receptor (TGFr) complex of human endothelial cells was put forward as a proliferating marker that is up-regulated on endothelial cells in

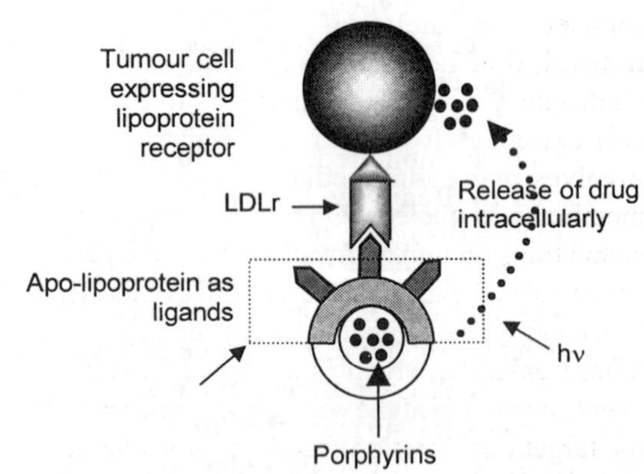

Fig. 2-16. Porphyrin Loaded Lipoproteins Bind to Tumour Site Through Specific LDL Receptors Expressed on the Surface

Table 2-17. Review of Studies Carried out using Vasoactive and Angiogenic Peptides as Endogenous Targeting Ligand*

Target cell/ site	Delivery system	Receptor
Tumour cells	Anti-EGF receptor antibody (B4G7) conjugated to poly(L-lysine)	EGFr
Human carcinoma cell lines (KB cells)	VEGFr antisense oligonucleotides in PEG-grafted liposomes	VEGFr
Cultured rat pheochromocytoma and human melanoma cells	'Sandwich' modules consisted of biotinylated NGF and liposome coupled streptividin	NGFr
Human brain cancer	Radiolabeled EGF-Ox 26 Mabs conjugate	Transferrin receptor
Blood brain barrier	Radiolabeled NGF-Ox 26 Mabs conjugate	Transferrin receptor
Tumour cell line	EGF peptides and anti-receptor antibody	EGFr
Tumour cells	Tumour necrosis factor conjugated with dextran based on metal chelation	TNFr
Tumour cells	Amylopectin hydrogel immobilized growth factor	EGFr
Tumour cells	TNF-interferon conjugates	TNfr

*Adopted from Vyas et al., 2001 with modifications

cases of miscellaneous human solid tumours. Various targeting strategies using vasoactive and angiogenic peptides are presented in Table 2-17.

FUTURE PERSPECTIVES

The innovation in the field of research on the targeted drug delivery in the coming years would be a shift from "receptor to nucleus" reflecting a desire to construct defined pathway linking the end points of different regulatory cellular events. However, for basic and technical reasons, research efforts have been focused overwhelmingly on receptor/ligand or transcription factor/DNA interactions. The task confronting molecular targeting is to link up these two extremes. It is clear that signal transduction involves many intermediate cellular events from membrane to nucleus. One of the simplest types of signal transduction pathway involves the generation of second messenger and cascade of events thereafter. A second type of signal transduction pathway is the kinase cascade, which is activated in response to events occurring at the cell surface. In each of these, the target transcription factors appear related to the nucleus under most circumstances giving an insight of the communication of the signals across the nuclear membranes. A number of studies are carried out in which the transcription factors themselves are actually located in the cytoplasm prior to activation and become relocated in the nucleus as a consequence of response to appropriate signals/ligands.

In the future, targeted drug-delivery systems may also prove particularly valuable to enable the use of a drug seems to be ineffective or toxic, if delivered systemically [e.g., neural growth factor (which need to cross blood-brain barrier) or vaccines (which need to be taken up by antigen presenting cells)]. At the current pace of gene cloning and recombinant-protein production within biopharmaceutical industry, many more site-specific drug-delivery products will be clinically investigated and implemented in near future.

REFERENCES

Allen T.M. (1997) *J. Liposome Res.* **7**, 315.

Annemiek J. M. L., Van Rensen Wauben M. H. M., Stulemeyer M. C. G., Van Eden W. and Cromelin, D. J. A. (1999) *Pharm. Res.* **16**, 198.

Balley M. B., Ansell S. M., Tardi P. G. and Harasym T. O. (1997) *J. Liposome Res.* **7**, 331.

Bangham A. D., Standish M. M. and Watkins J. C. (1965) *J. Mol. Biol.* **13**, 238.

Bigsterbosch M. K. and Van Berkel T. J. C. (1990) *Adv. Drug Deliv. Rev.* **5**, 231.

Castignolles N., Betbeder D., Ioualalen K., Merten O.,

Leclerc C., Samain D. and Perrin P. (1994) *Vaccine* **12**, 1413.

Chowdhury N. R., Wu C. H., Wu G. Y., Yerneni P. C., Bommineni V. R. and Chowdhury J. R.(1993) *J. Biol. Chem.* **268**, 11265.

Czop J. K. and Austen K.F. (1985) *J. Immunol.* **134**, 2588.

Davis S. S. and Hansrani P. (1985) *Int. J. Pharm.* **23**, 69.

Dumont S., Muller C. D., Schuber F. and Bartholeyns J. (1990) *Anticancer Res.* **10**, 155.

Ehrlich P. (1902) In: Collected papers of Paul Ehrlich: Immunology and cancer research, Pergamon Press, London, 442.

Feener E.P. and King G.L. (1998) *Adv. Drug Deliv. Rev.* **29**, 197.

Gregoriadis G. (1981) *Lancet* **2**, 241.

Gregoriadis G. and Florence A. T. (1993) *Drugs* **45**, 15.

Harashima H., Sakata K., Funato K. and Kiwada H. (1994) *Pharm. Res.* **11**, 402.

Illum L., Davis S. S., Muller R. H., Mak E. and West P. (1987) *Life Sci.* **40**, 367.

Illum L., Davis S. S., Wilson C. G., Frier M., Hardy J. G. and Thomas N. W. (1982) *Int. J. Pharm.* **12**, 135.

Illum L., Thomas N. W. and Davis S. S. (1986) *J. Pharm. Sci.* **29**, 53.

Illum L., Wright J. and Davis S. S. (1989) *Int. J. Pharm.* **52**, 221.

Jaitely V. and Vyas S. P. (1999) *J. Drug Target.* **6**, 315.

Jansen R. W., Molema G., Pauwels R., Schols D., De Clercq E. and Meijer D. K. F. (1991) *Mol. Pharmacol.* **39**, 818.

Jinnouchi Y., Sano H., Negai R., Hakamata H., Kodama T., Suzuki H., Yoshida M., Ueda S. and Horiuchi S. (1998) *J. Biochem.* **123**, 1208.

Khaw B. A., Torchilin V. P., Vural I. And Narula J. (1995) *Nature Med.* **1**, 1195.

Kinsky S. C. (1972) *Biochim. Biophys. Acta.* **265**, 1.

Lazo J. S. and Hacker M. P. (1986) *Fred. Proc.* **44**, 2335.

Lee M. J., Lee M. H. and Shim C. K. (1995) *Int. J. Pharm.* **113**, 175.

Liu D., Hu Q. and Song Y. K. (1995) *Biochim. Biophys. Acta.* **1240**, 277.

Lundberg B., Hong K. and Papahadjopoulos D. (1993) *Biochim. Biophys. Acta.* **1149**, 305.

Mew D., Lum V., Wat C. K., Towers G. H. N., Sun C., Oh C., Walter R. J., Wright W., Berns M. W. and Levy J. (1985) *Cancer Res.* **45**, 4380.

Mew D., Wat C. K., Towers G. H. N. and Levy J. (1983) *J. Immunol.* **130**, 1473.

Molema G. and Meijer D. K. F. (1994) *Adv. Drug Deliv. Rev.* **14**, 25.

Okuno K., Nakamura K., Tanaka A., Yachi K. and Yasutomi M. (1998) *Surg Today* **28**, 64.

Oseroff A. R., Ohuoha D., Hasan T., Boomer J. C. and Yarmush M. L. (1986) *Proc. Natl. Acad. Sci. USA* **83**, 8744.

Petit D. K. and Gombotz (1998) *Trend. Biotechnol.* **16**, 343.

Reddy J. A. and Low P. S. (1998) *Crit. Rev. Ther. Drug Carrier Syst.* **15**, 587.

Rensen P. C., Oosten M., Bilt E., Eck M., Kuiper J. and Berkel T. J. (1997) *J. Clin. Invest.* **99**, 2438.

Rosenberg M. B., Breakfield X. O. and Hawrot E. (1987) *J. Neurochem.* **48**, 865.

Sato J., Hamaguchi N., Doken K., Gotoh K., Ootsu K., Iwasa S., Ogawa Y. and Toguchi H. (1993) *Biotherapy* **6**, 225.

Spanjer H. H., van Berkel T. J. C., Scherphof G. L. and Kempen H. J. M. (1985) *Biochim. Biophys. Acta.* **816**, 396.

Tomlinson E. and Burger J. J. (1987) In: Polymers in controlled drug delivery, L. Illum and S.S. Davis (Eds.) Wright, Bristol, 25.

Van Berkel T. J. C., Kruijt J. K. and Kempen H. J. M. (1985) *J. Biol. Chem.* **260**, 12203.

Vyas S. P. and Dixit V. K. (1998) In: Pharmaceutical Biotechnology, First Edition. CBS Publishers and Distributors, New Delhi, 395.

Vyas S. P. and Sihorkar V. (2000) *Advanced Drug Delivery Reviews* **43**, 101.

Vyas S. P., Jaitely V. and Kanaujia P. (1997) *Pharmazie* **52**, 259.

Vyas S. P., Singh A. and Sihorkar V. (2001) *Critical Reviews in Therapeutic Drug Carrier System* 18,1.

Weinstein J. N., Magin R. L., Yatwin M. B. and Zaharko D. S. (1979) *Science* **204**, 188.

Wilson J. M., Grossman M., Wu C. H., Chowdhary N. R., Wu G. Y. and Chowdhary J. R. (1992) *J. Biol. Chem.* **267**, 963.

Yatwin M. B., Kreutz W., Horwitz B. and Shinitzky M. (1980) *Biophys. Struct. Mech.* **6**, 233.

CHAPTER 3

Bioconjugates

- Introduction
- Bioconjugation techniques
- Characterization of bioconjugates
- Applications of bioconjugates
- Bioconjugates in drug delivery and targeting
- Antibody conjugates (immunoconjugates)
- Antibodies conjugates developed against angiogenic peptides
- Bioconjugates of immunotoxins/ chimeric proteins
- Transferrin based bioconjughates
- Folic acid (folate) based bioconjughates
- Insulin based bioconjugates
- Bioconjugates with cytokines
- Glycoconjugates
- Polyethylene glycol (PEG) conjugates
- Poly-L-lysine conjugates
- Future perspectives
- References

Bioconjugation involves the linking of two or more molecules to form a novel complex having the combined properties of its individual components. Natural and synthetic compounds with their individual activities can be chemically combined to create unique drug carriers, which possess carefully engineered characteristics.

Essentially, proteins (anti-target or target specific) are used in bioconjugation technique as one of the handles, which are conjugated to other molecules or carriers capable of being detected by target site(s). It has now been recognized that delivery of many of the new therapeutic biotechnology products, recombinant proteins, oligonucleotides and their analogues can potentially benefit by the protection from enzymatic degradation, decreased uptake by reticuloendothelial system (RES)-rich organs, or from reduction of other unwanted manifestations of biological recognition. This can be achieved through their conjugation with macromolecules or carrier systems (Hermanson, 1996).

BIOCONJUGATION TECHNIQUES

Modification and conjugation techniques are dependent upon two inter-related chemical reactions: the reactive functional groups present on the various cross-linking or derivatizing agents and the functional groups present on the target macromolecules or delivery system to be modified. It is the aim that determines the type of conjugation technique to be implemented. The labeling, tagging, cross-linking, or targeting of small ligands, peptides, proteins, carbohydrates, nucleic acid, oligonucleotides, lipids with target molecules (or delivery device) can be accomplished by using various covalent and non-covalent conjugation techniques. Whether it be tagging proteins to target molecule to render them chromogenic or fluorescent, labeling molecules with biospecific ligands for subsequent affinity interactions, or cross-linking two or more moieties to create site specific active conjugates, the choice of cross-linking and derivatizing reagents is pivotal. The endogenous or exogenous ligands can be conjugated with either the drug or drug bearing delivery systems using various non-covalent and covalent techniques.

Covalent Conjugation

Covalent conjugation can be achieved by using cross-linking reagents which make the terminal functional groups of one molecule active which can subsequently be conjugated with another target molecule (Table 3-1). Generally three different cross-linking reagents are used :

- Zero-length cross-linkers,
- Homobifunctional cross-linkers, and
- Hetero-bifunctional (bifunctional and trifunctional) cross-linkers

The smallest available reagent systems are "zero-length cross-linkers". These compounds mediate the conjugation of two molecules by forming a bond containing no additional atoms, and thereby avoiding intervening linker or spacer. Most frequently used zero-length cross-linkers are carbodiimides and specially N-hydroxysuccinimide (NHS) (Chu et al., 1986; Ghosh et al., 1990). They are used to mediate the formation of amide linkages between a carboxylate and an amine or phosphomidate linkage between a phosphate and an amine. They are the most efficient zero-length cross-linkers in use, being efficient in forming conjugates between two protein molecules, between a protein and a peptide, between oligonucleotides and proteins, between a protein and a delivery system like liposomes and a combination of these with small molecules. A method of NHS ester mediated protein-carrier conjugation is to create sulpho-NHS esters directly on the carboxylate of the carrier protein using the EDC (Fig. 3-1). A carbodiimide reaction in the presence of sulpho-NHS activates the carboxylate group on the carrier to form amine reactive sulpho-NHS esters. The activation reaction is conducted at pH 6, since the amines on the protein get protonated and therefore tend to be less reactive towards sulpho-NHS esters that are formed. In addition, the hydrolysis rate of the esters is dramatically slow at acidic pH. Subsequent coupling with an amine-containing carrier creates conjugates through amide bond formation.

"Homobifunctional cross-linkers" are used for modification and conjugation of macromolecules consisted of bioreactive compounds containing the same functional group at both ends (Hartman and Wold, 1966). Most of these homobifunctional cross-linkers could tie one protein to another macromolecule or delivery system by covalently reacting with the same common groups on both the molecules (Fig. 3-2). Two protocols are generally used for the conjugation using these cross-linkers : single step protocol and two step protocol (Hermanson, 1996). Single step protocol involves the simultaneous addition of all reagents to the reaction mixtures. This protocol however, provides the least control over the cross-linking process and invariably leads to multiple products, only a small percentage of which represents the desired conjugates. In two step protocols, one of the proteins to be conjugated is reacted with the homobifunctional cross-linker and byproducts are removed. In the second stage, the activated protein is mixed with the other protein or molecule to be conjugated, and the final conjugation process occurs. The most commonly employed homobifunctional cross-linkers are NHS esters. They activate carboxylate groups on the proteins or other moieties to be conjugated with other molecules having amine nucleophiles.

"Hetero-bifunctional conjugation reagents" are most frequently used in anchoring ligands to the carrier or in constructing ligand-carrier conjugates covalently (Carlson et al., 1978). The most popular covalent conjugation reagents have terminal amine/carbonyl/sulphydryl reactive/photoreactive ends. In the process of conjugation with protein, haptens, immunotoxins, antibodies, liposomes or synthetic carriers, these cross-linkers with their bifunctional reactive ends are coupled to ligands and carriers in a selective manner (Hermanson, 1996). Various covalent coupling based approaches for the conjugations of ligands to the carrier of either endogenous or exogenous origin are shown in Figure 3-3.

A common method for coupling macromolecules and carriers with proteins or other macromolecules involves the use of a heterobifunctional cross-linker containing an NHS-ester and a maleimide group (Fig. 3-4). This type of cross-linker allows better control over the conjugation process than homobifunctional or zero-length conjugation methods by incorporating a two- or three- step reaction strategy directed against

Table 3-1. Various Cross-Linking Reagents Used in Bioconjugation of Proteins and Macromolecules with Other Target Macromolecules or Delivery Systems

Zero-length cross-linkers	Homobifunctional cross-linkers	Heterobifunctional cross-linkers
Carbodiimide	NHS esters	Bifunctional cross-linkers
EDC	Imidoesterases	Amine reactive and sulphydryl reactive
EDC and sulpho-NHS	Sulphydryl reactive cross-linkers	SPDP, LC-SPDP, sulpho-LC-SPDP
DCC	Aldehydes	SMCC and sulpho-SMCC, MBS and sulpho MBS
Woodward's reagent K	Bis epoxides hydrazides	Carbonyl reactive and sulphydryl reactive
N,N'-Carbonyldiimidazole	Bis-diazonium derivatives	MPBH, PDPH
Schiff base formation and reductive amination	Bis-alkylhalides	Amine or sulphydryl or carboxylate or arginate reactive and photoreactive
		NHS-ASA, APDP, ABH, APG
		Trifunctional cross-linkers
		ABNP, Sulpho-SBED

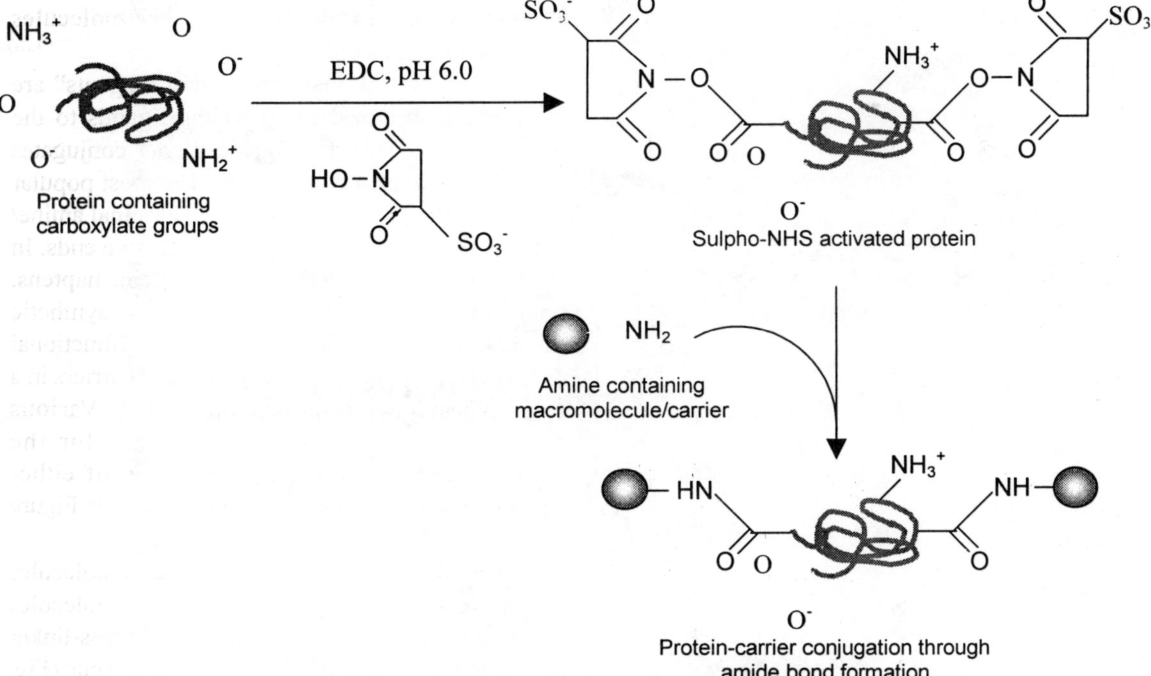

Fig. 3-1. Carbodiimide EDC can be Used in the Presence of Sulpho-NHS to Create Reactive Sulpho-NHS Ester Groups on Proteins, Which Subsequently Couple with Amine-containing Carrier (or Macromolecule) to Create Conjugates Through Resultant Amide Linkage

two different functional targets (Kitagawa and Aikawa, 1976; Edwards et al., 1989; Swanson et al., 1991). In this approach, the first molecule (a protein or a macromolecule) is first activated with the cross-linker through its amino group, and then cross-linked to a carrier (or another macromolecule) containing a sulphydryl group (Fig. 3-4). The use of sulpho-SMCC over other maleiimide containing cross-linkers such as MBS or SMPB provides the advantage of water stability of the maleiimide group prior to conjugation with a peptide.

The most intensively studied carrier system for the covalent ligand anchoring is liposomes. In two different strategies adopted for ligand anchoring to liposomes, the ligand is conjugated to a hydrophobic lipid anchor, typically a PE (phosphatidylethanolamine) which provides an accessible reactive amine (Wright and Huang, 1989). The two strategies

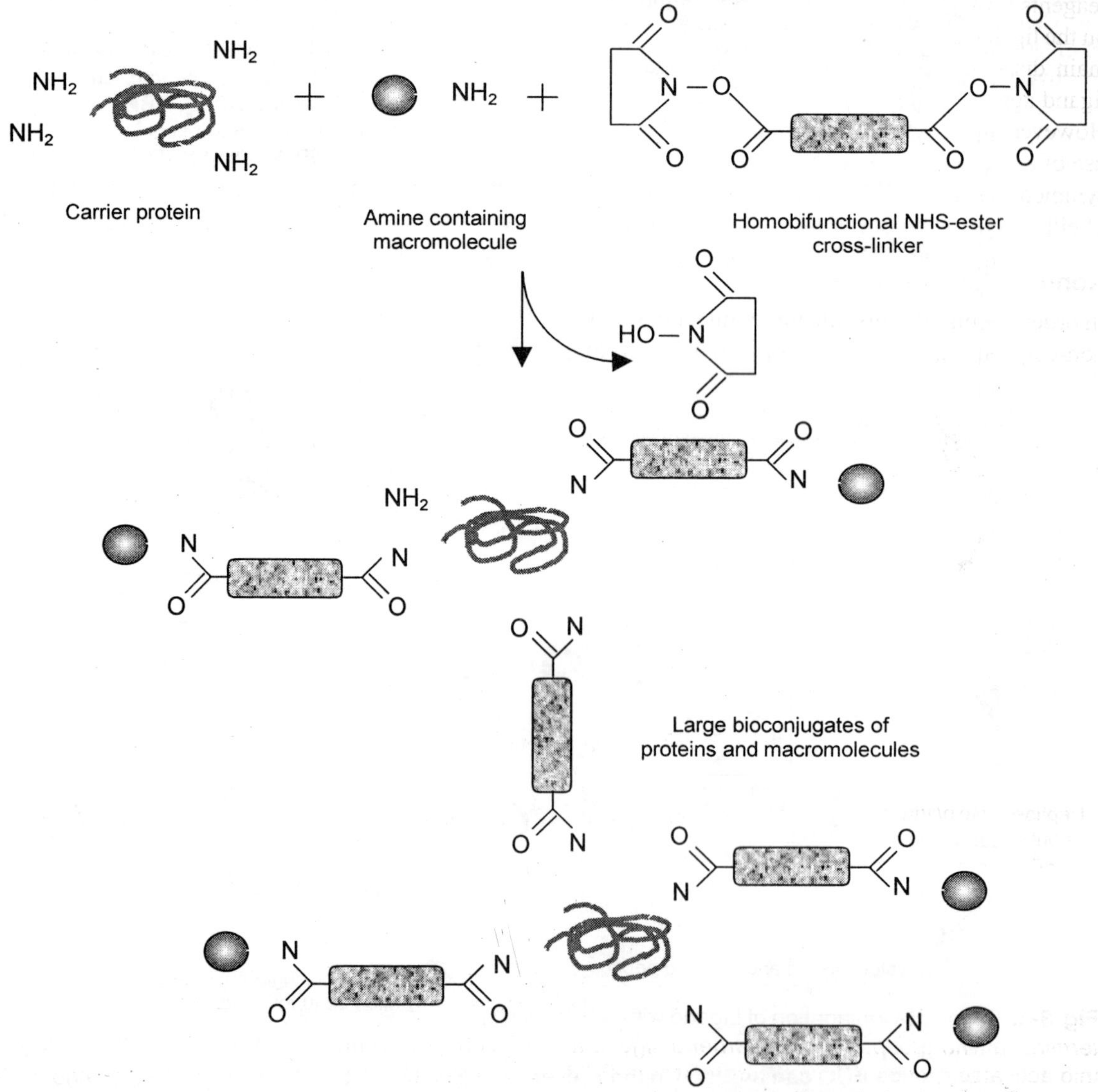

NH2 NH2 NH2 NH2 + NH2 +
Carrier protein
Amine containing macromolecule
Homobifunctional NHS-ester cross-linker
HO—N
Large bioconjugates of proteins and macromolecules

Fig. 3-2. Protein Carrier-Macromolecule Conjugate can be Formed Using Homobifunctional NHS Ester Cross-Linkers

differ in the manner of ligand conjugation to the lipid anchor. The first strategy involves the conjugation of ligand to PE before liposome formation. The ligand-lipid conjugate is then inserted in the mixed micellar solution of detergent and other lipids by detergent dialysis technique. This approach has been adopted to incorporate antibodies based ligands that have been already modified with fatty acids. The second strategy involves attachment of the targeting ligand onto preformed liposomes *in situ*. Hetero-bifunctional reagents form covalent bond between amino groups on the ligand and PE in the liposomes (Fig. 3-5). The main disadvantages with covalent conjugation are ligand aggregation and intervesicular cross-linking. However, these problems can be sorted out by the use of asymmetric bifunctional reagents rather than symmetric reagents that cause homo-polymerization of either ligand or liposomes.

Non-covalent Conjugation

In order to obtain a versatile targeting methodology, non-covalent anchoring of site directing ligands have been appreciated. An interesting observation of labeling of macromolecules with gold particles could simulate the non-specific interactions for non-covalent anchoring of ligand to macromolecular drugs or delivery systems (Gee et al., 1991). Non-specific interactions may include the electronic interactions between the negatively charged colloidal particles and the abundant positively charged sites on the protein molecules. An adsorption phenomenon involving hydrophobic pockets on the protein binding to the carrier surface can also be involved (Fig. 3-6). The potential for non-specific covalent binding of carrier to free sulphydryl/amine/carboxyl groups (dative binding), if present on ligand, can not be ruled out.

One of the most popular methods of non-covalent conjugation is to utilize natural strong binding of avidin or streptividin to small molecule biotin (Ross et al., 1986; Bayer and Wilchek, 1990). Biotinylated molecules can be targeted in complex mixtures by using appropriate avidin or streptividin conjugates. If the biotinylated component has affinity for binding to a particular antigen or receptor, then the same can

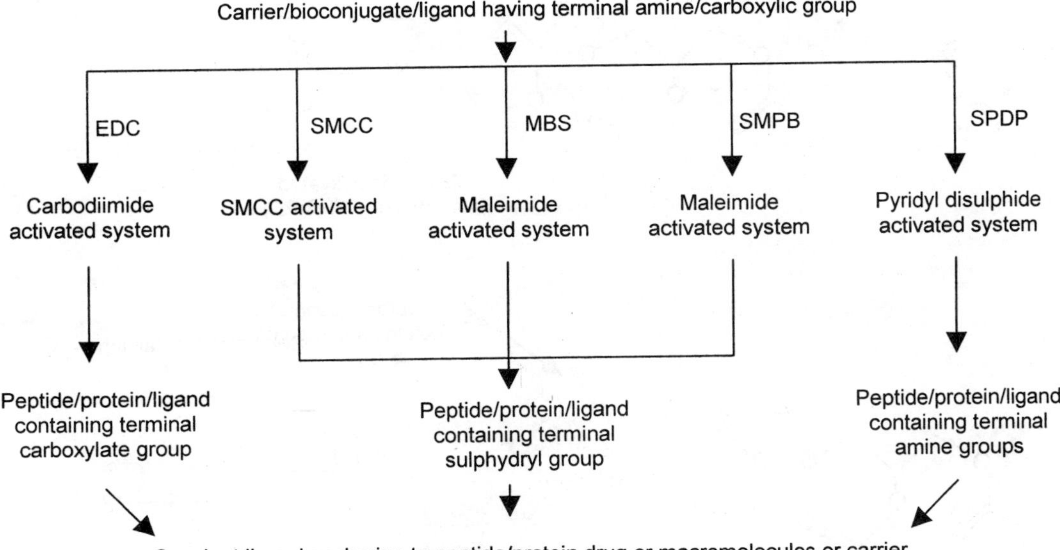

Fig. 3-3. Covalent-Conjugation of Ligand with Carrier Using Bi-Functional Reagents. These reagents activate terminal amino groups in either carrier or ligand and form covalent conjugation with maleimide activated or thio activated groups in ligand/carrier, where EDC=1-ethyl-3-(3-dimethylaminopropyl) carbodiimide; SMCC = succinimidyl-4-(n-maleimidomethyl) cyclohexane-1-carboxylate; MBS= m-maleimidobenzoyl-n-hydroxysuccinimide ester; SMPB= succinimidyl-4-(p-maleidophenyl)butyrate; SPDP=n-succinimidyl-3-(2-pyridylthio) propionate

be located by the use of an avidin/streptividin conjugate containing a detecting molecule. A series of avidin or streptividin-biotin interactions can be built upon each other by utilizing the multivalent nature of each tetrameric avidin/streptividin molecule to enhance further the detection capability for the target (Yoshikawa and Pardridge, 1992; Kang et al., 1994; Li et al., 1999). The same concept could be exploited with drug carriers as well. Liposomes with biotin modified lipids are prepared and used to attach a variety of avidin/streptividin linked targeting proteins/ligands (Plant et al., 1989). Non-specific protein based binding ligands (for example, avidin, streptividin, protein A or protein G) are attached to liposomes using covalent conjugation methods. However, the site directed targeting ligands, more often an antibody or biotinylated antibody, can then be non-covalently conjugated to the liposomes via specific affinity interactions with the non-specific binding ligands. This however, restricts the use of

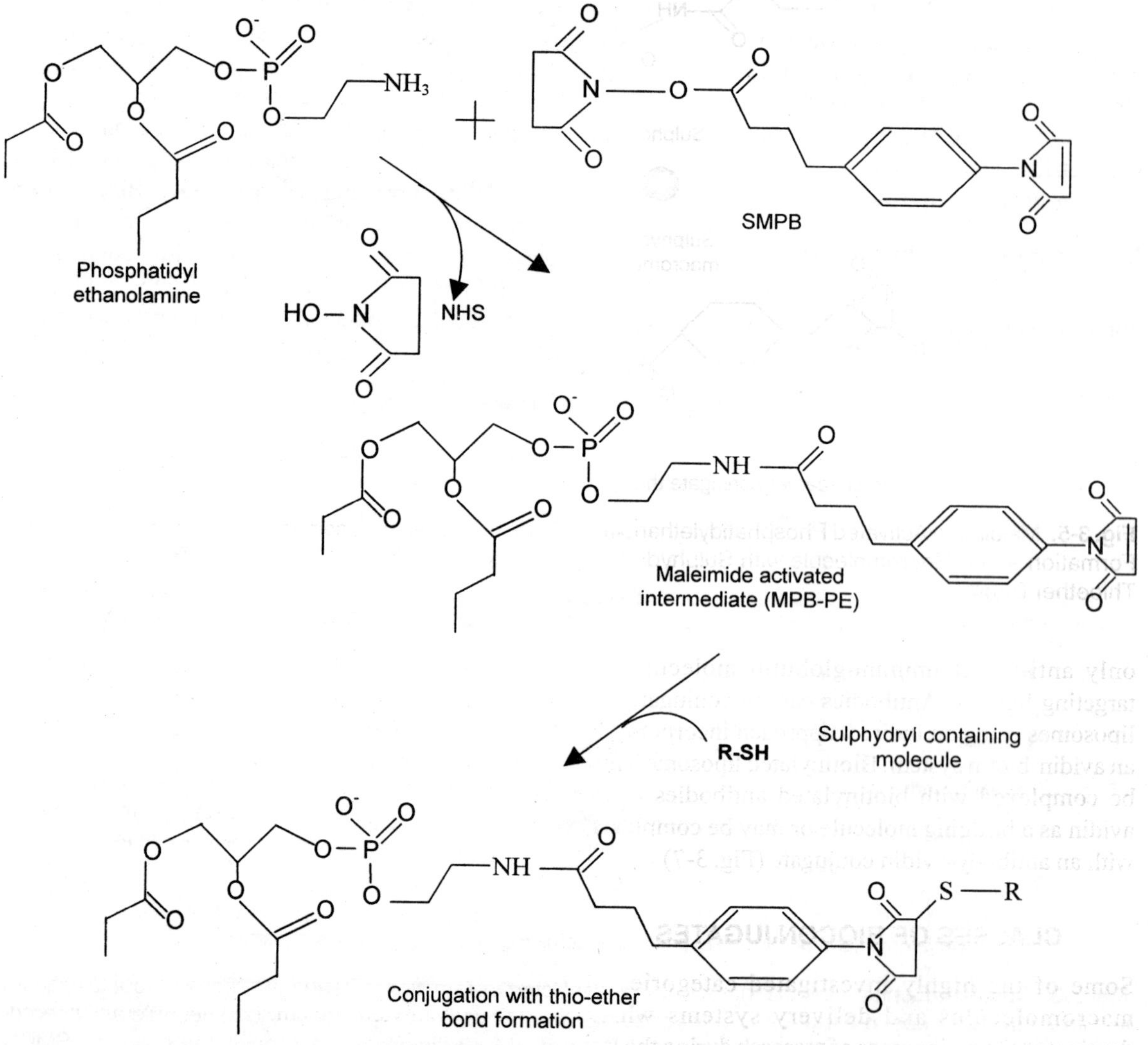

Fig. 3-4. Conjugation of Sulphydryl Containing Carrier (or Macromolecule) to a Protein (or Carrier). The first step is the activation of carrier with sulpho-SMCC to create an intermediate maleimide derivative, which is then coupled to thiols to form thioether bonds

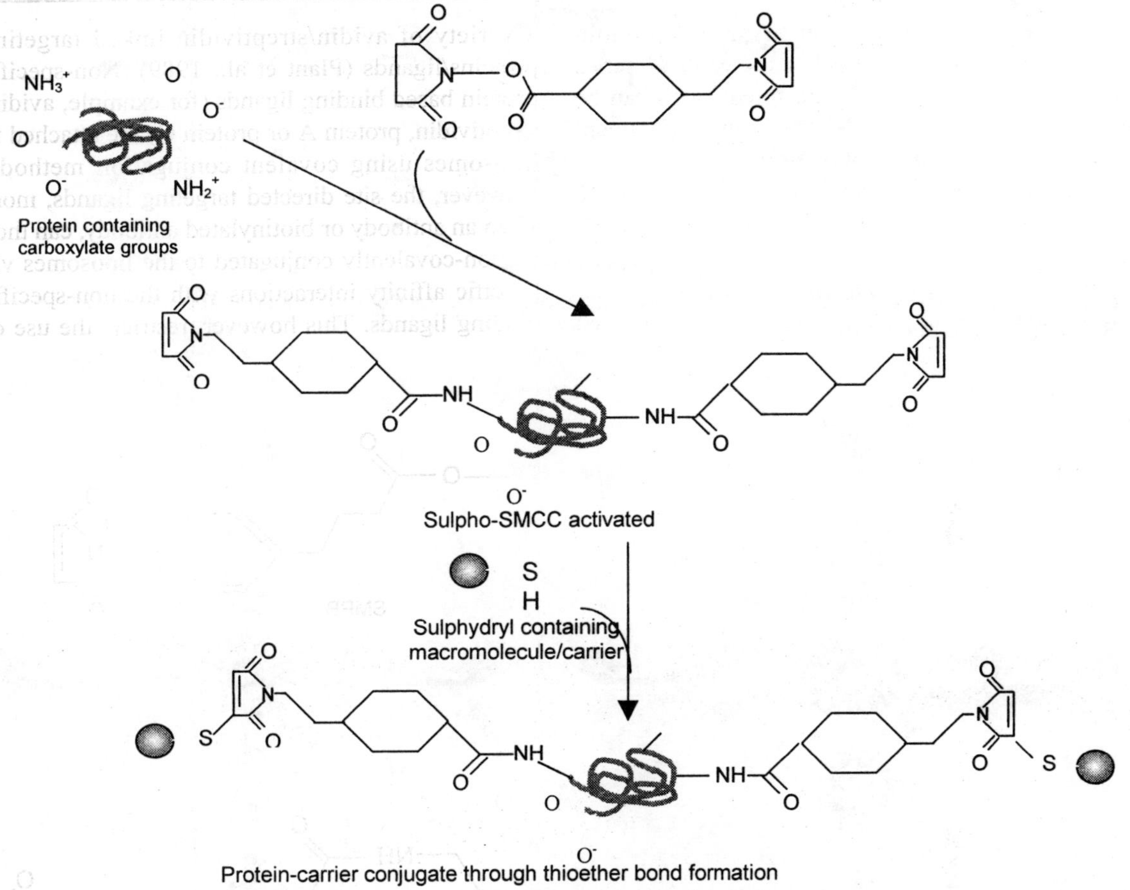

Protein containing carboxylate groups

Sulpho-SMCC activated

Sulphydryl containing macromolecule/carrier

Protein-carrier conjugate through thioether bond formation

Fig. 3-5. Maleimide Activated Phosphatidylethanolamine (MPB-PE) can be Used as a Component in Liposome Formation and a Macromolecule with Sulphydryl Group to these Liposomes may be Conjugated via Stable Thioether Bond

only anti-target immunoglobulin molecules as targeting ligands. Antibodies can be conjugated to liposomes using an indirect approach incorporating an avidin-biotin system. Biotinylated liposomes may be complexed with biotinylated antibodies using avidin as a bridging molecule or may be complexed with an antibody-avidin conjugate (Fig. 3-7)

CLASSES OF BIOCONJUGATES

Some of the highly investigated categories of macromolecules and delivery systems which dominated the major areas of research during the last decade include :

- Macromolecules
  - Antibody
  - Immunotoxins
  - Oligonucleotides
  - CD4
  - Interleukins and interferons
  - Transferrins
  - Folic acids and folate
  - Insulin
- Enzymes
- Glycoproteins and glycosylated polymers
- Polyethylene glycol, poly-l-lysine and related polymers
- Vesicles especially liposomes

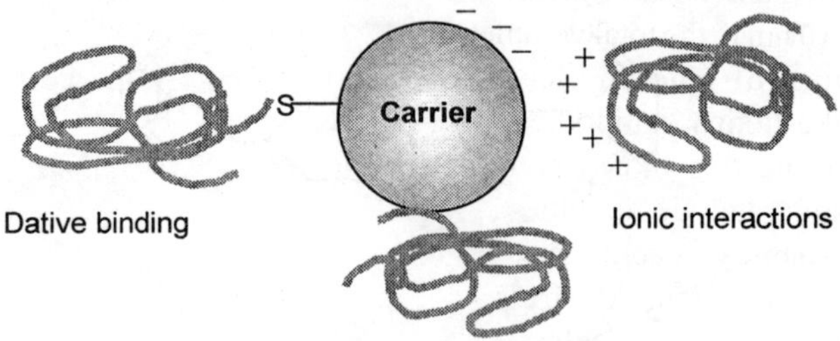

Fig. 3-6. Hypothetical Model to Depict Non-Specific and Non-Covalent Interactions that could Occur Between Ligand and Carrier

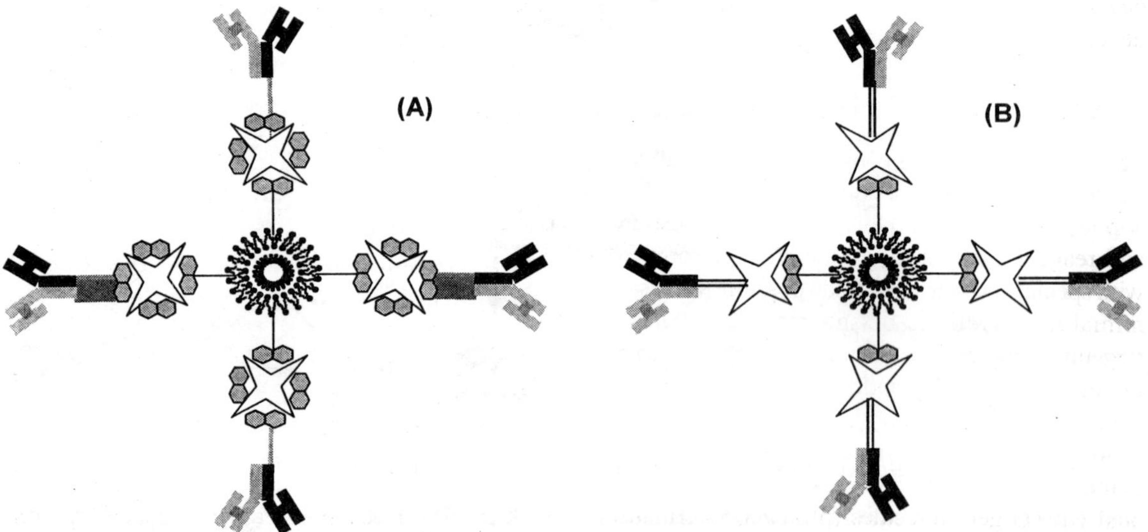

Fig. 3-7. Methods of Conjugation of Proteins/Macromolecules/Antibodies to Liposomal Surface. Method A depicts the conjugation of biotinylated antibody with biotinylated liposomes using avidin as a bridging molecule. Method B depicts conjugation of biotinylated liposomes with an antibody-avidin conjugate

These macromolecules may form bioconjugates with other proteins or between themselves for example, antibody and enzyme (antibody-enzyme conjugates) or antibody and toxins (immunotoxins) or by conjugation with drug carriers like conjugates of antibody and liposomes (immunoliposomes).

CHARACTERIZATION OF BIOCONJUGATES

Bioconjugates are particularly characterized for the specific purpose for which they are constructed and most of these studies are *in vivo* or *ex vivo* in nature. However, they are characterized in general for changes in shape using various microscopy (transmission electron, scanning electron or atomic force microscopy) and size using gel-exclusion chromatography. While practically any gel medium can separate drug conjugates from non-encapsulated molecules, gel media with larger porosities, such as Sepharose 4B or 2B, and Sephacryl S500 and S1000, allow fractionation of these conjugates in the working volume of the column. The largest inclusion volume is found in Sephacryl 1000, which separates in its elution volume particles with diameters between 0.4 μm in the void volume and ~10 nm in the total volume. Depending upon the nature of macromolecule selected for conjugation like toxins, antibodies or enzymes, their specific properties like toxicity, antigen binding capacity and catalytic activities is determined. Moreover, the stability of conjugates in various simulated or *in vivo* biological fluids (from a biological point of view) and in the accelerated storage conditions (from a pharmaceutical point of view) are also determined. Since, generally drug or toxin conjugates are studied for tumour targeting, their *in vivo* evaluation on *in vitro* or *ex vivo* developed tumour cell lines or in the experimentally developed tumour models can be assessed.

APPLICATIONS OF BIOCONJUGATES

The technology of bioconjugation has influenced nearly every discipline in the life sciences. The application of the available cross-linking reactions and reagent systems for creating novel conjugates with special activities has made possible the assay of miniature quantities of substances, the *in vivo* targeting of molecules, and the monitoring of specific biological processes. Modified or engineered conjugates have been used for purification, for detection or localization of specific cellular components, and in the treatment of infections as drug carriers conjugated with target molecules (proteins) (Hermanson, 1996). Some of the fields where bio-conjugates have been exploited are :

- Antibody-enzyme conjugates for use in enzyme immunoassay systems and in drug therapeutics.
- Antibody-toxin conjugates for use as targeted therapeutic agents.
- Hapten-carrier conjugates for immunization, antibody production and vaccine research.
- Lipid and liposome conjugates with proteins and antibodies for use in drug delivery and drug targeting.
- Conjugates of avidin or streptividin for use in avidin-biotin assays and in labeling of marker molecules.
- Labeling molecules with colloidal gold for sensitive detection processes.
- Polymer conjugates with PEG or dextran to modulate bioactivity or stability of macromolecules.

BIOCONJUGATES IN DRUG DELIVERY AND TARGETING

The current problems of controlling the viral and bacterial infections and managing tumour conditions as well as the lack of effective and safe pharmacotherapeutic measures have renewed interest in the options of targeting of drugs, antisense and genes to various blood cell types. Modifications of proteins, peptides, hormones, immunomodulators, growth factors, cytokines, vitamins and other macromolecules with drug, toxins, antibodies or other therapeutically potential moieties, result in the formation of bioconjugates, which exhibit an exquisite specificity and reproducibility. Bioconjugates have been appreciated in drug delivery and targeting for last 10 years as systems, which are either macromolecular or particulate in nature and *en route* the drug, enzyme, antibody or toxin to the desired site of action. They have been appreciated in site specific delivery of drugs, tumour targeting, viral targeting, gene and antisense oligonucleotide delivery. Some of the important bioconjugate systems studied and used in the field of drug delivery and targeting are described in this chapter.

ANTIBODY CONJUGATES (IMMUNOCONJUGATES)

Immunoglobulins clustered on the surface of the target cell expose their tail region (Fc) for recognition and subsequent interaction with the Fc receptors (FcR) present on the surface of the macrophages and neutrophils (Cline and Sumner, 1972; Garagiola et al., 1979). Largely by means of such Fc receptors the phagocytic cells of mononuclear phagocytic system negotiate tumour cell killing with the help of ligand-associated anti-receptor or chimera antibodies.

A new trend in the development of antibody-antigen (epitope) based targeting is the use of antibody fragment instead of whole immunoglobulin molecule (Fig. 3-8). Instead of using complete IgG portion, immunologically active fragments, $F(ab)_2$ and Fab′, have been used to improve access to the receptor-

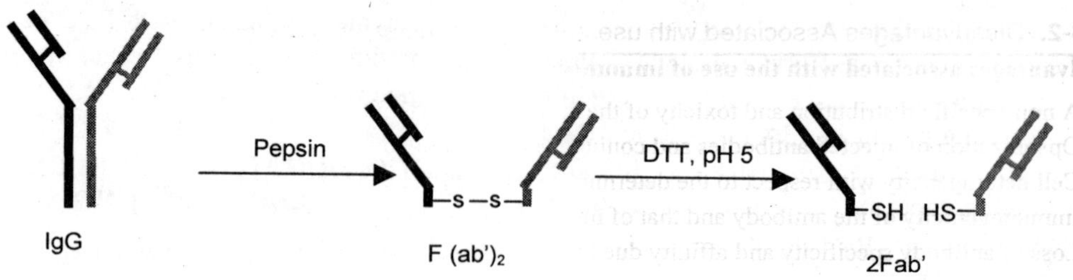

Fig. 3-8. Formation of Antibody Fragment. Preparation of $F(ab')_2$ Fragments by Pepsin Digestion of IgG Molecule. Fab' Monomers are Generated from these Fragments by Reduction with Dithiothreitol (DTT) at Low pH

bearing cells (Unkeless et al., 1981; Fleit et al., 1982). The molecular size decreases from 150 kD for an IgG via 50 kD for a Fab′ fragment to 27 kD for a single chain Fv protein (ScFv) (Cho et al., 1997). The greatest potential of ScFv is in antibody mediated ligand targeting, since they can be readily incorporated into fusion proteins with therapeutic entities. It was recently shown that anti-CEA ScFv located on all known tumour deposits, in patients with CEA-producing cancers are exploited in tumour imaging studies (Begnet et al., 1996). Tumour site accumulation was slightly reduced as compared to IgG and anti-CEA antibody. This was probably due to the monovalent antigenic nature of ScFv which, allowed for their rapid removal from circulation and hence restricted tumour accumulation. In mouse tumour model, antibodies against the basement membrane component fibronectin could deliver vasoactive agents to tumour tissue (Epstein et al., 1995). Stroma component fibrin has been identified as a tumour epitope and an antibody was developed, since in tumour tissues fibrin deposition is a pre-requisite for stroma deposition and extracellular matrix formation (Kairemo et al., 1993).

Antibody Conjugated Delivery Systems

Bioconjugated systems have been appreciated as delivery systems, which themselves act as targeting ligand due to the presence of targeting components that recognize either a component or a whole determinant (or receptor) present on the target cell. Monoclonal antibodies (Mab) directed against tumour antigens may be used as targeting agents for conducting certain cytotoxic substances to target cells for selective killing. This leads to the formation of a hybrid molecule with the specificity of the immunological ligand and the therapeutic activity of the drug or cytotoxic substance. Numerous cell surface markers are now known to proliferate solid tumours in human. The possibility to raise monoclonal antibodies against these markers allows tumour site targeting discretely. However, to make these antibodies a 'magic bullet", conjugation with toxic or cytotoxic components is required that, leads to the formation of immunoconjugates, which can be another antibody molecule (bispecific antibody), an enzyme (antibody-enzyme conjugates), toxins (immunotoxins), chemo-therapeutic agents (drug conjugates), biological modulators such as lymphokines or growth factors. Some immunoconjugates utilize intermediate carrier systems consisting of polymeric molecules such as polysaccharides, particularly dextran (Hermanson, 1996). The activated dextran is cross-linked to both the monoclonal antibody and a cytotoxic agent, providing multivalent conjugation sites to create larger complexes. However, some of the disadvantages noticed and anticipated with the use of immunoconjugate therapy are presented in Table 3-2. Hence, proper attention and effective measures should be taken to ensure the advantages associated with immunoconjugate delivery. Liposomes have been used in a similar fashion for conjugation of monoclonal antibodies (immunoliposomes) to their outer surfaces and cytotoxic agents contained in aqueous domains or intercalated within lipid domains.

Anti-receptor (target) monoclonal antibodies are well established for their role in tumour targeting.

Table 3-2. Disadvantages Associated with use of Immunoconjugates and Solutions Offered

Disadvantages associated with the use of immunoconjugates

- A non-specific distribution and toxicity of the antibodies due to their cross-reactivity with non-target cells
- Opsonization of injected antibodies and conjugates with circulating antigens
- Cell heterogeneity with respect to the determinant to which the antibody is directed
- Immunogenicity of the antibody and that of immunoconjugates
- Loss of antibody specificity and affinity due to coupling with another drug/cytotoxic molecule

Solutions offered with the use of immunoconjugates

- Purification of the antibody, using affinity techniques, can be used to minimize the cross-reactivity
- The use of antibody fragment instead of whole immunoglobulin molecule [Fab′, F(ab′)$_2$ and ScFv]
- The use of homologous antibody to prevent immunogenicity

The conjugation of these targeting ligands (antibodies developed against a specific tumour determinant) with another recognition component provides them dual specificity to target the drug or toxin intracellularly.

Antibody Enzyme Conjugates

A novel strategy for the delivery of cytotoxic and antiviral agents to specific cell types is the prodrug activation by antibody-enzyme conjugates. Such antibody-coupled enzyme can be specifically delivered to the cell types that express antigenic determinant (Senter, 1990). In fact, the need for antibody internalization, which is one of the problems associated with immunoconjugates, is addressed. The strategy is known as ADEPT (antibody directed enzyme prodrug therapy). The formation of active compounds in the close proximity of the target cells leads to higher cellular and lower systemic concentration of the active drug. Haisma and co-workers, 1992 described a Mab-β-glucuronidase conjugate as an activator of the prodrug epirubicin for the specific treatment of cancer.

An interesting strategy, Enzymosomes has been developed. Enzymosomes are basically liposomal constructs engineered to provide a mini bio-environment at the site of clinical significance. Enzymes are covalently immobilized or coupled to the surface of liposomes, therefore, when a nontoxic prodrug is administered simultaneously, it is converted by the immobilized enzyme to a potent anti-tumour agent in the vicinity of tumour cell lines. The specificity of enzyme reaction provides a means to limit prodrug activation at the tumour site, through prior enzyme targeting of enzymosomes, or via enzyme expressing gene delivery to the tumour cells (VDEPT). Figure 3-9 provides a schematic presentation of the concept of targeted delivery of anticancer prodrug activating enzymes with immunoliposomes (ADEPT based liposomal system), also known as immunoenzymosomes (Vingerhoeds et al., 1993).

The enzyme bearing immunoliposomes were first targeted to tumour cell lines with the help of appropriate Mabs. After binding of the immunoenzymes to target, a prodrug is administered, which is activated by cell bound immunoenzymes in the close proximity of the tumour cells. Vingerhoeds and co-workers, 1993 reported the coupling of the enzyme β-glucouronidase, capable of activating the prodrug epirubicin-glucouronide, to epirubicin. It was found that treatments with enzymosomes (bearing no specific anti-tumour antibodies) or immunoliposomes (bearing no enzymes) were ineffective, but pre-incubation with immunozymes (enzymosomes) resulted in an enhanced antitumour activity of the prodrug.

It is the options available in regard to choice of enzymes for ADEPT/GDEPT (Antibody/Gene Directed Enzyme Prodrug Therapy) and the range of tumour antigen-targets that makes these enzyme/prodrug/carrier seemingly a complex concept exploitable in cancer chemotherapy and gene therapy in the near future. Many ADEPT systems have been developed using alkylating agents, a class of anti-tumour drugs which include some of the most widely used clinical agents (Table 3-3). There is a wide spectrum of antigen specific targets available, which provide opportunities of targeting a range of tumours using Mab-enzyme conjugates (ADEPT). Similarly,

Table 3-3. ADEPT Systems Using Prodrugs Based upon Alkylating Agents

Enzyme system	Prodrug for
Carboxypeptidase	Benzoic acid mustard, phenol mustard
Alkaline phosphatase	Phenol mustard, Mitomycin derivatives
β-glucuronidase	Phenol mustard
β-lactamases	Phenylenediamine mustard, Carboplatinum derivatives, Mitomycin C
Penicillin V/G amidase	Melphalan
Nitroreductase	Nitrogen mustard

Compiled from Sherwood, 1996

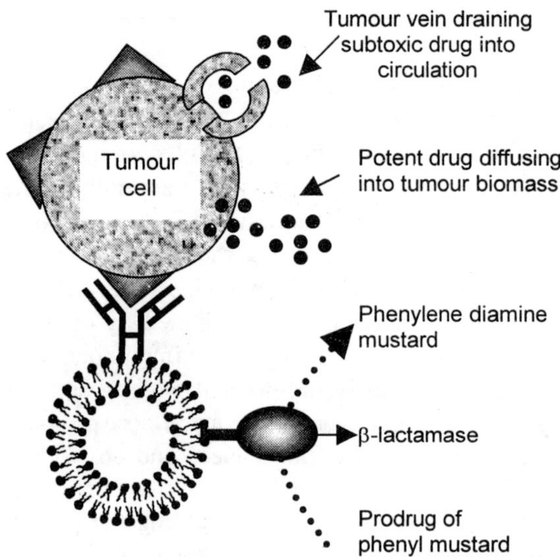

Fig. 3-9. Schematic Presentation of the Concept of Antibody Directed Enzyme Prodrug Therapy (ADEPT)

a range of antigen markers are available which might be used for selective accumulation and expression of prodrug activating enzymes delivered using enzymosomes.

Sherwood, 1996 reported several enzyme-prodrug systems and proposed carboxypeptidase G2 enzyme and a nitrogen mustard prodrug based enzymosomes for further clinical trials. Herpes simplex virus-thymidine kinase (HSV-tk) has been a leading and promising candidate for VDEPT (virus directed EPT), based on large differential insensitivity to GCV (Gancyclovir) between cells expressing HSV-tk and parental cells. Figure 3-10 presents two prodrugs of phenylenediamine mustard, which is converted into the active drug via the enzyme β-lactamases and in the process the cytotoxicity of the parent drug ($IC_{50\%}$) is reduced by a factor of 25-50% by prodrugs.

Recently, Reddy and Low, 1998 have suggested the ADEPT approach based on folic acid in place of monoclonal antibody. In their studies, penicillin-V-amidase (a fungal enzyme known to hydrolyse the prodrug, doxorubicin-N-p-hydroxyphenoxy-acetamide (DPO) to free doxorubicin) was conjugated to folic acid and tested for *in vitro* cytotoxicity. These workers suggested the use of this folate targeted enzyme prodrug therapy *in vivo*, where factors such as tumour selectivity and immunogenic behaviour can be more accurately assessed.

Bispecific Antibodies

This is an attractive strategy for target orientated site-specific drug delivery. The approach has been mainly suggested for immunotherapy of immunological disorders specially related to lack of MHC restricted recognition by immune effector cells (Staerz et al., 1985). Fanger and co-workers, 1992 reported a chimeric combination of an anti-tumour antibody with an anti-lymphocyte antibody as a bispecific protein that could redirect T-lymphocytes to lyse tumour cells. A similar approach was suggested for cytotoxic T-lymphocytes for killing of HIV infected cell. In this case, bispecific antibodies were produced that direct cytotoxic T-lymphocyte to cells expressing gp120 of HIV thus specifically targeting the infected cell lines (Burg et al., 1991). By cross-linking effector cells (CTLs) and tumour cells, the CTLs were found to be capable of lysing the tumour cells *in vitro* and *in vivo* (Kroesen et al., 1995). In carcinoma patients, the combination treatment of interleukin-2

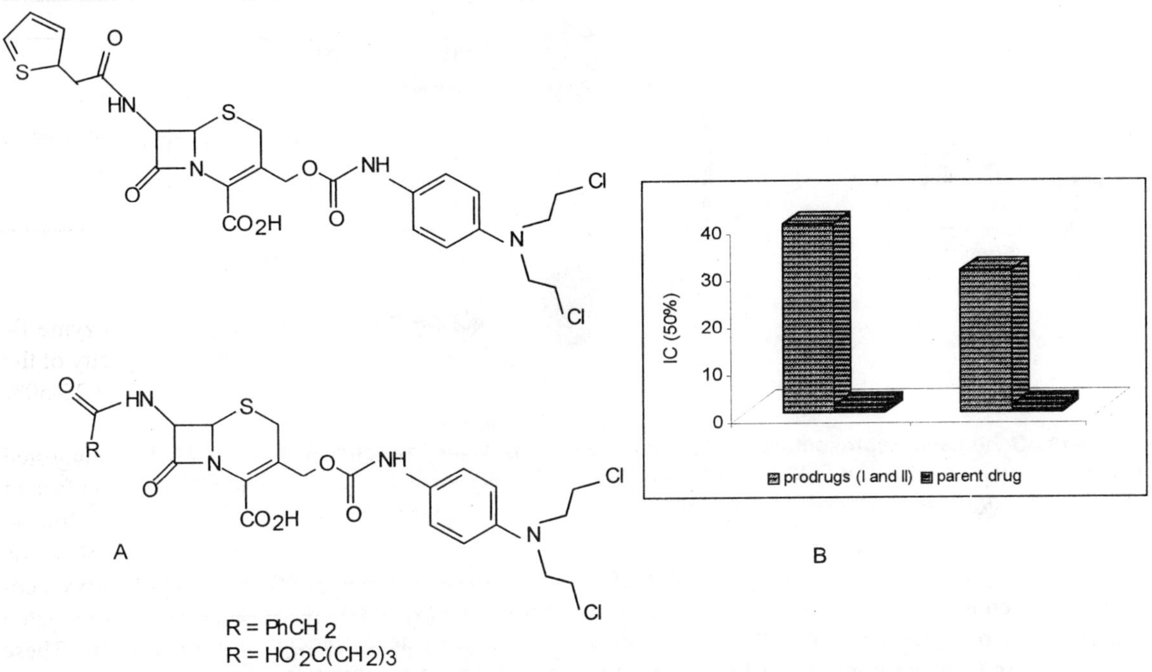

Fig. 3-10 Prodrugs of Phenyl Mustard, which Utilize β-Lactamase System for Active Conversion to Phenyl Mustard (A), Reduction in Cytotoxicity of Phenyl Mustard Prodrugs as Compared to Plain Drug (B)

(subcutaneous) and BIS-1 F $(ab')_2$ (intravenous) bispecific antibody directed against epithelial glycoprotein-2 (EGP-2) and the TcR/CD3 complex on T-lymphocytes could recruit T-lymphocytes and subsequently elicit an immune response as measured by elevated plasma levels of tumour necrosis factor-∝ and interferon-γ. However, these studies indicated that the accumulation levels of bispecific antibody loaded CTLs were not sufficient for an absolute therapeutic effect (Fig. 3-11).

Further, to improve tumour site targeting, strategies are being developed to selectively direct and deliver CTLs against tumour endothelium, followed by site activation or site specific coagulation (Molema et al., 1997). Interference with tumour blood flow can inhibit tumour growth. This was achieved either by damaging the endothelial lining resulting in the formation of thrombi (Molema et al., 1997) or by directly manipulating anti-coagulant activity (Burrow et al., 1995). Bispecific antibodies against tumour endothelium on one hand and tissue factors (the initiator of the extrinsic pathway of blood coagulation) on the other hand were combined for the synergistic effects. *In vivo* application of the bivalent antibody and a truncated form of tissue factor could directly induce thrombotic occlusion of the tumour blood vessels and facilitate targeting through such antibody conjugates (Burrow et al., 1995). Yet another option to obstruct blood flow is through direct lysis of endothelial cells by immune effector cells. This may be achieved by cross-linking of CTLs and tumour vascular endothelium with the help of bispecific antibodies directed against specific epitopes located on either of cell types.

Antibody Conjugated Liposomes (Immunoliposomes)

One of the fastest growing domains in bioconjugate technology is the use of liposomes and their conjugated versions. They function as macro-molecular carrier for nearly every application of bio-conjugate chemistry. They are used as delivery

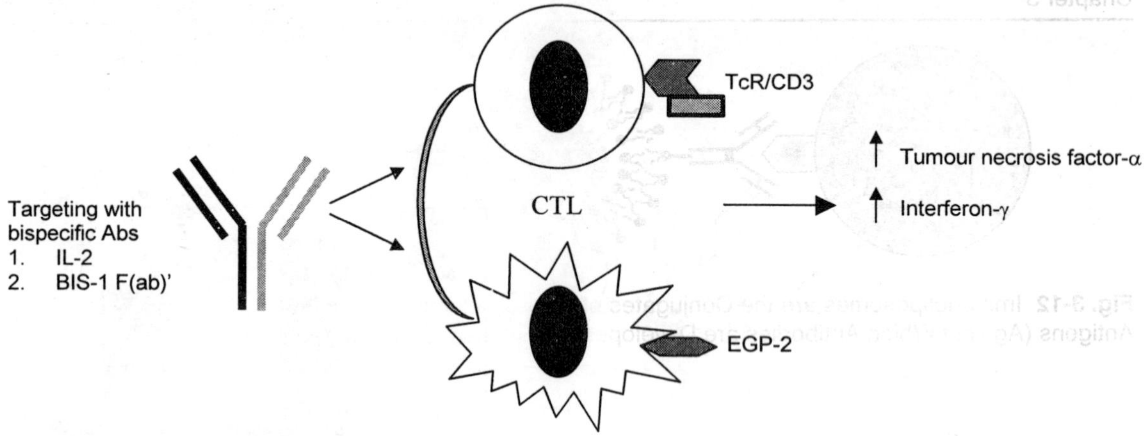

TcR/CD3

Tumour necrosis factor-α

Targeting with
bispecific Abs
1. IL-2
2. BIS-1 F(ab)'

CTL

Interferon-γ

EGP-2

Fig. 3-11. Schematic Representation of Bispecific Antibody Mediated Lysis of Target Cells. Through cross-linking of T cell receptor and CD3 complex on cytotoxic T-lymphocytes (CTLs) and epithelial glycoprotein-2 (EGP-2) on target cell, lymphocyte is capable of actively lysing target cells

devices to encapsulate drugs, cosmetics, and fluorescent detection markers and as vehicles to transport nucleic acids, peptides and proteins to cellular sites *in vivo*. Targeting components like antibodies (immunoliposomes), non-fusogenic proteins and peptides (proteo-liposomes) and fusogenic proteins (virosomes) can be conjugated to the liposome surface. These can be used to create specific bioconjugates that can be used to target cancer cells *in vivo*, to deliver proteins and nucleic acids and enhance gene delivery, as vaccine carriers, or to enhance detectibility in immunoassay systems, and as multivalent cross-bridge in avidin-biotin based assays.

However, one of the most extensively studied liposomal bioconjugates is immunoliposome (Norley et al., 1986). Antibodies can be covalently conjugated to liposome surface to create large antigen-specific conjugates that will deliver the entrapped drug (or toxins) specifically to the target cells expressing their counter recognition domains, i.e., surface-associated antigens (Fig. 3-12). Immunoglobulin developed against a surface determinant after immobilization on particulate or colloidal delivery systems could be targeted to the cells bearing Fc receptors via its Fc region or to the target antigen on the cell surface via its Fab′ region followed by internalization and release of the encapsulated bioactives (Fig. 3-12). Immunoglobulin fragments Fab′ and F(ab′)$_2$ or chimeric IgG developed against surface antigens or antigenic determinants are well negotiable strategies for Fc receptor mediated drug/gene therapy.

Recent developments in liposome technology make it possible to explore therapeutic applications involving site specific delivery using Mabs or antibody fragments like Fab′ or F(ab)$_2$ (Fig. 3-13). Anti-target monoclonal antibody anchored on liposomes (immunoliposomes) with specific avidity directed to carbohydrate containing antigens have been investigated to deliver the drugs like Idoxyuridine and Acyclovir in the treatment of Herpes Simplex Virus (HSV) infected cell lines (Norley et al., 1986)

A well-engineered immunoliposome has been ameliorated by coating the surface of large oligo-lamellar vesicles of egg PC with the polysaccharide pullulan as a targeting ligand (Sunamoto et al., 1987). The liposomes carry both cholesterol as the hydrophobic anchor and the monoclonal antibodies fragment (anti-sialosyl Lewis x : IgMs) as a site directing sensory device. The system showed better *in vivo* targetability and specific binding when tested with a range of tumour cell lines.

Antibody-associated liposomes containing anti-sense oligomer provide dual specificity : the antibody mediated selection of the particular cell lines along with the selectivity of the chosen mRNA sequence which is complementary to the liposome delivered oligomer (Leonetti et al., 1990). Khaw and co-

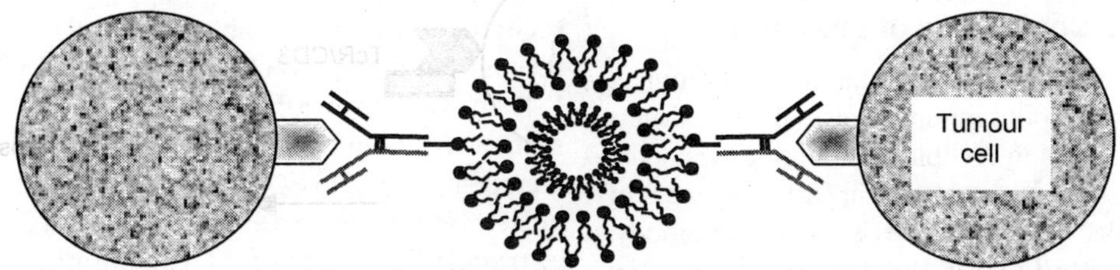

Fig. 3-12 Immunoliposomes are the Conjugates of Liposomes and Antibodies and Specifically Bind to the Antigens (Against Which Antibodies are Developed) Expressed by Target (Mainly Tumour Cells)

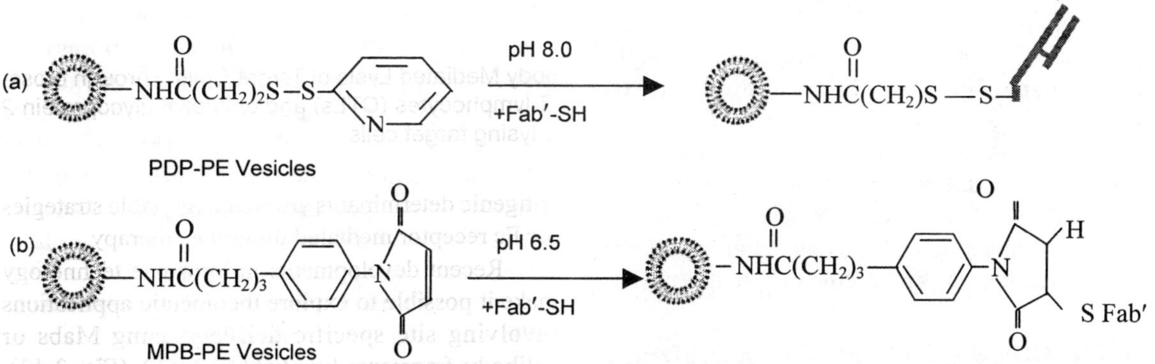

(a) $-NHC(O)(CH_2)_2S-S-$(2-pyridyl) —pH 8.0, +Fab′-SH→ $-NHC(O)(CH_2)S-S-$Fab′

PDP-PE Vesicles

(b) $-NHC(O)(CH_2)_3-$(p-phenyl)$-N$(maleimide) —pH 6.5, +Fab′-SH→ $-NHC(O)(CH_2)_3-$(p-phenyl)$-N$(succinimide, H, S Fab′)

MPB-PE Vesicles

Fig. 3-13. Immunoliposomes with Fab′ Fragments as Targeting Ligands. (a) Fab′ Fragments with Free Sulphydryl Groups React with Liposomes Containing 3-(2-pyridyldithio) Propionate-PE (PDP-PE) or (b) with Liposomes containing 4-(p-maleimidophenyl) butyrate-PE (MPB-PE)

workers, 1995 have also designed and discussed a novel adjunctive approach to seal the membrane lesions associated with acute myocardial infarction, using antimyosin Mab directed immunoliposomes. In this strategy, an antigen on intracellular cytoskeletal myosin in hypoxic embryonic cardiocytes, was used as an anchoring site, and a specific antibody on immunoliposomes was anchored as a sensing ligand to *'plug and seal'* the membrane lesions. The study indicated that selective cell membrane sealing can prevent cell death in hypoxic cardiocytes, and this concept holds exploitable promises in different immunological consequences.

Stealth Immunoliposomes

Recent developments related to sterically stabilized liposomes (SSL), renewed interest in systemic application of immunoliposomes due to their low RES uptake (reverse targetability) and long circulation half-life. This is due to their hydrophilic, opsonin repelling and sterically stabilized surface. The categories of these systems include liposomes that incorporate GM1 gangliosides or that coated with PEG polymers (protein PEGylation), i.e., hydrophilic polymer grafted immunoliposomes, or hydrophilic polymer grafted microparticulates. The development of new technologies for an efficient attachment of Mab at the surface of PEG containing liposomes permits the resulting sterically stabilized immunoliposomes not only to exhibit greater recognition and target binding characteristics but also allows them to remain in circulation for a longer time relative to classical immunoliposomes. SSL mediated targeting of anticancer drug, doxorubicin, has been reported in the treatment of murine solid tumours, human solid tumour xenografts and human haematological cancers (Allen, 1994; Lasic, 1994; Lasic, 1996). The surface immobilized Mabs directed to tumour associated antigens for immunospecific binding produce better therapeutic effect (Emanuel et al., 1996).

Haptenated Conjugates of Liposomes

The haptenated liposomes are based on biological target sensor and pilot module. Vesicular constructs were developed using PE lipids, containing the hapten linked to the liposome surface via carbon spacers of various lengths, in the presence of a specific antibody. It can be exploited for the fixation of hapten conjugates to target cells that express surface immunoglobulin with specific affinity for the hapten (Kinsky, 1972; Lewis et al., 1980). Avrilionis and Boggs, 1996 reported specific targeting of phototoxic haptenated liposomes to a hapten specific B lymphoma cell lines. The photosensitizer coupled to a phospholipid was incorporated into tri-nitrophenol (TNP) bearing lipid vesicles to target the photosensitizer to B-lymphoma IgM receptors (Fig. 3-14). These workers demonstrated the potential of antigen (hapten) anchored liposomal system for the purpose of targeting and selective elimination of B cells expressing antigen-specific surface Ig receptors.

ANTIBODIES CONJUGATES DEVELOPED AGAINST ANGIOGENIC PEPTIDES

Tumour endothelial cells are suitable targets for targeted drug delivery and immunotherapy as they are accessible through the blood. The epitopes present on the tumour endothelial vasculature in the form of angiogenic peptides and adhesion molecules that interplay between cells, soluble factors and extracellular matrix components could be exploited to negotiate targeting. At least 20 angiogenic peptides have been found on tumour vasculature that influence the endothelial cells directly (e.g., EGF and VEGF) or indirectly by inducing host cells to produce endothelial cell growth factors e.g., TNF and TGF (Table 3-4). Attempt has been made to target tumour cell lines using anti-epidermal growth factor (EGF) receptor antibodies. Fab′ fragment of anti-EGF receptor antibody (B4G7) is conjugated with poly-L-lysine to form an affinity complex with DNA. The system was found excellent for targeted delivery of therapeutic genes to EGF-receptor expressing tumour cells. Novel antibodies directed against the extracellular domain of the human vascular endothelial growth factor receptor (VEGFr) type II have shown specificity as reflected by immunohistochemistry and ELISA techniques. Antisense to mRNA for vascular endothelial growth factor receptor (VEGFr) has shown to block expression of VEGFr and thereby suppress the transforming phenotype of human carcinoma cell lines, KB cells (Molema et al., 1997). However, the uptake of folate conjugated liposomes bearing VEGFr antisense oligonucleotides (ODNs) has been reported to be nine times than the uptake of plain liposomes and 16 times higher than soluble or non-encapsulated ODNs. Recently, the over-expression of EGF receptors has been exploited to direct the radiolabeled EGF as a ligand and peptide radiopharmaceutical for imaging human brain tumours. This EGF peptide was made transportable through the blood brain barrier (BBB) by conjugating it with BBB drug delivery vectors such as the OX-26 monoclonal antibody, which undergoes receptor-mediated transcytosis through the BBB via the brain capillary transferrin receptors (Huwyler et al., 1996). Two different strategies including the one based on avidin-biotin complex and the other using extended poly(ethylene glycol) were adopted for making bifunctional conjugates, and both the strategies were able to retain the bifunctionality of the conjugate for binding to both EGF and transferrin receptors. In a further development, the same group of workers developed a vector mediated brain delivery system based on radiolabeled EGF (Penichet et al., 1999). Similar

Table 3-4. A Review of Studies Carried Out Using Vasoactive and Angiogenic Peptides Conjugates

Target cell/ site	Delivery system	Receptor
Tumour cells	Anti-EGF receptor antibody (B4G7) conjugated to poly(L-lysine)	EGFr
Human brain cancer	Radiolabeled EGF-Ox 26 MoAb conjugate	Transferrin receptor
Blood brain barrier	Radiolabeled NGF-Ox 26 MoAb conjugate	Transferrin receptor
Tumour cell line	EGF peptides and anti-receptor antibody	EGFr
Tumour cells	TNF-interferon conjugates	TNfr

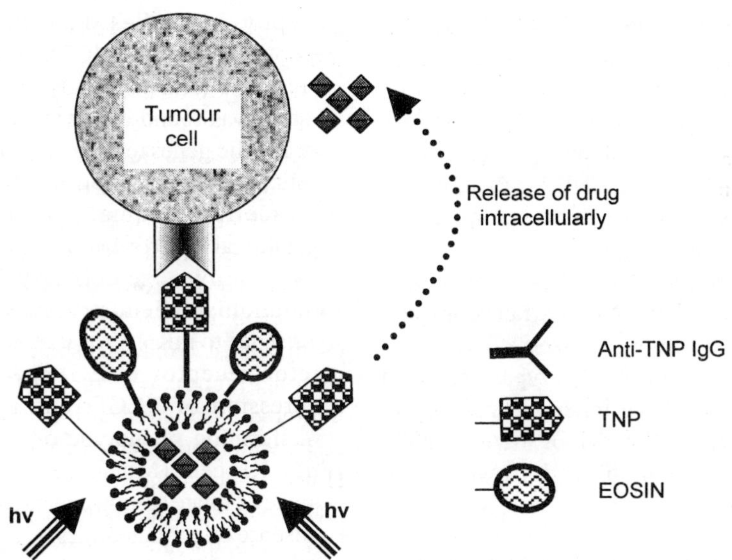

Fig. 3-14. Haptenated (TNP)-liposomes with Phototoxic Eosin Released upon Irradiation Following Specific Interaction of TNP with Anti-TNP IgG of the Target Cell

studies were performed for nerve growth factor delivery across the BBB using vector mediated process (OX-26 Mab). It is known that the EGF receptors and their ligands participate in triggering a number of biological responses in the tumour cells including EGF receptor phosphorylation and stimulation of DNA synthesis leading to cell proliferation. An attempt was made to construct EGF peptides and anti-EGF receptor antibodies and their fragments that specifically bind to over-expressed EGF receptors in different tumour models. The authors suggested that these EGF ligands can be used for immunotherapy and after labeling with an appropriate radionucleotide, also for radioimmunotherapy (Molema et al., 1997). The Fab′-immunogen is a novel gene transfer vehicle in which the Fab′ fragment of antihuman epidermal growth receptor antibody B4G7 is conjugated with poly-L-lysine to form an affinity complex with DNA. It was suggested that these antibodies in the soluble conjugated or as carrier immobilized forms could be developed to target the therapeutic genes into EGF-receptor expressing tumour cells.

Rosenberg and associates, 1987 targeted a liposome sandwich system to the cultured rat pheochromocytoma and human melanoma cells expressing nerve growth factor receptors (NGFr). In their study, the cells were incubated with biotinylated NGF and they were subsequently treated with streptividin-coupled liposomes. Tumour necrosis factor exhibits cytotoxic and cytostatic activity on a wide range of animal and human transformed cell lines. A series of studies was conducted to demonstrate that instead of using therapeutic activity of an individual cytokine, a synergistic activity of different cytokines in combination could enhance the immunotherapeutic and immunomodulatory activities of each component. These combinations include TNF and interferon (IFN-α, IFN-β and IFN-γ) (Depraetere and Joniau, 1995). The basic principle of targeting of TNF and similar vasoactive peptides to the tumour site is based on the anatomical feature of the tumour tissue where hyper-permeability of the vasculature and immature lymph systems offers optimally large-sized substances to be accumulated and retained at tumour site preferentially. Endoglin, an essential component of the tumour growth factor receptor (TGFr) complex of human endothelial cells was put forward as a proliferating marker that is up-regulated on endothelial cells in miscellaneous human solid tumours (Burrow et al., 1995). Recently, Tabata and co-workers, 1999 reported targeting of TNF through conjugation with dextran having metal chelating, diethylene-triaminepentaacetic acid (DTPA) residues co-ordinated and complexed with metal (Cu^{2+}). Intravenous injection of the TNF-DTPA-Dextran conjugate to tumour bearing mice revealed that tumour growth is greatly suppressed in comparison to free TNF injection, probably due to preferable tumour accumulation of the TNF-dextran conjugate. This conjugation technology based on Cu^{2+} co-ordination could be applied to other types of growth factors as well, if they have inherent tendency to chelate metal ions as earlier demonstrated for the amylopectin hydrogel immobilized growth factor (Tabata et al., 1998).

BIOCONJUGATES OF IMMUNOTOXINS/ CHIMERIC PROTEINS

Toxins are molecules that inactivate viral cytosolic components of the protein synthesis machinery in a catalytic manner. A major requirement of the toxins, therefore is to reach the cytosol of the target cells. Immunotoxins (ITs) are conjugates of antibodies (Mab) or Fab′ fragments and toxins (ricin) in which the cell binding moieties of the toxins are replaced by the binding specific chain of Ab (Fig. 3-15). Once endowed with specificity, toxin molecules inactivate vital cytosolic components of the protein synthesis machinery of viral infections in a specific and catalytic manner. The $F(ab)_2$ handled immunotoxins may be anchored to the surface of carrier systems, which provide better projection to them and effectively present and place them to recognition sites, leading to receptor mediated endocytosis and eventually killing of cells which express Fc receptors.

For the targeting of HIV infections, immunotoxins directed to specific viral antigens or aimed at the highly conserved CD4 receptors on T-lymphocytes and several other cell types have been developed (Zarling et al., 1990; Annemiek et al., 1999). Immunotoxin constructs of ricin A toxin or *Pseudomonas* endotoxin and Mab against gp 120 (Kim et al., 1990; Matsushita et al., 1990) or against fusion glycoprotein gp41 (Pincus et al., 1989) inhibited production of infectious virus in infected cells while non-infected cells remained unaffected. However, due to the heterogeneity of gp120 in various HIV isolates and an additional antiviral effect of anti-gp41 Mab, the latter are preferred in designing anti-gp41 based targeting devices. Anti-gp41-dgA (dgA=deglycosylated ricin A-chain) conjugates were shown to have selective targetability towards HIV-infected H9 and U937 cells (Pincus et al., 1989). The reason for this marked cytotoxic potency may be the proximity of the target epitope relative to the plasma membrane. This may facilitate internalization of dgA and routing of dgA to intracellular compartments that are instrumental in translocation of the A-chain into the cytosol. In a significant development, Pincus and McClure, 1993 have explored that the therapeutic efficacy of anti-receptor immunotoxins may be further enhanced by the coadministration of the free receptor ligand (CD4) in the soluble form. This may be due to the increased expression of gp41 on the cell surface of infected cells or altered internalization/

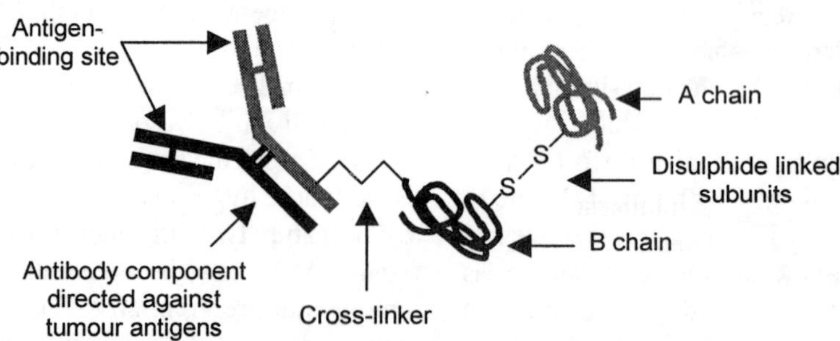

Fig. 3-15. The Design of an Immunotoxin Conjugate that Consists of an Antibody-targeting Component Cross-linked to a Toxin Molecule. The complexation typically includes a disulphide bond between the antibody portion and the cytotoxic component of the conjugate to allow the release of the toxin intracellularly

intracellular routing of the enveloped protein. On the contrary, novel conjugates of recombinant CD4 (rCD4) molecules and toxins are developed with the same degree of specificity and affinity as inhered by their antibody counterparts (immunotoxins). rCD4 has been exploited for its high affinity for the HIV envelope gp120. Although gp120 shows a distinct variability among different HIV strains, yet its CD4 binding site is highly conserved. Therefore, rCD4 may exhibit an exquisite affinity for gp120 comparable to cellular CD4 and could potentially deliver the coupled antiviral drugs to HIV-infected cells (Till et al., 1988). It is interesting to note that gp120 expression is required for rCD4-toxin conjugates to bind specifically to HIV-infected cells, and this is the reason that non-infected cells expressing MHC class-II antigens (natural ligand for CD4) remain unaffected.

Liposomes equipped with immunotoxins were prepared for the treatment of various tumours and the concept is documented for antiviral therapy (Vitteta, 1990). Diphtheria toxin (DPT) is a potent cytotoxic, however its selective and effective delivery has been an illusive goal. Liposomes could entrap and skip diphtheria toxin to deter them from immunoglobulin pool and eventually present them to the site of action. DPT inactivates vital cytosolic components of the protein synthesis machinery and can be effectively used in selective killing of target cell lines (Fig. 3-16). However, due to DPT anti-Mab pool (generated through immunization) diphtheria toxins are sequestered and thus obstructed for their access to the cytosol of the target cell lines (Nassander et al., 1992). The immobilization of liposomal DPT could deter them from anti-DPT-Mab and present them safely to the tumour cell lines. Thus, such engineered Diphtheriosomes may be a potential future strategy in 'pick and hit therapy'.

CD4 Bioconjugates

The CD4 molecule is a target molecule for human immunodeficiency virus (HIV) gp120 and oligo-saccharide side chains in gp120 (Singh et al., 2000). CD4 could also serve as a target molecule for, neoglycoproteins (mannose terminating) or recombinant gp120 (*r*gp120) conjugated with antiviral drugs. Though gp120 and gp 41 are not endogenous compounds, they are regularly expressed/ shedded from HIV-I infections. MHC-II^{+ve} T-lymphocytes are capable of internalizing, processing and presenting these antigenic ligands. Two regions of CD4 have been described as possible sites for the interaction of the HIV envelope protein gp120 with its cellular receptor. These include the use of liposomes, immunotoxins and glyco-conjugates (Fig. 3-16). Some of these blood cell-specific carrier-

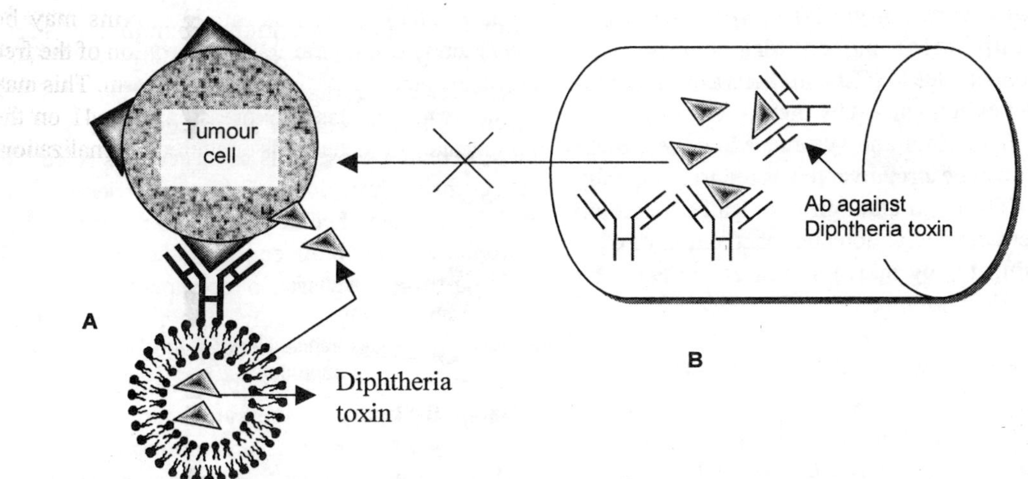

Fig. 3-16. Immobilization of DTA in Immunoliposome Presents them Safely to the Tumour Cell Lines to Affect Cytosolic Delivery (A). On the other hand, Diphtheria toxin antibody pool encountered *in vivo* sequesters diphtheria toxin A (DTA) *en route* to cytosol of target cell (B).

conjugates developed and studied for tumour/viral tropic cells targeting are discussed later in this chapter.

Recombinant CD4 Toxin Conjugates

In the search of more effective antiviral agents, a plethora of studies has been conducted, which report the use of recombinant CD4 (rCD4) as a promising carrier for toxins. It is assumed that rCD4 possesses the same degree of cell specificity as cell specific antibodies. rCD4 is used due to its high affinity for HIV envelope gp 120. Various strategies for the targeting of viral surface determinants (gp 120 and others) with bioconjugated CD4 have been described following the conclusion that viral gp 120 and other molecular targets serve as ligands for the CD4 molecules (Vyas and Sihorkar, 2000) (Fig. 3-17). Therefore, rCD4 may exhibit the same high affinity to gp 120 as cellular CD4 and therefore could preferentially target the conjugated antiviral drugs to HIV-infected cells.

Pronounced antiviral activity of a conjugate of rCD4 with deglycosylated ricin A-chain has been reported in an HIV-infected human T-cell line. Non-infected cells expressing MHC class-II antigens (the natural ligand for CD4) however, remained unaffected. A recombinant protein, containing the HIV-binding portion of the human CD4 molecule was linked to the active regions of Pseudomonas exotoxin A (PE-A) and displayed selective toxicity towards infected cells expressing gp 120. Nevertheless, CD4-toxin conjugates suffer drawbacks like immunogenicity due to rCD4 products as well as bio-detrimental effects caused by their interactions with elements of the immune system. Moreover, these limitations can be circumvented as reported recently by using CD4 toxin-albumin conjugates. Albumin may prevent the interaction and inactivation of CD4 toxin conjugates by native serum components by offering steric hindrance.

Liposome Conjugated CD4 Fragments

Liposomes have been used to conjugate CD4 or other peptidic segments for delivery of contained bioactives to HIV-infected cells. A peptide from CDR3 region was coupled to dimyristoyl-phosphatidylcholine/phosphatidylcholine/cholesterol liposomes. The system demonstrated enhanced cytotoxic effect specifically against HIV-infected cells *in vitro* (Kumagai et al., 1992). Specific binding of liposomes to HIV-1 infected cells was achieved by either reconstituting transmembrane CD3 receptor in the liposomal membrane (Cudd et al., 1990) or by covalently coupling recombinant soluble CD4 to the liposomal surface (Flasher et al., 1994).

Slepushkin and co-workers, 1996 investigated the potential of synthetic peptides for their use as ligands for targeting liposomes to HIV infections. A synthetic peptide from the complementary determining region 2 (CDR-2)-like domain of CD4 could bind specifically to HIV-infected cells and mediate the binding of peptide-coupled liposomes to these cells. A peptide from the CDR3-like domain of CD4 inhibited HIV-induced syncytia formation, but failed to target liposomes to infected cells This apparent discrepancy may be due to the requirement for a conformational change in the CD4 receptor for the CDR3 region to interact with the HIV-enveloped protein. These results suggest for the feasibility of targeting of liposomes or similar drug carriers containing anti-viral agents to HIV-infected cells. The same degree of specificity and affinity as of antibodies are shown by recombinant CD4 molecules and has been estimated for toxins based carriers (recombinant CD4 toxin conjugates).

TRANSFERRIN BASED BIOCONJUGATES

Transferrin (Tf) is a major mammalian serum glycoprotein, transporting iron from sites of absorption and storage to tissue cells. Tf cell surface receptors are present on all the growing cells and thereby render these cells as target sites selectively approachable through transferrins as carrier molecule. A diverse range of cell types including hepatocytes, fibroblasts, blood brain endothelial cell lines and T4 cells express the transferrin receptors (TfR). TfR are present on actively dividing cell types implicating a role in growth and differentiation of a variety of cells. Transferrin may be widely applied either as a carrier or targeting ligand in the active targeting of anti-cancer agents, proteins and genes to primarily proliferating malignant cells that over-express transferrin receptors (TfR).

Transferrin has been utilized as an endogenous cellular transport system for the delivery of

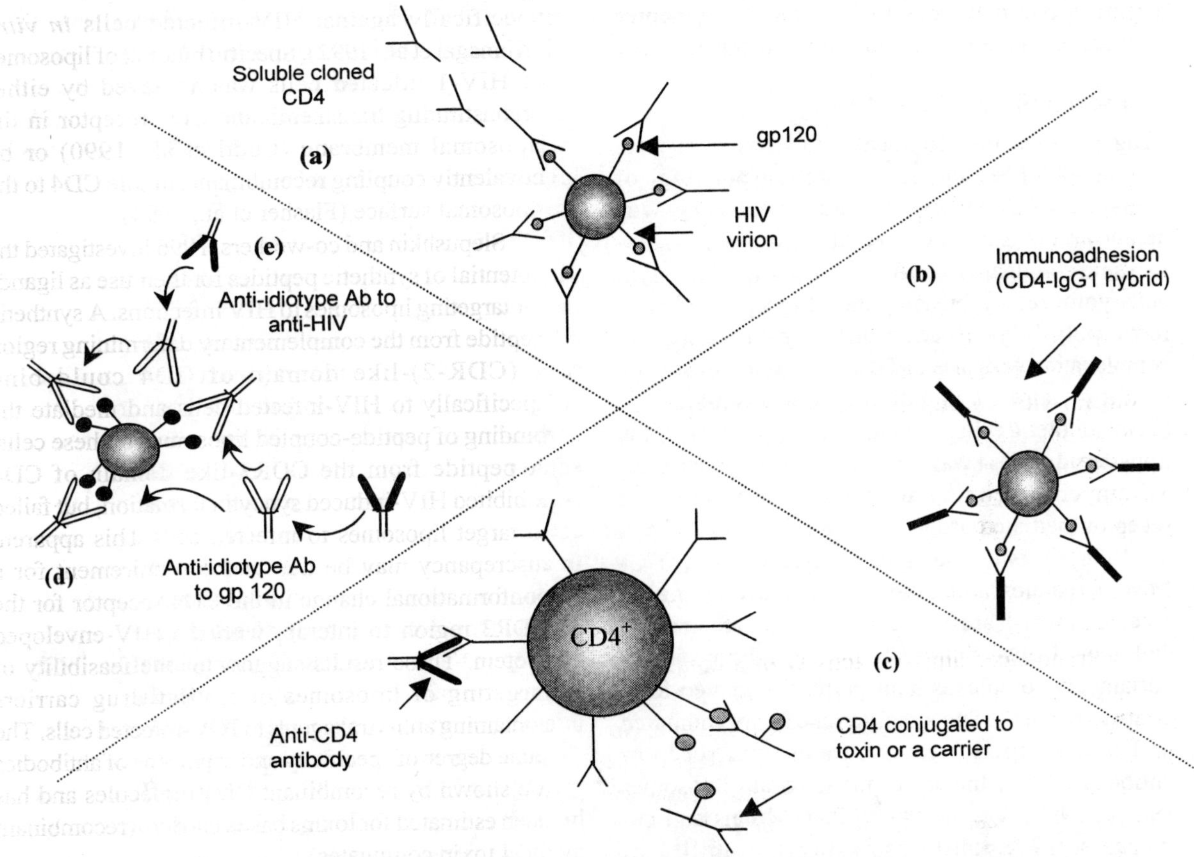

Fig. 3-17. Possible Mechanisms by which Soluble, Recombinant or Bioconjugated gp120 may Induce Depletion of Uninfected CD4 Positive T Cells. (a) Soluble cloned CD4 binds to gp120 on HIV virions. (b) CD4 and IgG1 hybrid (immunoadhesion) binds to gp120 on HIV Virions. (c) CD4-toxin conjugate binds to gp120 on HIV-infected cells. (d, and e) Both anti-CD4 antibody (d) and anti-idiotype antibody (e) Specific for paratope on anti-HIV antibody can induce production of Ab that bind to gp120 without exposing individual to HIV components

therapeutics across the blood-brain barrier (Wagner et al., 1994). The studies indicate the presence of definite transcytosis pathway for transporting iron across brain capillary endothelial cells (BBB) via transferrin receptor. In contrast to brain, capillary endothelial cells of non-brain tissues have very low-levels of transferrin receptors, presumably because the endothelium in these tissues is sufficiently leaky and allow transferrin to passively enter the extracellular fluid. This heterogenous distribution of transferrin receptor makes it an endogenous ligand for the site-specific delivery to brain. However, the successful results obtained with *in vitro* and *in vivo* evaluation of this system are limited. This is probably due to competition of the administered system with endogenous transferrin, or due to the ubiquitous distribution of transferrin receptor and frequently encountered *en route* anatomical barriers. In some of the reviews, the possibilities of expression of TfR on proliferating cells and intracellular delivery of antivirally active drugs/antisense oligomers have been documented (Wagner et al., 1994; Singh, 1999). Transferrin has been exploited as an endogenous carrier/ligand either in the form of drug conjugates, hybrid systems with macromolecules and as liposomal coated systems. Nevertheless, active targeting could be achieved using anti-receptor antibody directed against transferrin receptor.

Transferrin-Drug Conjugates

Drug or polycation conjugates of transferrin were evaluated for endogenous targeting potential of transferrin. A successful gene delivery was demonstrated using a carbohydrate linked Tf-poly-L-lysine conjugate for efficient gene introduction in eukaryotic cells expressing the Tf receptors. Transferrin-poly-L-lysine and transferrin-protamine on complexation with plasma DNA demonstrate efficient binding and subsequent endocytosis by haematopoietic cells, leading to the expression of the transferred genes (Wagner et al., 1992). Transferrin-Mitomycin C conjugates were investigated for receptor mediated drug-targeting system (Tanaka et al., 1996). This tumour specific drug carrier (Tf-G-MMC) reaches and binds specifically to the Tf receptors, which are over-expressed on Sarcoma 180 cell lines. Transferrin-methotrexate and transferrin-adriamycin complexes both in the conjugated form or anchored to the liposomal surfaces were compared and found superior to anti-transferrin receptor antibody (7D-3) linked to methotrexate liposomes (Singh, 1999). On the other hand, Munns and co-workers, 1998 while assessing the ability of transferrin-adriamycin complex for targeting of TfR-positive cancer cells, reported that Tf-ADR conjugates failed as cytotoxic delivery system as it neither prevented toxicity to the Tf-R negative cells nor could overcome the resistance of the adriamycin-resistant cells. Park and co-workers, 1998 recently characterized a novel fusion protein (ligand) containing transferrin and nerve growth factor (NGF). The workers demonstrated the ability of the novel conjugates to maintain both biologically active nerve growth factor and transferrin as part of the fusion protein. The conjugate offers enormous opportunities for the targeting of NGF or neurotrophic factors to the central nervous system. In a recent study, Uike and associates, 1998 reported the hybrids of transferrin with poly-L-lysine (PL) and cross-linked them to a DNA-binding protein as gene delivery vehicle, which operate through Tf receptors. Tf-PL hybrids were prepared using different cross-links, i.e., Tf-ss-PL (cross-linked by a cleavable disulphide bonds) and Tf-Schiff-PL (cross-linked by cleavable Schiff's base). The binding affinity of hybrids to HeLa cells was not different, however, expression of reporter gene (for luciferase) bound to these hybrids in HeLA cells transfected with Tf-Schiff-PL was greater than that of Tf-ss-PL.

Transferrin-Liposome Conjugates

Transferrin-liposome conjugates have been investigated for the delivery of drugs. The conjugation was carried out using hetero-bifunctional reagent SPDP with sulphydryl activated liposomes (Fig. 3-18). Stavridis and co-workers, 1986 demonstrated that transferrin-appended liposomes could be exploited to transport exogenous DNA to bone marrow erythrocytes in anaemic rabbits, as these cells express transferrin receptors on their surface. In an interesting study, Hege and co-workers, 1989 reported a comparison of liposome immobilized Anti-Tac (a monoclonal antibody directed against the IL-2 receptor) and Anti-TfR (a monoclonal antibody against transferrin receptor) for specific binding, internalization and intracellular drug delivery to adult T-cell leukaemia. The workers reported the better growth inhibition profile of Anti-TfR coupled liposomes over Anti-Tac coupled liposomes bearing methotrexate-γ-aspartate, a liposome-loaded cytotoxic drug. Sarti and co-workers, 1996 developed a liposomal carrier system that interacts specifically with HL60 leukaemia cell lines. The small unilamellar vesicles made up of pure phospholipid were chemically cross-linked to human transferrin. The modified liposomes interacted specifically with the cells and were subsequently internalized by active-receptor-mediated endocytosis, as demonstrated by the full inhibition of internalization by circulatory free ligand. Egea and co-workers, 1994 incorporated hydrophobic derivative of transferrin (with ceramide) into liposomes of various phospholipids, cholesterol and ceramide compositions and compared the efficiency of protein association with native transferrin. The surface activity of both native and hydrophobized transferrin was determined with monomolecular layers as a membrane model. The results suggested that endogenous proteins must be hydrophobically derivatized to attain efficient level of incorporation into the surface of liposomes. Ishida

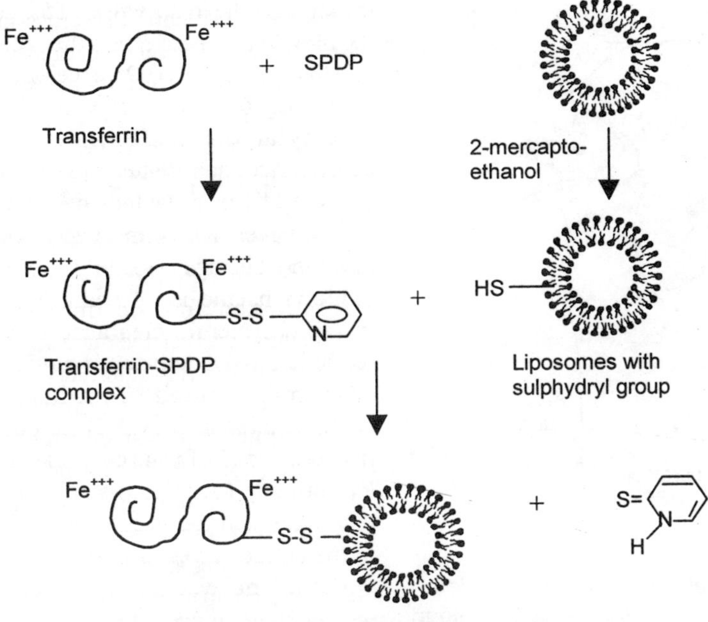

Fig. 3-18. Transferrin-liposome Conjugate Prepared Using Amine Reactive and Sulphydryl Reactive Hetero-bifunctional Cross-linker, SPDP

and Maruyama, 1998 reported transferrin conjugated to the PEG-grafted liposomes at the distal ends of PEG chains. The biodistribution and intracellular uptake studies revealed the localization of the Tf-PEG liposomes at the tumour cell surface, coated pits and endosomes. The results suggested endocytic pathway as internalization route of Tf-PEG liposomes, which retain specificity in tumour. Liposomes appended with anti-transferrin receptor antibody (a bioligand) were more efficiently internalized by a number of human T-cell leukaemic cell lines than liposomes carrying antibodies against surface antigens of these cells.

Anti-transferrin Antibody Conjugates

Active targeting to the brain has also been attempted using a monoclonal antibody directed to the transferrin receptor, since the brain micro-vessel endothelial cells express this receptor in abundance (Yoshikawa and Pardridge, 1992). The monoclonal antibody has been designated as anti-transferrin receptor antibody (OX-26) that binds to an extracellular projecting epitope of the receptor and undergoes receptor-mediated transcytosis (Fig. 3-19). Such antibodies have been used as a carrier for drugs, peptides, oligonucleotides, and peptide nucleic acids (Singh, 1999). The usefulness of this carrier has been realized in terms of absolute activity in penetrating the blood brain barrier as well as modified pharmacokinetics at systemic level.

In a further development, Huwyler and co-workers, 1996 anchored anti-transferrin antibody to the liposomal systems (immunoliposomes) for the delivery of anti-neoplastic drug daunomycin to the rat brain. Optimal brain targeting was achieved mediated through the OX26 monoclonal antibody to the rat transferrin receptor. The latter is selectively expressed in excess at the brain microvascular endothelium that mainly comprises the blood-brain barrier *in vivo*. Several attempts have been made to simplify the coupling of therapeutics to anti-transferrin receptor antibody (OX-26) by using avidin/streptividin-biotin systems (Watanabe et al., 1998; Penichet et al., 1999; Li et al., 1999) (Fig. 3-20). These workers have established the biotin binding capacity of the avidin coupled OX-26 and determined

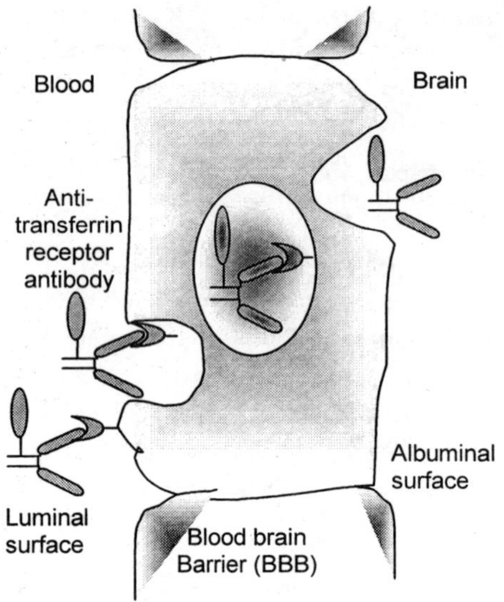

Fig. 3-19 Receptor Mediated Entry of Anti-transferrin Receptor Antibody Conjugates Across the Blood Brain Barrier (BBB). The antibody conjugate binds to transferrin receptors present on the luminal membrane of brain capillary endothelial cells. After RME, the antibody conjugates are eventually transported to and released from the abluminal surface of the capillary endothelial cells and, once released into the brain, diffuse and target the parenchymal cells

the rates for the transcytosis of the conjugates through the blood brain barrier. On the same lines, Watanabe and his colleagues, 1998 developed a simple method to conjugate biotinylated double strand DNA to biotinylated transferrin via streptividin and demonstrated successful transduction of the conjugate into the TfR-positive human cancer cells.

However, Kang and his associates, 1994 have discovered using co-loading or pre-loading of avidin or biotin that the use of avidin-based vectors resulted in rapid systemic clearance causing quantitative reduction in the delivery of biotin to brain, despite a comparable blood brain barrier permeability coefficient for avidin-OX 26 conjugates (OX-26-Av). In a recent study, Li and co-workers, 1999 synthesized Fv antibody (of OX26)-streptavidin fusion protein that facilitated the attachment of biotinylated drugs to the antibody vector (single chain Fv analogue of OX26). The workers revealed the potential of genetically engineered single chain Fv antibody (of OX26)-streptividin fusion proteins for non-invasive neuro-therapeutic delivery to the brain using endogenous transport system (Tf receptor).

Penichet et al., 1999 have constructed a novel Ab-avidin fusion protein (Ab genetically fused to avidin) to deliver biotinylated compounds across the blood brain barrier. This Ab-avidin fusion protein (anti-TfR-

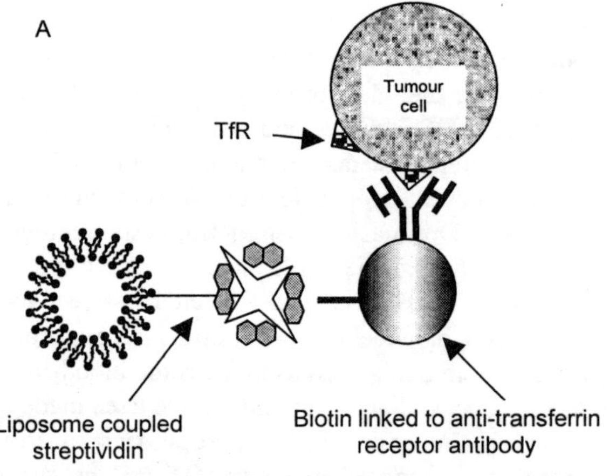

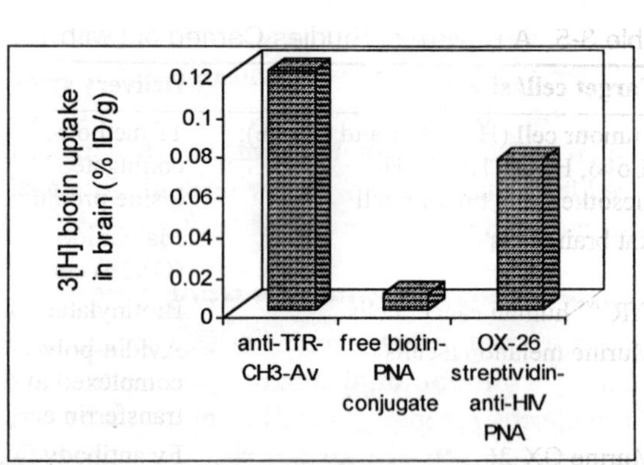

Fig. 3-20. Biotin-Avidin/Streptavidin Conjugated Carriers, Where Avidin/Streptavidin Links Delivery Systems and Biotinylated Targeting Ligand (A). Brain Targeting Achieved using Transferrin Ab-Streptividin-Fusion Protein as Compared Against Anti-Transferrin Receptor Antibody (B).

C_H3-Av) was different from OX-26-SA conjugate (Ab chemically conjugated to streptividin) and in animal models showed much longer half life than the chemical conjugate between OX26 and streptividin. Most importantly, this fusion protein demonstrated superior [^{3}H] biotin uptake into brain parenchyma as compared to the chemical conjugate. The fusion protein demonstrated a 15-fold increase (0.12% ID/g) compared to free biotin-PNA conjugate (0.0083% ID/g) and nearly 1.6 fold increase compared to OX-26 streptividin-anti-HIV PNA conjugate (0.075% ID/g). However, a marginal decrease in brain uptake was observed when the biotin-PNA was used in place of biotin for the conjugation with fusion protein. This reflects the poor intrinsic intracellular permeability of the PNA moiety in the complex. Even though the results indicate variations in carrier potential of novel anti-transferrin receptor antibody fusion proteins and conjugates, these serve as a universal vehicle to specifically deliver and target biotinylated compounds across the blood brain barrier. Receptor targeted lipid formulations appended with transferrin as a targeting ligand find their applications in gene therapy of haematopoietic/cancer cells (Table 3-5).

FOLIC ACID (FOLATE) BASED BIOCONJUGATES

The vitamin folic acid (FA) enters cells through a carrier protein, termed as the reduced folate carrier, or via receptor-mediated endocytosis facilitated by the folate receptor (FR). Since folate-drug conjugates can not serve as substrates of the former, they penetrate cells exclusively via FR-mediated endocytosis (Reddy and Low, 1998). The receptor for folate, also known as the folate-binding protein, is a glycosyl-phosphatidylinositol (GPI)-anchored membrane protein with an average molecular weight of 38 kDa. It mediates the cellular uptake of folate and the related coenzymes via receptor-mediated endocytosis occurring at non-coated membrane regions termed as caveolae (Rothberg et al., 1990). Ligand binding to folate receptors stimulates their endocytic uptake by a clathrin-independent pathway (potocytosis) that has been exploited to negotiate a non-specific uptake of macromolecules and particulate drug delivery systems (Anderson, 1993). In the potocytosis model of folate internalization, folate is proposed to bind receptor clustered around caveolae, i.e. specialized regions of the cell membrane enriched in cholesterol and other GPI anchored proteins. These caveolae then invaginate, forming a membrane-linked or cabled compartment within the cytoplasm. An integral proton gradient is then proposed to facilitate the release of the bound folate, allowing its movements across the caveolae membrane by an integral membrane anion carrier (Lisanti et al., 1994). In contrast, some reports suggest that FR exhibits no accumulation tendency in caveolae unless they are cross-linked with bivalent antibodies and also suggested the main involvement

Table 3-5. A Review of Studies Carried out with Transferrin Bioconjugates

Target cell/ site	Delivery system	Activity (investigated)
Tumour cell (Hela, KB and colone); (Lovo, HL60, Hep2); H-mesothelioma tumour cell	Tf-methotrexate, Tf-adriamycin conjugate; Tf-polycation (poly-L-lysine/protamine) conjugate	Receptor mediated targeting to tumour cells
Rat brain cells	Maleimide grafted and MoAb (OX26) conjugated liposomes	Selective brain targeting
TfR^{+ive} human cancer cells	Biotinylated Tf-DNA conjugate	Gene delivery to human cancer cells
Murine melanoma cells	Avidin-poly-L-lysine conjugate complexed to biotinylated transferrin and DNA	Anti-HIV antisense delivery to brain
Murine OX-26	Fv antibody (Murine OX-26) streptividin fusion protein	Receptor mediated tumour targeting
Bladder cancer cell line (MGH-U1)	Tf-adriamycin conjugate	Receptor mediated targeting to bladder cancer cell lines

Reproduced from Vyas and Sihorkar, 2000

of coated pits rather than caveolae (Wu et al., 1997a, b). Three receptor subtypes, α, β and γ, have been identified in humans. The γ-subtype is a rarely expressed form, whereas the most common subtypes, α and β are membrane bound and have a high affinity for folic acid (Ross et al., 1994). Folic acid retains its receptor-binding activity even after conjugation to a macromolecule via its γ-carboxyl group. Therefore, folate derivatization can equivocally be used to deliver foreign molecules into folate-receptor bearing cells.

Conjugates to FA linked to virtually any molecule or molecular complex of diameter <150 nm bind to the receptor possessing high binding affinity and enter the cell via receptor-mediated potocytosis. Since the same FA conjugates could not bind to FR negative cells even though they express the reduced folate carrier, the FA conjugates display significant selectivity for tumour cell *in vivo*. Reddy and Low, 1998 have revised and summarized the role of folate receptor-mediated tumour targeting approaches for the delivery of protein complex, low-molecular weight chemotherapeutic agents, radioimaging agents, MRI contrast agents, genes, antisense oligonucleotides, ribozymes and immunotherapeutic agents.Proteins, drugs and imaging agents were effectively delivered to the folate receptor bearing cells by derivatization of endogenous folate with the therapeutic active modules. Liposomes conjugated to FA were also tested for targeting to neoplastic diseases (Table 3-6). Unfortunately, poly(ethylene glycol) when used as a coating, interfered with receptor recognition when the folate was directly linked to a PEG-linked phospholipid head group. To circumvent this problem, FA was attached to the distal ends of a few lipid conjugated PEG-molecules, allowing the targeting ligand for better exposition and to reach the receptor sites far from the liposomal surface (Gabizon et al., 1999). Folate has been coupled to distearoyl-phosphatidylethanolamine (DSPE) using a PEG2000 linker (folate-PEG2000-DSPE) to deliver liposome encapsulated doxorubicin to epithelial cancer cells. A 45-fold higher uptake of encapsulated doxorubicin has been recorded over that observed for non-targeted vesicles (Lee and Low, 1994; Lee and Low, 1995). The same folate-PEG2000-DSPE construct was used to deliver a poly-L-lysine DNA complex to KB cells *in vitro* using a formulation based on dioleoyl-phosphatidyl-ethanolamine and cholesteroyl hemi-succinate. FR-expressing cells sequestered circulating FA-PEG-liposomes, however problems in regard to slow release of entrapped drug were encountered after RME. A useful alternative suggested by Reddy and Low, 1998 is to either incorporate a fusogenic peptide or to include in liposomal formulation a lipid that acquires fusogenic properties only after entry into target cells. Although the fusogenic peptide can either be entrapped free within the FA-PEG-liposomes or covalently ligated to the liposomal surface. The former protocol is preferred, since it avoids induction of immune response against fusogenic peptides. Various studies carried out to achieve folate mediated site-specific targeting is presented in Table 3-6.

Table 3-6. A Review of Studies Carried with Folate Conjugates

Target cell/ site	Delivery system	Activity (investigated/ proposed)
KB and HeLa cells	Folate-PEG-PE (Doxorubicin)	Tumour targeting expressing FR
KB cell lines	Folic acid-Penicillin-V-amidase (FA-enzyme conjugate)	Folate-targeted enzyme prodrug therapy
Tumour cell lines	Folic acid-single chain Fv conjugate	Folate-mediated immunotherpay (lysis of tumour cells by CTL in vitro)
CHO cells lacking folate receptor	Folic acid-PEG-PE (poly-L-lysine-DNA complex)	Folate-mediated non-viral gene therapy
HeLa cells	Folic acid-Cys^{287} (Pseudomonas exotoxin) conjugate	Efficient intracellular delivery and cytotoxicity of folate-linked toxins
Folate receptor expressing cancer cells (KB, HeLa, LoVo, SKOV3, SW620)	Folic acid-maytansinoid (DM1) conjugate	Selective killing of cancer cells expressing FR and non-toxic to normal cells

INSULIN BASED BIOCONJUGATES

Insulin receptors are over-expressed and up regulated in some cases and thus could be exploited either through endogenous insulin or an anti-insulin receptor antibody as targeting modules. Lai , 1988 suggested that the surface conjugated insulin could serve as a transporting molecule and selectively transport the liposomes and entrapped drugs to insulin-receptor rich tissues or cell lines. However, first reports of insulin immobilized on carrier surfaces were mere efforts to explain the thermal unfolding behaviour of insulin and aggregation kinetics of the carrier. Weissner and Hwang, 1982 reported the anchoring of insulin on the external surface of liposomes and evaluated the effects of the surface curvature, temperature, and lipid composition on the coupling efficiency, dynamics of liposome membrane and conformation of insulin. It was observed that the stability and unfolding of insulin is highly sensitive to changes in the environmental conditions, i.e. pH and hydrophobicity (Tokihiro et al., 1997) whereas insulin caused only minor changes on the transitional properties of one-component phospholipid vesicles (Sui et al., 1988). However, much work has been carried out on sulphatide-containing liposomes, which can be used as micro-carrier systems for insulin. Sulphatide is a glycosphingolipid that contains a sulphated monoglyco-group attached to the ceramide part. It is predominantly found in the extracellular leaflet of cell membranes, where it plays important roles in cellular signaling. It was argued that sulphatide-enriched lipid domains exist in the phospholipid-sulphatide lipid membranes and that the presence of sulphatides in the lipid membranes may facilitate a preferential interaction and binding with insulin that is important for its physiological response (and may be its exploitation as a targeting ligand?). Pedersen and co-workers, 1999 in contrast to earlier reports (indicating the insulin induces aggregation of sulphatide containing liposomes at acidic pH) revealed that only minor changes in the unfolding characteristics and thermal stability of the native conformations of insulin take place in the presence of sulphatide containing liposomes. Moreover, the lipid-membrane thermodynamics and phase behaviour of the vesicles remains unchanged. Still a deep understanding on the stability of endogenous protein and peptides structures in the presence of liposomes is of interest in order to use liposomes as either a micro-carrier of insulin or as a system appended with insulin as a transporter molecules.

Various approaches based upon the formations of hybrid proteins are developed to exploit the receptor-mediated localization/targeting using one of the conjugate components as site-directing ligand. These hybrid systems have the combined or re-ordered features of one or more proteins, in order to express effector functions as well as protection and recognition properties. Intracellular recognition signal structures have been used for the designing of synthetic peptides capable of mimicking endogenous biomolecules and bioevents derived from them. Site specific hybrid proteins may be produced by either synthetically linking protein fragments, or by using ligated gene fusion processes. In one study insulin, acylated with dimethylmaleic anhydride, was conjugated to transferrin (Tf) via a disulphide linkage (molar insulin:Tf ratio in the conjugate was 3:1) (Shah and Shen, 1996). The insulin-Tf conjugate (insulin-Tf) was tested for the transport of insulin across enterocyte-like Caco-2 cell monolayers by the process of transferrin receptor (TfR)-mediated transcytosis. The uptake of insulin-Tf in Caco-2 cells was TfR-mediated but negligible through insulin receptor-mediated endocytosis. Brefeldin A (BFA), an agent that causes an increase in TfR transcytosis, further enhanced the transport of the conjugated insulin 3-fold in both directions; thus, a combination of the conjugate and BFA can produce a nearly 45-fold increase in the apical-to-basolateral transport of insulin across Caco-2 cell monolayers. A procedure for synthesizing NB1-palmitoyl insulin for incorporation into liposomes to target the contents to hepatocytes was developed recently (Tsai et al., 1997). The amino group of the first amino acid phenylalanine on the B chain (B1) of insulin was selected for conjugation with palmitic acid assuming that binding site of insulin that corresponds to the insulin receptor would be preserved. Two other free amino groups present in insulin, the first amino acid glycine on the A chain (A1) and the 29th amino acid lysine on the B chain (B29), were first protected with a t-butoxycarbonyloxy (t-Boc) group to yield NA1, B29-di-(t-Boc) insulin. NA1, B29-Di-(t-Boc) insulin was then reacted with N-hydroxysuccinimide ester of palmitic acid, followed by deprotection of the t-Boc groups, to yield NB1-palmitoyl insulin. NB1-palmitoyl insulin was found to interact with the insulin receptor on fat cells, thereby catalyzing the conversion of [^{14}C] glucose into lipids

Insulin-like growth factor I (IGF-I), a 7.65 kD protein which has variety of metabolic functions, is being evaluated for its therapeutic benefit in several diseased states. Pierre et al., 1997 hypothesized that very low doses of IGF-I in liposomes will have positive wound-healing effect on local administration as higher doses of growth hormone (GH) plus IGF-I produce on systemic administration.

Pardridge and co-workers, 1995 examined the affinity of monoclonal antibody to the human insulin receptor and its ability to transcytose through the BBB. This was considered as a promising strategy that utilizes specific influx transporters existing at BBB for glycoproteins, which pump out cytotoxic and/or lipophilic drugs. The same group of workers explored the drug targeting of a peptide radiopharmaceutical through the primate BBB *in vivo* using a monoclonal antibody to the human insulin receptor that could be used for imaging amyloid and other brain disorders (Wu et al., 1997a). In these studies, ^{125}I-Abetal1-40 was mono-biotinylated (bio) and conjugated to a BBB drug delivery and brain targeting system comprised of a complex of the 83-14 monoclonal antibody (Mab) to the human insulin receptor tagged with streptividin (SA). A marked increase in the brain uptake of peptide radiopharmaceutical given as a conjugate with endogenous transporter system reveals that these systems could be used as future handles for the effective presentation of cytotoxic drugs to the brain tumours.

BIOCONJUGATES WITH CYTOKINES

Interleukin (IL) and interferon constitute a family of bio-ligands, which have their specific recognition portals on the various cell types in the body and participate in the activation of the immune system and/or in the anti-viral modalities. Endogenous antiviral protein ligands like interferons (α and β) play an important regulatory role in the antiviral effect. On the other hand, γ-interferon activates neutrophils and may participate in the immune responses or may lead to macrophage activation (Tortora et al., 1998). Even γ-interferon enhances expression of cellular receptors for other regulatory molecules like tumour necrosis factor. Incubation of several human tumour cell lines with human interferon-γ (IFN-γ) increased the specific binding of subsequently added ^{125}I-labeled recombinant human tumour necrosis factor (TNF) (Depraetere and Joniau, 1995). Interferon has been investigated largely for their controlled delivery rather than site-specific delivery. However, some reports of the active targeting are documented where the conjugated recognition ligand like asialofetuin (specific for galactose specific receptors of hepato-cytes), monoclonal antibody (against glioma associated antigen), and pullulan (non-specific affinity towards hepatic receptors) fortified the receptor specificity and activity of the interferon. Interleukins constitute a family of potent lymphokines/cytokines that activate cells of the immune system (Kuby, 1994). IL-2 is secreted by T-lymphocytes and upon activation by antigens becomes circulatory serum component. Similarly, other cytokines and non-specific mitogen equivocally stimulate the T-lymphocytes, which in turn secrete IL-2. IL-2 has been recognized as a possible therapeutic and adjuvant agent in the treatment of several diseases, including tumours, immuno-deficiency infections and for vaccination. Recently, it has been demonstrated that at least two classes of receptor for IL-2 exist with markedly different affinity for ligand (Weissman et al., 1986). All known biological actions of IL-2 have been correlated with occupancy of high affinity binding sites; the function of low-affinity sites however remains unknown. Expressed receptors bound to immobilize pure recombinant IL-2 or monoclonal anti-Tac antibody. These studies were the basis for the designing of different target oriented delivery systems in order to understand the regulation of IL-2 receptor expression and their clearance from the surface of the target or activated cells. Various other IL receptors including IL-4, IL-6, IL-7 and IL-12 are reported to be present on blood cells, which endocytose bound ligand and mediate lymphopoietic activities (Totpal and Aggarwal, 1991; Dittrich, 1994). IL-6 (an immuno bioligand) induces acute phase protein synthesis and augments cytotoxic T-cell generation in addition to B-cell IgG secretion. Cellular targets and receptors for IL-6 and hence receptor binding and biological activity of IL-6 could be negotiated by a diverse range of molecular isoforms having specific glycosylation patterns. They could become a tool for future research and in field of ligand mediated targeting to desired receptor units.

Despite their pleiotropic properties, immunotherapy with the respective cytokine ligands is restricted because these cytokines are rapidly cleared from the circulation and require high doses at which they induce toxic side effects (Nakamura et al., 1994; Okada et al., 1997). There have been various attempts to resolve the problems associated with the delivery of cytokines (Table 3-7). Recombinant cytokines are developed to circumvent unfavourable effects associated with endogenous IL-2. Sato and co-workers, 1993 investigated biological properties of an immune complex of recombinant interleukin-2 (rIL-2) and a monoclonal antibody against rIL-2 in mice for induction of killer cells and for anti-tumour activity. The results demonstrated that immune complex exerted a higher killer cell activity against YAC-1 cells and significant anti-tumour activity in a dose-dependent manner in Meth-A fibrosarcoma mice. In another development, polymer-conjugated cytokines (hybrid-cytokines), for instance PEG-modified IL-2 (Katre et al., 1987) and PEG-modified IL-6 (Tsunoda et al., 1998) were able to increase selectivity in their function but could not curtail the unfavourable functions. Targeted drug delivery using conjugates of cytokines with a variety of delivery systems including liposomes, micro-spheres, microcapsules, supramolecular biovectors, ceramics, and chimeric proteins, stabilizes the cytokines and potentiates only the selective functions *in vivo*. To further control the pharmacokinetics and pharmacodynamics *in vivo*, drug delivery systems using hybrid cytokines have been devised with increased stability (Tsunoda et al., 1998). Though cytokines are investigated mainly in encapsulated or entrapped forms yet they maintain their ligand specificity and bind selectively to their specific receptor portals.

In an attempt to enhance the therapeutic efficacy of IL-2, rIL-2 was encapsulated either in conventional or in long circulatory extravasating liposomes (sterically stabilized liposomes, SSL-IL-2) (Kedar et

Table 3-7. Conjugates of Cytokine Molecules

Target cell/ site	Delivery system	Activity
YAC-1 tumour cells/Meth A fibrosarcoma	Recombinant IL-2 immunocomplexed with MoAb against rIL-2	Induction of killer cells for anti-tumour activity
Murine CTLL-2 T cell line / human mitogen activated PBLs	IL-2 chemically coupled to liposomes	Receptor mediated immunotherapy
Human tumour xenograft/ Severe combined immuno-deficiency (SCID) mouse	IL-2 loaded poly(lactic acid) microsphere	Suppression of implanted tumour
IL-2 receptor bearing T cells (*in vitro*)	IL-2 in sterically stabilized liposomes	Anti-tumour activity in mice
Metastatic liver tumour	IL-2 in galactose containing liposomes	Enhancement of anti-tumour activity of lymphocytes
Hepatic sinusoidal lymphocytes/ hepatic metastasis in C3H/Me mice	IL-2 in galactose containing liposomes (Gal-lip-IL-2)	Activation of hepatic sinusoidal lymphocytes and local anti-tumour activity in liver
IL-6 transgenic mice	Alginate-poly-L-lysine-alginate membrane microencapsulating SK2 hybridoma cells	Suppression of IgG1 plasmacytosis in the IL-6 transgenic mice
Liver sites in BALB/c mice	Recombinant human interferon-pullulan conjugates	Enhancement of IFN-induced enzyme (2-5A) activity

Reproduced from Vyas and Sihorkar, 2000

al., 1994). The latter were found to bind selectively to IL-2 receptor bearing T-cells *in vitro*, indicating that the domain of the cytokine molecule involved in binding to the receptor is exposed to the outer liposomal membrane. An improved immuno-modulatory and anti-tumour activity of SSL-IL-2 in mice, suggested the targetability of the system as compared to soluble IL-2. In a further development, human rIL-2 as site directing ligand has been chemically coupled to external surface of liposomes containing methotrexate, a candidate immunosuppressive agent. The system specifically directs the immunoliposomes to activated T-cells expressing the high affinity IL-2 receptor (Konigsberg et al., 1998). IL-2 was chemically conjugated using succinimidyl-4-[p-maleidophenyl butyrate] (SMPB) while receptor binding domain on IL-2 was protected by monoclonal anti-IL-2 antibody bound to protein-A Silica gel. Antibody recognizes the receptor-binding domain of the IL-2 molecules. SMPB-IL-2 was covalently coupled to the external surface of small unilamellar vesicles constructed with DSPC:CHOL:SATA-PE (1.5:1:0.26 molar ratio). IL-2 bearing immunoliposomes presented a new class of cell-specific systems whose entry into the cytoplasm is regulated by cell surface receptor and associated cellular events. In order to increase the targetability of the liposome encapsulate IL-2, a galactose receptor specific ligand was appended to facilitate their selective uptake by liver parenchymal cells bearing galactose-specific receptors (Okuno et al., 1998). Gal-Lip-IL-2 lipo-somes were administered to C3H/He mice and *in vitro* anti-tumour activity of hepatic sinusoidal lymphocytes and hepatic metastases measurements were made. The results confirmed and subscribed to earlier reports of Nakamura and co-workers, 1994 in which they demonstrated highest accumulation and the highest localized anti-tumour activity of the lymphocytes at the liver sites. The system with enhanced IL-2 presentation activated the hepatic sinusoidal lymphocytes and increased the local anti-tumour activity in the liver. IL is also exploited as a bioligand for better antigen presentation. An antigen (dinitrophenylated bovine serum albumin) containing cytokine (IL-5 and IL-6) delivery system based on biodegradable micro-particle was evaluated for its role in potentiation of mucosal immune responses at both target and distal effector sites as well as in elicitation of circulating antibodies. IL is gaining extensive research attention for its inherent therapeutic roles and as a bioligand for site-specific targeting of conjugated or anchored bioactives (Table 3-7).

GLYCOCONJUGATES

Glycoconjugates, mainly glycoproteins (asialo-orosomucoids, asialofetuin, β-glucuronidase, etc.), neoglycoproteins (lactosaminated albumin, mannosylated and other glycosylated albumin) and galactosylated hydrophilic polymers are used as drug delivery or targeting systems. They are the pilot molecules which could be exploited for their intrinsic ability to specifically recognize soluble or membrane bound lectins and pilot the conjugated pharmacologically active moiety to the intended target cells (Molema and Meijer, 1994; Molema et al., 1997). Furthermore, neoglycoprotein and their drug conjugates have also been well studied as suitable carriers to target drugs, oligonucleotides and genes.

The classical approach of "dual targeting" employs intrinsic antiviral effect from carrier molecule, which synergies the antiviral effect of the loaded active drug (Meijer et al., 1992; Molema and Meijer, 1994). Based on this approach, drug conjugates were developed with a fortified activity profile against the viral replication process. In this approach, a carrier molecule that carries its own intrinsic antiviral effect is combined with the antiviral effect of the entrapped drug. The carrier-conjugates possess dual activity, i.e. coupled drug (intracellular action) and that of the carrier itself (extracellular action). A major advantage of using dual targeting complexes may be the prevention of development of resistant viral strain. Furthermore, the virus replication process can be attacked at multiple points, leading to synergistic effects (Fig. 3-21).

Neoglycoprotein-Drug Conjugates

Neoglycoproteins are artificial carrier systems consisted of protein backbones chemically modified with sugars. In this way they mimic the geometric organization of sugar groups in the naturally occurring

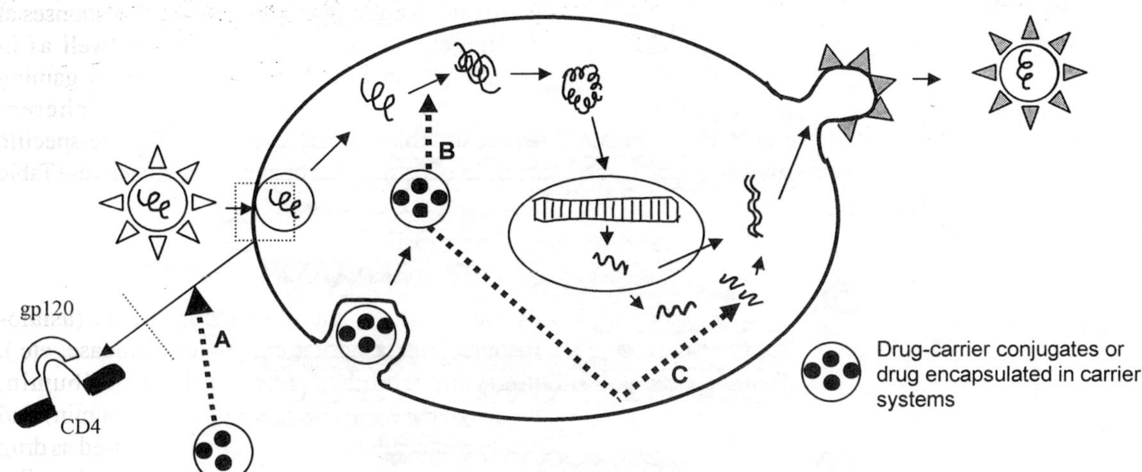

Fig. 3-21. The concept of dual targeting using antiviral drug conjugates. The carrier inhibits virus/cell binding and fusion extracellularly (A). After internalization of the drug-carrier composites encapsulated antiviral drugs such as nucleoside analogues (B) and glycosylation inhibitors (C) are released for intracellular inhibition of virus replication.

glycoproteins. Plasma proteins such as albumin and apoprotein B can be conjugated with sugars to produce neoglycoconjugates. Many enzymes, acute phase proteins and most plasma proteins (apart from albumin and lysozyme) have been investigated as a glycoprotein drug carrier (Steer and Ashwell, 1986). A major problem of naturally occurring plasma protein is the presence of non-terminal sugars in the oligosaccharide chain that invites unwanted interactions with other receptors in the body. To overcome these glycoprotein associated problems "neoglycoproteins" are designed, which consist of protein backbone, chemically modified using sugars, thereby mimicking the geometric organization of sugar groups of the naturally occurring glycoproteins. Molema and Meijer, 1994 investigated the specific delivery of anti-HIV drug azathioprene (AZT) to T-lymphocytes using neo-glycoprotein as drug carrier (neoglycoproteins-AZTMP conjugates) (Fig. 3-22). These workers synthesized neoglycoproteins with human serum albumin (HAS) as the protein backbone and varied the type of sugar molecule to prepare a variety of glycosylated albumin-AZTMP conjugates (mannosylated, galactosylated and fucosylated). Among the mechanisms of action discussed for the anti-HIV activity of these glyco-conjugates, the most striking was the sugar-specific recognition and internalization of the AZTMP conjugates by the MT-4 human T-lymphocyte cell line as the target cells, followed by the intracellular release of the drug.

Another interesting speculation for the anti-HIV activity was the co-endocytosis of virus and AZTMP conjugates following sugar specific interaction between virus and neo-glycoprotein-AZTMP conjugate. In this respect, it is of interest to note that gp120 serves as a mannose-binding lectin and that recombinant gp160 exhibits N-acetyl-β-D glucosaminyl-binding sites. Since neo-glycoprotein carrier contains a high ratio of mannose-terminating proteins, they could be proposed to have their own intrinsic activity against HIV-infections. Further a charge-based anti-viral activity of the neoglycoproteins have been demonstrated to inhibit virus/cell fusion and synctia formation (fusion of two or more infected cells to an infected cells resulting in the formation of a giant cell) (Molema and Meijer, 1994). This was hypothesized to be a result of interaction of negatively charged albumin with gp41 envelope glycoprotein or with V3 loop of gp 120. These carriers coupled with AZT-like drugs could form conjugates having dual targetability and a preferential activity against synctium-inducing variants of HIV-1, which are predominant in the terminal phase of HIV infection. Neoglycoconjugates (mannosylated BSA) upon

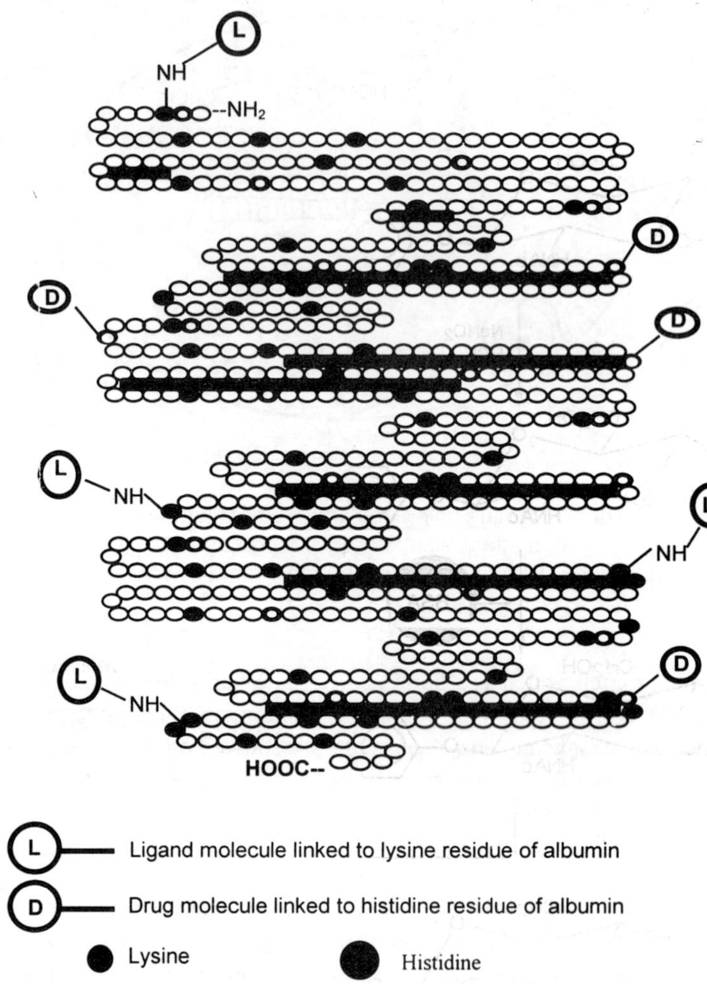

Fig. 3-22. Schematic Representation of a Neoglycoprotein-AZTMP Conjugate. In the conjugate, p-aminophenyl-mannose is conjugated to lysine groups of human serum albumin and AZTMP is conjugated to lysine and histidine residues (Adopted from Molema and Meijer, 1994)

conjugation with biological response modifiers, such as muramyl dipeptide (MDP) demonstrated *in vivo* cytostatic activity and macrophage activation and allowed targeting to macrophages or monocytes.

Neoglycoprotein-Liposomes Conjugates

The conjugation of neoglycoproteins with liposomes has been recently realized. Liposomes can be prepared using neutral glycolipids, gangliosides or lipid-anchor containing glycan derivatives, also known as neoglycolipids. A neoglycoprotein - liposome conjugate can be engineered by combining phosphatidylethanolamine anchor with matrix and ligand part of a neoglyco-conjugate, thus creating carbohydrate as an integral part of the liposomal membrane. Figure 3-23 demonstrate the general mechanism of preparation of neoglycoprotein-liposome conjugate. Conjugation was carried out in two steps :

- First, by coupling a diazo derivative of a p-aminophenyl glycoside (N-acetylneuraminic acid) preferentially to tyrosine residues of the carrier protein to the liposome surface exploiting periodate-mediated generation of

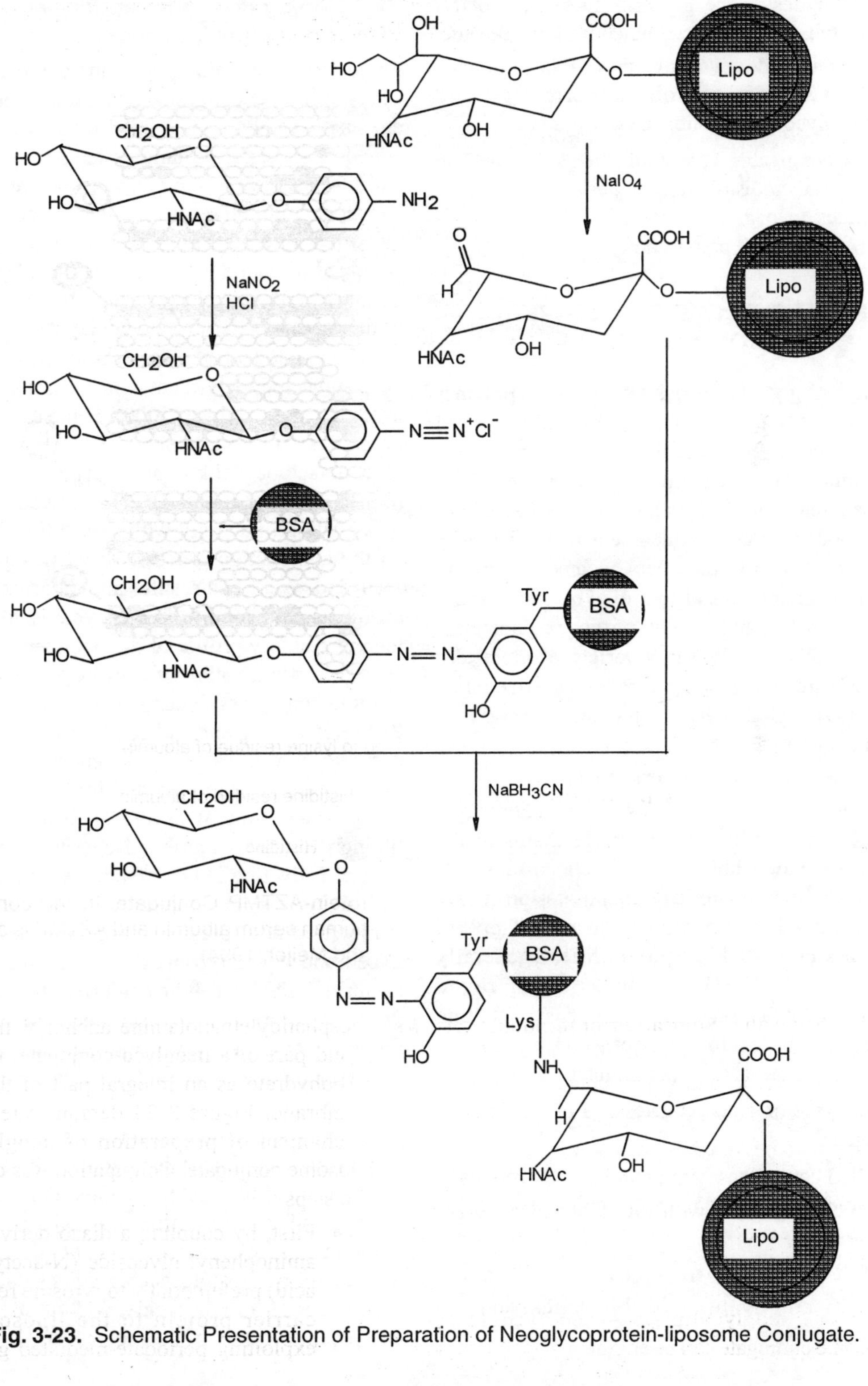

Fig. 3-23. Schematic Presentation of Preparation of Neoglycoprotein-liposome Conjugate.

aldehydes in the glycerol side chain of N-acetylneuraminic acid moieties of ganglioside.

- Second, reductive amination of the conjugate with sodium cyanoborohydride to yield neoglyco-protein-liposome conjugate.

These conjugates were studied for lectin binding specificity and biodistribution studies and quantitative differences in organ retention was observed as compared to control preparation.

POLY ETHYLENE GLYCOL (PEG) CONJUGATES

Polyethylene glycol (PEG) is a widely used polymer and functions as a covalent modifier of biological macromolecules and particulates as well as a carrier for low molecular weight drugs (Delgado et al., 1992; Ramchandran et al., 1996; Tan et al., 1998; Mehvar et al., 2000). Covalent attachment of biologically active compounds to polymers became one of the methods for alteration and control of biodistribution, pharmacokinetics and toxicity of these compounds. PEG is readily available in a variety of molecular weights and have a general structure HO-$(CH_2CH_2O)_n$-CH_2CH_2OH and molecular weights in the range of 100-20000 Da.

Monomethyl ether of PEG (mPEG) is often used for conjugation to biologically relevant materials. It is particularly useful when multiple chains of the polymer have to be linked to the intended substrate. Due to its structural simplicity and possession of only one derivatizable end group, the use of mPEG minimizes cross-linking possibilities (generally associated with PEG) and leads to improved homogeneity of the conjugates. Thus, it is the starting material of choice for covalent conjugation of proteins, biomaterials and particulates.

Four types of bioconjugates of PEG have been investigated :

- PEG conjugates with peptides and proteins
- PEG conjugates with low molecular weight drugs
- PEG conjugates with lipids
- PEG conjugates with biological macro-molecules

PEG Conjugates with Peptides and Proteins (mainly Enzymes)

There are three main area of applications of PEG-polypeptide conjugates : (1) therapeutics, (2) enzymatic catalysis in organic solvents and (3) two-aqueous phase partitioning systems for purification and analysis of various biologically derived mixtures. Covalent coupling reactions between amino groups (or other nucleophiles) of proteins and mPEG equipped with an electrophilic functional group (also termed as "activated PEGs") have been used in most of the cases of PEG-protein conjugates.

The single largest class of proteins, which have been subjected to covalent modifications with PEG, is of enzymes (Mehvar, 2000). Some enzymes, e.g., peroxidase, L-asparaginase, alkaline phosphatase, gluconolactone oxidase and superoxide dismutase (SOD), in conjugation with PEG showed remarkable preservation of activity with very little dependence on the conjugation process. PEG-L-Asparaginase recorded excellent results and pharmacokinetic profile as compared to free enzyme, signifying the long circulatory profile of the polymer (Fig. 3-24). However, preservation of enzyme activity of PEG-enzyme conjugates depends upon the chemistry of PEG activation and subsequent conjugation to enzymes as well as on the extent of modification. Similar results were recorded in the case of PEG-tissue plasminogen activator conjugates. The fibrinolytic activity was found to be independent from type of activating reagent employed but decreased with an increase in the extent of modification. PEG-conjugated acyl-plasmin-streptokinase, elastase, trypsin and chymotrypsin exhibited a similar decrease in fibrinolytic, hydrolytic and proteolytic activities. Some of the reasons for the decrease in enzyme activities of PEG-enzyme conjugates and the methods to overcome them are listed in Table 3-8.

Site-specific PEG grafting (pegylation) of proteins is a recent innovation to avoid random protein modification that leads to steric hindrance into essential binding sites of proteins. For example, in the case of glycoproteins (ovalbumin, immuno-globulins, glucose oxidase) it is possible to utilize the reactivity of oligosaccharide residues for the attachment of mPEG chains, without affecting the polypeptide portion of the molecules.

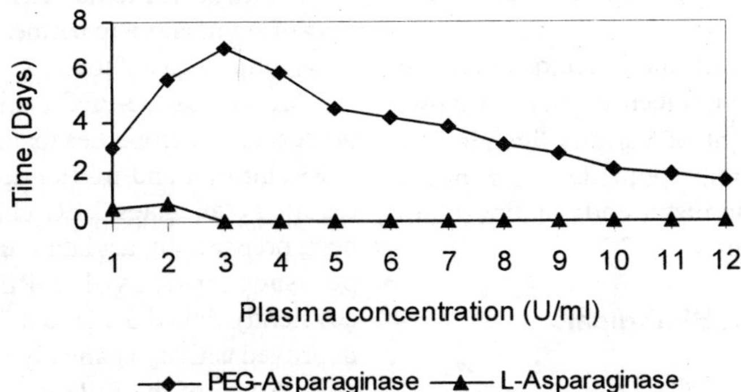

Fig. 3-24. PEG-L-Asparaginase Versus Free L-Asparaginase Plasma Levels in Non-immunized Mice

Table 3-8. Reasons for Decreased Enzyme-PEG Activities and Methods to Overcome them

Reasons for decreased enzyme-PEG activities
- Conformational change due to PEG conjugation
- Steric hindrance caused by grafted PEG chains to exclude proteins from their proximity

Methods to overcome decreased enzyme-PEG activities
- PEG conjugation in the presence of a macromolecular inhibitor of the protein (site protective)
- Site-specific PEG grafting (pegylation) of proteins
- Site specific mutagenesis

PEG Conjugates with Low Molecular Weight Drugs

There are three main areas of applications of PEG-low molecular weight drug conjugates : (1) PEG ligands in aqueous two phase partitioning, (2) bioreactor use of PEG cofactors and/or PEG catalysts and (3) PEG-drug conjugates for controlled delivery of biologically active substances. In contrast to the polypeptidic modifications with PEG, most low molecular weight drug molecules are hydrophobic in nature and allow the construction of conjugates in organic solutions. Maximum approaches are based upon the conjugation of PEG-OH with free carboxylic acid (formation of PEG esters) present in the low molecular weight drugs (Ibuprofen, penicillin V, aspirin). The use of succinate spacer can allow the use of PEG esters of a larger selection of drugs. For example, atropine and quinidine were successfully linked via ester linkages to PEG-succinate of various molecular weights (Mehvar, 2000). Direct attachment of drugs to hydroxyl groups of the polymer can also be achieved by forming ether (5-fluorouracil), amide (5-fluorouracil), carbonate (hydrocortisone and dexamethasone) and urethane (doxorubicin) bonds via the appropriate alkylation and acylation reactions (Mehvar, 2000).

PEG Conjugates with Lipids

Conjugation of lipids with PEG permits these conjugates to avoid quick recognition and their clearance *in vivo*. PEG-lipids are mainly utilized for the preparation of long circulatory (Stelath®) liposomes. Derivatization of phosphatidylethanolamine (PE) and the amino functional group of polymer leads to the formation of PEG-lipids. These can then be used as constructive components of the long circulatory liposomal formulations. Instead of using PEG-lipid conjugates to form liposomes, modified surface amino groups of DSPE-DPPE-cholesterol vesicles were modified with mPEG-tresylate. These PEG-PE derived liposomes (Stelath) offer several advantages over conventional liposomes like :

- Extended blood circulation ($t_{1/2}$ 48 h in humans)
- Reduction in the immunogenicity and antigenicity

- Avoidance of serum protein adsorption and opsonins
- Low accumulation in the reticuloendothelial system organs (liver, spleen and bone marrow)
- Ease of attachment of various ligands like immunoglobulins, peptides and polysaccharides to the distal ends of liposome-grafted PEG chains

PEG Conjugates with Biological Macromolecules

Several biological macromolecules like interleukins, interferons, oligonucleotides, polysaccharides and their analogues are conjugated with PEG and their *in vitro* and *in vivo* behaviour are well documented. Polymer-conjugated cytokines (hybrid-cytokines), for instance, PEG-modified IL-2 and PEG-modified IL-6 were able to increase selectivity in their function but could not curtail the unfavourable functions. Urethane-linked PEG-β interferon demonstrated a noticeably longer circulation lifetime. Conjugation of PEG to oligonucleotides or their backbone-modified analogues can improve some of the *in vivo* properties of these materials like :

- Resistance to nucleases
- Cell membrane permeability
- Improved solubility

Polysaccharide-PEG conjugates are expected to possess useful properties for their use as drug carriers. PEG-chitosan and mPEG-dextran are some of the reported conjugates. PEG-chitosan conjugates have been prepared by acylating the amino group on the polysaccharide with mPEG-carboxylate, and covalently linked 5-FU to it. The conjugate showed improved activity against lymphocytic leukaemia in mice. Some of the PEG-conjugated substrates, i.e., proteins, liposomes, blood-contact materials, are already launched in the market. Some of the applications of the PEG-conjugates in drug delivery and therapeutics are listed in Table 3-9.

POLY-L-LYSINE CONJUGATES

Poly-L-lysine conjugates have been investigated mainly for their role as non-viral gene vector (polycation conjugates) and for antiviral properties of the conjugated nucleoside analogues (Derrien et al., 1989). In order to reduce the extrahepatic side effects of antiviral nucleoside analogues in the treatment of

Table 3-9. Some of Applications of PEG-conjugates in Drug Delivery and Therapeutics

Protein/drug	Purpose
Enzymes and proteins	
Superoxide dismutase (SOD)	Anti-inflammatory, long circulation half lives
Alkaline phosphatase	Increased enzyme activity *in vivo*
L-Asparaginase	Increased amidolytic activity and reduction in antigenicity
Peroxidases	Increased enzyme activity *in vivo*
Gluconolactone oxidase	*In vitro* stability of the conjugate
Elastase	Increased hydrolyzing activity
Trypsin	Improved proteolytic activity
Chymotrypsin	Superior proteolytic activity than the native enzyme
Ribonucleases	Increased enzyme activity *in vivo*
Tissue plasmin activator	Long circulation half lives
Interferons	Anti viral
Interleukins	Mediator of immune responses
Drugs	
Ibuprofen	Longer lasting anti-inflammatory activity
Penicillin V	Conjugate on hydrolysis releases active antibiotic
Aspirin	Anti-inflammatory and anti-gout
5-Fluorouracil	Anti cancer
Ursodeoxycholic acid	Bile salts

Compiled from Mehvar, 2000

chronic viral hepatitis, these drugs were conjugated with galactosyl-terminating macromolecules. Adenine arabinoside mono-phosphate (ara-AMP), conjugated with lactosaminated human serum albumin (L-HAS, neoglycoconjugate) and administered to hepatitis B virus (HBV)-infected patients for 28 days, exerted an antiviral activity to the same extent as the free drug without producing any clinical side-effects (Molema and Meijer, 1994). However, when lactosaminated poly-L-lysine (Lac-poly(Lys)) was used as the hepatotropic carrier for ara-AMP and ribavirin, these conjugates demonstrated advantages over those prepared with L-HAS. Poly-L-lysine can be easily conjugated with biological response modifiers, such as muramyl dipeptide (MDP) and with sugar derivatives such as mannoside or 6-phosphomannoside to allow targeting of biological response modifiers to macrophages or monocytes.

Advantages of poly-L-lysine conjugated antiviral drugs as compared against neoglycoprotein drug conjugates are :

- They can be administered by the intramuscular route
- They are obtained entirely by chemical synthesis, thus eliminating the problems associated with the use of haemo-derivatives
- They have a heavy drug load, which permits administration of smaller quantities of conjugate that are more easily digested in lysosomes
- They enable higher quantities of drug to be introduced into hepatocytes.

However, the major role of poly-L-lysine conjugates is their ability to act as a non-viral gene vector. These polycation form stable polyelectrolyte complexes with DNA (or plasmids) (Wagner et al., 1992; Uike et al., 1998). Based on this property, various polylysine-plasmid conjugates were prepared using recognition portals such as transferrin, insulin, asialo-orosomucoid, asialoglycoprotein, epidermal growth factor, to help the polylysine-plasmid conjugate to enter into cells expressing the related receptors. Several non-viral gene vectors including fusogenic liposomes, genosomes (DNA-liposomes/lipid complexes), Lipofectin™ (lipid-DNA complex) and recently, cochleates are investigated as the major gene vectors. Poly-L-lysine has been used along with DC-Chol/DOPE liposomes to condense DNA and form a self-assembled vector system named as LPD1 (a lipopolyplex) (Gao and Huang, 1996). LPDI is currently used in a clinical trial for gene therapy of Canavan's disease, an autosomal recessive leukodystrophy. In a recent development, Lee and Huang, 1996 reported a lipid vector (LPDII) for gene transfer, where poly-L-lysine condensed DNA is entrapped into folate targeted anionic liposomes via charge interactions (LPDII differs from LPDI in that anionic lipids instead of cationic lipids are used).

Recently, glycosylated polymers (glycosylated poly-L-lysine) are reported to *en route* the conjugate due to its specific uptake thorough sugar terminals via specific lectin receptors (Meijer et al., 1992). Figure 3-25 explains the conjugate structure in which ε-amino groups are partially acylated by reacting with δ-gluconolactone, while the other amino groups are substituted by recognition signals (e.g., carbohydrate residues) and by drugs (antiviral drug, succinyl-5′-azathioprene). However, the research on glycosylated polymers is confined mainly to gene delivery and gene therapy. Lactose was conjugated through a PEG spacer to poly-L-lysine (PLL) to customize a gene carrier (lactosylated PLL) capable of condensing plasmid DNA (Meijer et al., 1992). This cationic polymer targeted Hep G2 cells preferentially in culture. The inclusion of a lactose-targeting moiety greatly increased the efficacy of the gene carrier over PEG-PLL and Lipofectin™.

A biodegradable nanoparticle gene carrier, polysaccharide-graft-PLL and poly(D,L-lactic acid), was synthesized and characterized. The nanoparticle size was classically controllable by changing the copolymer concentration, where the particles could be as small as 60 nm. When polysaccharide was used in the copolymer, the nanoparticle became more DNA adsorbent. This gene carrier targets the antigen confined to stage II immature cortical thymocytes for leukaemia therapy. A 20,000 mol. wt. PLL backbone was sufficient for compaction of DNA. Folic acid linked to PLL through a PEG spacer is currently being studied for DNA condensation and delivery to membrane associated folate binding protein positive endothelial cancer cells. A new DNA delivery vector (the TERPLEX system) based on a balanced hydro-

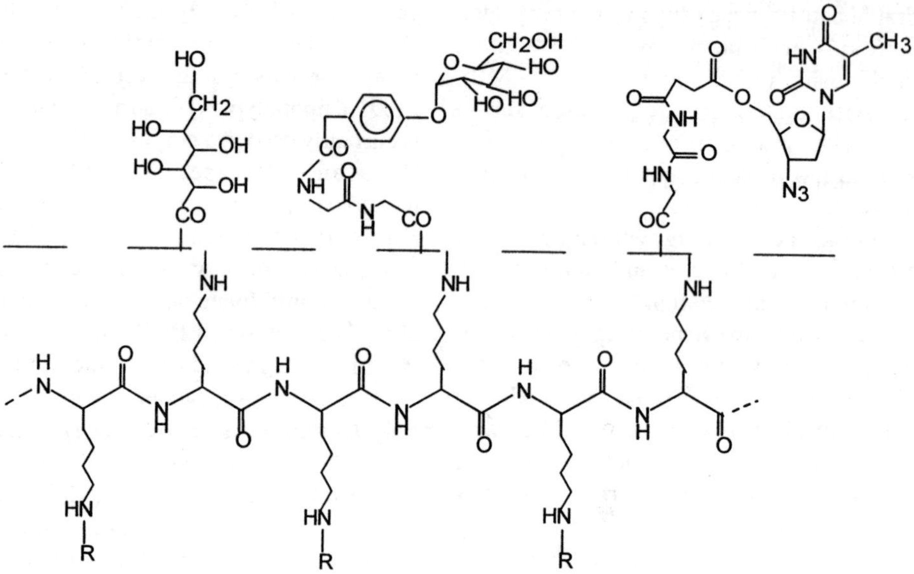

Fig. 3-25. Glycosylated Poly-L-lysine Based Carrier of Azathioprene (AZT)

phobicity and net surface charge between stearyl-poly-L-lysine, low density lipoprotein (LDL), and genetic material (i.e. plasmid DNA or antisense oligonucleotide) was designed for a more efficient and safer DNA delivery and effective gene therapy.

FUTURE PERSPECTIVES

Recent advances in drug delivery, genomics and antisense therapy have paved the way for an enormous potential for the bioconjugates in designing and tailoring the specific needs of therapeutics. The fields like drug delivery and gene therapy have already received utmost attention as far as the bioconjugation chemistry is concerned, but recent introduction of bio-conjugates of oligonucleotides makes the research still more attractive and challenging. Antisense oligonucleotides are putative antitumour and antiviral agents and their *in vitro* and *in vivo* survival has been exceptionally improved by their conjugation with macromolecules. To date, oligonucleotide-neoglyco-protein (man-BSA or man6P-BSA), oligonucleotide-biotin with glycosylated streptividin, oligonucleotide (streptavidin)-OX26-biotin conjugates, oligo-nucleotide-asialoglycoprotein, poly-L-lysine-asialoorosomucoid antisense oligonucleotides conjugates and lipid-oligonucleotide (cholesterol-oligonucleotide) conjugates are well defined.

The future role of gene gun, pharmacogenomics, aptamers and the biochemistry of receptor and ligands may explore future possibilities of the bioconjugates in drug delivery and therapeutics.

REFERENCES

Allen T. M. (1994) *Trends Pharmacol. Sci.* **15**, 215.

Anderson R. G. W. (1993) *Trends Cell Biol.* **3**, 69.

Annemiek J. M. L., van Rensen, Wauben M. H. M., Stulemeyer M. C. G., van Eden W. and Cromelin D. J. A. (1999) *Pharm. Res.* **16**, 198.

Avrilionis K. and Boggs J. M. (1996) *Cell. Immunol.* **168**, 13.

Bayer E. A. and Wilchek M. (1990) In: Methods in Enzymology, Vol. 184, Wilchek M. and Bayer E. A. (Eds.), Academic Press, San Diago, 174.

Begnet R. H. J., Verhaar M. J., Chester K. A., Casey J. L., Green A. J., Napier M. P., Hope-Stone L. D., Cushen N., Keep P. A. and Johnson C. J. (1996) *Nature Med.* **2**, 979.

Burl J., Lotscher E., Steimer K. S., Capon D. J., Baenziger J., Jick H. M. and Wabl M. (1991) *Proc. Natl. Acad. Sci. USA* **88**, 4723.

Burrow F. J., Tazzari P., Amlot P., Gajdar A. F., Derbyshire

E. J., King S. W., Vitetta E. S. and Thorpe P. E. (1995) *Clinical Cancer Res.* **1**, 1623.

Carlsson J., Drevin H. and Axen R. (1978) *Biochem. J.* **173**, 723.

Cho B. K., Roy E. J., Patrik T. A. and Kranz D. M. (1997) *Bioconjug. Chem.* **8**, 338.

Chu B. C. F., Kramer F. R. and Orgel L. E. (1986) *Nucleic Acid Res.* **14**, 5591.

Cline H. J. and Sumner H. A. (1972) *Blood* **40**, 62.

Cudd A., Noonan C. A., Tosi P. F., Melnick J. L. and Nicolau C. (1990) *J. AIDS* **3**, 109.

Delgado C., Francis G. E. and Fisher D. (1992) *Crit Rev Ther Drug Carr. Syst.* **9**, 249.

Depraetere S. and Joniau M. (1995) *Leuk. Res.* **19**, 803.

Derrien D., Midoux P., Petit C., Negre E., Mayer R., Monsigny M. and Roche A. C. (1989) *Glycoconjugate J.* **6**, 241.

Dittrich E. (1994) *J. Biol. Chem.* **269**, 19014.

Edwards R. J., Singleton A. M., Boobis A. R. and Davies D. S. (1989) *J. Immunol. Methods* **117**, 215.

Egea M. A., Garcia M. L., Alsina M. A. and Reig F. (1994) *J. Pharm. Sci.* **83**, 169.

Emanuel N., Kedar E., Bolotin E. M., Smorodinsky N. I. and Bareholz Y. (1996) *Pharm. Res.* **13**, 861, 1996.

Epstein A. L., Khawli L. A., Hornick J. L. and Taylor C. R. (1995) *Cancer Res.* **95**, 2673.

Fanger M. W., Morganelli P. M. and Guyre P. M. (1992) *Crit. Rev. Immunol.* **12**., 101.

Flasher D., Konopka K., Chamow S. M., Dazin P., Ashkenazi A., Pretzer E. and Duzgunes N. (1994) Biochim. Biophys. Acta. **1194**, 185.

Fleit H. B., Wright S. D. and Unkeless J. C. (1982) *Proc. Natl. Acad. Sci USA.* **79**, 3275.

Gabizon A. T., Horowitz D., Goren D., Tzemach D., Mondelbaum-Shavit F., Qazen M. M., Zalipsky S. (1999) *Bioconjugate Chem.* **10**, 289.

Gao X. and Huang L. (1996) *Biochemistry* **35**, 1027.

Garagiola D. M., Huard T. K. and Lo Buglio A. F. (1979) *Blood* **54**, 84a.

Gee B., Warhol M. J. and Roth J. (1991) *J. Histochem. Cytochem.* **39**, 863.

Ghosh S. S., Kao P. M., McCue A. W. and Chappelle H. L. (1990) *Bioconjugate Chem.* **1**, 71.

Haisma H. J., Boven M., Vanmuijen M., Dejong J., Vander Vijgh W. J. F. and Pinedo H. M. (1992) *Br. J. Cancer* **66**, 474.

Hartman F. C. and Wold F. (1966) *J. Am. Chem. Soc.* **88**, 3890.

Hege K. M., Daleke D. L., Waldmann T. A. and Matthay K. K. (1989) *Blood* **74**, 2043.

Hermanson G. T. (1996) In: Bioconjugate techniques, Academic Press, New York, 1.

Huwyler J., Wu D. and Pardridge W. M. (1996) *Proc. Natl. Acad. Sci. USA* **93**, 14164.

Ishida O. and Maruyama K. (1998) *Nippon. Rinsho.* **56**, 657.

Kairemo K., Ljunggren K., Strand S. E., Hiltunen J., Penttila P., Nicula T., Laine A. and Wahlstrom T. (1993) *Acta. Oncol.* **32**, 801.

Kajihara J., Shibata K., Nakano K., Nishimuro S. and Kato K. (1998) *Biochim. Biophys. Acta* **1199**, 202.

Kang Y. S., Bickel U. and Pardridge W. M. (1994) *Drug Metab. Dispos.* **22**, 99.

Katre N., Knauf M. and Laird W. (1987) *Proc. Natl. Acad. Sci. USA* **84**, 1487.

Kedar E., Rutkowski Y., Braun E., Emanuel N. and Barenholz Y. (1994) *J. Immunother. Emphasis Tumor Immunol.* **16**, 47.

Khaw B. A., Torchilin V. P., Vural I. and Narula J. (1995) *Nature Med.* **1**, 1195.

Kim Y. W., Fung M. S. C., Sun N. C., Sun C. R. Y., Chang N. T. and Chang T. W. (1990) *J. Immunol.* **144**, 1257.

Kinsky S. C. (1972) *Biochim. Biophys. Acta.* **265**, 1.

Kitagawa T. and Aikawa T. (1976) *J. Biochem.* **79**, 233.

Konigsberg P. J., Godtel R., Kissel T. and Richer L. L. (1998) *Biochim. Biophys. Acta* **1370**, 243.

Kroesen B. J., Helfrich W., Bakker A., Wubbena A. S., Bakker H., Kal H. B., The T. H. and Dleij L. (1995) *Int. J. Cancer* **61**, 812.

Kuby J. (1994) Immunology, IInd edition. W.H. Freman and Company, New York.

Kumagai K. and Ikuta K. (1992) In: Membrane interaction of HIV, Aloia R. C. and Curtain C. C. (Eds.), Washington DC, Wiley-Liss, 305.

Lai J. Y. (1988) *J. Pharm. Sci.*. **77**, 432.

Lasic D. D. (1996) *Nature* **380**, 56.

Lasic D. D. (1994) *Angew. Chem. Int. Ed. Eng.* **33**, 1785.

Lee R. J. and Huang L. (1996) *J. Biol. Chem.* **271**, 8481.

Lee R. J. and Low P. S. (1994) *J. Biol. Chem.* **269**, 3198.

Lee R. J. and Low P. S. (1995) *Biochim. Biophys. Acta* **1233**, 134.

Leonetti J. P., Degols G. and Lebleu B. (1990) *Bioconjugate. Chem.* **1**, 149.

Lewis J. T., Hafeman D. G. and McConnell H. M. (1980) *Biochemistry* **19**, 5376.

Li J. Y., Sugimura K., Jboado R., Lee H. J, Zhang C., Duebel S. and Pardridge W. (1999) *Protein Eng.* **12**, 787.

Lisanti M. P., Scherer P. E., Vidugiriene J., Tang Z. L., Hermanowski-Vesatka A., Tu Y. H., Cook R. F. and

Sergiacomo M. (1994) *J. Cell Biol.* **126**, 111.

Matsushita S., Koito A., Maeda Y., Hattori T. and Takatsuki K. (1990) *AIDS Res.Hum. Retroviruses* **6**, 193.

Mehvar R. (2000) *J. Pharm. Pharmaceut. Sci.* **3**, 125.

Meijer D. K. F., Jansen R. W. and Molema G. (1992) *Antiviral Res.* **18**, 215.

Molema G. and Meijer D. K. F. (1994) *Adv. Drug Deliv. Rev.* **14**, 25.

Munns J., Yaxley J., Coomer J., Lavin M. F., Gardinger R. A. and Watters D. (1998) *Br. J. Urol.* **82**, 284.

Nakamura K., Okuno K., Hirohata T., Shigeoka H., Jinnai H. and Yasutomi M. (1994) *Gan To Kagaku Ryoho* **21**, 2105.

Nassander U. K., Steerenberg P. A., Poppe H., Storm G., Jap P. H. K., Poels L. G., de Jong W. H. and Cromellin D. J. A. (1992) *Cancer Res.* **52**, 646.

Norley S. G., Huang L. and Rouse B. T. (1986) *J. Immunol.* **136**, 681.

Okada N., Miyamoto H., Yoshioka T., Katsume A., Saito H., Yorozu K., Ueda O., Itoh N., Mizuguchi H., Nakagawa S., Ohsugi Y. and Mayumi T. (1997) *Biochim. Biophys. Acta.* **1360**, 53.

Okuno K., Nakamura K., Tanaka A., Yachi K. and Yasutomi M. (1998) *Surg Today* **28**, 64.

Pardridge W. M., Kang Y. S., Bucialk J. L. and Yang J. (1995) *Pharm. Res.* **12**, 807.

Park E., Starzyk R. M., McGrath J. P., Lee T., George J., Schultz A. J., Lynch P. and Putney S. D. (1998) *J. Drug Target.* **6**, 53.

Pederson T. B., Frokjaer S., Mouritesen O. G. and Jorgensen K. (1999) *J. Liposome Res.* **9**, 261.

Penichet M. L., Kang Y. S., Pardridge W. M., Morrison S. L. and Shin S. U. (1999) *J. Immunol.* **163**, 4421.

Pierre E. J., Perez-Polo J. R., Mitchell A. T., Matin S., Foyt H. L. and Herndon D. N. (1997) *J. Burn Care Rehabil.* **18**, 287.

Pincus S. H. and MaClure J. (1993) *Proc. Natl. Acad. Sci. USA* **90**, 332.

Pincus S. H., Wehrly K. and Chesebro B. (1989) *J. Immunol.* **142**, 3070.

Plant A. L., Brizgys M. V., Lacasio-Brown L. and Durst R. A. (1989) *Anal. Biochem.* **176**, 420.

Ramchandran R., Katzenstein D. A., Winters M. A., Kundu S. K. and Merigan T.C. (1996) *J. Infect. Dis.* **173**, 1005.

Reddy J. A. and Low P. S. (1998) *Crit. Rev. Ther. Drug Carrier Syst.* **15**, 587.

Rosenberg M. B., Breakfield X. O. and Hawrot E. (1987) *J. Neurochem.* **48**, 865.

Ross J. F., Chaudhury P. K. and Ratnam M. (1994) *Cancer* **73**, 2432.

Ross S. E., Carson S. D. and Fink L. M. (1986) *Bio. Techniques* **4**, 350.

Rothberg K. G., Ying Y. S., Kolhouse J. F., Kamen B. A. and Anderson R. G. (1990) *J. Cell Biol.* **110**, 637.

Sarti P., Ginobbi P., D'Agostino I., Arancia G., Lendaro E., Molinari A., Ippoliti R. and Citro G. (1996) *Biotechnol. Appl. Biochem.* **24**, 269.

Sato J., Hamaguchi N., Doken K., Gotoh K., Ootsu K., Iwasa S., Ogawa Y. and Toguchi H. (1993) *Biotherapy* **6**, 225.

Senter P. D. (1990) *FASEB J.* **4**, 188.

Shah D. and Shen W. C. (1996) *J. Pharm. Sci.* **85**, 1306.

Sherwood R. F. (1996) *Adv. Drug Deliv. Rev.* **22**, 269.

Singh M. (1999) *Cur. Pharm. Res.* **5**, 443.

Singh P., Sihorkar V., Jaitely V., Kanaujia P., Mishra V. and Vyas S.P. (2000) *Indian Drugs* **37**, 259.

Slepushkin V. A., Salem I. I., Andreev S. M., Dazin P. and Duzgunes N. (1996) *Biochim. Biophys. Res. Commun.* **227**, 827.

Staerz U. D., Kanagawa O. and Bevan M. J. (1985) *Nature* **314**, 628.

Stavridis J. C., Deliconstantinos G., Psallidopoulos M. C., Armenakas N. A., Hadjiminas D. J. and Hadjiminas J. (1986) *J. Exp. Cell Res.* **164**, 568.

Steer C. J. and Ashwell G. (1986) In: Progress in Liver Diseases, Popper H. and Schaffner F. (Eds.) Vol. VIII, New York: Grune and Stratton, 99.

Sui S. F., Urumow T. and Sachmann E. (1988) *Biochemistry* **27**, 7463.

Sunamoto J., Sato T., Hirota M., Fukushima K., Hiratani K. and Hara K. (1987) *Biochim. Biophys. Acta.* **898**, 323.

Swanson S. J., Lin B. F., Mullenix M. C. and Mortensen R. F. (1991) *J. Immunol.* **146**, 1596.

Tabata Y., Matsui Y. and Ikada Y. (1998) *J. Control. Rel.* **56**, 135.

Tabata Y., Noda Y., Matsui Y. and Ikada Y. (1999) *J. Control. Rel.* **59**, 187.

Tan Y., Sun X., Xu M., An Z., Tan X., Han Q., Miljkovic D. A., Yang M. and Hoffman R. M. (1998) *Protein Extra. Puruf.* **12**, 45.

Tanaka T., Kaneo Y., Miyashita M. (1996) *Biol. Pharm. Bull.* **19**, 774.

Till M. A., Ghetie V., Gregori T., Patzer E. J., Porter J. P., Uhr J. W., Capon D. J. and Vitetta E. S. (1988) *Science* **242**, 1166.

Tokihiro K., Irie T. and Uekama K. (1997) *Chem. Pharm. Bull. Tokyo* **45**, 525.

Tortora G. J., Funke B. R. and Case C. L. (1998) Microbiology: An introduction, 6th edition. Addison Wesley Longman, California, 456.

Totpal K. and Aggarwal B. B. (1991) *Cancer Res.* **51**, 4266.

Tsai Y. J., Rottero A., Chow D. D., Hwang K. J., Lee V. H., Zhu G. and Chan K. K. (1997) *J. Pharm. Sci.* **86**, 1264.

Tsunoda S., Tsutsumi Y. and Mayumi T. (1998) *Nippon. Rinsho*. **56**, 573.

Uike H., Sakakibara R., Iwanaga K., Ide M. and Ishiguro M. (1998) *Biosci. Biotechnol. Biochem*. **62**, 1247.

Unkeless J.C., Fleit H. B. and Mellman, I. S. (1981) *Adv. Immunol.* **31**, 247.

Vingerhoeds M. H., Haisma H. J., van Muijen M., van de Rijh, Cromellin D. J. A. and Storm G. (1993) *FEBS Lett.* **336**, 485.

Vitetta E. S. (1990) *J. Clin. Immunol.* **10**, 515.

Vyas S. P. and Sihorkar V. (2000) *Adv. Drug Del. Rev.* **43**, 101.

Wagner E., Curiel D. and Cotton M. (1994) *Adv. Drug Deliv. Rev*. **14**, 113.

Wagner E., Zatloukal K., Cotton M., Kirlappos H., Mechtler K. and Curiel D. T. (1992) *Proc. Natl. Acad. Sci. USA* **89**, 6099.

Watanabe N., Sato Y., Yamauchi N. and Nitsu Y. (1998) *Nippon Rinsho* **56**, 724.

Weissman A. M., Harford J. B., Svetlik P. B., Leonard W. L., Depper J. M., Waldmann T. A., Greene W. C. and Klausner R. D. (1986) *Proc. Natl. Acad. Sci. USA* **83**, 1463.

Weissner J. H. and Hwang K .J. (1982) *Biochim. Biophys. Acta.* **689**, 490.

Wright S. and Huang L. (1989) *Adv. Drug Deliv. Rev.* **3**, 343.

Wu D., Yang J. and Pardridge W. M. (1997) *J. Clin. Invest.* **100**, 1804.

Wu M., Fan J., Gunning W. and Ratnam M. (1997) *J. Membr. Biol.* **159**, 137.

Yoshikawa T. and Pardridge W. M. (1992) *J. Pharmacol. Exp. Ther.* **263**, 897.

Zarling J. M., Moren P. A., Haffar O., Sias J., Richman D. D., Spina C. A., Myers D. E., Kuelbelbeck V., Ledbetter J. A. and Uckun F. M. (1990) *Nature* **347**, 92.

CHAPTER 4

Chemical Drug Delivery

- Introduction
- Prodrugs and chemical delivery systems
- Soft drug approach
- Membrane transporters as targeting site
- Conclusion
- References

Many therapeutically active drugs have undesirable properties that may become pharmacological, pharmaceutical or pharmacokinetic barriers in clinical drug application. Among various means of minimizing the undesirable drug properties while retaining the desirable therapeutic activity, the chemical approach using drug derivatization offers perhaps the highest flexibility and has been proved as an important approach of improving drug efficacy. The prodrug approach involving reversible derivatives, can be utilized for optimization of the clinical application of a drug. The prodrug concept was initiated for improving drug therapy in the early 1970s and since then numerous prodrugs have been designed and developed to overcome pharmaceutical and pharmacokinetic barriers like low oral drug absorption, specificity, lack of site, toxicity, chemical instability and poor patient compliance due to bad taste, odour, pain at injection site, etc. Albert, 1958 has introduced the term "Prodrug" or "Proagent" to signify pharmacologically inactive chemical derivatives that could be used to alter the physicochemical properties of bioactives in a temporary fashion to increase their usefulness and/or to retard associated toxicity. Prodrugs have also been called "Latentiated drugs", "Bioreversible derivatives" and "Congeners", however "prodrug" is now the most commonly accepted term (Sinkula and Yalkowsky, 1975; Stella et al., 1985). Usually prodrug implies a covalent link between a drug and a chemical moiety though some researchers also use this term to characterize some salts of the active drug. Although there is no strict definition for a prodrug, generally they are defined as pharmacologically inert chemical derivatives that can be converted *in vivo* to the active drug molecules, enzymatically or non-enzymatically to express its therapeutic efficacy. Ideally a prodrug should be broken down to parent active form at the target site with subsequent elimination of the released derivatizing group (Banerjee and Amidon, 1985).

A more advanced version of prodrugs is chemical delivery system (CDS) in which the drug is transformed into an inactive derivative, which will then undergo sequential enzymatic transformations to deliver a drug at its site of action. Another term called soft drugs, which are designed to have highly improved therapeutic indices and are isosteric/

isoelectronic analogs of lead drug, is included in broader term "Retrometabolic Drug Design" with chemical delivery systems (CDS) and prodrugs as its branches. The retrometabolic drug design approaches simultaneously incorporate structure activity (SAR) and structure metabolism (SMR) relationships in the design process. Two major approaches were developed, CDS, which allow chemical-enzymatic targeting of drugs via strategic sequential enzymatic activation of the inactive CDS and the soft drug (SD), with improved therapeutic indices by controlling their metabolism after they achieve their therapeutic role. In essence, retrometabolic approaches represent a complex collection of chemical-enzymatic means for the design of safer drugs and for their controlled release.

PRODRUGS AND CHEMICAL DELIVERY SYSTEMS

Prodrug approach and chemical delivery system (CDS) involve chemical modification of the drug. This promoiety essentially has the same pharmacological features as the lead drug but possesses different pharmacokinetic properties. The prodrug concept implies to improve the drug delivery through a chemical transformation of the active drug substances into inactive derivatives, which convert to the parent compounds due to their enzymatic chemical lability, within the body before or after reaching the site(s) of action. Prodrugs are usually activated in a single step enzymatic attack, however chemical delivery system involves a cascade of enzymatic reactions for activation. Chemical delivery systems (CDSs) are utilized for sustained drug delivery as well as site specific targeted drug delivery. These chemically modulated systems can be designed to target specific enzymes or carriers by considering enzyme-substrate specificity or carrier-substrate specificity in order to overcome various undersirable drug properties. This type of chemically modulated targeted drug design requires considerable knowledge of particular enzymes or carrier systems, including their molecular and functional characteristics. In chemically modulated prodrug design, enzymes can be recognized as presystemic metabolic sites or promoiety *in vivo* reconversion sites. The enzyme targeted prodrug approach can be broadly used to improve oral drug absorption vis-à-vis site specific drug delivery. Oral drug absorption can be improved by using gastrointestinal enzymes as the main targets, moreover use of a nutrient moiety as a derivatizing group gives more specific targeting to gastrointestinal enzymes (Amidon et al., 1980). There are three factors that should be optimized to achieve the site-specific delivery of drugs through promoiety approach:

1. The promoiety must be rapidly transported to the site of action and uptake to the site must be rapid and preferably via perfusion process.
2. After reaching the site of action promoiety should be selectively dissociated to the active drug relative to its cleavage at other body sites.
3. Once selectively cleaved at the site of action the active drug must be retained at the site.

In this approach, site specific delivery can be achieved from tissue-specific activation of a promoiety, which is the result of metabolism by an enzyme system that is either unique of the tissue or present in higher concentrations compared with other tissues. This causes an efficient activation of promoiety like glycosidase activity of colonic microflora, which provides an opportunity to design a colon-specific drug delivery system (Bohme et al., 1974). Glycoside derivatives are hydrophilic and therefore, poorly absorbed from the small intestine, however, once they reach the colon, they can be effectively cleaved by bacterial glycosidases to release the free drug or be absorbed by the colonic mucosa.

Eye as a Target Organ

The details of anatomy and physiology of eye is described by Ueno and Refojo, 1983. The eyelids are covered externally by skin and internally by conjunctiva, which is reflected over the globe of the eye. The lacrimal glands, which are compound racemose glands, are situated at the ocular upper angle of the orbit. The globe of the eye is composed of 3 layers: the cornea sclera, choroid iris and retina. The cornea consists of stratified epithelium, which may be regarded as continuation of the conjunctiva over the cornea. The sclera is composed of dense fibrous tissue, which is thickest at the back of the eyeball. The choroid is the vascular membrane in contact with the sclera and iris is the continuation of the choroid, which extends in front of the lens. The retina is part of the central nervous system and corresponds in extent to the choroid, which it lines. The lens is the biconvex mass of laminated tissue with transparent elastic capsule. The anterior chamber is the space filled with the aqueous humour, and is bounded by the cornea of the lens exposed in the pupil. The posterior chamber containing aqueous humour is the triangular space between the back of the iris, the anterior surface of the lens and ciliary body forming its apex at the pupillary margin. The vitreous chamber is the large space behind the lens containing gelatinous material, the vitreous humour.

The eye has earlier not been considered seriously for site-targeted drug delivery due to its direct accessibility to topical treatment. The cornea acts as a stern barrier against foreign substances including drugs for entry to various intraocular sites. Tears that are flowing continuously take part of an applied dose, which passes unabsorbed through the nasal-lacrymal canal and subsequently into the nasal and gastric mucosa. These mucosal sites are excellent areas for drug trafficking to the general circulation.

Currently, the drugs used for ophthalmologic therapy have not been optimized for the eye, but are basically systemic drugs as β-adrenergic agonists or antagonists, which are having profound effect when enter into the systemic circulation, thereby many dangerous systemic side effects can be precipitated after topical dosing of drugs in the eye. When β-blockers such as betaxolol or timolol are used for glaucoma treatment, peripheral bronchial β-adreno-receptor blockade can be precipitated, which may cause respiratory distress and even death (Schoene et al., 1984; Richards and Tattersfield, 1985; Franunfelder and Barker, 1985). Therefore, a selective drug delivery to eye can conceal many of these untoward effects and in turn greatly increase the safety of drugs. One of the leading method for this selective delivery to eye is a reduction/hydrolysis dependent chemical delivery systems (CDS).

Chemical Delivery Systems for Eye

A keto-derivative of epinephrine, adrenalone has in itself no sympathomimetic property, when applied topically on eye as a potential mydriatic agent. However, the esterified derivative of adrenalone with lipophilic carboxylic acids, the diesters exert profound mydriatic effects (Bodor et al., 1978). Studies have shown that the adrenalone esters undergo an initial ketone reduction *in vivo* in the eye followed by hydrolysis of ester resulting in epinephrine release (Bodor and Visor, 1984) (Fig. 4-1). The adrenalone esters appear to be reduced at the site of their action, the iris-ciliary body, while at all other sites of eye only inactive adrenalone is generated. It has been suggested that adrenalone, itself is not a reductase substrate as administration of adrenalone didn't lead to elevation of epinephrine levels. This epinephrine CDS provides potent mydriatic effects useful for diagnostic and various surgical procedures such as virectomy lens implantations or lens removal.

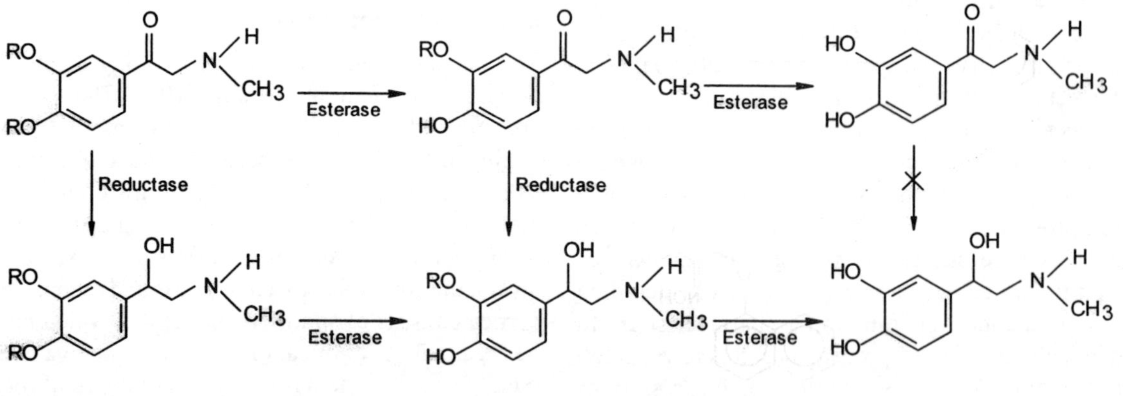

Fig. 4-1. Ketone Reduction of Adrenalone Esters followed by Ester Hydrolysis Results in Release of Epinepherine

Another approach has been made to conceal the undesirable side effects associated with β-blocking agents used in the treatment of glaucoma. Ketone analogues of β-hydroxyamino β-blockers have been proposed, which would undergo iris-ciliary reduction releasing the active drug. However, due to chemical instability such requisite precursors of propranolol, carteolol, timolol, etc. have not been synthesized. Nevertheless, a relatively stable intermediate, a hydrolytically stable oxime was considered (Bodor et al., 1978). This CDS undergoes oxime hydrolysis to yield the intermediate ketone, which subsequently undergoes reduction in the iris-ciliary body to yield the active β-blocker. As this drug activation occurs selectively in the eye no systemic toxicity has been noted from the CDS, which escapes the ocular sites.

The CDS of propranolol has been prepared as shown in Figure 4-2. The oximes of the β-blockers have been similarly synthesized. There is a generalized opinion that β-blockers with high degrees of lipophilicity give rise to more active CDSs (El-koussi and Bodor, 1989).

The oxime compounds are mixtures of E/Z isomers that are stable in aqueous solutions, however upon separation of this isomeric mixture showed that Z and E isomers are equipotent and these oximes also lack any irritating property when applied topically to eye. On application of the propranolol or alprenolol ketamine derivative to eye, a series of enzymatic reactions occurs as illustrated in Figure 4-3. Both the E/Z isomers of oximes remain in equilibrium in the eye. The intermediate ketone and parent drug are produced in the eye from both E and Z isomers that are hydrolyzed to give a unitary ketone, which subsequently undergoes reduction to yield the more potent S (–) isomer (Howe and Shanks, 1966). Thus the hydrolysis/reduction sequences mediated by intraocular enzymes give an optically active drug from CDS. The CDS thus generated are more potent and manifest lesser side-effects compared to the parent β-blockers. The CDS liberates the drug only at the site of action, i.e. eye and systemic administration of the CDS results in no change in heart rate or any other cardiovascular effect.

Skin

Skin is the most easily accessible route of drug administration, however, due to presence of stratum corneum and other cell layers it becomes challenging for drugs to pass through this stern barrier into systemic circulation. Prodrugs have been extensively utilized as tools for enhancement of transdermal absorption. Various new types of promoieties or masking groups have been synthesized that enable one to incorporate a particularly desirable property into the prodrug.

α-Acyloxyalkyl Prodrugs

This class of prodrugs is most extensively studied derivatives used for optimizing dermal delivery.

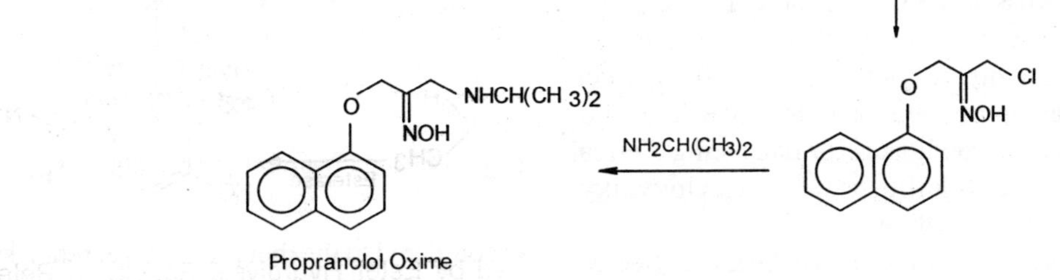

OH
CH_3
O
Cl
OH
DCC
DMSO
Pyridine
O
Cl
O
$NH_2OH.HCl$
O
Cl
NOH
$NH_2CH(CH_3)_2$
O
$NHCH(CH_3)_2$
NOH
Propranolol Oxime

Fig. 4-2. Synthesis of Propranolol Oxime

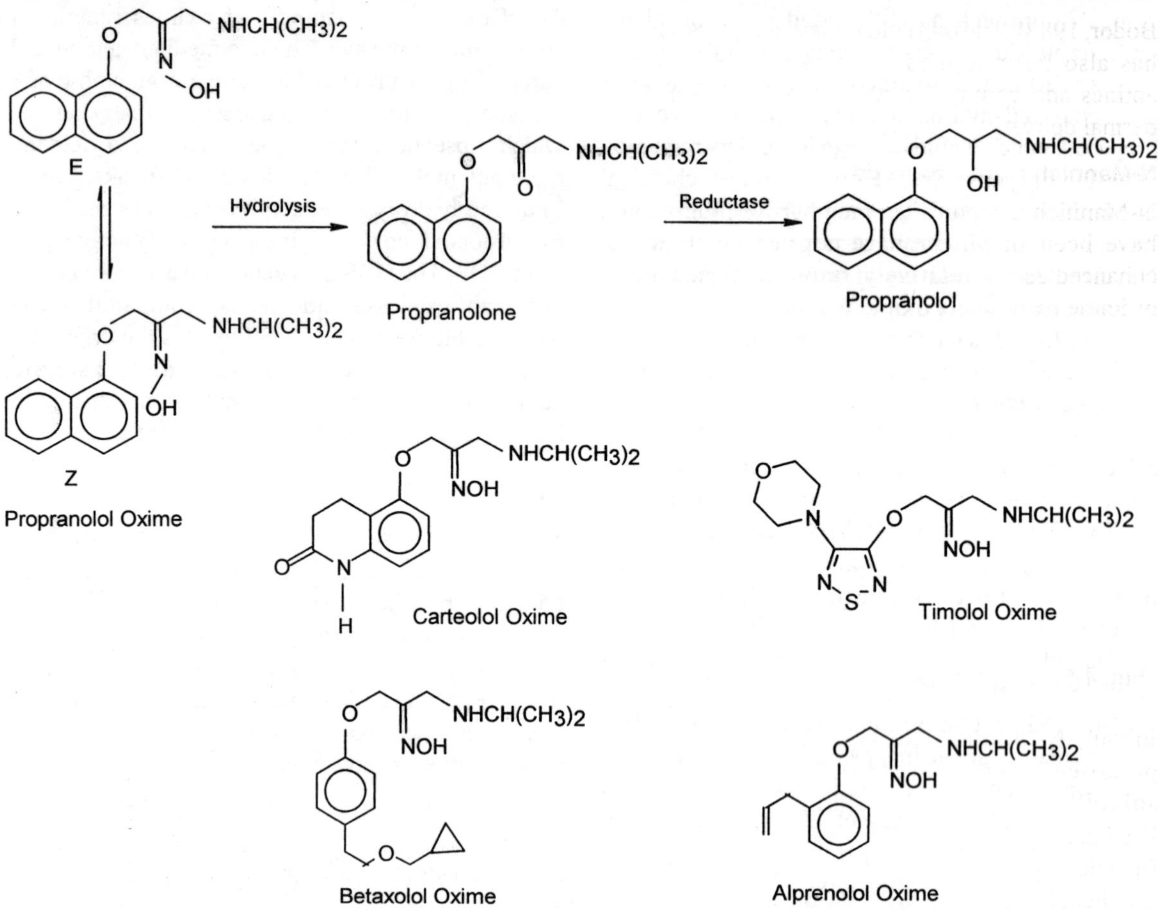

NHCH(CH3)2
E
Hydrolysis
Propranolone
Reductase
Propranolol
Z
Propranolol Oxime
Carteolol Oxime
Timolol Oxime
Betaxolol Oxime
Alprenolol Oxime

Fig. 4-3. Enzymatic Events occurring after Local Application of Propranolol or Alprenolol Ketoxime Derivatives to the Eye

Although the α-Acyloxyalkyl derivatives are alkyl derivatives, they are very similar to the O-acyl prodrug derivatives.

α-Acyloxyalkyl derivative of nitrofurantoin was the first prodrug in this class (Spencer and Michaels, 1964), followed by benzyl penicillin prodrug in 1965 (Jansen and Russell, 1965). Bodor and Sloan, 1977 extensively studied theophylline prodrugs and provided an important information based on which subsequent attempts were made for the selection of optimum prodrug candidates for enhancing dermal delivery. Figure 4-4 illustrates α-Acyloxyalkyl derivatives of theophylline.

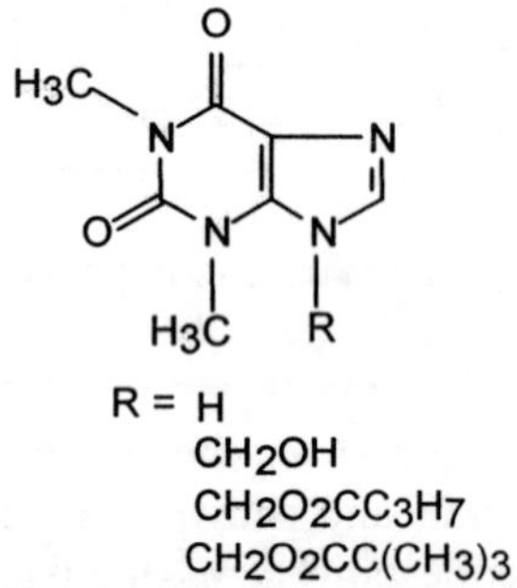

$R = H$
CH_2OH
$CH_2O_2CC_3H_7$
$CH_2O_2CC(CH_3)_3$

Fig. 4-4. Acyl oxymethyl derivative of Theophylline

All the derivatives are known to be more effective than theophylline, since they are more lipid soluble as compared to the theophylline yet retain significant hydrophilicity compared to theophylline (Sloan and

Bodor, 1982). The α-Acyloxyalkyl prodrugs strategy has also been applied to amides, thiols, imides, amines and carboxylic acids to achieve enhanced dermal delivery.

N-Mannich Base Prodrugs

N-Mannich base or amino methyl type derivatives have been shown to possess great potential for enhanced dermal delivery of drugs containing amide or imide functional groups (Fig. 4-5).

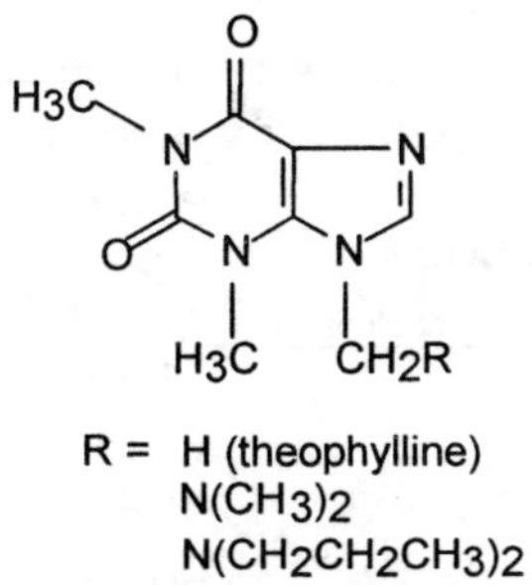

R = H (theophylline)
$N(CH_3)_2$
$N(CH_2CH_2CH_3)_2$

Fig. 4-5. Mannich Base Prodrugs of Theophylline

Initially N-Mannich base type derivatives had been proposed to improve the dissolution and water solubility of amide and imide (Johansen and Bundgaard, 1980). The first report of the use of N-Mannich bases for enhanced dermal delivery has been for theophylline and 5-fluoro uracil (Sloan et al., 1984). In addition to N-Mannich base prodrugs of the usual amides and imides, N-Mannich bases of the exocyclic amino group are also suggested as well as prodrugs of purine and pyrimidine nucleosides have been synthesized (Koch and Sloan, 1987; Sloan and Silver, 1984).

Acyl Prodrugs

Acyl prodrugs have been used to improve the dermal delivery of some drugs, especially steroids (Schlagel, 1965). Yu et al., 1980, demonstrated the effect of 51-acyl derivatives of Ara-A on the delivery of Ara-A through mouse skin and shown that the prodrug possess higher permeability across the skin compared to parent drug molecule.

(Bisalkyl Hetero) Alkyl Prodrugs

This prodrug strategy has been exploited for enhanced dermal delivery of drugs possessing ketone or aldehyde functional groups. The cysteine ethyl ester and β-amino ethyl thiol thiazolidine derivatives of hydrocortisone 21-acetate have shown relatively more activity and less toxicity compared to parent steroids (Bodor et al., 1982). 3,4-dimethyl-5-phenyl oxazolidine has been shown to be 90 times more effective than ephedrine for delivering ephedrine across human skin (Pitman et al., 1986).

CDS for Kidney

Kidney possesses high concentrations of L-glutamyl transpeptidase and L-amino acid decarboxylase. Selective delivery of dopamine in kidney has been obtained after administration of L-γ-glutamyl dopa produces almost 5 times higher concentrations of dopamine in kidney compared with equivalent dose of L-dopa (Mizoguchi et al., 1979). L-γ-glutamyl dopa is cleaved to dopamine in two steps catalyzed by γ-glutamyl transpeptidase followed by L-amino acid decarboxylase. Initially, γ-glutamyl linkage of promoiety is cleaved by γ-glutamyl transpeptidase producing L-dopa, which is further converted to dopamine by the L-amino acid decarboxylase. This leads to a selective activation of promoiety in kidney achieving a desired renal vasodialatation in kidney, while avoiding the systemic hypotension (Fig. 4-6). N-acyl-γ-glutamyl prodrug of sulphmethoxazole has also been synthesized with high efficiency of selective delivery. These promoieties are used for treating renal and urinary tract infections.

Lung as a Target Organ

The lung possesses the next highest levels of nearly all the metabolic enzymes found in liver (Damani, 1987) and in some cases even higher specific activities in certain cell types. Additionally, in contrast to all other tissues, the lung receives total venous return first, so it is in an ideal position to regulate the concentration of substrates in the blood before they reach the arterial circulation (Alabaster, 1977), hence avoiding problems that may be associated with a hepatic first pass and permitting a more efficacious sequestration of a drug entity in the lung. Lipoic acid (1,2-dithiolane-3-pentanoic acid or thioctic acid) has a potential to form disulfide linkages and has been investigated as targeting moiety in a CDS for selective drug delivery to lung tissue. Lipoic acid is non-toxic and it is a coenzyme for acyl transfer and redox

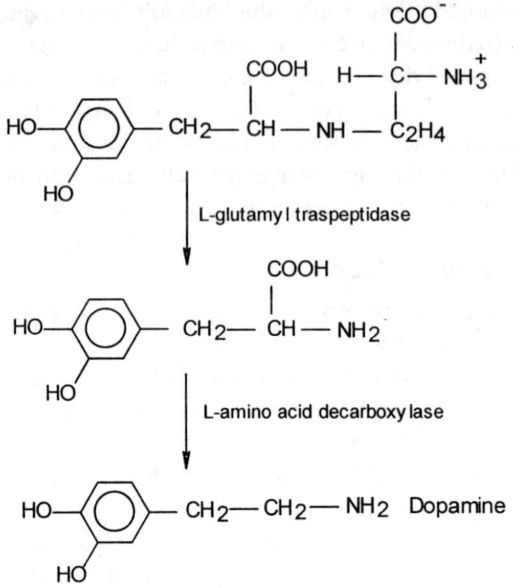

Fig. 4-6. Breakdown of L-γ Glutamyl Prodrug of DOPA by Kidney Enzymes

reactions in living systems (Kijima et al., 1984). Chlorambucil (4-[p-[bis(2-chloroethyl)amino]-phenyl] butyric acid), is a bifunctional nitrogen mustard alkylating agent that has shown wide clinical activity as an antineoplastic agent particularly against chronic lymphocytic leukaemia and malignant lymphomas (Oppitz et al., 1989; Greg et al., 1990), primarily due to its aldylation reaction with DNA. There are some problems associated with its use, which include a wide variety of major but usually dose limiting toxicity effects involving haematologic (e.g., Myelosuppression and anemia), gastrointestinal (nausea, anorexia), neurological (CNS effects like seizures, ataxia, etc.), dermatologic, immunologic (immunosuppression) and even mutagenic and carcinogenic effects. Introduction of the lipoyl groups to mask the ionizable carboxylic acid group will increase its lipophilicity and hence enhance its bioavailability in addition to the desired targeting capability and ultimately reduce its systemic toxicity. Figure 4-7 illustrates the pathway of chlorambucil CDS synthesis. Cromoglyn or disodium cromoglycate, DSCG, is a bis-chromone, the sodium salt of 1,3-bis[(2-carboxychromon-5-yl]-2-hydroxypropane. It is used primarily in the prophylactic treatment of asthma and allergic rhinitis. Although DSCG is the safest antiasthma drug currently in use (Kuzemko, 1989), it has very poor bioavailability as it is too polar and very water-soluble. It is thus poorly absorbed and rapidly cleared from the body. Figure 4-8 shows the steps of DSCG CDS. It has been observed CDS of DSCG and chlorambucil provided a significant and sustained released of the active drug over a protracted period of time.

Colon Targeting

Colon specific drug delivery can be accomplished by producing a polar promoiety with retarded

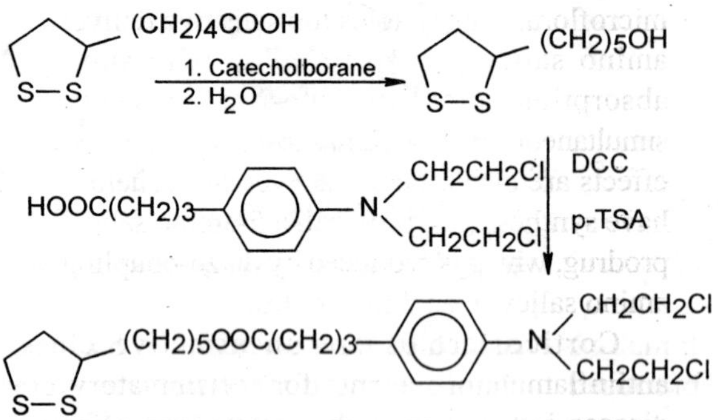

Fig. 4-7. Synthesis of Chlorambucil Prodrug

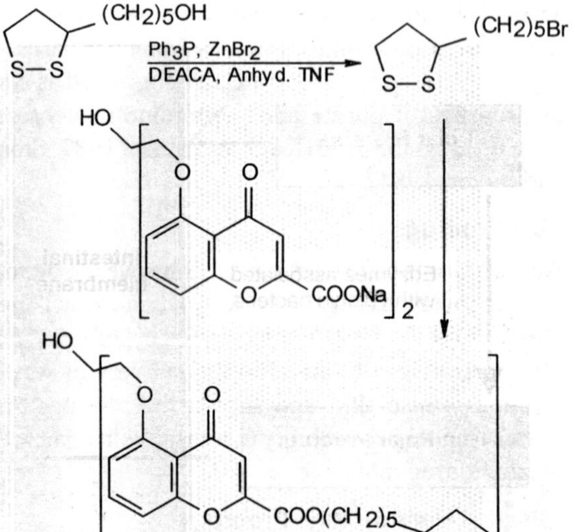

Fig. 4-8. Synthesis of Cromoglyn Prodrug

intestinal absorption, however, when it reaches colon it will be cleaved to a lipophilic entity, which can readily be absorbed (Fig. 4-9). Colonic microflora possesses many enzymes that offer an opportunity to design colon-specific chemical drug delivery systems. Sulphasalazine represents a typical example of colon specific prodrug approach, it is synthesized by coupling of diazotized 2-sulphanilamide pyridine and 5-amino salicylic acid (Pappercorn and Goldman, 1973). On oral intake a huge amount of sulphasalazine reaches colon due to non-absorption by small intestine and biliary excretion. After reaching the colon the prodrug is cleaved into active species 5-amino salicylic acid by azoreductase associated with colonic microflora. This enables the selective delivery of 5-amino salicylic acid to colon with subsequent absorption across the intestinal epithelium and simultaneously pre-colonic absorption associated side effects are also retarded. Jewel and Truelove, 1981 have synthesized azodiazal, a 5-amino salicylic acid prodrug, which is produced by diazo-coupling of two amino salicylic acid molecules.

Corticosteroids are an effective class of antiinflammatory agents for inflammatory bowel disease but due to their serious side effects and ineffective concentration, when given orally or systemically led to development of prodrugs.

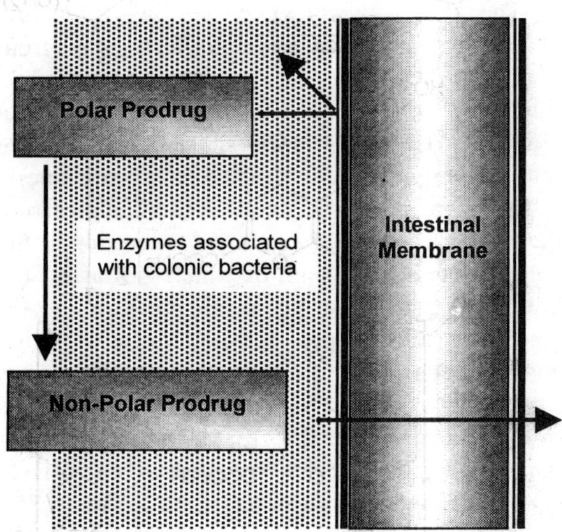

Fig. 4-9. Fate of Polar Prodrug in Colon

Glucuronidic (Nolen and Friend, 1994) and Glycosidic (Friend and Chang, 1985) prodrugs of dexamethasone and naloxone utilizing the activities of glucuronidases and glycosidases present in colon are reported. Poly-L-aspartic acid prodrug of dexamethasone also shows greater hydrolysis in colon compared to small intestine and therefore can be considered for drug targeting (Leopard and Friend, 1995).

CDS for Liver Targeting

Liver is an important organ and is considered to be focal point of metabolic activities in body. Targeted drug delivery to liver is achieved using bile acid transport system associated with the sinusoidal membrane of the hepatocytes (Anwer et al., 1976). Kramer et al., 1992 developed bile acid prodrug of chlorambucil for liver targeting. Thyroid hormone (L-T3) has been targeted to liver using bile acids as navigator units (Stephan et al., 1992). Hepatic asialoglycoprotein receptor mediated endocytosis has been exploited for antiviral drugs targeting to liver parenchymal cells (Wall et al., 1980).

Lymphatic Targeting

The lymphatic system is regarded as an integral and necessary part of the vascular system. Its main function is to collect the excessive tissue fluid and return it back to the blood. Lymphatics are numerous in number and distributed throughout the body. Their major physiological function is to maintain the body's water balance, thus acting as body's drainage system. The intestinal lymphatic system consists of a network of vessels distributed throughout the small and large intestine. They play a major role in the absorption of variety of nutrients, lipids including long chain fatty acids, triglycerides, cholesterol esters (Shiau, 1987), fluids, lipid soluble vitamins (Yeung and Vonsaigent, 1972), some xenobiotics (e.g. DDT) (Sieber, 1976) and drugs (Charman and Stella, 1991).

The intestinal lymphatic system offers a potential route for drug molecules to enter systemic circulation subsequent to oral administration. The physiology of the intestinal lymphatic system is such that drug transported from the intestinal lumen by the intestinal lymph gains an access directly to the general circulation of the body at the junction of the left internal jugular and left subclavian vein, thereby avoiding initial liver contact (Youmans, 1962).

The potential advantage of transporting drug through the intestinal lymphatic system includes :

1. Avoidance of hepatic first-pass metabolism.
2. Selective treatment of diseases and infections of the mesenteric lymphatic system.
3. Directing the delivery of appropriate agent to various sites of the intestinal and thoracic lymphatic system.
4. Enhancement of the absorption of large macromolecules such as peptides and particulates.
5. Inhibition of cancer cell metastasis.
6. Lymphocytic targeting and receptor mediated targeting via the low density lipoproteins receptor to regions of the lymphatics that are directly supplied by lymph from mesenteric lymphatics (these regions are often poorly perfused by the systemic circulation making it difficult to attain adequate drug concentration at the target organ/cell after the compound has absorbed via the portal blood)
7. Reduction in local gastrointestinal irritation and toxicity and
8. An overall modulation in the rate of drug input, thus providing a sustained delivery.

Anatomical and Physiological Considerations

The lymphatic vessels in the small intestine originate as elongated blind-ended vessels known as lacteal, in the center of each villus (Fig. 4-10). The finger-like villi host one central lacteal, whereas flattened villi, such as those found in rats, host several vessels (Kvietys et al., 1981). The lacteals are approximately 20 μm in diameter and are located at a distance of about 50 μm from the epithelial cells. The lacteals join a plexus of the lymphatic capillaries in the glandular layer of the mucosa and then pass down to a submucosal network of collecting lymphatics.

Numerous anastomoses exist between the lymphatics of mucosa and the submucosa. The superior mesenteric collecting lymphatic vessel drains the small intestine and the ascending and transverse colon, while the inferior mesenteric vessel drains the descending and sigmoid colon. The mesenteric lymph drains into the cisterna chyli and is returned to general circulation via the thoracic duct thus avoiding the liver

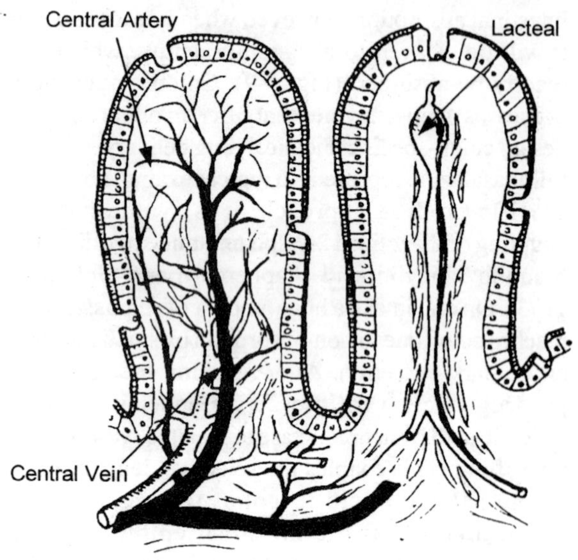

Fig. 4-10. Vessels of the Intestinal villus

and potential first pass metabolism (Granger, 1981; Barrowman, 1978; Granger and Kvietys, 1984) (Fig. 4-11). Intestinal lymph flow rates vary between species and are influenced by fluid and food intake. A large difference exists between intestinal lymph and blood flow rates. The relative flow of portal blood to intestinal lymph is approximately 500:1.

The intestinal lymphatic system plays a vital role in removing fluids and proteins, which escape from the blood circulation and in transporting, absorbed fluids and some nutrients from the lamina propria (Taylor and Granger, 1984; Granger et al, 1984). The rate of lymph formation in the small intestine is influenced mainly by the rate of fluid filtration across the capillaries and the rate of fluid absorption by the mucosal membrane, both of which will affect the interstitial hydrostatic and oncotic pressure.

As a result of lipid digestion and absorption, chylomicrons are synthesized within the enterocytes. The chylomicrons are released from the enterocytes by exocytosis and as their size is large enough to enter the blood capillaries, they are taken up exclusively via lymphatic system (Sabesin and Frase, 1977). Removal of chylomicrons from the mucosal interstition is one of the major functions of intestinal lymphatic. The transport of lipophilic compounds via

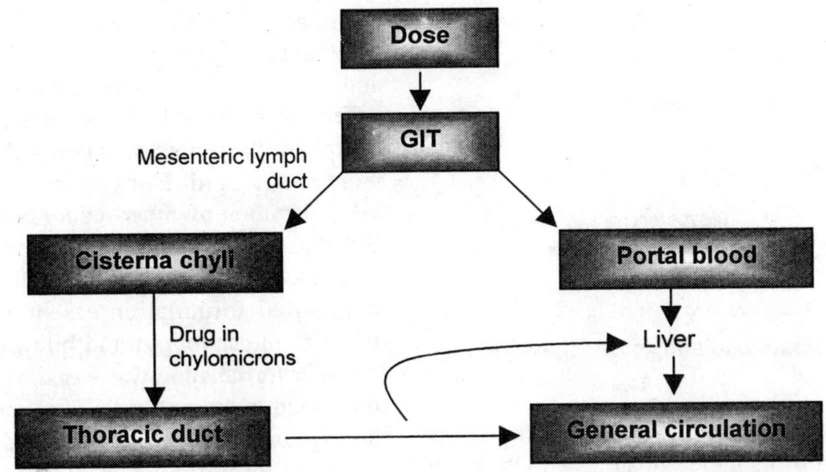

Fig. 4-11. Entry of Drug into Systemic Circulation after Oral Administration

intestinal lymphatics occurs primarily in association with the chylomicrons of the intestinal lipoproteins produced by enterocytes. Therefore, it is the chylomicron flux that at large determines lymphatic transport (Charman and Stella, 1986).

There is an increased intestinal or thoracic duct lymph flow following a meal or fluid ingestion (Barrowman, 1978). During net fluid absorption, the increase is 5-20 times higher than normal lymph flow in the non-absorptive state (Granger et al., 1980). The magnitude of increase is quite variable, due to the factors such as tonicity of the fluid ingested, portal vein pressure, intraenteric pressure and GI mobility. In any event, the overall lymphatic absorption rate in the absorptive state usually does not exceed 15-20 % (Granger, 1981). There have been two major prodrug approaches explored for increasing the overall lipophilicity of compounds. The first approach involves the lipophilic derivatization of compounds via simple ester or ether linkages.

The second approach is based on promoieties (prodrug/candidate), which particularly involve either passively or actively formation of chylomicrons by the enterocytes.

Simple Ester or Ether Prodrugs

Prodrugs to Avoid Presystemic Metabolism

Early works on prodrugs involve the evaluation of lipophilic of steroidal compounds and lipophilic vitamins for their improved oral bioavailability.

Testosterone

Testosterone is used in the treatment of androgen deficiency syndrome in men. It undergoes nearly complete hepatic first pass metabolism after oral dosing (Dagett et al., 1978). Depot parenteral formulations of testosterone esters are available, which provide for prolonged therapy, but oral therapy offers the advantages of patient compliance, convenience and better control over dosing profile. Coert et al., 1975 prepared the undecanoate ester of testosterone (Fig. 4-12) for improved oral bioavailability. It is a long chain alkyl ester of testosterone. It is preferentially and exclusively transported via the intestinal lymphatics, whereas the plain testosterone is not transported through lymphatics (Sieber et al., 1974). Kishimoto, 1973 has reported that testosterone esters may have intrinsic pharmacological activity of their own. Noguchi et al., 1985 determined the lymphatic transport of a series of testosterone esters (heptanate, undecanoate, palmitate and oleate) in a conscious rat model. A linear correlation between degree of lymphatic transport of the ester and free testosterone and logarithm of the heptane/water partition coefficient was also established. Tauber et al., 1980 reported comparative bioavailability of testosterone and its undecanoate ester in human. The absolute oral bioavailability of testosterone is 3.6±2.5% of the administered dose, which is apparently low due to consistent high first pass effect whereas the systemic

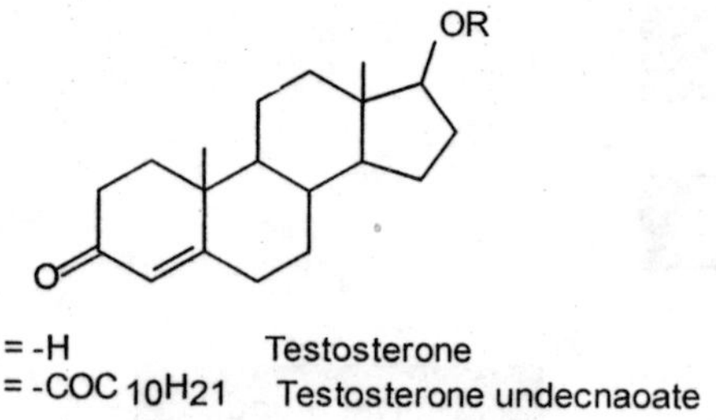

Fig. 4-12. Testosterone and its Undecanoate Ester

availability was doubled to 6.8±3.3 % in case of oral administration of its undecanoate ester. Obviously, the higher bioavailability accounts for hydrophilic prodrug, which transported through lymphatic avoiding major first pass metabolism.

Epitiostanol and Mepitiostane

Epitiostanol (EP) is a lipophilic epithiosteroid with anti-oestrogenic activity, and used in the treatment of breast cancer. It is administered intramuscularly, because of its extensive hepatic first pass metabolism when administered orally. Mepitiostane (MP), the 17 substituted methylglycopentane derivative of EP was designed as a prodrug for avoiding the extensive first metabolism associated with oral administration of EP (Ichihashi et al, 1992) (Fig. 4-13). The clinical profile of orally administered MP compared well with intramuscularly administered EP in terms of anti-estrogenic activity. Ichihashi et al., 1991 and Ichihashi et al., 1992 conducted a series of studies to determine the extent of lymphatic absorption of MP and effect of various lipid vehicle and bile salts on its lymphatic uptake. The extent of lymphatic absorption was determined using a thoracic duct fistulated rat model and approximately 35% of the administered dose of ^{14}C labeled MP (2 mg/kg in sesame oil) was recovered in lymph, where more than 90% of the radioactivity was found associated with the lipid core of the chylomicrons and VLDL fraction of lymph, suggesting active involvement of VLDL/ chylomicron indigenous biovectors in lymphatic transportation of MP.

Vitamin A

Vitamin is commonly available as an alcohol (retinol) or as an esterified form such as retinyl acetate or palmitate. It is absorbed from the gastrointestinal tract and transported to systemic circulation via the intestinal lymphatics (Blomhoff et al., 1984). The effect of various lipid vehicle on the extent of lymphatic transport of vitamin A was studied by Fernandez and Borgstrom, 1990 after oral administration of either retinol or retinyl palmitate. Retinol and its fatty acid ester were administered contained in emulsion and micellar solutions. The emulsified formulation essentially consisted of triolein, phospholipid and bile salts, whereas the micellar formulation was based on a 2:1 mixture of oleic acid and monolein. The extent of lymphatic absorption of vitamin A was independent of the chemical form of vitamin A when administered in the micellar formulation as approximately 50% of the administered dose was recovered in, lymph after oral administration of either retinol or its palmitic acid ester. In the case of emulsified formulation, the lymphatic transport of retinyl palmitate was approximately 50% of the administered dose, whereas transport after administration of emulsified retinol was estimated approximately 20% of the administered dose.

Berr and Kern, 1984 studied the lymphatic utake of retinyl palmitate in healthy human subjects and concluded that retinyl palmitate present in the chylomicron and intestinal VLDL stays associated with the lipoproteins in both *in vitro* and *in vivo*. They suggested that retinyl palmitate could be used as marker for the disposition of chylomicrons and chylomicron remmants. The preferential association

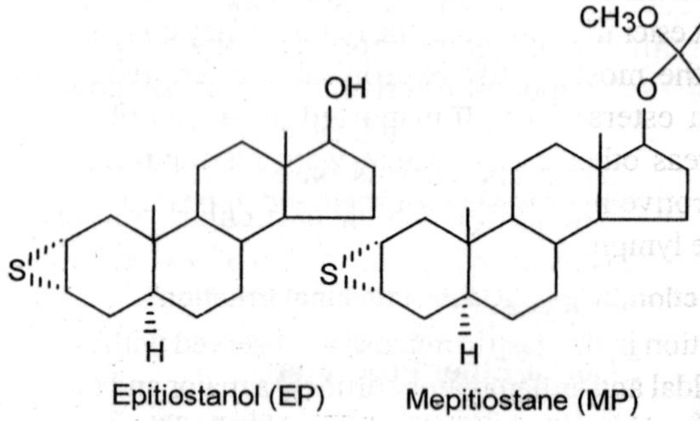

Fig. 4-13. Epitiostanol and its Prodrug Mepitiostane (MP)

of retinyl palmitate with chylomicron is responsible for its higher lymphatic transportation and as a result systemic availability.

Vitamin E

Most of the prodrugs studies, which have demonstrated better pharmaceutical and absorption properties especially pertaining to lipid soluble vitamins have focussed on the vitamin E, because of two reasons :

1. Vitamin E (α-tocopherol) is chemically unstable due to oxidation of the phenolic group (Nakamura et al., 1975). The preparation of simple esters prevents oxidation of the phenolic group thereby enhances the stability profile of the administered compound.
2. Vitamin E, a oil soluble vitamin is poorly absorbed on its oral administration. It therefore offers spectrum of possibilities of improved bioavailability if judiciously opted method is adapted. The methods essentially involve prodrug approaches or formulation based approaches (Kuksis, 1986).

Nakamura et al., 1975 prepared and evaluated a series of α-tocopheryl esters, which include straight chain, and branched alkyl esters as well as succinic and aromatic esters such as benzoate and nicotinate (Fig. 4-14). Higher lymphatic transport was recorded after oral administration of simple straight chain acetate and palmitate esters (approx. 50% of the dose administered), with the majority of the vitamin E related species being present as α-tocopherol. For the branched and aromatic esters of α-tocopherol, lymphatic transport estimated to be about 10% of the administered dose with a larger proportion of the intact ester transported in the lymph. They concluded that the most readily hydrolysable esters (straight chain esters) were transported as α-tocopherol, whereas other esters, which were resistant to pre-absorptive hydrolysis absorbed and appeared intact in the lymph.

R = H alpha-Tocopherol
R = $COCH_3$ alpha-Tocopheryl acetate
R = (nicotinoyl) alpha-Tocopheryl nicotinate

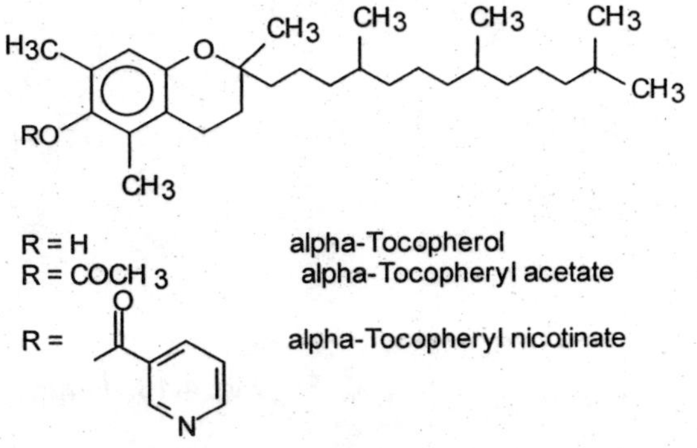

Fig. 4-14. α-Tocopherol and its Esters

Reduction in Local Gastrointestinal Irritation

Irritation in the gastric mucosa as observed with non-steroidal anti-inflammatory drugs is a major and often limiting side effect. Relatively simple alkyl lipophilic esters of a variety of anti-inflammatory agents have been evaluated for their gastrointestinal irritation effect. Indomethacin is an anti-inflammatory agent having severe gastrointestinal side effects. Kobayashi et al., 1988 and Mishima et al., 1990 evaluated the farnesyl ester of indomethacin (Fig. 4-15) for its ability to deliver indomethacin systemically with low degree of gastric irritation. When farnesyl ester of indomethacin administered orally to rats, approximately 12% of the ester prodrug was transported via the intestinal lymphatics over 8-hour period. Analysis of the intestinal lipoproteins indicated that more than 90% of the lymphatic transported drug transversed as intact prodrug associated with the chylomicrons fraction of lymph. There was no unchanged prodrug detected in portal blood. Nevertheless, indomethacin related compounds in the liver and plasma were estimated. These are the metabolic products of indomethacin formed during pre-absorptive hydrolysis of the prodrug. The prodrug and indomethacin both were orally available and pharmacodynamically active as estimated in a carrageenan-induced rat paw oedema model (Kumakura et al., 1990). The ulcerogenic potential of indomethacin farnesyl was found to be low, when assessed in humans. It was considerably less potent too than indomethacin in inducing damage to mucosa of the stomach and intestine of the rat (Murukami et al., 1988).

Functionally Designed Promoieties

Because of the metabolic liability associated with the simple ester-based promoieties limited their use, therefore attempts have been made to evaluate other functional approaches as a means for enhancing lymphatic transport. These functional approaches

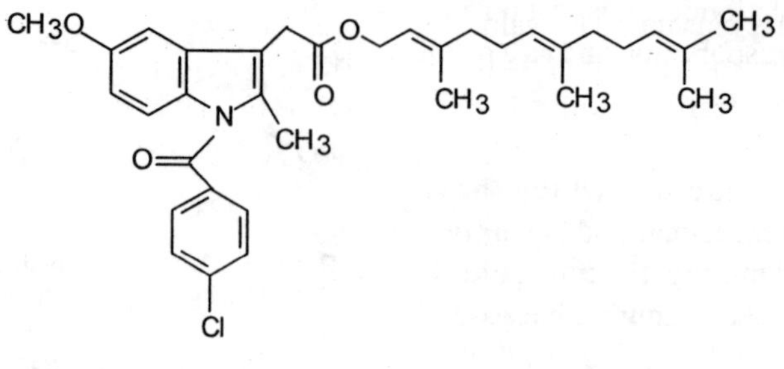

Fig. 4-15. Farnesyl Ester of Indomethacin

have been essentially inseminated by the understanding of the process associated with the absorption and subsequent intracellular processing of absorbed lipid digestion products involving high degree of intestinal lymphatic transport, as is the case of lipid soluble vitamins.

The most common functionally designed promoiety, which has been extensively studied is glyceride prodrug, where the drug is appropriately conjugated to either mono- or di-glyceride(s). Recently, a phospholipid prodrug mimic designed for preferential incorporation in the phospholipid-processing pathway, which supports lipoprotein biosynthesis (Sakai et al., 1993).

Glyceride Prodrug for Systemic Delivery

Orally administered triglycerides are first enzymatically hydrolyzed within the intestinal lumen to produce two fatty acids and the corresponding 2-monoglyceride. These digestion products are then absorbed by the enterocytes and sufficiently resynthesized into further triglyceride, which becomes incorporated into the lipid core of the intestinally derived lipoproteins. When drugs are conjugated in the 2-(or β-) position, the triglyceride mimic serves as a potential substrate for lipase-catalyzed hydrolysis, which would cleave the fatty acid at the 1- and 3- position (α- and α′- positions) releasing the 2-monoglyceride version of the prodrug. Once absorbed the 2-monoglyceride version of the prodrug may become subsequently substrate for the standard reacetylation pathway, which operates in the cell to convert naturally occuring 2-monoglycerides into diglycerides and eventually triglycerides. If the prodrug version of the 2-monoglyceride becomes associated with the lipid transport pathway, it can potentially and preferentially transported via the intestinal lymphatics to the systemic circulation owing to its triglyceride mimic character (Charman and Poster, 1996).

L-DOPA

L-Dopa undergoes significant presystemic metabolism through conjugation reaction as well as metabolism via other routes, including decarboxylation to dopamine. Grazon-Aburbeh et al., 1986, have reported the diglyceride prodrug of L-dopa for enhanced bioavailability via intestinal lymphatic transportation (Fig. 4-16). After the oral administration of L-dopa, only 0.19% of the administered dose was transported via intestinal lymphatics. When administered in its diglyceride prodrug form, 8.3% of the administered dose recovered present in lymph as parent diglyceride prodrug and 14.9% of the administered dose as related diglycerides. Additionally, no detectable amount of L-dopa or dopamine was present in lymph after administration of prodrug suggesting that the prodrug is not metabolized in gut. The oral administration of the diglyceride prodrug in the rat

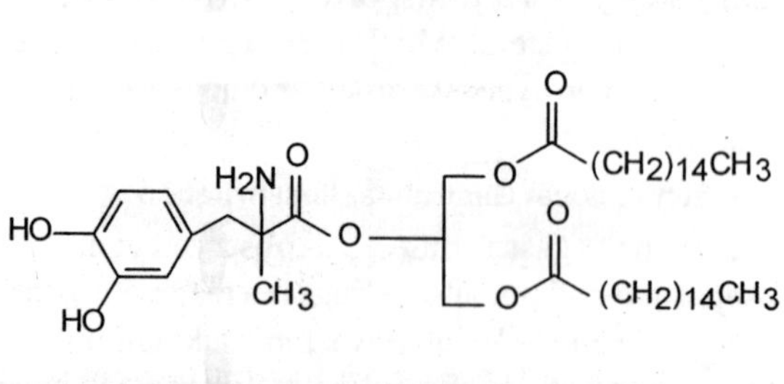

Fig. 4-16. Diglyceride Prodrug of L-DOPA

approximately doubled the plasma AUC values as compared with oral administration of L-dopa. Furthermore, oral administration of the L-dopa diglyceride prodrug produced a more favorable L-dopa/dopamine plasma profile ratio as compared to oral administration of parent L-dopa. Comparative brain uptake studies of L-dopa or diglyceride prodrug demonstrated a prolongation and slower increase of brain L-dopa levels after oral administration of diglyceride prodrug (Grazon-Aburbeh et al., 1986).

Naproxen

Sugihara and co-workers, 1988 have evaluated the utility of monoglyceride prodrugs of naproxen and nicotinic acid for enhanced lymphatic delivery. The effect of conjugating carboxyl group of drug to either the 1- or 2- position of the glycerol, and the role of an ether spacer group between the 1- or 2- hydroxyl group of the glycerol moiety and the carboxyl group was studied. Figure 4-17 depicts the structure of various prodrugs of naproxen studied. The lymphatic transport of the radioactivity after administration of (3H) naproxen as either a 1-glyceryl ester, 1-glyceryl octyl ester (octyl spacer group between the glycerol hydroxy group and the carboxyl group of naproxen), 2-glyceryl dodecyl ester (dodecyl spacer group between the glycerol hydroxy group and the carboxyl group of naproxen), or the 1,3-dipalmitoyl-2-glyceryl ester of naproxen was studied in thoracic duct cannulated rat after oral administration.

The lymphatic transport associated with administration of either parent naproxen or the simple monoglyceride prodrug was approximately 2% of the administered dose. This could be due to the cleavage of the prodrug to the parent drug in the lumen by the action of lipase or esterases. When an octyl or dodecyl spacer was incorporated between the glyceryl hydroxy group and the carboxyl function of naproxen, lymphatic transport of radioactivity improved significantly as up to 20% of the administered dose was recovered in the lymph. The distribution of radioactivity in thoracic lymph after oral administration of either the 1-or 2- substituted naproxen compounds was followed. A 70% proportion of triglyceride based analogs was observed in the case of 2-substituted derivatives, whereas for 1- substituted derivatives it was 50%. However, there was a corresponding lower proportion of diglyceride based analog after administration of 2- substituted derivatives compared with 1- substituted derivatives (approximately 20% vs 40%). The maximum lymphatic uptake was reported in the case of 1-monoglyceride derivative with octyl spacer (28.3%). The lymphatic transport of 1,3-dipalmitoyl-2 glycerol ester of naproxen was surprisingly low. The pharmacokinetic profile of naproxen after oral administration of either the conjugated or free naproxen were similar, thereby indicating little advantage with these monoglyceride conjugated system. This study indicates the potential utility of substituted 1- or 2- monoglyceride derivative for facilitating corresponding drug lymphatic transport.

LK-A and LK-903

LK-A and LK-903 are the hypolipidemic compounds that represent useful and successful examples, where

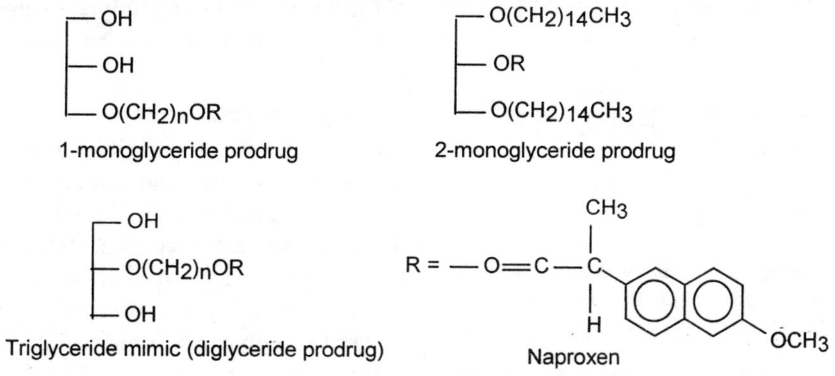

Fig. 4-17. Prodrugs of Naproxen

intestinal lymphatic transport play a major role in the absorption and bioavailability of the orally administered drug (Mizobe et al., 1983). Structurally LK-A is a carboxylic group containing hypolipidemic agent and LK-903 is the 1- monoacylglyceryl ester of LK-A (Fig. 4-18). Lymphatic uptake studies of various formulations of LK-A and LK-903 were conducted in beagle dogs. After oral administration of a lipid solution or LK-A or a tablet formulation of LK-903, analysis of the plasma radioactivity profile indicated the presence of LK-A, LK-903, as well as the mono- and di-acylated derivatives of LK-903.

In oral bioavailability studies, the different formulations of LK-A or LK-903 were administered. The total concentration of LK-related compounds in plasma was similar, however, the proportional distribution of mono- and di-acylated LK-903 derivatives and the parent LK-A and LK-903 forms was different.

The intestinal lymphatic transport studies conducted in rats revealed that orally administered LK-903 was essentially absorbed intact with only minimal conversion to parent LK-A within the gastrointestinal lumen. Once absorbed as the monoacyl form (LK-903), the free hydroxyl groups at the 2- and 3- positions were subsequently esterified and a triacylated form (LK-903 diglyceride) so formed was substantially transported via intestinal lympahtics into the systemic circulation. It was also demonstrated that the orally administered LK-A (or LK-A formed via hydrolysis of LK-903 in the intestinal lumen) was sebsequently esterified as significant proportions of the di-acylated and mono-acylated compounds appeared in the intestinal lymph (Sugihara and Furuchi, 1988).

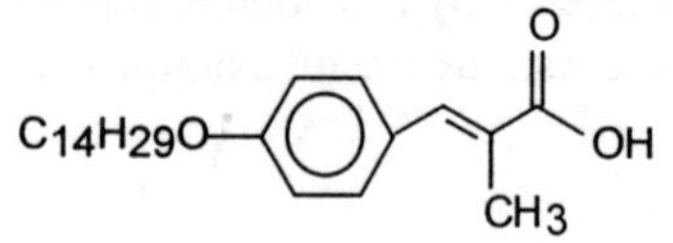

$C_{14}H_{29}O$ O OH CH_3

LK-A

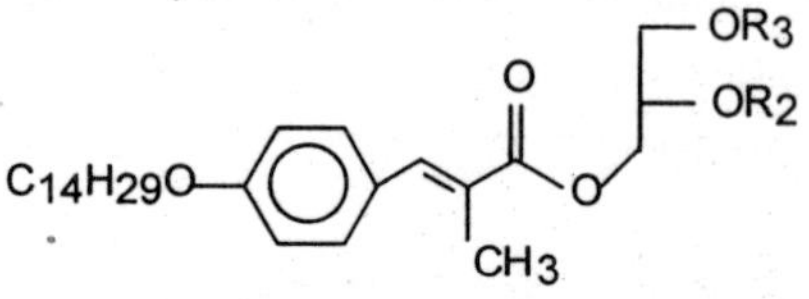

OR_3 O OR_2 $C_{14}H_{29}O$ O CH_3

$R_2 = R_3 = H$	LK-903
$R_2 = R_3 = -COC_{14}H_{29}$	LK-903 dipalmitate
$R_2 = H$, $R_3 = -COC_{14}H_{29}$	LK-903 monopalmitate

Fig. 4-18. LK-A, LK-903 and various Glyceride Prodrugs

Glyceride prodrug for targeted delivery

The selective drug delivery of chemotherapeutic agents e.g., anticancer drugs to the lymphatic system would be valuable in those cases where tumour cells spread via lymphatics or metastasize within the lymph nodes and also in the cases of bacterial and viral infection localized in lymph.

Chlorambucil

Chlorambucil is an effective, drug used in the treatment of Hodgkin's disease and other lymphomas. Garzon-Aburbeh et al., 1983, prepared a 1,3-palmitoyl-2-[4{bis(2-chloroethyl)amino} benzene butanoyl]-glycerol, which is a diglyceride of chlorambucil (Fig. 4-19). When evaluated orally in P383 leukaemic cells bearing mice, the diglyceride prolonged the survival time of the mice relative to the chloroambucil and the level of toxicity was also reduced. In a pharmacokinetic study conducted on rats, lymphatic transport of radioactivity after oral administration of diglyceride prodrug was 26% of the administered dose, as compared with 3.4 % after administration of parent chloroambucil.

TLC analysis of the lymphatically transported radioactivity after the administration of diglyceride prodrug, revealed that it was only associated with diglyceride prodrug. There was no parent chlorambucil detected in lymph after administration of diglyceride prodrug. Further, it was concluded on the basis of above study that the diglyceride prodrug of chlorambucil may have its own anticancer activity.

γ-Amino butyric acid (GABA)

Filariasis is the major parasitic disease prevailing in tropical and subtropical countries. The use of prodrug to deliver GABA and inhibitors of GABA trans-aminases, e.g. γ-vinyl-GABA to the brain and lymph for the treatment of parasite residing in the lymph has been studied. Deverre et al., 1989 have prepared a diglyceride prodrug of GABA for the lymphatic delivery of GABA. The study conducted in *in vitro* has been reported to be highly promising.

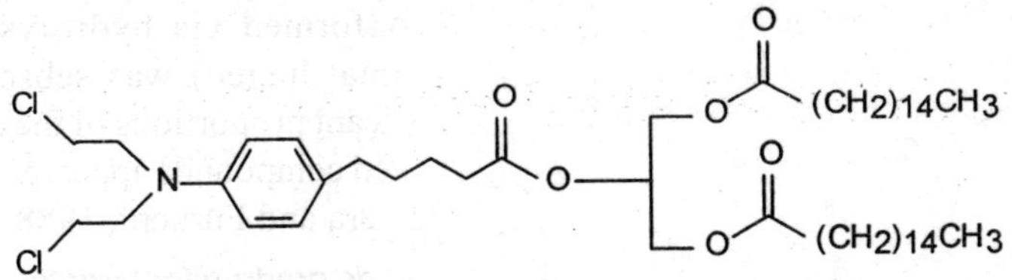

Fig. 4-19. Diglyceride Prodrug of Chlorambucil

Melaphalan

Deverre et al., 1992 have prepared a microfilaricidal prodrug of melaphalan, which upon oral administration concentrates in the lymphatic system. The esterification of melaphalan with 1,3 di-palmitin resulted into a chemically stable prodrug. The filaricidal activity of the prodrug was compared with that of melaphalan *in vitro* against adult infected larvae and microfilariae of *Molinema disseetae* and evaluated *in vivo* on *Molinema disseetae* infected Proechimy oris. The *in vitro* data indicated that the prodrug and melaphalan were equally effective, although the diglyceride prodrug exhibited a delayed onset of action. The *in vivo* data from infected rodents indicated effective oral activity of the diglyceride melaphalan prodrug.

Niclosamide

Elkihel and co-workers, 1994 have evaluated the macrofilaricidal activity of different prodrugs of niclosamide. The prodrugs were based on the glyceride mimic approach, where niclosamide was esterified at the 2-position of glycerol, but a variety of linkages were used for attachment of palmitic acids at 1- and 3-positions of glycerol. These linkages include standard ester, thiol ester and amide linkages. The *in vivo* evaluation of the compounds, after oral administration as carboxylmethyl suspension to infected rodents, indicated maximum activity after administration of the amide linked fatty acids substituted compounds.

Glyceride Prodrugs for Reduced Gastrointestinal Irritation

Glyceride prodrugs of anti-inflammatory agents have been extensively evaluated to potentially reduce gastrointestinal irritation. Kumar and Billimorai, 1978 have prepared glyceride prodrug of ^{14}C-aspirin and studied the extent of lymphatic transport. Similarly, glyceride prodrugs of indomethacin and naproxen were reported and evaluated for lymphatic transport, anti-inflammatory activity and reduced gastric ulceration (Sugihara et al., 1988). The overall activity profile of these prodrugs suggests that the compounds are biologically viable and the gastric irritation was less as compared to parent compound.

Phospholipid Prodrugs

Sakai and co-workers, 1993 synthesized a lymphtrophic prodrug of fluorouridine for targeing to intestinal lymphatic system. The phospholipid prodrug of fluorouridine (dipalmitoyl phosphatidyl-fluorouridine, DPPF) (Fig. 4-20) was designed to target the normal phospholipid processing pathways involved in lipid/phospholipid digestion and transport after oral administration.

After oral administration of aqueous solution of prodrug (30 mg/ml) to rats (dose 300 mg/kg); the lymph collected from thoracic duct contained parent DPPF and fluorouridine as well as other fluorouridine related compounds in much higher concentrations. They were identified as fatty acid congeners of DPPF, where the palmitic acid at the 2-position had been substituted with either arachidonic acid to produce PAPF or linoleic acid to produce PLPF. These could be due to the preabsorptive hydrolysis of DPPF to form LPF (lysopalmitoyl phosphatidyl fluorouridine) which is subsequently reacetylated within the enterocytes. Table 4-1 summarizes different lymphotropic prodrugs

Brain as a Target Organ for CDS

The brain is a vital and delicate organ and with the passage of time evolution built very efficient ways to protect it. Unfortunately, the mechanism that protects it against harmful chemicals also frustrates therapeutic interventions. Treatment of cerebral

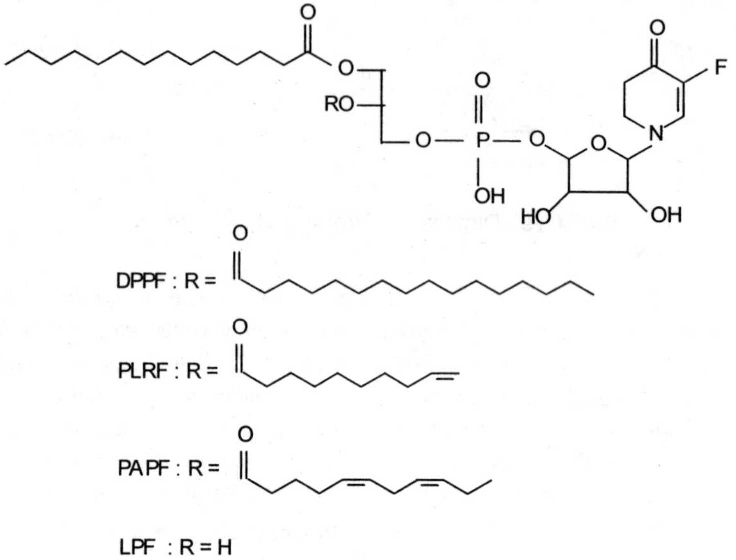

Fig. 4-20. Phospholipid Prodrugs of Fluorouridine

disorders is very difficult using existing pharmaceuticals due to their inability to effectively deliver the active agent and sustain it within the brain. Blood brain barrier (BBB) is a strong hurdle that has to be crossed for efficient delivery of any bioactive agent into the brain.

Structural and Enzymatic Aspects of BBB

The BBB is a unique membranous barrier that tightly segregates the brain from the circulating blood (Crone and Thompson, 1970; Oldendorf, 1974; Bodor and Brewster, 1983; Begley, 1996). Capillaries of the vertebrate brain lack the small pores that allow movement of solutes from circulation into other organs. In fact these capillaries are guarded by a layer of special endothelial cells that lack fenestration and are sealed with tight junctions. These endothelial cells along with astrocytes and pericytes constitute the blood brain barrier (BBB). Figure 4-21 gives a schematic representation of BBB. Almost 95% of the total surface area of the BBB is made up of microvessels, which represents the principal route for entry of chemicals into the brain (Smith, 1989). However, vessels in brain were found to have somewhat smaller diameter and thinner walls than vessels in other organs (Stewart and Tuor, 1994). Moreover, the mitochondrial density in brain microvessels was found to be higher than in other capillaries. Intercellular cleft, pinocytosis and fenestrae are virtually absent in brain capillaries, hence any substance must pass transcellularly. Therefore, only lipid soluble solutes, which can freely penetrate the capillary endothelial membrane by passive diffusion, can cross the BBB. The blood brain barrier is also equipped with a bucket of enzymes (Crone, 1986; Ghersi-Egea et al., 1994) and any solute crossing the cell membrane is exposed to these degrading enzymes present in large numbers in the endothelial cells that contain large densities of mitochondria, Metabolically highly active organelles. Some of the enzymes found in the BBB are adenylate cyclase, guanylate cyclase, Na^+-K^+ ATPase, alkaline phosphatase, catechol O-methyl transferase (COMT), monoamine oxidase (MAO), GABA transaminase, DOPA decarboxylase, etc.

In addition to lipid solubility, many other factors also govern the transportation of a solute across BBB. A few special solutes have access to BBB through specific, catalyzed transport, i.e. glucose transporter ensures that glucose, an essential nutrient, reaches

Table 4-1. Various Lymphotropic Prodrugs

Parent drug	Prodrug	Objective	References
Simple ester or ether prodrugs			
Testosterone	Testosterone undecanoate heptanoate, palmitate and oleate	Avoidance of hepatic first pass metabolism, thus increasing oral bioavailability	Coert et al., 1975; Noguchi et al., 1985
Epitiostanol (EP)	Mepitiostane (MP) (17-substituted methylcyclo pentane derivative of EP)	Avoidance of hepatic first pass metabolism, thus increasing oral bioavailability	Ichihashi et al., 1992a
Retinol (Vitamin A)	Retinyl palmitate	Enhanced oral absorption	Berr and Kern, 1984
α-Tocopherol (Vitamin E)	α-Tocopherol acetate and α-tocopherol nicotinate	Enhancement of stability *in vivo* by preventing oxidation of the phenolic group Increase in oral bioavailability	Nakamura et al., 1975
Indomethacin	Farnesyl ester of indomethacin	Reduced gastric irritation	Kobayashi et al., 1988; Mishima et al., 1990
Functionally designed prodrugs			
L-Dopa	Di-palmitoyl glyceride prodrug of L-dopa	Avoidance of hepatic first pass metabolism thus increasing oral bioavailability Preventing decarboxylation to dopamine thus reducing peripheral side effects and elevated brain level of the drug	Grazon-Aburbeh et al., 1986
Naproxen	Monoglyceride prodrug, Monoglyceride prodrug with octyl and dodecyl spacer group between the glycerol hydroxy group and the carboxyl group of naproxen and Di-palmitoyl prodrug of naproxen	Increased oral bioavailability due to enhanced intestinal lymphatic delivery	Sugihara et al., 1988
LK-A	1 mono acylglyceryl ester of LK-A (LK-903)	Increased oral bioavailability due to enhanced intestinal lymphatic delivery	Sugihara and Furuchi, 1988
Chrolambucil	Di-palmitoyl glyceride prodrug	Targeting to intestinal lymphatics for the treatment of Hodgkin's disease	Garzon-Aburbeh et al., 1983
γ-Amino butyric acid	Di-palmitoyl glyceride prodrug	Lymphatic targeting of GABA for the treatment of Filariasis	Deverre et al., 1989
Melaphalan	Di-palmitoyl glyceride prodrug	Lymphatic targeting of melaphalan for the treatment of Filariasis	Deverre et al., 1992
Niclosamide	Di-palmitoyl glyceride prodrug	Increased anthelmintics activity after oral administration	Elkihel et al., 1994
Aspirin	Di-palmitoyl glyceride prodrug	Reduced gastric ulceration, and irritation	Kumar and Billimorai, 1978
Fluorouridine	Dipalmitoyl phosphatidyl fluorodine	Lymphatic targeting for the treatment of cancer	Sakai et al., 1993

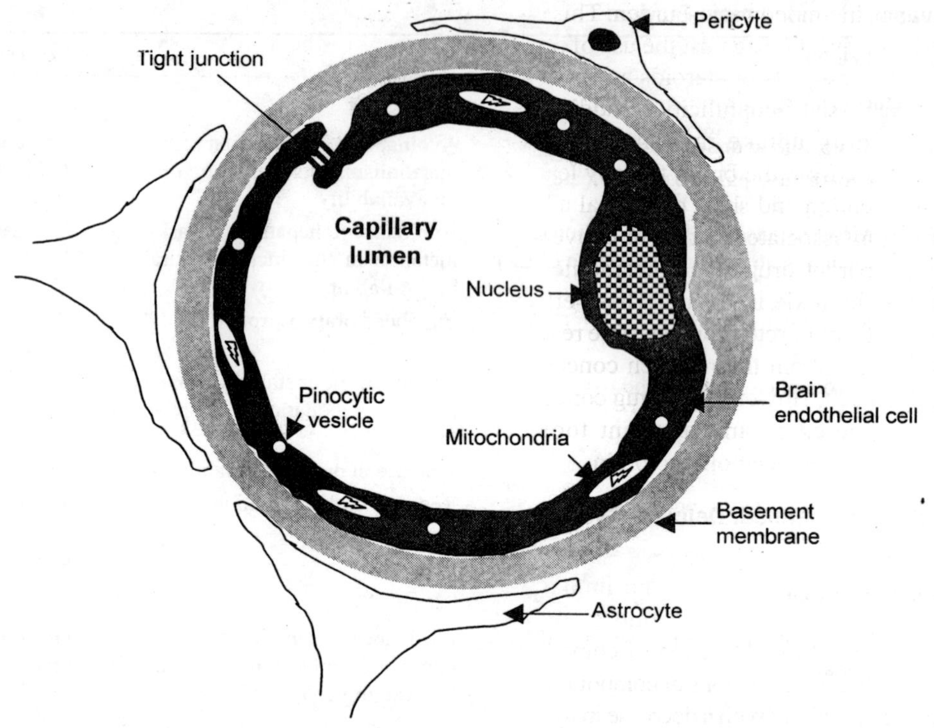

Fig. 4-21. Schematic Representation of Blood-Brain-Barrier (BBB), A Blood Capillary

the brain despite its low lipid solubility (Crone, 1965; Andersen, 1979). Carriers are facilitative in nature and help transport the solute against the concentration gradient, these carriers have been identical for hexoses, acidic, basic, monocarboxylic acids, choline and other biologically important molecules. Recently, probenecid-sensitive, active pumps for organic anions such as β-lactam drugs or valproic acid has been suggested (Barza, 1993). P-glycoprotein a multidrug transporter is also present in the BBB, which has relatively low substrate specificity and actively excludes a number of lipophilic compounds from cerebral endothelial cells (Tsuji and Tamai, 1997). Research is on to exploit these transport systems for delivering drug across the BBB.

Drug Delivery to Brain

Various possible strategies used for drug delivery across BBB are transient osmotic opening of the BBB, exploiting natural chemical transporters, high-dose chemotherapy or biodegradable, however, these suffer from various limitations as they are invasive procedures, have toxic side effects and low efficiency and are also not sufficiently safe.

One of the better options to smuggle drugs across BBB is prodrug approach in which drugs are transported as their lipophilic precursors (Stella, 1975; Bodor and Kaminski, 1984). Prodrugs are pharmacologically inactive compounds that result from transient chemical modifications of biologically active species. The chemical change in any parent drug is usually designed to improve some physicochemical property as lipid solubility or membrane permeability. The prodrug after administration, by virtue of its improved characteristics is brought closer to the receptor site and is maintained there for longer duration of time. Here it can be converted into an active form usually through a single activation step. Nevertheless, these simple prodrugs suffer from many limitations like increase in lipophilicity enhances the BBB crossing property, which in turn also increases the uptake into other tissues causing an increased tissue burden. This non-selectivity raises a question against the use of potent drugs like cytotoxic agents or steroids as prodrugs. Furthermore, increased lipophilicity in addition to facilitating the drug uptake into the CNS also enhances the efflux from the brain, thereby leading to poor tissue retention and short biological action. Another limitation associated is that in conversion of prodrug into parent drug some metabolites are formed that may be toxic in nature. These effects, i.e. poor selectivity, poor retention, possible reactive metabolites may constrain the research concerning the prodrug approach. However, prodrug concept is still being considered as an important tool for targeting of drug/active metabolite to brain.

Dihydronicotinate Chemical Delivery Systems (CDSs)

Prodrug approach suffers from certain limitations raised due to the fact that only one chemical conversion is required for activation of compound. In many cases multiple conversions of compound may lead to enhanced selectivity with a decrease in toxicity as well as sustained action. A CDS is defined as a biologically inert compound, which requires multiple steps for its conversion to an active molecule and which subsequently leads to enhanced drug delivery to a particular organ or site (Bodor and Brewster, 1983; Bodor et al., 1981). Analogous to prodrug a CDS should be sufficiently lipophilic to allow for brain uptake and subsequently, the molecule should undergo enzymatic conversions to promote retention within CNS vis-à-vis it should be eliminated as early as possible. Furthermore, the intermediate should degrade releasing the active compound in a sustained manner (Fig. 4-22). The figure indicates that CDS possesses a carrier molecule, which imparts a lipophilic character to the molecule. While many moieties may serve this function, 1,4-dihydro-trigonellinates are the best alternative. In this approach, an amine, carboxylic acid or hydroxy group containing drug is amidated, esterified or covalently linked to nicotinic acid or a nicotinic acid derivative. Subsequently, this compound is quaternized to produce 1-methynicotinate salt or trigonellinate and this is further reduced to generate 1,4-dihydrotrigonellinate or CDS. This reduced moiety strongly enhances the lipophilic character of the drug to which it is joined. When this CDS is administered systemically it can be partitioned to several body compartments due to its lipophilicity, which suggests that the CDS is working simply as a lipoidal prodrug, however the carrier molecule is designed in such a fashion that it undergoes enzymatic oxidation reaction, which leads to conversion of the membrane impermeable dihydrotrigonellinate salt. This new oxidized carrier drug conjugate, which is polar in nature is trapped within the BBB and therefore in CNS. When this reaction occurs in periphery it forms polar compound, which is readily eliminated from the body, hence reducing the systemic toxicity, on the other hand in CNS the conjugate is slowly hydrolyzed to give the active species at a slow and sustained rate, thereby avoiding any central toxicity. This approach allows for reduced toxicity and delivery of drug selectively to the target site. Furthermore, it also reduces the frequency of drug administration. The CDS technology has been particularly applied for delivery of neurotransmitters and amino acids, antiviral agents and estrogenic steroids for brain delivery.

Brain Targeting of Neurotransmitters and Aminoacids

Deficiency of various neurotransmitters and amino acids in brain causes many CNS disorders. Parkinsonism, which affects approximately 1% of population over the age of 60, is associated with selective depletion of striatal dopamine (Jankovic, 1988). Deficiency of inhibitory neurotransmitter, γ-aminobutryric acid (GABA) leads to Huntington's disease (Martin and Gusella, 1986). Replacement of these deficient neurotransmitters may be of use in treatment of these debilitating diseases. Hypertension, which affects a large percentage of population can be treated with tryptophan. Improved CNS delivery of tryptophan via chemical delivery systems may help treat hypertension.

Dopamine

Dopamine as such cannot cross BBB and therefore is not useful for replacement therapy (Roos and Steg, 1964). However, a prodrug, L-Dopa has been used clinically for treating parkinsonism but this suffers from severe peripheral toxicities, which limit its use.

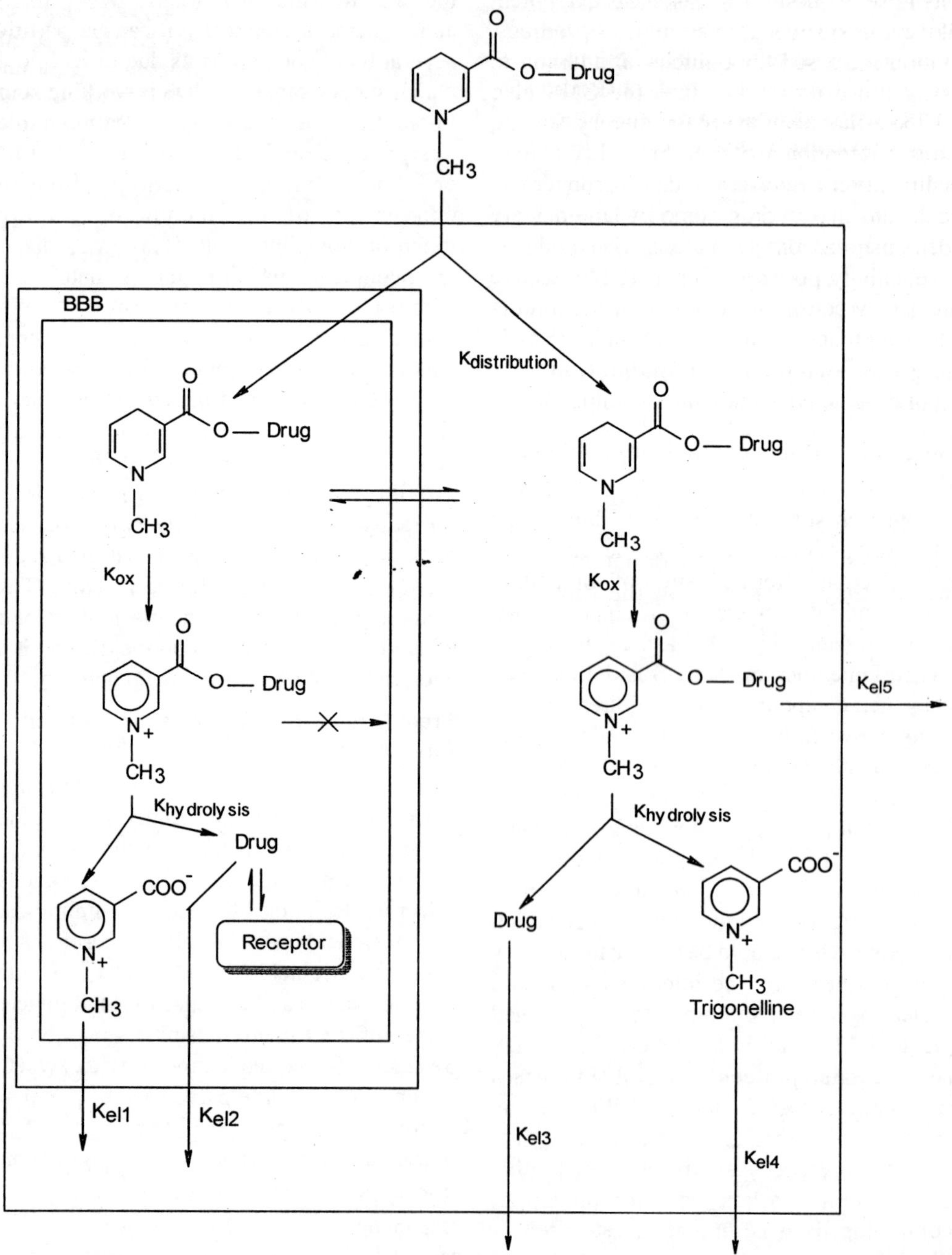

Fig. 4-22. Schematic Diagram showing Retention of CDS within the CNS and Accelerated Elimination

Therefore, a need for dopamine CDS was realized and a system was designed and synthesized by firstly condensing nicotinic acid and dopamine hydrobromide to produce the catechol nitotinamide derivative, as illustrated in Figure 4-23 (Bodor and Farag, 1983). Pivaloylation of the resultant compound yields the bis ester, which was subsequently quaternized and reduced to produce the protected dopamine delivery system (DCDS). *In vitro* studies demonstrated that DCDS was converted to the corresponding quaternary salt (P-D-Q$^+$), which subsequently underwent sequential ester hydrolysis to yield 1-methylnicotinamide of dopamine (D-Q$^+$), the ultimate dopamine prodrug. High levels of DA-Q$^+$ have been observed on systemic administration of DCDS to rats, while their blood levels declined down rapidly. This uncoupling of brain and blood concentration is the attractive feature of this CDS approach.

Another CDS approach for dopamine uses carbamate as the bridge linking the dihydronicotinamide and the dopamine nitrogen. The CDS was prepared by treating the dipivaloate of dopamine with chloromethyl chloroformate to yield the chloromethyl carbamate derivate. This intermediate when reacts with the triethylammonium salt of nicotinic acid produces the acyloxyalkyl carbamate, which is subsequently methylated to generate the CDS. *In vitro* studies suggested that this delivery system is rapidly converted to quaternary salt followed by dopamine release.

γ-Aminobutyric acid (GABA)

γ-Aminobutyric acid is an inhibitory neurotransmitter and is involved in the etiology of Huntington's disease and epilepsy (Fonnum, 1978). Unfortunately, GABA is the only neurotransmitter that passes the BBB least efficiently. Several CDSs were tried for GABA, however two of them are more popular and hence being described here. These GABA-CDSs are derivatives of GABA amides and analogues of GABA (Woodard et al., 1990). The cyclohexyl and Benzyl esters of GABA were condensed with

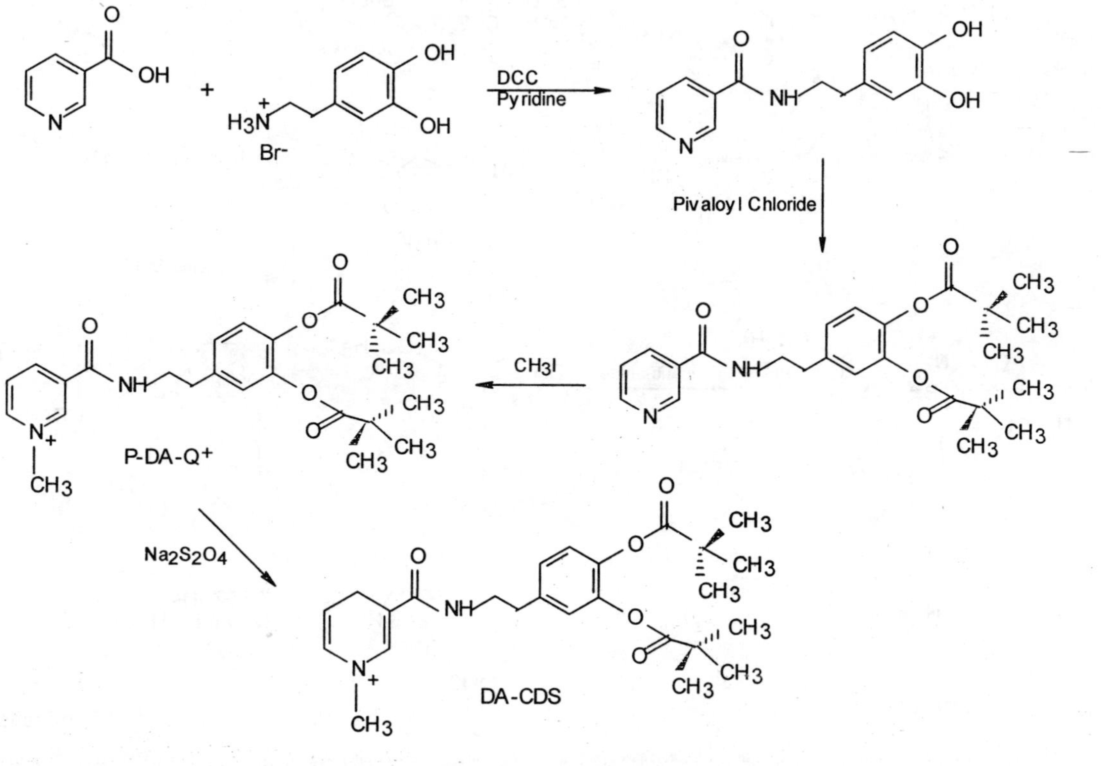

DCC Pyridine

Pivaloyl Chloride

CH_3I

P-DA-Q+

$Na_2S_2O_4$

DA-CDS

Fig. 4-23. Preparation of Dopamine CDS

nicotinic acid to produce corresponding GABA ester nicotinamide (Fig. 4-24). These intermediates were further quaternized with methyliodide to produce the nicotinate salts, which on subsequent reduction gave Benzyl-GABA-CDS (BZ-GABA-CDS) and Cyclohexyl-GABA-CDS (CH-GABA-CDS). GABA analogues were produced by including the GABA nitrogen into the pyridine of the delivery system. Quaternization of nicotinamide was affected with the ethylester of 4-bromobutyric acid, giving the nicotinamide salt, which was further reduced in aqueous basic sodium dithionite to produce GABA-CDS-1 (Fig. 4-24). Another ana-logue was synthesized using an agent that assists the conversion of primary amines to nicotinamide quaternary salts, 1-(2,4-dinitrophenyl)-nicotinamide chloride. The salt was further treated with diethylacetal of 4-amino butyraldehyde to yield the nicotinate salt, which was subsequently reduced to produce GABA-CDS-2. *In vivo* studies revealed that systemic administration of these GABA CDSs produced sustained concentration of the pyridinium salt in the brain.

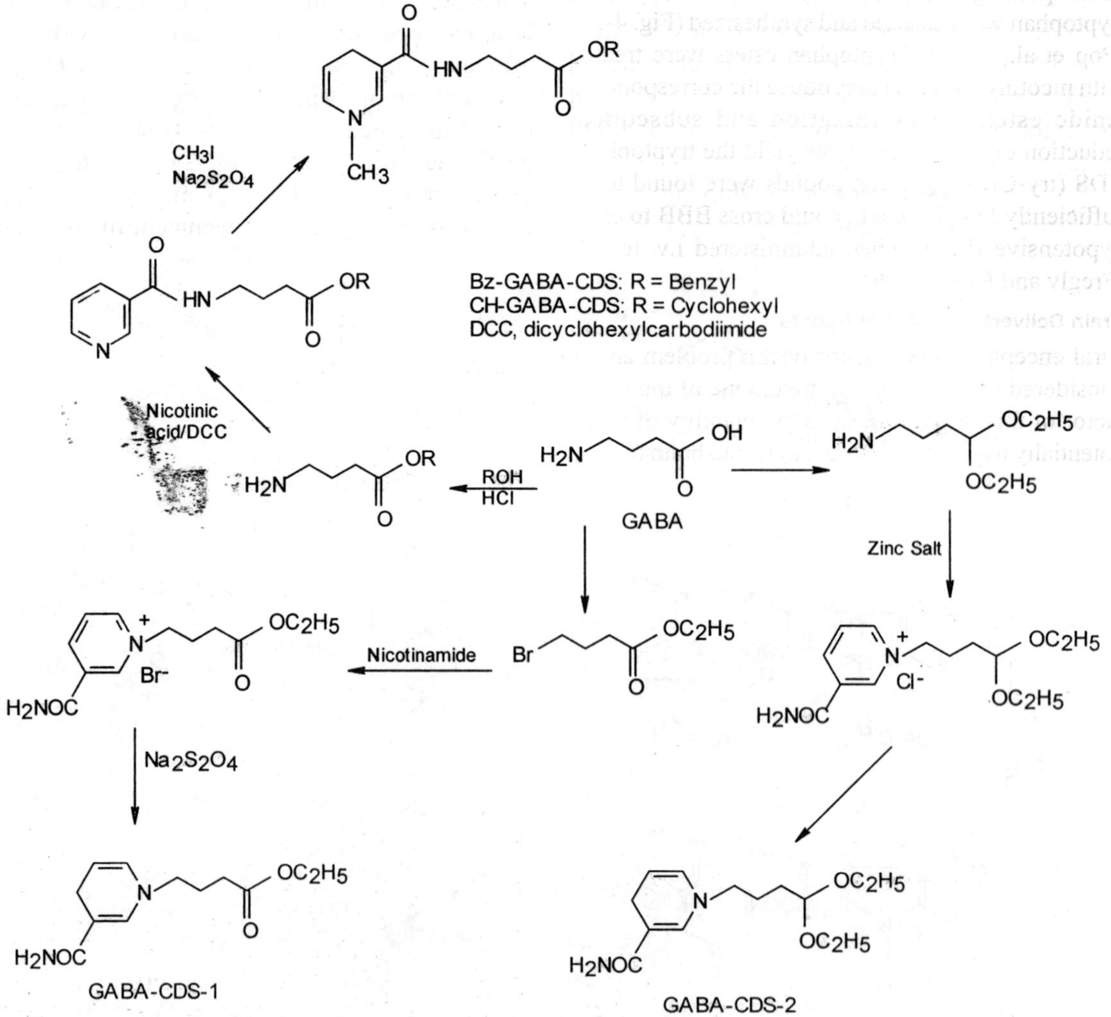

Bz-GABA-CDS: R = Benzyl
CH-GABA-CDS: R = Cyclohexyl
DCC, dicyclohexylcarbodiimide

Fig. 4-24. Synthesis of CDS for GABA and its Analogues

Tryptophan

L-tryptophan is an essential amino acid and usually administered as a nutrient or against depression. Recently, it has been reported that tryptophan lowers the blood pressure and studies suggested that the hypotensive effect is mainly due to action of tryptophan in CNS (Wolf and Kuhn, 1984; Sved et al., 1982). Tryptophan is delivered to brain inefficiently due to its high binding to serum albumin and to achieve higher brain levels the dose has to be increased manifolds. Unfortunately, it has been reported that large oral doses of tryptophan cause bladder cancer and blood dyscariasias especially eosinophilia (Caterall, 1988). Therefore, CDS of tryptophan was designed and synthesized (Fig. 4-25) (Pop et al., 1990). Tryptophan esters were treated with nicotinyl chloride to produce the corresponding amide esters. Quaternization and subsequent reduction of these derivatives yield the tryptophan-CDS (try-CDS). The compounds were found to be sufficiently lipophilic and could cross BBB to exert hypotensive effect, when administered i.v. to rats (Fregly and Fater, 1986).

Brain Delivery of Antiviral Agents

Viral encephalitis is a major health problem and is considered to be difficult to treat. One of the major factor of this refractoriness is the inability of many potentially useful drugs to penetrate into brain tissues. This section deals with the CDS of antiviral agents especially antiAIDS drugs, drugs for treatment of Japanese encephalitis, Cytomegaloviral encephalitis and Herpes encephalitis. Viral diseases are very difficult to cure by conventional means of therapy. CDS may provide a better way to treat these diseases.

Zidovudine (AZT)-CDS

AZT, the first drug approved for the treatment of AIDS, has been useful in improving the neuropsychiatric symptoms associated with AIDS encephalopathy. However, the doses required to elicit this improvement cause severe anemia that usually leads to the termination of AZT therapy. Although, AZT enters the cerebrospinal fluid (CSF) and achieves significant concentrations after oral or intravenous administration. The CSF levels may exceed brain tissue levels because the agent is capable of only poor penetration of the BBB (Balin et al., 1989, Klecker et al., 1987). This antiviral agent has a single primary alcohol function in the 5′-position that is available for the attachment of the redox targetor, conventionally nicotine (Fig. 4-26). AZT was treated with nicotinyl chloride hydrochloride in pyridine to produce the 5′ nicotinate. This ester was further quaternized with methyl iodide to give the 5′-trigonellinate (1-methyl nicotinate) and reduced in basic aqueous sodium dithionate to yield the 5′-(1,4-dihydrotrigonellinate (AZT-CDS) (Little et al.,

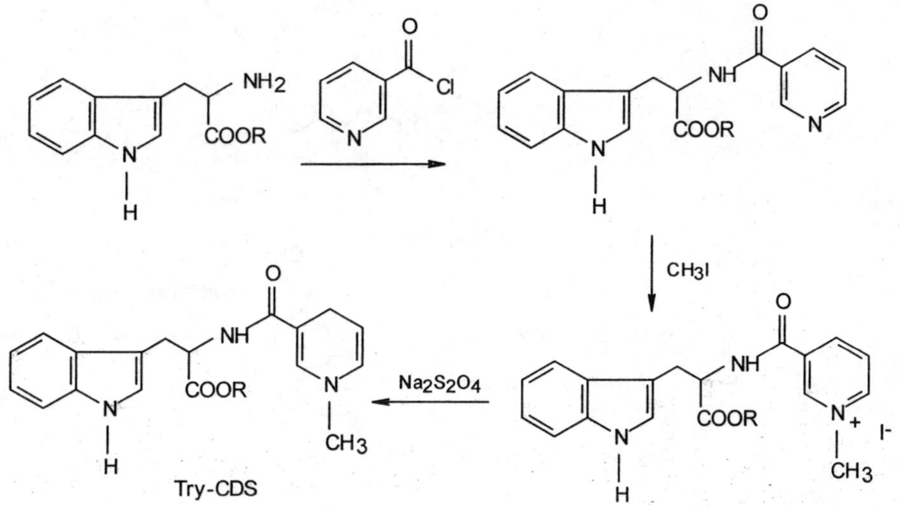

Fig. 4-25. Synthesis of Tryptophan CDS

1990; Goger et al., 1989). The mechanism for targeting of the brain by this CDS essentially relies on the changes in the lipophilicity caused by metabolism, therefore lipophilicity is an important factor that determines the efficacy of CDS. In brain AZT-CDS is converted to a pyridinium ion (AZT-Q^+) by NAD(P) NAD(P)H-dependent oxido-reductase (Fig. 4-26). There is approximately 4000 fold decrease in the lipid solubility of the conjugate after this metabolic step. The sustained release of AZT from AZT-Q^+ retained in the brain occurs via hydrolysis by ubiquitous esterases. *In vivo* studies were conducted on animal models to evaluate the performance of AZT-CDS. The concentrations of parent drug and the CDS were compared in brain and blood after administration of AZT-CDS i.v. Half-life in blood was approximately 20 min and no AZT was detected after two hours. The AZT distribution profiles in the two tissues studied were also quite different. In the blood, the initial high level of CDS rapidly disappeared, while no CDS was detected in brain. The AZT-Q^+ concentration in the brain, however, had a sustained level, reaching the maximum value after 15 min of administration and then slowly declining. The CDS was found to exert anti-HIV activity *in vitro* and to be less toxic to hematopoietic cells in culture than the parent drug itself, therefore, it may be a useful addition in the therapy of AIDS-related encephalopathy.

Antiherpetic Agents

Acyclovir (ACV) is an analogue of guanine, which efficiently destroys *Herpes simplex* virus and *Varicella zoster* virus. ACV is relatively harmless to host since it only gets activated in the virally infected cells (Elion et al., 1977). However, its poor penetration into the brain restricts its application for *Herpes simplex* encephalitis. Therefore, a CDS to ACV has been considered and synthesized as illustrated in Figure 4-27 (Venkatraghavan et al., 1986). As ACV is susceptible to alkylation, the

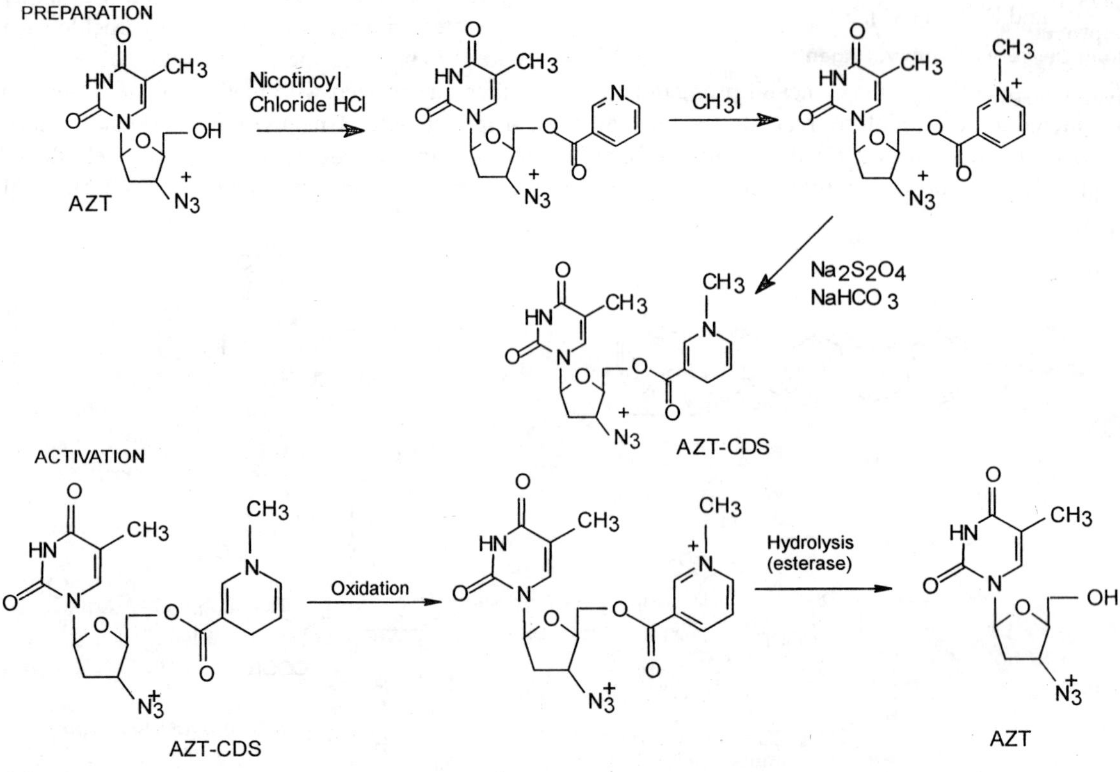

PREPARATION

AZT — Nicotinoyl Chloride HCl → — CH_3I → — $Na_2S_2O_4$, $NaHCO_3$ → AZT-CDS

ACTIVATION

AZT-CDS — Oxidation → — Hydrolysis (esterase) → AZT

Fig. 4-26. Preparation of Zidovudine CDS and Activation of AZT-CDS

trigonellinate unit should be attached in a single step in place of conventional acylation/alkylation method. This was achieved via the development of a trigonellinating reagent, trigonelline anhydride. When ACV is treated with activated anhydride trigonellinate salt (ACV-Q^+) was produced. Finally reduction of this intermediate produced the dihydro trigonellinate CDS (ACV-CDS) (Brewster et al., 1987).

When ACV and ACV-CDS were administered i.v. to rat, ACV produced a tissue distribution consistent with its polar structure. The ACV-CDS produced a different tissue distribution pattern, with the CDS easily penetrating the BBB, produced sustained levels of the ACV-Q^+ in the brain was nearly 2 days, while the compound was rapidly eliminated from liver and kidney. This system is one of the best examples of brain selective delivery using a CDS concept.

Trifluorothymidine (TFT) is used against herpes infection to the eye, however, its high systemic toxicity made its use intravenously difficult, therefore CDS of this compound was considered, which improved the toxicological profile of the agent vis-à-vis enhanced its CNS delivery. The TFT-CDS was prepared as shown in Figure 4-28. TFT was pivaloylated using pivaloyl chloride. Then this was treated with nicotinoyl chloride to yield 5′-pivaloyl-3′-nicotinoyl derivative. This intermediate was then methylated to give TFT-Q^+ and subsequent reduction produced the TFT-CDS. This delivery system undergoes many transformations to release TFT (Fig. 4-29). The TFT-CDS crosses the BBB and enters into the brain parenchyma. The CDS appeared to be present in the form of depivaloated TFT-Q^+ in brain. Treatment of animals with the TFT-CDS significantly reduced viral titers.

Ribavirin

Ribavirin (RV) is a broad spectrum antiviral agent and inhibits the cytopathicity of various RNA viruses. It is useful in the treatment of respiratory syncytial virus and lasser virus (Rodriguez and Parrott, 1987; McCormick et al., 1986). However, its highly water soluble nature with poor lipophilicity, renders it useless in the treatment of RNA viral encephalitic diseases like Japanese B encephalitis, Dengue fever and Raft valley fever. Therefore, CDS approach was applied to RV and 3-hydroxy groups present on the molecule were exploited for derivatization. The brain targeting moiety (1,4-dihydrotrigonellinate) can be joined at any or all of these loci. Moreover, the underivatized hydroxy groups can be used for tagging lipophilicity-modifying ester. The CDS was prepared, as illustrated in Figure 4-30. RV was protected as the 2′-3′-acetonide and deprotected using formic acid. So prepared 5′-nicotinate was then methylated and subsequently reduced to produce RV-5′-CDS. This CDS was found quite effective in brain with a sustain action.

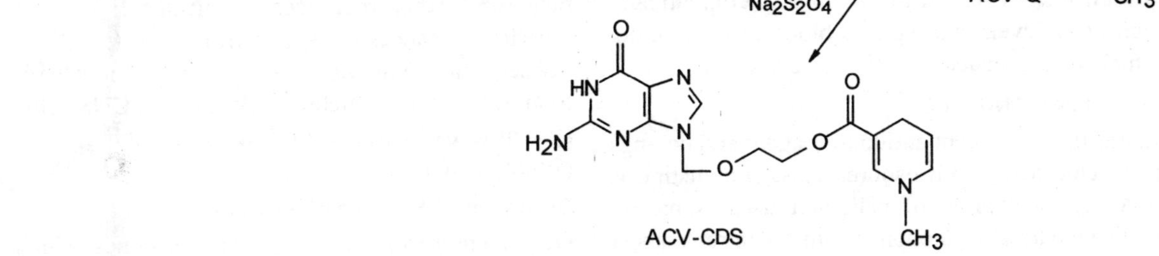

Acyclovir + Trigonelline Anhydride —(Pyridine, DMAP)→ ACV-Q^+ —($Na_2S_2O_4$)→ ACV-CDS

Fig. 4-27. Synthesis of Acyclovir-CDS

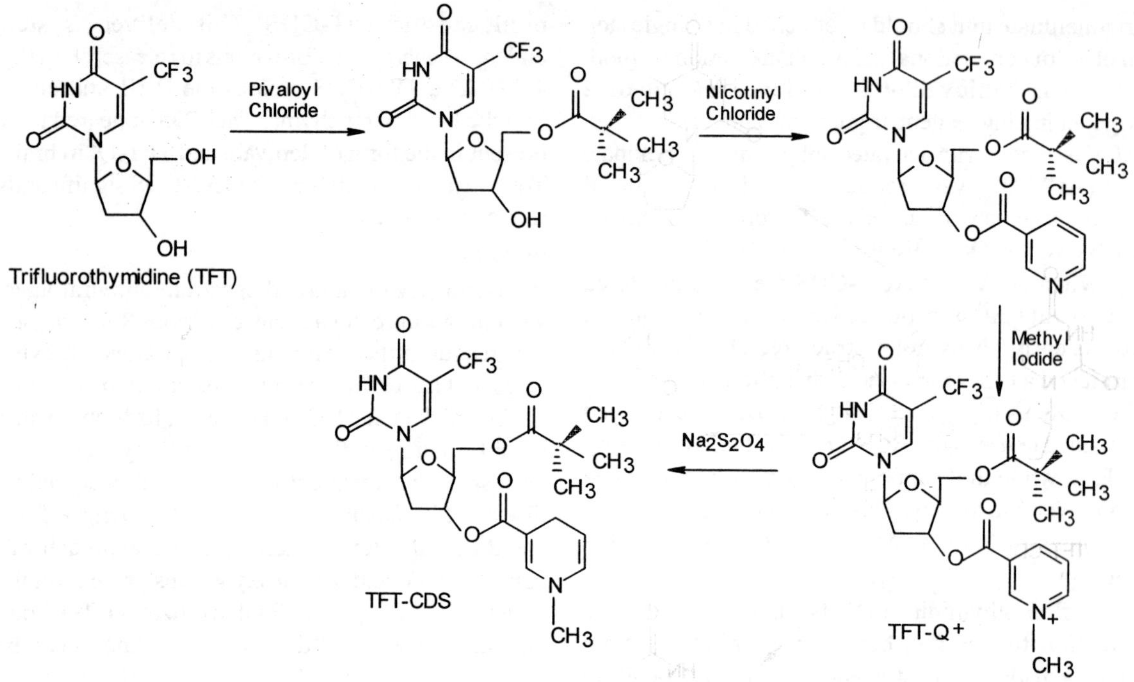

Trifluorothymidine (TFT)

Pivaloyl Chloride

Nicotinyl Chloride

Methyl Iodide

$Na_2S_2O_4$

TFT-CDS

TFT-Q+

Fig. 4-28. Synthesis of Brain Targeting TFT-CDS

Ganciclovir-CDS

Ganciclovir is a potent antiviral agent useful in treatment of human encephalitic and cytomegalovirus (CMV) infection (Brewster et al., 1994). CMV infections are common and usually benign, however human CMV occurs in 94% of patients suffering from AIDS. While some positive results were achieved in the treatment of the associated retinitis, but treatment of encephalitic cytomegalic disease is difficult with ganciclovir. The brain-targeted CDS was therefore designed to enhance brain selectivity. This CDS (Fig. 4-31) increases the brain exposure of ganciclovir 6 folds and simultaneously reduces the blood exposure approximately 8 times. Therefore, the CDS can sustain drug levels in the brain at therapeutically significant levels and reduced blood concentration, which are associated with systemic toxicity.

Lomustine (CCNU)-CDS

Lomustine is a potent antitumour agent and belongs to (2-chloroethyl) nitrosourea class. Lomustine is used against a variety of malignant diseases, mostly brain tumours and lymphomas. Most of the anticancer agents are lipophilic in nature and are capable of crossing BBB, however their poor CNS retention and peripheral toxicity prevent their use in the treatment of central cancers. Therefore, a CDS approach that can offer a 'lock-in' mechanism was designed (Raghavan et al., 1987; Raghavan et al., 1992). Lomustine (CCNU) has no functional group that would allow easy attachment of a targetor function, however, it has an active hydroxy metabolite, N-(2-chloroethyl)-N'-(trans-4-hydroxy cyclohexyl)-N-nitrosourea (CCNU(OH)), that can be exploited for CDS design. Figure 4-32 illustrates the 'lock-in' mechanism for this drug. The parent drug CCNU(OH), is sufficiently lipophilic to cross BBB, however attachment of the 1, 4,-dihydrotrigonelline targetor further increases the lipophilicity and therefore enhances transport diffusion across BBB. Subsequently, oxidation of the targetor moiety leads to an ionic form, which is locked in the CNS. This system leads to enhanced drug effectivity and low peripheral toxicity.

Oestrogen CDS for Brain Targeting

Oestrogens are lipophilic steroidal hormones, which can readily cross BBB. Unfortunately, they are poorly

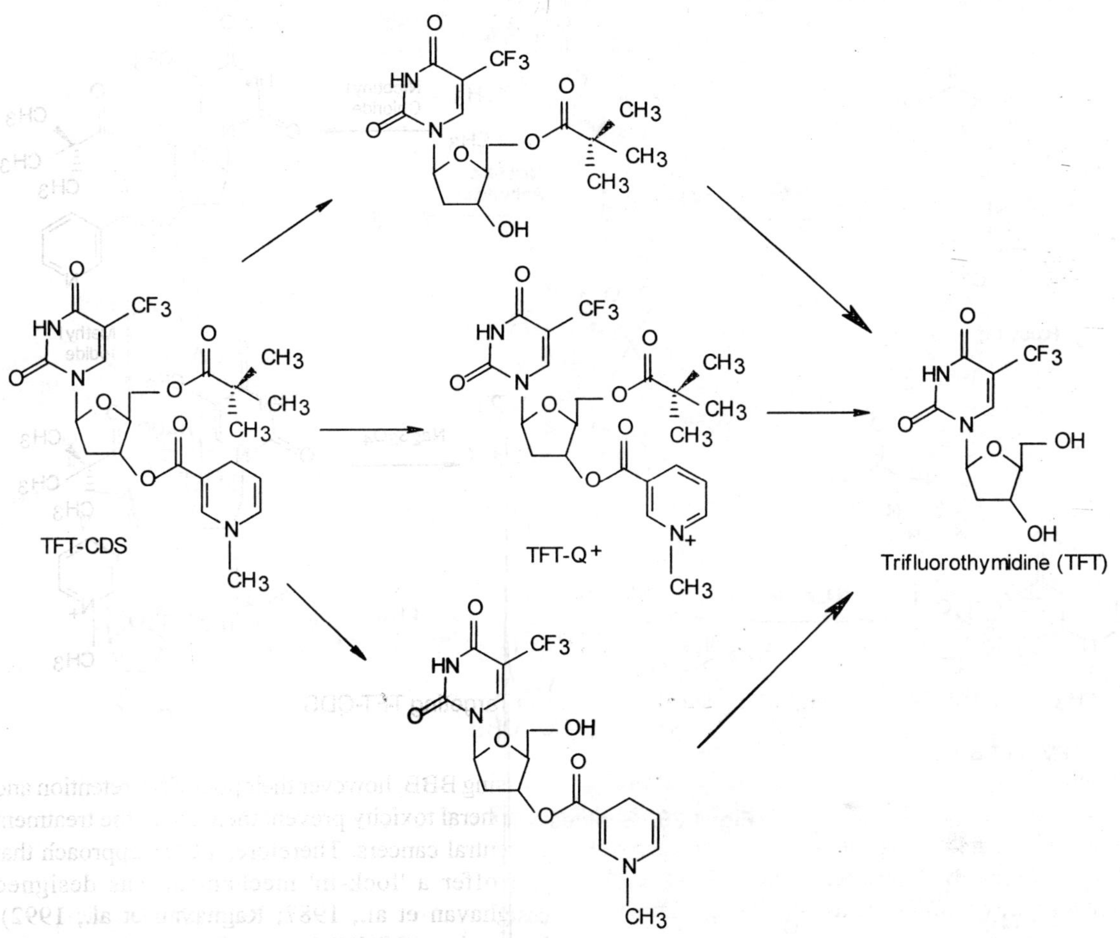

Fig. 4-29. Transformations of the TFT-CDS Required for Release of TFT

retained in brain. Therefore, they require frequent dosing to maintain therapeutic levels. It has been reported that constant peripheral exposure of oestrogen is related to a number of pathological conditions such as cancer, hypertension and altered metabolism (Kaplan, 1978). CNS is the major target site for estrogens and a brain-targeted CDS may provide a safer and more effective alternative. Synthesis of oestrogen CDS is illustrated in Figure 4-33. An oestrogen CDS (E-CDS) could be utilized to reduce the secretion of leutienizing hormone releasing hormone (LHRH) and in process leutinizing hormone (LH) and gonadal steroids. ECDS could also be employed for safe contraception devoid of any cancer related with simple steroid therapy. Other important uses of ECDS are in depression, dementia including Alzheimer's disease etc.

Cyclodextrin complexes

The physicochemical properties that enhances the brain delivery in turn implicates the development of acceptable pharmaceutical formulations. The increased lipophilicity allows partition into deep brain tissues but it also confers poor aqueous solubility. The oxidative lability, which is required for the 'lock-in' mechanism and the hydrolytic instability, which releases the modifier functions or the active drug, combined to limit the shelf life of the CDS. Cyclodextrin may provide a possible answer to such complications. Cyclodextrins are torus-shaped oligosaccharides that contain various number of α-

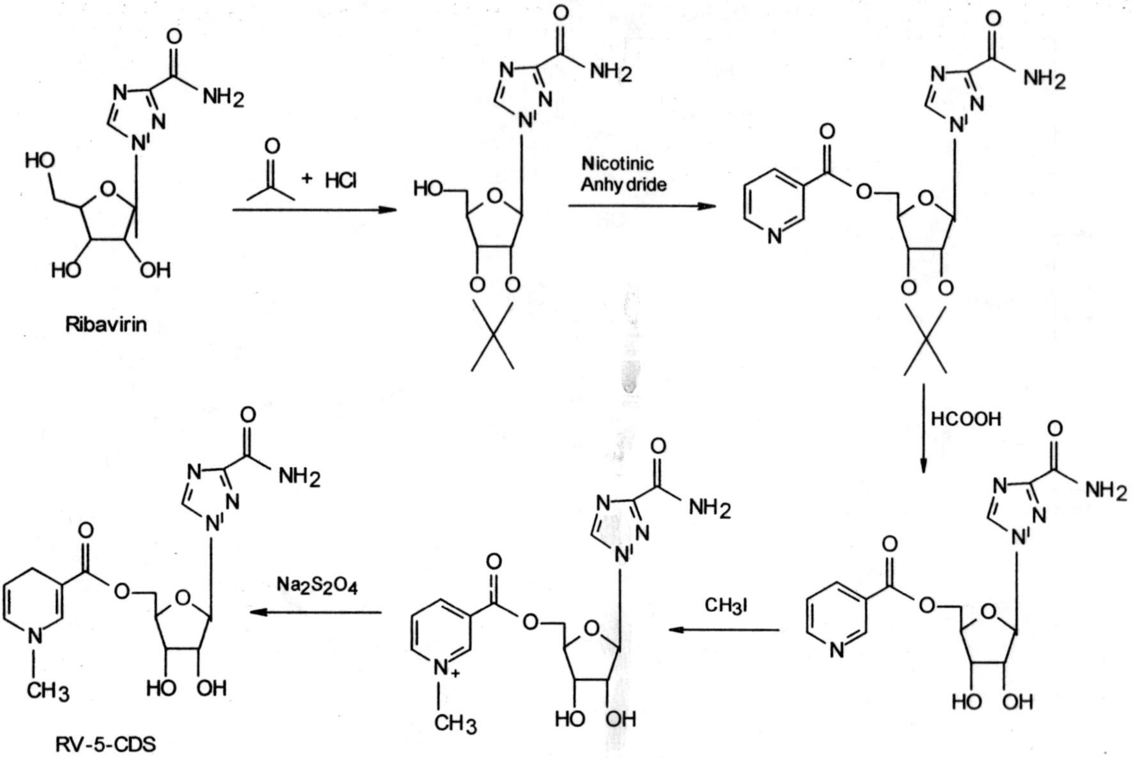

Fig. 4-30. Synthesis of RV-5′-CDS

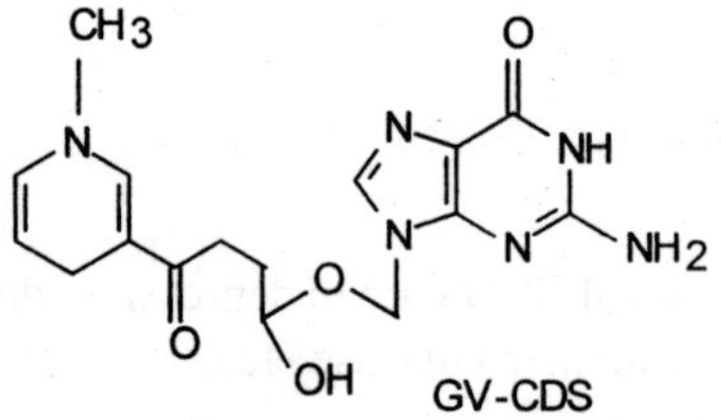

Fig. 4-31. Ganciclovir CDS

1,4-linked glucose units (6,7 and 8 for α-,β- and γ-cyclodextrin, respectively). There are number of advantages such as enhancement of solubility, stabilization of unstable drugs, enhancement of bioavailability, improvement of smell and taste, reduction of possible stomach injury, inhibition of haemolysis, transformation of liquids into powders etc (Szejtli, 1994). Inclusion complex of E2-CDS with 2-hydroxypropyl-β-cyclodextrin solved all the essential problems associated with CDS vis-à-vis it increased the stability of E2-CDS (Brewster et al., 1988). Similarly, promising results were obtained from lomustin CDS inclusion complexes with cyclodextrins.

Molecular Packaging of Neuropeptides

The CDS approach has been recently expanded to include various neuropeptides to achieve successful deliveries of enkephalin, TRH and kyotrophin analogues (Bodor et al., 1992; Prokai-Tatrai et al., 1996; Chen et al., 1998). Neuropeptides that act on the brain or spinal cord represent the largest class of transmitter substances and possess tremendous therapeutic potential, however, delivery of these peptides through the BBB is more complex as they can be rapidly inactivated by ubiquitous peptidases (Kastin et al., 1987). Therefore, for a successful delivery of peptides, lipophilicity of the molecule should be increased to enhance passive transport,

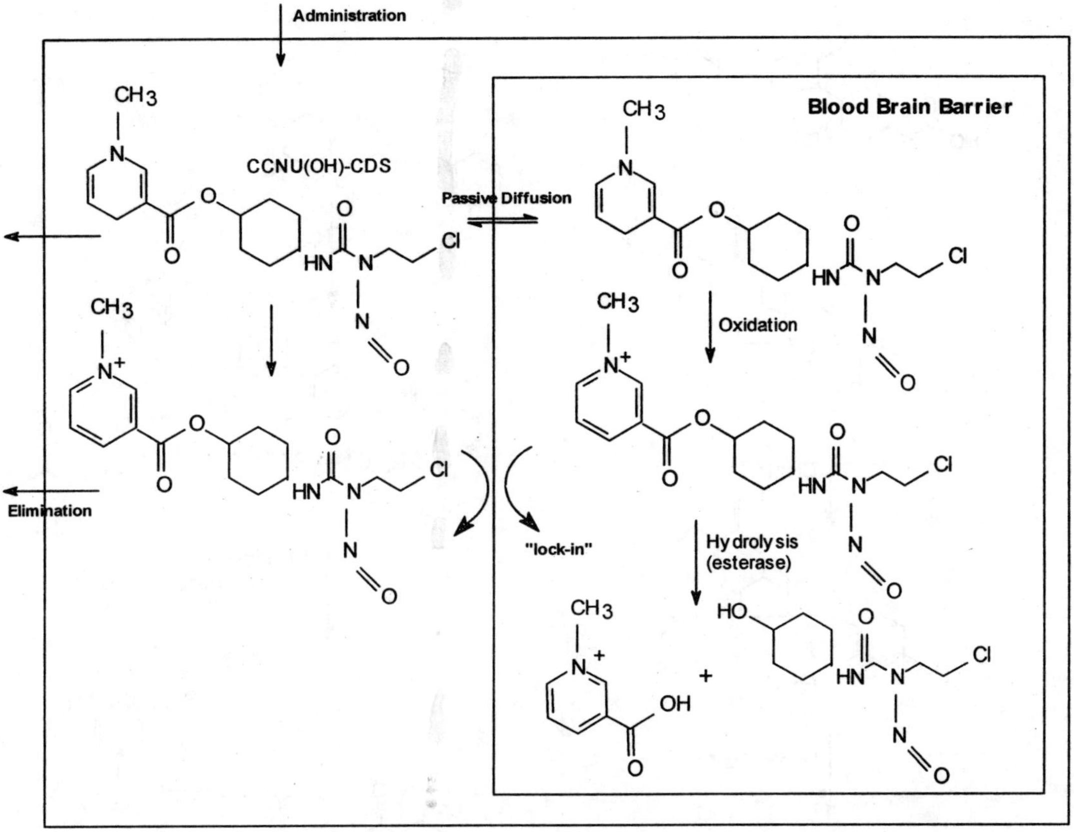

Fig. 4-32. Schematic Representation of the 'Lock-In' Mechanism for CCNU(OH) -CDS

should be protected from enzymatic attack and CNS retention should be increased. This CDS system comprises of a peptide unit that is part of a bulky molecule, dominated by lipophilic modifying groups that direct BBB penetration and prevent peptidases recognition (Bodor and Prokai, 1995). This CDS system contains following components: the redox targetor (T), a spacer function (S), the peptide (P), a bulky lipophilic moiety (L) attached to adjuster (A) (Fig. 4-34). After administration of CDS the first step must be the conversion of targetor to allow for 'lock-in'. This is followed by removal of lipophilic function (L), followed by cleavage of the targetor spacer moiety ultimately leading to the active neuropeptide (Fig. 4-34).

Leu-enkephalin analogues are used for the treatment of opiate dependence and numerous other CNS-mediated dysfunctions (Hughes et al., 1975). These peptides are implicated in stress responses, alcoholism, schizophrenia, eating disorders and in modulating memory functions, sexual behaviour, gastrointestinal function, heart rate and blood pressure. However, analgesia remains the prime use for these peptides. For effective analgesic action intracerebroventricular (i.c.v.) dosing is required and i.v. injection produced no effect. Therefore, CDS approach was applied. Four different CDSs were synthesized by segment coupling method and it was observed that their i.v. injection produced a significant and long lasting response in rats monitored by a tail-flick latency test. Studies conducted revealed that the peptide CDS successfully delivered, retained and released the peptides in the brain.

A similar strategy has also been employed for delivery of thyrotropin-releasing hormone (TRH) analogues to the CNS (Prokai et al., 1994). These

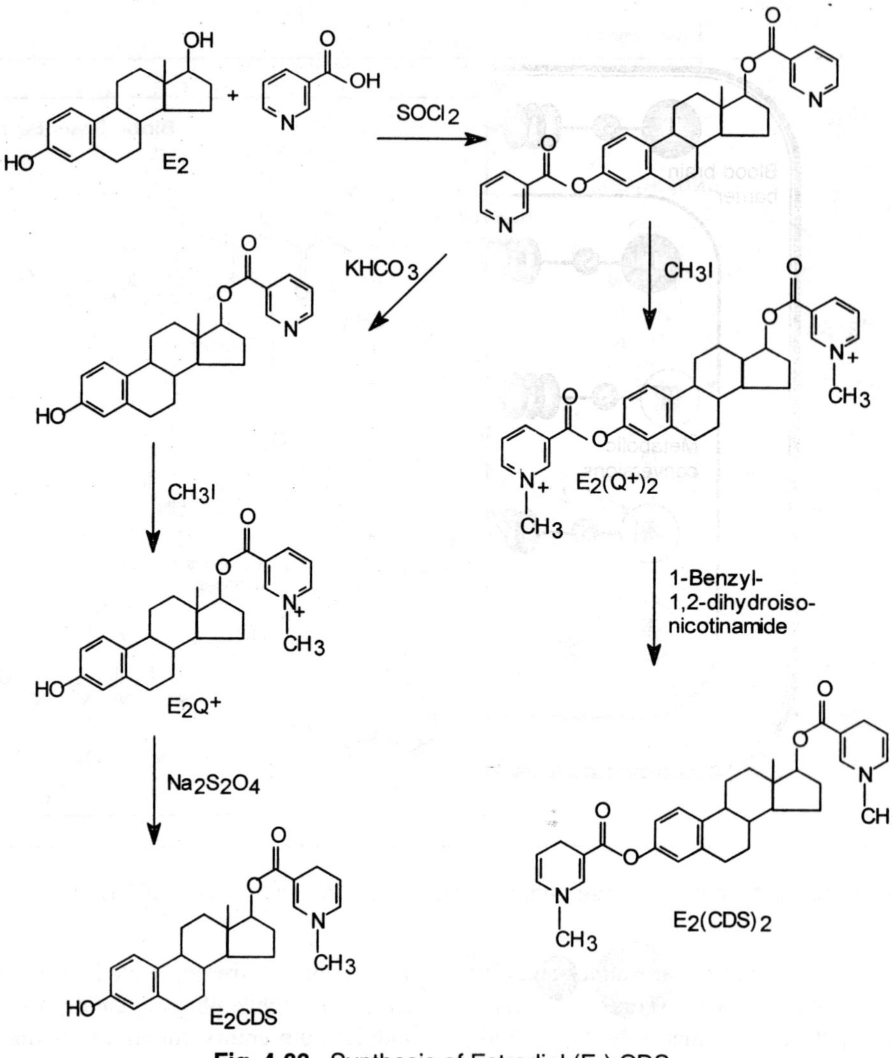

Fig. 4-33. Synthesis of Estradiol (E_2) CDS

analogues are used for treating neurodegenerative disorders like Alzheimer's disease. The efficacy of TRH-CDSs was measured by the decrease in the barbiturate induced sleeping time in mice. After i.v. injection TRH analogue itself produced a marginal decrease, whereas CDS produced a significant decrease in barbiturate induced sleeping time.

Kyotrophin, an endogeneous analgesic that produces analgesia through the release of endogenous enkephalin, is an important neuropeptide (Bodor and Buchwald, 1998). Its analogues contain free amine residue and studies indicated that these ionizable functional groups impede the successful delivery of peptides. Therefore, this free amine group was additionally covered by attaching Boc(tert-butyl oxycarbonyl) group. It was suggested that this liaison is bioconvertible and is reverted back after the lock in the peptide. Figure 4-35 illustrates chemistry of synthesis of various CDSs for kyotorphin analogues. It was found that these CDS showed good activity in the rat tail-flick latency test compared to free peptide. The molecular packaging of neuropeptides provides a rational drug design approach that leads to the first documented non-invasive brain delivery of these

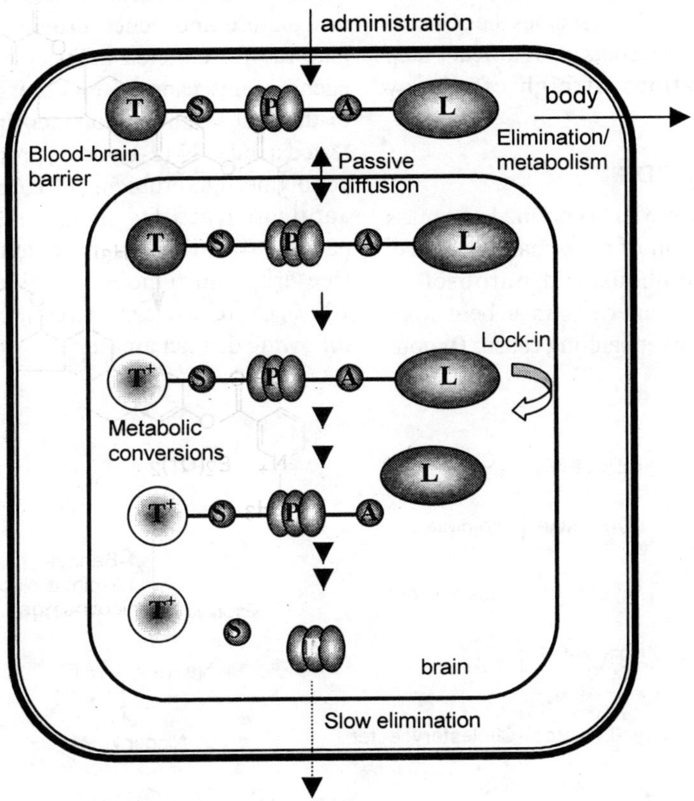

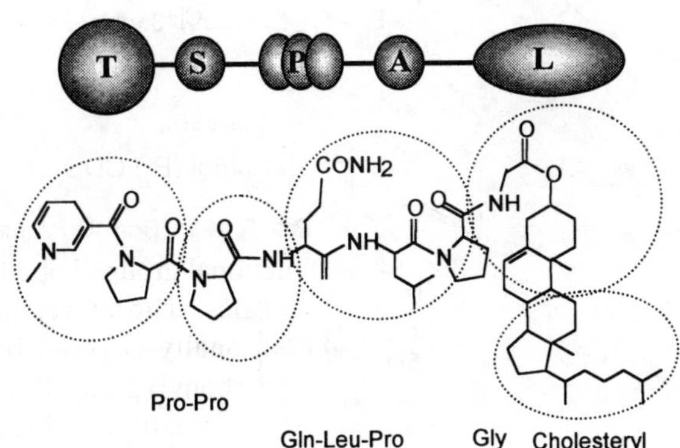

Fig. 4-34. Illustration of the Molecular Packaging and Sequential Metabolism used for Brain Targeting of Neuropeptides. TRH-CDS is included to provide a concrete illustration for the Targetor (T), Spacer (S), Peptide (P), Adjuster (A) and Lipophilic (L) moieties

important biomolecules in therapeutically effective concentrations. This approach overcomes the obstacle imposed by BBB and represents a significant step toward future generations of high efficiency neuropharmaceuticals.

Tumour Targeting by CDS

Cancer is a dreadful disease and is defined as a mass of tissue formed as a result of abnormal, excessive, uncoordinated, autonomous and purposeless proliferation of cells. For centuries human beings are trying hard to get rid of this appaulling cause. Tumour capillaries are hyperpermeable compared to normal vasculature and hence provide much sought after gateway for targeted delivery of chemotherapeutic agents against cancer. Reports of phase I clinical trials of the first synthetic polymer-drug conjugate to be tested in man, N-(2-Hydroxypropyl)methacrylamide copolymer-doxorubicin (FCE 28068) demonstrated antitumour activity in chemotherapy-refractory patients, significantly reduced toxicity compared with free drug and tumour selective targeting (Vasey, 1999). Currently, cancer research is being done in following distinct areas:

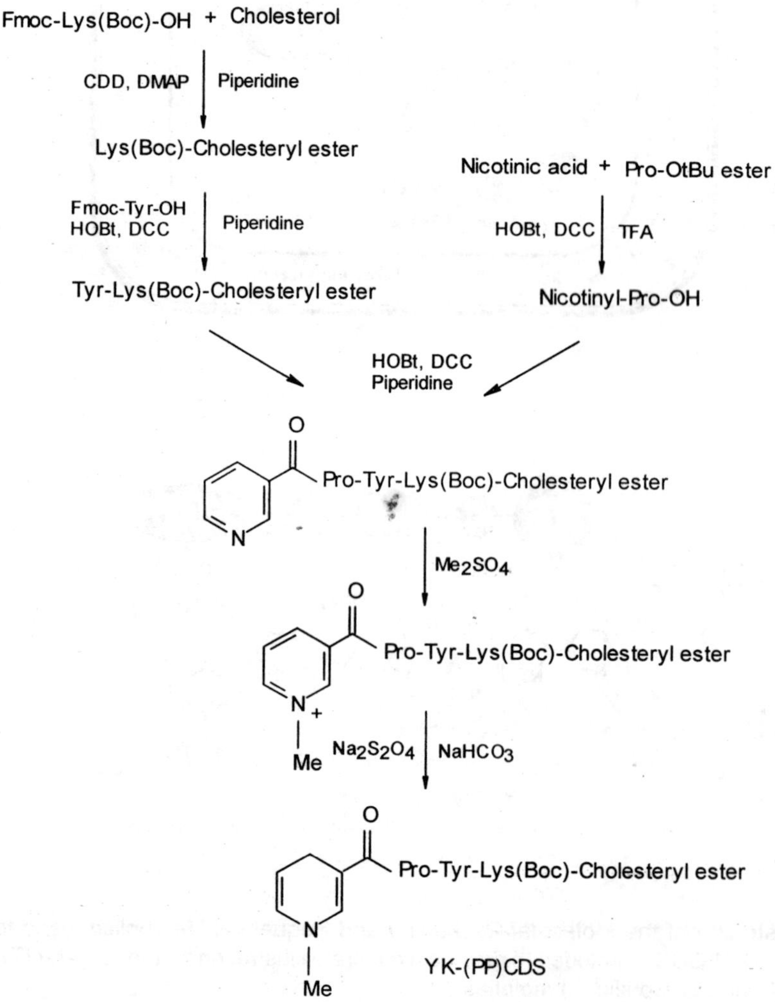

Fmoc-Lys(Boc)-OH + Cholesterol

CDD, DMAP | Piperidine

Lys(Boc)-Cholesteryl ester

Fmoc-Tyr-OH, HOBt, DCC | Piperidine

Tyr-Lys(Boc)-Cholesteryl ester

Nicotinic acid + Pro-OtBu ester

HOBt, DCC | TFA

Nicotinyl-Pro-OH

HOBt, DCC, Piperidine

O

Pro-Tyr-Lys(Boc)-Cholesteryl ester

N

Me_2SO_4

O

Pro-Tyr-Lys(Boc)-Cholesteryl ester

N^+

Me

$Na_2S_2O_4$ | $NaHCO_3$

O

Pro-Tyr-Lys(Boc)-Cholesteryl ester

N

Me

YK-(PP)CDS

Fig. 4-35. Synthesis of Kyotrophin Analogue CDS

1. Development of low molecular weight, more effective, anticancer agent from the knowledge of new pharmacological targets arising from the increased understanding of the molecular basis of cancer (Hill, 1996).
2. Recognition and identification of new targets for chemotherapy like apoptosis, signal transduction pathways, tumour vasculature vis-à-vis angiogenesis (Folkman, 1995; Lundberg and Weinberg, 1999).
3. Development of antisense oligonucleotides and gene therapy to introduce antitumour vaccines cytokines or enzymes that can be exploited for activation of low molecular weight prodrug (Sandhu et al., 1997; Crooke, 1998).
4. Drug delivery systems offer more potential area for targeted chemotherapy of cancer. Localized and selective delivery can be achieved using liposomes, immunoconjugates, proteins and polymer therapeutics (Robert et al., 1989).

Nevertheless, these delivery systems provide controlled release of an antitumour agent thus improve patient compliance by alleviating the need for repeated daily or weekly injections.

Tumour Vasculature

A single abnormal cell is capable of generating primary and secondary metastable tumours. As the tumour grows, oxygen and nutrients are initially obtained from adjacent normal blood vessels, but once the cellular mass exceeds 150-200 μm in size vascularization must proportionally be increased (Folkman, 1990). New tumour blood vessels originate by the sprouting of exciting host vessels or formation of completely new vessels by angiogenesis (Maragoudakis, 1998). Tumour vessels are consisted of basement membrane and endothelial cells. Vessels may have a wider lumen and devoid of normal innervation. This in addition to the absence of smooth muscle cells in the vessel wall can result in irregular blood flow and sometimes neovasculature itself could be considered as target for the design of innovative chemotherapy. There is approximately one endothelial cell per hundred tumour cells so any drug like combrestatin that can selectively destroy tumour endothelial cells will have the advantage of easier access to its target site and fewer target cells to destroy (Chaplin et al., 1999). Fumagillin analogue TNP 40, an antiangiogenic compound is under clinical trial and may hit the market in near future (Ingber, 1997). Although induction of vascular shutdown can cause tumour shrinkage and limits further growth, it is widely accepted that the remaining viable/dormant cells must be destroyed in order to obtain a complete cure. It has been suggested that disordered state of tumour vessels including their inherent leakiness provides an important gate-way for passive targeting of long circulating macromolecular therapeutics vis-à-vis particulate carriers to tumours using a phenomenon, enhanced permeability and retention (EPR) (Maeda and Malsumura, 1989).

Enhanced Permeability and Retention (EPR) Effect

Polymer-drug conjugates and vesicular carrier systems such as liposomes facilitate significant solid tumour targeting of commonly used chemotherapeutic agents such as doxorubicin in both animal models and man via phenomenon that is termed as Enhanced Permeability and Retention (EPR) effect (Muggia, 1999). The EPR effect is shown schematically in Figure 4-36. The EPR effect can be attributed to mainly two factors; leaky tumour vessels allowing macromolecular extravasation unusual in normal tissues and lack of effective tumour lymphatic drainage, preventing clearance of the penetrant macromolecules and promoting their accumulation. Although the contribution of EPR mediated targeting in clinical setting is still to be quantified in regard to features of the vector and tumour characteristics that can determine the extent of tumour targeting (Table 4-2).

The maximum size of drug navigating moiety either polymer-drug conjugate or liposomes that can extravasate intratumourally is still not defined however, experiments using ^{125}I-labelled HPMA (Hydroxy propyl methacrylamide) copolymer fractions of molecular weight 20-800 kDa as probes demonstrated that all molecular weight fractions had equivalent access to B16F10 and sarcoma 180 tumours, irrespective of molecular weight (Seymour, 1995). The blood clearance rates (blood concentration) of co-polymer was identified as the most important factor governing tumour levels. The

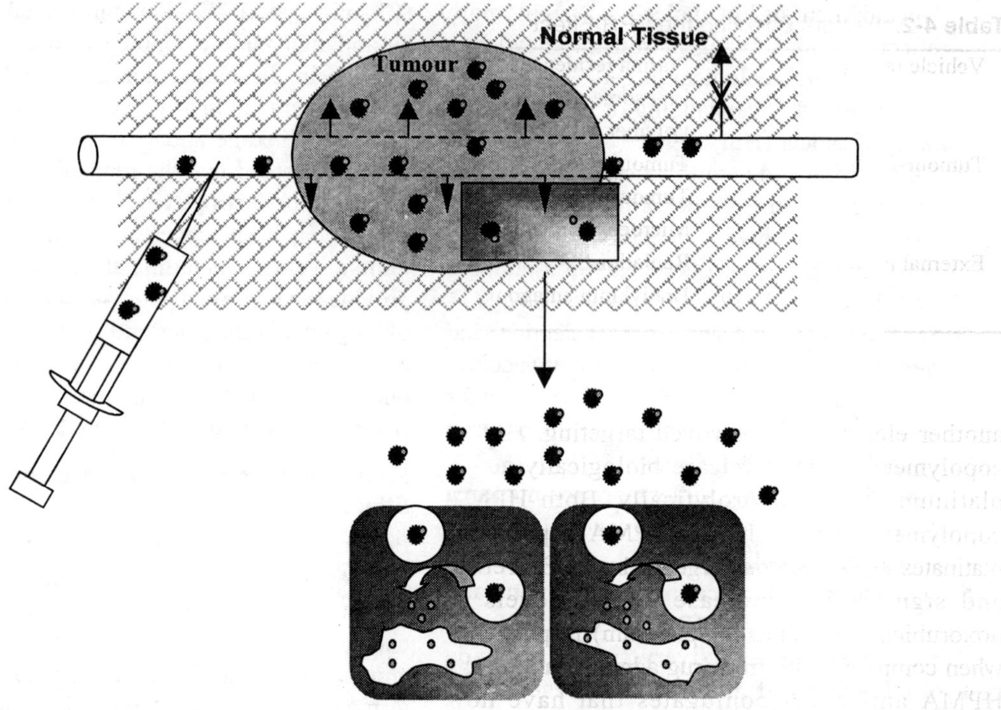

Fig. 4-36. Schematic Diagram Showing the Fate of Long Circulating Polymer-Drug conjugate. Figure Shows the Selective Uptake of the Polymer Conjugate by the Enhanced Permeability and Retention (EPR) Effect and the Uptake of Polymer Conjugates by Endocytosis and the Release of Drug Intracellularly

effectiveness of the EPR effect is not only limited by the extent of extravasation, but also by the extent of intra-tumoural retention. Comparison of the tumour levels attained after intraveneous administration of proteins, polymeric conjugates with a loose coiled structure and more compact synthetic polymers like dendrimers illustrates that loosely coiled polymers are better retained intratumourally than more globular proteins and polymers (Gianasi, 1999).

Polymer-anticancer Conjugates

Polymer anticancer conjugates were proposed to enhance the physicochemical properties of drug and to navigate the drug specifically to the tumour site. The ideal polymeric carrier should impart hydrophilic character to the drug and also should be equipped with the functional groups needed to permit covalent linkage of drug. Many times a biodegradable spacer is inserted to insure stability in the systemic circulation and subsequently to facilitate specific enzymatic or hydrolytic intratumoural drug release. Most of the polymeric carriers are selected on the basis of their inertness in the body. However, some of biologically active polymers have also been explored including N-(2-Hydroxy propyl) methacrylamide copolymer-doxorubicin (HPMA) copolymer conjugates for antitumour activity (Fig. 4- 37) (Duncan, 1992; Duncan et al., 1996; Brocchini and Duncan, 1999). The antitumour conjugates were prepared for daunomycin (Duncan, 1988), doxorubicin (Duncan, 1992), melphalan (Duncan, 1991), mesochlorin E6 (Krinick, 1994), emitine (Dimitrijevic and Duncan, 1998) and platinates (Gianasi, 1999). In general these anticancer agents bound to the polymer backbone using peptidyl spacers designed for cleavage by the lysosomal thiol-dependent (cytsteine) proteases (Freidrich, 1999). These enzymes are known to be elevated in many human tumours and high levels have been correlated with poor prognosis, so this may fortuitously provide

Table 4-2. Factors Effecting the EPR Effect

Vehicle related factor	Plasma residence time
	Liposome or particle size
	Polymer architecture
Tumour-related	Tumour size
	Tumour type
	Microenvironment
External mediators	Radiation
	Bradykinin antagonist, cyclooxygenase inhibitor and NO scavenger

another element for improved targeting. HPMA copolymer platinates release biologically active platinum species hydrolytically. Both HPMA copolymer-doxorubicin and HPMA copolymer-platinates showed tumour targeting by the EPR effect and significantly increase tumour levels of doxorubicin and cisplatin (platinum) respectively, when compared with free drug administration. The HPMA anticancer conjugates that have now progressed to the clinical trials are composed of a non-biodegradable HPMA copolymer main chain of molecular weight 30 kDa, a Gly-Phe-Leu-Gly peptidyl polymer drug linker and a drug content of 5-10 wt% (Pimm, 1996; Julyan, 1999). Figure 4-37 shows the doxorubicin conjugates where the drug is linked to the peptidyl linker via a peptide bond. On the other hand the HPMA copolymer-paclitaxel and campothecin conjugates contain drug bound to the carrier via a terminal ester linkage.

Phase I clinical trials of HPMA copolymer-Gly-Phe-Leu-Gly-doxorubicin (PK1, FCE 28068) showed that when it was given once every three weeks, it greatly reduced toxicity, compared with free doxorubicin and activity in chemotherapy refractory patients is also enhanced (Vasey, 1999). Currently, PK1 is undergoing phase II evaluation for treatment of breast, lung and colon cancer. HPMA copolymer-doxorubicin containing additional galactosamine (PK2, FCE 28069) and HPMA copolymer-paclitaxel are undergoing phase I/II clinical testing and another compound in the series HPMA copolymer camptothecin is recently been introduced into phase I trials (Fig. 4-38).

Antibody and Enzyme Based Tumour Targeting

Prodrugs have been found to be effective in the treatment of animal tumours possessing high levels of an activating enzyme (Cobb et al., 1969; Connors, 1986). However, clinical results were disappointing when it was found that human tumours containing appropriately high levels of the activating enzymes were rare and that the high levels of activating enzymes were not associated with any particular type of tumour (Bagshawe, 1993). Recently, new therapies have been proposed to overcome this limitation of chemically modulated delivery systems. These new approaches include antibody conjugates, ADEPT (antibody directed enzyme prodrug therapy) and GDEPT (gene directed enzyme prodrug therapy).

Antibody-drug conjugates or immunoconjugates are macromolecular prodrugs produced by covalently linking cytotoxic agent to monoclonal antibodies against tumour associated antigens. These immuno-conjugates binds and subsequently taken up by specific cells possessing surface antigens followed by breakdown of the immunoconjugate intracellularly by lysosomal enzymes. This approach suffers from certain drawbacks like heterogeneity of antigens present on cancer cells, inefficient internalization of the antigen-antibody complex and/or insufficient release of drug intracellularly.

Another approach referred to as ADEPT (antibody-directed enzyme prodrug therapy) attempts the localization of prodrug activation enzymes onto specific cancer cells prior to prodrug administration. Enzymes that activate prodrug can be directed to human tumour xenografts by conjugating them to

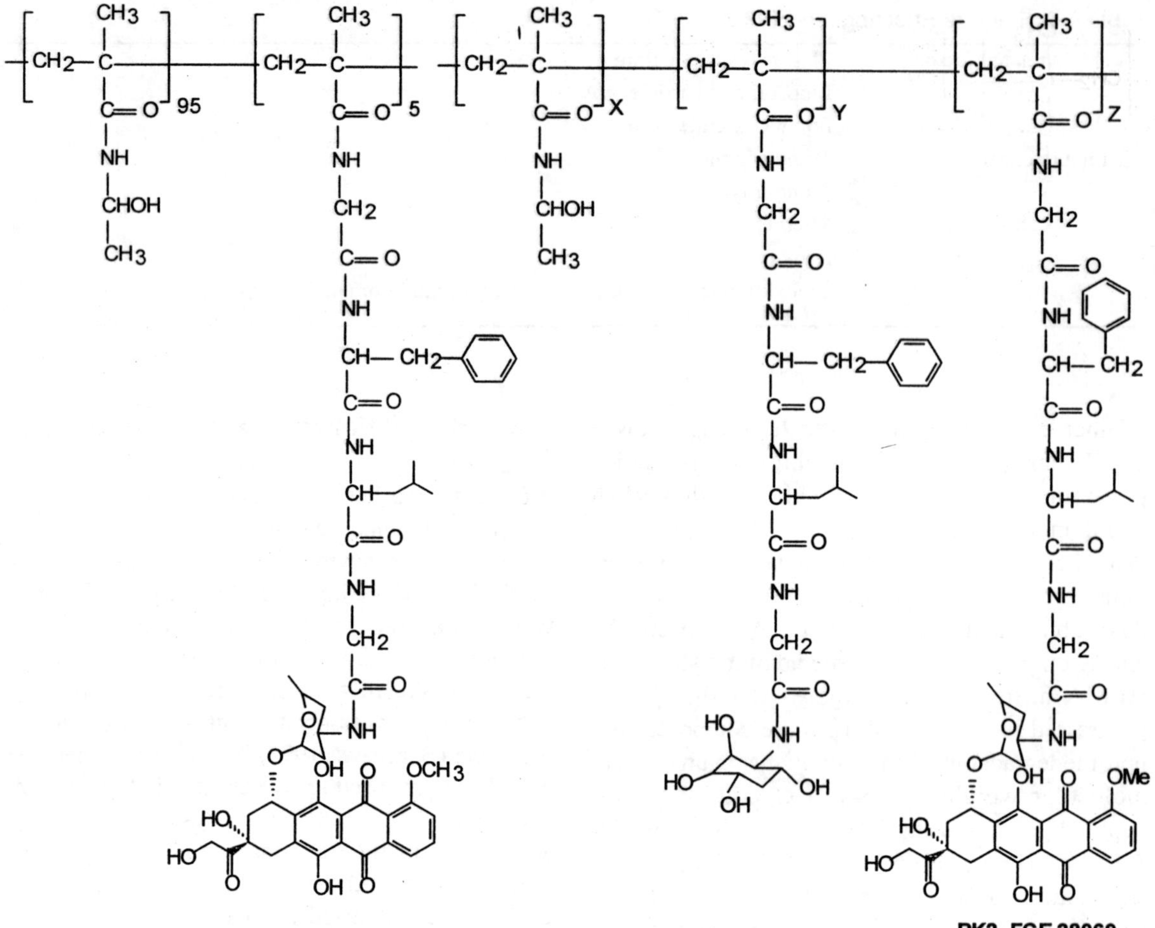

PK1, FCE 28068

PK2, FCE 28069

Fig. 4-37. HPMA Copolymer with Doxorubicin (PK1 and PK2)

tumour-selective monoclonal antibodies (Bagshawe, 1987; Connor and Knox, 1995; Sharma et al., 1992). As shown in Figure 4-39, an antitumour antibody is conjugated to an enzyme not normally present in extracellular fluid via intravenous infusion. After elimination of the conjugate from the blood, a prodrug is administered that is normally inert but is activated by the enzyme delivered to the tumour. Using different combinations of antibody enzyme and prodrug many classes of human tumour xenografts have been shown to be very sensitive to ADEPT procedure. Early clinical trials are promising and indicate that ADEPT may become an effective treatment for solid cancers for which tumour-selective antibodies are known (Springer et al., 1993; Harris et al., 1999).

Another novel approach of tumour targeting employes genes encoding prodrug-activating enzymes (Huber et al., 1994; culver et al., 1992), this approach utilizes viral vectors (eg., retroviral or adenoviral) to carry a prodrug-activating enzyme gene into both tumour and normal cells, however by linking the foreign gene downstream of tumour-specific trascription units, tumour specific expression of the foreign enzyme gene can be achieved (Huber et al., 1994), this approach is referred to as virus directed enzyme prodrug therapy (VDEPT) or more generally gene-directed enzyme prodrug therapy

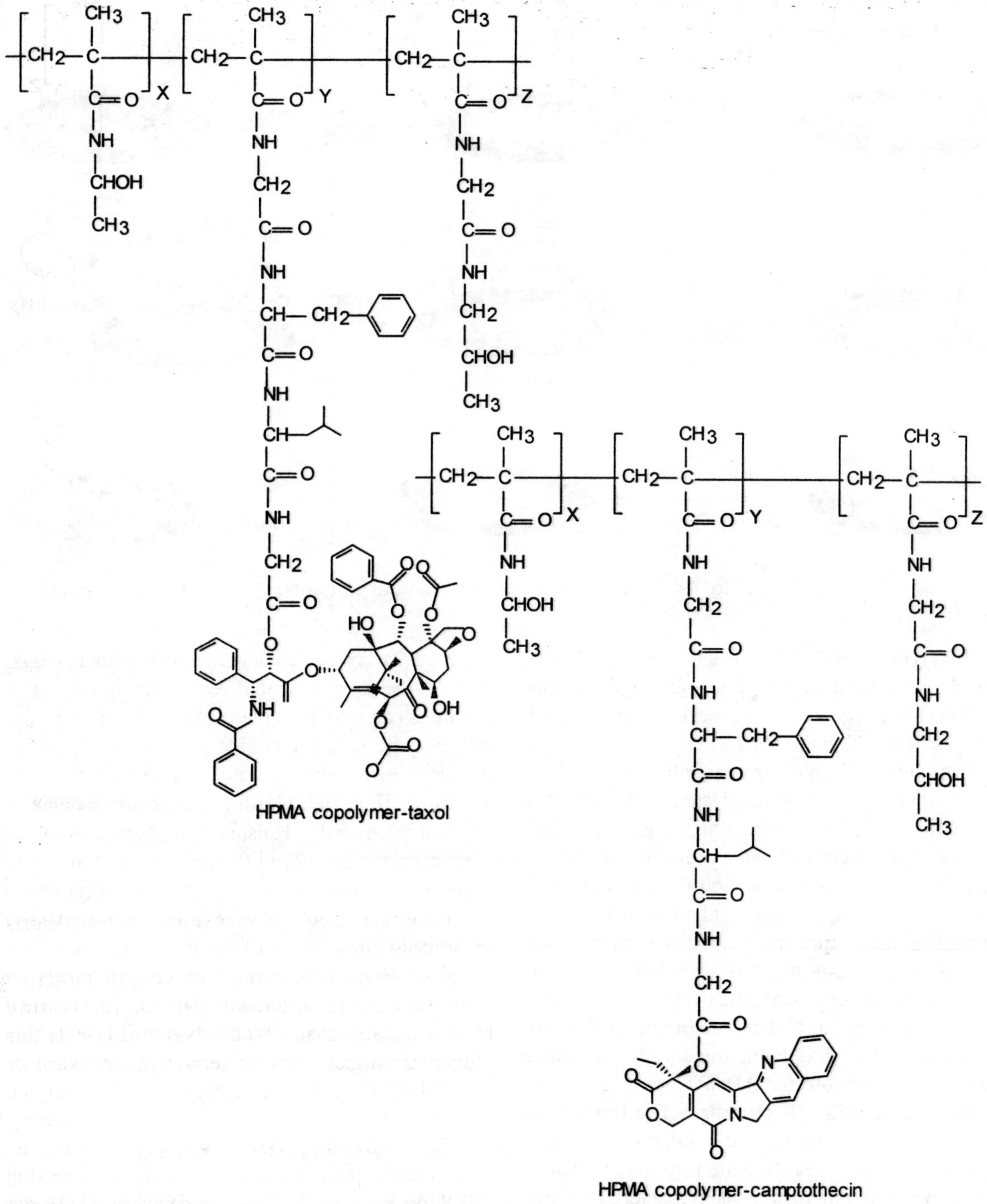

HPMA copolymer-taxol

HPMA copolymer-camptothecin

Fig. 4-38. Chemical Structure of HPMA Copolymer Conjugates of Taxol and Camptothecin

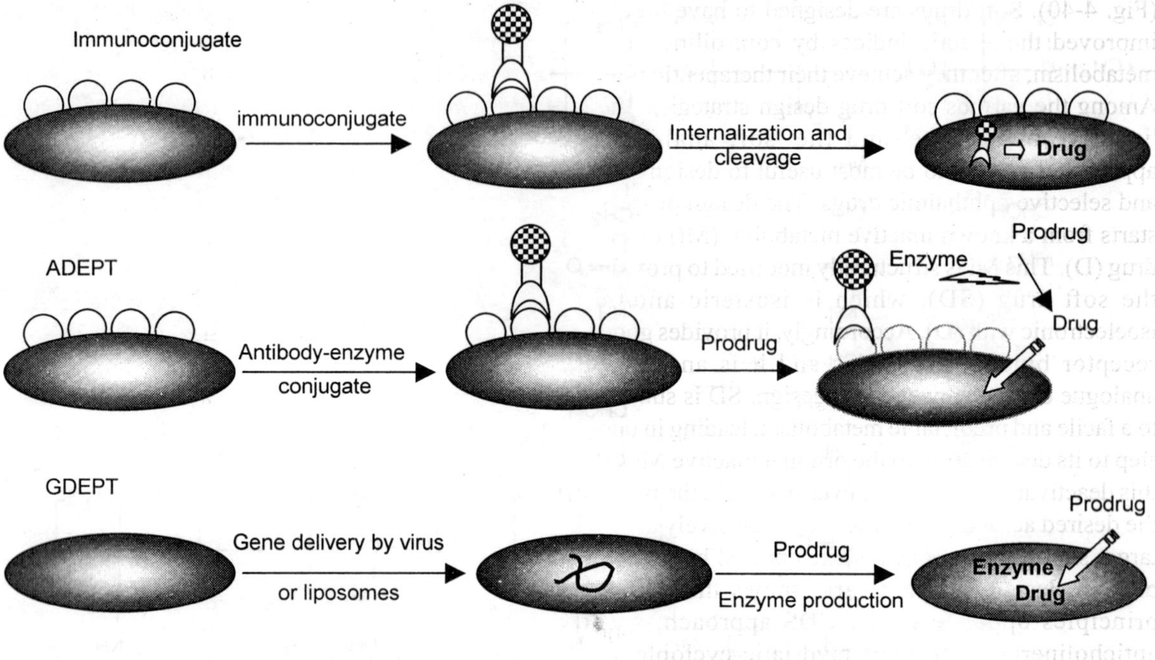

Fig. 4-39. Novel Techniques of Tumour Targeting

(GDEPT) (Barda et al., 1993; Deonarain et al., 1995). In addition to viral vectors, liposomes and cationic lipids have been proposed for gene delivery to tumour cells (Tsuji and Tamai, 1996).

The choice of enzyme is very critical for ADEPT as well as GDEPT procedure. Usually enzymes that are monomeric, low molecular weight and lack glycosalytion for activation are preferred for ease of handling and possible protein modification (Anlezark et al., 1992). Mostly enzymes of non-human or non-mammalian origin that could catalyze substrates not normally activated in humans are utilized. Thus in terms of specificity, enzymes from non-human sources especially those of microbiological origin are advantageous. It has been observed that some enzymes are sutitable for ADEPT, whereas others for GDEPT, in ADEPT, prodrug activation occurs extracellularly, whereas in GDEPT it occurs intracellularly. An ideal enzyme for GDEPT would appear to be monomeric enzyme of bacterial or viral origin with wide substrate specificity like bacterial nitroreductase that can convert a relatively non-toxic monofunctional alkylating agent into a 10,000 times more cytotoxic difunctional alkylating agent (Haisma et al., 1992). As nitoreductases require either NADH or NADPH as an essential reductant, activation of prodrugs can only take place intracellularly making this enzyme a better choice for GDEPT than for ADEPT. On the other extreme, charged prodrugs that are bifunctional alkylating agents are especially suitable for ADEPT (Haisma et al., 1992), as due to their charge they will not enter cells and are non-toxic because the essential target for alkylating agents is intracellular DNA. After extracellular activation of prodrugs in vicinity of tumour cells, the active drugs will freely diffuse and attain a high intracellular concentration. Thus, alkylating prodrugs activated by β-glucuronidase or carboxypeptidase G2 as glucuronic or glutamic acid derivatives are excellent for ADEPT (Eccles et al., 1994).

SOFT DRUG APPROACH

Retrometabolic drug design approaches simultaneously involve structure activity and structure metabolism relationship in the design process. Retrometabolic drug design includes both chemical delivery systems (CDSs) and soft drugs (SD)

(Fig. 4-40). Soft drugs are designed to have highly improved therapeutic indices by controlling their metabolism, after they achieve their therapeutic role. Among the various soft drug design strategies, the 'inactive metabolite' and the 'soft analogue' approaches proved to be most useful to design safe and selective ophthalmic drugs. The design process starts from a known inactive metabolite (Mi) of the drug (D). This Mi is structurally modified to provide the soft drug (SD), which is isosteric and/or isoelectronic with (D). Accordingly, it provides good receptor binding properties and it is an active analogue of (D). However, by design, SD is subject to a facile and predictable metabolism, leading in one step to its deactivation to the original inactive Mi. as this deactivation takes place everywhere in the body, the desired activities are produced exclusively at the target site. This approach is exemplified by soft β-blocker design, which clearly shows the design principles opposite to the CDS approach, soft anticholinergics for short mydriatic-cycloplegic activity and soft corticosteroids, which have the major benefit of providing good anti-inflammatory activity in the eye but essentially lack side effects like elevation of intraocular pressure or cataract formation.

Inactive metabolic approach can be summarized in following steps:

1. The design process starts with a known inactive metabolite of a drug which is then used as a lead compound.
2. Novel structures are generated from inactive metabolite, which are isosteric and/or isoelectronic with the drug from which the lead inactive metabolite was derived. This is referred to as activation stage.
3. The structure of the new soft analog is designed in such a way that its metabolism will yield the same starting inactive metabolite in one step (predictable metabolism)
4. The specific binding, transport properties vis-à-vis the rate of metabolism of the new soft drugs will be controlled by molecular manipulations in the activation stage (controllable metabolism).

β-adrenergic blockers are currently most important drugs for the treatment of glaucoma, the opthalmic soft β-blockers were designed based on specific β-blockers such as metoprolol and atenolol (Fig. 4-41), which are known to undergo various metabolic conversions involving the β-amino alcohol pharmacophore, but are also metabolized to a significant extent on the remote para position of the phenol ring, yielding the corresponding phenylacetic acid. This metabolite was shown to be inactive as a β-adrenergic antagonist, and it is actually eliminated as such. Therefore, it is a good lead compound to develop new soft β-blockers which have their metabolism directed exclusively to this para substituted phenylacetic site. A large number of ester derivatives were reported (Bodor et al., 1984), but for opththalmic use more lipophilic functions were

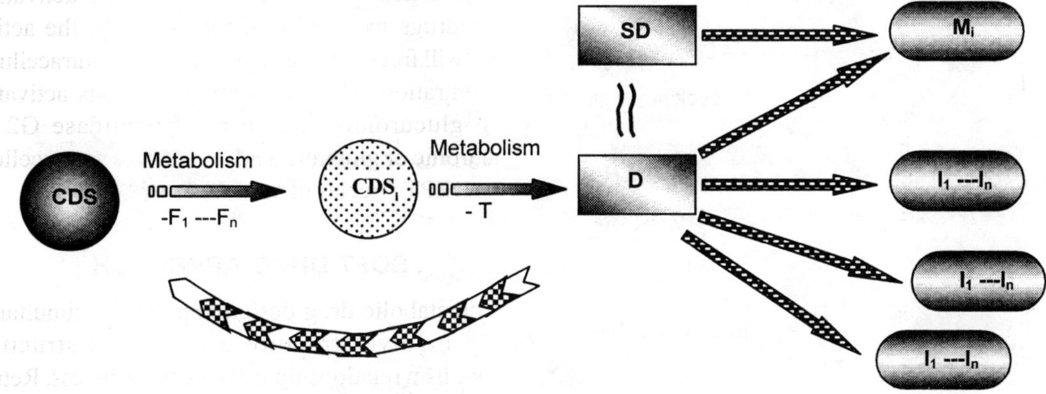

Fig. 4-40. Retrometabolic Drug Delivery Approach

used at it is important to retain integrity of the ester until they penetrate the cornea. The ester derivative of phenyl acetic acid analogue of β-blocker are active, however, they undergo a predictable singular metabolism by ester hydrolysis leading to the starting inactive phenyl acetic acid derivative of β-blocker. It has been observed that applications of soft β-blocker to rabbit eyes provided prolonged and significant reduction in the intraocular pressure (IOP) with reduced systemic side effects.

Prednisolone acetate is the drug of choice for ophthalmic application, although effective in a variety of inflammatory conditions, it causes significant elevation in the IOP, a debilitating side effect. Loteprednol etabonate is derived from prednisolone, its design and deactivation is shown in Figure 4-42. It has been shown that although it is not a fluorinated steroid still it has a relatively high intrinsic activity as well as good activity in the human vasoconstrictor test. Human studies revealed that loteprednol etabonate is very effective in various inflammatory diseases of the eye, such as giant papillary conjunctivitis or allergic conjunctivitis. Animal studies have shown that as compared to dexamethasone, which causes significant elevation of IOP, however, loteprednol elabonate did not show

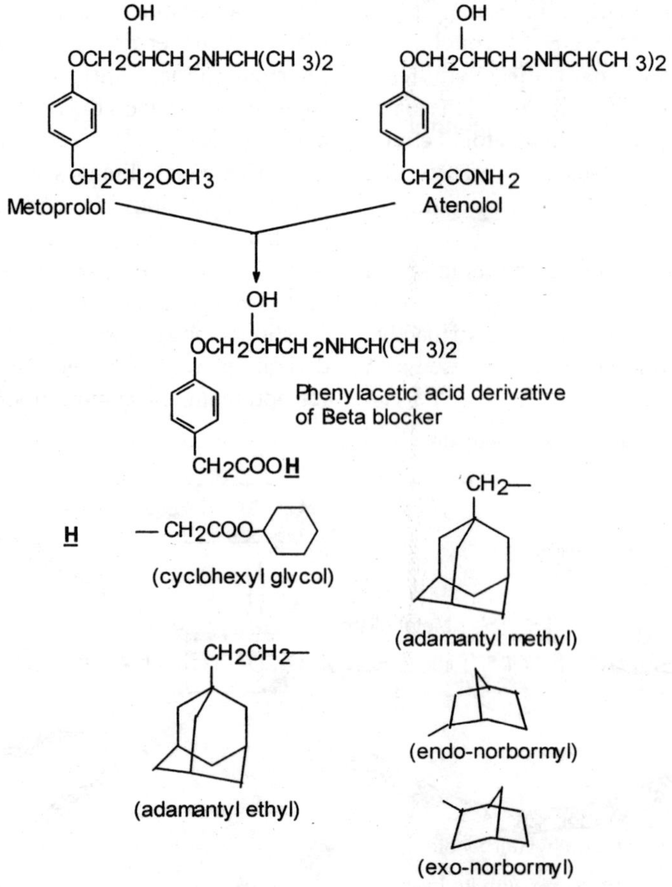

OH
$OCH_2CHCH_2NHCH(CH_3)_2$
$CH_2CH_2OCH_3$
Metoprolol

OH
$OCH_2CHCH_2NHCH(CH_3)_2$
CH_2CONH_2
Atenolol

OH
$OCH_2CHCH_2NHCH(CH_3)_2$
CH_2COO**H**
Phenylacetic acid derivative of Beta blocker

H — CH_2COO–
(cyclohexyl glycol)

CH_2—
(adamantyl methyl)

CH_2CH_2—
(adamantyl ethyl)

(endo-norbormyl)

(exo-norbormyl)

Fig. 4-41. Some Soft Drugs of β–Blockers

any effect. It was shown that topical application of dexamethasone for 2 days causes significant elevation of IOP, both in the unilaterally treated and the counter lateral eye. This is consistent with systemic absorption and activity. A similar regimen of dosing of equimolar loteprednol etabonate, did not cause any elevation in the IOP in either eyes. It can be concluded that soft corticosteroids offer significant advantages over the conventional steroids for local/topical use and in paticular in ophthalmology.

MEMBRANE TRANSPORTERS AS TARGETING SITE

Classically membrane permeability of polar drugs are enhanced by derivatizing them with lipophilic moieties to increase membrane penetration, however, targeted prodrug approach uses transporters designed for facilitating membrane transport of polar nutrients such as aminoacids and peptides. Studies have confirmed the participation of carrier mediated transport mechanisms, which enable efficient absorption of many hydrophilic compounds via specific transporters (Mizuma et al., 1993). Therefore, targeting specific membrane transporters are particularly important when prodrugs are polar or charged. Use of intestinal epithelial transporters to facilitate the absorption of appropriately modified drugs seems to be an attractive strategy for improving the bioavailability of poorly absorbed drug molecules. Prodrugs can be designed to resemble the intestinal nutrients structurally and are expected to be absorbed by specific carrier proteins, moreover, this strategy gives additional advantage of producing non-toxic nutrient byproducts in which prodrugs are converted to active form.

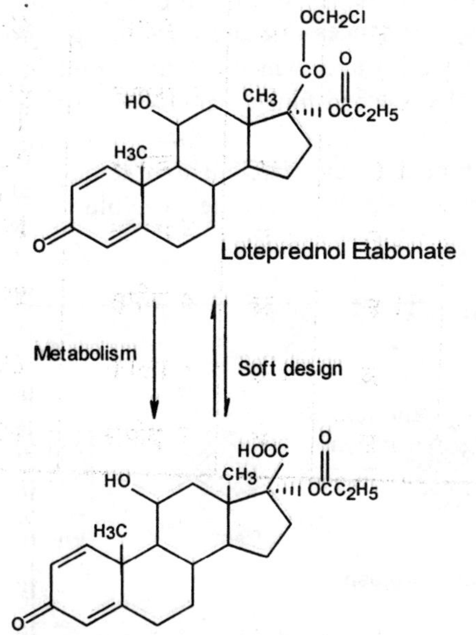

Many membrane transporters such as amino acids, peptides and glucose transporters have been targeted for improving drug absorption. Mizuma et al., 1993 studied the intestinal absorption of the β- and α- anomers of the glucoside and galactoside of p-nitrophenol to find a more suitable prodrug for poorly absorbed drugs. It has been observed that p-nitro-phenyl-β-D-gluco pyranoside was actively absorbed by glucose transporters and its permeation was comparable with that of D-glucose.

Hu et al., 1989, found that brain uptake of the potent glycine NMDA receptor antagonists, such as 7-chloro kynurenic acid and 5,7-dichlorokynurenic acid, was significantly improved by their respective prodrugs, L-4-chlorokynurenine an dL-4,6-dichlorokynurenine, which are amino acids. L-4-chlorokynureine has been shown to be rapidly transported to brain by the large neutral amino acid transporter of the blood brain barrier and is converted intracellularly to its parent drug, 7-chlorokynurenic acid. Furthermore, there are prodrug based strategies towards peptide transporters, which have also been exploited for delivery of methyldopa, alafosfalin and foscarnet (Swaan and Tukker, 1995; Grappel et al., 1985; Oh et al., 1999).

Among various membrane transporters, peptide transporters are attractive targets in prodrug design to improve oral drug absorption because they have broad substrate specificity and high capacity, secondly, they are more extensively studied than any other transporters, therefore considerable information is available about them.

Fig. 4-42. Loteprednol Etabonate with its Inactivation Steps

Peptide Transporter Associated Prodrug Therapy

Amidon et al., 1980 described a prodrug strategy referred to as Peptide Transporter Associated Prodrug Therapy (PTAPT). In this therapy a polar drug with low membrane permeability through passive diffusion is converted to a prodrug that is absorbed by peptide transporter in the cells of intestinal mucosa. After membrane transport, the prodrug may be hydrolyzed by enzymes in the mucosal cells, blood or liver. This prodrug strategy bas been demonstrated to be effective for improving the membrane permeability and systemic availability of the polar α-methyl dopa through peptidyl derivative (Fig. 4-43).

Recently applications of PTAPT have been broadened to non-peptidyl type prodrugs, such as amino acid ester prodrugs. Several amino acid ester prodrugs of the nucleoside antiviral drugs acyclovir and AZT have been synthesized and studied for intestinal absorption. It has been observed that amino acid ester prodrugs significantly (~3-10 fold) increased the intestinal absorption of their parent drugs via a peptide transporter mediated mechanism, even though they do not have a peptide bond in their structure (Han et al., 1998; Bai et al., 1992). These results established a new rationale for non-peptidyl prodrug design for targeting peptide transporters with great flexibility in structural modification. Studies revealed that L-Valyl ester prodrug of acyclovir is being transported by membrane bound peptide transporter-mediated mechanism and this shows high potential of PTAPT, in non-peptidyl as well as peptidyl drug design (Sinko and Balimane, 1998; de Vrueh et al., 1998). This supported the belief that PTAPT is a very useful strategy for improving absorption of polar drugs across intestinal membrane.

CONCLUSION

Various chemical means of achieving targeted and sustained delivery of bioactives have been discussed. The prodrug approach has been used to overcome various undesirable drug properties and to optimize the clinical effects. A number of novel retrometabolic drug delivery approaches have been developed. The particular advantage of these approaches is to enhance drug targeting to the site of action. The major classes include the CDSs and the SDs, which are opposite in terms of how they achieve the drug targeting. CDS is more sophisticated approach than prodrugs, the drug is designed to be inactive and to undergo strategic enzymatic activation in order to essentially provide the drug only at the site of action. On the other extreme, the SDs are intrinsically potent new drugs that are strategically deactivated after they achieve their therapeutic role. These approaches are general in nature and can essentially be applied to any drug. Advances in molecular biology provide easy availability of enzymes and carrier proteins with their molecular and functional characteristics. This chemical design of targeted promoiety for development of an efficient and selective drug delivery system has become possible task. The

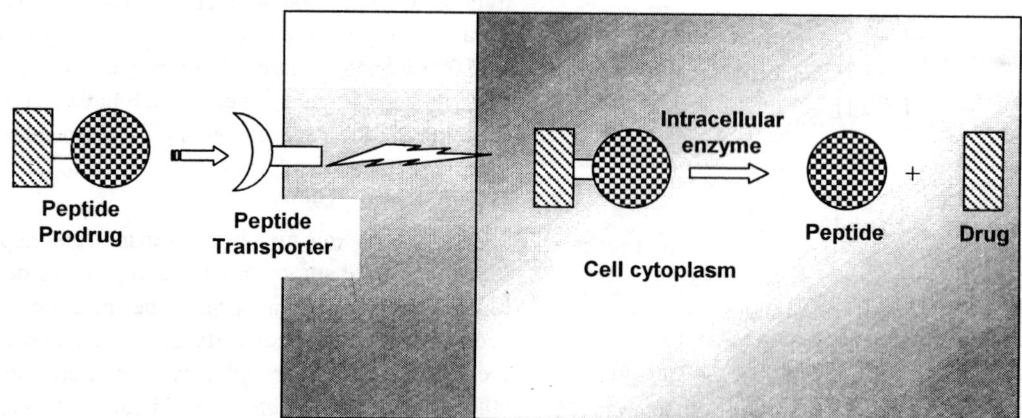

Fig. 4-42. Schematic Diagram showing Membrane Penetration of Prodrug by Peptide Transporter

chemical means of targeting, which can be combined with gene delivery and controlled expression of enzymes and carrier proteins, is a promising strategy for precise and efficient drug delivery and the enhancement of therapeutic efficacy.

REFERENCES

Alabaster V. A. (1977) In: Metabolic Functions of the Lung, Bakhle Y. S. and Vane J. R. (Eds.), Marcel Dekker Inc. New York, 3.

Albert A. (1985) *Nature* **182**, 421.

Alexander H. L., Shirley K. and Allen D. (1936) *J. Clin. Invest.* **15**, 163.

Amidon G. L., Leesman G. D. and Elliott R. L. (1980) *J. Pharm. Sci.* **69**, 1363.

Andersen H. L. (1979) *Physiol. Rev.* **59**, 305.

Anlezark G. M., Melton R. G., Sherwood R. F., Colos B., Friedlos F. and Knox R. J. (1992) *Biochem. Pharmacol.* **44**, 2289.

Anwer M. S., Kroker R. and Hegner D. (1976) *Physiol. Chem.* **357**, 1477.

Armstrong N. A. and James K. C. (1980) *Int. J. Pharmaceut.* **6**, 185.

Asperen J. V., Mayer V., Telliogen O. V. and Beijnen J. H. (1997) *J. Pharm. Sci.* **86**, 881.

Bagshawe K. D. (1987) *Br. J. Cancer* **56**, 531

Bagshawe K. D. (1993) *Adv. Pharmacol.* **24**, 99.

Bai J. P., Hu M., Subramanian P., Mosberg H. I. and Amidon G. L. (1992) *J. Pharm. Sci.* **81**, 113.

Balin F., Pizzo P., Murphy R., Eddy J., Jarosinski P., Fallon J., Broder S. and Poplock D. (1989) *Ann. Intern. Med.* **110**, 279.

Banerjee P. K. and Amidon G. L. (1985) In: Design of Prodrugs, Bundgaard H. (Ed.), Elsevier, New York, 93.

Barda D., Hardin J., Ray J. and Gage F. H. (1993) *J. Neurosurg.* **79**, 729.

Barrowman J.A., (1978) In: Physiology of the Gastrointestinal Lymphatic System, Cambridge University Press, Cambridge, 58.

Barza M. (1993) *Eur. J. Clin. Microbiol. Infect. Dis.* **12** (Suppl. 1), S31.

Begley D. J. (1996) *J. Pharm. Pharmacol.* **48**, 136.

Berr F. and Kern F. (1984) *J Lipid Res.* **25**, 85.

Blomhoff R., Helgerud P., Dueland S., Berg T., Pederson J. I., Norum K. R. and Drevon C. A. (1984) *Biochim. Biophys. Acta* **772**, 109.

Bodor N, Kaminski J. J. and Roller R. (1978) *Int. J. Pharm.* **1**, 189.

Bodor N. and Brewster M (1983) *J. Med. Chem.* **26**, 528.

Bodor N. and Brewster M. E. (1983) *Pharmacol. Ther.* **19**, 337.

Bodor N. and Buchwald P. (1998) *Chem. Br.* **34**, 36.

Bodor N. and Farag H. (1983) *J. Med. Chem.* **26**, 528.

Bodor N. and Kaminski J. J. (1984) *Med. Res. Rev.* **22**, 303.

Bodor N. and Prodai L. (1995) In: Peptide-Based Drug Design: Controlling Transport and Metabolism, Taylor M. and Amidon G. (Eds.), American Chemical Society, Washington DC, 317.

Bodor N. and Visor G. (1984) *Pharm. Res.* **1**, 168.

Bodor N., El-Koussi A., Kano M. and Nakamura T. (1988) *J. Med. Chem.* **31**, 100.

Bodor N., Farag H. and Brewster M. (1981) *Science* **214**, 1370.

Bodor N., Prokai L., Wu W. M., Farag H. H., Jonnalagada S., Kawamura M. and Simpkins J. (1992) *Science* **257**, 1698.

Bodor N., Sloan K. B., Little R., Selk S. H. and Coldwell L. (1982) *Int. J. Pharm.* **10**, 307.

Bohme H., Ahrens K. H. and Hotzel H. H. (1974) *Arch Pharm.* (Weinheim) **307**, 748.

Brewster M. E., Estes K. E., Loftsson T., Perchalski R., Derendorf H., Mullersman G. and Bodor N. (1988) *J. Pharm. Sci.* **77**, 981.

Brewster M. E., Raghvan K. Pop E. and Bodor N. (1994) *Antimicrob. Agents Chemother.* **38**, 817.

Brewster M. E., Venkatraghavan V., Shek E. and Bodor N. (1987) *Synthetic Commun.* **17**, 451.

Brocchini S. and Duncan R. (1999) In: Encyclopedia of Controlled Release, Mathiowitz E. (Ed.), Wiley, NewYork, USA, 786.

Bundgarrd, H. (1958) *Design of Prodrugs*, New York, 25.

Carey M. C., Small D. M. and Bliss C. M. (1983) *Am. Rev. Physiol.* **45**, 651.

Caterall W. C. (1988) *Biol. Psychiatry* **24**, 733.

Chaplin D. J., Pettit G. R. and Hill S. A. (1999) *Anticancer Res.* **19**, 189.

Charman W. N. and Stella V. J. (1986) *Int. J. Pharm.* **33**, 165.

Charman W. N. and Stella V. J. (1991) *Adv. Drug deliv. Rev.* **7**, 1.

Charman W. N. A. and Poster C. J. H. (1996) *Adv. Drug Deliv. Rev.* **19**, 174.

Charman W. N. A. and Steall V. J. (1986) *Int. J. Pharmaceut.* **34**, 175.

Chen P., Bodor N., Wu W. M. and Prokai L. (1998) *J. Med. Chem.* **41**, 3773.

Cobb L. M., Connors T. A., Elson L. A., Khan A. H., Mitcheley B. C. and Ross W. C. (1969) *Biochem. Pharmacol.* **18**, 1519.

Coert A., Geelen J., DeVissier J. and VanderVies, J. (1975) *Acta Endocrinol*. **79**, 789.

Connors T. A. (1986) *Xenotiotica* **16**, 975.

Connors T. A. and Knox R. J. (1995) *Stem Cells* 13, 501.

Crone C. (1965) *J. Physiol*. **181**, 103.

Crone C. (1986) In: The Blood-Brain-Barrier in Health and Disease, Suckling A. J., Rumbsby M. G. and Bradbury M. W. B. (Eds.), Ellis Horwood, Chichester, 17.

Crone C. and Thompson A. M. (1970) In: Capillary Permeability: The Transfer of Molecules and Ions between Capillary Blood and Tissue, Crone C. and Lassen N. A. (Eds.), Munksgaard, Coperhangen, 447.

Crooke S. T. (1998) *Biotechnol. Engineer. Rev.* **15**, 121.

Culver K. W., Ram Z., Wallbridge S., Ishii H., Oldfield E. H. and Blaese R. M. (1992) *Science* **256**, 1550.

Dagett P. R., Wheelaer M. J. and Naborro J. D. N. (1978) *Hormone Res*. **9**, 121.

Damani L. A. (1987) In: Drug Delivery to the Respiratory Tract, Ganderton D. and Jones T. (Eds.), Ellis Harwood Ltd., Chichester U.K., 47.

De Vrueh R. L., Smith P. L. and Lee C. P. (1998) *J. Pharmacol. Exp. Ther.* **286**, 1166.

Deonarain M. P., Spooner R. A. and Epenetos A. A. (1995) *Gene Ther.* **2**, 235.

Deverre, J.R., Loiseau, P., Gayral, P., Letourneux, Y., Couverur, P. and Benoil, J.P. (1989) *J. Pharm. Pharmacol*. **41**, 191.

Deverre, J.R., Loiseau, P., Gayral, P., Letourneux, Y., Couverur, P. and Benoil, J.P. (1992) *Arzneimittelforschung* **42**, 1153.

Dimitrijevic S. and Duncan R. (1998) *J. Bioact. Compat. Polym*. **13**, 165.

Dimm M. V. (1996) *J. Drug Targeting* **3**, 375.

Ducan R. (1992) *J. Control. Rel*. **19**, 331.

Duncan R. (1988) *Br. J. Cancer* **57**, 147.

Duncan R. (1991) *J. Control. Rel*. **16**, 121.

Duncan R. (1992) *Anticancer Drugs* **3**, 175.

Duncan R., Dimitrijevic S. and Evagoroa E. G. (1996) *STP Pharma Sci.* **6**, 237.

Eccles S. A., Court W. J., Box G. A., Dean C. J., Melton R. G. and Springer C. J. (1994) *Cancer Res*. **54**, 5171.

Elion G., Furman P., Fyfe J., deMiron da P., Beauchamp L. and Scharffer H. (1977) *Proc. Natl. Acad. Sci. USA* **74**, 5716.

Elkihel, L., Loiseau, P.M., Bourass, J., Gayral, P. and Letourneux, Y. (1994) *Arzneimittelforschung* **44**, 1259.

El-Koussi A. and Bodor N. (1989) *Int. J. Pharm.* **53**, 189.

Fernandez, E. and Borgstrom, B. (1990) *Lipids* **25**, 549.

Folkman J. (1990) *J. Natl. Cancer Inst*. **82**, 4.

Folkman J. (1995) *Adv. Cancer Res.* **43**, 175.

Fonnum F. (1978) In: Aminoacids as Chemical Transmitters, Fonnum F. (Ed.), Plenum, New York, 143.

Fraunfelder F. T. and Barker A. F. (1985) *N. Engl. J. Med.* **311**, 1441.

Fregly M. J. and Fater D. C. (1986) *Clin. Exp. Pharmacol. Physiol*. **13**, 767.

Freidrich M. E. (1999) *Eur. J. Cancer* **35**, 138.

Friend P. R. and Chang G. W. (1985) *J. Med. Chem*. **28**, 51.

Gans, H. and Mastumoto, K. (1974) *Proc. Soc. Exp. Biol. Med.* **147**, 736.

Ghersi-Egea J. F., Muller B. L., Suleman G., Siest G. and Minn A. (1994) *J. Neurochem.* **62**, 1089.

Gianasi E. (1999) *Eur. J. Cancer* **35**, 994.

Goger S. R., Aggarwal S. K., Rangan S. R. and Agrawal K. C. (1989) *Biochem. Biophys. Res. Commun.* **160**, 656.

Granger D. N. (1981) *Am. J. Physiol.* **240**, 343.

Granger D. N. and Kvietys P. R. (1984) In: Digestive system, small and large intestine, in Blood vessels and Lymphatics in Organ system, Abramson, P.I. and Dorbin, P.B. (Eds.), Academic Press, Orlando, 336.

Granger D. N., Mortillaro N. A., Kvietys R., Rutili G., Parker J. C. and Taylor A. E. (1980) *Am. J. Physiol*., **238**, G183.

Granger D. N., Ulrich M., Parks D. A. and Harper S. L. (1984) In: Physiology of the Intestinal Circulation, Shephard, A.P. and Granger, D.N. (Eds.), Raven Press, New York, 478.

Grapple S. F., Giovenella A. J. and Nishet L. J. (1985) *Antimicrob. Agents Chemother*. **27**, 961.

Grazon-Aburbeh, A., Poupert, J.H., Claesen, M. and Dumont, P. (1986) *J. Med. Chem.* **29**, 687.

Grazon-Aburbeh A., Poupert J. H., Claesen M., Dumont P. and Atassi G. (1983) *J. Med. Chem.* **26**, 1200.

Greig N. H., Genka S., Daly E. M., Sweeney D. J. and Stanley I. R. (1990) *Cancer Chemother. Pharmacol*. **25**, 311.

Haisma H. J., Boven E., van Muijen M., de Jong J., van der Vijgh W. J. and Pinedo H. M. (1992) *Br. J. Cancer* **66**, 474.

Han H-k, Oh D. M. and Amidon G. L. (1998) *Pharm. Res.* **15**, 1382.

Harris J. D., Gutierrez A. A., Hurst H. C., Sikora K. and Lemoine N. R. (1994) *Gene Ther.* **1**, 170.

Hill B. T. (1996) *Anticancer Drugs* **7**, 1.

Hoffman A. F. (1978) *Gastroenterology* **75**, 530.

Hoffman N. F. (1970) *Biochim. Biophys. Acta* **196**, 193.

Howe R. and Shanks R. G. (1966) *Nature* **210**, 1336.

Hu M., Subramanian P., Mosberg H. I. and Amidon G. L. (1989) *Pharm. Res.* **6**, 66.

Huber B. E., Richards C. R. and Austin E. A. (1994) *Ann N Y Acad Sci.* **716**, 104.

Hughes J., Smith T. V., Kosterlitz H. W., Fothergill L., Morgan B. A. and Morris H. R. (1975) *Nature* **258**, 577.

Hunt J. N. and Knox M. T. (1967) *J. Physiol.* **194**, 327.

Ichihashi T., Kinoshita H., and Yamada H. (1991) *Xenobiotica* **21**, 873.

Ichihashi T., Kinoshita H., Takagishi Y. and Yamada H. (1992) *J. Pharm. Pharmacol.* **44**, 560.

Ingber D. E. (1997) In: Cancer Therapeutics: Experimental and Clinical Agents, Teicher B (Ed.), Humana Press, Totowa, NJ, USA. 76.

Jankovic J. (1988) *South Med. J.* **81**, 1021.

Jansen A. B. A. and Russell T. J. (1965) *J. Chem. Soc.* **42**, 2127.

Jewel D. P. and Truelove S. C. (1981) *Lancet* **2**, 1168.

Johansen M. and Bundgaard H. (1980) *Arch. Pharm. Chem. Sci.* **8**, 141.

Julyan P. J. (1999) *J. Control. Rel.* **57**, 281.

Kamp J.D. and Neuman H.G. (1975) *Xenobiotica* **5**, 717.

Kaplan N. M. (1978) *Annu. Rev. Med.* **29**, 31.

Kastin A. J., Ehrensing R. H., Banks W. A. and Zadina J. E. (1987) In: Progess in Brain Research Neuropeptides and Brain Function, deKloet E., Wiegant V. M. and deWied D (Eds.), Vol. 72, Amsterdam, 223.

Katayama K. and Grass G. M. (1972) *Biochim. Biophys. Acta* **288**, 181.

Kijima M., Nambu Y., Endo T. and Okawara M. (1984) *J. Org. Chem.* **49**, 1434.

Kishimoto Y. (1973) *Arch. Biophys. Biochem.* **159**, 528.

Klecker R., Collins J., Yarchoan R., Thomas R., Jenkins J., Broder S. and Myer C. (1987) *Clin. Pharmacol. Ther.* **41**, 407.

Kobayashi S., Shirota H., Katoh Y., Hoshida R., Nagaoka J., Abe S. and Yamatsu I. (1988) *Pharmacometrics* **36**, 91.

Koch S. A. M. and Sloan K. B. (1987) *Int. J. Pharm.* **38**, 244.

Kramer W., Wess G., Schubert G., Bickel M., Girbig F., Gutjahr U., Kowalewski S., Baringhaus K. H., Enhsen A., Glembick H., Mullner S., Neckermann G., Schulz S. and Petzinger E. (1992) *J. Biol. Chem.* **267**, 185.

Krinick N. L. (1994) *J. Biomet. Sci. Polymer Ed.* **5**, 303.

Kuksis A. (1982) In : Fat absorption, Kuksis A. (Ed.) Vol. II, CRC Press, Boca Raton FL, 126.

Kumakura S., Mishima M., Kobayashi S., Shirota H., Abe S., Yamada K. and Teurufuji S. (1990) *Agents Actions* **29**, 286.

Kumar R. and Billimoria J. P. (1978) *J. Pharm. Pharmacol.* **30**, 743.

Kuzemko J. A. (1989) *Repir. Med.* **83**, (Suppl. A), 11.

Kvietys P. R., Wilborn R. J. and Granger D. N. (1981) *Gastroenterology* **81**, 1080.

Lamanna C. and Carr C. J. (1967) *Clin. Pharmacol. Ther.* **8**, 286.

Leopard Ç. S. and Friend D. R. (1995) *J. Pharm. Sci.* **126**, 139.

Little R., Bailey P, Brewster M., Estes K., Clemmons R., Sahb A. and Bodor N. (1990) *J. Biopharm. Sci.* **1**, 1.

Lundberg A. S. and Weinberg R. A. (1999) *Eur. J. Cancer* **35**, 531.

Maeda H. and Matsumura Y. (1989) *Crit. Rev. Ther. Drug Carrier Sys.* **6**, 193.

Maragoudakis M. E. (1998) Angiogenesis: Models Modulators and Clinical Applications, Plenum Press, New York, USA, 1.

Martin J. B. and Gusella J. F. (1986) *N. Engl. J. Med.* **315**, 1267.

May A. J. and Whaler B. C. (1958) *Br. J. Exp. Path.* **39**, 307.

Mayerson H. S., Wolfram C. G., Shirley H. H. and Waserman K. (1960) *Am. J. Physiol.* **198**, 155.

McCormick J., King I., Webb P., Scribner C., Craven R., Johnson K., Elliot L. and Belmont Williams R. (1986) *N. Engl. J. Med.* **314**, 20.

Mishima M., Kobayashi S., Abe S. and Yamato C. (1990) *Xenobiotica* **20**, 135.

Mizobe M., Matsuda S., Yoneyama T. and Kohno K. (1983) *Chem. Pharm. Bull.* **1031**, 2424.

Mizoguchi H., Orlowski M., Wolk S., Green J. P. (1979) *Eur. J. Pharmacol.* **57**, 239.

Mizuma T., Ohta K., Hayashi M. and Awazu S. (1993) *Biochem. Pharmacol.* **45**, 1520.

Muggia F. M. (1999) *Clin. Cancer Res.* **5**, 7.

Muranishi S. (1985) *Pharm. Res.* **2**, 108.

Murukami M., Oketani K., Fujisak H., Wakabayashi, T. Sano N., Watanabe R. and Katoh Y. (1988) *Oyo Yakuri* **36**, 433.

Nakamura T., Aoyama Y., Fujita T. and Katsii G. (1975) *Lipids* **10**, 627.

Nankervis R., Davis S. S., Day N. H., and Shaw P. N. (1995) *Int. J. Pharmaceut.* **119**, 173.

Nankervis R., Davis S. S., Day N. H., and Shaw P. N. (1996) *Int. J. Pharmaceut.* **130**, 57.

Noguchi T., Charman, W. N. A. and Stella V. J. (1985) *Int. J. Pharm.* **24**, 173.

Nolen H. W. and Friend D. R. (1994) *Pharm. Res.* **11**, 1707.

O'Hagen D.T. (1990) *Adv. Drug deliv. Rev.* **5**, 265.

Oh D. M., Han H-k and Amidon G. L. (1999) In: Membrane Transporters as Drug Targets, Amidon G. L. and Sadee W. (Eds.), Plenum Press, New York, 59.

Oldendrorf W. H. (1974) *Proc. Soc. Exp. Biol. Med.* **147**, 813.

Oppitz M. M., Musch E., Malek M., Rub H. P., Unruh G.

E., Loos U. and Mahlanbruch B. (1989) *Cancer Chemother. Pharmacol.* **23**, 208.

Palin K. J., Davis S. S. and Phillips A. J. (1980) *J. Pharm. Pharmacol*. **32**, 62.

Peppercorn M. A. and Goldman P. (1973) *Gastroenterology* **64**, 240.

Pitman I. H., Rae I. D. and Harwey J. A. Y. (1986) *Int. J. Pharm*. **30**, 151.

Pop E., Anderson W., Prokai-Tatrai K., Brewster M., Fregly M. and Bodor N. (1990) *J. Med. Chem*. **33**, 2063.

Porter C. J. H., Charman S. A., Humberstone A. J. and Charman W. N. A. (1996) *J. Pharm. Sci.* **85**, 357.

Prokai L., Ouyang X. D., Wu W. M. and Bodor N. (1994) *J. Am. Chem. Soc.* **116**, 2643.

Prokai-Tatrai K., Prokai L. and Bodor N. (1996) *J. Med. Chem*. **39**, 4775.

Raghavan K., Loftsson T., Brewster M. E. and Bodor N. (1992) *Pharm. Res*. **9**, 743.

Raghavan K., Shek E. and Bodor N. (1987) *Anticancer Drug Des*. **2**, 25.

Renkin, E.M. (1964) *Physiology* 7, 13.

Renkin E. M. and Curry F. E. (1978) In: Handbook of Epitelial Transport, Vol. 4, Springer, New York, 3.

Richards R. and Tattersfield E. (1985) *Br. J. Clin. Pharmacol.* **20**, 459.

Robert K. Y., Cheng Z. and Cheng C. C. (1989) *Meth. and Find Exp. Clin. Pharmacol*. **11**, 439.

Rodriguez W. and Parrott R. (1987) *Infect. Dis. Clin. North Am*. **1**, 425.

Roos B. E. and Steg G. (1964) *Life Sci*. **3**, 351.

Rubas, W. and Grass, G.M. (1991) *Adv. Drug Deliv. Rev*. **7**, 15.

Sabesin S. M. and Frase S. (1977) *J. Lipid Res.* **18**, 496.

Sakai A., Mori N., Shuto S. and Suzuki T. (1993) *J. Pharm. Sci*. **82**, 575.

Sandhu J. S., Keating A. and Hozumi N. (1997) *Crit. Rev. Biotechnol*. **17**, 307.

Schlagel C. A. (1965) *J. Pharm. Sci*. **54**, 335.

Schoene R. B., Ward R., Abuan T. and Beasley C. H. (1984) *Am. J. Ophthalmol.* **97**, 86.

Seymour L. W. (1995) *Eur. J. Cancer* **5**, 766.

Sharma S. K., Bagshawe K. D., Melton R. G. and Sherwood R. F. (1992) *Cell Biophys*. **2**, 109.

Shiau Y. (1987) In: Physiology of the Gastrointestinal Tract, Johnson L. R. (Ed.) Raven press, New York, 78.

Sieber S. M. (1976) *Pharmacology* **14**, 443.

Sieber S. M., Cohn V. H. and Wynn W. T. (1974) *Xenobiotica* **4**, 265.

Sinko P. J. and Balimane P. V. (1998) *Biopharm. Drug Dispos*. **19**, 209.

Sinkula A. A. and Yalkowsky S. H. (1975) *J. Pharm. Sci.* **64**, 181.

Sloan K. B. and Bodor N. (1982) *Int. J. Pharm.* **12**, 299.

Sloan K. B. and Silver K. G. (1984) *Tetrahedron* **40**, 3997.

Sloan K. B., Koch S. A. M. and Silver K. G. (1984) *Int. J. Pharm*. **21**, 251.

Smith Q. R. (1989) In: Implications of the Blood-Brain-Barrier and its Manipulation, Neuwelt E. A. (Ed.), Plenum, New York, 85.

Spencer C. F. and Michaels J. G. (1964) *J. Org. Chem*. **29**, 3416.

Springer C. J., Poon G. K., Sharma S. K. and Bagshawe K. D. (1993) *Cell Biophys.* **22**, 9.

Stella V. J. (1975) In: Prodrugs as Novel Drug Delivery Systems, Higuchi T. and Stella V. J. (Eds.), American Chemical Society, Washington DC, 1.

Stella V. J., Charman W. N. and Naringrekar V. H. (1985) *Drugs* **29**, 455.

Stephen Z. F., Yurachek E. C., Sharif R., Wasvary J. M., Steele R. E. and Howes C. (1992) *Biochem. Pharmacol.* **43**, 1469.

Stewart P. A. and Tuor U. I. (1994) *J. Comp. Neurol.* **340**, 566.

Sugihara J. and Furuchi S. (1988) *J. Pharmacobio-Dyn.* **11**, 121.

Sugihara J., Furuuchi S., Ando H., Takashima K. and Harigaya S. (1988) *J. Pharmacobio-Dyn.* **11**, 555.

Sved A., Van Itallie C. M. and Fernstrom J. D. (1982) *J. Pharmacol. Exp. Ther.* **221**, 329.

Swaan P. W. and Tukker J. J. (1995) *J. Pharmacol. Exp.* Ther. **272**, 242.

Szejtli J. (1994) *Med. Res. Rev.* **14**, 353.

Taube U., Schroda K., Dusterberg B. and Mathes H. (1980) *Eur. J. Drug Metab. Pharmacokinet*. **11**, 145.

Taylor A. E. and Granger D. N. (1984) In: Handbook of Physiology, Renkin E. M. and Michel C. C. (Eds.), American Physiological Society, Washington DC, 473.

Thomson A. B. R., Keelan M., Garg M. L. and Clandinin M. T. (1989) *Can. J. Physiol. Pharmacol*. **67**, 179.

Tso P. (1994) In: Physiology of Gastrointestinal Tract, Johnson, L.R. (Eds.), Raven press, New York, 186.

Tsuji A. and Tamai I (1996) *Pharm. Res*. **13**, 963.

Tsuji A. and Tamai I. (1997) *Adv. Drug Delivery Rev.* **25**, 287.

Ueno N. and Refojo M. F. (1983) In: Controlled Drug Delivery, Bruck S. D. (Ed.), Vol. II, CRC Press Inc., Boca Raton, Florida, 89.

Vasey P. (1999) *Clin. Cancer Res.* **5**, 83.

Venkatraghavan V., Shek E., Perchalski R. and Bodor N. (1986) *Pharmaclologist* **28**, 145.

Wall D. A., Wilson G. and Hubbard A. L. (1980) *Cell* **21**, 79.

Wolf W. A. and Kuhn D. M. (1984) *Brain Res.* **295**, 356.

Woodard P., Winwood D., Brewster M. E., Estes K. and

Bodor N. (1990) *Drug Design Delivery* **6**, 15.
Wrshaw A. L., Walker W. A. and Isselbacher K. J. (1971) *Lab. Inv.* **25**, 675.
Yeung D. L. and Vonsaigent M. J. (1972) *Can. J. Physiol. Pharmacol.* **50**, 753.
Youmans W. B., (1962) Human Physiology, Macmillan, New York, 642.
Yu C. D., Fox I. L., Higuchi W. I. and Ho N. F. H. (1980) *J. Pharm. Sci.* **69**, 777.
Zilvermist D. B. (1965) *J. Clin. Invest.* **44**, 1610.

SECTION II

CARRIER CONCEPTS IN DRUG DELIVERY

CHAPTER 5

Liposomes

- Introduction
- Mechanism(s) of liposome formation
- Classification of liposomes
- Methods of liposome preparation and drug loading
- Passive loading techniques
- Mechanical dispersion methods of passive loading
- Solvent dispersion methods of passive loading
- Detergent depletion (removal) methods of passive loading
- Remote (active) loading
- Microencapsulation or locus of drugs In liposomes
- Removal of unentrapped drug from liposomes
- Characterization of liposomes
- Stability of liposomes
- Interactions of liposomal drug delivery systems with cells
- Liposomal pharmacokinetics
- Commercial development and scale up
- References

Rational research in drug delivery began in 1950's with the advent of polyclonal antitumour antibodies developed for tumour targeting of cytotoxic drugs to experimental tumours. This had triggered a series of concerted efforts evolved with the emergence of a plethora of delivery systems. Liposomes were discovered in the early 1960's by Bangham and colleagues (Bangham et al., 1965) and subsequently became the most extensively explored drug delivery system. However, it took several years from the early to the late 60's before the system was realized as a potential drug carrier. At first they were used to study *in vivo* simulated biomembrane behaviour. Subsequent to that liposome has become an essential therapeutic tool most notably in drug delivery and targeting. Not surprisingly, liposomes have covered predominantly medical, albeit some non-medical areas like bioreactors, catalysts, cosmetics and ecology. However, their predominance in drug delivery and targeting has enabled them to be used as therapeutic tool in fields like tumour targeting, gene and antisense therapy, genetic vaccination, immunomodulation, lung therapeutics, fungal infections, and skin care and topical cosmetic products (Gregoriadis et al., 1971; Gregoriadis, 1976; Szoka and Papahadjopolous, 1978; Kirby and Gregoriadis, 1984; Gabizon and Papahadjopolous, 1988; Lasic, 1991; Janoff, 1993; Gregoriadis and Florence, 1993; Clerc and Barenholz, 1995; Lasic et al., 1995, Storm and Crommelin, 1998; Drummond et al., 1999; Vyas and Sihorkar, 2001).

Structurally, liposomes are concentric bilayered vesicles in which an aqueous volume is entirely enclosed by a membranous lipid bilayer mainly composed of natural or synthetic phospholipids. This chapter deals with the formulation, characterization, *in vitro* and *in vivo* disposition and therapeutic applications of this versatile delivery system.

Some of the advantages of liposome are as follows:

- Provides selective passive targeting to tumour tissues (liposomal doxorubicin).
- Increased efficacy and therapeutic index.
- Increased stability via encapsulation.
- Reduction in toxicity of the encapsulated agent.
- Site avoidance effect.
- Improved pharmacokinetic effects (reduced elimination, increased circulation life times)
- Flexibility to couple with site-specific ligands to achieve active targeting.

MECHANISM (S) OF LIPOSOME FORMATION

In order to understand why liposomes are formed when phospholipids are hydrated, it requires a basic understanding of physicochemical features of phospholipids.

Phospholipids are amphipathic (having affinity for both aqueous and polar moieties) molecules as they have a hydrophobic tail and a hydrophilic or polar head. The hydrophobic tail is composed of two fatty acid chains containing 10-24 carbon atoms and 0-6 double bonds in each chain. The polar end of the molecule is mainly phosphoric acid bound to a water-soluble molecule. The hydrophilic and hydrophobic domains/segments within the molecular geometry of amphiphilic lipids orient and self organize in ordered supramolecular structure when confronted with solvents (Lasic, 1988).

In aqueous medium the molecules in self-assembled structures are oriented in such a way that the polar portion of the molecule remains in contact with the polar environment and at the same time shields the non-polar part. Among the amphiphiles used in the drug delivery, viz. soaps, detergents, polar lipids, the latter (polar lipids) are often employed to form concentric bilayered structures. However, in aqueous mixtures these molecules are able to form various phases, some of them are stable and others remain in the metastable state (Lasic, 1993). At high concentrations of these polar lipids, liquid-crystalline phases are formed that upon dilution with an excess of water can be dispersed into relatively stable colloidal particles. The macroscopic structures most often formed include lamellar, hexagonal or cubic phases dispersed as colloidal nanoconstructs (artificial membranes) referred to as liposomes, hexasomes or cubosomes, respectively (Lasic, 1998).

The most common natural polar phospholipids are phosphatidylcholine (PC). These are amphipathic molecules in which a glycerol bridge links to a pair of hydrophobic acyl hydrocarbon chains with a hydrophilic polar head group, phosphocholine (Fig. 5-1). Figure 5-1 explains that the fatty chains are embedded in the hydrophobic inner region of the membrane, oriented at an angle to the plane of the membrane surface, the hydrophilic head group, including the phosphate portion, points out towards the hydrophilic aqueous environment.

Molecules of PC are not soluble (rather dispersible) in aqueous milieu in the physical chemistry sense, as in aqueous media they align themselves closely in planer bilayer sheets to minimize the unfavourable interactions between the bulk aqueous phase and long hydrocarbon fatty acyl chain. Such interactions are completely eliminated when the sheets fold over themselves to form closed, sealed and concentric vesicles. The large free energy change between an aqueous and hydrophobic environment explains the most favoured orientation of lipids to assemble as concentric bilayer structures that exclude confrontation between aqueous and hydrophobic domains. This distinctive behaviour derives in the lowest free energy state and hence ensures the maximum stability to a self-assembled structures (Lasic, 1993). The phosphatidylcholine and its synthetic analogues differ markedly from amphiphilic molecules of other origin (soaps, detergents, lysolecithin) in that they preferably orient to form bilayer sheets rather than micellar structures. This presumably attributed to the double fatty acid chain that imparts the molecule an overall tubular shape, more suitable for assemblage in planer sheets (Table 5-1). In contrast, the detergent molecules with a polar head and single acyl chain has a conical shape and facilitate the formation of spherical micellar structures. Depending on the hydrophobic environment and aqueous phase, homogenous smectic phases of parallel lipid bilayers (lyotropic phases) or heterogenous dispersion of multilamellar or single-walled liposomes can be observed. At lower water

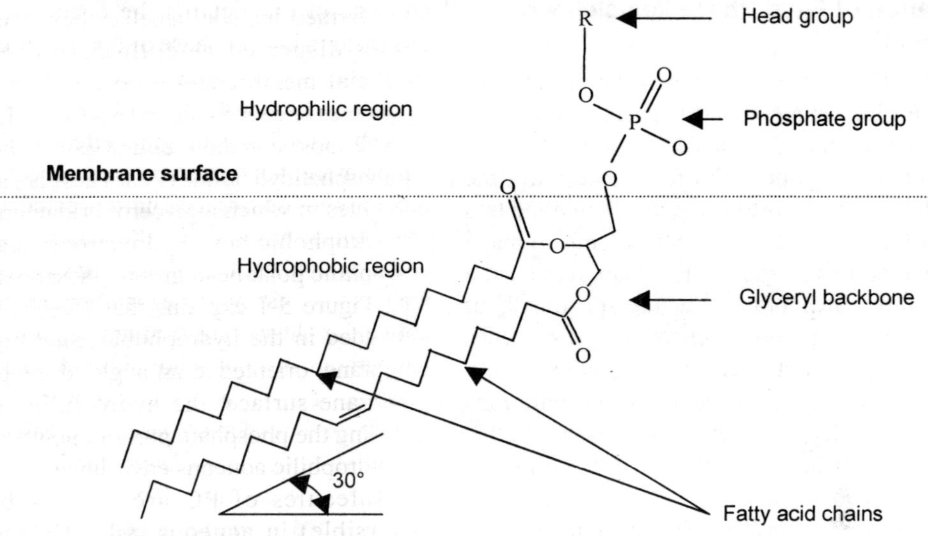

Fig. 5-1. Structure of a Typical Phospholipid Within Lipid Bilayer

Table 5-1. Some of the Parameters Affecting Bilayer Formation

- The large free energy difference between the aqueous and hydrophobic environment promotes the bilayer structures in order to achieve the lowest free energy level.
- The driving force for bilayer configuration of liposomes is the hydrophobic interaction coupled with the amphiphilic nature of the principal phospholipid molecules.
- Supramolecular self-assemblages mediated through specific molecular geometry

content and higher temperature, other lyotropic liquid crystalline phases exist, such as the hexagonal, the cubic and the ribbon phases (Fig. 5-2). Phase transition of lipids form a rather closely packed, relatively ordered state (gel phase) to a more loosely packed, less ordered liquid crystal state (fluid phase) where the side chains are capable of more rotational motion that occurs at a very narrow temperature range. Some of the physicochemical forces responsible for bilayer orientation are discussed (Table 5-1). Table 5-2 presents different liposome forming lipids with their molecular weights and phase transition temperatures (Tc°). The structures of these lipids are presented in Figure 5-3.

Thus the amphipathic (amphiphilic) nature of phospholipids and their analogues render them the ability to form closed concentric bilayers in the presence of water. Liposomes (lipid vesicles) are formed when thin lipid films or lipid cakes (of amphiphilic nature) are hydrated and stacks of liquid crystalline bilayers become fluid and swell. The hydrated lipid sheets detach during agitation and self close to form large, multilamellar vesicles (MLVs) which prevent interaction of water with the hydrocarbon core of the bilayer at the edges. Once these vesicles are formed, a change in the vesicle shape and morphology requires energy input in the form of sonic energy (sonication to get small unilamellar vesicles, SUVs) and mechanical energy (extrusion to get large unilamellar vesicles, LUVs) (Juliano and Lyton, 1980; Deamer and Uster, 1983) (Fig. 5-4). In order to explain the mechanisms or factors involved in the formation of concentric bilayers, the relationships between self-assemblages of amphiphiles, cholesterol and energy balance is pivotal.

Rigidization of Fluid Phase Vesicles with Cholesterol

Cholesterol is known to have important modulatory effect on the bilayer membrane (Papahadjopoulos et al., 1973; Kirby and Gregoriadis, 1980; New, 1989). Cholesterol acts as "fluidity buffer", since below the phase transition it tends to make the membrane less ordered while above the transition it tends to make the membrane more ordered, thus suppressing the tilts and shift in membrane structure specifically at the phase transition. Though cholesterol it self does not form bilayers, but it can be incorporated into phospholipid membrane in very high concentrations upto 1:1 or even 2:1 molar ratio of cholesterol to PC. Being an amphipathic molecule, cholesterol inserts into the membrane with its hydroxyl group oriented towards the aqueous surface, and the aliphatic chain aligned parallel to the acyl chains in the centre of the bilayer. Above a certain concentration of cholesterol, the membrane area occupied by combination of acyl chains and cholesterol is greater than (or equal to) that taken by phosphocholine head-group (Fig. 5-5). This could be the possible mechanism for phospholipid membranes with high levels of cholesterol that retards the chain tilt. The tilt is observed in the gel phase of liposomes composed of pure PC to maximize lipid chain interactions. Addition of cholesterol to PC membranes at lower concentration has a marginal effect on the transition temperature, but with increased concentration (~50 mole % cholesterol) it eliminates evidence of a phase transition at original Tc° altogether by reducing the enthalpy of phase change to zero value. In doing so, it alters the fluidity of the membrane both below and above the phase transition temperature. Below this temperature, the phospholipids are pushed apart, the packing of the head groups is weakened, and the fluidity of the ordered phase is increased. Above the transition temperature, the reduction in freedom of acyl chains causes the membrane to remain condensed and rigidized, with a reduction in area through closer packing and resultant decrease in fluidity. These changes in the fluidity are paraleled by changes in the permeability of the membrane, i.e., depressed by high cholesterol at temperatures higher than the Tc° but increased at lower temperatures. At a ratio of 1:1 of cholesterol to PC, space filling models show consistent and efficient packing of components in

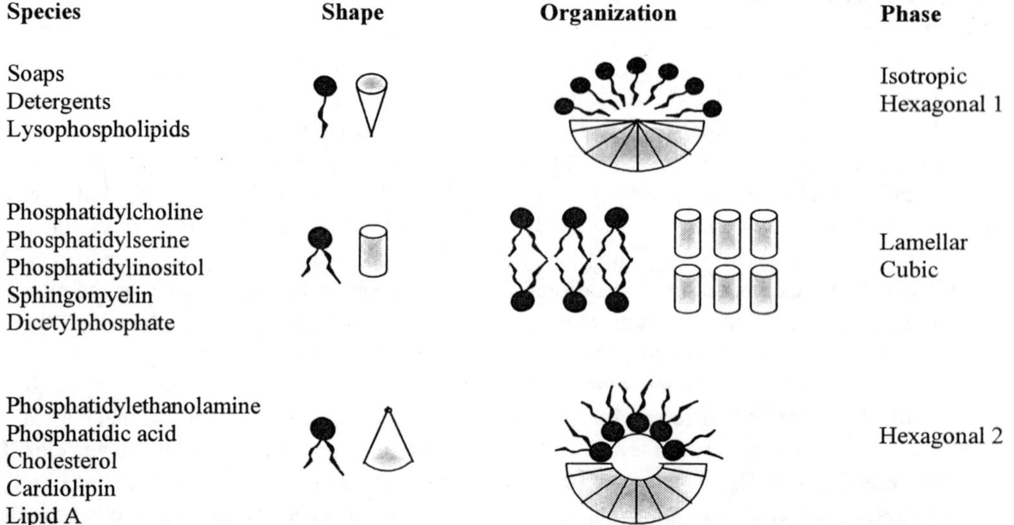

Fig. 5-2. The Effect of Molecular Geometry on the Structure of Amphiphilic Aggregates. Cone Like Molecules Tend to Pack into Structures with High Radii of Curvatuer and Inverse Cone-Like Molecules Form Structures with Large Negative Curvatures. Cylindrical Molecules Organize into Flat Lamellar Bilayered Structures.

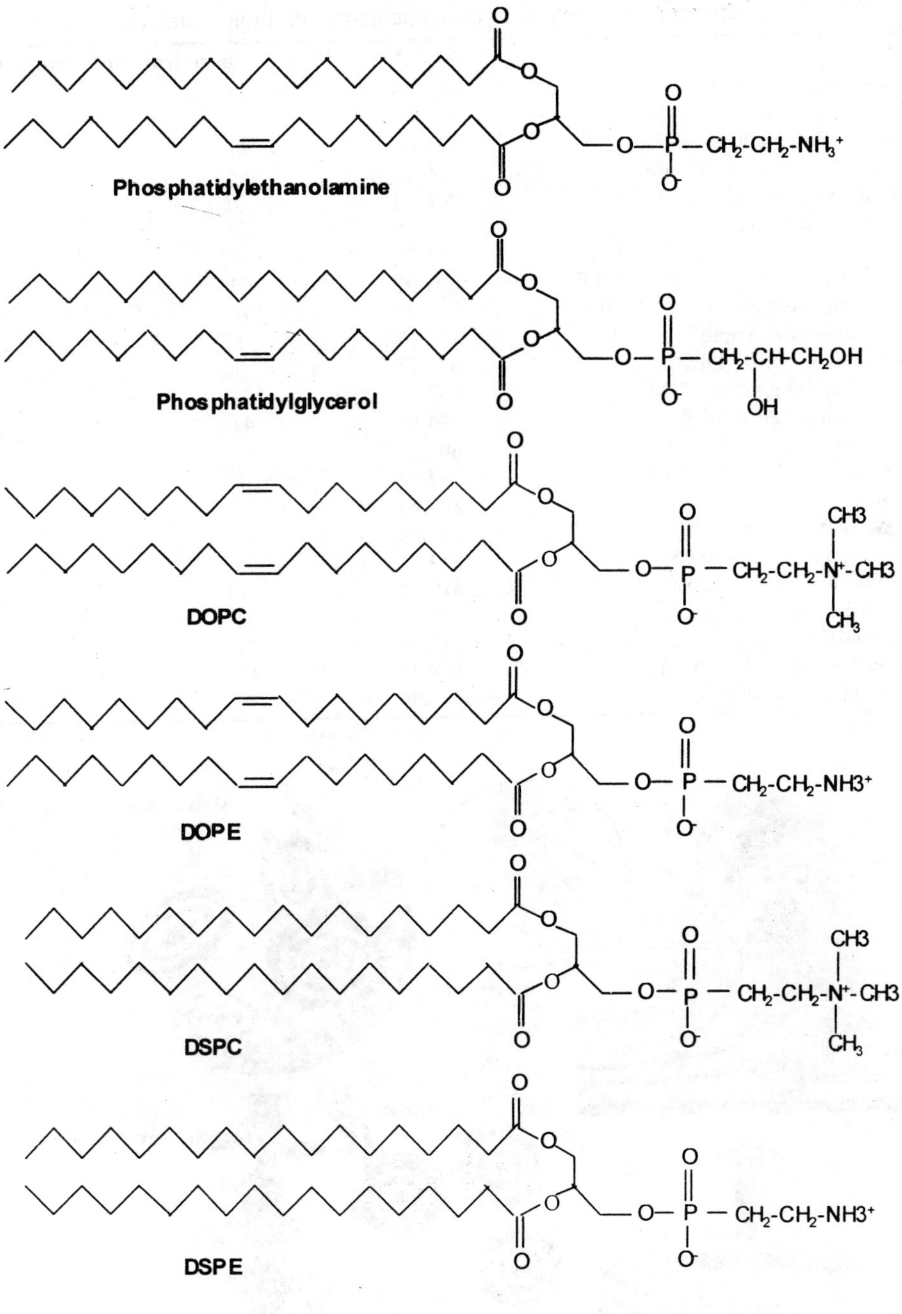

Phosphatidylethanolamine

Phosphatidylglycerol

DOPC

DOPE

DSPC

DSPE

DOPC=Dioleoylphosphatidylcholine; DOPE=Dioleoylphosphatidylethanolamine; DSPC=Distearoylphosphatidylcholine; DSPE=Distearoylphosphatidylethanolamine

Fig. 5-3. Some of The Commonly Used Synthetic Phospholipids.

Table 5-2. Phase transition temperatures of various phospholipids with their molecular weights

Lipids	Mol. Wt.	Phase transition temp. (°C)
Dilauryl phosphatidylcholine (DLPC)	621.83	-1
Dimyristoyl phosphatidylcholine (DMPC)	677.94	23
Dipalmitoyl phosphatidylcholine (DPPC)	734.05	41
Distearoyl phosphatidylcholine (DSPC)	790.15	55
Dioleoyl phosphatidylcholine (DOPC)	786.12	-20
Dilauryl phosphatidylethanolamine (DLPE)	579.75	29
Dimyristoyl phosphatidyl ethanolamine (DMPE)	635.86	50
Dipalmitoyl phosphatidyl ethanolamine (DPPE)	691.97	63
Distearoyl phosphatidyl ethanolamine (DSPE)	748.07	74
Dioleoyl phosphatidyl ethanolamine (DOPE)	744.04	-16
Dilauryl phosphatidyl glycerol (DLPG)	632.75	-3
Dimyristoyl phosphatidyl glycerol (DMPG)	688.85	23
Dipalmitoyl phosphatidyl glycerol (DPPG)	744.96	41
Distearoyl phosphatidyl glycerol (DSPG)	801.07	55
Dioleoyl phosphatidyl glycerol (DOPG)	797.04	-18
Dimyristoyl phosphatidyl serine (DMPS)	701.85	50
Dipalmitoyl phosphatidyl serine (DPPS)	757.96	63
Distearoyl phosphatidyl serine (DSPS)	814.06	74
Dioleoyl phosphatidyl serine (DOPS)	810.03	-11
Dilauryl phosphatidic acid (DLPA)	557.65	31
Dimyristoyl phosphatidic acid (DMPA)	613.76	50
Dipalmitoyl phosphatidic acid (DPPA)	669.87	67
Dioleoyl phosphatidic acid (DOPA)	721.94	-8

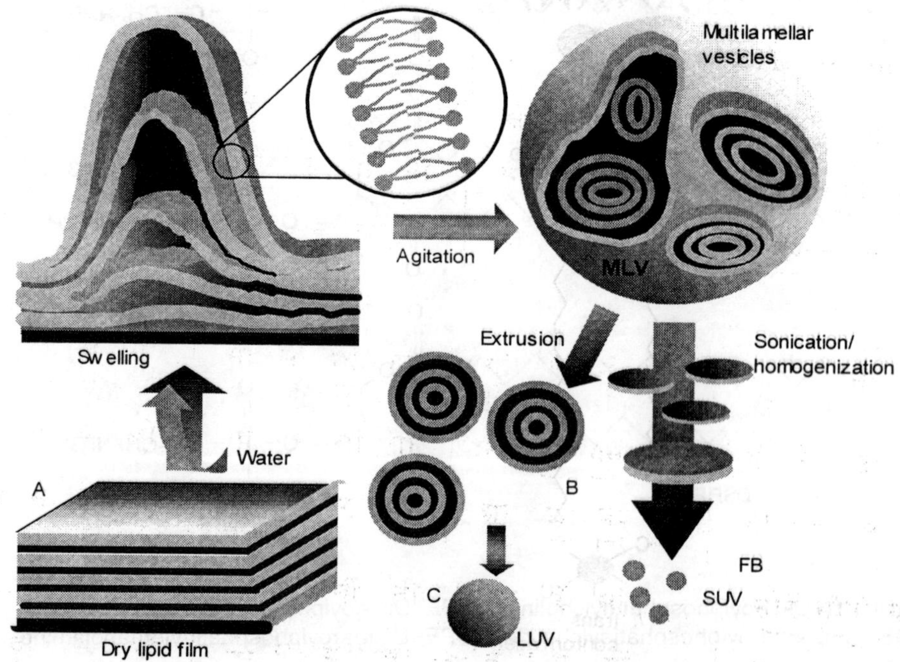

Fig. 5-4. Mechanism of Liposome Formation and Subsequent Processing to Generate Various Types of Vesicles

two-dimensional lattice in the form of linear arrays, with rows of cholesterol molecules alternating with rows of phospholipids, such that both cholesterol-cholesterol and cholesterol-PC interactions are favourably possible (Fig. 5-5A). Thus cholesterol interacts preferentially with the component having the lower transition temperature, i.e., with more fluid phase (and presumably in *gauche*-confirmation) which is rigidized in the gel phase with a resultant restriction of the transformations of *trans*- to *gauche*-conformations (New, 1989) (Fig. 5.5B). It should be emphasized however, that concentration of cholesterol above 50 mole % is difficult to incorporate without disrupting the bilayer configuration and conventional linear structure as it reduces the number of specific intermolecular interactions. The addition of cholesterol to membranes composed of heterogenous lipids abolishes the phase transitions and alters permeability and fluidity characteristics in the same way. Some of the roles of cholesterol and mechanisms involved in bilayer orientation are discussed in Table 5-3.

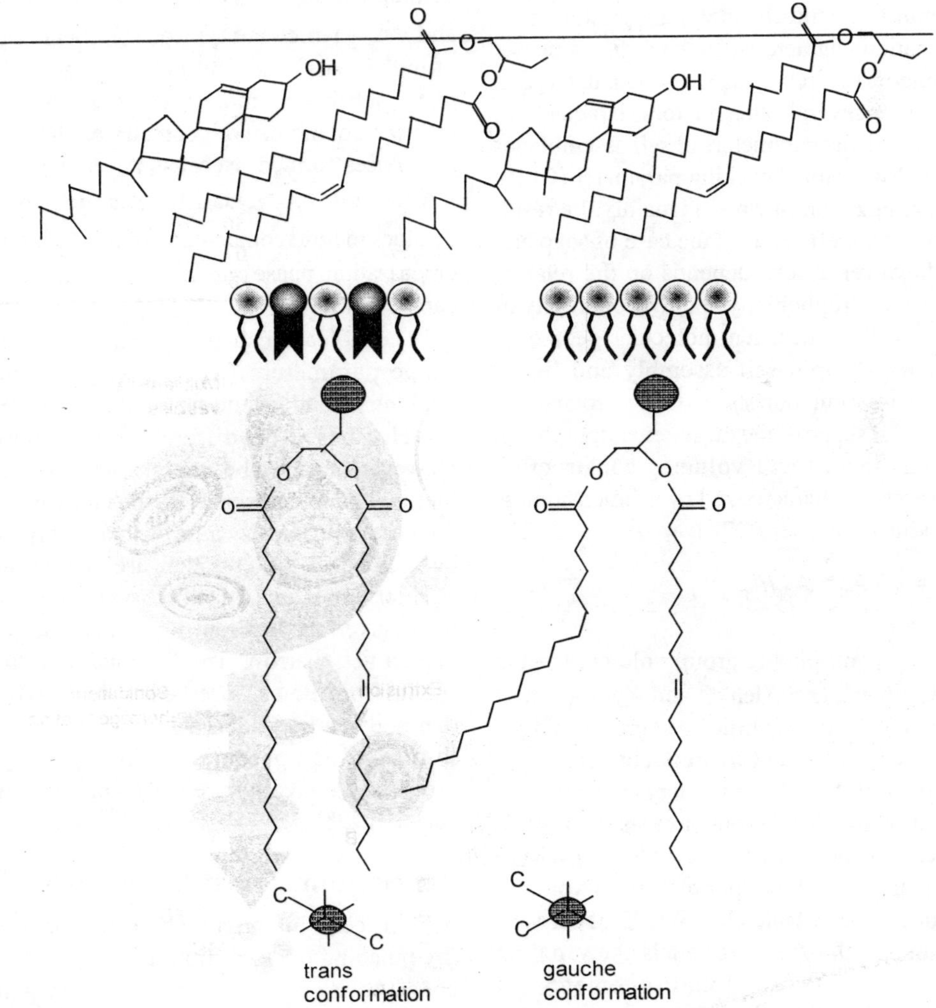

Fig. 5-5. The Orientation of Cholesterol in Phospholipid Bilayers (A). Transformations of *Trans*- to *Gauche*-Conformations (B)

Table 5-3. Role of Cholesterol in Bilayer Formation

- Acts as a fluidity buffer.
- After intercalation with phospholipid molecules alters the freedom of motion of carbon molecules in the acyl chain
- Restricts the transformations of *trans-* to *gauche-* conformations

Molecular Geometry and Liposome Formation (Israelachvili Hypothesis)

The micelle-forming amphiphiles show relatively high solubility in water (CMC about 10^{-3} mol L^{-1}). The concentration corresponds to CMC in case of membrane forming lipids is significantly low (CMC about 10^{-8} mol L^{-1}). Unfortunately, the prediction of vesicle formation characteristics is not just a matter of HLB numbers (as in the case of soaps, detergent, etc.), it involves several other factors. Israelachvili (1991) suggested that parameters of self assemblages are governed by a critical packing parameter (CPP). Their self-organization in water is mainly the result of the hydrophobic effect, as in the case of soap and detergent, however, it also depends on the relative proportions of hydrophobicity and hydrophilicity of the lipid, as well as mesogen molecular geometry. The symmetry of lipid self-assembly and liquid crystalline-phase formation show strong dependence on the molecular shape of the mesogen/amphiphiles. The different shapes and volumes constructing different phases are characterized by a dimensionless critical packing parameter (CPP):

$$CPP = \nu/l_c A_p = A_{hp}/A_p \quad (5\text{-}1)$$

Where, ν= hydrophobic group volume, l_c = the critical hydrophobic group length and A_p = the cross-sectional area of the hydrophilic head group, and A_{hp} = the cross sectional area of hydrophobic group.

A CPP below 0.5 (indicating a large contribution from the hydrophilic head group area) is reported to give spherical micelles and above 1 (indicating a large contribution from the hydrophobic group volume) should produce inverted micelles. A CPP of between 0.5 and 1 indicates that the surfactant is likely to form vesicles. The cross sectional geometry of hydrophobic and hydrcphilic domains suggests for geometric configuration that is most stable. For $A_{hp}>A_p$, structures with high curvature (such as micelles) are formed. When the areas are comparable $A_{hp}\cong A_p$, a bilayered configuration is the most stable form, while for $A_{hp}<A_p$, inverse micelles (with negative surface curvature) are formed. Furthermore, in self assembled multi-component systems, one can define an average value for the two parameters, $\langle A_{hp}\rangle$ and $\langle A_p\rangle$ which are typically a linear combination of individuals areas multiplied by the mole fraction of a contributing molecule. Figure 5-2 shows the influence of molecular geometry on the symmetry of the phases formed. Because A_{hp} and A_p, as well as $\langle A_{hp}\rangle$ and $\langle A_p\rangle$, can be changed by adopting changes in lipid compositions for $\langle A\rangle_s$, temperature or ionization, phase transition between various phases can be induced.

The molecular shape analysis and the concept of shape parameters (A_{hp}/A_p) are very useful for qualitative understanding of the topology of lipid vesicles based on different lipid compositions. However, one must be careful not to attempt accurate thermodynamic analysis of liposomal models based on these concepts, because such an analysis can only be applied to systems that are at thermodynamic equilibrium. If applied to liposomes containing lipids with a given shape parameter, such an analysis should yield a very narrow size distribution, rather a quite shallow profile as observed in real practice. Such thermodynamic models also predict the spontaneous formation of liposomes, however, a high-energy process is typically needed to produce liposomes (Lasic, 1998).

Vesicle Formation in Living Cells

In living cells, billions of vesicles are being generated (by pinching off from lipid tubules, exocytosis and endocytosis) and readsorbed (fusion with plasma membrane) constantly. The energy for this process comes from various proteins and their conformational changes. It has been speculated that this excess energy can be conserved in living cells, where the fusion of the vesicles is constantly occurring (Lasic, 1991; Abeles, 1992). The excess energy, e, associated with each vesicles is around 10-15 kT, which corresponds approximately to the energy provided by the hydrolysis of several adenosine triphosphate (ATP) molecules (~15 kT per reaction). This analysis points to the possibility that some of the energy in the cell can be stored in the curvature of various vesicles and may eventually be bioavailable upon vesicle fusion with the membrane.

CLASSIFICATION OF LIPOSOMES

Liposomes may be produced by a wide variety of methods. Their nomenclature also depends upon the method of preparation, structural parameters or special functions assigned to them (Table 5-4). One way of their classification relies upon the number of bilayers formed and diameters of the resultant vesicles. Liposomes are classified into small unilamellar vesicles (SUV, single bilayer, 10-100 nm), large unilamellar vesicles (LUVs, single bilayer, 100 nm-1μm), multilamellar vesicles (MLVs, several bilayers, 100 nm-20μm), oligolamellar vesicles (OLVs, more than one but not as many as MLVs, 0.1-1 μm) and intermediate-sized unilamellar vesicles (IUVs, ~100nm). Other terms are also used in the literature, which mainly relate to the method of manufacture. These include, multivesicular vesicles (MVVs, 100 nm-20μ), dried-reconstituted vesicles (DRVs, uni-or oligolamellar, <1μm), reverse-phase evaporation vesicles (REVs, unilamellar, ~0.5μm), micro-emulsification liposomes (MEL, multilayered, 0.1-0.2μm), large unilamellar vesicles prepared by extrusion (VET, single bilayer, 100nm-1μm) and stable plurilamellar vesicles (SPLVs, multilayered, 100 nm-2μm).

METHODS OF LIPOSOME PREPARATION AND DRUG LOADING

Liposomes are manufactured in majority using various procedures in which the water soluble

Table 5-4. Liposome Classification Based on Pharmaceutical and Therapeutical Aspects

Type	Specifications
Based on structural parameters	
MLV	Multilamellar large vesicles- >0.5 μm
OLV	Oligolamellar vesicles-0.1-1 μm
UV	Unilamellar vesicles (all size range)
SUV	Small unilamellar vesicles-20-100 nm
MUV	Medium sized unilamellar vesicles
LUV	Large unilamellar vesicles- >100 nm
GUV	Giant unilamellar vesicles- >1μm
MV	Multivesicular vesicles- >1μm
Based on method of liposome preparation	
REV	Single or oligolamellar vesicles made by reverse-phase evaporation method
MLV-REV	Multilamellar vesicles made by reverse-phase evaporation method
SPLV	Stable plurilamellar vesicles
FATMLV	Frozen and thawed MLV
VET	Vesicles prepared by extrusion technique
DRV	Dehydration-rehydration method
Based upon composition and applications	
Conventional liposomes (CL)	Neutral or negatively charged phospholipids and Chol
Fusogenic liposomes (RSVE)	Reconstituted Sendai virus envelopes
pH sensitive liposomes	Phospholipid such as PE or DOPE with either CHEMS or OA
Cationic liposomes	Cationic lipids with DOPE
Long circulatory (stealth) liposomes (LCL)	Neutral high Tc°, Chol and 5-10% of PEG-DSPE or GM1
Immuno-liposomes	CL or LCL with attached monoclonal antibody or recognition sequence

(hydrophilic) materials are entrapped by using aqueous solution of these materials as hydrating fluid or by the addition of drug/drug solution at some stage during the manufacturing of the liposomes (Ostro, 1987; New, 1989; Talsma and Crommelin, 1992a,b). The lipid soluble (lipophilic) materials are solubilized in the organic solution of the constitutive lipid(s) and then evaporated to a dry drug containing lipid film followed by its hydration. These methods involve the loading of the entrapped agents before or during the manufacturing procedure (passive loading) (New, 1989). However, certain types of compounds with ionizable groups, and those which display both lipid and water solubility, can be introduced into the liposomes after the formation of intact vesicles (remote loading) (Fig. 5-6) (Lasic et al., 1995).

PASSIVE LOADING TECHNIQUES

Passive loading techniques include three different groups of methods working on different principles namely, mechanical dispersion, solvent dispersion and detergent solubilization.

MECHANICAL DISPERSION METHODS OF PASSIVE LOADING

All methods covered under this category begin with a lipid solution in organic solvent and end up with lipid dispersion in water. The various components are typically combined by co-dissolving the lipids in an organic solvent and the organic solvent is then removed by film deposition under vacuum. When all the solvent is removed, the solid lipid mixture is hydrated using aqueous buffer. The lipids spontaneously swell and hydrate to form liposomes. At this point methods incorporate some diverge processing parameters in various ways to modify their ultimate properties. These post-hydration treatments include vortexing, sonication, freeze thawing and high-pressure extrusion.

Thin film hydration using hand shaking (MLVs) and non-shaking methods (ULVs)

In these methods, the lipids are casted as stacks of film from their organic solution using flash rotary evaporator under reduced pressure (or by hand

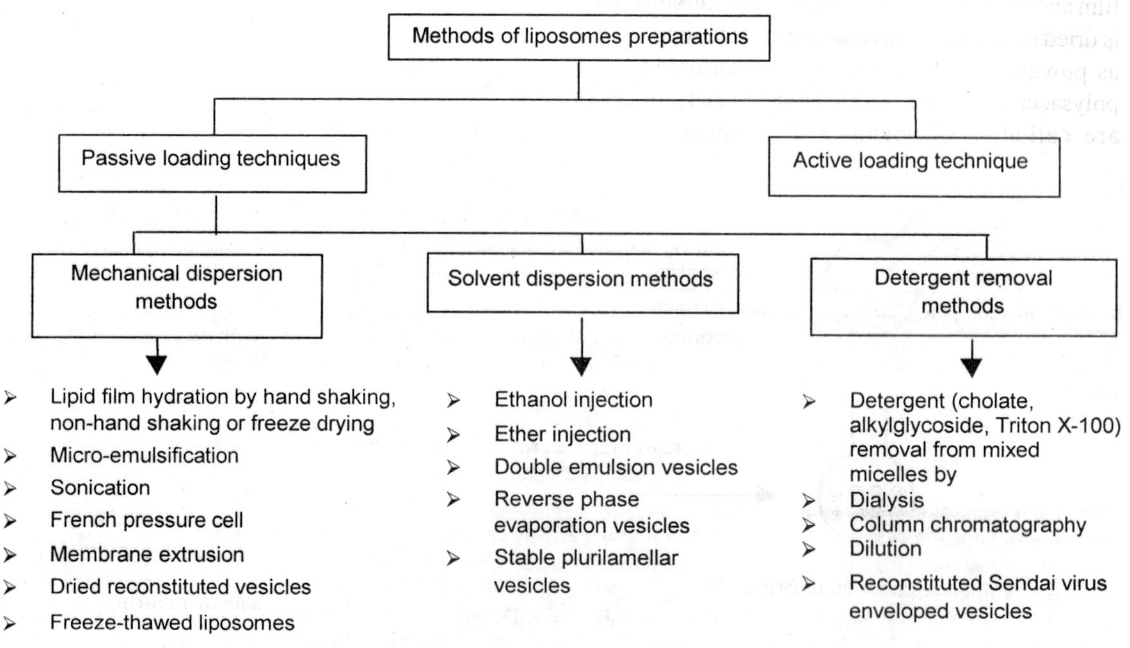

Fig. 5-6. Various Methods Used for the Preparation of Liposomes

shaking) and then the casted film is dispersed in an aqueous medium. Upon hydration the lipids swell and peel off from the wall of the round bottom flask and vesiculate forming multilamellar vesicles (MLVs) (Fig. 5-7). The mechanical energy required for the swelling of lipids and dispersion of casted lipid film is imparted by manual agitation (hand shaking technique) or by exposing the film to a stream of water-saturated nitrogen for 15 min followed by swelling in aqueous medium without shaking (non-shaken vesicles). It is interesting to note that as compared to hand-shaking method (that produces MLVs) the vesicles produced by non-shaken methods are large uni-lamellar vesicles (LUVs). The percent encapsulation efficiency as high as 30% (at 100 mg lipid ml^{-1}) is achieved. However, large amounts of water-soluble compounds are wasted during swelling as only 10-15% of the total volume gets entrapped. On the other hand, lipid soluble compounds can be encapsulated at 100% efficiency, provided they are present in adequate quantities, and does not disturb structural composition of the membrane.

Pro-liposomes

In order to increase the surface area of dried lipid film and to facilitate instantaneous hydration, the lipid is dried over a finely divided particulate support, such as powdered sodium chloride, or sorbitol or other polysaccharides. These dried lipid coated particulates are called pro-liposomes. Pro-liposomes form dispersion of MLVs on adding water into them, where support is rapidly dissolved and lipid film hydrates to form MLVs. The size of the carrier influences the size and heterogeneity of the liposomes. This method also overcomes the stability problems of liposomes encountered during their storage as dispersion, dry or frozen form. It is ideally suited for preparations where the material to be entrapped incorporates into lipid membrane. The method is applicable in cases where 100% entrapment of components is not a requirement rather the stability is preferred.

Mechanical Treatment of MLVs

Multilamellar vesicles formed on hydration of dried lipids could be further engineered or modified for their size and other characteristics. A large number of methods are devised to reduce their size and to convert liposomes of the large size range into smaller homogenous vesicles. These include techniques such as microemulsification, extrusion, ultrasonication and use of French pressure cell. A second set of methods is designed to increase the entrapment volume of hydrated lipids, and/or reduce the lamellarity of the vesicles formed. These include procedures such as freeze-drying, freeze thawing, or induction of vesiculation by ions or pH change.

Sonicated Unilamellar Vesicles (SUVs)

At high energy level, the average size of the vesicles is further reduced. This was first achieved on

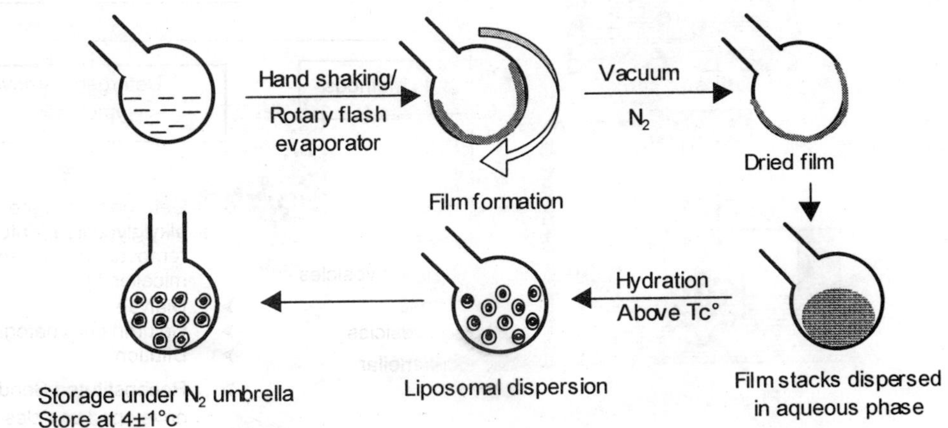

Fig. 5-7. Multilamellar Vesicles (MLVs) Formed by either Hand Shaking Technique or Using Rotary Flash Evaporator

exposure of MLVs to ultrasonic irradiation and still remains the method most widely used for producing small vesicles (Huang, 1969). There are two methods of sonication based on the use of either probe or bath ultrasonic disintegrators (Fig. 5-8). The probe is employed for dispersions, which require high energy in a small volume (e.g. high concentration of lipids, or a viscous aqueous phase) while the bath is more suitable for large volumes of diluted lipids. Probe tip sonicators supply a high-energy input to the lipid dispersion but suffer from overheating of the liposomal dispersion causing lipid degradation. Sonication tips also tend to release titanium particles into the liposome dispersion, which must be removed by centrifugation prior to use. For these reasons, bath sonicators are the most widely used for the preparation of SUVs. Sonication of an MLV dispersion is accomplished by placing a test tube containing the dispersion in a bath sonicator (or placing the tip of the sonicator in the test tube in a probe sonicator) and sonicating for 5-10 min (1,00,000 g) above the Tc° of the constituent lipid. The lipid dispersion should begin to clarify to yield a slightly hazy transparent solution. The haze is due to light scattering induced by residual large particles remaining in the dispersion. These particles can be removed using centrifugation to yield a clear SUV dispersion.

Liposome dispersion after sonication is placed in clear plastic walled ultracentrifuge tube. Th dispersion is generally centrifuged at 100,000g (3(min, 20° C) to sediment titanium particles and larg MLVs followed by higher speed centrifugatio (1,59,000g for 3-4 h). After spinning the tube i carefully removed from the rotor and with the hel of a Pasteur pipette, the liquid with top clear layer i decanted leaving the central opalescent laye (containing small multilamellar vesicles) and a pelle behind. The top layer constitutes pure dispersion o SUVs with varying diameters (in nanometric range) as the size and distribution is influenced by composition and concentration, temperature, sonication time and power, volume and sonication tuning.

French Pressure Cell Liposomes

The ultrasonic radiation not only degrades the lipids but also macromolecules and other sensitive compounds, which are to be entrapped in liposomes. One of the first and still very useful method developed is extrusion of preformed large liposomes in a French press under very high pressure (Barenholtz et al., 1979; Hamilton et al., 1980). This technique yields rather uni- or oligo- lamellar liposomes of intermediate size (30-80nm in diameter depending on the applied pressure). These liposomes are more stable as compared to sonicated liposomes. The

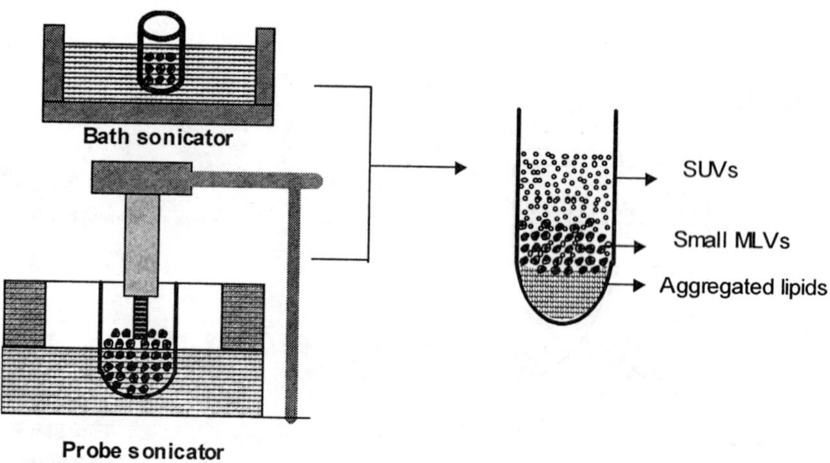

Fig. 5-8. Preparation of Small Unilamellar Vesicles (SUVs) by Bath/Probe Sonication Processes From MLVs

method however, suffers some drawbacks, which include high initial cost of the press that consists of an electric hydraulic press and pressure cell (Fig. 5-9).

The sizes of resulting French press extruded liposomes (FPL) are variable, depending on the lipid composition, the temperature and most important, on

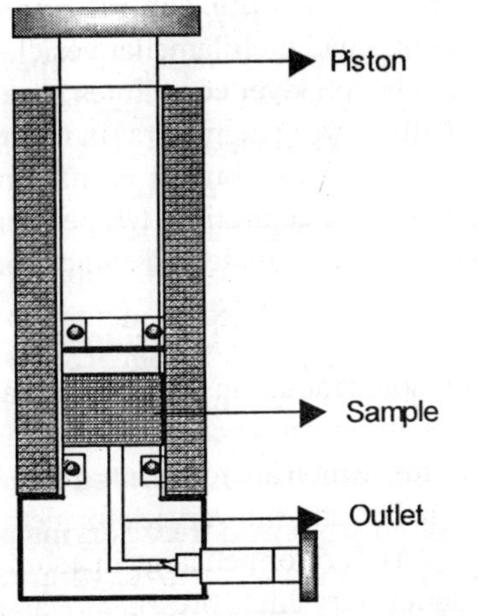

Fig. 5-9. French Pressure Cell and Parts Used for Pre-paration of Uni- or Oligo-Lamellar Vesicles

the pressure. The liposomes prepared by this technique are less likely to suffer from the structural defects and instabilities as observed in sonicated vesicles. Leakage of contents from liposomes prepared using French press is slower and lower than sonicated liposomes. French press has also been used to reduce the heterogeneity of populations of proteoliposomes obtained by detergent dialysis technique.

Micro Emulsification Liposomes (MEL)

"Micro fluidizer" is used to prepare small MLVs from concentrated lipid dispersion (Mayhew et al., 1984). Microfluidizer pumps the fluid at very high pressure (10,000psi, 600-700 bar) through a 5 μm orifice. Then, it is forced along defined micro channels, which direct two streams of fluid to collide together at right angles at a very high velocity, thereby affecting an efficient transfer of energy. The lipids can be introduced into the fluidizer, either as a dispersion of large MLVs, or as slurry of unhydrated lipid in an organic medium. The fluid collected can be recycled through the pump and interaction chamber until vesicles of the spherical dimension are obtained (Fig. 5-10).

After a single pass, the size of vesicles is reduced to a size 0.1 and 0.2 μm in diameter. The exact size

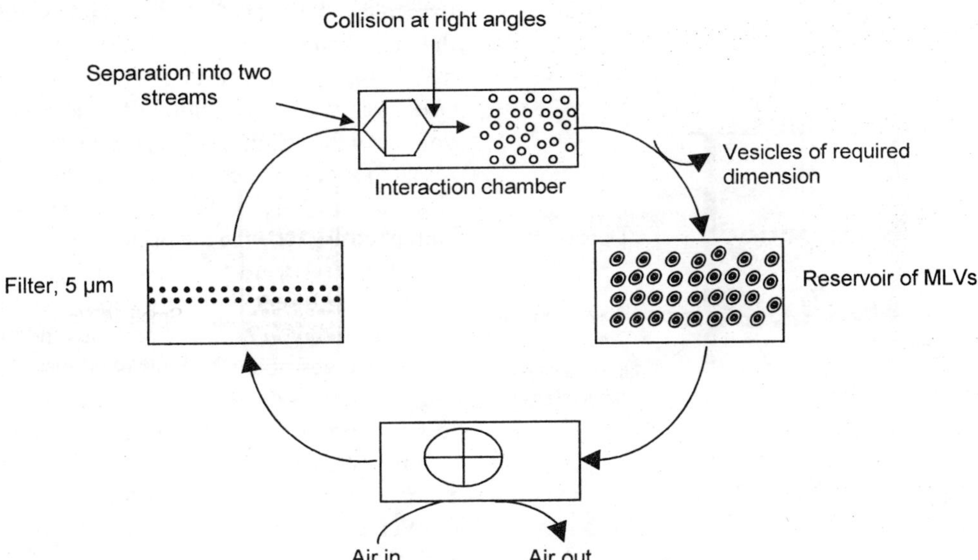

Fig. 5-10. Representation of Use of Micro-Fluidizer to Prepare Small Unilamellar Vesicles (SUVs) From MLVs

distribution, however depends on the nature of the components of the membrane and hydration medium. The presence of negative lipids tends to decrease their size, while increasing cholesterol concentration gives larger liposomes. In addition to the high rate of production, this method has the advantage of being able to process samples with a very high proportion of lipids (20% or more by weight). This process is efficient for encapsulation of water-soluble materials. Percentage capture values up to 70% have been reported, starting with lipid concentration of approximately 200mg/ml.

Vesicles Prepared by Extrusion Techniques (VETs)

In membrane extrusion method, the size of liposomes is reduced by gently passing them through membrane filter of defined pore size (Hope et al., 1985). This can be achieved at much lower pressure (<100psi.) than required in case of French pressure cell (Fig. 5-11).

The membrane extrusion technique can be used to process LUVs as well as MLVs. In this process, the vesicle contents are exchanged with the dispersion medium during breaking and resealing of phospholipid bilayers as they pass through the polycarbonate

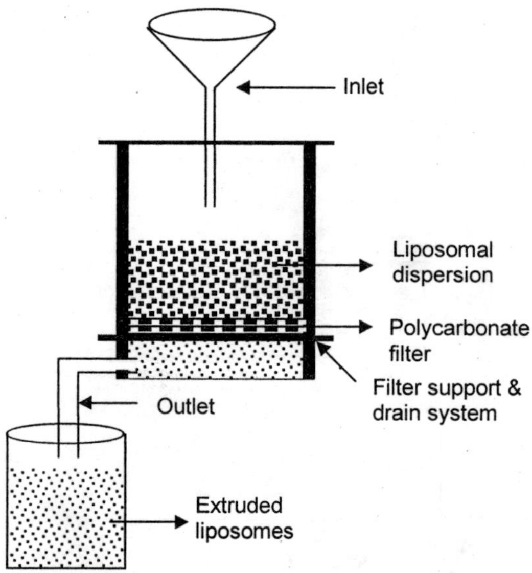

Fig. 5-11. Liposomes Preparation Using Extrusion Technique Based on Polycarbonate Filters

membrane. In order to achieve high entrapment, the water-soluble compounds should be present in suspending medium during the extrusion process. The material, which is not entrapped, can be removed subsequently. The liposomes produced by this technique have been termed LUVETs. The 30% capture volume can be obtained using high lipid concentration (300 mM PC). The trapped volume in this process is 1-2 litre/mol of lipids.

Extrusion technique is the most widely used method for SUV and LUV production for *in vitro* and *in vivo* studies. It is due to their ease of production, readily selectable vesicle diameter (dictated by the nominal pore size of the track-etch membranes used for extrusion, typically between 50-120 nm for *in vivo* experiments), batch-to-batch reproducibility, and freedom from solvent and/or surfactant contamination.

Dried-reconstituted Vesicles (DRVs)

This method starts wtih freeze drying of a dispersion of empty SUVs and then rehydrating it with the aqueous fluid containing the material to be entrapped (Kirby and Gregoriadis, 1984). This leads to a dispersion of solid lipids in finely subdivided form. However, the step of freeze-drying is used to freeze and lyophilize a preformed SUVs dispersion rather than to dry the lipids from an organic solution (as in the case of other methods). This leads to an organized membrane structure as compared to random matrix structure, which on addition of water (one tenth the volume of the original SUVs) can rehydrate, fuse and reseal to form vesicles with a high capture efficiency (Fig. 5-12). The water-soluble materials to be entrapped are added to the dispersion of empty SUVs and they are dried together, so the material for inclusion is present in the dried precursor lipid before the final step of addition of aqueous medium.

Liposomes obtained by this method are usually uni- or oligo- lamellar of the order of 1.0 μm or less in diameter. Entrapment yield can vary, but 40% is fairly standard compared with 2-10% for MLVs prepared by hand-shaking method.

Various advantages proposed for the DRV technique are high entrapment of water soluble component and the use of mild conditions for the preparation and loading of bioactives (Gregoriadis et al., 1990). However, this method is suitable only for unilamellar vesicles (i.e., SUVs), i.e., the liposomes to be freeze-dried should be in the form of unilamellar vesicles as the incorporation rates with multilamellar vesicles are quite low.

Freeze Thaw Sonication (FTS) Method

The FTS method is an extention of classical DRV method (Mayer et al., 1985, Ohsawa et al., 1985). The method is based upon freezing of a unilamellar (mainly SUV) dispersion and then thawing by standing at room temperature for 15 min (cf. DRV method where the freeze-dried lipids are rehydrated with aqueous buffer) and finally subjecting to a brief sonication cycle. Thus the process ruptures and refuses SUVs during which the solute equilibrates between inside and outside, and the liposomes themselves fuse and increase markedly in size.

The entrapment volume can be up to 30% of the total volume of the dispersion (10μl/mg phospholipids). Similar to DRV, the starting preparation of empty liposomes is made by sonication and after thawing, the liposomes are subjected to brief sonication again (Fig. 5-12). The second step sonication considerably reduces the permeability of the liposome membrane, perhaps by accelerating the rate at which packing defects are eliminated. In order to prepare giant vesicles of diameter between 10 and 50 μm, the freeze thaw technique has been modified to incorporate a dialysis step against hypo-osmolar buffer in place of second step sonication (Oku and MacDonald, 1983). In this case, SUVs (prior to freeze-thawing step) are first mixed with salt solution followed by freeze thawing several times. During subsequent dialysis, the large vesicles formed by freeze thawing swell and rupture as a result of osmotic lysis whereupon they fuse with each other to yield a large number of giant vesicles.

The inclusion of some negatively charged lipids gives yet higher trapped volume (20 μl/mg as compared to 10 μl/mg for neutral phospholipids). The FTS method has several disadvantages compared to

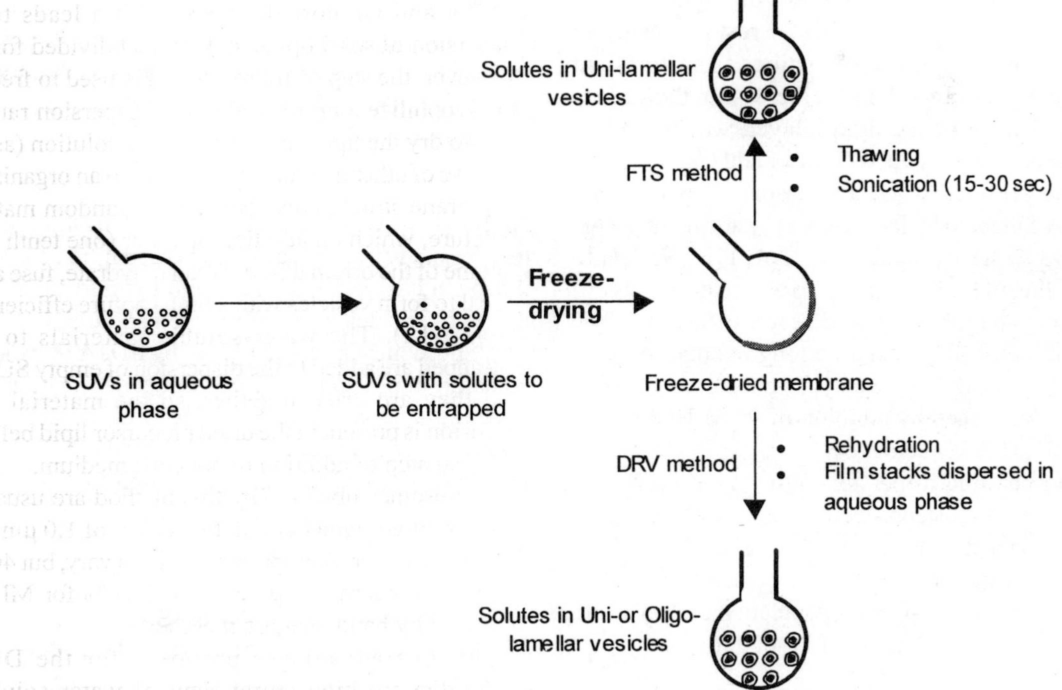

Fig. 5-12. Preparation of Dried-Reconstituted Vesicles (DRVs). Membrane Restructures Enclosing a Proportion of Solute, which was Originally Present in Extra-Liposomal Medium

DRVs in regard to encapsulation efficiency. Since the presence of charge is required for the formation of ice crystals to aid in the rupture/fusion process, neutral liposomes can not be subjected to freezing and thawing method. For similar reasons sucrose (a cryo-protectant), divalent metal ions (which can neutralize the surface charge) and high ionic strength salt solutions can not be entrapped efficiently. Nevertheless, the method is simple, rapid and mild for entrapped solutes, and results in a high proportion of large unilamellar vesicles formation, which are useful for study of membrane transport phenomenon.

Liposomes from Preformed Vesicles

Several methods of liposome preparation use preformed vesicles and are intended mostly to increase the encapsulation efficiency of the preformed vesicles by using fusion of SUV's by fusogenic agents or by change in the microenvironment of the system.

pH Induced Vesiculation

This method is used to transform MLVs to LUVs using a change in the pH of the dispersion thus avoiding the use of sonication or high-pressure application. The process is an electrostatic event and termed "pH induced vesiculation". The transient change in pH brings about an increase in the surface charge density of the lipid bilayer, which induces spontaneous vesiculation (Hauser and Gains, 1982).

The preformed MLVs (prepared using hand shaking followed by freeze-thawing and having a pH of 2.5-3.0) are exposed to high pH (1M NaOH) to bring the pH 11.0. The period of exposure of liposomes to high pH should be less than 2 min. The exposure time should not be long enough to cause any detectable degradation of the phospholipid. Then the pH is reduced by addition of 0.1M HCl until a value of pH 7.5 is achieved.

Phospholipid dispersion with similar properties is obtained if concentrated NaOH solution is added directly to the dry lipid film to give dispersion without freeze thawing. The resultant dispersion is consisted of a relatively homo-genous population of SUVs with an average outer diameter of 20-60nm.

Calcium Induced Fusion

Calcium induced fusion method is principally based upon the concept of aggregation and fusion of acid phospholipid vesicles in the presence of calcium (Papahadjopoulos et al., 1975).

In this method, SUVs are formed using sonication buffer (NaCl 0.385g, histidine 31.0 mg, Tris-base 24.2 mg, EDTA 3.72 mg, water 100 mL, pH 7.4) as the hydrating fluid. The large liposomes and lipid particles are removed by centrifugation at 100,000g. Equimolar proportion of calcium solution ($CaCl_2$) is added to phospholipids in the supernatant resulting in the formation of a white flocculent precipitate. It is incubated for 60 min at 37 °C and the precipitate (pellet) is separated by spinning the contents at 3000g for 20 min at room temperature where the supernatant is discarded. The pellet is resuspended in a buffered saline containing the material to be entrapped, and incubated at 37 °C for 10 min. The addition of EDTA to the pellet suspension with mixing, results in the formation of a cloudy dispersion, which clears rapidly and incubated for 15 min at 37 °C and further 15 min at room temperature. Finally, the Ca-EDTA complex is removed by dialyzing the dispersion overnight against a litre of phosphate saline buffer.

The method has the advantage that it does not expose lipids or entrapped materials to deleterious chemical or physical conditions. Its principal drawback is the requirement of acidic phospholipids and the presence of calcium inside the liposomes, even after dialysis.

Cochleate Method

Cochleates are formed when small unilamellar vesicles made from negatively charged lipids mainly phosphatidylserine (PS) fuse into cylindrical rolls, termed as cochleate cylinders, upon addition of Ca^{++} ions. Subsequent removal of Ca^{++} by EDTA or by ion exchange or precipitation, results in the formation of large unilamellar vesicles. Concentration of Ca^{++} required to repoduce such effects vary for the nature of lipids used, for PS, it should be slightly above the half of the lipid concentration, while cardiolipin (CL) and especially PG require higher overages.

SOLVENT DISPERSION METHODS FOR PASSIVE LOADING

In solvent dispersion method, lipids are first dissolved in an organic solution, which is then brought into contact with an aqueous phase containing materials to be entrapped within the liposomes. The lipids align themselves at the interface of organic and aqueous phase forming monolayer of phospholipids, which forms the half of the bilayer of the liposome. Methods employing solvent dispersion can be categorized on the basis of the miscibility of the organic solvent and aqueous solution. These include the conditions where the organic solvent is miscible with the aqueous phase; the organic solvent is immiscible with the aqueous phase, the latter being in excess; and the cases where the organic solvent is in excess, and immiscible with the aqueous phase.

Ethanol Injection

This method has been reported as one of the alternatives used for the preparation of SUVs without sonication (Batzri & Korn, 1973). An ethanol solution of lipids is injected rapidly through a fine needle into an excess of saline or other aqueous medium. The rate of the injection is usually sufficient to achieve complete mixing, so that the ethanol is diluted almost instantaneously in water, and phospho-lipid molecules are dispersed evenly throughout the medium (Fig. 5-13). This procedure yields a high proportion of SUVs (~25 nm), although lipid aggregates and larger vesicles may form if the mixing is not thorough enough. This method is extremely simple and has low risk of degradation of sensitive lipids. The vesicles of 100 nm size may be obtained by little modification in this method, i.e. by varying the concentration of lipid in ethanol or by changing the rate of injection of ethanol solution in preheated aqueous solution.

The major shortcoming of the method is the limitation of the solubility of lipids in ethanol and volume of ethanol that can be introduced into medium (7.5% v/v maximum), which in turn limits quantity of lipid dispersed, so that resulting liposomal dispersion gets diluted. Another drawback is difficulty to remove residual ethanol from phospholipid membrane.

Ether Injection

Ether injection method is similar to the ethanol injection method however, it contrasts markedly with ethanol injection in many respects. It involves injecting the immiscible organic solution very slowly into an aqueous phase through a narrow needle at the temperature of vapourizing the organic solvent (Fig. 5-13). This method may also treat sensitive lipids very gently. It has little risk of causing oxidative degradation provided ether is free from peroxides. The disadvantages of the technique are the long time

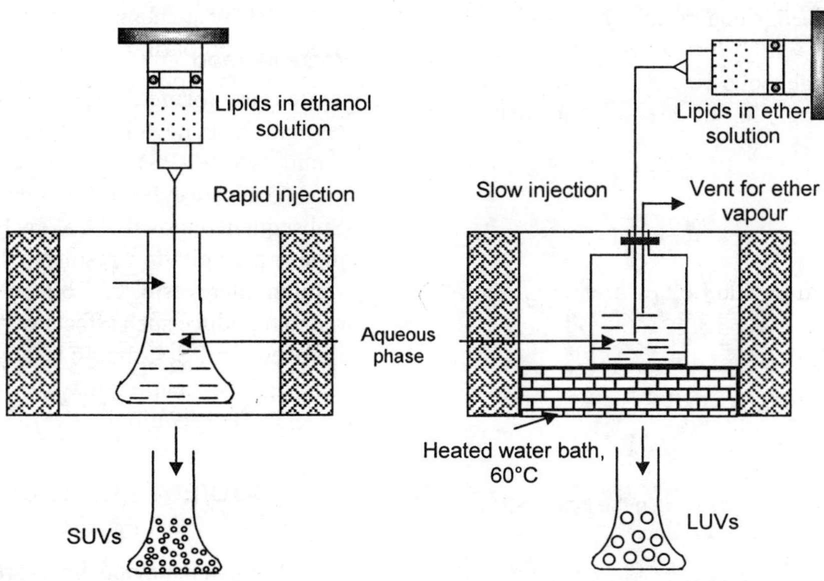

Fig. 5-13. Principle of Vesicle Formation by Solvent Dispersion Methods in which Two Phases (Aqueous and Organic) are Miscible with Each Other and Forms Different Types of Vesicles

taken to produce a batch of liposomes and a careful control needed for introduction of the lipid solution, requiring a mechanically operated pump. If substances are degraded at elevated temperature (60 °C), then the fluorinated hydrocarbons (Freons) may be used instead of ether. The efficiency of encapsulation is relatively low, although the captured volume per mole of lipid remains high, 8-17 l/mol.

Rapid Solvent Exchange Vesicles (RSEVs)

Rapid solvent exchange method has been a recent addition to the field of methodology of liposome preparation (Buboltz and Feigenson, 1999). In this method principally, the lipid mixture is quickly transferred between an essentially pure solvent environment and a pure aqueous environment. This method is specifically designed to form compositionally homogenous dispersion by sudden precipitation of a lipid mixture in an aqueous buffer. Phospholipid/cholesterol dispersion turns to be free of artifactual crystals when prepared by rapid solvent exchange method.

The method involves passing the organic solution of the lipids through the orifice of blue-tipped syringe (injection needle) under the vacuum in to a tube containing aqueous buffer. The tube is mounted on the vortexer. Bulk solvent vaporizes and is removed within seconds before coming in contact with aqueous environment, while the lipid mixture rapidly precipitates in aqueous buffer. Since the method is devised specifically for the fast and efficient removal of organic solvent, it does not require a highly volatile solvent. RES liposomes require not more than a minute for preparation and manifest high entrapment volumes with a high fraction of external surface area with no evidence of artifactual demixing as observed with conventional solvent dispersion methods.

De-emulsification Methods

This method requires two steps for the preparation of liposomes, first the inner leaflet of the bilayer, then the outer half (Fig. 5-14). The common feature of this method is the formation of "water in oil" emulsion by introduction of a small quantity of aqueous medium containing material to be entrapped into a large volume of immiscible organic solution of lipid. This was followed by mechanical agitation to break up the aqueous phase into microscopic water droplets. These droplets are stabilized by the presence of phospholipid monolayer at the interface. The size of droplets is determined by the intensity of mechanical energy used to form the emulsion and amount of lipid relative to the volume of aqueous phase, since each droplet requires a complete monolayer of phospholipid covering its surface in order to prevent the possible coalescence with other droplets. The aqueous solution surrounded by the monolayer of phospholipid forms the central core of the final liposome. There are number of methods, which could be used for preparing droplets including double emulsion, reverse phase evaporation and sonication methods.

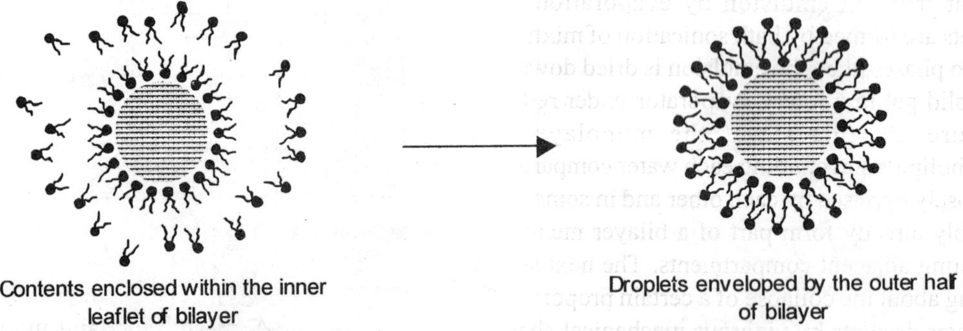

Fig. 5-14. Principle of Vesicle Formation by Solvent Dispersion Methods in Which the Two Phases (Aqueous and Organic) are Immiscible with Each Other and Form the Vesicles in Two Steps: First, the Inner Half of the Monolayer and Second, the Outer Half of the Bilayer

Double Emulsion Vesicles

In this method, the outer half of the liposome membrane is created at a second interface between two phases by emulsification of an organic solution in water. If the organic solution, which already contains water droplet, is introduced into excess aqueous medium followed by mechanical dispersion, multi compartment vesicles are obtained. The ordered dispersion so obtained is described as a W/O/W system (i.e., double emulsion). These vesicles with aqueous core are suspended in aqueous medium, the two aqueous compartments being separated from each other by a pair of phospholipid monolayers whose hydrophobic surfaces face each other across a thin film of organic solvent. Removal of this solvent clearly results in an intermediate sized unilamellar vesicle. The theoretical entrapment may reach upto 90%.

The double emulsion is prepared by rapidly injecting the dispersion of micro-droplets into hot aqueous solution of Tris-buffer with the help of 22-gauge hypodermic needle under vigorous stirring. The organic solvent is evaporated using strong jet of nitrogen thus forming double emulsion. The last traces of organic solvent are removed by evaporation and finally the volume is adjusted by adding extra-distilled water and then the product is centrifuged at 20 °C for 30 min at 37,000g to remove lipid aggregates.

Reverse Phase Evaporation Vesicles

The essential feature of this method, established by Szoka & Papahadjopoulos (1978), is the removal of solvent from an emulsion by evaporation. The droplets are formed by bath sonication of mixture of the two phases, then the emulsion is dried down to a semisolid gel in a rotary evaporator under reduced pressure. At this stage, the monolayers of phospholipids surrounding each water compartment are closely opposed by each other and in some cases probably already form part of a bilayer membrane separating adjacent compartments. The next step is to bring about the collapse of a certain proportion of the water droplets by vigorous mechanical shaking using a vortex mixer. In these circumstances, the lipid monolayer, which enclosed the collapsed vesicle, is contributed to adjacent intact vesicle to form the outer leaflet of the bilayer of a large unilamellar liposome. The aqueous content of the collapsed droplet provides the medium required for dispersion of these newly formed liposomes. After conversion of the gel into a homogenous free flowing fluid, the dispersion is dialyzed to remove the last traces of solvent. The vesicles formed are unilamellar and have an average diameter of 0.5 μm (Fig. 5-15). The encapsulation percentage is found to be nearly 50%.

Stable Plurilamellar Vesicles (SPLVs)

The method of plurilamellar vesicle formation involves preparation of water-in-organic phase dispersion with an excess of lipid followed by drying under continued bath sonication with an intermittent stream of nitrogen. The redistribution and equilibration of aqueous solvent and solute occurs in between the various bilayers in each plurilamellar vesicle. The internal structure of SPLVs is different from that of MLV-REVs, in that they lack a large aqueous core, the majority of the entrapped aqueous medium being located in the compartment in between adjacent lamellae. The percent entrapment normally ranges around 30% (compared with > 60% for MLV-REVs).

DETERGENT DEPLETION (REMOVAL) METHODS OF PASSIVE LOADING

In these methods, the phospholipids are brought into intimate contact with the aqueous phase via detergents, which associate with phospholipid molecules and serve to screen the hydrophobic portions of the molecule from water. The structures formed as a result of this association are known as micelles, and can be composed of several hundreds of component molecules. Their shape and size depend on chemical nature of the detergent, the concentration and other lipids involved. The concentration of detergent in water at which micelles just start to form is known as the 'critical micelle concentration' (CMC). Below the CMC, the detergent molecules exist entirely in free solution. As detergent is dissolved in water in concentration higher than the CMC, micelles form in more and more numbers, while the concentration of detergent in the free form remains essentially the same as it is at the CMC. Micelles containing other participating components

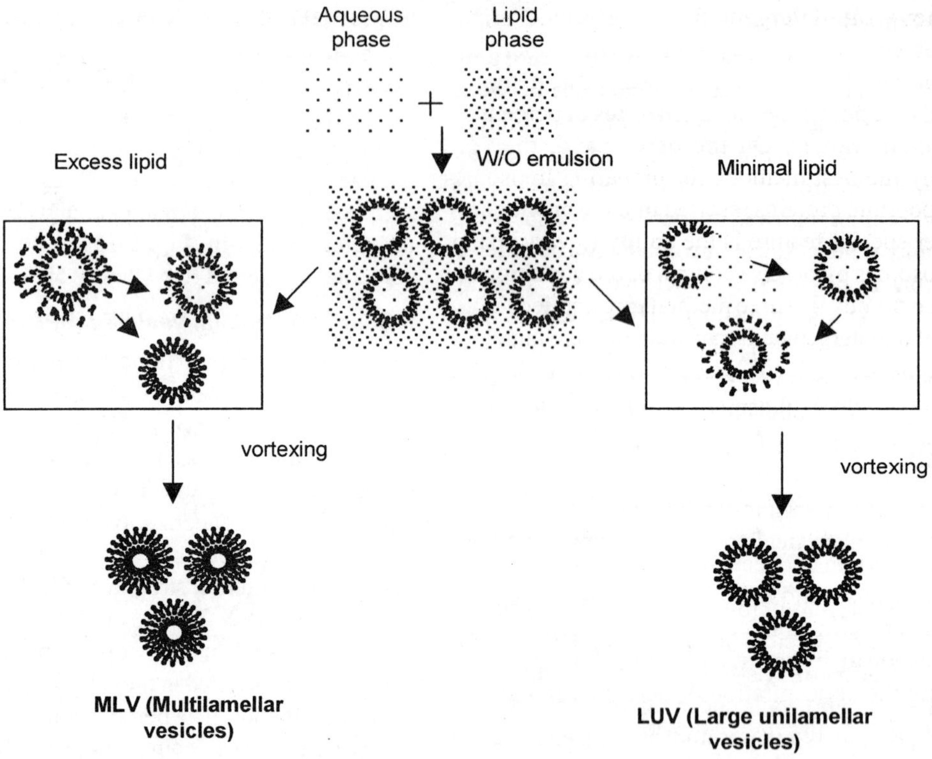

Fig. 5-15. Formation of Different Liposomes Using Reverse Phase Evaporation Method. MLV-REVs are Formed in Presence of Excess Phospholipids, whereas LUV-REVs are Formed in Absence of Extra Lipid

in addition to the detergent (or composed of two or more detergents) in their formation, are known as "mixed micelles".

As a general rule, membrane solubilizing detergents have a higher affinity for phospholipid membranes than for the pure detergent micelles. Thus, as detergent is added in increasing amounts to the membrane preparation, more and more detergent gets incorporated into the bilayer, until a point is reached where a transition from the lamellar to the spherical micellar phase configuration takes place. As the detergent concentration increases further, the micelles are reduced in size until they become saturated with detergent, whereupon the concentration of free molecules equals the CMC and simple detergent micelles are formed. It is usually found that a high concentration is advantageous for solubilizing membrane phospholipids although one might expect the converse, since a high affinity for lipid membranes should be reflected by a low CMC. A three-stage model of the interaction for detergents with the lipid bilayers with increasing detergent/lipid radius was proposed.

- At low (sublytic) concentrations detergent equilibrates between vesicular lipid and water phase (stage-I). At this stage, mean vesicle size increases and functional properties of the bilayer change.
- After reaching a critical detergent concentration ('saturation' of the bilayers), membrane structure tends to be unstable and transforms gradually into micelles (stage-II). In this stage detergent saturated bilayers coexist with lipid-saturated micelles.
- At stage-III, all lipid exists in mixed micelle form.

Invariably in all methods, which employ detergent in the preparation of liposomes, the basic feature is to remove the detergent from preformed mixed micelles containing phospholipid, whereupon unilamellar vesicles form spontaneously. The detergent methods are not very efficient in terms of percentage entrapment values. On the other hand, they are certainly the best methods for preparing liposomes with lipophilic proteins inserted into the membranes. Another special feature is the ability to vary size of the liposomes by precise control of the conditions of detergent removal. Three methods are applied for the removal of detergent and transition of mixed micelles to concentric bilayered form. These include, dialysis, column chromatography and the use of biobeads.

Dialysis

In contrast to phospholipids, detergents are highly soluble in both aqueous and organic media and there is an equilibrium between the detergent molecules in the water phase, and in the lipid environment of the micelle. The critical micelle concentration can give an indication to the position of this equilibrium. Upon lowering the concentration of detergent in the bulk aqueous phase, the molecules of detergent can be removed from mixed micelle by dialysis. A higher CMC indicates that the equilibrium is strongly shifted towards the bulk solution, so that removal from the mixed membrane by dialysis becomes relatively easy.

Detergents commonly used for this purpose exhibit reasonably high CMC (~10-20 mM) so that their removal is facilitated. They include the bile salts sodium cholate and sodium deoxycholate and synthetic detergents such as octylglucoside. The treatment of egg PC with a 2:1 molar ratio of sodium cholate followed by dialysis results in the formation of vesicles (~100 nm). A commercial version of the dialysis system is available under the trade name LIPOREP™

Column Chromatography

Phospholipids in the form of either sonicated vesicles or as a dry film, at a molar ratio of 2:1 with deoxycholate form unilamellar vesicles of 100 nm on removal of deoxycholate by column chromatography (Enoch and Strittmatter, 1976). This could be achieved by passing the dispersion over a Sephadex G-25 column pre-saturated with constitutive lipids and pre- equilibrated with hydrating buffer.

Detergent Adsorption using Bio-beads

Detergent (non-ionic)/phospholipid mixtures can form large unilamellar vesicles upon removal of non-ionic detergent (Triton X-100) using appropriate adsorbents for the detergent (Levy et al., 1990). The ability of Bio-beads SM-2, to adsorb Triton X-100 selectively and rapidly, makes them a suitable candidate for LUV preparation by detergent solubilization method. On hydrating the casted lipid film with 0.5-1.0 % Triton X-100, washed Bio-beads are added to the dispersion (0.3 g wet Bio-beads per ml of dispersion) and rocked for about 2 h at 4±1°C.

REMOTE (ACTIVE) LOADING

A general scheme describing various types of liposomes is presented with their formation methodology (Fig. 5-16). The utilization of liposomes as drug delivery systems is stimulated with the advancement of efficient encapsulation procedures. The membrane from lipid bilayer is in general impermeable to ions and larger hydrophilic molecules. Ions transport can be regulated by the ionophores while permeation of neutral and weakly hydrophobic molecules can be controlled by concentration gradients. Some weak acids or bases however, can be transported through the membrane due to various transmembrane gradients, such as electrical, ionic (pH) or specific salt (chemical potential) gradients. Several methods exist for improved loading of the drugs, including remote (active) loading methods which load drug molecules into preformed liposomes using pH gradients and potential difference across liposomal membranes (Fig. 5-16). A concentration difference in proton concentration across the membrane of liposomes can drive the loading of amphipathic molecules. Active loading methods have the following advantages over passive encapsulation techniques:

- A high encapsulation efficiency and capacity
- A reduced leakage of the encapsulated compounds
- "Bed side' loading of drugs thus limiting loss of retention of drugs by diffusion, or chemical degradation during storage
- Flexibility for the use of constitutive lipids, as

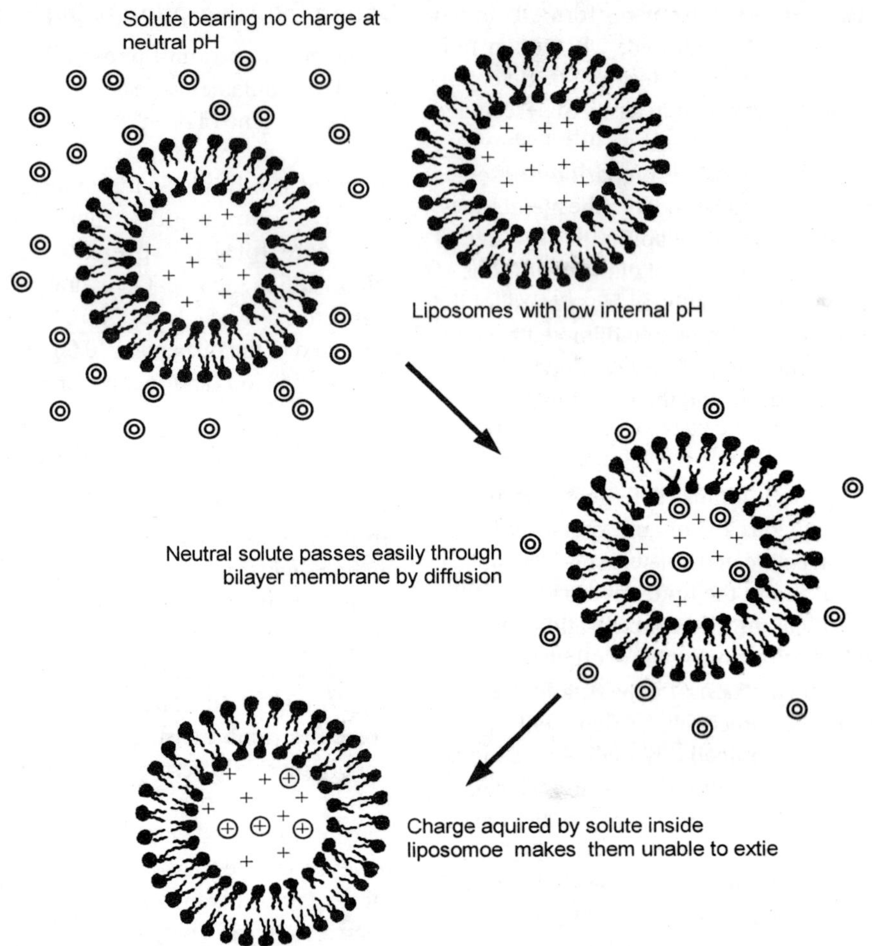

Fig. 5-16. Active Loading of Drug into Preformed Liposomes by pH Gradient Obtained by $(NH_4)_2SO_4$ Gradient. Solid Arrows Indicate Shifts in Equilibria Resulting in Increased Entrapment of Drug

drug is loaded after the formation of carrier units

- Avoidance of biological active compounds during preparation steps in the dispersion thus reducing safety hazards
- The transmembrane pH gradient can be developed using various methods depending upon the nature of the drug to be encapsulated
- For amphipathic weak bases by remote loading procedures such as using a proton gradient or an ammonium sulphate gradient
- For amphipathic weak acids by remote loading procedures using a calcium acetate gradient

Weak amphipathic bases accumulate in the aqueous phase of lipid vesicles in response to a difference in pH between the inside and outside of the liposomes (pH_{in} <pH_{out}). The pH gradient is created by preparing liposomes with a low pH inside and outside the vesicles, followed by the addition of the base to the extraliposomal medium. Usually, a two step process generates this pH imbalance and remote loading: first, the vesicles are prepared in a low pH solution, thus generating a low-pH within the liposomal interiors, followed by the addition of the base to the extraliposomal medium. Basic com-pounds, carrying amino groups are relatively lipo-philic at high pH and hydrophilic at low pH. In a two chambered aqueous system separated by a membrane (liposomes), accumulation occurs at the low pH side, under dynamic equilibrium conditions. Thus the unprotonated form of basic drug can diffuse through the bilayer. At the low-pH side the molecules are predominantly protonated, which lowers the concentration of the drug in the unprotonated form, and thus promote the diffusion of more drug molecules at the low-pH side of the bilayer. The second step involves the exchange of external medium by gel-exclusion chromatography with a neutral solution. Weak bases like doxorubicin, adriamycin and vincristine which co-exist in aqueous solutions in neutral and charged forms have been successfully loaded into preformed liposomes via the pH gradient method. Similarly, short modified peptides and insulin (FITC-insulin) were also loaded successfully in large unilamellar vesicles through pH gradients (inside acidic). Recently, the approach has been further modified using transmembrane differences in salt concentrations, such as ammonium sulphate (amine gradient method) or calcium acetate (acetate gradient method). This technique takes advantage of the large differences in the permeability coefficients across lipid bilayer of the sulphate anion (P<10-12 cm/s) and of the ammonia molecule (P=0.13 cm/s), generated by the dissociation of the ammonium cation. This results into an increase in liposomal internal pH. In addition, the sulphate salt of this molecule has a very low solubility and aggregates inside the liposomes, resulting in even larger encapsulation efficiencies and the stabilization of the loading.

MICROENCAPSULATION OR LOCUS OF DRUGS IN LIPOSOMES

Liposomes due to their biphasic environment can act as carriers for both lipophilic and hydrophilic drugs (Fig. 5-17). Highly hydrophilic drugs (log P<-0.3) are located exclusively in the aqueous domains, whereas highly lipophilic drugs (log P<5) are entrapped within the lipid bilayers of the liposomes (Fresta et al., 1993; Vadiei et al., 1989). It is interesting to note that the loss of drug (drug leakage) on long term storage is maximal with former and minimal or none with latter. Drugs with intermediary partition coefficients (i.e., 1.7< log P< 4) impose problem for loading as they equilibrate between lipid and aqueous domains and are prone to leakage on storage of liposomes (Sasaki et al., 1984). However, drugs with poor biphasic insolubility mostly anticancer drugs like 6-mercaptopurine, azathioprene and allopurinol are most problematic due to their immiscibility with both aqueous and lipidic domains (Gulati et al., 1998). One good way of approaching the economic viability of liposomal formulations is

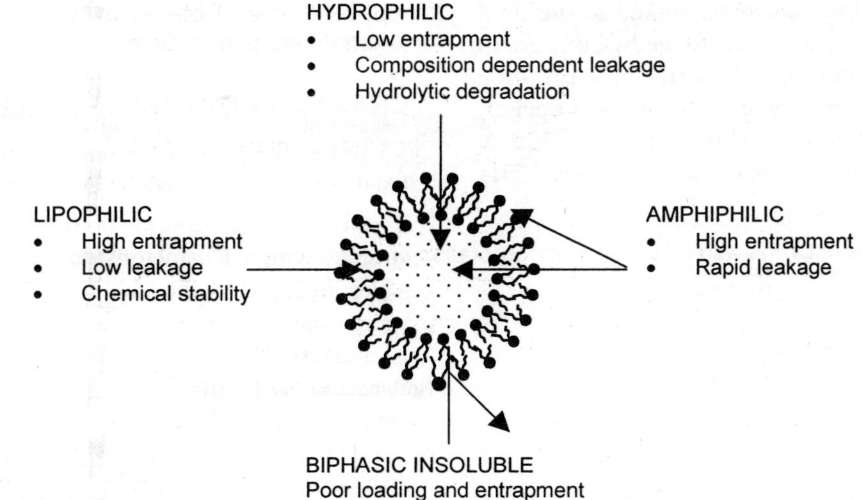

Fig. 5-17. Scheme Showing Various Drugs and their Confinement in Different Domains of Liposomes

to keep the drug:phospholipid ratio maximum in the favor of the drug. However, this is always not feasible as the extent of incorporation of a drug in the lipid vesicle strongly depends upon its solubility in aqueous milieu and/or the lipid bilayer. Based on whether the drug is hydrophilic, lipophilic, amphiphilic or biphasic insoluble, the degree of entrapment may range from nil to 100%. The partitioning characteristics, site of entrapment and examples of various categories of drugs are given in Table 5-5 and presented schematically in Figure 5-17.

Three approaches have emerged during last decade for increasing the lipophilicity of the drugs with the purpose of enhancing their liposomal encapsulation. These include preparation of prodrug and non-prodrug lipophilic derivative (Gulati and Singh, 2001), formation of lipophilic complexes and formation of pharmacosomes. The preparations of lipophilic drug derivatives are at different stages of development with several of them having already reached the stage of clinical trials.

Lipophilic Transformation of Drugs: Pharmacosomes

Pharmacosomes are colloidal dispersion where the drugs are covalently anchored to lipid components. They are designed to avoid the usual problems associated with the liposomal entrapment of polar drug molecules like low drug incorporation, leakage and poor stability. This approach of forming vesicles by the use of drug molecules linked to the lipid directly or through the spacer to the hydroxy group of a lipid molecule was utilized to produce pharmacosomes of pindolol (Vaizoglu and Speiser, 1986), azidothymidine (Hostetler et al., 1990), fenoprofen (Muller-Goymann and Hamann, 1991) and most recently for propranolol (Vyas et al., 2000). Problems like poor entrapment efficiency and physical as well as chemical instability have been found to be associated with the liposomal entrapment of drug molecules, other than those that are highly lipophilic. Lipophilic drugs show very high degree of entrapment, which sometimes reaches 100%. Over the last three decades, large number of drugs that are not lipophilic by themselves have been structurally altered to impart lipophilicity (Gulati and Singh, 2001). A large number of drug molecules belonging to the category of anticancer, antiviral, steroids and diagnostic aids with varying solubility behaviour have been structurally altered to maximize their liposomal encapsulation.

REMOVAL OF UNENTRAPPED DRUGS FROM LIPOSOMES

It is important to estimate the amount of drug encapsulated within liposomes. This is easier in the case of MLVs compared to LUVs and SUVs. MLVs due to their large size settle at the bottom and form the pellet when centrifuged at high speed, while the non-encapsulated drug remains in the supernatant. However, LUVs and SUVs do not settle upon centrifugation. It is therefore, important to accurately estimate the encapsulation of drugs in LUVs and SUVs using appropriate, rapid and economical processes. Table 5-6 provides a brief account of various methods used for the separation of unentrapped drugs with their merits and demerits.

CHARACTERIZATION OF LIPOSOMES

Liposomal formulations after their formulation and processing for a specified purpose are characterized

Table 5-5. Types of Drugs with Site of their Incorporation and Entrapment Characteristics

Type of drug	Log P_{oct}	Site of entrapment	Candidate
Lipophilic	>5	Lipid bilayer	Cyclosporine
Hydrophilic	<-0.3	Aqueous domain	CDP Choline
Amphiphilic	1.7<log P<4	Both aqueous and lipid phases	Mitomycin C, Actinomycin D, Vinblastin
Biphasic Insoluble		–	6-Mercaptopurine, Azathioprine, Allopurinol

to ensure their predictable *in vitro* and *in vivo* performances (Ostro, 1987, New 1989, Weiner et al., 1989). The liposomes produced by different techniques may have different physicochemical characteristics. These differences do have an impact on their behaviour *in vivo* (disposition) and *in vitro* (e.g. sterilization and shelf life). The characterization parameters for the purpose of evaluation could be classified into three broad categories, which include physical, chemical and biological parameters. Physical characterization evaluates various parameters, including size, shape, surface features, lamellarity, phase behaviour and drug release profile. Chemical characterization includes those studies which establish the purity and potency of various liposomal constituents. Biological characterization parameters are helpful in establishing the safety and suitability of the formulations for the *in vivo* use or for therapeutic applications.

Some of the parameters characterized in liposome product development are size and size distribution, surface topology, encapsulation efficiency, capture volume, lamellarity and *in vitro* drug release profile (Talsma and Crommelin, 1992b; Barenholz and Cromellin, 1994).

Vesicle Shape and Lamellarity

Vesicle shape can be assessed using various electron microscopic techniques, which can also be extended to determine the average size of the vesicles. The lamellarity of MLVs is heterogeneous and usually it is unilamellar as well as multilamellar. Earlier lamellarity calculations were based on techniques that detected proportion of lipids exposed to the external medium (New, 1989). This led to approximately half of the total lipid in LUVs and an even smaller fraction in MLVs. Labeling or binding studies are now employed to determine the proportion of outer monolayer lipid. However, lamellarity of the vesicles, i.e., the number of bilayers present in the liposomes is determined using Freeze-fracture electron microscopy (Ostro, 1987) and ^{31}P nuclear magnetic resonance analysis (Hope et al., 1985).

Freeze-fracture and freeze-etch Electron Microscopy

Freeze-fracture electron microscopy can be used not only to assess the shape and lamellarity but also the surface morphology (topology) of the liposomes (Mandal and Downing, 1993). In this technique the fracture plan passes through the vesicles, which are randomly positioned in the frozen state. Thus, the fracture plan may not necessarily passes through the mid-plane and thus non-mid plane fracture may result in erroneous readings. The observed distribution profile thus depends on the distance of vesicle centre from the plane of fracture. Furthermore, heterogenous populations require a careful monitoring before analysing the final results (Fig. 5-18). However, quick freeze and deep etching techniques give much better lamellarity evaluation (Nakata et al., 1990). It is reported that ethching of freeze-fractured specimen can provide information about fractures of vesicles that are unilamellar in a given population. After 5 min of etching, cross-fractured

Table 5-6. Summary of Advantages and Disadvantages of Various Methods Used to Separate Non-Encapsulated Drugs from Liposomes

Method	% Loading	Advantages	Disadvantage(s)
Dialysis	26	Sample recovery	Inaccurate
Minicolumn centrifugation	34	Economical; sample recovery	Tedious; Small sample volumes
Ficoll Density gradient	34	Economical; rapid; sample recovery	Small sample volume (0.5 ml)
Protamine aggregation	34	Economical; applicable to MLVs and LUVs	Slow with neutral and positively charged liposomes; Causes contamination of liposome sample
Gel chromatography	28-29	Sample recovery	Slow and tedious; Tends to dilution of samples
Centifree filtration	31	Rapid; Small sample volume	Expensive; Applicable only to ULVs; Lipid concentrations can not exceed 5 mg ml^{-1}

vesicles are clearly seen and the number of lamellae can readily be determined.

^{31}P Nuclear Magnetic Resonance Analysis

^{31}P nuclear magnetic resonance analysis has been one of the most accurate and straightforward techniques that determines the lamellarity of liposomes (Arica et al., 1995). The technique exploits ^{31}P nuclear magnetic resonance (NMR) to monitor the phospholipid phosphorus signal intensity. In particular, adding an impermeable paramagnetic shift or nonpermeable broadening agent (such as Mn^{++}) to the external medium will decrease the intensity of the initial ^{31}P NMR signal by an amount proportional to the fraction of lipid exposed to the external medium. Manganese ions interact with the outer leaflet of the outermost bilayer. Thus, a 50% reduction in NMR signal intensity indicates a unilamellar whereas subsequent reductions indicate a multilamellar vesicular preparation.

Vesicle Size and Size Distribution

The average vesicle size and size distribution are important parameters as far as *in vitro* characterization of the liposomal product is concerned. This is because they influence the physicochemical properties and biological fate of the liposomes and/or entrapped materials after *in vivo* administration. Various techniques are described in the literature for the determination of size and size distribution. These include light microscopy, fluorescent microscopy (if a fluorescent probe is included in either lipid or aqueous domain), electron microscopy (specially transmission electron microscopy and freeze-fracture microscopy), laser light scattering, photon correlation spectroscopy, field flow fractionation, gel permeation and gel exclusion and zetasizer. Most of the methods used in the size, shape and distribution analysis can be grouped into various categories, namely microscopic, diffraction and scattering and hydrodynamic techniques.

Microscopic Techniques

Optical Microscopy

The microscopic methods include the use of Bright-field, phase contrast microscope and fluorescent microscope (if liposomes are loaded with fluorescent probes) and are useful in evaluating the vesicle size of large vesicles (>1 μm) particularly the upper end of the size distribution for multilamellar vesicles. Vesicular dispersion appropriately diluted are wet mounted on a haemocytometer and photographed with a phase contrast microscope. The negatives then can be projected on a piece of calibrated paper using a photographic enlarger at ×1250 (Vyas and Katare, 1991). Diameters of approximately 500 vesicles are measured and thus this method is tedious and coupled with the limitation of resolution, hence electron microscopic methods with greater resolutions are preferred.

Negative Stain Transmission Electron microscopy (TEM)

Electron microscopic techniques used to assess liposome shape and size are mainly negative-stain transmission electron microscopy (New, 1989) and

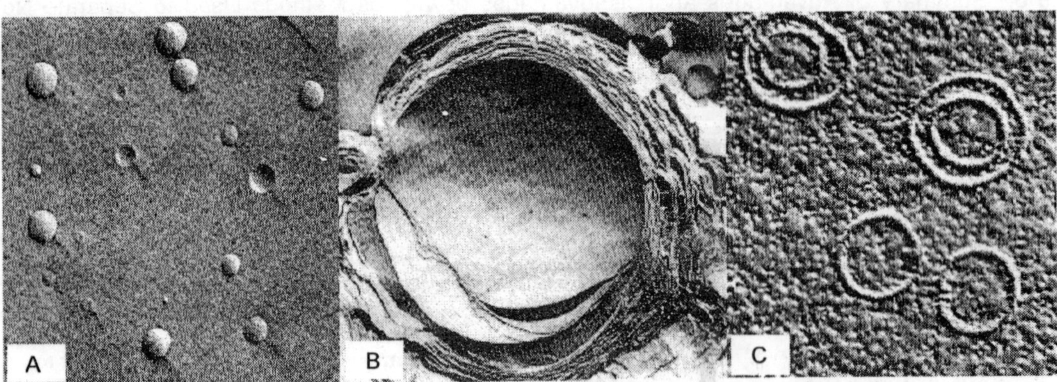

Fig. 5-18. Freeze-Fracture (A &B) and Freeze-Etch (C) Electron Microscopy Photographs of Liposomes

scanning electron microscopy (Barenholz and Cromellin, 1994). However, the latter technique requires dehydration of the sample prior to examination and is less preferred. Negative stain electron microscopy visualizes relatively electron transparent liposomes as bright areas against a dark background (hence termed as negative stain) (Fig. 5-19). Liposomes are embedded in this method in a thin film of electron-dense heavy metal (salt) stain.

The negative stains used in the TEM analysis are ammonium molybdate ($(NH_4)_6Mo_7O_{24}$, AM, 0.5-2%) or phosphotungstic acid ($H_3PO_4.12WO_3.24H_2O$, PTA, 0.5-2.0%) or uranyl acetate ($UO_2(CH_3COO)_2.2H_2O$, 0.2-0.5%). Both PTA and AM are anionic in nature and thus do not bind to liposomes composed of either neutral (PC) or negatively charged phospholipids (e.g., PA, PG or PS) However, they may precipitate or aggregate liposomes composed of positively charged lipids. In the latter case, cationic uranyl acetate should be used. However, it should be noted that uranium salts are precipitated by phosphate ions, and therefore, liposomes prepared in phosphate buffer should be washed before being stained with uranyl acetate (New, 1989).

The use of negative stain electron microscopy facilitates estimation of the liposome size range at the lower end of the frequency distribution. For SUVs, sizing by negative staining compares favourably with measurements determined by coulter counter or by freeze-fracture techniques. However, for larger sizes, or for heterogenous populations of liposomes, negative staining electron microscopy offers real advantage over freeze- fracture technique. In the latter technique, the fracture plane passes through liposomes, oriented randomly in the frozen specimen, hence non-midplane sectioning is a possibility which will result in an observed diameter of vesicles different from real diameter of liposome (Ostro, 1987).

Negative staining electron microscopy alleviates this drawback in that complete structure is observed, although the liposome morphology may be deformed from spherical. Irregular or ellipsoid shapes can be treated mathematically to correct for perimeter irregularities thus estimations of original spherical diameters can be calculated.

Cryo-Transmission Electron Microscopy Technique (Cryo-TEM)

Cryo-TEM has been used to elucidate the surface morphology and size of the vesicles. This method is also used to characterize liposomal formulations where the drug is loaded by remote loading in order to ensure their stability. The method involves freeze fracturing of samples followed by their visualization using transmission electron microscopy (Fig. 5-19). Thin sample films are prepared under controlled temperature (25 °C) and humidity conditions within a custom-built environment chamber. The films are thereafter vitrified by quick freezing in liquid ethane and transferred to TEM analysis. To prevent sample preparation and formation of ice crystals, specimens are kept below 108K during both transfer and reviewing procedures.

Schmidtgen et al., 1998 used cryo-TEM to examine the morphology of vesicles formed from

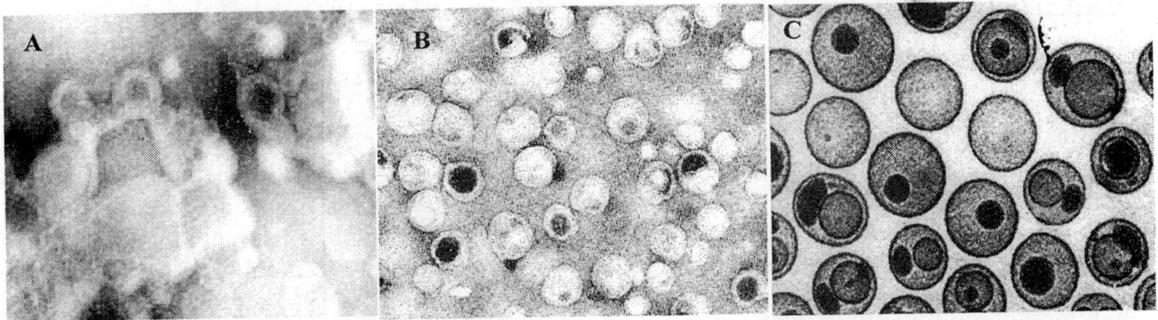

Transmission electron microscopy of liposomes
A. Multilamellar vesicles. B. Unilamellar vesicles

Cryo- Transmission electron microscopy

Fig. 5-19. TEM and Cryo-TEM Photographs of Liposomes

lipids of the human stratum corneum (hSC). Gustafsson et al., 1995 studied the association structures formed by cationic liposomes and DNA-plasmids based gene carriers by cryo-TEM (cryo-transmission electron microscopy).

Freeze-fracture Electron Microscopy

Freeze-fracture electron microscopy though is used mainly to assess the surface features and lamellarity, it can also be used to calculate the true vesicle diameter. If the angle of disposition of the shadowing material is 45° to the fracture plane, then vesicle faces that are 50% shadowed are cleaved equatorially and thus may reflect the true vesicle diameter.

Scanning Electron Microscopy (SEM)

Scanning electron microscopy is less frequently used, although SEM has been reported in the literature. The distortion during sample preparation can be cited as the reason of non-acceptability of SEM as one of the evaluation method. Scanning tunneling microscopy (or atomic force microscopy) on the other hand offers excellent improvisation in resolution. Monolayers under water can be resolved at the level of individual lipid molecules using these techniques.

Diffraction and Scattering Techniques

Laser light Scattering

Light scattering techniques, particularly laser-based, quasi-elastic light scattering techniques are useful in analyzing the homogeneous colloidal particulate populations (Kolchens et al., 1993; Barenholz and Cromellin, 1994). The technique is based on the time-dependent coherence of light scattered by a vesicle, sensitive to vesicle diffusion, which in turn is dependent upon the viscosity of the aqueous medium and vesicle size. This technique can be applied to unimodel systems (homogeneous or monodisperse) with mean diameters less than 1 µm. Moreover, its application in case of heterogenous systems exhibiting bimodal or more complex size distributions should be crosschecked using other methods. This is because light scattering methods rely on algorithms to determine the vesicle size distributions and the results obtained thus are not well correlated with hetero-dispersed systems. Furthermore, such techniques can not distinguish between a large particle and a flocculated mass of smaller particles. Most importantly, it is imperative in these methods to remove micron-sized (or beyond µm) particles that are present in the dispersion prior to analysis. Recently, multi-angle quasi-elastic light scattering based (QELS) methods are used to avoid errors due to the angular dependence of the scattering function of the particles. The experimentally determined auto-correlation function was analyzed by multiple mathematical procedures, i.e. single exponential, CUMULANT, exponential sampling, non-negatively constrained least square and CONTIN, in order to select suitable models for vesicle characterization (Barenholz and Cromellin, 1994).

Photon correlation spectroscopy is the major technique based upon laser scattering analysis that exploits the time dependence of intensity fluctuations in scattered laser light due to the different Brownian motions of the particles in liposomal dispersion. This differential diffusion profile of the particles of small and larger dimensions accordingly influences the rate of fluctuations of scattered light intensity, which is a function of the mean hydrodynamic radius of the particles (vesicles) determined using Stokes-Einstein equation.

Hydrodynamic Techniques

Field-Flow-Fractionation (FFF) Techniques

The applicability of hydrodynamic method like FFF for characterization of liposomes is recently introduced (Moon and Giddings, 1993). Because of fundamental differences in their driving forces, sedimentation FFF and flow FFF measure different vesicle properties. Sedimentation FFF, although used to measure vesicle sizes and size distributions, is fundamentally a technique that measures the effective mass and mass distribution of particles. It is sensitive to small changes in the effective mass of either the biomembrane or its encapsulated load. It is useful in characterizing properties such as drug loading, biomembrane volumes and areas, and distributions of these properties. Size characterization by sedimentation FFF can only be done by deducing size from effective mass. Flow FFF, in contrast, provides a direct measurement of vesicle size and size distribution. The effect of ionic strength and pH of carrier solutions on the separation of liposomes by flow field-flow fractionation (flow FFF) has been studied for the determination of accurate vesicle size distribution of liposomes.

Gel Permeation

Gel permeation or gel-exclusion chromatography are preferably used techniques for the size distribution determination of liposomes. The ability to separate various components of heterodispersed preparations could be exploited to estimate various sized particles present in the dispersion. However, it is also used for the separation of unentrapped drug or separation of various heterodispersed liposomal preparations (Lesieur et al., 1991; Andrieux et al., 1998). While practically any gel medium can separate liposomes from non-encapsulated molecules. Gel media with larger porosities, such as Sepharose 4B or 2B, and Sephacryl S500 and S1000, allows fractionation of liposomes in the working volume of the column.

The largest inclusion volume is found in Sephacryl 1000, which separates particles with diameters between 0.4 μm in the void volume and ~10 nm in the total volume. A proper calibration of the gel column offers valuable data for size distribution of liposomes, as well as interactions such as fusion, lipid mixing and size growth.

Ultracentrifuge

Ultracentrifuge can yield valuable data on size-distribution of liposomes. It is however, used for the analytical purposes. The density of egg PC bilyer is 1.0135 g/ml (with 50 mol% of cholesterol it increases to 1.0142 g/ml), and since physiologic saline is having a density of 1.0048, liposomes can be pelleted. Because of the small differences in density, SUV's have very small sedimentation coefficient.Therefore, to pellet SUV's, centrifuge at 2,00,000 g for 10-12 h is required.

Surface Charge

Liposomes are usually prepared using charge imparting constituting lipids and hence it is imperative to study the charge on the vesicle surface. In general two methods are used to assess the charge, namely free-flow electrophoresis and zeta potential measurement. From the mobility of the liposomal dispersion in a suitable buffer (determined using Helmholtz-Smoluchowski equation), the surface charge on the vesicles can be calculated (Adamson, 1967).

Encapsulation Efficiency and Trapped Volume

Encapsulation efficiency and trapped volume determine the amount and rate of entrapment of water soluble agents in the aqueous compartment of liposomes (Fry et al., 1978; Gunter et al., 1982; Weiner et al., 1989; New, 1989; Barenholz and Cromellin, 1994).

Encapsulation Efficiency

The encapsulation efficiency describes the percent of the aqueous phase and hence the percent of water soluble drug that becomes ultimately entrapped during preparation of liposomes and is usually expressed as % entrapment/mg lipid. Encapsulation efficiency is assessed using two techniques including minicolumn centrifugation method and protamine aggregation method (Fig. 5-20).

Minicolumn centrifugation is generally used both as a means of purification and separation of liposomes on a small scale and analysis of a liposomal dispersion to determine encapsulation efficiency (Fry et al., 1978). A Sephadex or Sepharose column pre-saturated with the dispersion medium in 1.0 ml disposable syringe is run while applying liposomal dispersion (200 μl) first and saline (250 μl) thereafter and centrifuging the column at 2000 rpm for 3 min and assaying the elutes. Depending upon the different molecular weights of solutes entrapped, various medium and their cut off point should be chosen. The concentration of free or entrapped material in elutes can be assessed by disrupting liposomes using ethanol (2 ml ethanol for 10 μl of liposomes) or Triton X-100 (10 μl of 10% Trition X-100 for 10 μl of liposomes) and estimating the liberated contents using standard methods. The lipid concentration can be assessed using Barlett assay.

Protamine aggregation method may be used for neutral and negatively charged liposomes (Gunter et al., 1982). Liposomal dispersion (~100μl) can be precipitated with a protamine solution (100μl, 10 mg ml^{-1}) and subsequent centrifugation at 2000 rpm. By analyzing the material in the supernatant and in the liposome pellet (after disrupting liposomal pellet with

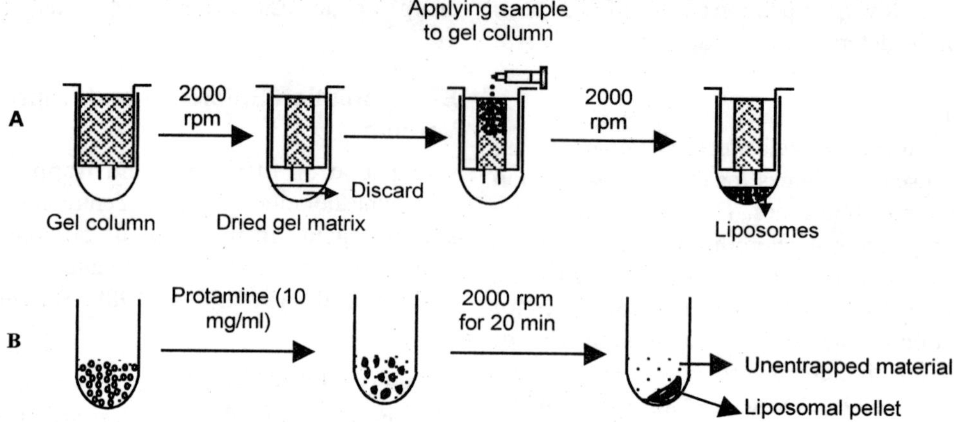

Fig. 5- 20. Determination of Entrapment Efficiency of Liposome Entrapped Material Using (A) Minicolumn Centrifugation Technique and (B) Protamine Aggregation Methods.

0.6 ml of 10% Triton X-100), the encapsulation efficiency of the entrapped material can be estimated.

Trapped Volume

Trapped volume is an important parameter that governs the encapsulation efficiency and morphology of the vesicles (Ostro 1987, Perkins et al., 1988; Weiner et al., 1989). Measurement of captured volumes by solute entrapment is pivotal for most types of vesicles. While estimating the encapsulation, it is assumed that no solute has leaked out of the liposomes after separation of unentrapped material. However, such assumptions sometime may prove invalid. For example in two phase methods of preparations, the aqueous phase (water) can be lost from the internal compartment during the drying down process that removes organic solvent or otherwise water can be expelled from the internal compartment as a result of unanticipated osmotic gradients. The measurement of the quantity of aqueous buffer is the best way to calculate trapped volume.

The internal or trapped volume is the aqueous entrapped volume per unit quantity of lipid and expressed as μl/μmol or μl/mg of total lipid. This can vary from 0.5 μl/μmol for some MLVs and SUVs to as much as 30μl/μmol for certain LUVs. Various materials including spectroscopically inert fluid, radioactive markers and fluorescent markers are used to determine the internal volume (entrapped volume) (Ostro, 1987).

The best way to measure internal volume is to measure the quantity of water directly, and this may be done by replacing the external medium (water, H_2O) with a spectroscopically inert fluid (deuterium oxide, D_2O), and then measuring the water signal, for example, using NMR. The permeability of the liposomal membrane to water is such that H_2O and D_2O equilibrate very rapidly throughout the whole volume of the medium. The NMR scan of this medium can be used to assess the peak height, which can be related to concentration by comparison with standards containing known amount of H_2O in D_2O.

The validity of atomic absorption spectrophotometry for measuring markers of trapped volume is also investigated and its superiority against determinations of markers with established optical spectrophotometry methods has been established (Yoss et al., 1985).

Trapped volumes are also determined experimentally by dispersing lipid in an aqueous medium containing non-permeable radioactive solute such as [^{22}Na] and [^{14}C] inulin. The proportion of solute trapped is determined by removing external radioactivity by centrifugation, dialysis or gel filtration and subsequently residual activity per lipid is determined. Another method is the use of entrapped water-soluble markers such as 6-carboxyfluorescein, ^{14}C or ^{3}H-glucose or sucrose and then lysing the liposomes by the use of detergent (Triton X-100). The trapped volume can then be back calculated using the amount of the marker that is entrapped (Barenholz and Cromellin, 1994). Gruber and co-workers (1995) reported a novel method of calculation of intravesicular volumes by salt entrapment.

Phase Response and Transitional Behaviour

Liposomes and lipid bilayers exhibit various phase transitions that are studied for their roles in triggered drug release or stimulus-mediated fusion of liposomal constituents with the target cells. Lipid bilayers can exist in a low-temperature solid-ordered phase and, above a certain temperature, in a fluid-disordered phase, the temperature of this phase transition can be tailored by selecting the proper lipids (Chapman, 1975). Various phase transition situations are studied in liposomal behaviour (Table 5-7). An understanding of phase transitions and fluidity of phospholipid membranes is important both in the manufacture and exploitation of liposomes, since the phase behaviour of a liposomal membrane determines such properties as permeability, fusion, aggregation, and protein binding. Moreover, these phase behaviours are important to characterize while formulating the liposomes with lipids having different phase transition temperatures and for polymer (PEG) grafted liposomes where polymer grafting as such provides a stealthing effect deterring them from macrophagic uptake (and hence long circulation) (Lasic, 1998).

Thermodynamic Methods

These phase transitions have been evaluated using freeze-fracture electron microscopy, They are more comprehensively verified by differential scanning calorimetry (DSC) analysis (Fig. 5-21) (New, 1989). In differential scanning microcalorimeter, the heat required by liposomes to maintain a steady upward rise in temperature is plotted as a function of temperature. In basic terms, two small aluminium paths are compared, one empty, and one containing a concentrated liposomal dispersion. Transmitter monitors the temperature of each pan, as the pans are heated up separately.

The heat input of the sample pan is adjusted so that its temperature matches those of the reference pan. At the phase transition point, extra heat is required to maintain the rise in temperature of the sample pan equal to that of the reference, and this is recorded directly (Fig. 5-21). The area under the peak is recorded as the enthalpy of the phase transition.

Vesicle Fusion Measurements

Liposomal fusion with cells and with intracellular contents has been a major area of research especially in the case of fusogenic liposomes, like pH sensitive liposomes, pH sensitive immunoliposomes, virosomes and cationic liposomes (Jones and Cossins, 1989). Fusion has been monitored using a fluorescence resonance energy transfer (RET) between two lipid analogues originally placed in

Table 5-7. Various Phase Transitions Reported in Liposomes

Phase transition	Initiating factor	Inferences
Gel-liquid crystal	Temperature, Ionic strength	Liposome leakage
Lamellar-micellar	Hydrolysis, ionization of weak amphiphilic bases, Protonation of surface attached polymer	Liposome leakage, disintegration
Lamellar-inverse hexagonal	Protonation of weak amphiphilic acids, PEG-PE linkage break in an unstable bilayer, PEG-PE dissociation from the bilayer	Liposome fusion, leakage
Steric destabilization	Removal of PEG from a stable bilayer (stealth-nonstealth)	Liposome destabilization, macrophage uptake
Collapse of a polymer brush	Temperature, presence of specific ions (random coil-helix)	Liposome destabilization, fusion
Precipitation or gelation of entrapped agents	Gradient loading	Stable encapsulation, shape changes
Solubilization of encapsulated gel, crystals	pH change, addition of ionophores	Leakage of encapsulated molecules

*Compiled from Lasic, 1998

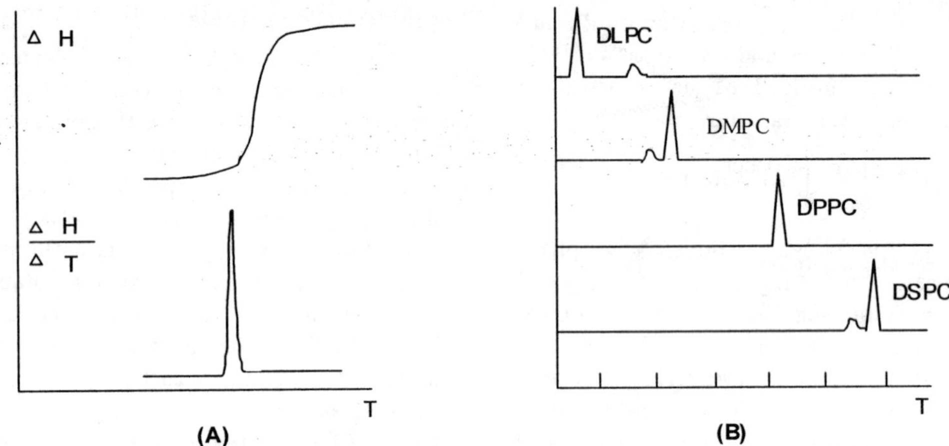

Fig. 5-21. (A) Phase Transition in Liposomes Triggered by Temperature and Recorded Using Differential Scanning Microcalorimeter. Upper Curve Records Extra Heat Required at Phase Transition. Lower Trace is Obtained From Upper By Mathematical Differentiation and Area Under Peak is Enthalpy of Phase Transition. (B) Microcalorimetry Curves Showing Phase Transitions of Membranes Containing Single Lipid Components

separate vesicle population or in the same vesicle population (termed as fluorescence probe dilution assay) that measures intermixing of membrane lipids (Uster and Deamer, 1981; Morgan et al., 1983). This technique depends upon an overlap in the emission spectrum of one fluorophore (the donor) and the excitation spectrum of a second fluorophore (the acceptor). Excitation of acceptor molecules can then occur by direct energy transfer of energy from the excited donor molecule, which is manifested as a reduction in the emission intensity of the donor fluorescence and a corresponding increase in emission intensity of the acceptor fluorescence. Thus, by incorporating donor and acceptor molecules into different liposome populations, the fusion could be detected by the onset of RET (Fig. 5-22). The relative change of RET on fusion is linearly related to the extent of fusion. The fluorescent lipid analogues most frequently used in the fusion assay are:

- N-(-7-nitro-2,1,3-benzoxadiazol-4-yl) phosphatidylethanolamine (N-NBD-PE), which acts as a donor
- N-(Lissamine rhodamine B sulphonyl) phosphatidylethanolamine (N-Rh-PE), which acts as an acceptor.

A variation in the RET method (also termed as probe dilution assay) is to premix the donor and acceptor lipid analogues in the same liposomes (0.5 mol %) and to induce fusion in the presence of an excess of unlabelled liposomes (Fig. 5-22).

The dilutions of the fluorophores as they disperse through the unlabelled membranes (increased distance between the NBD-PE and Rh-PE) then leads to a decrease in RET. Because RET decreases as the sixth power of distance between donor and acceptor molecules, it occurs only when the two molecules come into close contact, as in the case when both occupy the same bilayer. The maximum fluorescent intensity (F_{max}) in each sample can be calculated following the solubilization of vesicles with Triton X-100 to reach an infinite dilution of the probe. The percent of fusion can be calculated using the following equation:

$$\% \text{ Fusion} = \frac{F_t - F_0}{F_{max} - F_0} \times 100 \qquad (5\text{-}2)$$

Where, F_t is the fluorescence intensity at each time point and F_0 is the initial fluorescence intensity.

Chemical Characterization of Liposomes

Various chemical analysis methods used for quantitative and qualitative tests of liposomal components prior to and after the preparation are critical characteristics of liposomes (Barenholz and

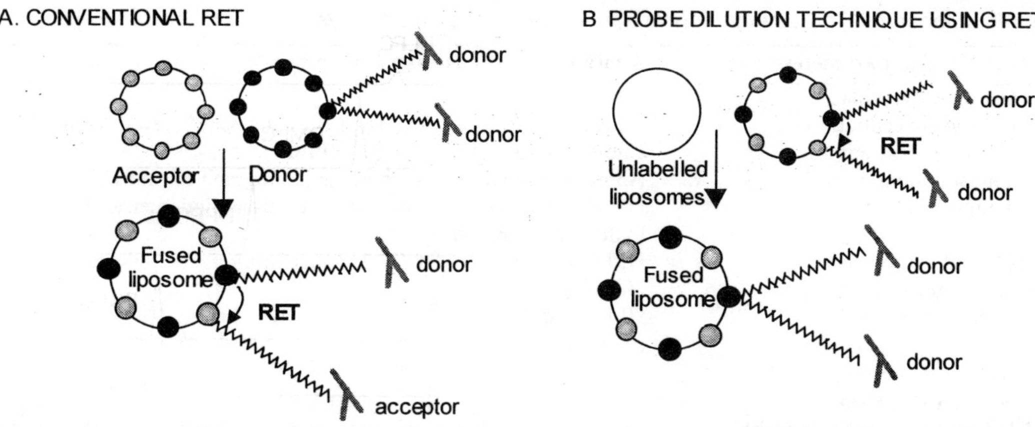

Fig. 5-22. Liposome Based Fusion Experiments, Where Acceptor and Donor Fluorophores are Used in Separate Liposome Population (A) and when Acceptor and Donor Fluorophores are Used in Same Liposome Population

Cromellin, 1994). These methods become more essential to characterize liposomes, which require lipid stability cropping up from oxidation, lipid peroxidation, hydrolysis and degradation in various environments used in their manufacturing.

Phospholipid concentration is determined in terms of lipid phosphorus content using Barlett assay/ Stewart assay (Barlett, 1959; Stewart, 1959) and thin layer chromatography (Terao et al., 1985); cholesterol concentration is determined using Cholesterol oxidase assay/Ferric perchlorate method (Wybenga et al., 1970) and GLC (Brooks et al., 1984); and drug concentration can be determined using appropriate methods given in the monograph. Lysolecithin, which is one of the major product of hydrolysis of lecithin (egg PC) is estimated using densitometry (New, 1989). However, phospholipid peroxidation is quantitatively determined using UV absorbance, TBA reagent (for endoperoxidase), iodometry (for hydroperoxidase) and GLC techniques (New, 1989). Phospholipid hydrolysis is determined using HPLC and TLC and cholesterol autooxidation can be assessed using HPLC and TLC (New, 1989). Various physical, chemical and related parameters and quality control assays are presented in Table 5-8.

STABILITY OF LIPOSOMES

The stability of any pharmaceutical product is the capability of the delivery system in the prescribed formulation to remain within defined or pre-established limits for a predetermined period of time (shelf life of the product). There is no established protocol for either accelerated or long-term stability studies for the liposomal formulations though many of them are now available in the market. However, the traditional guidelines that are generally observed for pharmaceutical dosage forms are followed while adopting the environmental conditions of the institutional set up. The stability studies could be broadly covered under two main sections (Grit et al., 1993; Grit and Crommelin, 1993; Zuidam and Crommelin, 1995; van Winden, et al., 1998). First, the stability *in vitro*, which covers the stability aspects prior to the administration of the formulation and with regard to the stability of the constitutive lipids. Second, the stability *in vivo*, which covers the stability aspects once the formulation, is administered via various routes to the biological fluids. These include stability aspects in blood (serum) if administered by systemic route or in gastrointestinal tract, if administered by oral or peroral routes.

Stability *In vitro*

Lipid vesicles (liposomes) are self-assemblages of amphiphiles into closed bilayer structures. Hydrated bilayer vesicles however, are not deemed to be thermodynamically stable and are thought to represent a metastable state in that the vesicles possess an

Table 5-8. Liposome Characterization with their Quality Control Assays

Characterization parameters	Analytical methods/Instrumentation
Chemical characterization	
Phospholipid concentration	Lipid phosphorus content using Barlett asssay/ Stewart assay, HPLC
Cholesterol concentration	Cholesterol oxidase assay and HPLC
Drug concentration	Appropriate methods given in the monograph for individual drug(s)
Phospholipid peroxidation	UV absorbance, TBA (for endoperoxidase), iodometric (for hydroperoxidase) and GLC
Phospholipid hydrolysis	HPLC and TLC and fatty acid concentration
Cholesterol auto-oxidation	HPLC and TLC
Anti-oxidant degradation	HPLC and TLC
pH	pH meter
Osmolarity	Osmometer
Physical characterization	
Vesicle shape and surface morphology	Transmission electron microscopy, freeze-fracture electron microscopy
Vesicle size and size distribution	
Submicron range	Dynamic light scattering, transmission electron microscopy, zetasizer
Micron range	Transmission electron microscopy, freeze-fracture electron microscopy, photon correlation spectroscopy, laser light scattering, gel permeation and gel exclusion
Surface charge	Free-flow electrophoresis
Electrical surface potential and surface pH	Zetapotential measurements and pH sensitive probes
Lamellarity	Small angle X-ray scattering, freeze-fracture electron microscopy, ^{31}P-NMR
Phase behaviour	Freeze-fracture electron microscopy, differential scanning calorimetry
Percent capture/Percent of free drug	Minicolumn centrifugation, gel exclusion, ion-exchange chromatography, protamine aggregation, radiolabelling
Drug release	Diffusion cell/ dialysis
Biological characterization	
Sterility	Aerobic or anaerobic cultures
Pyrogenicity	Rabbit fever response test or Limulus Amebocyte Lysate (LAL) test
Animal toxicity	Monitoring survival rates, histology and pathology

*Compiled from Lasic and Papahadjopoulos, 1998

excess of energy. Liposomal phospholipids can undergo chemical degradation such as oxidation and hydrolysis. Either as a result of these changes or otherwise, liposomes maintained in aqueous dispersion may aggregate/fuse and as a result may dump their contents.

Furthermore, method of formulation, nature of amphiphile and encapsulated drug/macromolecules, manipulate membrane fluidity/rigidity and permeability characteristics. The leakage of hydrophilic drugs from the aqueous domains of the liposomal bilayers upon storage is an area of considerable interest. The storage temperature of these dispersions must be strictly defined and controlled. A wide variability in the storage temperature of the system often leads to a change in the fundamental nature of the system. These vesicles are thus predicted to transform into bilayer stacks against the challenges of physicochemical and bio-environment stimuli.

Stability *in vitro* mainly covers the chemical stability of the constitutive lipids under the various accelerated or long-term storage conditions. Chemically, phospholipids are susceptible to hydrolysis. Additionally, phospholipids containing unsaturated fatty acids are vulnerable to oxidative degradation and peroxidation. Categorizing stability as physical or chemical is not sufficient, unless a detailed shelf life stability protocol is designed and conducted.

Lipid Oxidation and Peroxidation

Oxidative deterioration is a complex process involving free radical generation that results in the formation of cyclic peroxides and hydroxyperoxidase. Most of the procedures used to measure lipid peroxidation are non-specific, either based on the disappearance of unsaturated fatty acids (determined by lipid extraction techniques followed by GLC analysis) or the appearance of conjugated dienes. The latter technique is now well established as it is accompanied by increased UV absorption in the 230-260 nm range. However, the best way is to minimize either the use of unsaturated lipids, the use of argon or nitrogen environment to minimize the exposure to oxygen, use of anti-oxidants such as α-tocopherols or BHT or the use of light resistant containers for the storage of liposomal formulations.

Lipid Hydrolysis

The formation of lyso-phospholipid (lyso-lecithin) from phospholipid (lecithin) is a measure of the chemical instability of the lipid leading to the enhanced permeability of the liposomal contents. This results from the hydrolysis of the ester bond at the C-position of the glycerol moiety. Lyso-PC is usually analyzed by phospholipid extraction followed by separation of PC and lyso-PC by TLC.

To produce a system with an optimal stability, it is required that the predicted transformations be slowed down to such an extent as to produce a product with a reasonable shelf life. Methods to enhance the stability of liposomes abound in the literature (Fig. 5-23). The inclusion of a charged molecule in the bilayer shifts the electrophoretic mobility and makes it positive with the inclusion of stearylamine or negative with dicetyl phosphate, thus prevents liposomal fusion/swelling or aggregation.

Long Term and Accelerated Stability

Stability tests commonly stress the system to the limits, which the product generally encounters after it is released for the marketing and for patient use (Zuidam et al., 1996). Typical examples of stress tests include exposures of the product to high temperatures and large gravitational forces. High temperature testing (>25 °C) is almost universally used for heterogenous products. Various laboratories store their products at temperature ranging from 4 °C (refrigerator temperature) to 50 °C (or even higher in some cases). For liposomes, higher temperatures may dramatically alter the nature of the interfacial film, especially if the phase transition temperature is reached. If one expects the product to be exposed to a temperature of 45 °C for an extended period of time

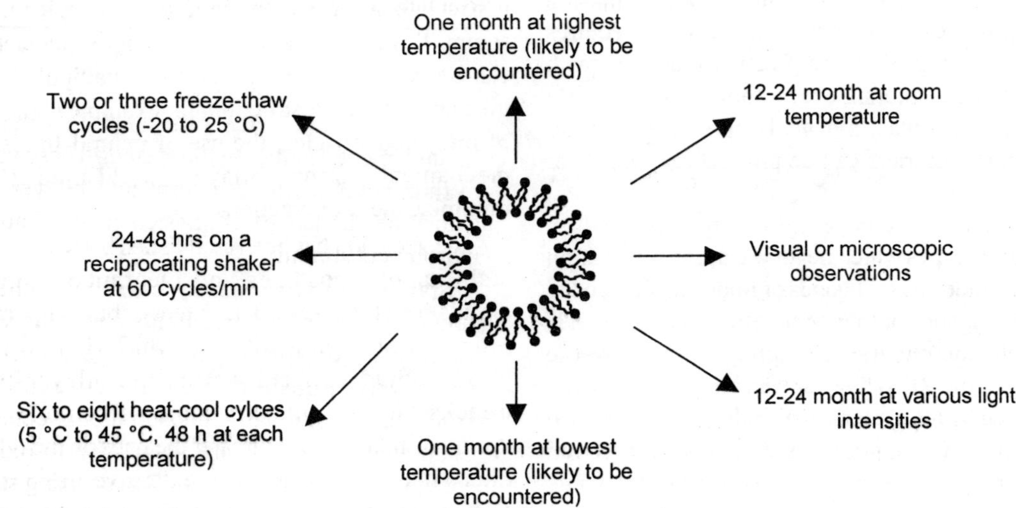

Fig. 5-23. Schemes Showing Different Stability Protocols that Assess Liposome Stability *In Vivo* and *In Vitro*.

or for short duration (shipping and warehousing storage), studies at 45-50 °C (long term and heat-cool cycling) are quite justified. If a liposomal dispersion is partially frozen and then thawed, ice crystals nucleate and grow at the expense of water. The liposomes may then be pressed together against the ice crystals under great pressure. If the crystals grow to a size greater than the void spaces, they lead to instability. As suggested by Weiner and associates (1989) stability testing protocols can be developed for liposomal formulations. The extreme storage and shipping and warehousing facilities should be documented on case by case basis.

Stability after Systemic Administration

A great deal has been written on the stability of liposomes after their intravenous administration (Gregoriadis and Senior, 1980; Weiner et al., 1989; van Winden et al., 1998). Following intravenous administration, the liposomes first confront with plasma/serum proteins before they come in contact with target cells. The two most frequently encountered biological events that the administered liposomal system undergoes are phagocytosis or antigen presentation via the macrophages of the reticulo-endothelial system. With this background, it is useful to understand various plasma/serum factors and components that affect the disposition and biofate of the liposomes *in vivo*. Most notably, the interaction of the liposomes with the phagocytes often requires these serum components for effective interaction with complement receptors, Fc receptors and sugar/lectin receptors on the macrophage, lymphocytes or other cells. Soluble carriers can be pinocytosed via Fc or lectin receptors.

A number of other receptors are expressed on different cell types which negotiate the transportation of various endogenous ligands or liposomes appended with these ligands or their synthetic bio-mimics. It is now well documented that phagocytosis by the elements of the RES (liver, spleen and bone marrow) is regulated by the presence and balance between two groups of serum components. One group of serum components promotes phagocytosis (opsonins), while the other group suppresses the process (dysopsonins) (Absolom, 1986). The former have been identified as proteinaceous components of the serum that adsorb onto the surface of liposomes (probably due to the surface hydro-phobicity) including liposomes and particulate systems, thereby making these exogenous material more 'palatable' and 'conducive' to phagocytes (Moghimi and Patel, 1989; Patel, 1992; Moghimi and Patel, 1998).

Among the host of opsonizing proteins that have been found to adsorb on the carrier composites are: complement components, blood coagulation factors, fibronectin, tuftsin, C-reactive proteins, serum amyloid P, serum albumin and immunoglobulins. These have also been shown to enhance recognition of various particulates by different macrophages. Dysopsonins, on the other hand, are thought to impart a high degree of hydrophilicity to the surface and this could explain their mechanistic role in RES-avoidance effects (Patel, 1992).

Immunoglobulin A (IgA) and secretory IgA (sIgA) are the best known dysopsonins. On the other hand, high density lipoprotein removes phospholipid molecules from the bilayered vesicular systems, leading to varying degree of vesicle disintegration and release of encapsulated solutes at rates dependent on the extent of bilayer damage.

The molecular origin of these interactions are mostly long range electrostatic, Vander Waals and short range hydrophobic interactions of colloidal/particulate surface with the macromolecules in the serum. The electrostatic and hydrophobic interactions can be minimized by the selective manipulation of the materials of construction, for example in the case of bilayered vesicles, the use of neutral lipids and mechanically strong bilayers could modify and minimize these interactions.

A correlation has been established between *in vivo* stability of liposomes and clearance from the circulation (Fig. 5-24). The extent of bilayer porosity is dependent on the ability with which HDL removes phospholipid molecules from the bilayer. HDL attacks "loose" bilayers more effectively than "packed" bilayers. The greater the gaps on the bilayer after HDL attack, the more extensive the opsonin adsorption occurs leading to their subsequent uptake by the reticuloendothelial system (Woodle and Lasic, 1992).

Stability *In Vivo* after Oral Administration

The stability of different liposomal constituents was tested under gastrointestinal conditions (Chiang and Weiner, 1987; Weiner and Chiang, 1989; Devissaguet et al., 1992):

- Low pH and pepsin for the gastric environment,
- Bile salts and lipases from the intestine

The protection of an entrapped drug from luminal degradation relies firstly on the physical integrity of the liposomes and secondly on the impermeability of the bilayers to the aggressive species of the gastro-intestinal fluids. However, in studies carried out in various laboratories, it was observed that liposomal entrapment may protect some labile drugs (like insulin) from luminal enzymatic or proteolytic activities, but only while the physical structure of the bilayered system is retained in harsh G.I. environment. In different studies however, no conclusive results could be drawn on the pharmacological or pharmacokinetic effectiveness of oral delivery of liposomes. Similarly, physical stability was found to be a function of the lipid composition, the number of bilayers and the surface charge However, they are always more or less sensitive to bile salts and lipases. Moreover, if liposomes escape destruction (as thought to be a rare event), the reports suggest that small proportion may be sequestered by digestive cells and contents are released intracellularly. Several studies are reported for the oral stability of liposomes (Table 5-9). Vyas and Katare reported oral administratin of stabilized versions of NSAID loaded proliposomes and the cell healing and cytoprotective nature of these liposomes (Katare and Vyas,1991). Two mechanisms were proposed: the classical mechanism of cell-cell interactions and the role of unsaturated fatty acids in the constitutive lipids as prostaglandin precursors, thus offering resultant cytoprotection. Similarly, the role of plain proliposomal systems for the cytorepairing and cytoprotection of NSAID induced GI ulceration sites was also documented.

INTERACTIONS OF LIPOSOMAL DRUG DELIVERY SYSTEMS WITH CELLS

Liposome mediated drug or gene delivery to selected tissues or cells is a highly promising approach for improving controlled or targeted delivery. An interaction of conventional liposomes with tissues at the cellular level is a highly complex phenomenon. The main interactions processes believed to operate independently or in a combination, are endocytosis, fusion, adsorption and lipid transfer (Fig. 5-25) (Juliano and Layton, 1980). With the advent of various specialized (ligand appended) liposomal versions, the role of coated or associated ligands in

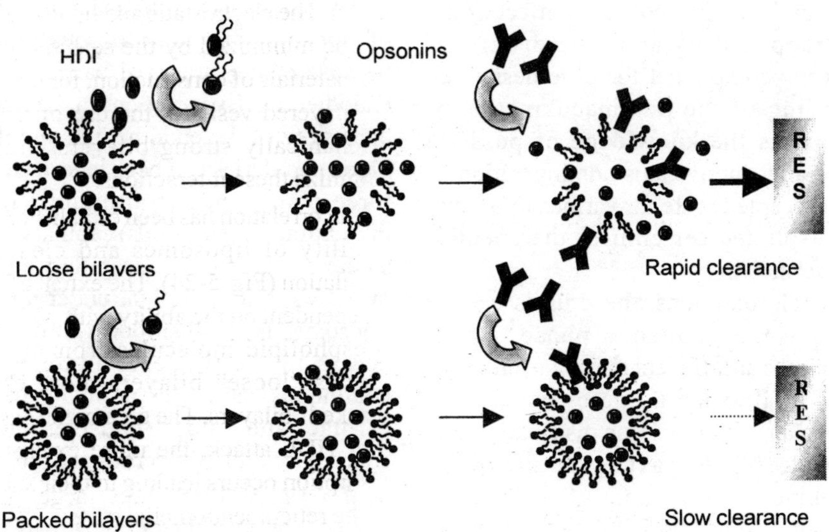

Fig. 5-24. Scheme Showing Role of Bilyer Configuration on *In Vivo* Stability of Liposomes

Table 5-9. Various Studies for Oral Stability of Liposomes

Liposomal version	Drug	Reference
Liposome entrapped NSAID	Indomethacin	Katare et al., 1991
Proliposomes NSAID	Indomethacin	Katare et al., 1991
Polymerized liposomes	Antigen	Chen et al., 1996
Lectin bearing polymerized liposomes	Antigen	Chen et al., 1996
Polysaccharide coated liposomes	Propranolol	Sihorkar and Vyas, 2000a
Sialic acid conjugated polysaccharide liposomes	Metronidazole	Sihorkar and Vyas, 2000b
Lectinized liposomes	Metronidazole	Vyas et al., 2001

triggering the cellular events like transcytosis, potocytosis and uptake through macropinosomes is now known (Vyas and Sihorkar, 2000; Vyas et al., 2001). Similarly, the intracellular microtubules and other vesicular motor proteins (kinesin, cytoplasmic dynein and myosin) and their decisive role in numerous membrane trafficking events including endocytosis and transcytosis, have revolutionized the approaches of liposome interactions with the target cells at the cellular or intracellular levels (Hamm-Alvarez, 1998).

LIPOSOMAL PHARMACOKINETICS

Liposome pharmacokinetics mainly deals with the time course of the absorption, distribution and degradation of the liposomal carriers *in vivo*. Pharmacokinetic information can be used to interpret the differences in the pharmacological effect of the liposome-entrapped drug and free drug, and subsequently can be exploited for dose designing. An understanding of the pharmacokinetics of liposomes requires the knowledge of possible accessible sites after intravenous administration as this is the most accepted route for various liposomal formulations exploited for clinical therapeutics except topical formulations.

Under optimal conditions, the drug is carried within the liposomal aqueous phase during circulation, but leaks at sufficient rate to become bio-available on arrival at the tissue or other sites. Liposomes can alter both the tissue distribution and the rate of clearance of a drug as they are affected by the pharmacokinetic parameters of the carrier. Bioavailability in case of liposomal carriers can be defined as the amount of free drug that is able to escape the confines of the carrier and thus becomes available for redistribution to neighbouring tissue. General outcome of liposomal delivery of drugs on biopharmaceutical and pharmacokinetic parameters are:

- Protection of drug from metabolism and inactivation in plasma
- Reduced volume of distribution and hence decrease in non-specific localization
- Higher therapeutic index
- Decrease in the amount and type of nonspecific toxicity
- Increase in concentration of drug at target site

Pharmacokinetics of Liposomes after Intravenous Administration

Based upon the size of liposomes that ranges from 190 Å to several microns in diameter, the accessibility of liposomes to some tissues may be restricted because of the structural barrier of capillaries and endothelium. By variations in the fine structures and continuity of the endothelium and its basal lamina, blood capillaries can be categorized (Fig. 5-26) into three main types: continuous, fenestrated and discontinuous (sinusoids) capillary beds. In different studies concerning transcapillary migration of SUVs or MLVs, it appears that under normal conditions, liposomes larger than 600Å in diameter have little access to the tissues containing primarily the continuous capillaries normally found in skeletal, cardiac, and smooth muscles, lung, skin, sub-cutaneous tissue, and serous and mucous membranes.

Similarly, liposomes larger than 0.5 μm in diameter are confined primarily to the intravascular space. As a result of intravascular confinement, most

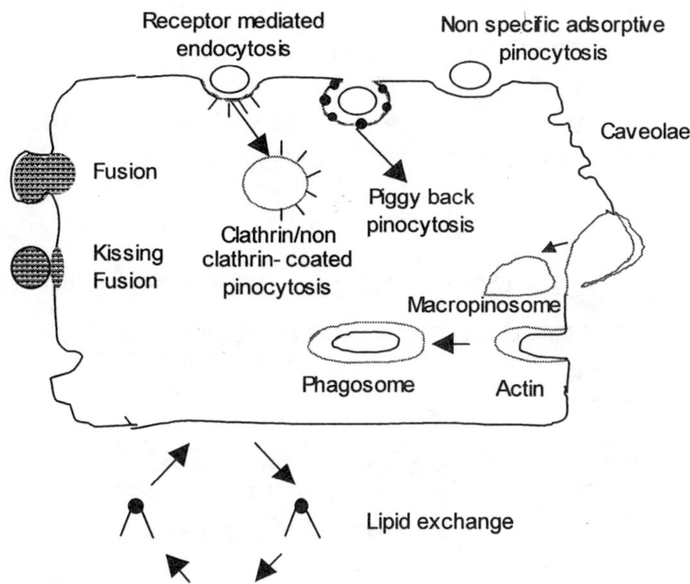

Fig. 5-25. Various Mechanisms of Liposomal Interaction with the Cell

of the studies have shown that the phagocytic cells in the blood and in the reticuloendothelial systems (RES), which are located primarily in liver, spleen, and bone marrow, are the major organs involved in the uptake of large liposomes (Abra and Hunt, 1981; Allen et al., 1989). Some, and usually a minor portion, ..ne large liposomes, reaches the extravascular space after being phagocytosed by blood macrophages (Hwang, 1987; Allen et al., 1995).

Many investigations have shown that after injecting an excess dose of liposomes into experimental animals, the blood levels of liposomes rise, and concomitantly, the extent of uptake of large liposomes by the liver and spleen is temporarily suppressed. This indicates that the uptake of large liposomes by tissues *in vivo* is primarily a saturable process (Allen et al., 1995; Allen and Stuart, 1999). The blood clearance kinetics of liposomes are compatible with a non-linear, saturable pathway of elimination. Mathematically, this can be described as a non-linear, capacity limited, Michaelis-Menten process:

$$V=\frac{V_{max}\,C}{K_m+C}+K'C \qquad (5\text{-}2)$$

Where, V is the rate of clearance or elimination of liposomes from the blood, V_{max} is the maximum velocity of elimination of liposomes from blood circulation by non-linear pathway, C is the concentration of liposomes in the blood. K_m is the Michaelis-Menten constant, which is equal to the concentration of liposomes in the blood at which the velocity of the elimination of liposomes from the blood is half-maximal. $K'_m C$ denotes a non-saturable process, such as clearance due to extravasation or uptake by liver hepatocytes. However, for large liposomes, the value of K'C is equivalent to zero. Similarly, the uptake of large liposomes by tissues may also be described by the sum of several such kinetic equations.

For small liposomes (less than 0.1μm in diameter), phagocytosis by RES and uptake by liver parenchymal cells are involved in their elimination from the blood (Hwang, 1987). Interestingly, two parallel pathways were found to operate in the pharmacokinetic distribution of small liposomes. One pathway is non-linear, capacity limited Michaelis-Menten process, the other pathway is a linear, non-saturable process that follows first order kinetics. It has been hypothesized that pinocytosis (fluid phase

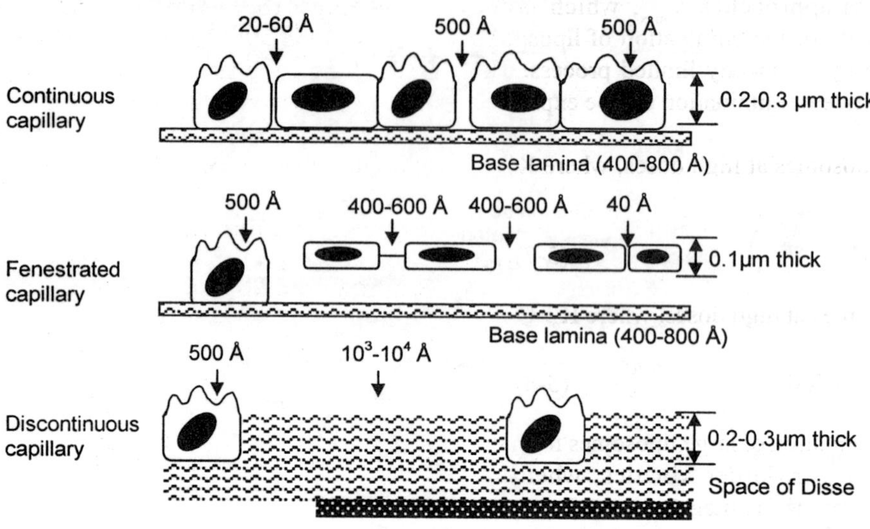

Fig. 5-26. Various States of Endothelial Membrane in Healthy (Continuous) and Tumorous (Discontinuous) Tissues

endocytosis) by the parenchymal cells of the liver represents the predominant non-saturable process in the hepatic uptake or the blood elimination of the small liposomes. On the other hand, the uptake of SUVs by phagocytic cells in the RES and blood occurs via a saturable pathway. Mathematically, this can be explained as follows:

$$V = V_1 + V_2 \qquad (5\text{-}3)$$

$$V = \frac{V_{max}\, C}{K_m + C} + K_2 C \qquad (5\text{-}4)$$

V is the rate of elimination from the blood or hepatic uptake of small liposomes, V_1 and V_2 are the rates of the elimination from the blood or hepatic uptake of small liposomes by the saturable and non-saturable processes, respectively. V_{max} is the maximum velocity of the elimination from blood or hepatic uptake of liposomes by non-linear pathway. K_m is the Michaelis-Menten constant. C is the concentration of liposomes in the blood. K_2 (replacing K' in the original equation) is the rate constant of the blood elimination or hepatic uptake of the liposomes by Classical pathway.

Effect of Dose on Pharmacokinetics

These equations can further be solved for the effect of liposomal dosage administered. One, if the injected dose and hence the concentration of liposomes in the blood is lower than Km, the pharmacokinetic equation can be written as follows:

For large liposomes at low dosage, where $K'_m = 0$, $K_m >> C$, the equation can be written as:

$$V = \frac{V_{max}\, C}{K_m} \qquad (5\text{-}5)$$

For small liposomes at low dosage, where $K_m >> C$

$$V = \frac{V_{max}\, C}{K_m} + K_2 C \qquad (5\text{-}6)$$

Therefore, at low dosage, the elimination of both the large and small liposomes from the blood follows the first order, linear kinetics as long as the condition of $C << K_m$ is met. This means that the time course of the concentration of large-sized liposomes in the blood should be linear on a semilogarithmic plot.

Second, if the concentration of liposomes in the blood is markedly higher than K_m, the Michaelis-

Menten process approaches V_{max}, which is the maximum velocity of the elimination of liposomes from the blood by a capacity limited process. The equation of the rate of elimination can be expressed as:

For large liposomes at high doses, where $K'_m = 0$, $C >> K_m$

$$V = V_{max} C \tag{5-7}$$

For small liposomes at high doses, where $K_2 > C$

$$V = V_{max} C + K_2 C \tag{5-8}$$

Thus the elimination of large liposomes from the blood follows a zero-order kinetics, when the requirement of $C >> K_m$ is met. On the other hand, the kinetic pattern of the elimination of small liposomes is dominated by first order kinetics when the blood concentration of liposomes is so high that V_{max} becomes insignificant relative to k_2C, i.e., $K_2C >> V_{max}$. When the injected dose of liposomes is neither too high nor too low, such that the concentration of liposomes in the blood is comparable with K_m, the blood clearance curve of liposomes is no longer linear on the semi-logarithmic plot prepared between concentration and time.

Pharmacokinetics of Release of Liposomal Contents in Tissues

Liposomal therapeutics is based upon the fraction of the drug that is released from the liposomes at any given time. This means that the extent of the release of a liposome-encapsulated drug at a target tissue determines the ultimate bioavailability of drug. Liver is the only organ that has been extensively and quantitatively analyzed using physiological models (Allen et al., 1995). The rate and extent of release of contents entrapped in liposomes in the liver can be estimated by kinetic analysis (Fig. 5-27). A_B and A_L denote the amount of intact liposomes, expressed as the percentage of administered dose in the blood and liver, respectively. The amount of degraded liposomes in the liver is denoted by D_L. K_1, k_{-1} and k_2 are the rate constants for intact liposomes to enter the liver from the blood, to re-enter to blood from the liver, and to enter other tissues from the blood, respectively. The rate constants for the degradation or elimination of intact liposomes in the blood and in the liver are denoted by k_3 and k_4 respectively. Based on the model, the rate equations for the three measurable variables namely the % of injected intact liposomes that remained in the blood and the liver and the % of the injected liposomes that were degraded in the liver can be estimated.

Pharmacokinetics of Long Circulatory Liposomes for Tumour Targeting/ Localization

Liposomes prevent the transport of large macromolecules and carriers across healthy endothelium and thus ensure a reduced toxicity (Working et al., 1994). However, discontinuous endothelium of the tumour vasculature results in an increased extravasation of large carriers (like liposomes) and in combination with an impaired lymphatics, an increased accumulation of liposomal drug at the tumour site. Pharmacokinetic parameters of the liposomes, such as size, surface charge, membrane lipid packing and steric stabilization, as well as the administered dose and route of administration govern and determine liposomal disposition kinetics. The pharmacokinetics of both conventional and sterically stabilized long circulatory liposomes have been extensively reviewed (Hwang, 1987; Allen et al.,

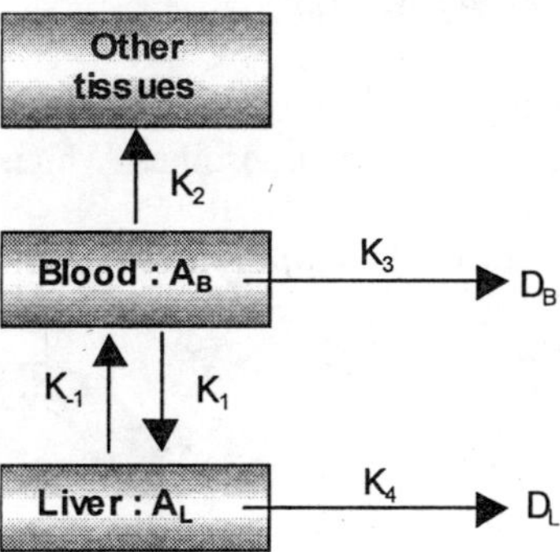

Fig. 5-27. Three-Compartment, Physiological Model for Fitting Kinetics of Uptake and Degradation of Liposomes in Liver

1995; Allen and Stuart, 1999).

Both slow release conventional liposomes and long circulatory (sterically stabilized) liposomes have a volume of distribution not significantly different from the total blood volume, indicating the drug is generally confined to the systemic circulation. However, after i.v. administration, conventional liposomes follow saturable, non-linear kinetics, whereas long circulatory liposomes follow non-saturable, non-linear kinetics (Allen et al., 1995).

The role of long circulatory properties and tissue uptake rates on the expected efficacy of a liposomal drug after i.v. bolus administration may be explored using a two compartment open pharmacokinetic model (Fig. 5-28).

The amount of liposomes in the blood compartment (A_b) and in the selected tissue, i.e., tumour (A_t) is defined by the following sets of equations and boundary conditions. These sets of linear differential equations with constant coefficients allow simple analytical solutions.

$$dA_t/dt = -(k_e+k_i)\, A_b + k_o A_t \quad (5\text{-}9)$$

$$dA_t/dt = k_i A_b - k_o A_t \quad (5\text{-}10)$$

$$A_b(0) = A_0;\ A_b(\infty) = 0 \quad (5\text{-}11)$$

$$A_t(0) = A_t(\infty) = 0 \quad (5\text{-}12)$$

Assuming that drug efficacy correlates with the tissue exposures to the liposomes, which, in turn, is characterized by AUC. AUC can be calculated for blood and tumour using following equations.

$$AUC_b = 1/Vb \int_0 A_b\, dt \quad (5\text{-}13)$$

$$AUC_t = 1/V_t \int_0 A_t dt \quad (5\text{-}14)$$

Where, V_b and V_t are physical volumes of the blood and tumour compartments, respectively. After integration of right and left parts of equations from zero to infinity and applying boundary conditions,

$$(k_e+k_i).\ V_b.AUC_b - k_0.V_t.\ AUC_t = A_0 \quad (5\text{-}15)$$

$$k_i.V_b.AUC_b - k_0.V_t.AUC_t = 0 \quad (5\text{-}16)$$

and finally,

$$AUC_t = A_0.\ k_i/(k_e.k_0.V_t) \quad (5\text{-}17)$$

$$T_e = (AUC_t)/(AUC_b) = (k_e.V_b)/(k_e.V_t) \quad (5\text{-}18)$$

In these equations, blood elimination first order rate constants k_e include all processes that lead to the removal of the carrier from the blood, including excretion, phagocytic clearance, and distribution into organs and tissues other than tumour. T_e termed as "tumour accumulation efficiency" does not include liposome longevity in the circulation (characterized by k_e) as a factor and is determined essentially by the liposome uptake rate into the tumour (Mayer et al., 1997; Mayer et al., 1998) .

On the contrary, tumour AUC correlates not only with the liposome uptake (uptake rate constant k_i)

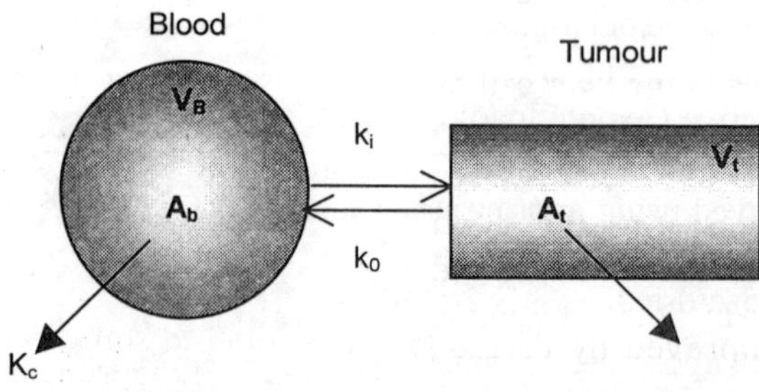

Fig. 5-28. Two Compartment-Open Model for Study of Rate and Extent of Accumulation of Long-Circulatory Liposomes in Tumors

but also with the liposome longevity in circulation (uptake rate constant k_i). Thus, within the framework of these models, circulation longevity of liposomes is not a factor in tumour accumulation efficiency, T_e, but rather is an important factor in the determination of overall tumour exposure to the drug carrier construct (Drummond et al., 1999).

COMMERCIAL DEVELOPMENT AND SCALE UP

Several liposome based products have been either approved or under the process of approval in the various parts of the world (Lasic, 1993; Janoff, 1993; van Winden et al., 1998). However, scaling up them as a conventional market product still remains to be successfully implicated. Problems generally encountered in the development of pharmaceutical liposomes are:

- Poor quality of the raw material mainly the phospholipids,
- Poor characterization of the physicochemical properties of the liposomes,
- 'Pay load' is too low,
- Shelf life is too short,
- Scale up related problems,
- Absence of any data on safety of these carrier systems on chronic use.

However, in recent years several pragmatic solutions are being worked upon to circumvent above-mentioned process related problems, which include:

- High quality products with improved purification protocols and validated analytical techniques are available.
- Quality control assay can be performed using sophisticated instruments and batch to batch variability can be checked.
- Payload problems can be sorted out using either lipophilic drug/lipophilic prodrug of hydrophilic drugs or using active (remote loading) techniques.
- Shelf life can be improved using appropriate cryoprotectant and lyoprotectant and product can be successfully freeze-dried.
- Scaling up can be improved by carefully selecting method of preparation (high shear homogenizer), sterilization by autoclaving or membrane filtration (0.2 μm) coupled with aseptic processing and pyrogen removal using properly validated LAL test.
- By choosing candidate potent drugs with narrow therapeutic window (e.g., cytotoxic drugs and fungicides) the drug related safety problems can be alleviated.

Freeze-drying and Cryoprotection/ Lyoprotection of Liposomal Products

The problems related to lipid oxidation and hydrolysis during shelf life of the liposomal product can be obviated by the storage of liposomal dispersion in the dry state. Freeze-drying (lyophilization) of liposomal dispersion may result in a cake with a large surface area, which can easily be reconstituted prior to patient use. The process consists of a freezing step and subsequent sublimation of the aqueous phase. However, liposomes can be damaged both by freezing and the drying process. In an aqueous liposomal dispersion, water interacts with the polar head-groups of the phospholipids by hydrogen bond formation. This, in combination with the hydrophobicity of the acyl chains, is an essential contribution for organization of these lipids in a bilayer. In addition, water may be considered as a spacer between the vesicles. Therefore, it is not surprising that removal of water affects the liposome integrity, resulting in changes in vesicle size and leakage of the encapsulated bioactives. Since both parameters are important for the therapeutic activity of a liposome formulation, some strategies have been adopted to avoid damage to the liposomal products during freeze- drying. Two processes commonly employed to achieve the above mentioned goals are cryo-protection (protection against damage by freezing) and lyoprotection (protection against damage by dehydration). However, there is a marginal line of difference in their functioning and their working mechanisms and hence these terms have been used interchangeably in the literature (Talsma et al., 1992; Crowe and Crowe, 1993; van Winden et al., 1998).

Cryoprotection

Freeze-drying (lyophilization) has great potential as a method to solve long-term (shelf) stability with respect to liposomes. For the long-term preservation of liposome, freeze-drying of liposomes has been studied and AmbiSome™ (Amphotericin B-containing liposomes) is available as a freeze-dried preparation (NeXstar Pharmaceuticals, Inc.). Saccharides (trehalose, maltose, maltriose, maltotetraose and glucose) have been effectively used as cryoprotectant for this purpose. They prevent aggregation and fusion upon reconstitution of the cake after lyophilization step. It is not always possible to avoid drug leakage from liposomes after a freeze drying-rehydration cycle, but recent insights into the mechanism of cryoprotection improve the chances for success. Two hypotheses have been proposed for the cryoprotection phenomena during lyophilization of liposomes. These are:

- Water replacement model
- Vitrification model

In the water replacement model, hydrated water molecules associated to the head group of lecithin are replaced by saccharide molecules, which protect them from aggregation and fusion. During the lyophilization process, water is removed from products in the frozen state at extremely low pressures. However, in the vitrification model, the glassy solid of saccharide surrounds liposome and the interaction between liposome surface and the glassy solid wall decreases the surface tension of liposome surface. In this way a spacer is provided between the vesicles which prevents fusion, and damaging crystallization processes of water or salts are also inhibited.

Lyoprotection

Lyoprotection is required to prevent damages that are caused during the drying and rehydration process. Damaging processes that may occur during drying from the frozen or unfrozen state until subsequent hydration include: fusion of the vesicles, loss of bilayer structures, phase separation and bilayer damage due to osmotic forces during rehydration. Currently used lyoprotectants are disaccharides, which also provide protection for the liposomes against freezing and thawing stresses. Lyoprotectants may exert their action by one or more of the following mechanisms:

- Water substitution
- Glass formation

The disaccharide molecules may interact with the phospholipid head groups (hydrogen bonding between the hydroxyl group of sugars and phosphate group of the phospholipids) in the dry state and thus replace the aqueous phase (water). The mechanism of glass formation signifies the formation of an amorphous matrix between the vesicles, which prevents fusion and bilayer damage due to crystal formation. In conclusion, using proper conditions, freeze-drying of a wide-range of liposomes loaded with hydrophobic, bilayer interacting drugs seems to be feasible. However, for successful freeze-drying of liposomes loaded with hydrophilic, non-bilayer interacting drugs, some constraints are defined which remain unresolved even in presence of lyoprotectants and cryoprotectants.

Commercial Manufacturing of Liposomal Drugs

After many encouraging preclinical data and safety studies the liposomal formulations entered in the clinical trial stages. In parallel the manufacturing process is scaled up and all the quality controls and analysis are defined and standardized (Fildes, 1981, Martin, 1990; Amselem et al., 1990; Sorgi and Huang, 1996; Lasic, 1998). In a typical large-scale method, production lipids are mixed and dissolved in officially approved organic solvent, i.e., chloroform, methylene chloride, methanol tertiary butanol and some other solvents. These solvents can be removed either by evaporation, vacuum drying or lyophilization (in case of t-butanol).

The dry lipid film, paste or cake is then hydrated. Alternatively, one can inject an ethanol or propylene glycol lipid solution into the aqueous phase and remove the solvent by chromatography, filtration or dialysis. Upon hydration of lipids, large multilamellar vesicles are formed. The size of the prepared vesicles is reduced by extrusion, homogenization or sonication. This is a critical step in the evaluation of the prepared liposomal formulation and their upscaling feasibility (Table 5-10). Hydrophilic drugs are normally added in the hydrating medium, while hydrophobic ones are co-dissolved in the organic phase. In the case of weak acids and bases, these molecules can be loaded in to preformed liposomes by pH or ammonium sulphate gradient technique. Free (non-encapsulated) drug can be removed either by dialysis, chromatography, filtration or

Table 5-10. Sizing Methods in Industrial Liposome Production and their Upscaling Feasibility

Method	Instruments	Upscaling feasibility	Disadvantages
Ultrasonic irradiation gives mainly SUV (~20 nm)	Sonicators: Bath or probe	Poor	Fractionation and homogeneity is required
High pressure extrusion (above 35 Mpa, ca. 5000 psi) gives unilamellar vesicles	French pressure cell; Micro-fluidizer; High-pressure homogenizer	Good to very good	Limited to vesicles ~100 nm
Low- or medium pressure extrusion (up to 14 Mpa, ca. 2000 psi) through pores of definite size	Polycarbonate membrane, Ceramic filters; Stainless steal filters	Very good	Complex process

centrifugation. For drug delivery, liposomes can be formulated as a suspension, as an aerosol or in a semisolid form such as a gel, cream or lotion, as a dry vesicular powder (proliposomes) for reconstitution or they can be administered orally, topically or parenterally.

In the case of Doxil™ constitutive lipids are mixed and dissolved in a FDA and safety committee approved organic solvent, which is injected into an aqueous solution of ammonium sulphate. Upon hydration the organic solvent is diafiltered away and large multilamellar vesicles are sized down, preferably by an extrusion technique. After the exchange of the external solution empty liposomes are loaded with doxorubicin which is added as a concentrated solution in the system. Loading is so high that free drug removal is not necessary. Some buffers may be added and the product is then purified, sterile filtered, filled into vials, sealed and labeled. Figure 5-29 schematically presents the manufacturing process and scaling up of liposomal doxorubicin (Doxil™) as an example.

THERAPEUTIC APPLICATIONS OF LIPOSOMES

Liposomes are used for the following range of therapeutic and pharmaceutical applications (Table 5-11):

1. Liposomes as drug/protein delivery vehicles
   - Controlled and sustained drug release *in situ*.
   - Enhanced drug solubilization
   - Altered pharmacokinetics and biodistribution
   - Enzyme replacement therapy and lysosomal storage disorders
2. Liposomes in antimicrobial, antifungal (lung therapeutics) and antiviral (anti-HIV) therapy
   - Liposomal drugs
   - Liposomal biological response modifiers
3. Liposomes in tumour therapy
   - Carrier of small cytotoxic molecules
   - Vehicle for macromolecules as cytokines or genes
4. Liposomes in gene delivery
   - Gene and antisense therapy
   - Genetic (DNA) vaccination
5. Liposomes in immunology
   - Immunoadjuvant
   - Immunomodulator
   - Immunodiagnosis
6. Liposomes as artificial blood surrogates
7. Liposomes as radiopharmaceutical and radiodiagnostic carriers
8. Liposomes in cosmetics and dermatology
9. Liposomes in enzyme immobilization and bioreactor technology

Liposomes as Drug Delivery Vehicles

Several modes of drug delivery applications have been proposed for the liposomal systems for some of the opportunistic pathogen caused diseases (Table 5-12). The major ones are enhanced drug solubilization (amphotericin B, minoxidil, paclitaxel, cyclosporin), protection of sensitive drug molecules (cytosine arabinose, DNA, RNA, antisense oligonucleotides, ribozymes), enhanced intracellular uptake (anticancer, antiviral and antimicrobial drugs), altered pharmacokinetics and biodistribution

Table 5-11. Potential Biomedical Applications of Liposomes with Predicted or Investigated Studies

Liposome associated drug/gene/macromolecule	Route	Application	Desired attributes
Plasmid DNA, Antisense oligonucleotides	i v, i a, i m, i t, topical and oral	Gene and antisense therapy	High yield DNA incorporation, Fusogenic (cationic, virosome, pH sensitive), targeted
Haemoglobin (Hb), synthetic oxygen transporters	i v	Blood surrogates	High yield Hb entrapment, stability, long circulating
Endogenous cytokines (IL, IFN, TNF, GM-CSF) Exogenous products (lipo-polysaccharide, lipid A trehalose, muramyl-dipeptide)	i v, i m, s c, i t	Immuno-modulation	High yield incorporation, stability, controlled clearance rates, targeted
Antigens and allergen extracts	i m, s c, oral	Desensitization	High yield allergen entrapment, stability
Anticancer and antimicrobial drugs	i t	Site specific lung therapeutics	Stability as aerosols, localized targeting within the respiratory tract

Table 5-12. Liposomal Drug Delivery Against Opportunistic Infections

Fungal	Protozoan	Viral	Bacterial
Histoplasmosis (Amphotericin B) Cryptococcoses (Amphotericin B)	Leishmaniasis (Antimonials, Amphotericin B) Malaria (Chloroquine) Toxoplasmosis	Herpes simplex virus (HSV) (Acyclovir) AIDS (Azathioprene)	Tuberculosis, Leprosy (Rifampicin) Salmonellosis (Gentamycin) Brucellosis

(prolonged or sustained release of drugs with short circulatory half-lives). Various advantages are cited for adopting liposomes as versatile delivery systems and include:

- The delivery of liposomes could be beneficial for drugs that are rapidly excreted or metabolized.
- An undesirable "saw-tooth" pattern of circulating drug levels observed in conventional dosage forms can be avoided.
- Like other colloidal carrier systems liposomes can provide relatively constant and sustained bloodstream levels of certain types of drugs.
- In contrast to sustained release formulations based on artificial polymers, liposomes can be injected into the circulation, and thus can serve as an "intravascular drug depot".
- The use of liposomal sustained release preparations may be of significant value for drugs with low "therapeutic windows" or low water solubility or which require administration by intravenous route.
- Passive macrophage targeting and RES-accumulation can be achieved for the treatment of ailments caused due to intracellular pathogens using conventional liposomes (Fig. 5-30).
- Surface engineered versions of liposomes circumvent passive uptake by RES-predominant organs and increase in circulation time and hence provide a better sustained action than conventional liposomes (active targeting) (Fig. 5-30).

Increased Therapeutic index

The delivery aspect of liposomes could also be exploited for drugs , which are required to penetrate the plasma membrane in order to be therapeutically beneficial. The use of liposomal carrier system offers a way of surpassing the membrane barriers (as they structurally mimic natural membrane) and of promoting the non-specific entry of drugs in to the cellular interiors. For example, in the case of anti-

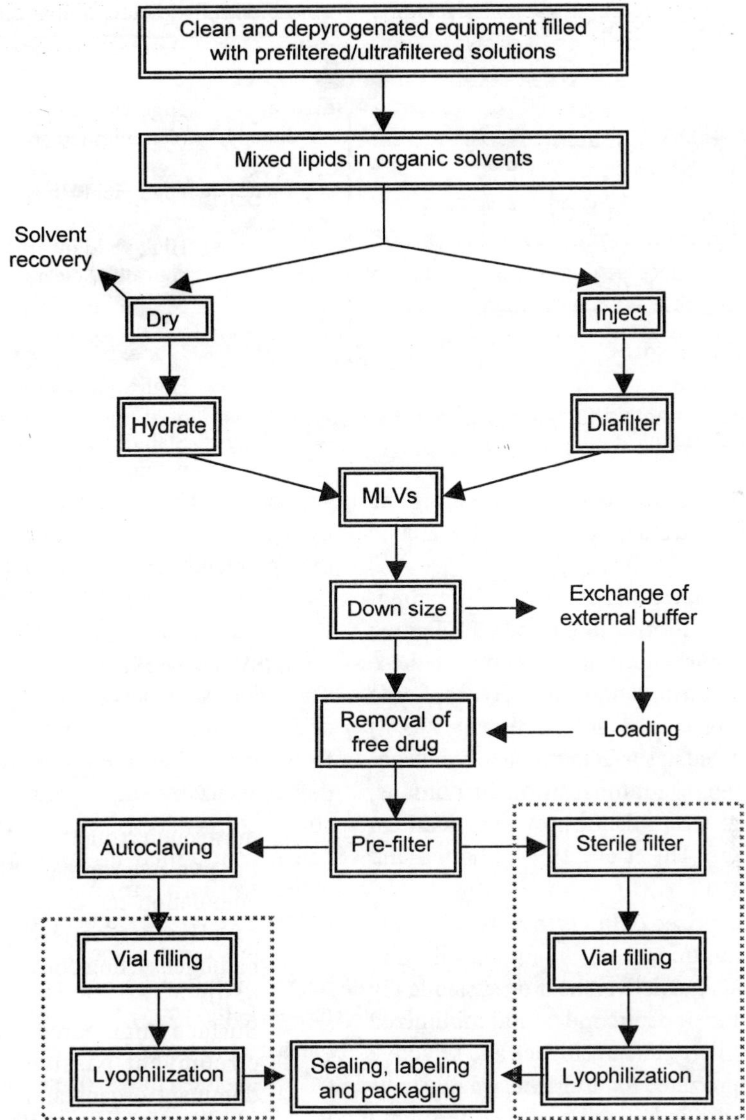

Fig. 5-29. Various Steps for the Commercial Manufacturing of Liposomes (Doxil^{TM}). Steps Indicated in the Box with Discontinuous Lines should be Performed under the Aseptic Conditions (Adopted with modifications from Lasic, 1998)

tumour drugs, i.e. cytosine arabinoside tri-phosphate (ara-CTP), the tumour cell population often acquires resistance by reducing the level of deoxycytidine kinase, the first enzyme in the pathway that activate the drug. The drug administered in the liposomal form alleviate the problem of reduced enzyme level (Rubas et al., 1986). Similar results were observed with actinomycin-D, where increased levels of drug permeation were recorded after being delivered in the liposomal form (Juliano and Layton, 1980). In fact, liposome encapsulation hinders the active transport or passive diffusion (general course of drug uptake of the cells). However, in cases of genetically determined resistance as in tumour cells, the

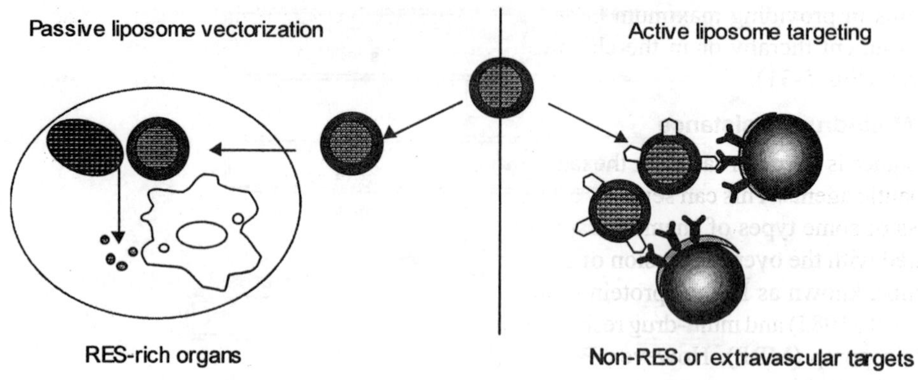

Fig. 5-30. Passive and Active Targeting Approaches Using Conventional and Ligand-Anchored Liposomes

liposomes are of immense value in overcoming the permeability barrier and thus negotiate the therapeutic effects.

Another field that utilizes use of liposomal delivery system is the formulation of better tolerated pre-clinical and clinical formulations, where these carriers serve as a formulation aid. Hydrophobic drugs such as cyclosporin A and paclitaxel (Taxol) are usually formulated in surfactants and organic co-solvents for systemic administration in humans, however, liposomal encapsulation provides maximum therapeutic benefits (Hu et al., 1994; Sharma and Straubinger, 1994).

Liposomes comprised of lipids that are relatively non-toxic, non-immunogenic, biocompatible and biodegradable lipids can deliver the drug systemically with an increased therapeutic index and minimized toxicity index. Similarly, site avoidance and selective delivery can be appreciated for drugs that usually have a narrow therapeutic index and that can be highly toxic to normal tissues. Liposome formulation may improve the therapeutic index by altering the biodistribution of drug away from drug sensitive normal tissues as in the case with drugs with dose-dependent pharmacokinetics.

Liposomes as a Lysosomotropic Carrier

There are many proposed therapeutic applications of liposomal delivery of bioactives and include enzyme replacement therapy of inherited metabolic disorders, hormone replacement therapy and detoxification of tissues that contain intracellularly deposited metals. Liposomes have been used as "lysosomotropic carriers" to *en route* the enzyme and supplement it therapeutically in enzyme deficiency diseases like Gaucher's disease (β-glucoisdase deficiency) or Pompe's disease (α-glucosidase deficiency) (Gregoriadis, 1984; Gordon and Rabinowitz, 1989). These diseases result from the genetically determined deficits of particular lysosomal hydrolytic enzymes. In order to affect the correction of the disease the deficient enzymes must be delivered to the lysosomal compartment of cells. A variety of lysosomal enzymes can be entrapped in liposomes and delivered to patients suffering from lysosomal storage disorders. Liposomes have also been used in the treatment of metal poisoning, since the liver is the major site of heavy metal and iron accumulation (Behari and Gregoriadis, 1992). The use of liposomal EDTA was measured to be far more effective than free drug in enhancing the removal of excess metal and promoting its secretion. The use of liposome-encapsulated desferrioxamine, an iron chelator, in the treatment of chronic haemosiderosis has also been documented (Juliano and layton, 1980). In recent years liposomes as a delivery systems have been used to administer a plethora of bioactives including drugs like genes, antisense oligonucleotides, antigens or haptens, proteins, macromolecules, dyes, metals, and radio-pharmaceuticals.The specific therapeutic applications are dealt in different sections of this chapter. Liposomes can also be used for micro-compartment-alization of catalysts including metallic catalysts and enzymes for permselectivity of action. This immobilization helps in providing maximum benefits in enzyme replacement therapy or in the chemical analysis processes (Fig. 5-31).

Liposomes in Multi-drug Resistance

Multi-drug resistance is the main cause for the failure of chemotherapeutic agents. This can severely affect the effectiveness of some types of chemotherapy. It is often associated with the over-expression of some drug efflux pumps, known as P-glycoprotein pump (PGP) (Kartner et al., 1985) and multi-drug resistance associated protein pump (MRP). However, PGP is the best-characterized efflux pump responsible for multi-drug resistance. PGP is a cell membrane glycoprotein of 170 kDa molecular weight and is a membrane spanning ATPase located in the plasma membrane. This multi-drug resistance transporter could act as an efflux pump and reject positively charged amphipathic drugs (mostly anticancer drugs) from the cells as shown for bacterial transport proteins.

Over-expression of P-glycoprotein in tumour cells can lead to a marked decrease in sensitivity to drugs. Thus multi-drug resistance is associated with a resultant low intracellular accumulation of these drugs. This is more pronounced with drugs which appear to enter the cell by passive diffusion through the lipid bilayer, for example, doxorubicin (an anticancer drug) (Endicott and Ling, 1989). Upon entering the cell, these drugs bind to P-glycoprotein, which forms transmembrane channels and uses the energy of ATP hydrolysis to pump these compounds out of the cell.

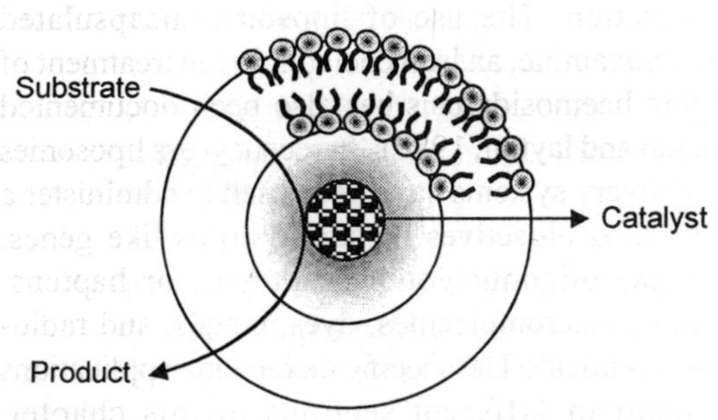

Fig. 5-31. Role of Liposomes for Immobilization and Micro-Compartmentalization of Catalysts

Various delivery systems including liposomes loaded drugs have resulted in the effective chemotherapy of a number of refractory cancers both in animal and clinical models results are well documented with anticancer drugs such as doxo-rubicin (Vaage et al., 1994; Muggia et al., 1997). Several mechanisms are proposed through which liposomes avoid multi-drug resistance of encapsu-lated drugs:

- Negatively charged phospholipids (phosphatidylserine or cardiolipin) used in the liposomal formulations may directly regulate the P-glycoprotein transporter.
- Liposomes may provide sustained and high levels of drug to resistant cells over long period of time.
- In combination with the above mechanisms, after endocytosis of drug loaded liposomes, the lysosomal localization of the drug protects it from the action of the P-glycoprotein, by avoiding immediate contact with P-glycoprotein transporter located at plasma membrane. (Fig. 5-32).
- Along with cell sensitization, liposomal drug delivery may help overcome a broader range of drug resistance due to favourable pharmacokinetics.

Though the stated mechanism(s) could circumvent the multidrug resistance problem to a considerable level yet the complete reversal of multi-drug resistance is difficult. Thus, to more effectively treat patients resistant to a particular type of chemotherapy, it is important to combine liposome encapsulated drug with other presently used chemotherapeutic agents or to develop additional liposomal chemotherapeutic agents with non-overlapping mechanisms of drug resistance.

Liposomes in Antimicrobial, Antifungal (Lung Therapeutics) and Anti-viral (Anti-HIV) Therapy

Intracellular pathogens (protozoal, bacterial and fungal) harbour in the liver and spleen and thus therapeutic moieties can be targeted to these organs using liposomes as a carrier system. Due to their intrinsic passive vectorization to RES-predominant organs, liposomes offer enormous potentials and

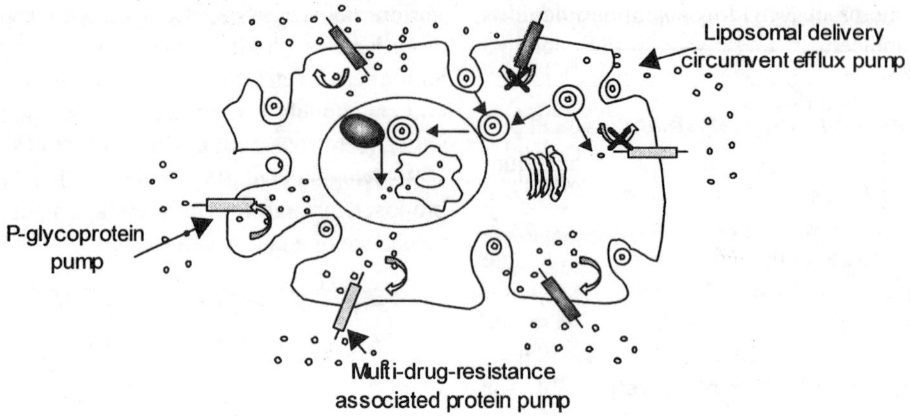

Fig. 5-32. Schematic Diagram of Supposed Trafficking Into Multi-Drug Resistant Cell of Free Drug and of Drug Associated With Liposomes

opportunities for targeted drug delivery to intracellular pathogens like leishmaniasis, candidiasis, aspergillosis, histoplasmosis, cryptococosis, girardiasis, malaria, and tuberculosis. Liposome mediated treatment of fungal, viral, bacterial and protozoal infections takes the advantage of the natural targeting of liposomes to the RES-predominant organs and their "lysosomotropism" as well as "parasitotropism" (Vyas, 2001) (Table 5-13).

Leishmaniasis infections in human are manifested in three forms: visceral leishmaniasis (Kala-azar caused by *L. donovani*), mucocutaneous leishmaniasis (*L. mexicana*) and cutaneous leishmaniasis (*L. tropica*). The drugs of first choice are the pentavalent antimonials, meglumine antimonate and sodium stilbogluconate and the second choice drug, amphotericin B, is dose-compromised because of hepatic, gastrointestinal, cardiac and renal toxicities. However, on administration of liposomal form of these drugs exceptional hepatosplenic accumulation of encapsulated drug was observed with minimal toxic side effects (Alving, 1982; Bakker-Wounderberg, 1994). Similarly, the existence of malaria parasite in the hepatocytes and possibly the Kupffer cells in its tissue stage, resulted in investigations on use of the liposomes in the treatment of malaria. The uptake of liposome-entrapped primaquine was shown to occur initially in the Kupffer cells as expected with subsequent intrahepatic redistribution of liposomal contents to hepatocytes.

The lysomotropic optional of liposomes also makes them a suitable carrier to target facultative intracellular bacteria (*Brucella, Listeria, Mycobacteria, Legionella, Salmonella, Klebsiella, Escherichia* sp.) with loaded antibiotics (Vyas, 2001). Fusion of liposomes and cell after their uptake by RES-predominant organs, sustained release of the antibiotic, protection of drug from *in vivo* enzymatic hydrolysis, and increased local concentration of drug. These are some probable mechanisms, which contribute to their better therapeutic effects. The potential for liposomal delivery in bacterial infections at sites other than RES organs is quite vogue (except where lipid-based delivery systems reduce the toxicity of the drug and provide a sustained release of the loaded antimicrobial agent). However, in recent years these problems have also been curtailed to a considerable extent with the use of ligand mediated liposomal targeting (active targeting) and inverse targeting approaches. These strategies either exploit any recognition port located on the target cell, where liposomes anchored through suitable site-directing ligands are destined to the target sites (active targeting), or provide them a long-circulatory or stealth behaviour, which permits targeting to sites other than RES (inverse targeting). Liposomes anchored with glycolipids having terminal galactose residues (Bacchawat et al., 1984) and liposomes constructed of mannosylated phospholipids (Barrat et al., 1986) (to be recognized by receptors present

Table 5-13. Applications of Passive and Active Targeting Approaches to Macrophages using Liposomes

Bioactive(s)	Applications
Passive targeting approaches	
Amphotericin B	Candidiasis, Leishmaniasis, Experimental cryptococcal meningitis, Cryptococcosis, Murine Histoplasmosis
MTPPE/ IFN-γ	Macrophage activation for protection against *Klebesiella pneumoniae*
MTP-PE	Macrophage activation for tumoricidal properties against spontaneous metastases
Dichloromethylene diphosphonate	Macrophage depletion
Praziquantel	Macrophage activation
Sparfloaxacin	*M. avium, M. intracellularlae* complex infection in mice
Gentamycin	*Staphylococcal pneumoniae*
Active targeting approaches	
Pentamidine	Leishmaniasis
Antisense oligonucleotide	Leishmaniasis
Aanamycin	Leishmaniasis
Idoxuridine/ acyclovir	Herpes simplex virus
Asiaticoside	Tuberculosis and leprosy
Rifampicin	Tuberculosis

*Adapted from Vyas, 2001

on Kupffer cells of the liver) were appreciated and documented for active targeting of the entrapped contents to the target site. However, the most important and commercially successful feature of therapeutics is their effectiveness as a carrier for antifungal agents for the treatment of systemic fungal diseases mainly candidiasis.

Amphotericin B Liposomes

Systemic fungal infections are associated with increasing frequency in the immuno-compromised patient. Although, restricted by a variety of side and toxic effects, parenteral amphotericin B (Amp B) is still the drug of choice in most invasive fungal infections. Recent advances has focused on the improvement of its therapeutic index, through reduction of Amp B toxicity by its incorporation in lipid carriers (Hiemenz and Walsh, 1996; Wasan and Lopez-Berestein, 1998). Several lipid formulations of Amp B are in the market (Table 5-14) and include Fungizone® (Bristol Myers-Squibb, Woerden, The Netherlands), AmBisome™ (Nexstar, Boulder, CO, USA), ABELECT™ (The Liposome Company, Princeton, NJ, USA) and AMPHOTEC™ (Sequus Pharmaceuticals, Merlo, CA, USA).

Amphotericin B manifests serious adverse complications related to dose dependent acute and chronic toxicity. For diseases of microbial aetiology, the intracellular localization of the pathogens necessitates the administration of relatively high doses of the cytotoxic drugs for the effective killing of the pathogens, thereby causing the side effects. The rationale approach to the problem requires that drugs should be targeted to the macrophages in such a way that the interaction of the free drug with non-target tissues could be minimized. Maximum tolerated dose of Amp B is considerably low in mice; LD_{50} is 1.2 mg/kg and doses higher than 1.6 mg/kg cause acute toxic reactions followed by cardiac-respiratory arrest (Lopez-Berestein et al., 1983). Treatment of disseminated fungal infections by liposomal Amp B results in a lower toxicity and significantly increased survival times. It has been proposed that increased concentrations of drug in macrophages through passive liposomal uptake improves its therapeutic index. Toxicological comparison of free and liposomally formulated Amp B in mice has revealed that maximum tolerated dose has been significantly increased. The LD_{50} has been found to increase from 1.2 mg/kg to more than 12 mg/kg in the case of mice. Liposomal formulations of Amp B could considerably reduce the toxicity of the drug and subsequently make it possible to enhance the therapeutic index. The marketed liposomal formulations, AmBisome™ (Nexstar, Boulder, CO,

Table 5-14. Various Liposomal Formulations of Amphotericin B either Approved or under Various Trials

System	Drug	Target disease	Status	Product
Liposomes (AmBisome) (Intravenous)	Amphotericin B	Systemic fungal infections, Visceral leishmaniasis	Approved in 18 countries including Europe and USA	NeXstar, USA
Liposomes (Amphocil) (Intravenous)	Amphotericin B	Systemic fungal infections	Approved in UK, Russia, Finland, Ireland and Europe	SEQUUS, USA
Liposomes (ABLC) (Intravenous)	Amphotericin B	Systemic fungal infections	Approved in UK	The Liposome Company, USA

USA), similar to other marketed lipid formulations of Amp B like Fungizone® (Amp B-desoxycholate complex), ABELECT™ (Amp B-lipid complex) and AMPHOTEC™ (Amp B colloidal dispersion) preferentially accumulate in the liver and spleen of animals (Hiemenz and Walsh, 1996). However, the rate of uptake of AmBisome by the reticuloendothelial system appears to be much slower than by ABELECT or AMPHOTEC. It is hypothesized that the larger lipid complexes and dispersions may be readily phagocytosed by the macrophages of the reticuloendothelial system than the small unilamellar vesicles of AmBisome (Hiemenz and Wlash, 1996). However, this may account for the higher peak plasma levels and prolonged circulation times compared with its larger counterparts. This creates a discrepancy that whether the chemotherapeutic effect of Amp B is due to the localization of the drug inside the intracellular pathogen infected macrophages or to the slow and sustained release of free Amp B in the circulation and tissues.

Recently, Vyas and co-workers, 2000 reported the role of anionic ligands and their subsequent receptor mediated uptake by coating Amphotericin B loaded liposomes with O-palmitoylated mannan (OPM) and p-aminophenyl-mannopyranoside (PAM) as specific ligand modules. Comparative *in vivo* distributions and targeting profiles of O-palmitoylated mannan and P-aminophenyl-mannopyranoside anchored liposomes as compared to plain liposomes were studied in terms of % drug localization indices. The extent of accumulation of plain and ligand anchored liposomal Amphotericin B in macrophage rich organs, especially liver, spleen and lungs was significantly higher than equivalent free drug administration. The rates and extents of accumulation were higher on ligand anchoring. In either of the cases, the macrophage uptake of ligand anchored liposomes was inhibited significantly on pre-injection of hydrolysed mannan, suggestive of receptor mediated uptake of ligand anchored liposomes. The comparison of bio-distri-bution patterns of ligand anchored MLVs revealed that PAM linked liposomes are subjected to higher hepatosplenic extraction leading to sebsequent accumulation. The drug accumulation in lungs was maximum in the case of OPM anchored liposomes. Thus, mannopyranoside is a specific ligand for targeting bioactives to the macrophages of liver and spleen while OPM could preferentially negotiate selective uptake of bioactives by alveolar macrophages.

Liposomes in Tumour Therapy

Most of the medical applications of liposomes that have reached the pre-clinical and clinical stages are in cancer treatments. Several clinical studies did not support the use of conventional liposomes in cancer treatment. It is however not clear whether such liposomes (especially the ones remote loaded with anthracyclines) can be beneficial in cancer therapy. It has been demonstrated that small and stable liposomes can passively target several different tumours because they can (owing to their biological stability) circulate for prolonged times and extravasate (owing to their small size, 50-150 nm) in tissues with enhanced vascular permeability, which is often the case with tumours (Gregoriadis et al., 1971; Gabijon and Papahadjopoulos, 1988). However, recent trends in research often frequently opt for the specially engineered long-circulatory liposomes (Stealth liposomes) for long circulation times and increased probability, so that they can extravasate to the tumour vascular endothelium (Woodle and Lasic, 1992; Allen, 1994; Gabizon et al., 1997). Targeting strategies using liposomes can be designed in three different ways:

- Natural targeting (lysosomotropism) of conventional liposomes (passive vectorization).
- Use of long-circulatory (stealth liposomes).
- Use of ligand mediated targeting (active targeting).
- The use of anti-receptor antibodies or antibodies developed against specific surface antigens on the tumour vascular endothelium;
- The use of angiogenic peptides and adhesion molecules as ligands against receptors expressed on tumour vascular endothelium.
- Use of stealth liposomes and ligand mediated targeting in combination.

Sterically Stabilized (Stealth) Liposomes (SSL)

The old dream of site specific drug targeting requires properly designed and intelligent delivery systems that avoid scavenging through receptor mediated uptake by mononuclear phagocytic cells of RES-rich organs. Moreover, several targeting strategies require the system to be placed either into tumour cells or their extravasation into non-RES cellular lineage. As a matter of fact, recently described approaches to avoid RES-uptake of the drug-carrier composites, lead to the concept of ligand-appended system long circulatory in nature (stealth systems), which resist opsonization and serum protein binding to their surface. Sterically stabilized liposomes thus avoid their recognition from RES uptake and this "stealthing" effect makes them long circulatory in nature.

Sialic Acid Conjugated Liposomes

Sialic acid and glyco-conjugates were anchored on liposome surface to provide them with long circulatory behaviour. Sialic acid has been thought to play a key role in prolonging the circulation time of serum proteins (Morell et al., 1968). Since then sialic acid residues on the liposomal surface have been incorporated and appreciated for their biodistribution and cell recognizability. The major glyco-conjugates, the glycophorin of the human erythrocyte membrane, has been found to carry numerous blood group antigens, however sialic acid (N-acetyl-neuraminic acid) present at the termini of the oligosaccharide side chains has been successfully exploited as a site directing molecules to avoid undesirable interaction with serum components and provide long circulation. The sialo-glycoconjugates include sialoglycoprotein of human erythrocytes (Utsumi et al., 1987), monosialoganglioside GM1 (Allen and Cohn, 1987), sialoglycopeptide derived fetuin (Saito et al., 1988), sialic acid conjugated cholesterol substituted pullulan (Sunamoto et al., 1988) and sialoglycolipid, a novel synthetic sialic acid derivative (Yamauchi et al., 1995).

GM1 and PEG Coated Liposomes

A plethora of research in the field of targeted drug delivery concentrated on exploration of the effects of glycolipids and gangliosides, primarily monosialogangliosides GM1 or phosphatidylinositol, in prolonging the circulation half-life and altering the biodistribution of liposomes (categorically known as first generation long circulatory liposomes). However, recent advances in the field of stealth systems have focused categorically on the evaluation of effect of hydrophilic polymers such as polyethyleneglycol (PEG) linked by various means to lipid molecules (second generation of long circulatory liposomes). The colloidal basis for this approach is referred to as classical 'steric stabilization' which due to osmotic and entropic effects of an inert, nonionic, hydrophilic, and flexible polymer coating, increases repulsive forces, which operate on these modified surfaces, resulting in the reduced levels of interaction and adsorption of plasma proteins. Several attempts have been made to understand the underlying mechanisms (Woodle et al., 1994; Marjan and Allen, 1996) Long circulatory behaviour demonstrated by first generation long circulatory liposomes could be ascribed to one of the following attributes, either independently or in combinations (Fig. 5-33).:

1. Glycocalyx similar to red blood cells (RBC), which is instrumental in providing ability to surface modified liposomes that mimics outer monolayer of RBC.
2. Hypothesis of shielded negative charge that proposes existence of screened negative

charge. This leads to increased surface hydrophilicity of the liposomes without imparting a negative charge binding site at the surface of the liposomes for the liver scavenger systems.

3. Hypothesis of dysopsonin, which proposes specific recognition of the GM1 by serum proteins (dysopsonin) that prevent the attack and recognition of opsonins and hence the phagocytosis.

Long circulatory behaviour imparted by second generation long circulatory liposomes could be ascribed to one of the following strategies, either independently or in combinations:

1. Hypothesis of steric barrier that proposes steric stabilization by the grafted polymer (polymer brush steric hindrance).
2. Increased surface hydrophilicity that avoids or inhibits specific opsonization of the lipid surface by immunoglobulins.
3. Inhibition of nonspecific adsorption of plasma proteins and lipoproteins.

However, literature is divided upon considering specific mechanisms of stealth and long circulatory behaviour to ganglioside GM1 and PEG-grafted liposomes. Increased surface hydrophilicity and steric hindrance however, remain as major mechanisms for long circulation imparted by GM1 and/or PEG coats (Gabizon and Papahadjopoulos, 1992; Allen, 1993; Woodle and Lasic, 1992; Allen, 1994; Allen et al., 1998). The hydrophilicity contributed by various glycolipids and hydrophilic polymers is realized to be the central dogma of the stealth behaviour of the liposomes and other colloidal systems. Opsonins and/or serum proteins recognize hydrophobic surfaces and scavenge hydrophobic particulate and vesicular systems. However, liposomes coated or appended with hydrophilic polymers present an opsonin repelling surface and thus become less susceptible to recognition (Fig. 5-34).

Rational and Concept of using Stealth Liposomes in Tumour Targeting

Major aims and benefits of sterically stabilized liposomes (SSL) or Stealth liposomes are as following:

- Making liposomal systems more stable in bio-environmental conditions
- Making them long circulatory (i.e., less recognizable to serum proteins specially opsonins and hence less recognizable to phagocytic cells of RES)
- Making them targeted along with long circulatory behaviour by anchoring site specific ligands
- Making them more sensitive towards external stimuli and signals like pH, substrates and temperatures
- Making them more suitable for tumour targeting

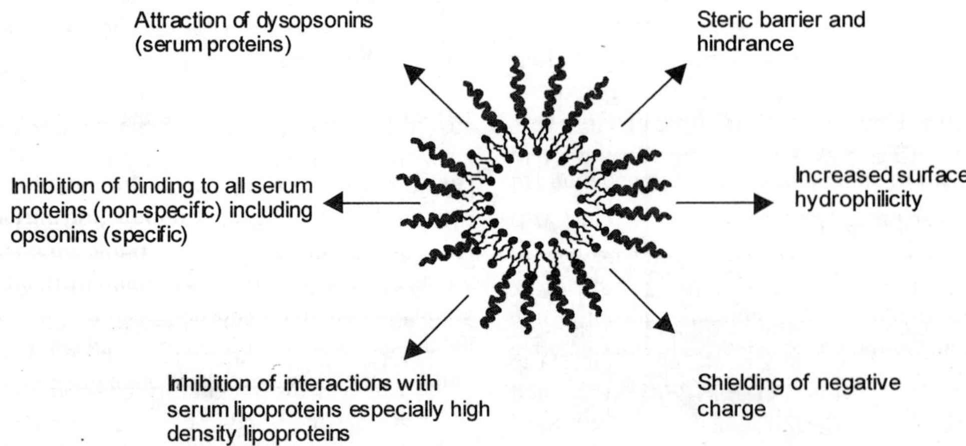

Fig. 5-33. Various Mechanisms Proposed for Stealth or Long Circulatory Behaviour of Polymer Graftec Glycolipid Anchored Liposomes

The potentials of stealth liposomes for tumour targeting can be realized by following attributes:

1. Long-circulatory liposomes with encapsulated anticancer drugs can reach sites other than RES (if tumour belongs to an extravascular site), either by extravasation through leaky blood vessels in tumours or directed through surface attached ligands (mostly antibodies).
2. They can serve as the sustained release micro-reservoirs for the anticancer drugs. This can be either long-circulatory systemic application, local injection to body cavities, such as intra-peritoneal, or intramuscular or subcutaneous drug depot with customized permeability or leakage characterisitcs.
3. They may be used in indirect applications, such as delivery of free radical oxygen to enhance radiotherapy or other photo- and radio-therapeutic substances.

Liposomal Anthracyclines

Some of the liposomal anticancer products either approved or under clinical trials are tabulated with major antineoplastic agents (Table 5-15). The highly investigated category for tumour therapy is the use of anthracyclines. Cytotoxic anthracycline antibiotics, daunorubicin and doxorubicin are approved anticancer agents for a range of tumour associated conditions like acute leukaemia, resistant Hodgkin's diseases, non-Hodgkin's lymphomas, sarcoma, neuroblastoma, ovarion and endometrial carcinoma, breast carcinoma, bronchogenic carcinoma, lung cancer and thyroid and bladder carcinoma (Billingham et al., 1984). AIDS-related Kaposi's sarcoma is somewhat responsive to anthracycline antibiotics used as a single agent or in combination regimens (Fischal et al., 1993). Conventional liposomal formulations bearing the anthracyclines are found to better the pharmacokinetic and dose-dependent toxicity profile (Gabizon et al., 1990). However, recognizing that rapid liposome clearance coupled with the release of encapsulated drug, severely limits the potential of conventional liposomes to transport encapsulated drug to systemic tumours. Strategies have been deviced to stabilize liposomes in plasma and prolong their circulation following administration. Similarly, efforts have been made to optimize liposome size to promote their extravasation at sites of tumour.

Two liposomal formulations namely, Doxil and DaunoXome, have been approved and are commercially available in USA, Europe, Japan and certain parts of Asia for the treatment of AIDS related Kaposi's sarcoma (Working et al., 1994; Forssen and Ross, 1994). Currently, both formulations are being used in the treatment of Kaposi's sarcoma, while some studies in solid tumour promise for their future use. DaunoXome was shown to be therapeutically more effective than conventional therapies, with reduced drug toxicity and improved quality of life-scores of

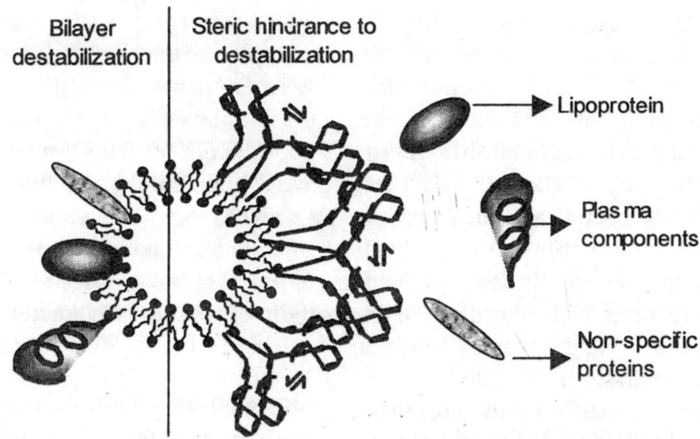

Fig. 5-34. Steric Barrier Hypothesis of Long Circulatory Liposome Behaviour

Table 5-15. Various Intravenous Liposomal Antibiotics/Antineoplastics either Approved or Under Various Clinical Trial Stages

System	Drug	Target disease	Status	Product
Liposomes (Doxil)	Doxorubicin	Kaposi's sarcoma	Approved by FDA	SEQUUS, USA
		Refractory tumours	Phase II	
Liposomes (TLC™ D-99) or EVACET™	Doxorubicin	Metastatic breast cancer	Phase III	The Liposome Company, USA
Liposomes (DaunoXome)	Daunosome	Advanced Kaposi's sarcoma	Approved UK, Sweden	NeXstar, USA
		Breast, small cell lung cancer, leukaemia, and solid tumours	Phase II	
Liposomes	Nystatin	Systemic fungal infections	Phase II	Aronex, USA
Liposomes	Anamycin	Kaposi's sarcoma	Phase II/III	Aronex, USA
		Refractory breast cancer	Phase I/II	
Liposomes (VincaXome)	Vincristine	Solid tumours	Preclinical development	NeXstar, USA
Liposomes (MiKasome)	Amikacin	Serious bacterial infections	Phase II	NeXstar, USA

the patients. The use of Doxil in Kaposi's sarcoma has shown a higher response levels in comparison to standard treatments. Doxil (Sequus) is essentially a formulation of doxorubicin (which is often referred to by its trade name Adriamycin) precipitated in sterically stabilized liposomes, while DaunoXome (NeXstar) is daunorubicin encapsulated in small liposomes with very strong intercalation in cohesive bilayers, which can be referred to as mechanical stabilization.

DaunoXome™ is comprised of small liposomes (small unilamellar vesicles consisting of distearoylphosphatidylcholine : cholesterol (2:1), total lipid concentration 7 mM) with daunorubicin (1 mg ml^{-1}) loaded by using a pH gradient technique. These liposomes are relatively stable in the circulation because they are small and their membrane is electrically neutral and mechanically very strong. However, their plasma stability is hampered due to reduced ability for charge induced or hydrophobic interactions with plasma proteins; they do not protect against Vander Waals adsorption of serum components (Forssen et al., 1996).

Doxil™ (also known as CAELYX in Europe) is a long-circulatory (Stealth™) dispersion of 80-100 nm liposomes (^{2000}PEG- distearoylphosphatidylethanolamine soya phosphatidylcholine:cholesterol, 20 mM) with doxorubicin HCl (2 mg ml^{-1}). The drug is encapsulated into preformed liposomes by an ammonium sulphate gradient technique and is additionally precipitated with encapsulated sulphate anions. These liposomes circulate in patients for several days, which increases their chances of extravasating at sites with a leaky vascular system (Gabizon et al., 1994). Their stability is due to their surface PEG coating and their mechanically strong bilayers. These liposomes were visualized by video microscopy extravasating into the gaps of interstitium of implanted tumours (Seymour, 1992). As the tumour vasculature has been shown to be leaky and the cut-off size of the gaps in the endothelial cell walls ranges 400-600 nm (average), smaller size (for both Doxil and DaunoXome) and long circulation times (for Doxil) favour their extravasation and make them suitable for tumour therapy. Some of current classes of antineoplastic drugs at clinical trial stages with their evaluation parameters are tabulated (Table 5-16).

Liposomes in Gene Therapy

Recombinant–DNA technology and studies of gene function and gene therapy all depend on the successful

Table 5-16. Antineoplastic Drugs Investigated for Liposome Encapsulation at Clinical Trial Stages with their Evaluation Parameters

Class/Drug	# of different liposomes	Pre-clinical evaluations	Clinical testing
Plant alkaloids			
Vincristine	<10	Extensive	Phase II
Vinblastine	<5	Very limited	-
Antibiotics			
Doxorubicin	<10	Extensive	Approved
Daunorubicin	<5	Extensive	Approved
Antimetabolites			
Methotrexate	<5	Limited	-
5-Fluorouracil	<5	Limited	-
Cytosine arabinoside	<5	Limited	-
Alkylating agents			
Cis-diammine-dicholorplatinum	<5	Limited	-
Other			
Mitoxantrone	<5	Extensive	Phase II

delivery of nucleic acids (genetic materials) into cells *in vitro* and *in vivo*. A variety of physical (e.g., electroporation, microinjection, particle bombardment), chemical (DEAE-dextran, polybrene-dimethyl sulphoxide, calcium phosphate precipitation, liposomes, poly-lysine conjugates) and biological (e.g. virus) methods have been developed for transferring genes into cells. The most widely used type of vehicles for gene delivery are: viral (e.g., adenovirus, retrovirus and adeno-associated virus) and non-viral (e.g., liposomes and lipid-based systems, polymers and peptides) (Storm and Crommelin, 1998). The relative advantages and disadvantages of viral and non-viral systems are discussed in Table 5-17.

Amongst the non-viral vector systems, liposomes and lipid complexes, especially engineered liposomes such as pH sensitive liposomes, cationic liposomes, fusogenic liposomes, genosomes, lipoplex, and lipopolyplex have extensively been investigated for their gene delivery potential (Fig. 5-35) (Ledley, 1995). Lipid based gene delivery is the focus of several specialized high-technology companies, of which Vical (San Diago, CA, USA), Genzyme (Farmington, MA, USA), GeneMedicine (The Woodlands, TX, USA) and Megabios (Burlingame, CA, USA) have products in clinical trials. Some of the engineered liposomal and non-liposomal versions like pH sensitive cationic and anionic liposomes, pH sensitive immunoliposomes, fusogenic liposomes, genosomes (DNA-liposomes/lipid_complexes), lipofection™ (lipid-DNA complex) and recently cochleates are being investigated as the major gene vectors. However, most of the commercially available non-viral gene vectors used for transfection are cationic liposome-DNA complexes (Liu et al., 1995). The cationic charge offers a template for electrostatic adsorption of DNA on to the surface and lipid-DNA complexation. The system is reportedly capable of consolidating the DNA molecule via electostatic comperassion *per se*. The cationic liposomes deliver the content through probably membrane fusion thus avoid lysosomal and nucleolus degradation of DNA. It is an efficient means of gene delivery. Some of the widely used cationic liposomes formulations are: lipofectin (DOTMA:DOPE::1:1), lipofectamine (DOSPA:DOPE::3:1), transfectase (DDAB:DOPE::1:3), cytofectin (DMRIE:DOPE) and transfectam (DOGS) (Fig. 5-35) (Table 5-18).

pH Sensitive Liposomes

Knowledge of lipid phases and membrane fusion has been used to design potentially more versatile pH sensitive liposomes that exploit the endosomal acidification to promote fusion with endosomal membranes (Conor and Hunag, 1985). Such an

Table 5-17. The Relative Advantages and Disadvantages of Viral and Non-Viral Systems

Type of vectors	Advantages	Disadvantages
Viral vectors (Adenovirus, retrovirus and adeno-associated virus)	• Relatively high transfection efficiency	• Immunogenicity, presence of contaminants and safety • Vector restricted size limitation for recombinant gene • Unfavourable pharmaceutical issue-large scale production, GMP, stability and cost
Non-viral vectors (Liposomes/ lipid-based systems, polymers and peptides)	• Favourable pharmaceutical issue-large scale production, GMP, stability and cost • Plasmid independent structure • Low immunogenicity • Opportunity for chemical/physical manipulation	• Relatively low transfection efficiency

Table 5-18. Liposome based Gene Delivery using Cationic Formulations

Name	Composition	Producer
Lipofectin	DOTMA:DOPE (1:1)	Life Technologies, Inc. (Gibco)
Lipofectamine	DOSPA: DOPE (3:1)	Life Technologies, Inc. (Gibco)
LipofectASE	DDAB:DOPE (1:2.1)	Life Technologies, Inc. (Gibco)
TransfectASE	DDAB:DOPE (1:3)	Life Technologies, Inc. (Gibco)
DOTAP	DOTAP	Boehringer Mannheim, Avanti
CellFectin	TMTPSp:DOPE (1:1.5)	Life Technologies, Inc. (Gibco)
Transfectam	DOGS	ProMega
TFX-50	TDA:DOPE (1:1)	ProMega
DC-Chol	DC-Chol:DOPE (3:2)	R-Gene, University of Pittsburgh

Abbreviations:

DOTMA: N-[1-(2,3-dioleoyloxy)propyl]-N,N,N-trimethylammonium chloride
DOTAP: N-[1-(2,3-dioleoyloxy)propyl]-N,N,N-trimethylammonium methylsulphate
DOSPA: 2,3-dioleoyloxy-N-[2(sperminecarboxamido)ethyl]-N,N-dimethyl-1-propanammonium trifluoroacetate
DDAB: Dimethyl-dioctadecylammonium bromide
DOPE: Dioleoylphosphatidylethanolamine
DOGS: Dioctadecyl amido glycyl spermine
DC: Chol-dimethylaminoethane carbamoyl cholesterol

approach is best exemplified by anionic, pH sensitive liposomes that have been designed to destabilize or fuse with the endosomal membrane at acidic pH (Fig. 5-36). The pH sensitive liposomes have been reported as plasmid expression vectors for the cytosolic delivery of DNA (Wang and Huang, 1987; Legender and Szoka, 1992; Lasic, 1997) and also as effective carriers for intracellular trafficking of antisense oligonucleotides (Ropert et al., 1992; Zelphati et al., 1996; deOliveria et al., 1998). Anionic, pH sensitive liposomes have delivered a variety of membrane-impermeant compounds includ-ing DNA (Budker et al., 1996; Chonn and Cullis, 1998). However, the negative charge of these vesicles limits them in regard to per cent DNA encapsulation and also prevents their cellular interaction, thus decreasing their utility for transfection.

pH sensitive cationic liposomes were found to mediate the efficient transfection of DNA into a variety of cells in culture as fusogenicity was offered by both the constitutive lipids, i.e., pH sensitive and cationic lipids (Lasic, 1997; Chonn and Cullis, 1998).

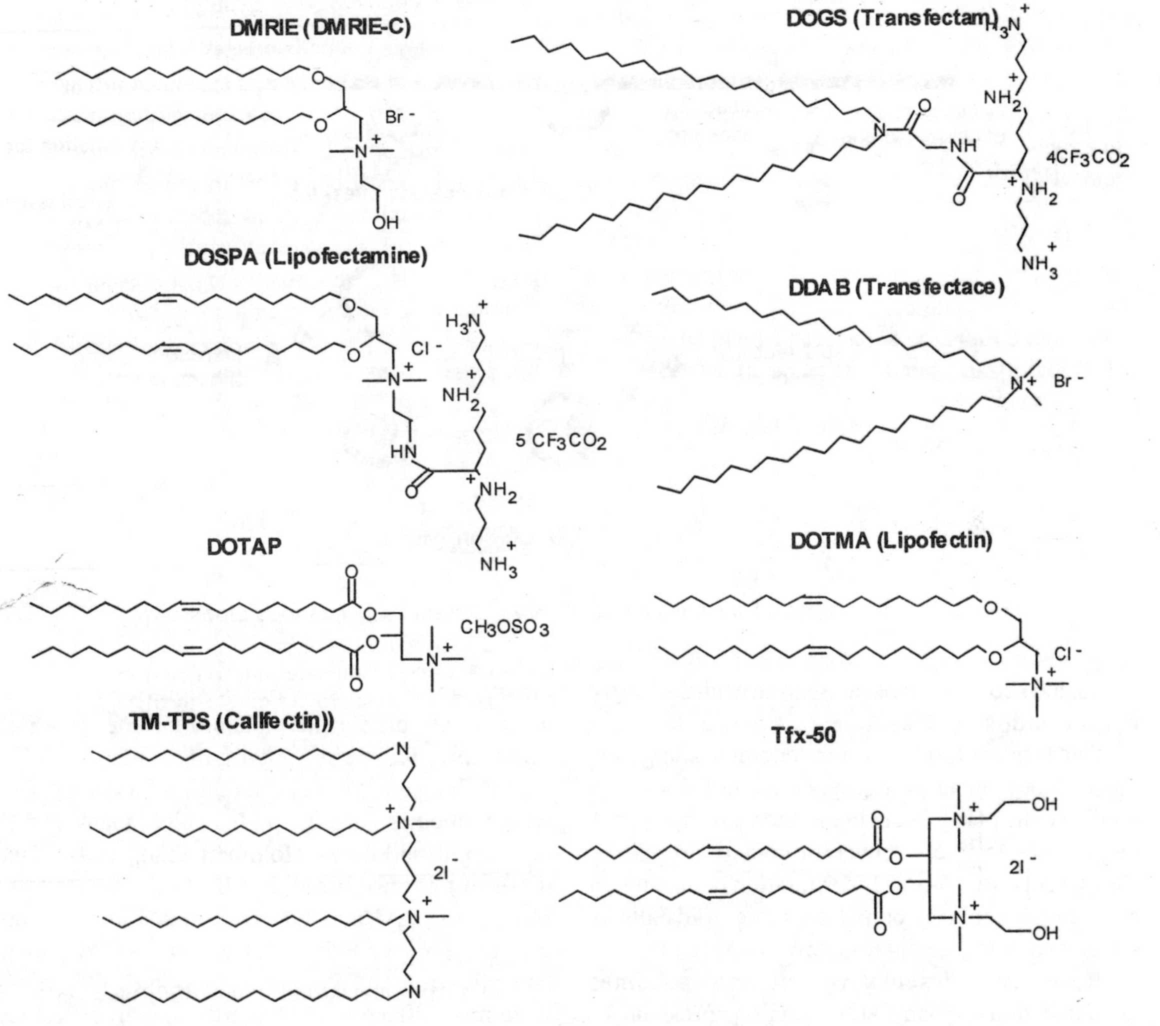
DMRIE (DMRIE-C)
Br -
OH
DOGS (Transfectam)
4CF3CO2
DOSPA (Lipofectamine)
Cl -
5 CF3CO2
DDAB (Transfectace)
Br -
DOTAP
CH3OSO3
DOTMA (Lipofectin)
Cl -
TM-TPS (Callfectin))
2I -
Tfx-50
OH
2I -
OH

Fig. 5-35. Structures of Some of the Commonly Used Cationic Lipids

Acid conditions promoted DNA binding, DNA incorporation and DNA induced fusion by cationic, pH sensitive liposomes (cationic lipid:DOPE in 1:1 molar ratio). Transfection efficiency in cultured cells by these liposomes was dependent on endosomal acidification in a manner akin to acid-induced endosomal release of viruses and hence been named as synthetic virus like vectors. Several mechanisms have been proposed for acid-induced fusogenicity of cationic liposomes (Lasic, 1997). With a decreased pH as would occur in the endosomal compartment, the polar head group of cationic lipid would become more strongly positive. This would increase the effective size of head group as a result of electrostatic repulsion. The increased positive charge of the cationic lipid would also increase its interaction with the DNA and with negative components of the endosomal membrane. These pH-dependent changes would cause dislocations in the liposomal membrane that lead to subsequent membrane fusion.

pH Sensitive Immunoliposomes

pH sensitive liposomes (Connor and Huang, 1985; Wang and Huang, 1987) have been developed to

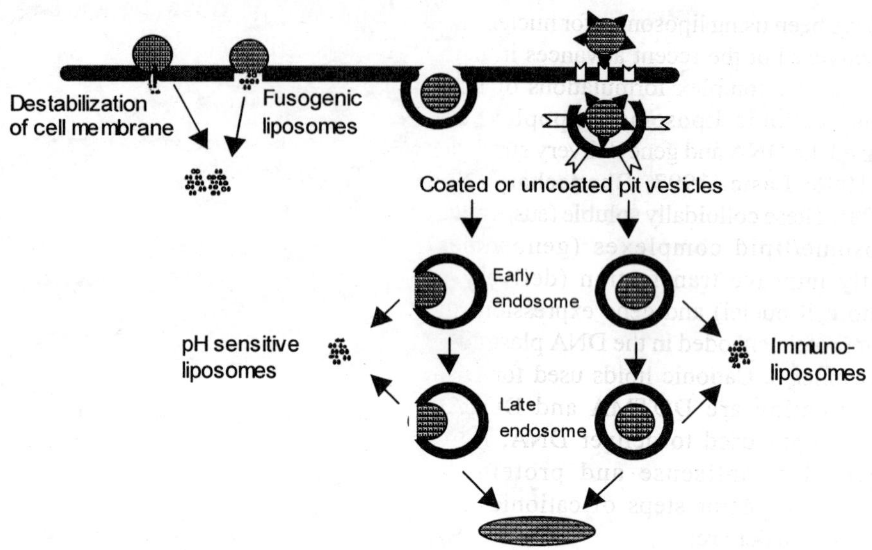

Fig. 5-36. The Uptake Pathways and Delivery Mechanisms of Various Liposomes

release their contents in response to an acid machinery within endosomal system following receptor mediated endocytosis of the immunological targeting ligand. They undergo transient destabilization at a mildly acidic pH as found in the endosomes and thus they could selectively deliver the contents to cellular components (Fig. 5-36). Incorporation of anti-target monoclonal antibody on pH sensitive lipids allows selective delivery to the respective target cells.

Recently, pH sensitive immunoliposomes mediated delivery and subsequent expression of exogenous genes in target cells have been reported. Some workers have also compared pH sensitive immunoliposomes to both, non pH sensitive immunoliposomes and pH-sensitive liposomes for their efficiency in transfecting the HSV-TK gene into the mouse lymphoma cells *in vitro* (Wang and Huang, 1989). Immunoliposomes were shown to adsorb DNA non-specifically on their surface and to transfer it directly into the cytoplasm, without being presented to lysosomes for degradation. pH sensitive immunoliposomes guided by MoAbs against a surface antigen on mouse L cells, were observed to fuse with endosomal membrane in response to acidic pH of the endosome. Specific gene delivery via this latter mode was found to express TK (thymidine kinase) genes at a statistically significant level as compared to pH sensitive plain liposomes (without immunological targeting ligand). pH sensitive immunoliposomes have been utilized for conjugation with antibodies specific to glial cells (gliasomes) to deliver plasmid DNA (Holmberg et al., 1994). Two different monoclonal antibodies of different subclasses, IgM and IgG, were examined for the transfection specificity against cultured C6 glioma (specific target cell type) using gliasomes. Gliasomes were more effective in their transfection efficiency than the cationic lipid complex methods using lipofectin and transfectase.

Results of these studies indicate a three-fold increase in % transfection with the use of IgM subclass ligand and an approximately two-fold increase in % transfection with IgG subclass ligand. Gliasomes were further tested for their transfection specificity by the addition of excess antibody to the cell culture in order to pre-saturate specific receptors on C6 glioma cells. Administration of pH sensitive immunoliposomes to theses glioma cells pre-saturated with excess antibody, showed a measurable reduction in transfection, signifying transfection efficiency and specificity to be dependent on receptor mediated endocytosis.

Genosomes

Scientists have been using liposomes for nucleic acid and gene delivery but the recent advances in terms of genosomes, i.e., complex formulations of DNA with various cationic liposomes (lipoplex) has revolutionized the DNA and gene delivery strategies (Flegner, 1996; Lasic, 1997; Bhattacharya and Huang, 1998). These colloidally soluble (suspended) DNA-liposome/lipid complexes (genosomes) significantly improve transfection (delivery of plasmid into cell nuclei) and gene expression (the synthesis of protein encoded in the DNA plasmid by the cell machinery). Cationic lipids used for DNA complex formation are DOTMA and DOTAP. Cationic lipids are used to deliver DNA, RNA, oligonucleotides, antisense and proteins to mammalian cells. Major steps of cationic lipid mediated gene transfer are:

- Complex formation by DNA condensation
- Binding with molecules in biological fluids such as serum
- Transport from the site of injection to target cell surface
- Complex binding to the cell surface
- Uptake into the cell by endocytosis
- Release of the complex from endosome
- Uncoating of DNA
- Uptake into the nucleus
- Expression of the gene

Lipopolyplex

For most of the formulations, the lipoplex formed by the complexation of cationic liposomes with DNA has some disadvantages especially *in vivo*. First, they have a tendency to aggregate with DNA to form large and heterogenous particles at high concentration. Second, cationic liposomes in general lack the ability of targeted delivery because of non-specific charge interactions with the cells. Third, opsonin or serum proteins or RES may remove them from the circulation. To avoid all the above stated problems lipopolyplex formulations composed of liposomes/polycation/DNA complex are devised. Poly-l-lysine has been used along with PC-Chol/DOPE liposomes to condense DNA and form a self-assembled vector system named as LPDI (a lipopolyplex) (Gao and Huang, 1996). LPDI is currently used in a clinical trial for gene therapy of canavan's disease, an autosomal recessive leukodystrophy. In a recent development, Lee and Huang (1996) reported a lipid vector (LPDII) for gene transfer, where poly-L-lysine condensed DNA is entrapped into folate targeted anionic liposomes via charge interactions (LPDII differs from LPDI in that anionic lipids instead of cationic lipids are used).

Liposomal DNA Immunization

DNA immunization is one of the most exciting fields of gene therapy. It arose from an unexpected observation that injected purified plasmid DNA containing encoding sequences for a protein immunogen transfects cells whereupon the expressed protein induces humoral and cell-mediated immunity (Mor et al., 1996). Selective antigen presentation by either ligand appended or engineered carrier systems can be appraised via major histocompatibility complex (MHC) molecules that process and present the antigen to the antigen presenting cells of the immune systems, such as macrophages, dendritic cells and B lymphocytes.

Major histocompatibility complex (MHC) molecules exist in two forms, class I (MHC-I) and class II (MHC-II). The mechanisms of antigen processing differ for the two classes. MHC-II molecules present antigens derived from extracellular proteins or proteins that target endocytic compartments, whereas MHC-I molecules present antigens that are synthesized in the cytosol or penetrate directly in to the cytosol. Gregoriadis and co-workers (1998) have recently revealed that DNA immunization with plasmid DNA immobilized/entrapped within the aqueous domains of artificial membranes (liposomes) and compared its potential for DNA immunization with naïve plasmid DNA. It was proposed that following vaccination with plasmid DNA the plasmid is taken up by the myocytes. These myocytes release the antigenic peptide, which is captured by antigen presenting cells and B cells. Stimulation of CD4+ and CD8+ T cells by antigenic peptides induces cytotoxic T cell response (CTL) and also induces B cells to produce antibodies. MHC-I expression may occur on the myocytes and MHC-II on APC. On the other hand, once liposome entrapped plasmid DNA are taken by endocytosis by antigen presenting cells such as dendritic cells, some unknown cellular events (other than MHC restriction) derive the pDNA to be released from the endosome and the liposome carrier (Fig. 5-37). The released pDNA may or may not become integrated with the master genome and results in transfection and MHC-I and MHC-II restricted presentation, which stimulates the CD4+and CD8+ T cells by antigenic peptide and induces cytotoxic T cell response and may induce B cells to generate antibodies.

A variety of plasmid DNAs can be quantitatively incorporated by DRV method into MLVs composed of PC and DOPE alone or supplemented with anionic and cationic lipids (Gregoriadis et al., 1996). *In vitro* studies indicate that DNA entrapped in such liposomes is capable of transfecting cells, with vesicles bearing a cationic charge being the most effective. DNA immunization experiments confirmed that plasmid DNA entrapped in cationic liposomes was much more effective in inducing humoral and cell-mediated immunity to encoded antigen than naked DNA or DNA entrapped in neutral or anionic liposomes (Gregoriadis et al., 1998). Thus immunization with liposomal DNA could have an important implication in human and veterinary immunization programs of future.

Liposomes in Antisense Oligonucleotide Therapy

Oligonucleotides are being developed as therapeutic agents to selectively deliver altered genetic functions through sequence specific interactions with intracellular RNA or DNA. This may involve a variety of mechanisms including antisense, ribozymes, triplex and decoy. The approaches halt DNA transcription or messenger RNA translation with code-blocking triplex forming or antisense oligomers (Marshall and Caruthers, 1993; Gold, 1995). Antisense oligonucleotides interact with specific mRNA sequences by Watson-Crick base pairing, resulting in the reduced synthesis of the proteins those RNAs encode. Liposomal delivery of these agents avoids the drawbacks associated with the other modes of administration including degradation by nucleases, increased toxicity and undesirable interactions with proteins.

Conventional liposomes are useful for the transport of either (a) natural phosphodiester oligonucleotides or (b) modified oligonucleotides i.e., phosphorothioate, phosphoroamidate, methyl phosphonate and C-5 propyne modification) by reducing the administered dose (Juliano and Akhtar, 1992) (Fig. 5-38). However, cationic liposomes, anionic liposomes, pH

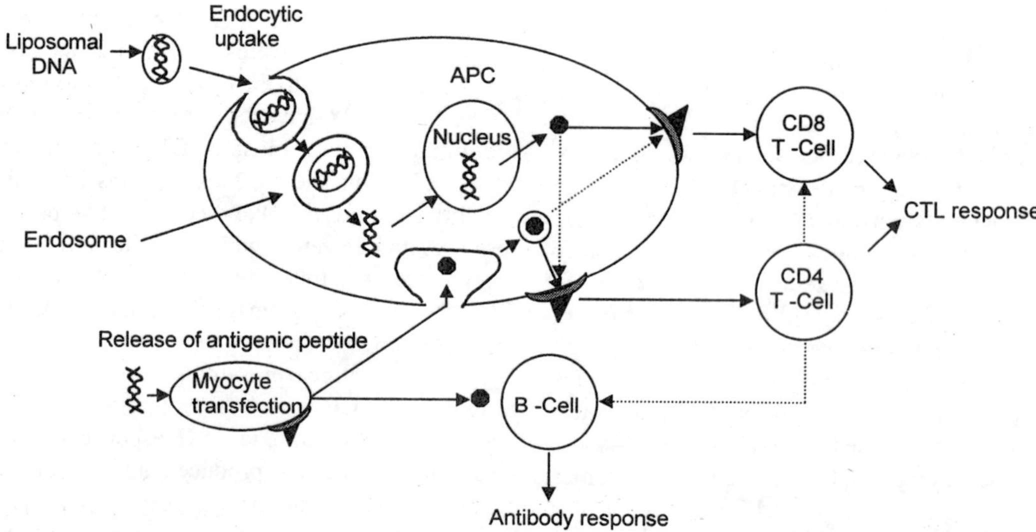

Fig. 5-37. Proposed Mechanism of DNA Immunization Via Endocytic Pathway. Vaccination with Plasmid DNA and Liposomal DNA are Compared for their Expression Through Various Routes

sensitive liposomes, antibody coated (immunoliposomes), fusogenic liposomes or PEG-grafted (sterically stabilized stealth liposomes) are more appropriate in designing an appropriate and defined biodistribution and pharmacokinetic profile (Woodle and Leserman, 1998). The encapsulation of oligonucleotides in liposomes is useful for several reasons:

- Protection of oligonucleotides from nucleases degradation
- Enhancement of cellular uptake in several cell types
- Improvement of oligonucleotide potency, especially *in vitro*
- Modification of their intracellular distribution
- Increased retention of oligonucleotides in cells
- Potential for slow release depots for modified oligonucleotides

Immunological Applications of Liposomes

Besides its potential applications in cancer chemotherapy, antifungal therapy and genetic applications, liposome as a delivery system has established itself in the area of immunology (Allison and Gregoriadis, 1975; van Rooijen, 1990; Alving, 1992; Gluck, 1995) and the major areas of interest from a therapeutic point of view are:

- Liposomes as an immunological (vaccine) adjuvant
- Liposomal vaccines
- Liposomes as a carrier of immunomodulators
- Liposomes as a tool in immunodiagnostics

Liposomes as an Immunological (Vaccine) Adjuvant

Liposomes have been firmly established as immunoadjuvants (enhancers of the immunological response), potentiating both cell-mediated (cytotoxic T lymphocytes) and humoral immunity (antibody production). In recent years, mucosal immunoadjuvant activity of liposomes, involving the induction of strong secretory IGA (s-IGA) responses by delivering the system in the gastrointestinal or respiratory tracts have been appreciated (de Haan et al.., 1995). Their main advantages against other adjuvants (detoxified cholera toxins, alum) can be summarized as:

- Liposomes are non-toxic, biocompatible and biodegradable

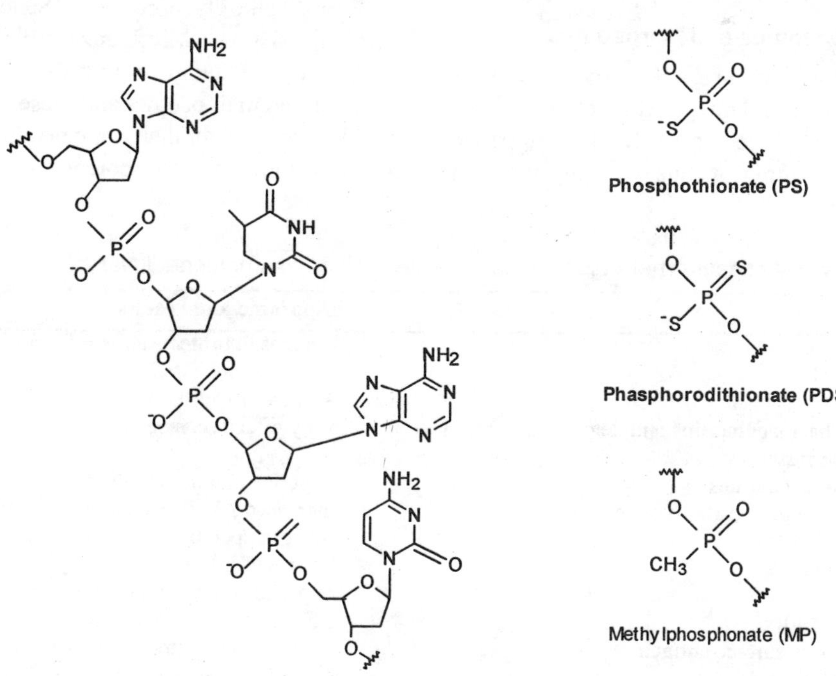

Fig. 5-38. Chemical Structure of Phosphorothioate and other Common Chemical Analogues of Oligodeoxynucleotides with each of Four Common Bases Found in DNA

- Non-immunologically inert in most of the cases and tailor made compositions
- May incorporate other adjuvants to provide strong immune response
- Convert loaded or anchored non-immunogenic substances into immunogenic ones with small amount of antigen
- Reduce or eliminate the toxicity of toxic antigens and allergic reactions to nontoxic proteins
- Modulate the immune system and may induce cell-mediated immunity
- Liposomal vaccines produce higher titres of functional antibodies as well as prolonged duration of these antibodies

Liposomal immunoadjuvants act by slowly releasing encapsulated antigen on intramuscular injection and also passively accumulating within regional lymph nodes. Liposomal vaccines can be made by incorporating microbes, soluble antigens, cytokines or deoxyribonucleic acid with liposomes, the latter stimulate an immune response on expression of the antigenic protein. Alternatively, antigens can be covalently coupled to liposomal membrane (Wassef et al., 1994) (Table 5-19).

Fusogenic Liposomes and "Virosomes"

Fusogenic liposomes are specially engineered liposomes that fuse and merge with cell membranes and directly introduce molecules (entrapped or anchored) into cytoplasm thus avoiding the route followed by conventional liposomes, i.e., internalization via endocytic compartments into lysosomes. The fusogenic liposomes mimic the way by which several viruses (HIV, Sendai virus) bind and merge with cell membranes at neutral pH and subsequently release their genome into the cytoplasm. The fusion between liposomes and cell membrane is not a spontaneous phenomenon and several methods have been used to facilitate this type of delivery (Table 5-20).

Fusion can be mediated by fusogenic agents like polyethylene glycol, glycerol and polyvinyl alcohol or by reconstituted viral membranes. These reconstituted fusogenic viral membrane based liposomes are also termed as virosomes (Gould-Fogerite et al., 1989). Virosomes are liposomes with virus spike glycoproteins incorporated into the liposomal bilayers. The spike glycoproteins of viral origin mediate the interaction of the virus with the target cell receptor. The interaction either results in the transfer of the virus genome into the host cell by an micro-injection mechanism (in the case of non-enveloped virus) or results in membrane fission or fusion (in case of enveloped virus).

Fusion spike glycoproteins of Sendai virus, rabies virus, measles virus, influenza virus, herpes virus, HIV-1 and vesicular stomatitis virus have been incorporated in liposomes and these virosomes have been investigated for their immunoadjuvant, gene and oligonucleotide delivery potentials (Jones, 1994).

Table 5-19. List of Antigens where Liposomes have been Used as Immunoadjuvants

Antigen	Liposome and results
Influenza subunit antigen	Intranasal, protects animal from virus
Tetanus toxoid	Mannose-mediated liposomal targeting, Increased Ab titre
Filamentous haemagglutinins and detoxified Pertussis toxin of *Bortella pertussis*	Very effective vaccine
Bacterial polysaccharides	Superior immunoadjuvants
Streptococcus mutant carbohydrate antigen	Increased Ab titre in salivary glands
Rabies Glycoprotein	Antigen specific interleukin-2 enhancement
Polio virus peptides	Enhanced Ab level
Cholera toxin	Superior immunoadjuvants
Diphtheria toxoid	PC/Chol/DCP, Higher Ab response
Hepatitis B virus surface antigen	PC/PA/Chol, humoral and cellular immunity
Herpes Simplex Virus	MLV with Lipid A, Enhanced Ab level

*Compiled from Gregoriadis, 1990

Table 5-20. Methods Used to Facilitate Fusogenic Drug Delivery

Viral spike glycoproteins	Target site/Function
Sendai virus haemagglutinin/neuraminidase glycoprotein	Negatively charged liposomes
Sendai virus glycoprotein HN and F	P815 and EL-4 cells
Rabies virus surface glycoprotein	Immune response in animals
Measles virus haemagglutinin and fusion glycoprotein	Murine macrophage cell lines
Influenza virus haemagglutinin/neuraminidase glycoprotein	Vaccine adjuvant
Herpes simplex virus glycoprotein D	Immune response in mice and guinea pigs
HIV-1 envelope glycoprotein	Immune response in mice lymphocytes

*Compiled from Jones, 1994

Liposomal Vaccines

New generation vaccines that are based on recombinant protein subunits and synthetic-peptide antigens are usually non-immunogenic hence the need of immuno-potentiation is well realized. Although, many structurally unrelated agents (immunological adjuvants) are capable of inducing immune responses to vaccine antigens, most of them are toxic. Apart from alum, which is the only immunological adjuvant used for last few decades (associated with problems like not capable of inducing cell-mediated immune response), others are not clinically useful. After being established the immunoadjuvant properties of liposomes, several liposome-based vaccines have been either approved or licensed for use in human (Table 5-21). Most of the liposomal vaccines investigated to date are based either on novasome or immunopotentiating reconstituted influenza virosome (IRIV). Vaccines based on novasomes (non-phospholipid, biodegradable pausilamellar vesicles formed from single-chain amphiphiles, with or without other lipids) have been licensed for the immunization of fowl against Newcastle disease virus and avian retrovirus (IGI, Vineland Laboratories, Vineland, NJ, USA) (Gregoriadis, 1995). However, the first liposome-based vaccine (against hepatitis A) that has been licensed for use in human is an IRIV vaccine produced by Swiss serum and vaccine institute, Berne, Switzerland known as "Epaxal-Berna Vaccine" is an IRIV vaccine (Gluck, 1995). IRIVs are spherical, unilamellar vesicles with a mean diameter of ~150 nm (Gluck et al., 1992). IRIVs are prepared by detergent removal of influenza surface glycoproteins and a mixture of natural and synthetic phospholipids containing 70% egg yolk phosphatidylcholine, 20% synthetic PE and 10% envelope phospholipids originating from H1N1 influenza virus. Thus IRIV combines several components that are known to contribute to immunostimulation and at the same time are harmless and bioacceptable.

Liposomes as a Carrier of Immunomodulators

Activation of the immune system for the management of certain types of tumours like micrometastases and osteosarcoma is a well accepted treatment modality. The main purpose is to activate macrophages and render them tumouricidal. If macrophages are activated to their tumouricidal state, they become an ideal modality for the treatment of metastatic diseases that are resistant to other forms of therapy. Tumouricidal macrophages acquire the ability to recognize and destroy neoplastic cells both *in vitro* and *in vivo*, while leaving normal cells unharmed by a non-immunological mechanism that requires cell-to-cell contact (Tucker et al., 1981). The ability of tumouricidal macrophages to discriminate between tumourigenic and normal cells has been demonstrated with syngeneic and allogeneic tumours of rodents and allogeneic human tumours. The problem of rapid clearance of systemically administered cytokines and macrophage activators (as immunomodulators) and pathogenicity of microorganisms and their products can be overcome by encapsulating activating agents into liposomes composed of phospholipids (Sone and Filder, 1980). Many of problems have been addressed with introduction of liposome based delivery systems. For immunopotentiation, immunomodulating agents such as muramyl dipeptide (MDP), lipopolysaccharide and lipid can be incorporated into liposomes (Schroit and Fidler, 1986; Fidler, 1992) (Table5-22).

Table 5-21. Liposome based Vaccines either Approved or Licensed for Use in Human

System	Drug	Target disease	Status	Product
Novasomes (New castle disease vaccine) (Intramuscular)	Killed New castle disease virus	New castle disease (Chicken)	Licensed	IGI, Vineland Lab, NJ, USA
Novasomes (Avian retrovirus vaccine) *(Intramuscular)	Killed avian retrovirus	Retrovirus infection (chicken); Breeder chicken vaccination	Licensed	IGI, Vineland Lab, NJ, USA
Novasome (*Escherichia coli* 0157:H7) (Oral)	*E coli* 0157:H7 (killed)	E coli 0157 infections	Phase I	Novavax, USA
Novasome (*Shigella flexneri* 2A vaccine) (Oral)	*Shigella flexneri* 2A	Shigella flexneri 2A infections	Phase I	Novavax, USA
IRIV liposomes (Epaxal-Berna vaccine) (Intramuscular)	Inactivated hepatitis A virions	Hepatitis A	Approved in Switzerland	Swiss Serum &Vaccine Institute, Switz.
IRIV liposomes (Trivalent influenza vaccine) (Intramuscular)	Haemagglutinin/ neuraminidase from influenza strains	Influenza	Phase III	Swiss Serum and Vaccine Institute, Switz.
IRIV liposomes (HAV/HB-IRIV combined vaccine) (Intramuscular)	Genetically engineered hepatitis B antigens (HAV)	Hepatitis A and B	Phase I	Swiss Serum and Vaccine Institute, Switz.
IRIV liposomes (Diphtheria/tetanus/hepatits A combined vaccine) (Intramuscular)	Diphtheria and tetanus toxoids; inactivated HAV virions	Diphtheria, Tetanus and Hepatitis A	Phase I	Swiss Serum and Vaccine Institute, Switz.
IRIV liposomes (Hepatitis A & B/ Diphtheria/ tetanus/hepatitis A combined vaccine) (Intramuscular)	Inactivated HAV virions; Diphtheria and tetanus toxoids	Hepatitis A and B, Diphtheria, Tetanus and Influenza	Phase I	Swiss Serum and Vaccine Institute, Switz.

Liposomes in Immunodiagnosis

Immunoassays such as ELISA, RIA or LILA are based on the selective interaction of an analyte antigen with corresponding antibodies. The concentration of antigens or antibodies is normally determined by competition of analyte with known concentration of radio- or fluorescent-labeled receptor in the binding to the immobilized antibody. Liposomes can be useful analytical reagents as they can encaspulate upto a million markers and can therefore, serve as signal amplifiers. Liposome is well recognized as a model membrane and its lytic ability inculcated through various lytic agents such as complement led to the development of an efficient assay system known as "liposome immune lysis assay (LILA)". The technique is based upon specially engineered liposomes constructed with a marker inside and either antigen/antibody appended to the liposomal surface (Yasuda et al., 1981; Ishimori et al., 1984). Addition of either antibody/antigen along with a lytic substance such as complement (an opsonin) will lyse liposomes with a release of marker, which can be monitored. The total lysis is dependent on the antigen/antibody binding and thus help to quantitate the test material. The marker could be a fluorescent dye such as carboxyfluorescein (CF), calcein or some markers that could be monitored enzymatically. LILA using fluorophores is based on the quenching phenomenon of fluorophores. The trapping efficiency of CF at high concentrations within liposomes results in the absence

Table 5-22. List of Immunomodulators where Liposomes have been Used as a Carrier

Antigen(s)
Macrophage activating factor (MAF)
N-acetyl-muramyl-L-alanyl-D-isoglutamine (muramyl dipeptide or MDP)
N-acetyl-muramyl-L-alanyl-D-isoglutamyl-L-alanyl-phosphatidylethanolamine (MTP-PE)
Lipopolysaccharide
Endotoxin derived lipid A

*Compiled from Schroit and Fidler, 1986; Fidler, 1992

of any fluorescent signal. Upon lysis, the dilution of the released test material markedly reduces quenching, allowing the determination of the fluorescent signal for titrating antibody or antigen.

LILA has certain advantages over the existing assay systems like enzyme immunoassay (EIA) and radio-immunoassay (RIA):

- Homogeneous assay, which does not require separation of free antigen/antibody from immune complex
- Avoidance of the hazardous chemicals such as radioisotopes in the assay
- Sensitivity is nearly same as that of EIA and RIA

However, the major drawback of LILA is that serum contains some non-specific factors, which can damage liposomes and subsequently the release of entrapped chromophore or fluorophore creating a non-reproducible background. Moreover, a judicious selection and concentration of marker can be executed to minimize the background error. LILA assay has been implicated in the detection of serum components such as α-fetoprotein, carcinoembryonic antigen, C-reactive protein and other serum proteins, which serve as diagnostic tools especially for cancer. LILA sandwich method has been used to detect many important antigens in serum, which are useful indicators of various abnormalities (Yasuda, 1986).

Liposomes in Dermatology and Cosmetology

Liposomes represent a model for biological membranes in biological and medical research because they mimic the lipid composition and structure of the human skin. In early studies, liposomes containing stratum corneum lipids have been tested in order to enable better skin penetration (Gray and White, 1976; Abraham et al., 1988). In order to gain more knowledge about the pharmacological potential of the topical liposomes (Dermosomes) the interactions between liposomes and epidermis and/or keratinocytes or reconstructed human skin were investigated by several groups (Abraham and Downing, 1990; Foldvari et al., 1990; Schreier and Bouwstra, 1994). Recently, two distinctive mechanisms are being explored for enhanced topical localization and/or targeting of liposome encapsulated bioactives: the trans-epidermal pathway (consists of skin layers) and trans-follicular pathway (consists of pilosebaceous units like hair follicles and glands) (Singh et al., 2000). The advantages of topical liposomes in dermatology or cosmetics are as follows:

- Similar to biological membranes they can navigate water soluble and lipophilic substances in different phases or domains.
- Mimic epidermis composition and structure, which enables them to penetrate the epidermal barrier to a greater extent as compared to other delivery vehicles.
- Liposomes are biodegradable and nontoxic, thus avoiding systemic/local side or toxic effects.
- Liposomes are thought to act not only as "drug transporters" but also as "drug localizers" thus avoiding systemic absorption and consecutively untoward effects.
- Moisturizing and restoring action of the constitutive lipids.
- Liposomes may act as localized drug depots in the skin and skin appendages, resulting in sustained release of dermatically active compounds, thereby improving the therapeutic index (T.I.) of the drug at target site while reducing the toxicity profile to its minimum.

Diverse ranges of substances are considered as

"candidates" for liposome encapsulation in the field of dermatology (Schmid and Korting, 1996). According to the patent literature almost every kind of active ingredients might be suitable to be encapsulated in topical liposomes (Table 5-23). However, among the great variety of candidates for liposome encapsulation, e.g. antibiotics, antifungals, disinfectant, immunosuppressive agents, monoclonal antibodies, DNA and several hydrophilic and hydrophobic peptides, the following groups are considered most often:

1. Those drugs that have severe side effects on either systemic administration or on conventional way of topical administration, e.g. topical glucocorticosteroides (Mazei and Gulasekharam, 1980; Lasch and Wohlrab, 1986).
2. Drug that are normally effective on systemic application and not by topical application, e.g., interferons (Weiner et al., 1989).
3. Drugs that show insufficient effects when applied topically, e.g. hamamelis distillate (Korting et al., 1991).
4. Drugs that on conventional topical application show local irritant effects and flare up reactions at the beginning of treatment, e.g., retinoids (tretinoin) (Korting et al., 1991).
5. Drugs which require prolonged application time and high drug concentrations to alleviate unpleasant sensations often associated with dermatological diseases or their treatment, e.g., local anaesthetics (tetracaine) (Gesztes and Mezei, 1988).

Liposomes based anti-ageing topical formulations (e.g., creams, lotions, gels and hydrogels) have been formulated and launched in the cosmetic market in 1986 by L'Oreal in the form of Niosomes and then by Christian Dior in the form of liposomes (Capture™). Similarly, liposomal preparations reduce the skin roughness because of its interaction with the corneocytes and of the intercellular lipids resulting in skin softening and smoothening (Moghimi

Table 5-23. Various Liposomal Products either Launched or Investigated in the Field of Dermatology and Cosmetics

Vesicular system	Marketed by	Liposomes and ingredients
Capture™	Christian Dior	Liposomes in gel with ingredients
Plenitude™	L'Oreal	Tanning agents in liposomes
Dermosome™	Microfluidics	Skin care, loaded liposomes
Inovita™	Pharm/Apotheke	Thymus extract, hyaluronic acid and vitamin E in liposomes
Penta™	Pentapharm	Humectant pentavitin R in liposomes
Coatsome NC™	Nichiya Liposome Co.	Liposomes with humectant (polyol, sugar and amino acid)
Nactosomes™	Lancome (L'Oreal)	Vitamins, retinolacetate, in liposomes
Sympathik 2000™	Biopharm GmbH	Thymus extract, vitamin A palmitate and soya phospholipid
Brookosome™	Brook's In's; Applied Genetics, Inc.	Genetic engineered enzymes (repair of DNA) in liposomes
Aquasomes™	Nikko Chemical Co.	Liposomes with humectant
Novasome I™	-	Liposomes with interferons, cyclosporin
Niosome™	-	Hydrating agents in non ionic liposomes
Bioadhesive liposomes	-	Gelatin or hyluronic acid bearing liposomes with Flucanazole
Transfersomes™	-	Liposomal corticosteroids, anaesthetics and analgesic agents
Depofoam™	-	Liposomes loaded with gentamycin
Pevaryl™	-	Liposomes loaded with econazole

*Compiled from Lasic, 1993; Weiner and Lieb, 1998; Lasic and Paphadjopoulos, 1998

and Patel, 1993). Presently, a variety of liposomes based anti-ageing creams and skin moisturizers are available in world market. Success rates of these products range between 83-98 % when parameters such as tightening and firming effects, texture, smoothness, softness, vitality, complexion, luminosity and clarity are considered. Currently, various liposome based formulations for facial and body care, make-up, mascara and foundations as well as hair care, self tanning and sun screen products and even perfumes are being launched in the cosmetic market.

Liposomes as Radiopharmaceutical and Radiodiagnostic Carriers

Liposomes loaded with the appropriate contrast agents have been shown to be suitable for all used imaging modalities (Seltzer, 1989; Lund et al., 1991; Torchilin and Trubetskoy, 1995). These imaging modalities are based on different physical principles and achieve appropriate signal intensity from an area of interest in order to differentiate certain structures from surrounding tissues. According to the physical principle involved, currently used imaging modality include:

- γ-scintigraphy (involving application of γ-emitting radioactive materials)
- Magnetic resonance (MR, phenomenon based on transition between different energy levels of atomic nuclei under action of radiofrequency signal)
- Computed tomography (CT, the modality, which utilizes ionizing radiation with the aid of computers to acquire cross-images of the body and 3-D images of area of interest)
- Ultrasound imaging or ultrasonography (US), the modality using irradiation with ultrasound and based on the different rates at which ultrasound passes through various tissues.

The imaging of different organs and tissues for early detection and localization of pathological states however, can not be achieved without using appropriate contrast agents. The problems of low or different attenuation (the ability of a tissue to adsorb a certain signal, such as X-ray, sound waves, radiation or radio frequency) of different tissues could be resolved using contrast agents. The contrast agents are substances, which are able to absorb certain types of signal (irradiation) much stronger than surrounding tissues. The contrast agents are specific for each imaging modality and as a result of their accumulation in certain sites of interest, those sites may be easily visualized when the appropriate imaging method is applied. To further facilitate the accumulation of contrast agents in the required tissue or area of interest liposomes have been used as their carriers (Table 5-24).

Liposomes (conventional and targeted including immunoliposomes and stealth liposomes) are used in different imaging modalities to locate the sites specifically (Reviewed by Tilcock, 1995). Their radio-diagnostic applications include liver and spleen imaging (Niesman et al., 1994), lymphatic imaging (Trubetskoy and Torchilin, 1994), tumour imaging (Gabizon, 1995), blood pool imaging (Tilcock et al., 1993), imaging cardiovascular pathologies (Torchilin et al., 1996), visualization of inflammation and infection sites (Goins et al., 1993), brain imaging (Shermatova, 1990), visualization of bone marrow and eye vasculature (Niesman et al., 1994).

However, the progression from experimental animals to human patients may proceed differently for different liposomal preparations. While liposomes for CT imaging and ultrasonic imaging still are the subject of laboratory research, the advantages of γ-scintigraphy and MR imaging with liposomes have been demonstrated in many clinical studies (Niesman et al., 1994).

Liposome based imaging agents have already been successfully used for γ-, MR, CT- and US imaging of tumours. ^{111}In-labelled liposomes for tumour imaging (VenCan®, Vester, Inc.) are already in phase II-III clinical trials. Liposomal uptake by RES, which is useful strategy in localization of contrast agents in RES-rich organs like liver, spleen and bone marrow, is not useful for localization to non-RES organs. The RES-avoidance of contrast agents can be successfully be achieved using targeted liposomes like immunoliposomes, long circulatory (PEG- and PEG-like polymer coated) liposomes and even by long circulatory immunoliposomes (Torchilin, 1998).

Table 5-24. Imaging Modality and Required Concentration of Diagnostic Moieties

Imaging modality	Diagnostic moiety	Concentration
γ-Scintigraphy	Diagnostic radio-nuclides such as ^{111}In, ^{99m}Tc, ^{67}Ga	10^{-10} M
Magnetic resonance imaging	Pro-magnetic ions such as Gd and Mn, and iron oxide	10^{-4} M
Computed tomography imaging	Iodine, Bromine and Barium	10^{-2} M
Ultrasound imaging or ultrasonography	Gas (Air, argon and nitrogen)	

Liposomes as Red Cells Substitutes and Artificial RBCs

Various semi-synthetic and synthetic blood-substitutes, which carry oxygen, i.e., red cell substitutes, are reported (Fig. 5-39). These include perfluorochemical emulsion (Flusol, USA), recombinant haemoglobin, glutaraldehyde cross-linked haemoglobin and inter-molecularly cross-linked (using chemical reagents), polyoxyethylene-bound haemoglobin and haemoglobin encapsulated liposomes (Hb-vesicles or liposomes encapsulated liposomes, LEH) (reviewed in Tsuchida, 1995; Rudolph, 1995). Protoheme moieties of haemoglobin and myoglobin are completely surrounded by hydrophobic residues of the globin chain and this hydrophobic environment effectively prevents the irreversible oxidation of iron to ferric states and promotes the reversible formation of oxygen adducts. In haemoglobin vesicles, this hydrophobic environment is provided by lipid bilayer and thus they mimic the red cells.

Liposome encapsulated haemoglobin products are being investigated as artificial RBCs (oxygen carrying RBC substitutes) (Sherwood et al., 1995). Tsuchida (1994) reported that the aggregation and fusion of haemoglobin vesicles (Hb-vesicles) and the leakage on long-term storage can be prevented by using either polymerized phospholipids or polyphospholipids (the stabilized polyphospholipid vesicles containing concentrated Hb are called ("artificial red cell") or by introduction of oligosaccharide type of glycolipid in the bilayer membrane. Recent studies suggest that the sterically stabilized liposome bearing haemoglobin (PEG-PE LEH) are even better than LEH as artificial blood substitutes as they manifest less toxicity, less platelet activation and aggregation and less haemostatic generation (Jato et al., 1998). Tsuchida (1995) reported completely synthetic amphiphilic heme derivative (lipid heme) and incorporated them into the hydrophobic centre of the bilayer membrane of the phospholipid vesicles. These lipid-heme vesicles demonstrated excellent oxygen carrying and transporting abilities

Miscellaneous Applications

Various liposome-based products are being investigated (Table 5-25) and are under clinical trial at various stages for the delivery of all-trans retinoic acid (Aronex, USA) and for prostaglandia E1 (Ventus, The Liposome Company, USA) (Lasic and Papahadjopoulos, 1998). Similarly, liposomes have been exploited in anti-asthma, anti-infective and antioxidant therapy and more recently in the gene therapy of the pulmonary diseases. Recently, ALEC™ (Artificial Lung Expanding Compound) has been

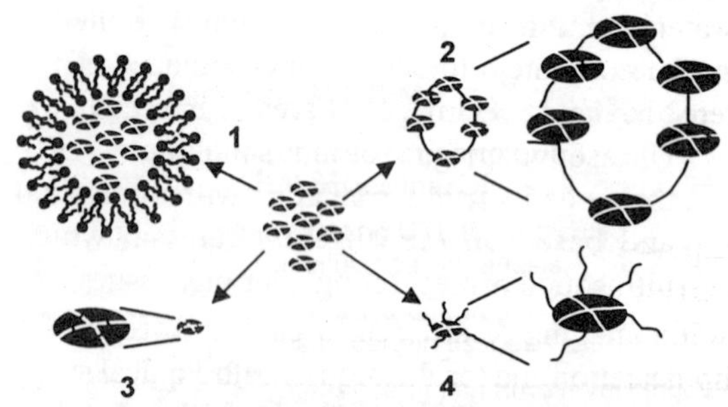

1. Liposome encapsulated haemoglobin;
2. Glutaraldehyde cross-linked haemoglobin;
3. Inter-molecularly cross-linked using chemical reagents; and
4. Polyoxyethylene-bound haemoglobin

Fig. 5-39 Various Synthetic Blood Substitutes.

Table 5-25. Some of Miscellaneous Products either Approved or Licensed for Human Use

System(s)	Drug	Target disease	Status	Product
Liposomes (Intravenous)	All-trans retinoic acid	Leukaemia	Phase II	Aronex, USA
Liposomes (D53) or VENTUS™ (Intravenous)	Prostaglandin E_1	Systemic inflammatory diseases (ARDC, AMI, SEPSIS/SIRS)	Phase II	The Liposome Company, USA
ALEC™	Dry powder of DPPC:PG	Expanding lung diseases in babies	Marketed in Europe	Britannia Pharm, UK

Table 5-26. Some of the Medical and Non-Medical Significance of Liposomes

Science domain(s)	Application(s)
Biophysics	Properties of cell membranes and channels
Biochemistry	Function of membrane proteins and their reconstitution in to artificial membranes
Physics	Characterization of soft and high mechanical strength materials
Chemistry	Catalysts, energy conversion, photosynthesis, biomineralization, compartmentalization of reactions
Physical chemistry and colloidal science	Colloidal behaviour and stability, thermodynamics of finite systems
Mathematics	Topology of 2-D surfaces in 3-D spaces and bilayer elasticity
Biology	Excretion, cell function, trafficking and cell signaling, gene delivery and function),
Ecology	Bioconversion of organic debris
Pharmacology	Studies of cell function and drug action
Pharmaceutical sciences	Drug delivery and targeting

administered as a reasonably good substitute for lung surfactant in very premature babies (Bangham, 1998). ALEC™ is a dry protein-free powder consisting of a 7:3 mole/mole mixture of DPPC and PG, and after administration reduces the burden of expanding air/water interface from 1 cm^2 to 2 cm^2 by lowering surface tension, which is most frequently administered in UK as a prophylactic lung surfactant.

CONCLUSION

Liposomes have been realized as extremely useful carrier systems, additive(s) and tools in various scientific domains. Some of the potentials of liposomes in the science domains are highlighted in Table 5-26. Thus, liposomes over the years have been investigated as the major drug delivery systems due to their flexibility to be tailored for varied desirable purposes. The flexibility in their behaviour can be exploited for the drug delivery through any route of administration and for any drug or material irrespective of its physicochemical properties. The uses of liposomes in the delivery of drugs and genes to tumour sites are promising and may serve as a handle for focus of future research.

REFERENCES

Abeles R. H., Frey P. A. and Jencks W. P. (1992) *Biochemistry* **24**, 235.

Abra R. M. and Hunt C. A. (1981) *Biochim. Biophys. Acta* **666**, 493.

Abraham W. and Downing D. T. (1990) *Biochim. Biophys. Acta* **1021**, 119.

Abraham W., Wertz P. W. and Downing D. T. (1988) *J. Invest. Dermatol.* **90**, 259.

Absolom D. (1986) *Methods in Enzymology* **132**, 28.

Adamson A. W. (1967) In: Physical Chemistry of Surface, II Ed., Interscience, New York, 223.

Allen T. M. (1993) *Adv. Drug Deliv. Rev.* **13**, 285.

Allen T. M. (1994) *Trends Pharm. Sci.* **15**, 215.

Allen T. M. and Cohn A. (1987) *FEBS Lett.* **223**, 42.

Allen T. M., Hansen C. and Rurledge J. (1989) *Biochim. Biophys. Acta* **981**, 27.

Allen T. M., Hansen C. B. and Lopez de Menezes D. E. (1995) *Adv. Drug Deliv. Rev.* **16**, 267.

Allen T. M., Hansen C. B. and Stuart D. D. (1998) In: Medical applications of liposomes, Lasic D. D. and Papahadjopoulos D. (Eds.), Elsevier, Oxford, 297.

Allen T.M. and Stuart D. D. (1999) In: Liposomes: Rational design, Janoff A. S. (Ed.), Marcel Dekker, New York, 63.

Allison A. C. and Gregoriadis G. (1975) *Nature* **252**, 252.

Alving C. R. (1992) *Biochim. Biophys. Acta* **1113**, 307.

Alving C.R. (1982) In: Targeting of Drugs, Gregoriadis G., Senior J. and Trouet A. (Eds.), Plenum press, New York, 285.

Amselem S., Gabizon A. and Barenholz Y. (1990) *Pharm. Res.* **79**, 1045.

Andrieux K., Lesieur S., Ollivon M. and Grabielle-Madelmont C. (1998) *J. Chromatogr. Biomed. Sci. Appl.* **706**,141.

Arica B., Ozer A.Y., Ercan M. T. and Hincal A. A. (1995) *J. Microencapsul.* **12**, 469.

Bacchawat B. K., Das P. K. and Ghosh P. K. (1984) In: Liposome Technology, Gregoiadis, G. (Ed.), CRC Press, Boca Raton, FL, 117.

Bakker-Wounderberg I. A., Storm G. and Woodle M. C. (1994) *J. Drug Target.* **2**, 363.

Bangham A. D. (1998) In: Medical applications of liposomes, Lasic, D. D. and Papahadjopoulos, D. (Eds.), Elsevier, Oxford, 455.

Bangham A. D., Standish M. M. and Watkins J. C. (1965) *J. Mol. Biol.* **13**, 328.

Barenholtz Y., Amselem S. and Lichtenberg D. (1979) *FEBS Lett.* **99**, 210.

Barenholz Y. (1998) In: Medical applications of liposomes, Lasic, D. D. and Papahadjopoulos, D. (Eds.), Elsevier, Oxford, 545.

Barenholz Y. and Cromellin D. J. A. (1994) In: Encyclopedia of pharmaceutical technology, Swarbrick J. (Ed.), Marcel Dekker, NY, 1.

Barlett G. R. (1959) *J. Biol. Chem.* **234**, 466.

Barrat G. M., Tenu J. P., Yapo A. and Petit J. F. (1986) *Biochim. Biophys. Acta* **862**, 153.

Batzri S. and Korn E. D. (1973) *Biochim. Biophys. Acta* **298**, 1015.

Behari J. R. and Gregoriadis G. (1992) *Int. J. Pharm.* **79**, 213.

Bhattacharya S. and Huang L. (1998) In: Medical applications of liposomes Lasic, D. D. and Papahadjopoulos, D. (Eds.), Elsevier, Oxford, 371.

Billingham M. and Bristow M. (1984) *Cancer Treat Symp.* **3**, 71.

Bisgaier C. L., Siebenkas M. V. and Williams K. J. (1989) *J. Biol. Chem.* **264**, 862.

Brooks C. J. W., MacLachlan J., Cole W. J. and Lawrie T. D. V. (1984) In: Proceedings of symposium on Analysis of Steroids, Szeged, Hungary, 349.

Buboltz J. T. and Feigenson G. W. (1999) *Biochim. Biophys. Acta* **1417**, 232.

Budker V., Gurevich V., Hagstrom J. E., Bortzov F. and Wolff J. A. (1996) *Nature* **14**, 760.

Ceve G., Schatzlein A. and Blume G. (1996) *J. Control. Rel.* **36**, 3.

Chapman D. (1975) *Quart. Rev. Biophys.* **8**, 185.

Chiang C. M. and Wiener N. (1987) In: Liposomes as drug carriers, Gregoriadis G. (Ed.), Wiley, Chichester, 599.

Chonn A. and Cullis P. R. (1998) *Adv. Drug Deliv. Rev.* **30**, 73.

Clerc S. and Barenholz Y. (1995) *Biochim. Biophys. Acta* **1240**, 257.

Conor J. and Huang L. (1985) *J. Cell Biol.* **101**, 582.

Crowe L. M. and Crowe J. H. (1993) In: Liposome Technology, Gregoriadis, G. (Ed.), Vol. I, Boca Raton, CRC Press, FL.

De Haan A., Tomee J. F. C., Huchshorn J. P. and Wilschut J. (1995) *Vaccine* **13**, 1320.

Deamer D. W. and Uster P. S. (1983) In: Liposomes, Ostro M.J. (Ed.), Marcel Dekker, New York, 25.

DeOliveria M. C., Fattal E., Couvreur P., Lesieur P., Bourgaux L, Ollivon M. and Dubernet C. (1998) *Biochim. Biophys. Acta* **1372**, 301.

Devissaguet J. P., Fessi H., Ammoury N. and Barratt G. (1992) In: Drug Delivery and Targeting: Concepts in dosage form design, Junginger H. E. (Ed.), Ellis Horwood, New York, 71.

Drummond D. C., Meyer O., Hong K., Kirpotin D. B. and Papahadjopoulos D. (1999) *Pharmacol. Rev.* **51**, 691.

Endicott J. A. and Ling V. (1989) *Annu. Rev. Biochem.* **58**, 137.

Enoch H. G., Stritamatter P. (1976) *Proc. Natl. Acad. Sci. USA* **76**, 145.

Felgner J. H., Kumar R., Sridhar R., Wheeler C., Tsai Y. J., Border R., Ramsay P., Martin M. and Felgner P. L. (1994) *J. Biol. Chem.* **269**, 2550.

Fidler I. J. (1992) *Res. Immunol.* **143**, 199.

Fildes F. J. T. (1981) In: Liposomes: From physical structure to therapeutic applications, Knight, K. (Ed.), Elsevier/North-Holland Biomedical press, UK.

Fischal M. A., Krown S. E. and O'Boyle K. P. (1993) *J. AIDS* **6**, 259.

FitzGerald D. J., Waldmann T. A., Willingham M.C. and Pastan I. (1984) *J. Clin. Invest.* **74**, 966.

Flegner L. P. (1996) *Human Gene Ther.* **7**, 1791.

Foldvari M., Gesztes A. and Mezei M. (1990) *J. Microencap.* **7**, 479.

Forssen E. A. and Ross M. E. (1994) *J. Liposome Res.* **4**, 481.

Forssen E. A., Male-Brune R., Adler-Moore J. P., Lee M. J. A., Schmidt, P. G., Krasieva T. B. and Shimizu S. (1996) *Cancer Res.* **56**, 2066.

Fresta M., Villiari A., Puglisi G. and Cavallaro G. (1993) *Int. J. Pharm.* **99**, 145.

Fry D. W., White C. and Goldman D. J. (1978) *Anal. Biochem.* **90**, 809.

Gabizon A. (1995) *Adv. Drug Deliv. Rev.* **16**, 285.

Gabizon A. Amselem S. and Goren D. (1990) *J. Lip. Res.* **1**, 491.

Gabizon A. and Papahadjopoulos D. (1988) *Proc. Natl. Acad. Sci. USA* **85**, 6949.

Gabizon A. and Papahadjopoulos D. (1992) *Biochim. Biophys. Acta* **1103**, 94.

Gabizon A., Catane R., Uziely B., Kaufman B., Safra T., Cohen R., Martin F. Hunag A. and Barenholz Y. (1994) *Cancer Res.* **54**, 987.

Gabizon A., Goron D., Horowitz A. T., Tzemach D., Lossos A. and Siegal T. (1997) *Adv. Drug Del. Rev* **24**, 337.

Gao X. and Huang L. (1996) *Biochemistry* **35**, 1027.

Gesztes A. and Mezei M. (1988) *Anesthesia and Analgesia* **67**, 1079.

Gluck R. (1995) *J. Liposome Res.* **5**, 467.

Gluck R., Mischler R., Brantschen S., Just M., Althaus B. and Cryz S. J. (1992) *J. Clin. Invest.* **90**, 2491.

Goins B., Klipper R., Rudolph A. S., Cliff R. O., Blumhardt R. and Phillips W. T. (1993) *J. Nucl. Med.* **34**, 2160.

Gold L. (1995) *J. Biol. Chem.* **270**, 13581.

Gordon S. and Rabinowitz S. (1989) *Adv. Drug Del. Rev.* **4**, 27.

Gould-Fogerite S., Mazurkiewicz J., Lehman J. and Mannino R. J. (1989) *Gene* **84**, 148.

Gray G. M. and White R. J. (1976) *Biochem. Soc. Trans.* **7**, 1129.

Gregoriadis G. (1976) *N. Eng. J. Med.* **295**, 704.

Gregoriadis G. (1984) In: Liposome Technology, Vol. 1, CRC Press, Boca Raton, FL.

Gregoriadis G. (1995) *Trends Biotechnol.* **13**, 527.

Gregoriadis G. and Florence A. T. (1993) In: Liposome Technology, Gregoriadis G. (Ed.), Vol. 1, CRC Press, Boca Raton, 37.

Gregoriadis G. and Senior J. (1980) *FEBS Lett.* **119**, 43.

Gregoriadis G., de Silva H. and Florence A. T. (1990) *Int. J. Pharm.* **65**, 235.

Gregoriadis G., Leathwood P. D. and Ryman B. E. (1971) *FEBS Lett.* **14**, 95.

Gregoriadis G., McCormack B., Perrie Y. and Saffie R. (1998) In: Medical applications of liposomes, Lasic D. D. and Papahadjopoulos D. (Eds.), Elsevier, Oxford, 61.

Gregoriadis G., Saffie R. and Hart S. L. (1996) *J. Drug Target.* **3**, 469.

Grit M. and Crommelin D. J. A. (1993) *Chem. Phys. Lipids* **64**, 3.

Grit M., Zuidam N. J. and Crommelin D. J. A. (1993) In: Liposome Technology, Gregoriadis G. (Ed.), Vol I, CRC Press, Boca Raton, FL, 455.

Gruber H. J., Wilmsen H. U., Schurga A., Pilger A. and Schindler H. (1995) *Biochim. Biophys. Acta* **1240**, 266.

Gulati M., Grover M., Singh S. and Singh M. (1998) *Int. J. Pharm.* **165**, 129.

Gunter K. K., Gunter T. E., Jarkowski A. and Rosier R. N. (1982) *Anal. Biochem.* **120**, 113.

Gustafsson J., Arvidson G., Karlsson G. and Almgren M. (1995) *Biochim. Biophys. Acta* **1235**, 305.

Hamilton R. L., Goerke J., Guo L. S. S., Williams M. C. and Havel R. J. (1980) *J. Lipid Res.* **21**, 981.

Hamm-Alvarez S. F. (1998) *Adv. Drug Deliv. Rev.* **29**, 229.

Hauser, H. and Gains, N. (1982) *Proc. Natl. Acad. Sci. USA* **79**, 1683.

Hiemenz J. W. and Walsh T. J. (1996) *Clin. Infect. Dis.* **22** (S-2), S113.

Holmberg E. G., Reuer Q. R., Geisert E. E. and Owens J. L. (1994) *Biochem. Biophys Res. Commun..* **201**, 888.

Hope M. J., Bally M. B., Webb G. and Culis P. R. (1985) *Biochim. Biophys. Acta* **812**, 55.

Hostetler K. Y., Stuhmiller L. M., Lenting H. B. M., van den Bosch H. and Richman D. D. (1990) *J. Biol. Chem.* **265**, 6112.

Hu Z., Niemiec S. M., Ramchandran C., Wallach D. F. H. and Weiner N. (1994) *STP Pharm. Sci.* **4**, 466.

Huang C. (1969) *Biochemistry* **8**, 344.

Hwang K. J. (1987) In: Liposome: From biophysics to therapeutics, Ostro M. J. (Ed.), Marcel Dekker, New York, 109.

Israelachvili J. N. (1991) In: Intramolecular and Surface Forces, Academic Press, New York.

Janoff A. S. (1993) *J. Liposome Res.* **3**, 451.

Jato J., Beissinger R., Zheng S., Shankey V., Fareed J., Sherwood R., McCormick D., Lasic D. and Martin F. (1998) In: Medical applications of liposomes, Lasic D. D. and Papahadjopoulos D. (Eds.), Elsevier, Oxford, 487.

Jones G. R. and Cossins A. R. (1989) In: Liposomes: A practical approach, New R. R. C. (Ed.), OIRL Press, Oxford, 184.

Jones M. N. (1994) *Adv. Drug Deliv. Rev.* **13**, 215.

Juliano R. L. and Akhtar S. (1992) *Antisense Res. Dev.* **2**, 165.

Juliano R. L. and Layton D. (1980) In: Drug delivery systems and biomedical application, Juliano R. L. (Ed.), Oxford University Press, New York.

Kartner N., Evernden,-Porelle D., Bradley G. and Ling V. (1985) *Nature* **316**, 820.

Katare O. P. and Vyas S. P. (1991) *J. Microencap.* **8**, 1.
Kirby C. J. and Gregoriadis G. (1980) *Life Sci.* **27**, 2223.
Kirby C. J. and Gregoriadis, G. (1984) *Biotechnol.* **2**, 979.
Kolchens S., Ramaswami V., Birgenheier J., Nett L. and O'Brien D. F. (1993) *Chem. Phys. Lipids* **65**, 1.
Korting H. C., Blecher P., Korting M. S. and Wendel A. (1991) *J. Am. Acad. Dermatol.* **25**, 1068.
Lasch J. and Wohlrab W. (1986) *Biomed. Biochim. Acta* **45**, 1295.
Lasic D. D. (1991) *Nature* **351**, 613.
Lasic D. D. (1988) *Biochem. Journal* **29**, 335.
Lasic D. D. (1993) In: Liposomes: From biophysics to applications, Elsevier, New York, 9.
Lasic D. D. (1997) In: Liposomes in gene therapy, CRC Press, Boca Raton, FL.
Lasic D. D. (1998) *Trends in Biotechnol.* **16**, 307.
Lasic D.D. and Papahadjopoulos, D. (1998) In: Medical Applications of liposomes, Elsevier, New York.
Lasic D. D., Ceh D. D., Stuart M. C. A., Guo L., Frederik P. M. and Barenholz Y. (1995) *Biochim. Biophys. Acta* **1239**, 145.
Ledley F. D. (1995) *Human Gene Ther.* **6**, 1129.
Lee R. J. and Huang L. (1996) *J. Biol. Chem.* **271**, 8481.
Legender J. Y. and Szoka Jr. F. C. (1992) *Pharm. Res.* **9**, 1235.
Lesieur S., Grabielle-Madelmont C., Paternostre M. T. and Ollivon M. (1991) *Anal. Biochem.* **192**, 334.
Liu Y., Liggitt D., Zhong W., Tu G., Gaensler K. and Debs R. J. (1995) *J. Biol. Chem.* **270**, 24864.
Lopez-Berestein G., Mehta R., Hopffer R., Mills K., Kasi L., Mehta K., Fainstein V., Luna M., Harsh E. N. and Juliano R. (1983) *J. Infect. Dis.* **147**, 939.
Lund P., Fuller L., Fritz T., Kulik B., Herres B. and Tilcock C. (1991) *J. Ultrasound Met.* **10**, S44.
Mandal T. K. and Downing D. T. (1993) *Acta Derm. Venereol.* **73**, 12.
Marjan M. J. and Allen T. M. (1996) *Biotechnol.* **14**, 151.
Marsh M. (1984) *Biochim. J.* **218**, 110.
Marshall W. and Caruthers M. (1993) *Science* **259**, 1564.
Martin F. J. (1990) In: Specialized drug delivery systems: Manufacturing and production technology, Tyle P. (Ed.), Marcel Dekker, 267.
Mayer L. D., Cullis P. R. and Balley M. B. (1998) In: Medical applications of liposomes, Papahadjopoulos D. and Lasic D. (Eds.), Elsevier Science BV, New York, 231.
Mayer L. D., Dougherty G., Harasym T. O. and Balley M. B. (1997) *J. Pharmacol. Exp. Ther.* **280**, 1406.
Mayer L. D., Hope M. J., Cullis R. P. and Janoff A. S. (1985) *Biochim. Biophys. Acta* **817**, 193.
Mayhew E., Lazo R., Vali W. J., King J. and Green A. M. (1984) *Biochim. Biophys. Acta* **775**, 169.
Mazei M. and Gulasekhram V. (1980) *Life Sci.* **26**, 1473.
Moghimi S. M. and Patel H. M. (1989) *Biochim. Biophys. Acta* **984**, 379.
Moghimi S. M. and Patel H. M. (1993) *J. Microencap.* **2**, 155.
Moghimi S. M. and Patel H. M. (1998) *Adv. Drug Deliv. Rev.* **32**, 45.
Moon M. H. and Giddings J. C. (1993) *J. Pharm. Biomed. Anal.* **11**, 911.
Mor G., Yamschikov G., Sedegah M., Takeno M., Wang R., Houghten R. A., Hoffman S. and Klinman M. (1996) *J. Clin. Invest.* **98**, 2700.
Morell A. G., Irrine R. A., Sternlieb I., Schinberg I. H. and Ashwell G. (1968) *J. Biol. Chem.* **243**, 155.
Morgan C. G., Thomas E. W. and Yianni Y. P. (1983) *Biochim. Biophys. Acta* **728**, 356.
Muggia F. M., Hainsworth J. D., Jeffers S., Miller P., Groshen S., Tan M., Roman L., Uziely B., Muderspach L., Garcia A., Burnett A. and Greco F.A. (1997) *J. Clin. Oncol.* **15**, 987.
Muller-Goymann C. C., Hamann H. J. (1991) *Eur. J. Pharm. Biopharm.* **37**, 113.
Nakata T., Sobue K. and Hirokawa N. (1990) *J Cell Biol.* **110**, 13.
New R.R.C. (1989) In: Liposomes: A practical approach, OIRL Press, Oxford, London, 1.
Niesman M. R., Khoobehi B., Magin R. L. and Webb A. G. (1994) *J. Liposome Res.* **4**, 741.
Ohsawa T., Miura H. and Harada K. (1985) *Pharm. Bull.* **33**, 2916.
Oku N. and MacDonald R. C. (1983) *Biochemistry* **22**, 855.
Ostro M. J. (1987) In: Liposomes: From biophysics to therapeutics, Marcel Dekker, New York.
Papahadjopoulos D., Cowden M. and Kimelberg H. (1973) *Biochim. Biophys. Acta.* **310**, 8.
Papahadjopoulos D., Vali W. J., Jacobson K. and Poste G. (1975) *Biochim. Biophys. Acta* **394**, 483.
Patel H. M. (1992) *Crit. Rev. Ther. Drug Carr. Syst.* **9**, 39.
Perkins W. R., Minchey S. R., Ostro M. J., Taraschi T. F. and Janoff A. S. (1988) *Biochim. Biophys. Acta* **943**, 103.
Ropert C., Lavingnon M., Dubernet C., Couvreur P. and Malvy C. (1992) *Biochim. Biophys. Res. Commun.* **183**, 879.
Rubas W., Suersaxo A., Weder H.G., Hartmann H.R., Hengartener H., Schott H. and Schwendener R. (1986) *Int. J. Cancer* **37**, 149.
Rudolph A. S. (1995) In: Liposomes in biomedical applications, Shek, P.N. (Ed.), Harwood Academic Publisher, UK, 217.
Saito K., Ando J., Yoshida M., Haga M. and Kato Y. (1988) *Chem. Pharm. Bull.* **36**, 4187.

Sasaki H., Takakura Y., Hashida M., Kimura T. and Sezaki H. (1984) *J. Pharm. Dyn.* **7**, 120.

Schmid M. H. and Korting H. C. (1996) *Adv. Drug Deliv. Rev.* **18**, 335.

Schmidtgen M. C., Drechsler M., Lasch J. and Schubert R. (1998) *J. Microsc.* **191**,177.

Schreier H. and Bouwstra J. (1994) *J. Control. Rel.* **30**, 1.

Schroit A. L. and Fidler I. J. (1986) In: Medical application of liposomes, Yagi, K. (Ed.), Japan Scientific Societies Press, Tokyo, 141.

Seltzer S. E. (1989) *Radiology* **171**, 19.

Seymour L. W. (1992) *Crit. Rev. Ther. Drug Carr. Syst.* **9**, 135.

Sharma A. and Straubinger R. M. (1994) *Pharm. Res.* **11**, 889.

Shermatova S. Z. (1990) *Br. J. Rhematol.* **27S**, 118.

Sherwood R. L., McCormick D. L., Zheng S. and Beissinger R. L. (1995) *Artificial cells, blood substitutes, and immobilization technology* **23**, 665.

Singh P., Sihorkar V., Jaitely V., Kanaujia P. and Vyas S.P. (2000) *Ind. J. Pharmacol.* **32**, 269.

Sone S. and Fidler I. J. (1980) *J. Immunol.* **125**, 2454.

Sorgi F. L. and Huang L. (1996) *Int. J. Pharm.* **144**, 131.

Stenseth K. and Thyberg P. (1989) *Eur. J. Cell Biol.* **49**, 326.

Stewart J. C. M. (1959) *Anal. Biochem.* **104**, 10.

Storm G. and Crommelin J. A. (1998) *Pharm. Science Technol. Today* **1**, 19.

Sunamoto J., Sakai K., Sato T. and Kondo H. (1988) *Chem. Lett.* **10**, 1781.

Szoka F. and Papahadjopoulos D. (1978) *Proc. Natl. Acad. Sci. USA* **75**, 4194.

Talsma H. and Crommelin D. J. A. (1992b) In: Liposomes as Drug Delivery Systems, Part II: Characterization, Pharmaceutical Technology, 16, 52.

Talsma H., van Steenbergen M. J. and Crommelin D. J. A. (1992) *Cryobiology* **29**, 80.

Talsma, H. and Crommelin D.J.A. (1992a) Liposomes as Drug Delivery Systems, Part I: Preparation, Pharmaceutical Technology, 16, 96.

Terao J., Asano I. and Matsushito S. (1985) *Lipids* **20**, 312.

Tilcock C. (1995) In: Liposomes as tools in basic research and industry, Philippot J. R. and Schuber F. (Eds.), CRC Press, Boca Raton, FL, 225.

Tilcock C., Ahkong Q. F. and Fisher D. (1993) *Biochim. Biophys. Acta* **1148**, 77.

Torchilin V. P. (1998) In: Medical applications of liposomes, Lasic D. D. and Papahadjopoulos D. (Eds.), Elsevier, Oxford, 515.

Torchilin V. P. and Trubetskoy V. S. (1995) *J. Liposome Res.* **5**, 795.

Torchilin V. P., Narula J., Halpern E. and Khaw B.A. (1996) *Biochim. Biophys. Acta* **1279**, 75.

Trubetskoy V. S. and Torchilin V. P. (1994) *J. Liposome Res.* **4**, 961.

Tsuchida E. (1994) *Artificial cells, blood substitutes, and immobilization technology* **22**, 467.

Tsuchida E. (1995) Liposomes in biomedical applications, Shek P.N. (Ed.), Harwood Academic Publisher, UK, 2241.

Tucker R.W., Meltzer M.S. and Sanford K.K. (1981) *Int. J. Cancer* **27**, 555.

Uster P.S. and Deamer D.W. (1981) *Arch. Biochem. Biophys.* **209**, 385.

Utsumi T., Aizono Y. and Funatsu G. (1987) *FEBS Lett.* **216**, 99.

Vaage J., Donavan D., Loftus T., Abra R., Working P. and Hunag A. (1994) *Cancer* **73**, 2366.

Vadiei K., Lopez-Berestein G., Parez-Soler R. and Luke D. R. (1989) *Int. J. Pharm.* **57**, 133.

Vaizoglu M. O. and Speiser P. P. (1986) *Acta Pharm. Suec.*, **23**, 163.

Van Rooijen N. (1990) *Adv. Biotechnol. Progresses* **13**, 255.

van Winden E. C. A., Zuidam N. J. and Crommelin D. J. A. (1998) In: Medical applications of liposomes, Lasic D. D. and Papahadjopoulos D. (Eds.), Elsevier, Oxford, 567.

Vyas S .P., Singh A. and Sihorkar V. (2001) *Crit. Rev. Ther. Drug Carr. Syst.* **18**, 1.

Vyas S. P. and Sihorkar V. (2000) *Adv. Drug Deliv. Rev.* **43**, 101.

Vyas S. P., Katare Y.K., Mishra V. and Sihorkar V. (2000) *Int. J. Pharm.* **210**, 1.

Vyas, S. P. and Sihorkar, V. (2001) In: Advances in liposomal therapeutics, Vyas S. P. and Dixit V. (Eds.), CBS Publishers, New Delhi, 230.

Wang C. Y. and Huang L. (1989) *Biochemistry* **28**, 9508.

Wang C.Y. and Huang L. (1987) *Biochem. Biophys. Res. Comm.* **147**, 980.

Wasan M. W. and Lopez-Berestein G. (1998) In: Medical applications of liposomes, Lasic D. D. and Papahadjopoulos D. (Eds.), Elsevier, Oxford, 165.

Wassef N. M., Alving C. R. and Richards R. L. (1994) *Immunol. Methods* **4**, 217.

Weiner N. and Lieb L. (1998) In: Medical applications of liposomes, Lasic D. D. and Papahadjopoulos D. (Eds.), Elsevier, Oxford, 493.

Weiner N., Martin F. and Riaz M. (1989) *Drug Dev. Ind. Phar.* **15**, 1523.

Weiner N., Williams N., Birch G., Ramchandran C., Shipman C. Jr. and Flynn G. (1989) *Antimicrob. Agents Chemother.* **33**, 1217.

Wiener N. and Chiang C. M. (1988) *Int. J. Pharm.* **37**, 75.

Woodle M. C. and Lasic D. D. (1992) *Biochim. Biophys. Acta* **1113**, 171.

Woodle M. C. and Leserman L. (1998) In: Medical applications of liposomes, Lasic, D. D. and Papahadjopoulos, D. (Eds.), Elsevier, Oxford, 429.

Woodle M. C., Newman M. S. and Cohen J. A. (1994) *J. Drug Target.* **2**, 397.

Working P. K., Newman M. S. and Hunag S. K. (1994) *J. Liposome Res.* **4**, 667.

Wybenga D. R., Pileggi V. J., Dirstine P. H. and Di Giorgio J. (1970) *J. Clin. Chem.* **16**, 980.

Yamauchi H., Yano T., Kato T., Tanak I., Nakbayashi S., Higashi K., Miyoshi S. and Yamda H. (1995) *Int. J. Pharm.* **113**, 141.

Yasuda T. (1986) In: Medical application of liposomes, Yagi K. (Ed.), Japan Scientific Societies Press, Tokyo, 155.

Yasuda T., Naito Y., Tsumita T. and Okada H. (1981) *Immunol. Methods* **44**, 153.

Yoss N. L., Popescu O., Pop V. I., Porutiu D., Kummerow F. A. and Benga G. (1985) *Biosci. Rep.* **5**, 1.

Zelphati O., Francis C. and Szoka Jr. F. C. (1996) *J. Control. Rel.* **41**, 99.

Zuidam N. J. and Crommelin D. J. A. (1995) *J. Pharm. Sci.* **84**, 1113.

Zuidam N. J., Talsma H. and Crommelin D. J. A. (1996) In: Handbook of nonmedical applications of liposomes: From design to microreactors, Barenholz Y. and Lasic D. D. (Eds.), CRC Press, London, 71.

CHAPTER 6

Niosomes

- Introduction
- Physicochemical aspects of non-ionic surfactant vesicles
- Methods of preparation
- Separation of free drug
- Characterization of niosomes
- Stability of niosomes
- Rheological properties of niosomal dispersion
- Solute release profile form niosomal formulations
- Colloidal properties of niosomal dispersion
- Discomes
- Nsvs reversed vesicles
- Non-ionic surfactant vesicle-in-water-in-oil (v/w/o) systems
- Non-ionic surfactant based organogels
- Polymer coated nonionic surfactant vesicles
- Proniosomes
- Non-ionic surfactant vesicles and their therapeutic potential
- References

Non-ionic surfactant vesicles (niosomes or NSVs) are now widely studied as an alternative to liposomes (Baillie et al., 1985). Non-ionic surfactant vesicle results from the self-assembly of hydrated surfactant monomers. Non-ionic surfactants of a wide variety of structural types have been found to be useful alternatives to phospholipids in the fabrication of vesicular systems (Florence, 1993). Though the terminology suggests that distinctions exist between niosomes and liposomes of which the former is having chemical differences in the monomer units, niosomes possess physical properties, which are similar to liposomes, which are formed from phospholipids. As the name indicates, generally, non-ionic surfactant vesicles are prepared by incorporation of components containing non-ionic surfactants (Kronberg et al., 1990). However, they may also be prepared with various ionic amphiphiles such as dicetylphosphate, stearylamine, etc., (Azmin et al., 1985; Florence et al., 1990) in order to achieve a stable vesicular suspension.

A schematic diagram of a niosome, formed with non-ionic surfactant and cholesterol is shown in Figure 6-1. Non-ionic surfactants form a variety of aggregates from micelles to large vesicles, which can be used as vehicles for drug delivery. These include, drug carriers in oncology (Rogerson et al., 1988; Kerr et al., 1988; Florence et al., 1990; Uchegbu et al., 1993; Azmin et al., 1985), for delivery of antiparasitic agents (Baillie et al., 1986; Carter et al., 1987), cosmetic formulations (Handjiani-Vila et al., 1979; Handjiani-Vila et al., 1993), topical vehicles (Mezei et al., 1993) and as potential diagnostic devices (Hillis, 1993).

Niosomes are essentially non-ionic surfactant based multilamellar or unilamellar vesicles in which an aqueous solution of solute(s) is entirely enclosed by a membrane resulted from the organization of surfactant macro-molecules as bilayers. Similar to liposomes, niosomes are formed on hydration of non-ionic surfactant film, which eventually hydrates imbibing or encapsulating the hydrating aqueous

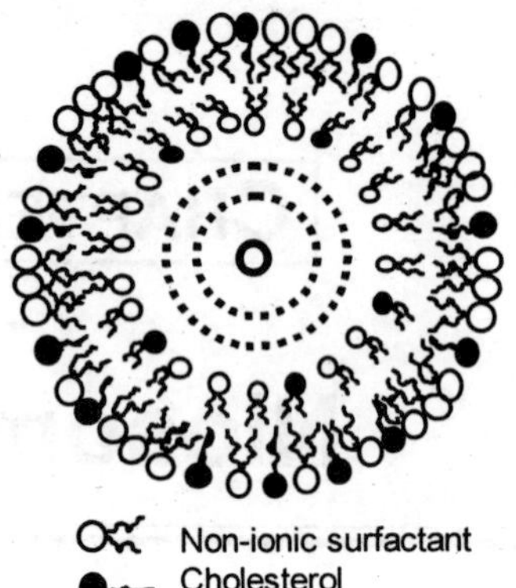

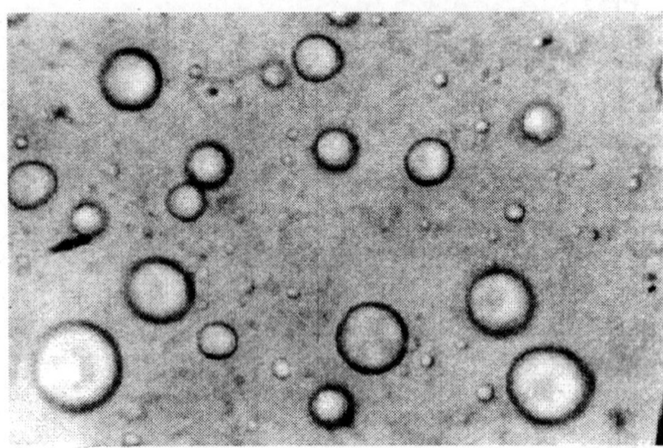

Fig. 6-1. Schematic Representation and Photomicrograph of Non-ionic Surfactant Vesicle (Niosome)

solution (Baillie et al., 1985; Stafford et al., 1988). The liposomes which, are highly organized lipoidal vesicles have been adopted well for extensive studies. However, their potential use as a carrier system appeared to limit at best, in treating lysosomal storage diseases owing to an quantitative and rapid interception of liposomes and their contents by reticuloendothelial system (RES). The enormous strides in the area of research pertaining to liposomes have been made, which provide informations on biofate and *in vivo* interactions of liposomes or vesicular drug carrier systems. The latter could be considered to be an important information, which may be harnessed to circumvent the physiological, and anatomical barriers encountered in a biosystem.

Nearly 25 odd years of continual and intensive research culminated the first liposomal formulation (AmBisome®) to be licensed for use in human beings. The natural lipid(s) used as principle constituents of liposomes are of biological origin and highly susceptible to oxidation and pH effects. Likewise, the purity of lipids used in the preparation of liposomes affects the size, shape and stability of liposomes significantly. Thus, the sequential consequences of deteriorative susceptibility, the cost of the lipids and specific handling procedures are some of the obstacles which come in way of practical adaptation of liposomes as drug carrier systems (Kempt and Crommelin, 1988). It has been proposed and suggested that niosomes could be used as an alternate version of liposomes to modify the biodistribution and activity profile of drug(s). Compared to phospholipids used in liposomes, the synthetic non-ionic surfactants used in the preparation of niosomes are chemically stable, precise in chemical composition and cheaper in cost (Baillie et al., 1985).

Amphiphiles other than natural phospholipids have also been studied and found to form vesicular system similar to liposomes in physical characteristics. The other amphiphiles noted to form vesicles include saturated (Gebicki and Hicks, 1976) and unsaturated fatty acids (Okahota et al., 1981), synthetic ionic and non-ionic surfactants (Handjani-vila et al., 1979) and lipid conjugated pharmacophores (Vaizoglu and Spieser, 1986).

Emphasis has been placed on slow release of drug, resulting into sustained activity, reduced toxicity, targeting and modifications of distribution profile of drugs as aims of vesicular systems development. Drug targeting is a process, which is accomplished through size and surface charge of the colloidal particles as drug carriers. However, targeting to specific cells such as macrophages is a consequence of vectoring process wherein chemical or biodeterminants are attached to or coated on vesicles surface in order to negotiate more specialized uptake of the vesicular system (Burkhnov et al., 1988).

PHYSICOCHEMICAL ASPECTS OF NON-IONIC SURFACTANT VESICLES

Structural Components and Niosomes Bilayer

L'Oreals reported alkyl and dialkyl polyglycerol ethers as vesicle forming non-ionic surfactant (Tanaka et al., 1990). Muller and Goymann, 1987 investigated bilayer-forming characteristics of PEG-polyglycols and polyethylene ethers systems. Dialkylpolyglycerol and dialkylpolyoxyethylene ethers (Vanlerbergh et al., 1978) are structurally similar to the natural phospholipids, yet free to acquire various configurations. Other bilayer forming amphipathic substances are steroidal oxyethylene ethers (Vanlerberghe and Handjani, 1975), laurat ethers (Echegoyan et al., 1988), alkyl galactosides (Yoshioka et al., 1990), sorbitan monooleate (Chandraprakash et al., 1991), and polyoxyethylated-hydrogenated castor oil (Tanaka et al., 1990).The hydrophilic and hydrophobic variations determined by HLB number and balance between hydrophilic and hydrophobic interaction resulted from forces of attraction and repulsion are crucial in determining the type of aggregates which could form in an aqueous environment, i.e. spherical or asymmetrical micelles, mesophases or vesicles.

Like lipids the non-ionic surfactants also orient in an aqueous medium as planner bilayer lattices wherein polar or hydrophilic heads align facing aqueous bulk (media) while hydrocarbon segments are so aligned that their interaction with aqueous media is minimized. Every bilayer for thermodynamic reasons folds over itself to be a continuous membrane, i.e. forms a vesicle so that hydrocarbon/water interface remains no more exposed. Obviously, every intracalated liquid compartment exists isolated from continuous phase. The alignment of amphiphiles in bilayer is mainly attributed to hydrophobic interaction in order to avoid or minimize unfavourbale thermodynamic state resulted due to the exposure of hydrocarbon segments to an aqueous bulk. Such interactions could be avoided effectively in closed/sealed vesicular shape as compared to planner bilayer orientation (Gregoriadis, 1993). An understanding of x-ray crystallography reveals that in a bilayer membrane the glycerol between the two segments of carbon chain orients approximately perpendicular to the plane of membrane. When the bilayer thickness calculated theoretically and compared with the actually determined one, it was noticed that the length of straight carbon segment was not in accordance with bilayer thickness. The variation in thickness may be attributed to a tilt in carbon chain at bridging carbon. The tilt may in turn affect the orientation and packaging of membrane components and as a consequence its thickness (New, 1990).

Various physicochemical aspects of non-ionic surfactants vesicles required for their behaviour as delivery vectors are being discussed in the preceding paragraphs.

Basic Structural Units of NSVs

It is important to identify and know the basic structural units of NSVs. While an amphiphilic nature is an inexplicable prerequisite for molecules to form vesicular assemblies (Israelachvili, 1985), variations are abound in the nature of facilitating hydrophilic head groups. Principal among vesicle forming non-ionic compounds are the alkyl ether lipids. These can be broadly divided into two classes based on the nature of their hydrophilic head group : alkyl ethers in which the hydrophilic head group essentially consists of repeat glycerol subunits, related isomers or larger sugar molecules, and those in which the hydrophilic head group consists of a repeat ethylene oxide subunits. In addition, alkyl esters, amides and fatty acids and amino acid compounds also form vesicles (Uchegbu and Vyas, 1998).

Alkyl Ethers

Alkyl glycerol ethers synthesized by L'Oreal, France (Vanlerberghe et al., 1972) were the first compounds reported to form NSVs (Fig. 6-2). L'Oreal non-ionic surfactants have been explored for a wide variety of drug delivery applications. Surfactant I to III and other surfactants are developed by L'Oreal, used for the preparation of niosomes containing sodium stibogluconate. Surfactant I (Mol. wt. 473). is C_{16} monoalkyl glycerol ether ether with average of 3 glycerol units. Surfactant II (Mol. wt. 972) is diglycerol ether with average of 7 glycerol unit and Surfactant III (Mol. wt. 393) is ester linked surfactant. Apart from the alkyl glycerol their analogues, alkyl

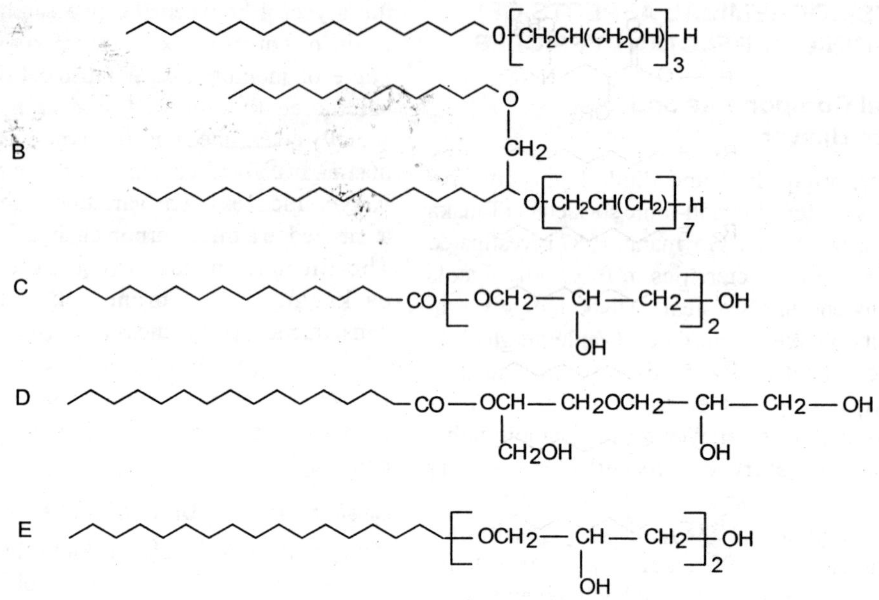

Fig. 6-2. Alkyl Glyceryl Ethers

glycosides have also been studied as drug carriers (Kiwada et al., 1985a; Kiwada et al., 1985b; Kiwada et al., 1988). In addition, a class of alkyl ethers bearing polyhydroxyl head groups is also reported as a group of vesicle forming surfactants (Fig. 6-3) (Assadullahi et al., 1991).

The second group of alkyl ether amphiphiles in which the hydrophilic head group consists of ethylene oxide units have also received considerable attention (Fig. 6-4) (Tanaka et al., 1990; Okahata et al., 1981; Chauhan and Lawence, 1989; Bowstra et al., 1990; Hofland et al., 1992).

Alkyl Esters

The widely used alkyl ester in food industry, the sorbitan esters (Fig. 6-5), have been studied as the basic building block of NSVs (Yoshioka and Florence, 1994; Yoshioka et al., 1994; Uchegbu, 1994; Chandraprakash et al., 1990; Chandraprakash et al., 1994; Udupa et al., 1993; Parthasarathi et al., 1994; Yoshioka et al., 1995).

Preparation of vesicles with polyoxyethylene sorbitan monolaurate (Polysorbate 20; Fig. 6-6) a relatively soluble surfactant has been reported (Murtas et al., 1994). Similarly, encapsulation of diclofenac sodium into polysorbate 60 has also been reported (Raja Naresh et al., 1994). A non-ionic surfactant vesicle formulation consisting of a mixture of alkyl ether and alkyl ester surfactants, namely polyoxyethylene-10-stearyl ether ($C_{18}EO_{10}$):glyceryl laurate ($C_{12}G_{1}$):cholesterol (27:15:57), has been used in the transdermal delivery of cyclosporin A (Niemiec et al., 1994).

Alkyl Amides

Alkyl galactosides and glucosides incorporating amino acid spacers have also been found to produce vesicles (Fig. 6-7)(Zarif et al., 1993; Guedj et al., 1994; Griener et al., 1993). While as a general rule, the alkyl groups in all vesicle forming amphiphiles consist of fully or partially saturated C_{12} to C_{22} hydrocarbons, certain novel amide compounds bearing fluorocarbon chains (Fig. 6-8) reported, form vesicles and small disk shaped structures which could have potential use as drug carriers.

Fatty acids and Amino acid Compounds

Amino acid moieties, when made suitably amphiphilic by the addition of hydrophobic alkyl side chains, form vesicles (Fig. 6-9) (Neumann and Ringsdor, 1986). Peptide liposomes were prepared using these amino acid vesicles in the presence of a water-soluble carbodimide condensing agent. Long

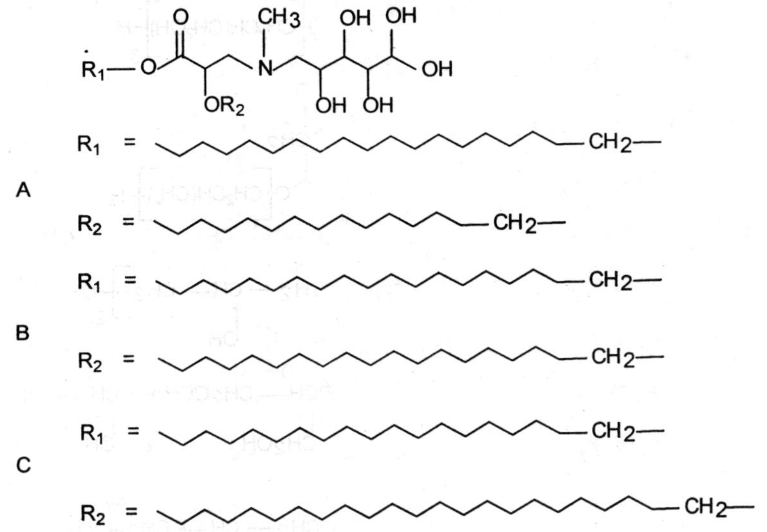

Fig. 6-3. Alky Glyceryls and their Analogues

chain fatty acids also form "Ufasomes", closed vesicles formed from fatty acid bilayers (Gebicki and Hick, 1976).

Other Structural Components

Cholesterol

Steroids are important components of cell membrane and their presence in membrane brings about discernible changes in regard to bilayer fluidity and permeability. Cholesterol can be incorporated in bilayers at significantly higher molar ratio, however, by itself it does not form bilayers. Thus, it could be used to ameliorate and manipulate the bilayer characteristics (Fig. 6-10).

Being amphipathic in nature cholesterol aligns itself in such a way that its OH group orients towards aqueous phase while aliphatic chain aligns parallel to the hydrocarbon chain of surfactant. Further, in a mixed molecular bilayer it occupies an alternate position. Thus, 3 β–hydroxyl group could be positioned with polar glycerol and hydroxyl group of surfactant molecules allowing very little vertical movements. The presence of rigid steroidal skeleton along side the carbon chain of surfactant could possibly restrict the freedom of movements of the carbons of hydrocarbon segment thus providing an absolute rigidization. The free space occupation of cholesterol minimizes the amphiphile carbon segment tilt vis a vis provides rigidization to the bilayer (New, 1990). As in the case of liposomes hydrophilicity, lipophilicity, temperature of hydration and phase transition temperature (Tc) are of importance similarly for non-ionic surfactants, the hydrophilic-hydrophobic segments and a balance between them are of paramount importance. It has been observed that glucosides of myristyl, cetyl and stearyl alcohols form the vesicles whilst glucosides of lauryl, decyl and octyl alcohols do not form vesicles. The surfactants once transformed into the vesicles their entrapping efficiency has been established to be related to the nature, size and polarity of the polar heads of surface active amphiphiles. In a well designed study Israelachvili has classically discussed the significance of dimensions of optimal head group area (Kiwada et al., 1985a). Israelachvili, 1985 in his study used an equation to compute critical packing parameter.

v/a. Ic = critical packing parameter

where, v = is hydrocarbon chain volume, a = is optimal head group area and Ic is hydrocarbon chain length.

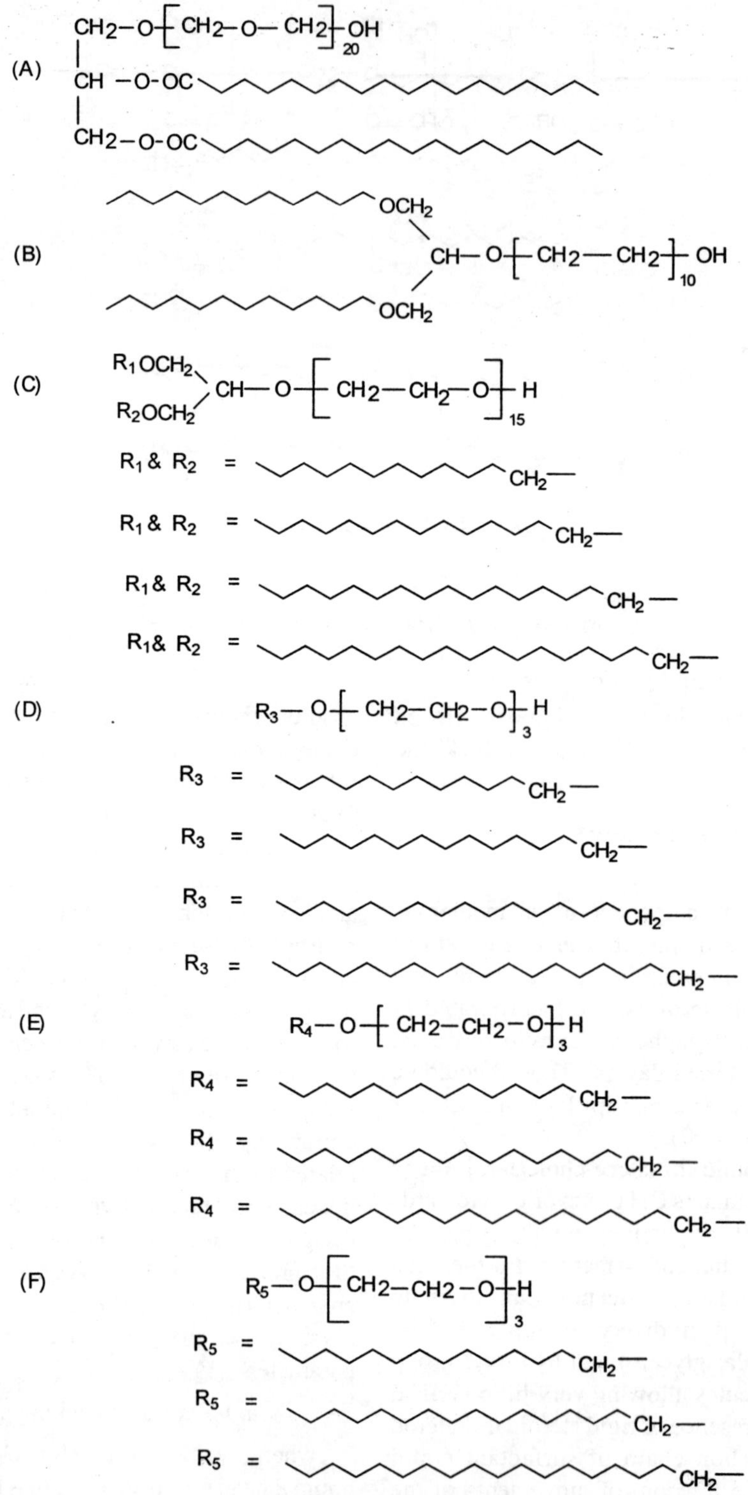

(A) $CH_2-O-[CH_2-O-CH_2]_{20}-OH$; $CH-O-OC$; CH_2-O-OC

(B) OCH_2; $CH-O-[CH_2-CH_2]_{10}-OH$; OCH_2

(C) R_1OCH_2, R_2OCH_2 $CH-O-[CH_2-CH_2-O]_{15}-H$

R_1 & R_2 = CH_2—

R_1 & R_2 = CH_2—

R_1 & R_2 = CH_2—

R_1 & R_2 = CH_2—

(D) $R_3-O-[CH_2-CH_2-O]_3-H$

R_3 = CH_2—

R_3 = CH_2—

R_3 = CH_2—

R_3 = CH_2—

(E) $R_4-O-[CH_2-CH_2-O]_3-H$

R_4 = CH_2—

R_4 = CH_2—

R_4 = CH_2—

(F) $R_5-O-[CH_2-CH_2-O]_3-H$

R_5 = CH_2—

R_5 = CH_2—

R_5 = CH_2—

Fig. 6-4. Alkyl Ether Amphiphiles with Hydrophilic Head Group consists of Ethylene Oxide (contd.)

(G)

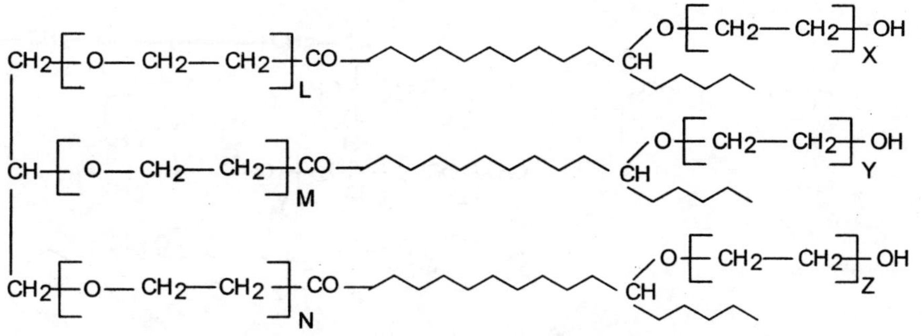

(H)

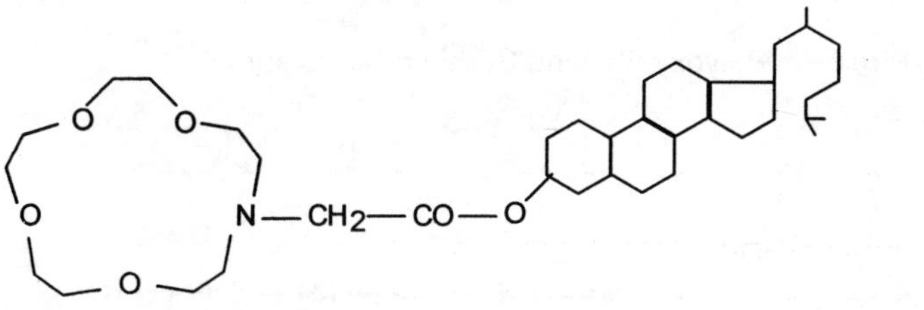

Fig. 6-4. Alkyl Ether Amphiphiles with Hydrophilic Head Group consists of Ethylene Oxide

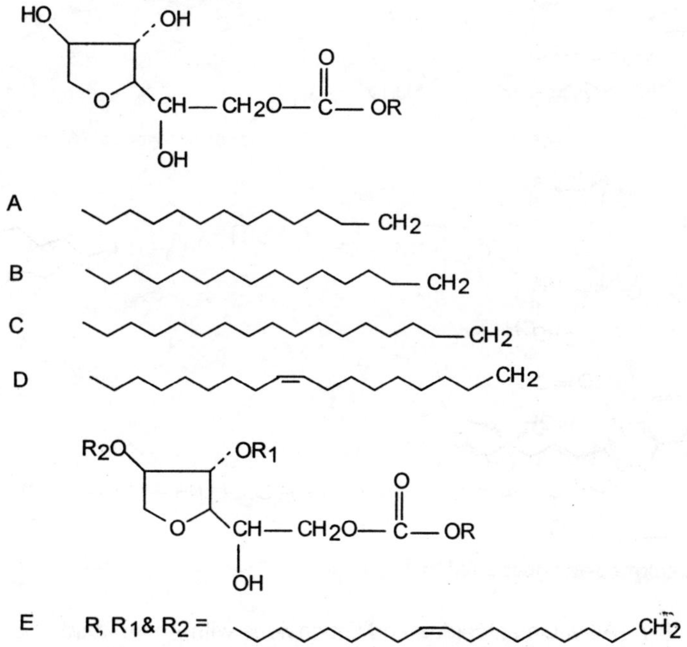

A

B

C

D

E R, R_1& R_2 =

Fig. 6-5. Sorbiton Esters

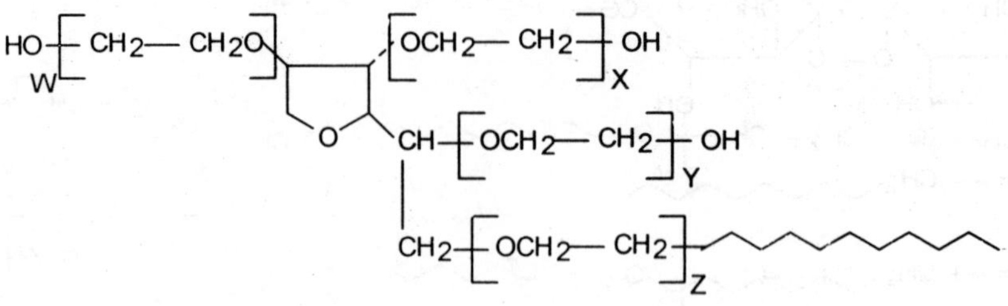

Polysorbate 20 (W+X+Y+Z = 20)

Fig. 6-6. Polyoxyethylene Sorbiton Monolaurate

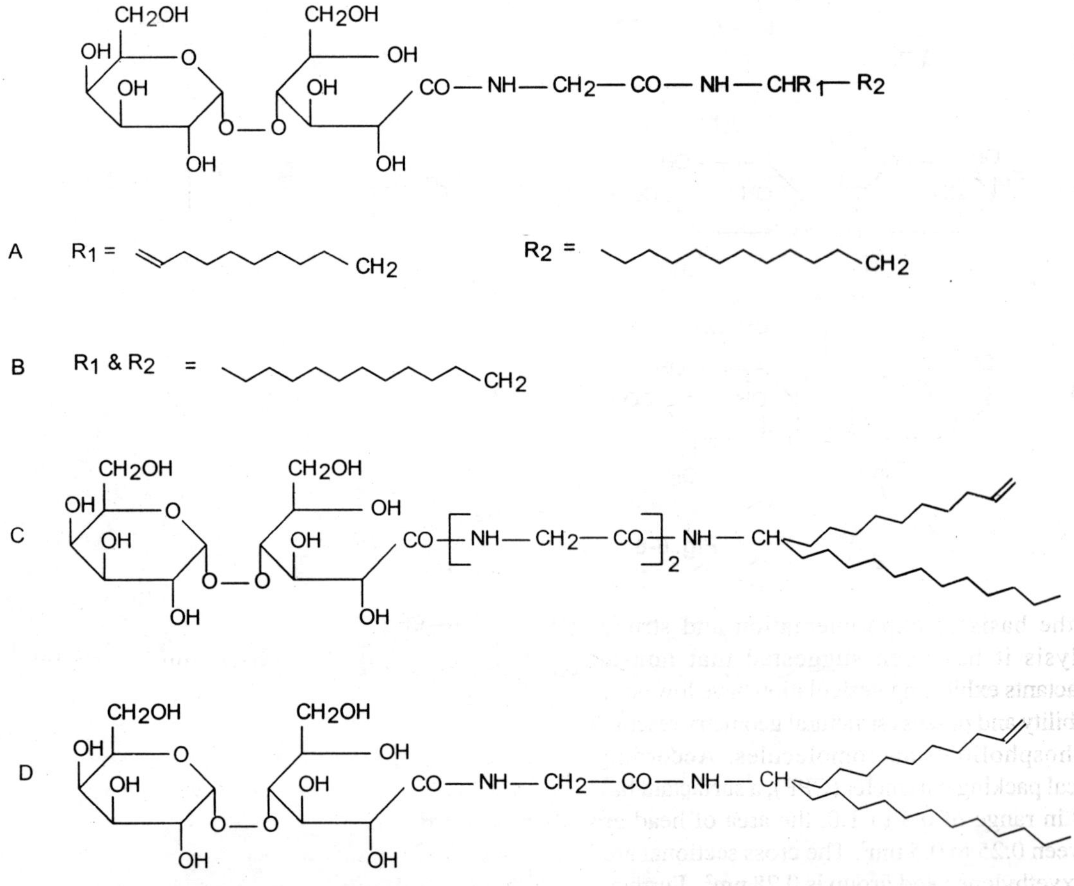

A R_1 = CH_2 R_2 = CH_2

B R_1 & R_2 = CH_2

C

D

Fig. 6-7. Alkyl Galactosides and Glucosides with Amino acid Spacer

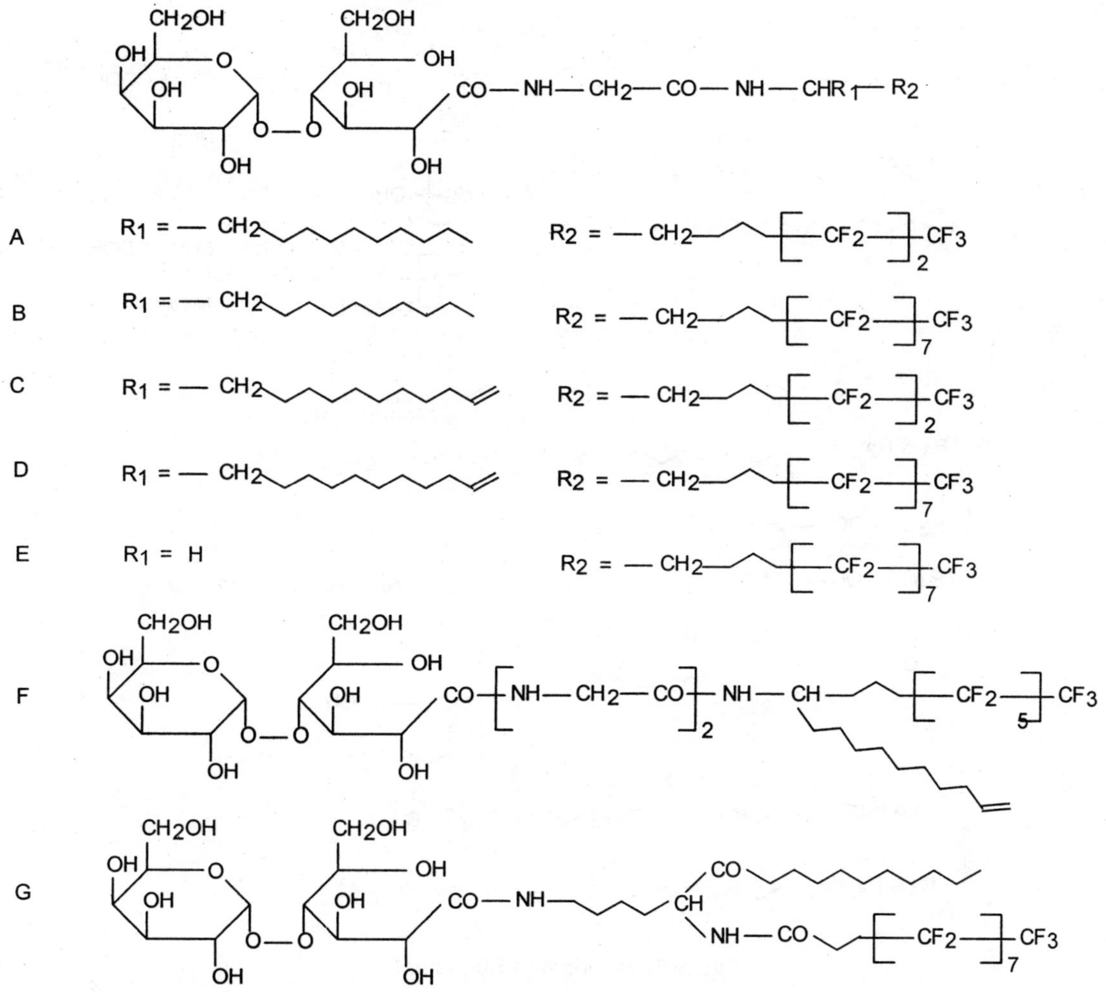

Fig. 6-8. Fluorinated surfactants

On the basis of experimentation and structural analysis it has been suggested that non-ionic surfactants exhibiting vesiculation have low aqueous solubility and possess structural geometry resembling to phospholipid macromolecules. According to critical packing parameter (CPP), a surfactant having CPP in range of 0.5 to 1.0, the area of head group between 0.25 to 0.5 nm^2. The cross sectional area of tri-oxyethylene head group is 0.28 nm^2. Further, the area of oxyethylene head group increases with increasing length (E=6, a=0.5, E=16, a=1.0 nm^2). It was observed that on increasing hydrophilic chain length of cholesteroyl ether a point is reached where the critical packing parameter (CPP) of molecules falls below 0.5 into a region which favours micellization rather than vesiculation. Like lipids, non-ionic surfactants form liquid crystals (mesophases) however, this behaviour has been observed above certain HLB values (Tanaka et al., 1990). Alkylpolyoxyethylene ethers demonstrated typical phase system displaying hexagonal(H1) lamella (La) liquid phases. It has been noticed that in a homologous series of L12 Ex surfactants La(lamella) phase grows on cost of H1 phase. The former is considered to be the precursor of the vesicular phase. Thus, it could be concluded that for

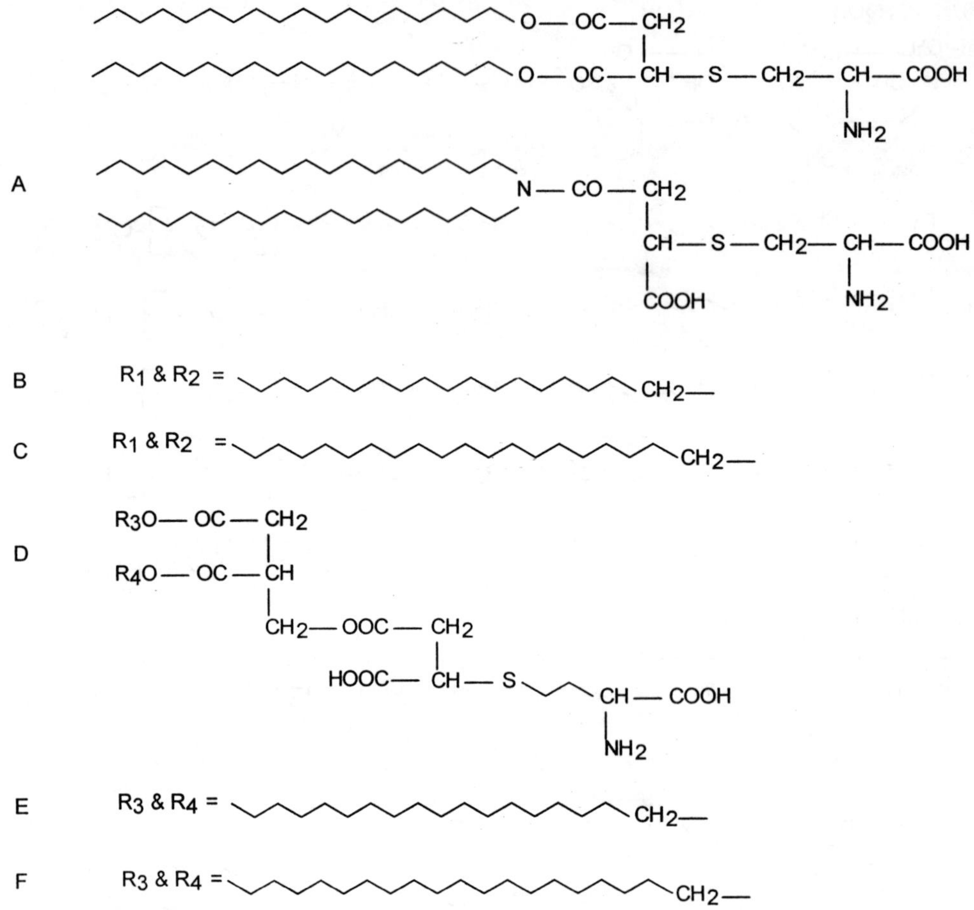

Fig. 6-9. Fluorinated Surfactants

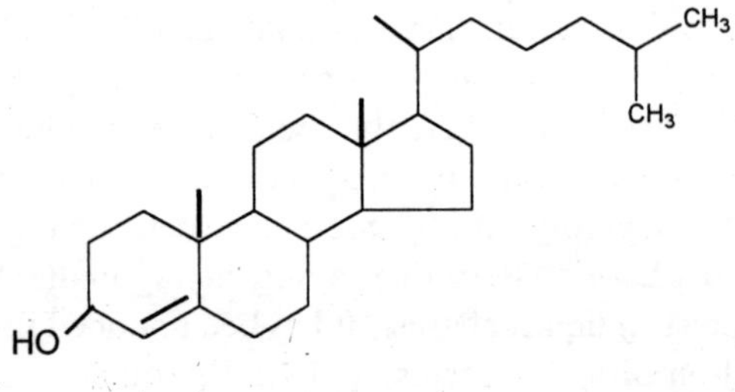

Fig. 6-10. Structure of Cholesterol

liquid crystal formation, a surfactant should have an appropriate HLB. An increase in HLB via chemical modification decreases the ability of surfactant to form vesicular structures. The hydrophilic surfactants owing to high aqueous solubility on hydration do not reach the stage of concentrated systems in order to allow free hydrated units to exist aggregates and coalesced to form lamellar structure (Jousma et al., 1988; Jousma et al., 1989).

METHODS OF PREPARATION

The various methods of preparation of niosomes are similar to those discussed under liposomes. However, to brush up them a few are discussed in brief below.

Ether Injection

The ether injection method is essentially based on slow injection of surfactant:cholesterol (150 μmol) solution in ether (20 ml) through a 14 gauge needle at rate approximately 0.25 ml/min into a preheated 4.0 ml aqueous phase maintained at 60 °C (Baillie et al., 1985). The mechanism whereby relatively larger unilamellar vesicles are formed however is not understood, presumably it could be ascribed to the slow vapourization of solvent resulting into a ether gradient extending across the interfacial lipid/ surfactant monolayer at ether-water interface. The latter subsequently may result into the formation of a bilayer sheet, which eventually folds on itself to form sealed vesicles. Fluorinated hydrocarbons evaporating at much lower temperature could susbstitute ether in cases where drug(s) to be incorporated are highly susceptible to temperature. The variation in vesicular size in aqueous phase may be varied via an additional addition of etherial solution of surfactants whilst effective volume of disperison remains to be constant (Deamer and Bangham, 1976; Deamer, 1978).

Hand Shaking Method

Surfactant and cholesterol mixture (150 μmol) is dissolved in 10 ml of diethylether in a round bottomed flask. The ether is evaporated under vacuum at room temperature in a rotary evaporator as discussed by Baillie et al., 1985. Upon hydration the surfactant swells and is peeled off the support in to a film, like lipids in lipid based film. Swollen amphiphiles eventually fold to form vesicles. The liquid volume entrapped in vesicles appears to be small, i.e. 5-10%. The entrapable volume seems to be unsuitable for water soluble solute(s) although the absolute yield/ ml of solution/gram of lipid/surfactant may be satisfactory for practical purposes.

Sonication

Niosomes using sonication method were prepared by Baillie et al., 1986, where in 150 μmol of surfactant-cholesterol mixture was dispersed in 2 ml of aquoues phase in a vial. The dispersion was probe sonicated for 3 min at 60 °C. Essentially, the method involves the formation of MLVs which are subsequently subjected to ultrasonic vibrations. The sonication may be accomplished using probe sonicator where sample size is a small volume. However, for larger sample volume bath sonicator is considered to be suitable. The finished product, i.e. vesicles are unilamellar in shape. Great care must be taken while working with a temperature sensitive solute (Baillie et al., 1985; Hofland et al., 1989).

Reverse Phase Evaporation

Surface active agents are dissolved in chloroform and 0.25 volume of phosphate saline buffer is emulsified to get W/O emulsion. The mixture is then sonicated and subsequently chloroform is evaporated under reduced pressure. The lipid or surfactant forms a gel first and subsequently hydrates to form vesicles. Free drug (unentrapped) is generally removed by dialysis (Jausma et al., 1988; Kiwada et al., 1985b; Kiwada et al., 1988).

Aqueous Dispersion

The method essentially based on microdispersion of surfactants in aqueous media containing solute(s) for encapsulation or entrapment. Continuous agitation under controlled temperature condition leads homogenous vesiculation. The dispersion may further be homogenized and ultracentrifuged (Handjani-Vila et al., 1979). Another variation of aqueous dispersion method has been attempted and reported by Talma et al., 1994 as a one step preparation method for liposomes and niosomes. The method deals with dispersion of vesicle forming substance and active drug which is subsequently homogenized at room temperature followed by continuous bubbling of nitrogen till the vesiculation or hydration is completed. The bubbles possibly provide spherical gas/air at interface for amphiphiles to get organized as per thermodynamic stability requirements. Nitrogen is released subsequently and allows subsequent hydration of amphiphiles to form vesicles.

Extrusion

Niosomes were prepared using $C_{16}G_2$ (from L'Oreal) a chemically defined non-ionic surfactant by extrusion through a polycarbonate membrane (0.1 μm nucleopore). The study not only demonstrated the effect of number of extrusion on vesicle size but also the effect of size on encapsulation of drug. It was found that using extrusion method vesicles of mean size diameter 136 nm could be prepared. However, on encapsulation of stilbogluconate and calcein in vesicles the resultant eventual mean size of niosomes increased significantly as it was measured to be 200 nm and 300 nm respectively (Stafford et al., 1988). Other methods such as reverse phase evaporation, double emulsion hydration etc. as discussed for liposomes (Chapter 5) can be used in the preparation of liposomes with adaptive modification.

SEPARATION OF FREE DRUG

The aqueous dispersions of solute bearing niosomes prepared by one of the method described above are exhaustively dialyzed using cellophane tubing against phosphate saline buffer (PBS) (pH7.4) or saline (Baillie et al., 1985; Okahota et al., 1981; Baillie et al., 1986; Azmin et al., 1985; Cable and Florence, 1988). The column chromatographic methods are also used for separation of free drug from niosomal suspension. For vesicular systems in order to make them free of free drug Sephadex G-50 is commonly employed. The column allows frequent separation of unentrapped drug from vesicular suspension as the drug is preferentially retained by Sephadex G-50 while vesicles percolate down with eluate. Incorporation of cholesterol however, provides an increase in the density of surfactant(s). Thus, the suspended vesicles in water, PBS, or saline are expected to sediment under the high gravitational field effect. The multilamellar vesicles (MLVs) may be spun down for an hour at 1,00,000 g depending on their size (Newman and Huang, 1975).

CHARACTERIZATION OF NIOSOMES

Size, Shape and Morphology

Vesicular structure of surfactant based vesicles has been visualized and established using freeze fracture electron microscopy while photon correlation spectroscopy could be successfully used to determine mean diameter of the vesicles. Electron microscopy can well be used for morphological studies of vesicles while master sizer based on laser beam is generally used to determine size distribution, mean surface diameter and mass distribution of niosomes.

Freeze Fractured Microscopy

Vesicles are freeze thawed (one cycle) and visualized using freeze fractured electron microscopy. The vesicular suspension is cryofixed in liquid propane. Some cryoprotectant like glycerol can be used. The cryofixed vesicles are fractured at an angle between 90-150 while low pressure is maintained (10^{-2} Pa). The surface obtained following fracturing is then shadowed using platinum or carbon vapours at an angel of 45 °C. Coating with carbon further strengthens so formed replica. After cleaning, the replica is observed and examined using transmission electron microscope. The niosomes have been observed 80 nm to 800 nm as larger unilamellar vesicles and they can be more 1 μm in size as MLVs. The size, shape of niosomes are found to be dependent on drug entrapment, nature of drug and nature of surfactant used. Cholesterol is used as one of the component of NSVs and which stabilizes the vesicular structure. Baillie et al., 1985 reported that in the case of polyglycol surfactant based vesicles the incorporation of cholesterol resulted in a decrease in latency of entrapped CF. It was found that in cases where surfactant concentrations used at significantly higher level, the incorporation of DCP about 50% was necessary in order to stabilize the vesicles (Yoshika et al., 1994; uchegbu, 1994; Chandraprakash et al., 1990; Zarif et al., 1993). The variation in shape of NSVs upon dispersion in phosphate buffer saline is well reflected in change in size of vesicles.

Effect of Entrapped Solute on Size of the Vesicles

Hexadecyldiglyceryl ether based vesicles demonstrated the effect of incorporated solution on the size of vesicles. It was observed on drug entrapment generally the size of niosomes increases. The effect is attributed to the interaction of solute molecules with the head group of surfactants. The net increase in resultant charge and force of repulsion thereby accounted for an increased vesicle size.

The mean size of extruded vesicles prepared employing extrusion method was recorded to be 136 nm where as on incorporation of solute (stilbogluconate and calcein), it tended to increase and eventually measured to be 200 nm and more than 300 nm respectively. It was thought to be an effect of complex formation between polar head of surfactant and solute molecule or presumably the consequence of salting out of surfactant polar heads due to complex formation, thus leading to local high energy built. The latter may cause thermodynamic instability, which in turn could promote vesicles to aggregate and to form larger vesicles (Yoshioka et al., 1994; Zarif et al., 1993).

Effect of Vesicle Forming Components on Size

In a well designed study it was noticed that mixed poly(glycerols), poly(oxyethylene) ether niosomes exhibited remarkable effect of solulan C24. Niosomes were prepared by sonication in the presence of increasing amount of solulan C24 and average diameter of resultant vesicles was determined. Solulan exhibited self-micellization of micellar size of 135 nm and 1.5 nm diameters while at higher concentration level solubilizes the niosomal contents preventing vesicle formation. The size of vesicles was recorded relatively smaller with increasing chain length of polyoxyethylene most probably due to reduction in radius of curvature of bilayers of surfactant I and II owing to a better interaction of polyoxyethylene ether segment of the surfactant (Gtiener et al., 1993).

Entrapment Efficiency

Entrapment efficiency may be determined using carboxyfluorescein (CF) as a marker and relative effect of method of preparation on entrapment could be compared. It is generally assumed that the concentration, i.e. 200 mM of CF used for hydration should be the concentration within vesicles (before disruption). The carboxyfluorescein at this concentration in vesicles is self-quenched and gives no fluorescence. Vesicle disruption using hydrophilic surfactant Solulan C24, Triton X-100, 0.2% desoxycholate or 50% propanol could be affected which increases the fluorescence by factor 100 owing to the release of entrapped CF. The ratios of CF before and after disruption of vesicles is calculated to determine entrapment efficiency and expressed as ml of CF per mole of surfactant (Florence, 1993).

Entrapment efficiency depends mainly upon the preparation method. Non-ionic surfactants prepared by ether injection method demonstrated higher entrapment efficiency as compared to those prepared by hand shaking method. The difference critically related to the vesicle type and size which in turn were found to be related to the method of preparation. Ether injection method produces conventional unilamellar vesicles more uniform in size resulting into higher drug entrapment compared to MLVs.

Baillie et al., 1985, Chauhan and Florence, 1989 prepared non-ionic surfactant vesicles (NSVs) with and without cholesterol using modified stable plurilamellar method. It was observed that gradual increase in cholesterol concentration results into relatively low entrapment efficiency. Cholesterol is however retards the afflux profile of the entrapped solute. A vesicle forming non-ionic surfactant having polyethylene glycol chain (Kiwada et al., 1985) was studied for entrapment efficiency and effect of method of preparation by Chauhan and Florence, 1989. Surfactant-I, polyoxyethylene 1 and 2 stearyl ether were mixed with cholesterol and NSVs were prepared by plurilamellar method (SPLV) of Gruner et al., 1985 by reverse phase evaporation method of Szoka and Papahadjopolous, 1978 or by hydration of thin film to form MLVs. Sodium stilbogluconate was used for entrapment. The hydrodynamic diameters (m) and entrapment efficiencies of vesicles prepared using different methods were determined. The study suggests that PEG chain length assists or reduces the radius of curvature of bilayer resulting into better packing and eliminates the effect of solute (stilbogluconate) on size of the vesicles.

The entrapment efficiency was also found to be linearly related to the length of carbon chain in alkylglycosides. In a study Kiwada et al., 1985b reported that an alkyl chain length of not less than myristyl could form stable vesicles. Cetylglycoside vesicles with glucose, galactose, and mannose showed encapsulation capacity practically comparable to the phosphatidylcholine liposomes. The shorter length alkyl chain (lauryl, decyl, and octyl) surfactants of alkylglycosed series however do not form the vesicular structure. It was noted that a vesicular system with optimum encapsulation capacity can only be produced by selection of alkylglycosed surfactant of an appropriate chain length (Table 6-1 and 6-2). Similarly, modification or alteration of hydrophilic head group of C_{16} surfactant demonstrated dramatic effect on encapsulation efficiency. It could be attributed to the associated water with sugars used as head group. However, more detailed studies are required to establish the mechanism via which head group dependent entrapment efficiency by NSVs could be demonstrated.

CF was determined spectrophotometrically following the disruption of vesicles mean value ± s.d. n, given in parenthesis.

Encapsulation Efficiency and Solute Release Rates

Numerous studies have been undertaken till date to investigate the encapsulation efficiency of hydrophilic and hydrophobic solutes within NSVs. However, no satisfactory theoretical correlation could be reached. This is partly due to the method of preparation and subsequent processing of the system. However, the encapsulation efficiency can be said as a product of the stability of the dispersion. That is, the encapsulated solute and the solute retention capability of the encapsulating membrane, together with the stability of both the surfactant and the vesicle structure, all contribute to the stability of the formulation. Encapsulation efficiency is governed by the method of loading, nature of solute and hydration temperature. Vesicles loaded by transmembrane ion gradient method show higher entrapment efficiency than those loaded during the hydration step (Uchegbu, 1994; Cullis et al., 1987; Harrigan et al., 1993; Montero et al., 1993; Uchegbu et al., 1994; Haran et al., 1993). As a rule, larger niosomes show higher entrapment efficiencies than smaller vesicles (Uchegbu, 1994; Vemuri et al., 1990). Encapsulation of water soluble solutes results in increased vesicle size, which can be attributed to the interaction of solutes with the amphiphile head groups. Thus increasing the mutual repulsion of surfactant bilayers (Stafford et al., 1988).

Table 6-1. Variation of NSVs Size with Composition and Method of Preparation

Method of preparation	Composition	Hydrodynamic diameter	Hydrodynamic diameter	% loading of drug
SPLV	100I	741±75	679±69	27%
SPLV	50I:50CH	571±52	608±69	22%
REV	100I	648±79	640±63	...
REV	50I:50CH	744±154	...	26%
MLV	100I	139±239	950±142	21%
MLV	50I:50CH	995±173	1127±125	32%

Table 6-2. CF Entrapment Efficiency of NSVs of Different Composition(s) Prepared using Different Methods of Prepartion

Preparation method	Composition mole %	Entrapment efficiency ($Lmol^{-1}$ surfactant)
Hand shaking	100I	0.124
	50I:50CH	1.06±0.065
Ether injection	100I	1.22±0.120 (n=5)
	80I:20CH	0.85±0.09 (n=3)
	70I:30CH	0.68±0.080(n=6)
	60I:40CH	0.86±0.130(n=3)
	50I:50CH	0.44±0.060(n=9)
Sonication	50I:50CH	0.65±0.24(n=6)
	50I:50CH	0.132±0.090

Effect of Cholesterol on NSVs

Encapsulation efficiency is a measure of the solute retention and cholesterol has been shown to assist solute retention. Investigations over the years have shown that cholesterol plays an important role in absolute encapsulation efficiency of a formulation and in turn the stability of the vesicles. The synthetic alkyl glycosides shown in Figure 6-8 are all capable of forming vesicles without the inclusion of cholesterol (Kiwada et al., 1985a). However, a threefold increase in encapsulation efficiency of C16-glucoside vesicles was observed after incorporation of 29 mole % cholesterol. Similarly, 50-100% increase in encapsulation efficiency was observed with vesicles formed by synthetic polyhydroxyl lipids with 20 mole % cholesterol content, and up to 50 mole % was reported with a series of sorbitan monoesters (Yoshioka et al., 1994).

The amount of cholesterol also decides the release rate and extent of solute from the vesicles. For example, Florence and co-workers, 1990 reported that the release of doxorubicin from vesicles containing surfactant and stearylamine with 8.5 mole % cholesterol was around 2% over a time period of 6 h. However, when the cholesterol content was increased to 47.5 mole % in the formulation only 0.1% release was recorded over the same time period. Nevertheless, there are some reports which show a decrease in entrapment on inclusion of cholesterol (Baillie et al., 1985). Similarly, vesicles prepared from polyoxyethylene (Florence 1993) 1,2 distearoyl ether did not show any significant influence on encapsulation efficiency on inclusion of cholesterol (Chauhan and Lawrence,1989).

Nature of Hydrophilic Head Group

One another factor governing the stability of niosomes is the nature of the hydrophilic head group. This is evidenced from the report by Kiwada and co-workers, 1985. As shown in Table 6-3, the entrapment efficiency of a series of alkyl glycoside based vesicles gave different entrapment efficiencies, C_{16}-glucoside and C_{16}-mannoside gave entrapments of above 7% where C_{16}-galactoside showed only 5%. This is attributed to the sugar moieties present in the glycoside, which differ in their orientation due to 4-hydroxyl group.

Non-ionic surfactant vesicles prepared using surfactants with identical alkyl groups but different hydrophilic groups (epoxy v/s glycerol moieties) revealed that the glycerol moieties had lower head group area measurements compared to ethoxy group. This gives an increased mobility to the poly-ethoxylated alkyl chains which in turn increases the fluidity of the corresponding bilayers and ultimately leads to leaky membranes as compared to alkylglycerol derivatives (Riber et al., 1984). A recent report has shown that the change from a poly-5-oxyethylene to a diglycerol head group resulted in two fold increase in encapsulation efficiency of a macromolecular prodrug (Uchegbu and Florence, 1995).

Nature of the Alkyl Side Chain

Kiwada and co-workers, 1985b have reported on the effect of alkyl side chain on percent encapsulation. They have reported the effect of alkyl chain length on the encapsulation efficiency of ^{14}C sucrose (Table 6-4)

It is evident from Table 6-4 that longer the alkyl chain glycolipids, better is the encapsulation efficiency. These workers suggested that the alkyl chain length cut off point for vesicle formation may be a 14 carbon chain. They also claimed that the dialysis procedure used to separate the encapsulated material from unencapsulated material would have

Table 6-3. Vesicle Formation with 100% Polyoxyethylene Alkyl Ethers (C_{10} EO_m) Surfactants

Surfactant	EO_3	EO_5	EO_7
C_{10}	+	-	-
C_{12}	+	-	-
C_{14}	+	+	-
C_{16}	+ (phase seperation)	+ (slightly viscous)	+ (viscous)
C_{18}	+ (phase seperation)	+ (phase seperation)	- (slightly viscous)

+ = formation of vesicles

resulted in the loss of C_8, C_{10} and C_{12} compounds. However, vesicles purification using gel filtration technique (using Sephadex G-50) is said to prevent the destabilization of vesicles prepared from low molecular weight sorbitan lauryl esters (C_{12}) (Yoshioka et al., 1994; Uchegbu, 1994).

One should know the effect of alkyl chain length on vesicle size. It was reported that a gradual decrease in size (3.4-0.9 μm) as the alkyl chain length increases is observed with 5(6)-carboxyfluorescein entrapped niosomes (Yoshioka et al., 1994). These vesicles are smaller than doxorubicin loaded vesicles which show a size of approximately 6 μm, irrespective of the sorbitan surfactant used (Uchegbu, 1994). The relationship observed between niosome size and sorbitan monoester monomer hydrophobicity has been attributed to the decrease in surface free energy with increasing hydrophobicity. Uchegbu, 1994 has reported that the size of doxorubicin niosome decreases with a decrease in hydrophilicity.

Nature of Encapsulated Solute

The effect of method of loading on retention of encapsulated doxorubicin within sorbitan monosterate vesicles was studied (Cullis et al., 1987; Harrigan et al., 1993; Montero et al., 1993; Uchegbu et al., 1994; Haran et al., 1993). It is found that when vesicles are loaded using ordinary pH gradients, approximately 50% of the drug is releases over 24 h at 37 °C. However, only 20% of the drug was released over the same period from vesicles loaded using ammonium sulphate gradients (Uchegbu and Florence, 1995). This is attributed to the nature of the counter-ion and ultimately the stability of the ionic association produced by the cationic drug ions and the intravesicular sulphate counter ions, which have a major influence on solute retention. From this, it can be understood that leakage of encapsulated solute due to membrane permeability can be overcome using a suitable intravesicular ionic trap. The release rate of a solute is affected by the nature of the solute, even when similar counter ions are considered. The release of 5(6)-carboxyfluorescein and doxorubicin from $C_{16}G_2$:cholesterol:Solulan C24 (30:80:40) vesicles were 3% and 10% over a time period of 6 h at 22 °C (Uchegbu, 1994). The slow release of 5(6)-carboxyfluorescein is attributed to the reason that they are fully ionized at the working pH (7.4) and thus require a high energy process to pass through the membrane as compared to the passage of the partially ionized doxorubicin molecule through the membrane.

Vesicle Surface Charge

The presence of surface charge in vesicular dispersions is critical. It has been found that aggregation of vesicles in isotonic saline solution occurs when the vesicles are prepared without the inclusion of a charged molecule in the bilayer (Haran et al., 1993). Aggregation is attributed to the shielding of the vesicle surface charge by ions in solution and there by reducing the electrostatic repulsion. However, a reduction in the formation of aggregates was observed when a charged molecule like dicetylphosphate was incorporated in C_nEO_m bilayer vesicles (Cable, 1989).

Vesicle surface charge can be estimated by measurement of particle electrophoretic mobility and is expressed as the zeta potential which is calculated using the Henry equation (Vanhal, 1994),

Table 6-4. Effect of Alkyl Chain on Encapsulation Efficiency

Surfactant	Encapsulation efficiency (%)
C_8 – glucoside	2.28 ± 0.57
C_{10} – glucoside	1.11 ± 0.20
C_{12} – glucoside	1.27 ± 0.73
C_{14} – glucoside	5.52 ± 0.35
C_{16} – glucoside	7.74 ± 1.57
C_{18} – glucoside	5.76 ± 0.67
Phosphatidyl choline	5.54 ± 1.56

Lipid composition – Surfactant:DCP:CH:: 4:1:2

$$\zeta = \frac{\mu E 4\pi\eta}{\Sigma} \qquad (6\text{-}1)$$

where, ζ = zeta potential; μE = electrophoretic mobility; η = viscosity of the medium; Σ = dielectric constant

STABILITY OF NIOSOMES

Stability in Buffer

The stability of alkyl glycoside vesicles was compared with phosphatidylcholine based (liposomes) vesicles both containing lipid:DCP:cholesterol 4:1:2. It was observed that the phosphatidylcholine based vesicles (liposomes) disintegrated *in vitro* after 22 week, while niosomes prepared using alkylglycoside endured at least for 25 weeks (Baillie et al., 1985). In regard to efflux profile of CF it was observed to be biphasic. The overall release in initial phase was faster, while after 4 h, invariably in all the preparations the release rate was slow which continued for 24 h. Cholesterol incorporation retarded efflux of entrapped solute significantly. The observed effect of cholesterol is in accordance with its membrane stabilizing effect (Demel and De Kruyff, 1976). Moreover, at constant cholesterol level in surfactant I and II based NSVs the variation in concentration of surfactant did not effect the efflux of CF significantly.

Stability in Hypertonic Media

Osmotic Shrinkage

Similar to liposomes on addition of hypertonic salt solution to the suspension in order to bring about osmotic gradient across NSVs bilayer (membrane) relatively higher absorbance of (CF) in hypotonic buffer was recorded. The efflux was described to be in accordance with the findings of Blok et al., (1975). It was interpreted that the osmotic gradient induces the reduction in vesicle size by effectively pumping out the vesicular contents. The latter could be attributed to the higher absorbance recorded. Intrestingly, cholesterol free niosomes were without osmotic sensitivity in contrast to vesicles containing this lipid. Thus, apparent resistance to osmotic shrinkage presumably be related to higher permeability efflux of solute(s). This is in general agreement of CF efflux profile as well as membrane stabilizing effect of cholesterol.

It could be drawn from the above study that osmogen borne reduction in niosomal vesicle diameter could result into an effective efflux of vesicular fluid. Baillie et al., 1985 quantified the efflux for the 50%I:50% cholesterol vesicles after addition of 10 μl of 1M NaI solution. The same change in term of entrapment volume of 0.106 l/mol of surfactant was recorded. The volume was calculated to be equivalent to 3.333 moles H_2O. Thus, in terms of water efflux it was 3.33 moles of water per mole of surfactant. The efflux profile and osmotic consequence recorded to occur over a period of 1 min, thus for surfactant I and surfactant II it was determined to be 3.33 moles and 4.52 mole/min/mol of surfactant I and II respectively.

Stability in Hypotonic Media

Unlike, osmotic shrinkage the vesicular system containing high load of solute(s) when diluted with demineralized water, a slow release of drug for 1 h period followed by a relatively faster drug release phase in water was observed. The release profile described to be related to osmotic response of vesicular system from Span 85 and cholesterol (75:25). The initial slow release phase may be explained on the basis of imbibition of eluting diameter from 645 nm to 650 nm. Owing to swelling a mechanical loosening of vesicular bilayer under osmotic stress could presumably be related to faster drug diffusion in eluting media (demineralized distilled water) (Jain, 1993).

Stability *In Vivo*

Plasma Component Interaction

Moser and colleagues, 1980 studied plasma protein interaction with haemoglobin containing NSVs. It was noticed that agglutinization with ABO blood group components did not occur in case of vesicles from DPPC:CH:DCP as a result plasma component mediated destabilization was not recorded. In case of NSVs albumin and transferrin were identified and determined to adsorb on vesicles without destabilizing them. Thus, haemoglobin containing niosomes were found to be stable, however chemical instability, i.e. oxidation of haemoglobin to methaemoglobin was recorded as a result haemoglobin content reached about 30% after 5 months at 4 °C.

Tucker and Florence, 1983 studied the interaction of non-ionic surfactant with low-density lipoprotein (LDL2). LDL2 is delipidized by high concentration of anionic, cationinc and non-ionic surface active agents (Helenus and Simons,1971). Zampighi et al., 1980 have shown that apoprotein B solubilized in dodecyl-octaethylene glycol solution and acquires rod shaped with dimensions 80.5 nm whereas surfactant phospholipid mixed micelle are typically spherical in shape (Helenus and Simons, 1971). Thus, LDL2 undergoes some dimensional changes in the presence of surfactants, which subsequently are manifested in its hydrodynamic properties. Non-ionic surfactant caused rapid increase in G50% in Stroke's radius upto surfactant/LDL2 molar ratio 1000:1. This was interpreted as a result of unfolding of LDL2 and its subsequent intercalation in surfactant micellar assemblages with lipoprotein surface layer. The absorption of protein such as albumin on vesicular surface following intravenous administration leads to changes in vesicular structure particularly its permeability. Hume, 1987 reported that surfactant III (L'Oreal) NSVs containing 50 mole % cholesterol bind quantitatively more protien as compared to DPPC liposomes containing the same proportion of cholesterol. The uptake of surfactant I and DPPC based liposomes of Tetrahymenaellioti has been found to be comparative, suggesting that chemical structure determines the pattern of plasma protein adsorption. However, protein coated vesicles are recognized and up taken selectively. *In vivo* there is a possibility that breakdown of liposomes and NSVs may differ. Phospholipase as might be expected, has more defined and profound effect on liposomes stability thus resulting into solute release than NSVs. The incorporation of cholesterol however, reduces the susceptibility of the system. Vesicles from surfactant I and II and egg lecithin were found relatively resistant and less susceptible to carboxylic ester hydrolase attack. *In vivo* fate of vesicles could not be generalized as it has a bearing, of other vesicular adjuvant i.e. cholesterol, PC, amphiphiles and incorporated drug molecules.

RHEOLOGICAL PROPERTIES OF NIOSOMAL DISPERSION

The rheological characteristics of NSVs-haemoglobin system have been evaluated. NSVs were found to be relatively more viscous than red blood cells suspension. However, overall rheological behaviour was comparable. The studies conducted suggest that it is rationale to determine hydrodynamic characteristics of niosomal suspension, which are relevant and pertinent to *in vivo* behaviour. Under a set of conditions, intrinsic viscosity of niosomal suspension was measured as an indication of the hydration of the vesicle.

System prepared by surfactant I/cholesterol (50:50 molar ratio), vesicles of 230 nm diameter, and the systems prepared following the addition of Solulan C24 (25%) have the intrinsic viscosities 16 and 12.6 ml/g respectively. It appears that the structure of niosomes undergoes some deformation during flow, thus it is not advisable to make direct interpretation of the results (Florence, 1993).

SOLUTE RELEASE PROFILE FROM NIOSOMAL FORMULATIONS

In regard to release of entrapped solute from niosomal system, cholesterol was noted to have distinct effect on release profile as well as on vesicle stability. It also determines and governs *in vivo* fate of vesicular systems and liposomes in particular. In a study the effect of cholesterol incorporation on $C_{16}G_3$ based niosomes has been well correlated with mixed monolayers consisted of surfactants and cholesterol. Cholesterol was found to retard release rate of solute and stabilize the system against degradation (Khand et al., 1987).

NSVs demonstrated temperature dependency on release of solute, which could successfully be utilized in therapeutics using local hyperthermia. The characteristics recorded was similar to the liposome. In case of liposomes it was related to some lipid component that brings down phase transition temperature of lipoidal system. Cholesterol, is however noted to abolish the clear temperature dependency of solute film. Similarly, incorporated drug may effect temperature dependent efflux profile of itself (Rogerson, et al., 1987).

Tanaka et al., 1990 studied and determined fluidity of bilayer using ESR spectrum of lipophilic probe (5-12 and 16 deoxy stearic acid, 5Ns, 12Ns and 1,6 Ns respectively). Order of parameters is a function of number of ethylene oxide units; the order however decreases with increasing HLB of surfactant used in the formation of bilayer or vesicles.

COLLOIDAL PROPERTIES OF NIOSOMAL DISPERSION

Stability of NSVs is maintained by entropic/enthalpic repulsion forces arise as vesicles approach close thus flocculation is prevented. Dehydration of surface hydrophilic groups generally leads to flocculation. Thus, salt addition or temperature rise, affect the stability particularly the dispersibility. In a study the mean hydrodynamic diameter of vesicular aggregates were measured as a function of time and it was observed that niosomes from surfactant I and cholesterol tended to aggregate. However, the nature of aggregation was recorded to be reversible. The vesicles redispersed on shaking. The addition of DCP in a low concentration prevented the aggregation.
Surfactants with smaller hydrophilic group as compared to surfactant I was noted to form relatively smaller vesicle redispersible with greater difficulty, possibly due to less prominent repulsion between the vesicles. The vesicles (NSVs) generally bear net negative charge due to absorbed hydroxyl ion from the solution. Incorporation of charge bearing drug may also impart and confer an effective charge over vesicular surface.

In an attempt to improve the stability of NSVs against flocculation, cholesteryl oxyethylene ether was added to NSVs based on surfactant I to increase the hydrophilicity of the exterior surface (Klibanov et al., 1990). The influence of cholesteryl oxyethylene ether addition on the surface properties was measured as its effect on electorphoretic mobilities or net surface charge. The effect of 5 mole % addition of Solulan C5, C16 and C24 was recorded in terms of electrophoretic mobilities as a function of pH. The increasing length of polyoxyethylene unit adsorbed on the surface pushes the plane of shear farther from the particle and decreases the resultant charge borne by vesicles, the latter attributes to the selective adsorption of OH ions from the bulk (Uchegbu et al., 1991).

DISCOMES

Uchegbu et al., 1991 have observed disc like structure based on non-ionic surfactants during niosomes to mixed micelles transitions. The structures were noted to exist under certain conditions of phase diagram of niosomes prepared from a hexadecyl diglycerol ether ($C_{16}G_2$), cholesterol and dicetylphosphate (DCP) in the molar ratio 69:29:2 by mechanical disruption and sonication method (Fig. 6-11) (Uchegbu et al., 1992). Among the other phases, a unique phase termed the "discome" phase was identified. The vesicles were incubated with polyoxyethylene cholesteryl ether and solulan C24 at 74 °C. Turbidity measurements were made at 350 nm. A plot between turbidity and solulan C24 corresponding to change in the phase, was observed specially in regard to lamellar, micellar and discome phase existence. Dispersion in discome phase was noted to be comprised of larger disc like structures (volume distribution diameter 12-60 μm). Discomes were found to entrap water soluble solute effectively. Carboxyfluorescien (CF) aqueous volume entrapment 1.209±0.97 L per mol of surfactant has been reported. From discomes, 50% of the entrapped CF was released in 24 hours when studied for diffusion study.

A $C_{16}G_2$:Cholesterol ratio 7:3 favoured the formation of discomes. Increasing concentration of cholesterol at the above stated level, prior to challenge with solulan C24, suppressed the formation of discomes. The low mole fraction of cholesterol in vesicular system prior to addition of solulan C24 facilitates the formation of discomes by lending bilayer relatively more permeable to the solulan molecules. Thus, solubilization of niosomes by addition of solulan probably proceeds involving dispersion and surfactant bilayer phases until a critical level of solulan in bilayer is reached with an eventual formation of discomes. Further, partitioning of solulan C24 beyond its critical phase concentration leads to the break down of discomes. Finally, solubilization of vesicles/discomes/aggregates is completed through mixed micellization.

Discomes differ from the bilayer sheets, which are formed during transition of vesicles to the micelles. The empty disocomes incubated with CF for 1 h immediately prior to *in vitro* release measurement were noted to have no CF adsorbed on their surfaces. Dialysis of discome system was found not to affect their morphology. Discomes were found to be stable upto 6 months when stored at 4 °C.

However, discome dispersion exhibited a decrease in turbidity when heated to 37 °C indicating their instability. The large volume carrying capacity and minimal opacity of discomes may present them as novel drug delivery system especially in ophthalmology. However, in order to stabilize discomes at 37 °C further formulation modification studies should be carried out. The nonuniform curvature of nonionic surfactant disc (discomes) could be related to heterogenous dispersion of disc components at molecular level. The same could be a possible explanation for $C_{16}G_2$ vesicles to micelles transition.

Niosomes are smectic mesophases of alternating layers of aqueous and non-aqueous phases. When these are solubilized by the non-ionic surfactant Solulan C24 (SC 24), in appropriate amounts, breakdown of vesicles takes place and transforms into a mixed micellar system with the formation of an intermediate phase referred to as "discome". Discomes are thus large (12-60 μm) structures derived from niosomes on addition of soluble surface active agents (e.g., SC 24). As discomes are capable of entrapping water soluble solutes, they could be explored as drug carriers (Uchegbu and Florence, 1993).

Discomes, in addition to their many advantages seem to have a special advantage for ocular route where in their large size may prevent their drainage into the systemic pool as well as the 'disc' shape could provide for better fit in the cul-de-sac of the eye. The use of discoidal niosomes for ocular delivery has been studied by Vyas et al., 1998. Timolol maleate, α β-blocker used in the treatment of open-angle glaucoma was entrapped in discomes and their use as delivery system in the treatment of open-angle glaucoma was studied (Fig. 6-11). Timolol maleate loaded discomes were found to release the drug in a controlled fashion over a prolonged period of time. The change in intraocular pressure (IOP) was reported to be high in discoidal formulation treated animals as compared to plain drug solution and niosomal timolol maleate treated animals.

Recently, Uchegbu and co-workers, 1992 have reported the solubilization of the lipophilic tubulin inhibitor paclitaxel by using $C_{16}G_2$: cholesterol: Solulan C24 in different ratios. This is the first of its kind, where the solubilization of an extremely hydrophobic compound by $C_{16}G_2$ discomes. It has been well documented by Uchegbu et al., 1992 that

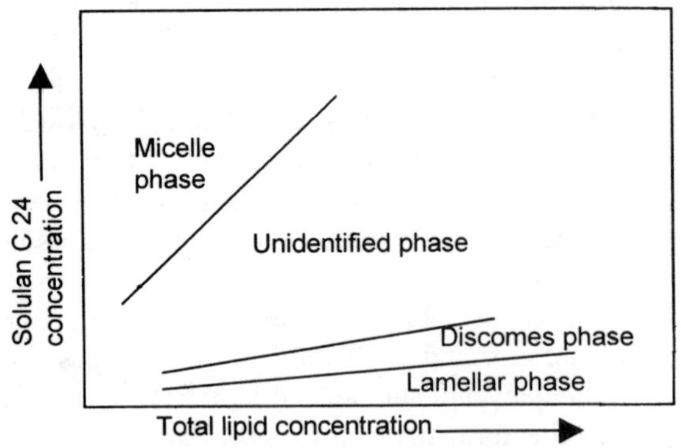

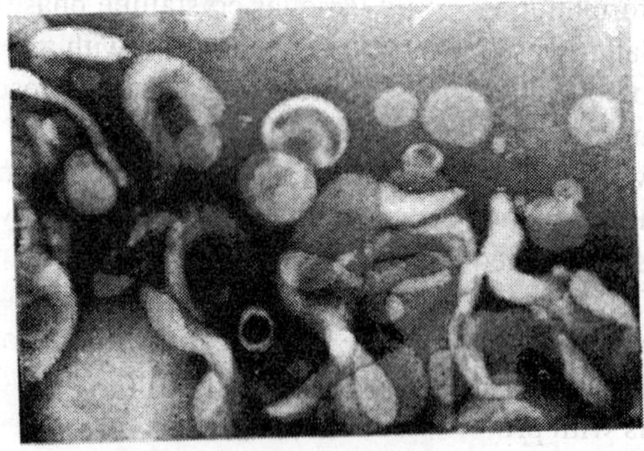

Fig. 6-11. Schematic of Vesicle to Micelle Transition Phase Diagram and TEM Photomicrograph of Discome

heating formulations containing discomes (>35 °C) resulted in loss of turbidity due to the transition from a discome phase that also contains spherical and tubular vesicles to a phase containing tubular and spherical vesicles and possibly mixed micelles. It is interesting to note that a change in the structure of the vesicles from discomes to mixed micelles was not accompanied by the precipitation of paclitaxel. This is likely due to the drug in the discome phase is solubilized in the bilayer(s) and becomes solubilized in the hydrophobic core of the mixed micelles at higher temperature.

NSVs REVERSED VESICLES

Reverse micelles and reverse emulsion, i.e. O/W and W/O are well known and accepted terms in expression of symmetrical pattern. One notable exception is reversed vesicles. Normal vesicles where in close hydrocarbon compartments separating aqueous interior and exterior was first described in 1964. These systems, as discussed earlier also were resulted from the hydration of phospholipids as lamellar liquid crystals dispersed in aqueous phase. The literature on normal vesicular systems, i.e. liposomes and niosomes is abound where as reverse vesicle formation is recently reported.

Non-ionic surfactant tetraethyleneglycol dodecylether ($R_{12}EO_4$) was dissolved in dodecane to form an isotropic solution. The binary system so constituted was without any crystal structure. However, addition of small amount of water resulted in to split of isotropic structures and as a consequence formation of liquid lamellar crystalline phase. The latter was found to be in equilibrium with an excess of oil phase. The system was noted to resemble normal vesicular system in which addition of water widens the spacing between hydrocarbon segments. Reversed vesicles are formed spontaneously by hand shaking method on addition of an excess of oil phase. The system exhibited common characteristics of colloidal system, i.e. aggregation on storage or separation of phases. The effective surface of vesicles is with projecting hydrocarbon chain, thus, they are expected to have better barrier penetration efficiency. The potential of such a system in therapeutics is still to be explored and established.

NON-IONIC SURFACTANT VESICLE-IN-WATER-IN-OIL (V/W/O) SYSTEMS

Modified versions of vesicular systems have always been the thought of researchers in order to explore their full potential as a drug delivery system. This led to the report of inverse vesicles (discussed earlier). However, there are limitations due to the structural constraints on formulation of both amphiphile and oil phase.

A newer system employing the use of NSVs in the vesicle-in-water-in-oil (V/W/O) system. The system and its potential as a drug delivery system has been studied exhaustively by Yoskioka et al. (Florence, 1993, Florence et al., 1996).

Generally, vesicular systems are used as aqueous suspensions, but there are potential uses for systems in which the external phase may be replaced with a nonaqueous. V/W/O systems are those in which the aqueous suspensions of vesicles are dispersed in a continuous oil phase. This type of a system has been studied as a potential immunological adjuvant and as a drug delivery system (Florence et al., 1996). The system has a dual advantage of not only capable of encapsulating water-soluble and insoluble agents but also the presence of an external nonaqueous vehicle through which the encapsulated solute must diffuse.

The system is an emulsion prepared by dispersion of niosomes in water, followed by reemulsification of an oil using a surfactant mixture of low HLB to achieve a stable W/O emulsion. The resulting vesicle-in-water-in-oil system (V/W/O) (Fig. 6-12) is a close analogue of O/W/O emulsions and microsphers(s)-in-oil-in-water dispersions (M/O/W) (Yoshioko and Florence, 1994) or W/O/W multiple emulsions (Hasida et al., 1980).

The major advantage of the system is the use of a non-ionic surfactant to form the vesicles (NSVs), which is also serve as a component of the stabilizing system used for W/O emulsion. Thus, the migration of the stabilizing surfactant from the O/W interface to the W/O interface and vice versa is arrested, hence W/O/W multiple emulsion (Florence et al., 1989) with an improved stability.

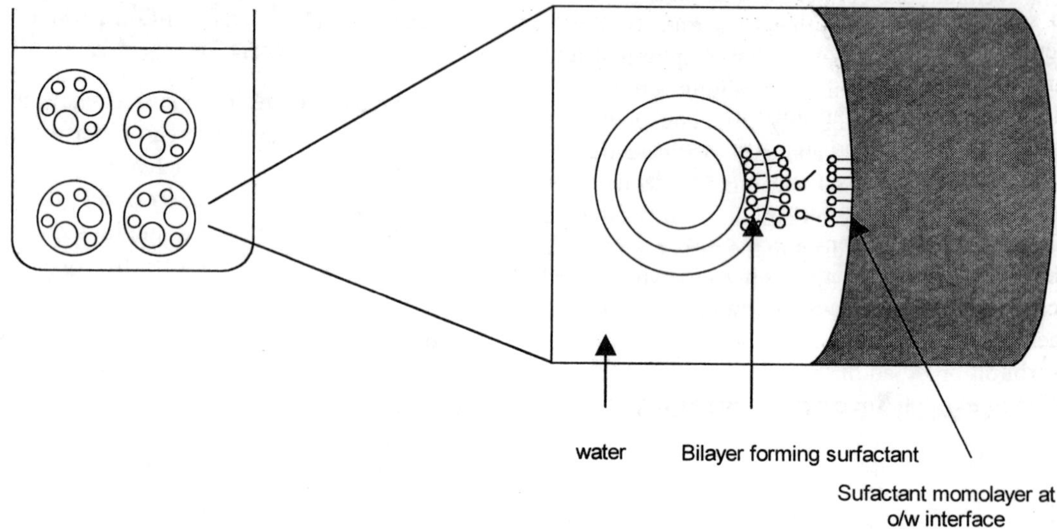

Fig. 6-12. Schematic Representation of the V/W/O formulation

NON-IONIC SURFACTANT BASED ORGANOGELS

A novel non-ionic organogel has been reported by Murdan and co-workers, 1996. A study on V/W/O with Span 60 showed that gelation of hexadecane at surfactant concentrations as low as 1% w/v occurred yielding a smooth white semisolid gel. *In vitro* release studies have shown a controlled release of 5(6)-carboxyfluorescein from the V/W/O based organogel as compared to simple solution, NSVs and anhydrous organogel.

POLYMER COATED NON-IONIC SURFACTANT VESICLES

Non-ionic surfactant vesicles are now well accepted as an alternative to liposomes, as liposomes pose certain stability problems. In order to improve the stability of multilamellar vesicular systems, a novel method has been recently reported by us (Vyas and Venkatesan, 1999). The multilamellar vesicles were coated with poly(phthaloyl-L-lysine). The coating was affected by interfacial polymerization technique using p-phthaloyl dichloride and L-lysine. The polymeric coat was brought about around each bilayer of the multilamellar vesicles. The polymer coated vesicles were found to be stable under various osmotic conditions and released the drug in a controlled fashion. The drug release rate was much retarded compared to plain uncoated MLVs.

A similar report for increasing the vesicle stability of unilamellar vesicles was reported by us earlier (Venkatesan and Vyas 1998). The method involved the use of butylcyanoacrylate to form a polymeric coat on individual discrete ULVs. The polymeric coat was brought about by a pH (5.8-5.5) change induced polymeization. The polymer coated vesicles were found to be osmotically stable. These vesicles can be used to increase the stability of the vesicles both *in vitro* and *in vivo*. The system is further being studied for the triggered delivery of drugs from the vesicles.

PRONIOSOMES

Proniosomes are dry formulations of surfactant-coated carrier, which can be measured out as needed and rehydrated by brief agitation in hot water (Hu and Rhodes, 1999). These 'proniosomes' minimize problems of niosome physical stability such as aggregation, fusion and leaking, and provide additional convenience in transportation, distribution, storage, and dosing. Proniosomes are normally prepared by spraying surfactant in organic solvent onto sorbitol powder and then evaporating the solvent. Because the sorbitol carrier is soluble in the organic solvent, it is necessary to repeat the process until the desired surfactant load has been achieved. The surfactant coating on the carrier comes out to be very thin and hydration of this coating allows multilamellar vesicles to form.

Drug-containing proniosome-derived niosomes can be prepared in manner analogous to that used for the conventional niosomes, by adding drug to the surfactant mixture prior to spraying the solution onto the sorbitol, or by addition of drug to the aqueous solution used to dissolve hydrate the proniosomes. Proniosomes-derived niosomes are superior to conventional niosomes in convenience of storage, transport, and dosing. Stability studies are still in progress, but it is expected that the dry proniosomes preparation will be more stable than a pre-manufactured suspension. In release studies, proniosomes appear to be equivalent to conventional niosomes. (Rhodes and Hu, 2000). Size distributions of proniosome-derived niosomes are somewhat better than those of conventional niosomes, so the release performance in more critical cases turns out to be superior. Proniosomes are dry powder, which makes further processing and packaging possible. The powder form provides optimal flexibility, unit dosing, in which the proniosome powder is provided in capsule could be beneficial. A slurry method is developed to produce proniosomes using maltodextrin as a carrier. The time required to produce proniosome by this method is independent of the ratio of surfactant solution to carrier material. In slurry method, the entire volume of surfactant solution is added to maltodextrin powder in a rotary evaporator and vacuum applied until the powder appears to be dry and free flowing.

NON-IONIC SURFACTANT VESICLES AND THEIR THERAPEUTIC POTENTIAL

Niosomes for the Treatment of Leishmaniasis

Niosomes with desirable release profile and stability characteristics can be prepared by tailoring surfactant chemically or via bilayer composition modification. However, the real therapeutic potentialities of a system can only be evaluated and established through *in vivo* experimentation in animals followed by clinical trials. *In vivo* studies on NSVs bearing stilbogluconate an antileishmaniasis agent were carried out on mice. The vesicular therapy originate organ specific drug delivery. Hunter et al., (1988) reported the proven ability of liposomal system in effective and radical eradication of visceral leishmaniasis.

NSVs prepared using surfactant I-III (L'Oreal) have been recorded to be effective carrier system for delivery of stilbogluconate to the visceral cells (Baillie et al., 1986; Hunter et al., 1988; Stafford et al., 1988). Croft, 1986 presented an exhaustive review on liposomal vesicular system in parasitic diseases. It was apparently reported that the magnitude of improved efficiency by the use of vesicular carrier systems is dependent on experimental conditions as well. The important variables reported include size of infective inoculum or challenge, to the host, route of administration, volume inoculated, timing profile of treatment in relation to the infection and strain of parasite and host used in the study. In addition, the variables that relate to the experimental therapy, such as number of doses and vesicular components may also affect the experimental results.

Hunter et al., 1988 suggested that niosomes are as effective as liposomes in delivery of loaded drug in experimental leishmaniasis. The NSVs containing stilbogluconate tested *in vivo* recorded a spectrum of activity between 10 to 100 μg antimony per mouse. For drug with high aqueous solubility it was assumed that the drug is entrapped in aqueous space of the vesicles (liposomes or niosomes). The ability of these aqueous compartments to accommodate and retain the drug may be a limiting factor of vesicular systems. Changes in absolute efficiencies with variation in vesicle forming components were recorded, however, they were between 10-100 μg per mouse.

Baillie et al., 1986 reported that NSVs prepared by ether injection method in which 450 μmols of surfactant-cholesterol (7:3) were dissolved in ether and NSVs were prepared by injecting the etherial solution into 5 ml of 300 μg/ml aqueous solution of stilbogluconate. The NSVs so prepared were tested in *Leishmaniasis donavani* infected male BALB/c mice. It was found that in regard to the biodistribution of stilbgluconate, the liposomes and niosomes were similar. It was further noticed that chemical characteristics of vesicular components are not of much importance as far as parasite hit or antileishmaniasis activity is concerned. This may be assumed related to passive delivery of vesicle and the contents through RES recognition and uptake.

In another study, Carter et al., 1988 evaluated various stilbogluconate preparations against *Leishmaniasis donavani*. The experiment was conducted on BALB/c mouse model of leishmaniasis. One or single dose therapy or multiple dosing with drug loaded vesicles prepared following sonication, liposomes and niosomes were found to be therapeutically effective against parasite(s). Reduction of vesicle size has little effect on over all efficacy of the system(s), whilst chances of their escape to Kupffer cells uptake increased since smaller vesicles could pass easily through the fenestration to accumulate in the sinusoidal spaces of epithelium.

Niosomes in Oncology

Investigations carried out with methotrexate reveal that NSVs containing methotrexate exhibited an effect comparable to its liposomal counter part. Much more consistent plasma levels were obtained, however, methotrexate levels in liver of mice were significantly higher at all sampling times than the liver methotrexate levels estimated in mice administered with methotrexate solution. The brain methotrexate level was significantly different in the case of methotrexate NSVs administration as compared against the level estimated following Tween 80-methotrexate administration. Furthermore, at 2,3,4 and 24 h sampling time, the levels estimated after methotrexate NSVs administration were significantly higher than those estimated following MTX-Tween 80 solution administration. The distribution of methotrexate administered as NSVs was noticeably different as compared to MTX-Tween 80 in aqueous solution of methotrexate did not affect its distribution pharmacokinetics.

The study thus suggested that MTX contained in NSVs could be useful in maintaining the blood MTX levels after intravenous administration. Similar re^ults were reported by many workers for methotrexate after its administration in liposomal form (Kimelberg, 1976; Kimelberg et al., 1976; Kimelberg and Atehison, 1978; Freise et al., 1981, Puisieux and Benita, 1982). It was concluded that large amount of MTX administered, accumulates in liver due to selective uptake of vesicular system. It is likely that similar to liposomes, niosomes are also taken up intact by liver. The vesicles subsequently are broken down to release their contents (MTX), the latter (liberated drug eventually reenters the blood circulation. Moreover, following administration of MTX in niosomes, minimizes the side effects significantly.

Rogerson et al., 1988 prepared and evaluated niosomes based doxorubicin (DOX) formulation. surfactant I:cholesterol (50:50 molar) was used as basic vesicular components. The formulation was administered as a bolus through tail caudal vein at a dose of 5 mg per Kg body weight. Following administration, the drug was estimated in serum, liver, heart, lungs and tumour. Doxorubicin was found to distribute rapidly after intravenous administration with concomitant rapid equilibration in heart and liver tissues. The plasma doxorubicin levels were considerably higher for entire period of study; confirming sustained release characteristics of niosomal preparation.

Contrary to the findings of Azmin et al., 1985 for NSVs-MTX uptake by liver cell, a negligible accumulation of doxorubicin was recorded in liver. Cholesterol containing DOX-NSVs produced relatively protracted blood levels probably as a consequence of slow release of entrapped drug.

Cardiac tissue concentration profile of doxorubicin for each of the reparation was monitored and found to be similar over the entire course of study. Cholesterol free niosomes were generally found to be more effective of the two other carrier systems as the reduced cardiac level was noted following its administration.

The doxorubicin levels determined in lungs were noticeably higher after NSVs-DOX administration as compared to free drug. It was conceivably assumed that NSVs are not completely sieved out by alveolar capillaries, thus retention of substantial number of NSVs could be accounted for higher drug tissue levels. The increase in drug levels may also be attributed to the rapidly proliferating alveolar phagocytic cells within the basement epithelium, which could effectively intercept the particulate carriers from the circulation. The drug level pattern recorded in spleen was similar to the liver, wherein no significant difference in doxorubicin levels was observed when compared amongst the formulations. It was observed that following NSVs-DOX administration, the doxorubicin level in S-1809 sarcoma increased significantly as recorded just after administration.

The higher tumour DOX concentration reflected an improved antitumour activity following a single 2.5 mg per Kg bolus to S-180 bearing mice. Study suggests that administration of NSVs-DOX increased the life span of tumour bearing mice and discernibly regressed the tumour. The prolonged circulation of drug, altered metabolism and maintenance of antitumour activity have been demonstrated. Cable et al., 1988 prepared DOX bearing niosomes using hexadecylpoly(3) glyceryl ether I (50%), cholesterol (25%) and cholesteryl poly (24) oxyethylene ether (solulan C-24) (25%) employing hand shaking technique. The surfactant thin film was hydrated using an aqueous DOX solution. Following hydration the vesicles were sonicated. The niosomes bearing DOX was injected in mice. NSVs-DOX resulted in sustained and higher plasma levels of doxorubicin. Drug levels estimated in heart, kidney and liver suggested that solulan C-24 enhanced the absorption of DOX.

Incorporation of methotrexate in Span 60 and Span 85 - cholesterol based NSVs has been reported. It was observed that in Span(s) with increased lipophilicity their entrapment efficiency increased. Unilamellar vesicles prepared using Span 80 showed maximum entrapment as well as improved antitumour activity when tested in S-180 sarcoma bearing mice and compared against free drug solution administration in equivalent dose (Chandraprakash et al., 1990).

Adriamycin loaded niosomes using monoalkyl triglycerol ether were prepared and their tumouricidal activity was compared against free drug solution. Human lung tumour cells were grown in monolayer cell lining and spheroidal culture and used in *in vitro* antitumour activity study. The activity of niosomal preparations was also determined in tumour xenografted nude mice. The activity of encapsulated adriamycin tested in *in vitro* was found to be maintained with similar clonogenic survival curve (Kerr et al., 1988).

Various doxorubicin particulate delivery systems have been found to circumvent the multi-drug resistance in tumour cells. In a study DOX resistant ovary cell lining produced via repeated exposure to the agent and subsequently incubated with free and niosome entrapped DOX. It was observed that survival curve after niosomal DOX exhibited improved performance, however cross resistance was recorded (Uchegbu et al., 1993).

The use of doxorubicin, a broad-spectrum antineoplastic agent is hampered by a dose limiting cardiomyopathy and myelosuppresion (Omotosho et al., 1986). To overcome this, PK1, a N-(2-hydroxypropul) methacrylamide (HPMA) copolymer conjugate containing doxorubicin and currently in early clinical development has been described (Chabner et al., 1996; Duncan, 1992). However, a i.v. injection of PK1 showed significant amount of excretion of glomerular filtration (Duncan et al., 1991; Seymour et al., 1990). This led to less accumulation at the toxicity site. To overcome this, encapsulation of PK1 within non-ionic surfactant vesicles have been studied (Pimm et al., 1996; Uchegbu et al., 1996a). The studies have shown encouraging results.

Uchegbu et al., 1996b reported the altered levels of niosomal doxorubicin in plasma along with the effect of encapsulation on metabolism. The clearance of doxorubicin released from the niosomes was about 10 fold greater (176.5 ml/h) than the clearance of niosomal doxorubicin (16.2 ml/h). The area under the tumour level-time curve increased by over 50% as compared to plain drug solution. Doxorubicin metabolites, namely doxorubicinol and the aglycones doxorubicinone, doxorubicinolone and 7-deoxyrubicinone were found associated with the niosomes in the plasma, possibly due to their adsorption on to the vesicle surface once formed outside the niosome or may be due to the degradation of the parent molecule within the bilayer.

Encouraging effects of niosome bearing doxorbuicin against ovarian cancer cell lines have been studied and reported by Uchegbu et al., 1996c.

Niosomes as Immunological Adjuvant

The ability of non-ionic surfactant based vesicles (niosomes) to enhance antibody production in response to bovine serum albumin (BSA) was compared with Freund's complete adjuvant (FCA) in the BALB/c mouse. The administration of niosomal-BSA as two subcutaneous inoculum induced antibody levels comparable to those produced by FCA by subcutaneous or intraperitoneal route of inoculation. Intraperitoneal administration however did not generate a stronger antibody response. The adjuvant activity of NSVs was found to be dependent on the BSA entrapped within the preformed vesicles. Analysis of the anti-BSA IgG subclasses induced by NSVs and FCA showed that NSVs are relatively better stimulant of IgG2 than FCA, whereas for IgG1 it was found to be a poorer stimulator. Thus, NSVs were realized as potentially better stimulant for Th1 lymphocyte subset than FCA and thus by inference, potent stimulator of cellular immunity. The NSVs are believed to be potentially advantageous adjuvant in terms of immunological selectivity, low toxicity and stability (Brawer and Alexender, 1992).

Hemoglobin containing niosomes were prepared and studied for functional and physical properties. Haemoglobin niosomes were prepared using Oreal's synthetic lipids (non-ionic surfactants) by reverse phase evaporation method. The niosomes were unilamellar and were found to be permeable to oxygen, with haemoglobin dissolution profile modifiable quite closer to nonencapsulated haemoglobin.

Moser et al., 1980 carried out study on niosomal haemoglobin for its compatibility and interaction with blood. The study mainly included the agglutination phenomenon with ABO blood group components as plasma extenders and erythrocyte phenotypes. Adsorption of plasma protein by immunoelectrophoresis, effect of niosomal haemoglobin on blood coagulation by thromboelastography, interaction of niosomes with phagocytes by electron microscopy, chemotaxis migration, oxygen consumption, superoxidase generation and oxidase function were also evaluated. It was concluded that agglutination with erythrocytes was dispersible on shaking. Albumin and eventually transferrin were found to adsorb on the surface, however, caused no destabilization of niosomes. With regard to coagulation, insignificant effect of niosomes on prothrombin time and coagulation was recorded. However, extended clotting time was noted which was considered essentially a consequence of blood dilution. Cellular oxygen consumption, oxygenated metabolite generation and oxidase activity were non responsive to the contained electric charge on the niosomes, and all recorded to be at acceptable levels and limits.

Non-ionic Surfactants and Oral Drug Delivery

Peptoidal ergot alkaloids are poorly absorbed after oral administration. The incomplete intestinal absorption of the alkaloids was increased significantly when administered in bile duct cannulated rats as micellar solution together with POE-24-cholesteryl ether. *In vitro* diffusion studies suggested that diffusion of ergot alkaloids across the mucous barrier is facilitated by micellar entrapment of the drug.

Yoshida et al., 1992 studied the potential of niosomal carrier system in oral delivery of peptide drugs. The absorption of 9-desglycinamide-8-arginine vasopressin (DGAVP) entrapped in $C_{12}EO_3$, $C_{12}EO_7$, $C_{18}EO_3$ and $C_{18}EO_7$ non-ionic surfactant based vesicles after oral administration was determined. The vesicles exhibited strong dependency on cholesterol concentration for CF release. The absorption studies were conducted in *in vitro*.

The stability of DGAVP was found to increase significantly in mucosal fluid on incorporation into the niosomes. No substantial difference between the absorptions of DGAVP was recorded. Thus, the possible penetration enhancing effect of surfactants was excluded. An entirely different serosal concentration profile of DGAVP was recorded when niosome encapsulated DGAVP was administered. The increased concentration of DGAVP found in acceptor phase was apparently assumed due to the protection of DGAVP against intestinal degradation due to an effective reduction in transport pathway owing to the attachment of intact niosomal vesicles to the intestinal wall. Another explanation proposed was the absorption and translocation of the vesicular system intact into the systemic circulation. The actual mechanism, which brings about an enhanced absorption of niosomal DGAVP is still to be explored. Nevertheless, niosomes have great potential, as carrier system in safe and successful delivery of peptoidal drugs, however extended studies to define toxicological behaviour and *in vivo* performance are desired before they can become clinical reality.

Niosomes for Transdermal Drug Delivery

Niosomes appear to have application in topical and transdermal products both containing hydrophobic and hydrophilic drugs. Besides, niosomes have also been used to encapsulate, lidocaine (Vanhal et al., 1996a), estradiol (Vanhal et al., 1996b), cyclosporin (Dowton et al., 1993), erythromycin (Jayaraman, 1996), alpha-interferon (Niemac et al., 1995), plasmid DNA for the human interleukin-1 receptor (Niemic et al., 1997) for topical and transdermal delivery.

Junginger et al., 1991 have observed small (100 nm) vesicular structures between the first and second layer of human cornecytes on 48 h incubation with niosomes prepared from dodecyl alcohol polyoxyethylene ether and cholesterol. Penetration by niosomes of this upper layer appears plausible as these layers are only loosely packed. However, the same study reports the presence of vesicular structures in the deeper layers seemingly inaccessible areas of the skin and concludes that there was a reorganization of the niosome membrane into individual monomers which on arriving at these deeper layers reformed into niosomes (Junginger et al., 1991).

Vanhal et al., 1996b have performed *in vitro* studies on the transdermal penetration of oestradiol using high phase transition sucrose ester niosomes or $C_{18}EO_7$ niosomes and low phase transition $C_{12}EO_7$ niosomes. They found that $C_{12}EO_7$ niosomes are better transdermal carriers. The higher flexibility of these bilayers is said to be responsible for this improved transdermal penetration. Reducing the cholesterol content of these niosomes also increases the transdermal delivery of oestradiol.

The intracellular route is the main route of vesicle penetration across the skin (Schatzlein and Ceve, 1993; Schatzlein and Ceve, 1998; Kuijk-Meuwissen et al., 1998). Ultraflexible vesicles penetrate along irregularities between the intracellular lipid lamellae and adjacent cornecyte envelops (Fig. 6-13). The combination of molecules with suitably differing molecular shapes (Fig. 6-14) can render a membrane flexible. The flexible membrane accommodates stress induced curvature changes and the vesicle changes shape easily. Consequently such vesicles require significantly less (deformation) energy to pass through small pores than rigid membranes. Sufficiently elastic vesicles can penetrate into deeper layers but rigid vesicles remain restricted to the

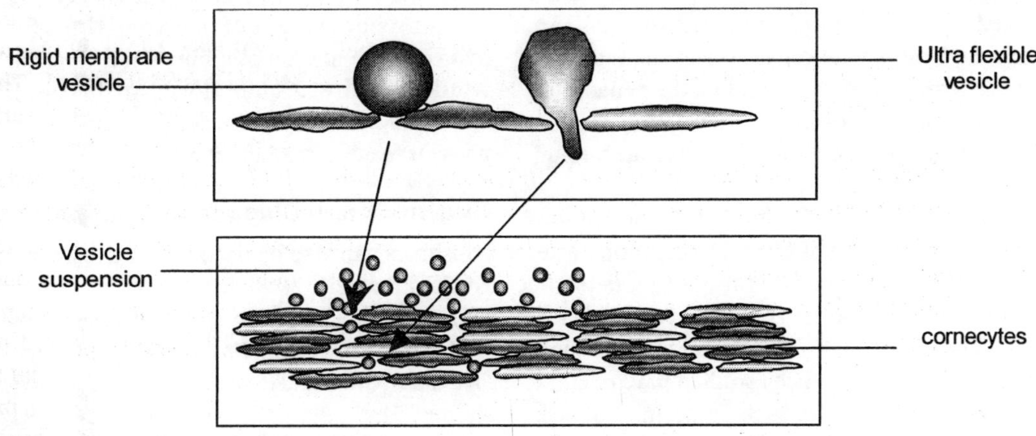

Fig. 6-13. Schematic Representation of Vesicle Penetration Across the Skin via Intracellular Route

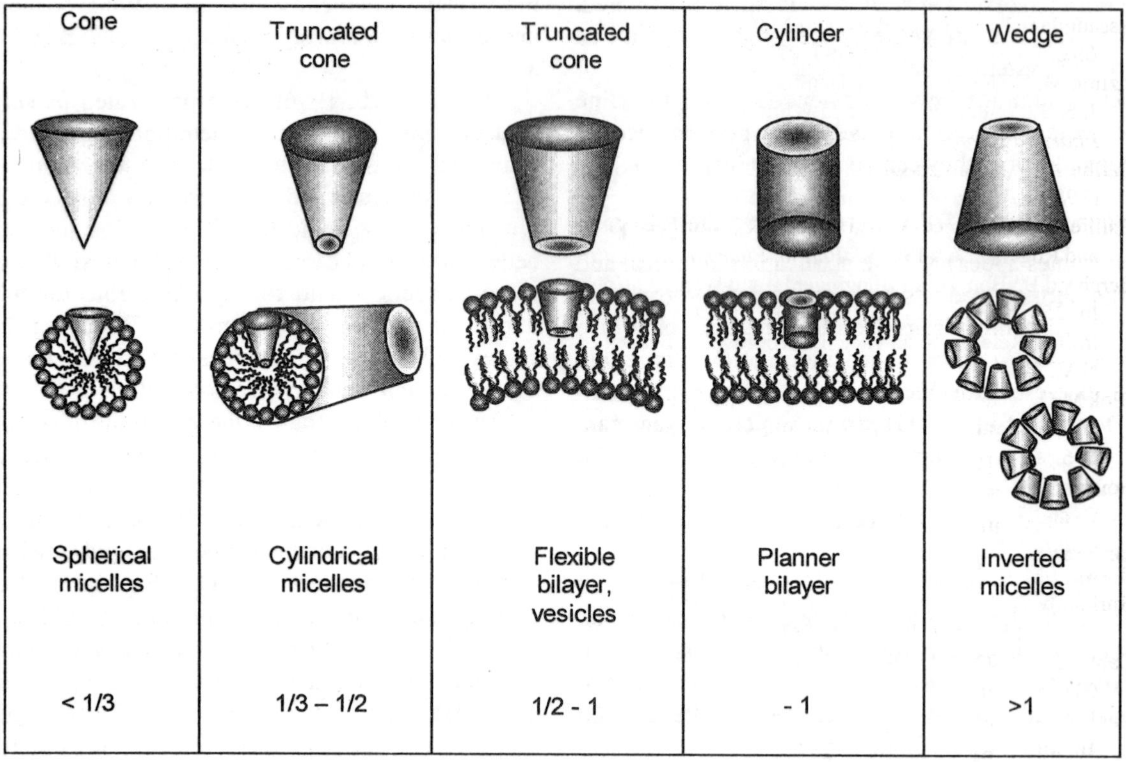

Cone	Truncated cone	Truncated cone	Cylinder	Wedge
Spherical micelles	Cylindrical micelles	Flexible bilayer, vesicles	Planner bilayer	Inverted micelles
< 1/3	1/3 – 1/2	1/2 - 1	- 1	>1

Fig. 6-14. Schematic Representation of the Effective Molecular Shapes of Amphiphiles and the Resulting aggregates. The shape of molecule will be determined by the ratio of chain volume to head group

loosely packed upper layers. Bergh et al., 1998 prepared flexible liquid state niosomes from polyoxyethylene laurate ester, sucrose laurate ester and cholesterol sulphate and studied the penetration behaviour of these niosomes. They found that the flexible niosomes can penetrate and permeate through skin.

Hu and coworker, 1994 studied the delivery of cyclosporin A in a number of formulations after topical application in hairless mouse model. The migration of cyclosporin A from cyclosporin A glyceryl dilaurate/$C_{16}EO_{10}$/cholesterol niosomes into the deeper strata has also been studied *in vitro* and it was found that the factors such as dosing volumes produce an increased uptake of the drug into deeper skin strata (Niemec et al., 1994). Based on above studies, it does appear that transdermal drug delivery with niosomes appears promising for both hydrophobic and amphiphilic drug molecules and would require higher doses to be applied by entrapping the drug in niosomes prepared from low phase transition surfactant mixtures.

Niosomes and Diagnostic Imaging

Niosomes can also be used for diagnostic purposes. Korkmaz et al., 2000 formulated DTPA carrying niosomes (hexadecyl triglycerol ether:chol:DTPA 10:1:4) to study the *in vitro* release, radiolabeling, *in vivo* distribution and to perform scintigraphic imaging studies. They found that niosomes can act as carrier for radiopharmaceuticals and site specific vehicle for spleen and liver imaging.

REFERENCES

Assadullahi T. P., Hidler R. C. and McAuley A. J. (1991) *Biochim. Biophys. Acta* **1083**, 271.

Azmin M. N., Florence A. T., Handjani-Vila R. M., Stuart J. F. B., Vanlerberghe G. and Whittaker J. S. (1985) *J. Pharm. Pharmacol.* **37**, 237.

Baillie A. J., Coombs G. H., Dolan T. F. and Laurie J. (1986) *J. Pharm. Pharmacol.* **38**, 502.

Baillie A. J., Florence A. T., Hume L. R., Murihead G. T. and Rogerson A. (1985) *J. Pharm. Pharmacol.* **37**, 863

Bergh v.d.B., Bouwstra J. Junginger H. and Wertz P. (1998) In: 25th Int. Sym. On Contrl. Rel. of Bioact. Mat., Controlled Release Soc., Inc., Deerfield I.L., Lasvegas, N.V., USA, 18.

Blok M.C., Vander E.C.M., Neutkot L., Van-Deenan L.M. and DeGier J. (1975) *Biochim. Biophys. Acta* **406**,187-196.

Bowstra J. A., Hofland H. E. J., Spies F., Ponec M., Verhoef C. and Junginger H. E. (1990) *Proc. Int. Symp. Control. Rel. Bioact. Mater.* **17**, 395.

Brawer J.M. and Alexander J. (1992) *Immunology* 75, 570.

Burkhnov S.A., Kosykh V.S., Saatov T.S. and Torchlin V.P. (1988) *Int. J. Pharm.* **46**, 31.

Cable C. (1989) Ph.D. Thesis, University of Strathclyde, Glasgow.

Cable C. and Florence A.T. (1988) *J. Pharm. Pharmacol.* **40**, 30.

Cable C., Cassidy J., Kaye S.B. and Florence A.T. (1988) *J.Pharm. Pharmacol.* **40**, Suppl.31.

Carter K. C., Baillie A. J., Alexander J. and Dolan T. F. (1988) *J. Pharm. Pharmacol.* **40**, 370.

Chabner B. A., Allegra C. J., Curt G. A. and Calabresi P. (1996) In: Goodman and Gilman's The Pharmacological Basis of Therapeutics, 9th edition. McGraw Hill's 1265.

Chandraprakash K. S., Udupa N., Umadevi P. and Pillai G. K. (1990) *Int. J. Pharm.* **61**, R1.

Chandraprakash K. S., Udupa N., Umadevi P. and Pillai G. K. (1994) *J. Drug. Target.* **1**, 143.

Chandraprakash K.S., Udupa N., Umadevi P. and Pillai G.K. (1991) *Int. J. Pharm.* **61**, 41.

Chauhan S. and Florence A.T. (1989) *J. Pharm. Pharmacol.* **41**, 6.

Croft S. (1986) *Pharm. Int.* **7**, 229.

Cullis P. R., Hope M. J., Bally M. B., Madden T. M., Mayer L. D. and Janoff A. S. (1987) In: Liposomes from Biophysics to Therapeutics. Ostro M. J. (Ed.) Marcell Dekker Inc. New York. 39.

Deamer D.W. (1978) *Ann. N.Y. Acad. Sci.* **308**, 250.

Deamer D.W. and Bangham A.O. (1976). *Biochem. Biophys. Acta* **443**, 629.

Demel R.A. and Kruyff B. (1976) *Biochim. Biophys. Acta* **457**, 109.

Dowton S. M. (1993) *STP Pharma Sciences*. **3**, 404.

Duncan R. (1992) *Anti Cancer Drugs* **3**, 175.

Duncan R., Bhakoo M., Riley M. L. and Tuboku-Metzger A. (1991) In: Progress in Membrane Biotechnology, Gomez-Fernandez J. C., Chapman D. and Packer L (Eds.) Birkhauser Verlag, Basel, 253.

Echegoyan L.E., Hernandez J.C., Kaifer A.E. Gokel G.W. (1988) *J. Chem. Soc. Chem. Communi.* **8**, 36.

Florence A. T. (1993) In: Liposome Technology, Vol. II. 2nd ed. Gredoriadis G. (Ed.), CRC Press, Boca Raton, FL., 157.

Florence A. T., Cable C., Cassidy J. and Kaye S. B. (1990) In: Targeting of Drugs, Gregoriadis G., Allison A. C. and Poste G. (Eds.) Plenum Pres, New York. 117.

Florence A. T., Omotosho J. A. and Whateley T. L. (1989) In: Controlled Release from Drug Polymers and Aggregate Systems. Rosoff M. (Ed.) VCH, New York.

Florence A.T. (1993) In: Liposome Technology, Gregoriadis G. (Ed.) Vol. II, 2nd edition, CRC Press, Boca Raton, London, 165.

Freise J., Muller W., Broelsch C.H. and Magerested P. (1982) *Hepato.Gastroenterol.* **28**, 90.

Gebicki J. M. and Hicks M. (1976) *Chem. Phys. Lipids* **16**, 142.

Gregoriadis G. (1993) In: Liposomes: Technology, Gregoriadis G. (Ed.) 2nd edition, CRC Press Inc., Boca Raton, London.

Griener J., Reiss J. G., Vierlungin P. (1993) In: Organofluorine Compounds in Medicinal Chemistry and Biomedical Applications. Filler R., Kobayashi Y. and Yagopolskii L. M. (Eds.) Elsevier, Amsterdam. 339.

Gruner S.M., Lenk R.P., Janoff A.S. and Ostro M.J. (1985) *Biochemistry* **24**, 2833.

Guedj G., Pucci B., Zarif L., Coulomb C., Riess J. G. and Pavia A. (1994) *Chem. Phys. Lip.* **172**, 153.

Handjani-Vila R. M., Ribier A. and Vanlerberghe G. (1993) In: Liposome Technology. Gregoriadis G. (Ed.) CRC Press, Boca Raton. 201.

Handjani-Vila R.M., Riber A., Randot B. and valenberghe G. (1979) *Int. J. Cosmo. Sci.* **1**, 303.

Haran G., Coben R., Bar L. K. and Barenholz Y. (1993) *Biochim. Biophys. Acta* **1151**, 201.

Harrigan P. R., Wong K. F., Redelmeier T. E., Wheeler J.

J. and Cullis P. R. (1993) *Biochim. Biophys. Acta* **1149**, 329.

Hashida M., Liao M. H., Muranishi S. and Sezaki H. (1980) *Chem. Pharm. Bull.* **28**, 1659.

Helenus A. and Simons K. (1971) *Biochem.* **10**, *2542.*

Hillis L. R., Handly J. D. and Babbitt B. P. (1993) In: Liposome Technology. Vol. III 2nd ed. Gregoriadis G. (Ed.) CRC Press, Boca Raton FL. 301.

Hofland H. E. J., Bouwstra J. A., Verhoef J. C., Buckton G., Chowdry B. Z., Ponec M. and Junginger H. E. (1992) *J. Pharm. Pharmacol.* **44**, 287.

Hofland H.E.F., Bouwstra J.A., Verhoef J. and Junginger H.E. (1989) *Procee. Int. Symp. Contrl. Rel. Bioact. Mater*. **16**,136.

Hu C. and Rhodes D.G. (1996) *AAPS Meeting*, New Brunswick, NJ.

Hu Z., Niemice S.M., Ramchandran C. Wallach D.F.H. and Weiner N. (1994) STP Pharm. Sci. **4**, 446.

Hume K. (1987) Comparative Study of Niosomes and Liposomes: Their stability in Biological Environment. Ph.D.Thesis,Uniiversity of strathclyde, Scottland.

Hunter J.A., Dolan G.H., Coombs A..Baillie, J. (1988) *J.Pharm.Pharmacol*. **40**, 161.

Israelachvili J. (1985) In: Intermolecular and Surface Forces. Academic Press, London, 246.

Jain C.P. (1993) Niosomal Drug Delivery Systems, Ph.D. Thesis, Dr.Harisingh Gour Vishwavidyalaya, Sagar, India.

Jayaraman C. S. (1996) *J. Pharm. Sci.* **85**,1082.

Jousma H., Joosten J.G.H., and Junginger H.E. (1988) *Coll. Polym. Sci.* **266**, 640.

Jousma H., Joosten J.G.H., Gooris G.S. and Junginger H.E. (1989) *Coll. Polym. Sci.* **267**,353.

Junginger H., Hofland H., Bouwstra J. (1991) *Cossmet. Tolilet* **106**, 45.

Kato Y., Hosokawa T., Okubo Y., Hayakawa and Ito K. (1993) *Biol. Pharm. Bull.* **16**, 965.

Kempt J.M.A. and Crommelin D.J.A.(1988) *Pharm. Weekbl* **123**, 457.

Kerr D., Rogerson A., Morrison G. J., Florence A. T. and Kaye S. N. (1988) *Br. J. Cancer* **58**, 432.

Khand L., Rogerson A., Halbert G.W., Baillie A.J. and Florence A.T. (1987) *J.Pharm.Pharmacol* **39**, 41.

Kimelberg H.K. (1976) *Biochem.Biophys.Acta*. **448**, 531.

Kimelberg H.K. and Atchison M.L. (1978) *Ann. New York. Acad. Sci.* **308**, 395.

Kimelberg H.K., Tracy T.F., Biddlecome T.F. and Bourke R.S. (1976) *Cancer Res*. **36**, 2949.

Kiwada H., Nakajima I., Matsuura H., Tsuji M. and Kato Y. (1988) *Chem. Pharm. Bull.* **36**, 1841.

Kiwada H., Nimura H. and Kato Y. (1985a) *Chem. Pharm. Bull.* **33**, 2475.

Kiwada H., Nimura H., Fujisaki Y., Yamada S. and Kato Y. (1985b) *Chem. Pharm. Bull.* **33**, 753.

Kiwada, H., Nakamura, T., Matsuura, H., Tsuji, M. and

Klibanov A.L., Maruyama K., Torchilin V.P. and.Huang L. (1990) *FEBS. Lett.* **268**, 235.

Korkaz M., Ozer A.Y. and Hincal A.A. (2000) In: Synthetic surfactant vesicles, niosomes and other non-phospholipid vesicular systems, Uchegbu I. F. (Ed.) Hardwood Academic press, Netherland, 83.

Kronberg B., Dahlman A., Carlfors J., Karlsson J. and Artusson P. (1990) *J. Pharm. Sci.* **79**, 667.

Kuijk-Mauwissen V. M., Junginger H. and Bouwstra J.A. (1998) *Biochem. Biophy. Acta* **1371**, 31.

lsraelachvili J.N. (1985) Intermolecular and surface forces, Academic Press, London, 246.

Mezei M. (1993) In: Liposomes in Drug Delivery. Gregoriadis G., Florence A. T. and Patel H. M. (Eds.) Harwood, Amsterdam. 125.

Montero M. T., Marti A. and Hernandez-Borrel J. (1993) *Int. J. Pharm.* **96**, 157.

Moser P., Marchand A.M., Labrude P., Handjanivila R.M. and Vigneron C. (1980) *Pharmaceutica Acta Helvetiae* **64**, 192.

Muller, C.C. and Goymann, P. (1987) *Acta. Pharma. Tech.* **33**,60.

Murdan S., Gregoriadis G. and Florence A.T. (1996) *STP Pharm. Sci.* **6**, 44.

Murtas E., Carafa M., Riccierei E., Santucci E. and Alhaique F. (1994) *Proc. Int. Symp. Control. Rel. Bioact. Mater.* **21**, 857.

Neumann R. and Ringsdor H. (1986) *J. Am. Chem. Soc.* **108**, 487.

New R.R.C. (1990) In: Liposomes: A practical approach, New R.R.C. (Ed.) Oirill Press, Oxford University Press, New York, 19.

Newman G.C. and Huang C. (1975) *Biochemistry* **14**, 3363.

Niemac S., *et al.*, (1995) *Pharmaceutical research* **12**, 1184.

Niemic S. M., Hu Z., Ramachandran C., Wallach D. F. H. and Weiner N. (1997) *J. Pharm. Sci.* **86**, 701

Niemiec S. M., Hu Z., Ramachandran C., Wallach D. F. H. and Weiner N. (1994) *S.T.A. Pharm. Sci.* **4**, 145.

Okahata Y., Tanamachi S., Nagai M. and Kunitake T. (1981) *J. Colloid Interface Sci.* **82**, 401.

Omotosho J. A., Law T. K., Whateley T. L. and Florence A. T. (1986) *Colloids Surf.* **20**, 133.

Parthasarathi G., Udupa N., Umadevi P. and Pillai G. K. (1994) *J. Drug. Target.* **2**, 173.

Pimm M. V., Perkins A. C., Strohalm J., Ulbrich K. and Duncan R. (1996) *J. Drug Target.* **3**, 375.

Puisieux F. and Benita S. (1981) *Biomedicine* **36**, 4.

Raja Naresh R. A., Singh U. V., Udupa N. and Pillai G. K. (1994) *Indian Drugs* **30**, 275.

Rhodes D.G. and Hu C. (2000) In: Synthetic surfactant vesicles, niosomes and other non-phospholipid vesicular systems, Uchegbu I. F. (Ed.) Hardwood Academic press, Netherland, 83.

Riber A., Handjani-Vila R. M., Bardez E. and Valeur B. (1984) *Colloids Surfaces* **10**, 155.

Rogerson A., Cummings J., Willmott N. and Florence A. T. (1988) *J. Pharm. Pharmacol*. **40**, 337.

Rogerson A., Cummings J., Willmott N. and Florence A.T. (1988) *J.Microencapsulation* **4**, 321.

Schatzlein A. and Ceve G. (1993) In: 6th International colloquium on phospholipids, Oct. 25-27, Ceve G. and Pathauf F. (Eds.) AOCS press, Champaign, Illinois, USA, 189.

Schatzlein A. and Ceve G. (1998) *Br. J. Dermatol.* **138**, 538.

Seymour L. W., Ulbrich K., Strohalm J., Kopecek J. and Duncan R.(1990) *Biochem Pharmacol*. **39**, 1125.

Stafford S., Baillie A. J. and Florence A. T. (1988) *J. Pharm. Pharmacol* **40**, 26P.

Szoka F. and Papahadjopoulos D. (1978) *Proc. Natl. Acad. Sci. USA* **41**, 48.

Talma H., Steenbergen M.J.V., Borchert J.C.H. and Crommelin D.J.A. (1994) *J. Pharm. Sci*. **83**, 276.

Tanaka M., Fukuda H. and Horiuchi T. (1990) *J. Am. Oil Chem. Soc.* **67**, 55.

Tucker I.G. and Florence A.T. (1983) *Pharm.Pharmacol.* **35**, 705.

Uchegbu I. F. (1994) Ph.D. Thesis. School of Pharmacy, University of London.

Uchegbu I. F. and Florence A. T. (1995) *Adv. Colloid Interface Sci.* **58**, 1.

Uchegbu I. F., Bouwstra J. A., Florence A. T. (1992) *J. Phys. Chem.* **96**, 10548.

Uchegbu I. F., Double J. A., Kelland L. R., Turton J. A. and Florence A. T. (1996a) *J. Drug Target*. **3**, 399.

Uchegbu I. F., Double J. A., Turton J. A. and Florence A. T. (1995) *Pharm. Res.* **12**, 1019.

Uchegbu I. F., Gianasi E., Cociancich F., Florence A. T. and Duncan R. (1996b) *Proc. Int. Symp. Control. Release Bioact. Mater.* **23**, 182.

Uchegbu I. F., McCarthy D., Schatzlein A. and Florence A. T. (1996c) *S.T.P. Pharma Sci.* **6**, 33.

Uchegbu I. F., Turton J. A., Double J. A. and Florence A. T. (1994) *Biopharm. Drug Dispos*. **15**, 691.

Uchegbu I.F., Bouwstra J.A. and.Florenece A.T (1991) *J.Phys.Chem.* **96**, 10548.

Uchegbu I.F., Kelland L.R., Turton J.A. and Florence A.T. (1993) *J.Pharm.Pharmacol.* **45**, 1112.

Uchegbu I.F. and Vyas S. P. (1998) *Int. J. Pharm.* 172, 33.

Udupa N., Chandraprakash K. S., Umadevi P. and Pillai G. K. (1993) *D rug Develop. Ind. Pharm.* **19**, 1331.

Vaizoglu M.O. and Spieser P.P. (1986) *Acta. Pharm. Soc.* **23**, 167.

Van Hal D. A. (1994) Ph.D. Thesis, Leiden University, Leiden.

Vanhal D. A., Junginger H. and Bouwstrg J.(1996) *European J. Pharm. Sci.* **4**, 147.

Vanhal D., Varensen A., Deveringer T., Junginger H. and Bouwstrg J. (1996b) *STP Pharm. Sci.* **6**, 72.

Vanlerbergh G., Handjani-Vila R.M. and Robber A.(1978) *Coll. Nationaux. C.R.N.S.* No. 938,303.

Vanlerberghe G. and Hanjani-Vila R.M. (1975) *French Patent* 2,358,991.

Vanlerberghe G., Handjani-Vila R. M., Berthelot C. and Sebag H. (1972) In: Chemie Physikalische Chemie and Anwendungstechnik der Grenzflachenaktiven Stoffe. Carl Hanser Verlag, Munchen. 139.

Vemuri S., Yu C. D., Wangsatorntanakun V. and Roosdorp N. (1990) *Drug Devel. Ind. Pharm.* **16**, 2243.

Venkatesan N. and Vyas S.P. (1998) *Pharma. acta Helv.* **74**, 51.

Venkatesan N. and Vyas S.P. (1999) *Drug Delivery* **5**, 251.

Vyas S.P., Mysore N., Jaitely V., Venkatesan N. (1998) *Pharmazie* **53**, 466.

Yoshida H., Lehr C.M., Kok W., Junginger H.E. and Verhoef J.C. (1992) *J.Contr. Rel.* **21**, 145.

Yoshioka T., Gursel M., Skalko N., Gregoriadis G. and Florence A. T. (1995) *J. Drug. Target.* **2**, 533.

Yoshioka H., Ohmura T., Goto A. and Fujita T. (1990) *Agri. Biol. Chem.* **54**, 1763.

Yoshioka T. and Florence A. T. (1994) *Int. J. Pharm.* **108**, 117.

Yoshioka T., Sternberg B. and Florence A.T. (1994) *Int. J. Pharm.* **105**, 1.

Yoshioko T. and Florence A. T. (1994) *Int. J. Pharm.* **108**, 117.

Zarif L., Gulik-Krzywicki T., Reiss J. G., Pucci B., Guedj C. and Pavia A. (1993) *Colloids Surfaces* **84**, 107.

Zampighi G., Renolds J. A. and Watt R. W. (1980) *J. Cell Biol.* **87**, 556.

CHAPTER 7

Submicron Emulsions

- Introduction
- Submicron lipid emulsions
- Microemulsions
- Microemulsion formation and phase behaviour
- Theoretical aspects of the preparation of microemulsions
- Characterization of microemulsions
- Advantages of microemulsion-based systems
- Applications of Microemulsions
- Solid colloildal systems prepared from microemulsions
- Self Emulsifying Drug Delivery Systems (SEDDS)
- References

Emulsions are heterogeneous systems in which one immiscible liquid is dispersed as droplets in another liquid. Such a thermodynamically unstable system is kinetically stabilized by addition of one further component or mixture of components that exhibit emulsifying properties. The present international union of pure and applied chemistry definition of an emulsion, including liquid crystalline phases: 'In an emulsion, liquid droplets and/or liquid crystals are dispersed in a liquid'.

Emulsions in which water is an internal phase dispersed in oil are termed as water-in-oil (W/O), whereas, emulsions in which the oil is dispersed and water forms the continuous phase are known as O/W emulsions. All pharmaceutically emulsions designed for parenteral administration are typically of O/W type. More complex systems, in which one emulsion is further dispersed into another continuous phase, are called double emulsion, multiple emulsions or emulsified emulsions (discussed in detail elsewhere in the book). The droplet-size distribution of emulsion droplets is 0.5 - 50.0 μm. A more common average droplet size is 0.5 - 5.0 μm. The inner droplet size distribution of the W/O emulsion in the multiple emulsion is usually smaller than 0.5 μm, where as the outer, external multiple emulsion is quite large and can exceed 10 μm. Another emulsion system is microemulsion and can be defined as 'a system of water, oil and amphiphile, which is a single optically isotropic and thermodynamically stable solution.' The droplets in a microemulsion are in the range of 0.1- 1.0 μm. Self-microemulsifying drug delivery systems (SMEDDS) are not microemulsions but they are closely related system. A SMEDDS typically comprises a mixture of surfactant, oil and drug (known as the concentrate) which when introduced into the body is rapidly dispersed to form droplets of approximately the same size range as those observed in microemulsion systems. Once dispersed such systems would be expected to behave *in vivo* much the same way as oil-in-water (O/W) microemulsions (Lawrence and Rees, 2000). This chapter mainly deals with submicron lipid emulsions and microemulsions.

SUBMICRON LIPID EMULSIONS

Submicron (O/W) lipid emulsions are potential drug carriers for lipophilic and amphiphilic drugs with many favourable properties; they are biocompatible, biodegradable, stable, and easy to prepare and handle. The basic structure is a neutral lipid core (i.e. triglyceride) stabilized by a monolayer of amphiphilic lipid (i.e. phospholipid). Such emulsions can solubilize considerable amounts of lipophilic drugs in the core or/and amphiphilic ones in the surface monolayer. Table 7-1 shows reasons for development of medicated emulsions.

There are three prerequisites to be met by lipid emulsions for the designing of a drug carrier system;

1. Methods of preparation for adequate lipid emulsions,
2. Drugs should be suitable for incorporation into such systems,
3. Ligands attach on to the surface of emulsion globules for targeting to special sites in the body.

After appropriate choice of the emulsifiers, the emulsification can be performed by applying brief sonication or by pressure homogenization. Phospholipids are generally weak emulsifiers, but by addition of a non-ionic detergent like polysorbate 80, emulsions with globules diameter down to 50 nm with good physical stability can be produced. Drugs for effective incorporation into lipid emulsions should be preferably oil soluble or amphiphilic. An interesting prospect is also to combine several drugs in the same carrier, i.e. with an oil soluble drug in the core while an amphiphilic one in the surfacial monolayer crown. Lipid emulsions are suitable for both passive and active drug targeting. Especially, coarse emulsions are rapidly taken up by the mononuclear phagocyte system (MPS) and can thus be used to deliver the drugs to macrophages. By coating emulsion droplets with a hydrophilic polymer like poly (ethyleneglycol) modified phosphatidyl-ethanolamine (PEG-PE), the uptake by MPS can be reduced, which results in prolonged circulation time.

Site specific delivery can be designed by attaching ligands specific for cellular receptors on to the surface of the emulsion globules. The system could be engineered to be long circulatory and site specific by binding of the ligands to the distal end of PEG chains. Such long circulating immunoemulsions have shown good immunochemical activity against target cells. The development of new effective ligands for site specific delivery is a challenging task in the future development of lipid emulsions as drug carriers.

Intravenously administered emulsions are excellent carriers for lipophilic drugs, which otherwise difficult to deliver. Emulsion systems are biodegradable, biocompatible, physically stable and relatively easy to produce on large scale. Lipid emulsion drug delivery systems seem to offer a wide variety of possibilities for preparing better tolerated intravenous formulations of poorly water soluble

Table 7-1. Rationale for Using and Developing Medicated Emulsions

Reason	Drug examples
Solubilization of poorly water soluble drugs	Diazepam, vitamin A, vitmin E, propofol, dexamethsone palmitate
Stabilization of hydrolytically susceptible compounds	Lomustine, physostigmine salicylate
Prevention of drug uptake by infusion sets	Diazepam, perilla ketone
Reduction of irritation, pain or toxicity of intravenously administered drugs	Amphotericin, diazepam, propofol
Potential for sustained release dosage forms	Barbiturates, dexamethasone palmitate, physostigmine salicylate
Site specific drug delivery to various organs	Cytotoxic agents

drugs while either maintaining the same characteristics engineered to pharmacokinetic and tissue distribution or enhancing the site specific delivery to target organs (Lovell et al., 1994; Tibell et al., 1995). Intralipid® was the first approved i.v. emulsion for parenteral nutrition and consists of an O/W emulsion of 10 or 20% soybean oil droplets (70-400 nm in size) stabilized by monolayer of egg yolk mixed phospholipids (1.2%) and glycerol (2.25%) as an osmotic agent. Some of the commercially available lipid emulsions are given in the Table 7-2 (Klang and Benita, 1998). Figure 7-1 describes the schemetic of the submicron lipid emulsion preparation.

MICROEMULSIONS

In the recent years microemulsions have attracted a great deal of attention not only because of their importance in industrial applications but also their intrinsic interest. They optimize the performance of a wide spectrum of products and processes. Microemulsions are isotropic and thermodynamically stable multicomponent fluids composed of water, oil, surfactant and/or cosurfactant. This unique class of optically clear solutions comprises of the colloidal systems that have attracted many scientific and technological interest over past decades. This wide interest stems from their properties, namely ultra low interfacial tension, large interfacial area and solubilization capacity for both water- and oil-soluble drugs. Microemulsions show diverse structural organizations due to the use of wide range of surfactant concentrations, water-oil ratios, temperatures etc. These and other properties render microemulsions intriguing from a fundamental point of view at the same versatile for industrial applications.

The basic difference between emulsions and microemulsions are that emulsions may exhibit excellent kinetic stability while fundamentally thermodynamically unstable and will in due time phases would separate out. In appearance emulsions are cloudy while microemulsions are clear and translucent. Emulsions require a large input of energy during their method of preparation but in the case of microemulsions energy requirement is considerably low.

Basic Aspects of Microemulsions

Microemulsions are fluid, transparent, thermodynamically stable oil and water systems, stabilized by a surfactant usually in conjunction with a cosurfactant, which may be a short chain alcohol, amine or other weakly amphiphilic molecule (Lawrence, 1994). An interesting characteristic of microemulsions is that the diameter of the droplets in a microemulsion is in the range of 100Å- 1000Å, whereas the diameter of droplets in a kinetically stable macroemulsion is 50 μm. This includes normal micellar solutions, reverse micelles, cores or droplets of water or oil and for some systems, even bicontinuous structures, in which neither oil nor water surrounds the other. Analysis of the thermodyna-

Table 7-2. Some Marketed available Lipid Emulsions Formulations (Klang and Benita, 1998)

Trade name	Oil phase (%)	Emulsifier (%)	Other components(%)
Intralipid® (Kabi-Pharmacia)	Soyabean 10 and 20	Egg lecithin 1.2	Glycerol 2.5
Lipofundin S® (Braun)	Soyabean 10 and 20	Soyabean lecithin 0.75 or 1.2	Xylitol 5.0
Lipofundin® (Braun)	Cottonseed	Soyabean lecithin 0.75	Sorbitol 5.0
Lipofundin N® (Braun)	Soyabean and MCT (1:1) 10 and 20	Egg lecithin 1.2	Glycerol 2.5
Liposys® (Abbott)	Safflower 10 and 20	Egg lecithin 1.2	Glycerol 2.5
Abbolipid® (Abbott)	Safflower and soybean (1:1) 10 and 20	Egg lecithin 1.2	Glycerol 2.5
Lipovenos® (Fresenius)	Soyabean 10 and 20	Egg lecithin 1.2	Glycerol 2.5
Travemulsion® (Travenol)	Soyabean 10 and 20	Egg lecithin 1.2	Glycerol 2.5

(adopted from Benita, 1998)

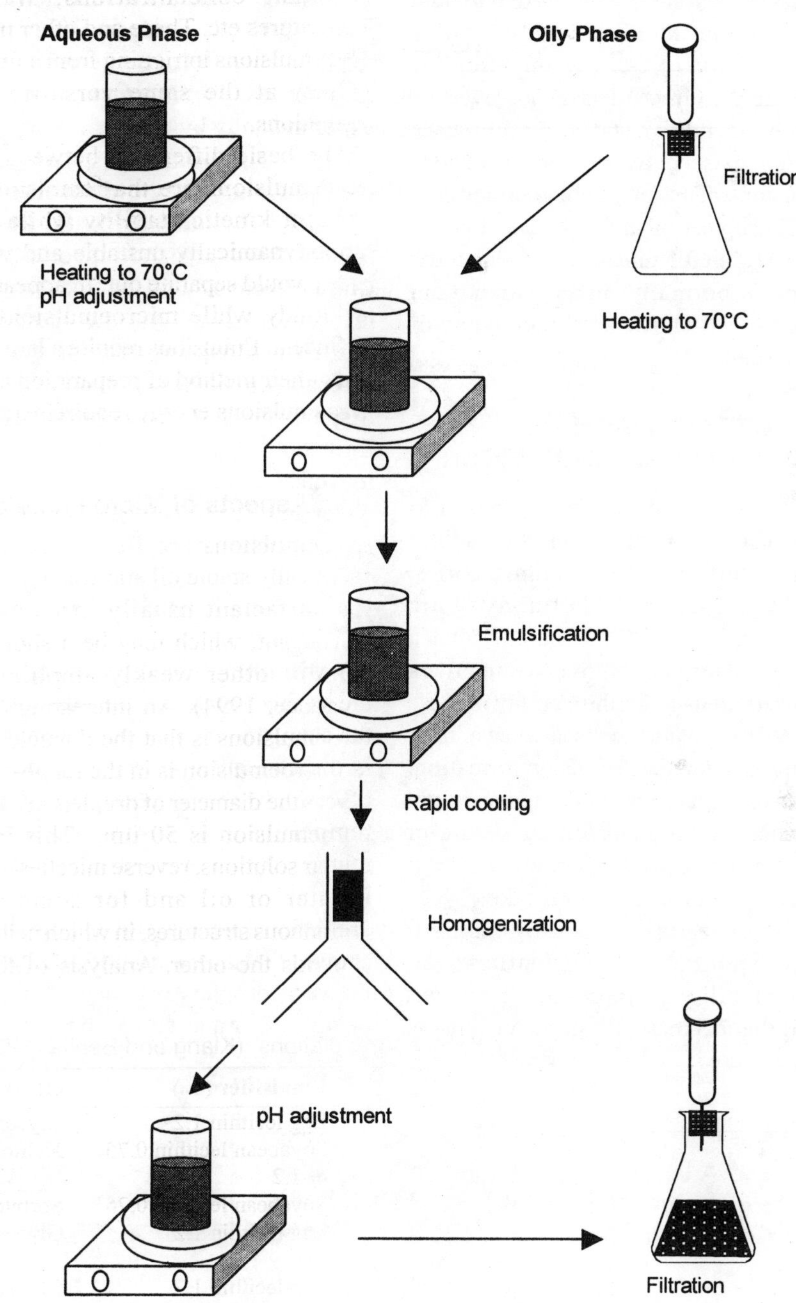

Fig. 7-1 Schematic Diagram of the Submicron LipidEmulsionPreparation

mically stability indicates that a microemulsion, being a liquid-liquid dispersed system, consists of two bulk phases separated by an interface region. In this respect microemulsion differs from micellar solutions; there are no direct means, however, of distinguishing between the two states. By contrast, a clear-cut distinction exists between microemulsions and coarse emulsions. The latter are thermodynamically unstable, droplets of their dispersed phase are generally larger than 0.1 μm, and, consequently, their appearance is normally milky rather than transparent. Figure 7-2 shows different types of microemulsion systems.

MICROEMULSION FORMATION AND PHASE BEHAVIOUR

Three different approaches have been proposed to explain microemulsion formation and the stability aspects. These are interfacial or mixed film theories, solubilization theories and thermodynamic treatments. Schulman et al., 1959 realized that a reduction in interfacial tension by three to four orders of magnitude is a requirement for the stability of these systems. This view was a natural consequence of their experimental approach to microemulsion formation. A typical experiment consisted of adding a medium chain length alcohol to an emulsion consisting of water, oil and soap as an emulsifier. At a certain concentration of alcohol a transition takes place spontaneously from a turbid to a transparent emulsion. The spontaneous formation and thermodynamic stability of microemulsion was attributed to a further decrease of interfacial tension between water and oil by the effect of added alcohol. The lowering of interfacial tension continued to proceed till it aquired a negative value. The requirement of transient negative interfacial tensions for microemulsion formation was theoretically and experimentally by different groups.

The understanding of basis for the thermodynamic stability of microemulsions was advanced considerably with the development of several thermodynamic theories. Ruckenstein and Chi, 1975 considered the free energy of formation of microemulsions to be consisted of three contributions; interfacial energy, energy of interaction between droplets, and entropy of dispersion. The free energy of microemulsion formation can be considered to depend on the extent to which surfactant lowers the surface tension of oil-water interface and the change in entropy of the system such that,

$$\Delta G_f = \gamma \Delta A - T \Delta S \qquad (7\text{-}1)$$

where ΔG_f is the free energy of formation, γ is the surface tension of the oil-water interface, ΔA is the change in interfacial area on microemulsion. ΔS is the change in entropy of the system, which is effectively the dispersion entropy, and T is the temperature. It should be noted that when a microemulsion is formed, the change in ΔA is very large as a the large number of very small droplets are formed. Analysis of the thermodynamic factors showed that the contribution of the interaction energy between droplets was negligible and that the free energy of formation can be zero or negative if the

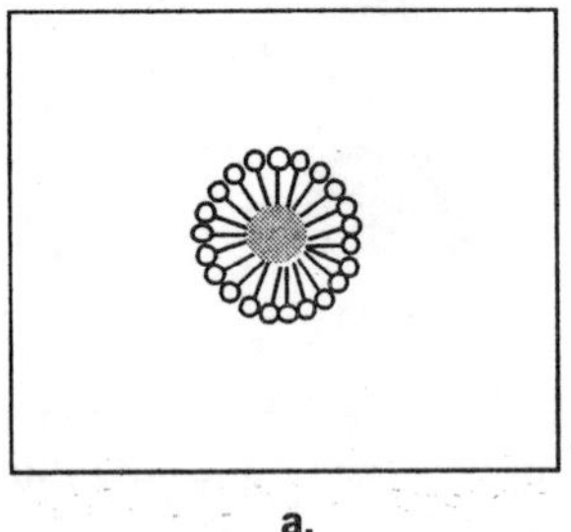

a.

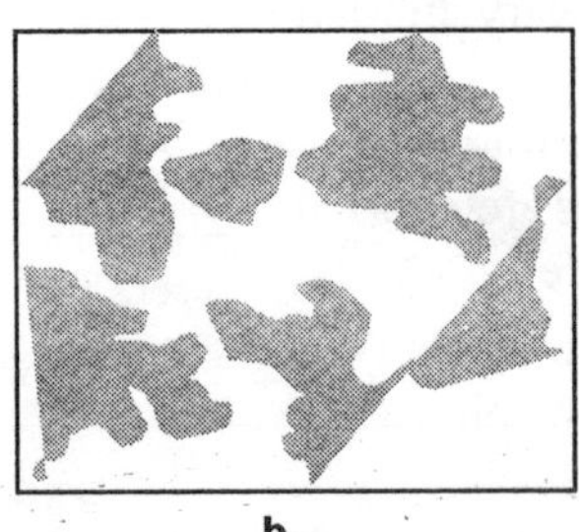

b.

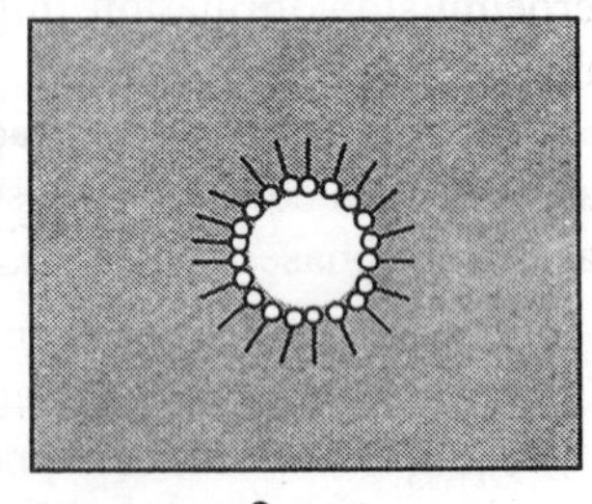

c.

Fig. 7-2. Schematic Representation of Different Microemulsion Systems: a. O/W Microemulsion; b. Bicontonuous Microemulsion; c. W/O Microemulsion

surface tension of oil-water interface is very low (of the order of 10^{-2} - 10^{-3} mN/m), although not necessarily negative.

Phase Behaviour

The phase behaviour of a mixture and its composition can be studied with the help of a phase diagram. The phase behaviour of simple microemulsion systems composing oil, water and surfactant can be studied with the aid of ternary phase diagram (at fixed pressure and temperature) in which each corner of the diagram represents 100% concentration of the particular component.

Generally, pharmaceutical microemulsions contain additional components such as a cosurfactant and/or drug. The cosurfactant is also amphiphilic with an affinity for both the oil and aqueous phases and partitions to an appreciable extent into the surfactant interfacial monolayer present at the oil-water interface. A wide variety of molecules can function as cosurfactant including non-ionic surfactant, alcohol, alkanoic acids, alkanoids and alkylamines. A large number of drug molecules are by themselves surface active and they are expected to influence phase behaviour. For four or more components, pseudo ternary phase diagrams are used to study the phase behaviour. In this diagram a corner will typically represent a binary mixture of two components such as surfactant/cosurfactant, water/drug or oil/drug. The number of different phases present for a particular mixture can be visually assessed. A schematic pseudo ternary phase diagram is shown in Figure 7-3. It should be noted that not every combination of components produce microemulsion over the whole range of possible composition, in some instances, the extent of microemulsion formation might be very limited (Table 7-3).

At low surfactant concentration, there are certain phases exists in equilibria, these phases are referred to as Winsor phases (Fig. 7-4). They are

1. Winsor I: With two phases, the lower (oil/water, O/W) microemulsion phase in equilibrium with the upper excess oil;
2. Winsor II: With two phases, the upper microemulsion phase (water/oil, W/O) in equilibrium with excess water;
3. Winsor III: With three phases, middle microemulsion phase (O/W plus W/O, called bicontinuous) in equilibrium with upper excess oil and lower excess water;
4. Winsor IV: In single phase, with oil, water and surfactant homogeneously mixed.

For microemulsions it is useful to consider the so-called critical packing parameter (Israelachvilli et al., 1976). The concept considers that the amphiphlic molecules can be regarded as two- piece structure: polar head and hydrophobic tail. The possible geometery of a film formed by the amphiphile molecules depends on their intrinsic geometery. The critical packing parameter (CPP) is calculated as

$$CPP = V/a_0 l \qquad (7\text{-}2)$$

where a_0 is the optimal area of the polar head, l the length of the hydrophobic tail, and V is volume. The area per polar head is usually measured at an air-water or oil-water interface using Gibbs isotherm (Ross and Morrison, 1988). The length of the hydrophobic tail can be calculated from the values obtained by Tanford (Tanford, 1980) and the volume of the hydrocarbon tail can be calculated from density of bulk hydrocarbon. Critical packing parameter lower than 1/3 give a tendency to form globular structures, values around 1/2 favour cylindrical structures, and values close to 1 favour planner layers. This parameter evaluates the natural geometery of the amphiphile itself. In microemulsions, hydrocarbon penetration and cosurfactant presence may completely change the structure to an alter form than which is predicted from the natural tendency of amphiphiles. Oil penetration in the hydrocarbon tail produces an increase in the apparent hydrophobic volume and thus an increase in the critical packing parameter. Cosurfactant, such as medium-chain alcohols, coabsorb at the interface, producing an overall reduction of the CPP. The concentration of the surfactant and the ratio of the pseudophases may play roles in the structure as well. High amounts of ionic surfactant produce a high ionic strength with a subsequent reduction of the polar head area and reduction of the CPP. High amounts of the internal

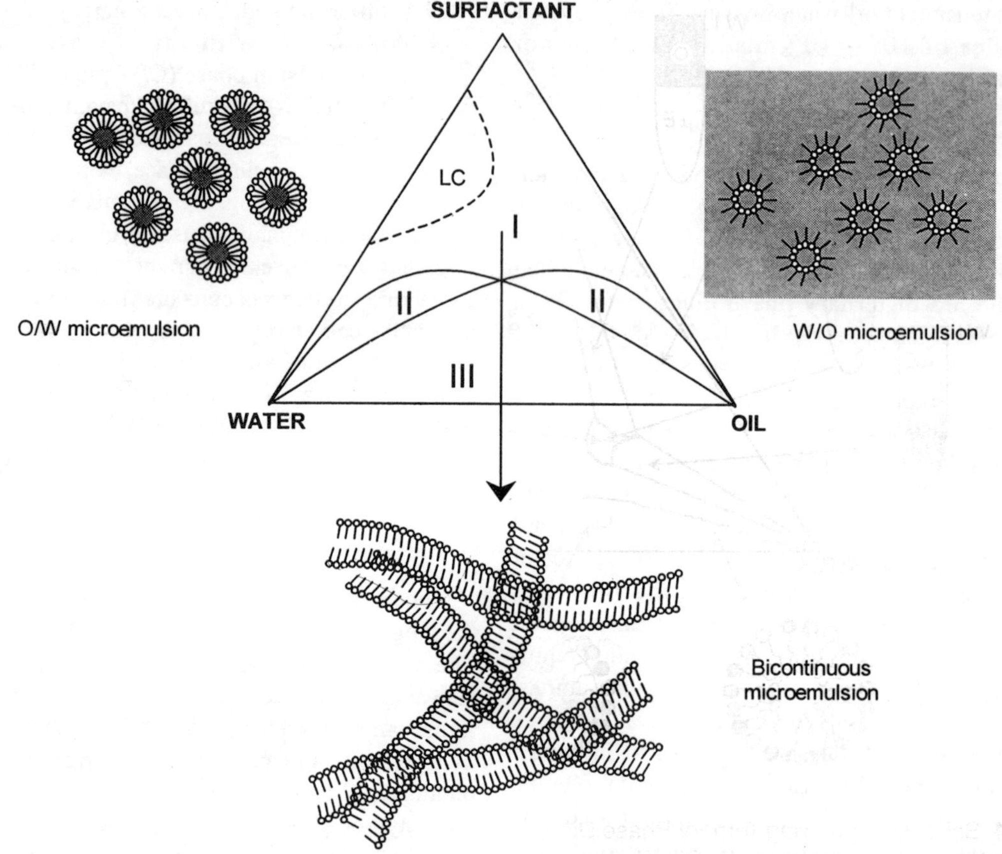

Fig. 7-3. Schematic Ternary Phase Diagram for a Typical Water/Nonionic Surfactant/Oil System at the HLB Temperature

pseudophase may produce phase separation if the total concentration of surfactant is low. Electrolyte concentration and temperature also affect the natural curvature of the amphiphile (Auvary et al., 1984; Kahlweit et al., 1987; Ravey and Buzier, 1984). Different structure depending on CPP are shown schematically in Figure 7-5.

Hydrophilic-lipophilic balance (HLB) also affects the surfactant behaviour (Carlford et al., 1991). The HLB takes into account the relative contribution of hydrophilic and hydrophobic fragments of the surfactant molecules. It is generally accepted that low HLB surfactants favoure for the formation of W/O microemulsions whereas surfactants with high HLBs are preferred for the formation of O/W microemulsion systems. Ionic surfactants such as sodium dodecyl sulphate which have HLBs greater than 20, often require the presence of a cosurfactant to reduce their effective HLB to a value within the range required for microemulsion formation.

THEORETICAL ASPECTS OF THE PREPARATION OF MICROEMULSIONS

For practical purposes, it is essential to form temperature-insensitive microemulsions of large solubilization potential. The use of hydrophilic surfactants oil-swollen-type or oil-in-water (O/W) microemulsions form, whereas lipophilic surfactants produce water-swollen-type or water-in-oil (W/O) microemulsions. When the hydrophilic-lipophilic types of surfactants are used in combination, a microemulsion (also called a surfactant phase or middle-phase microemulsion) coexists with an excess

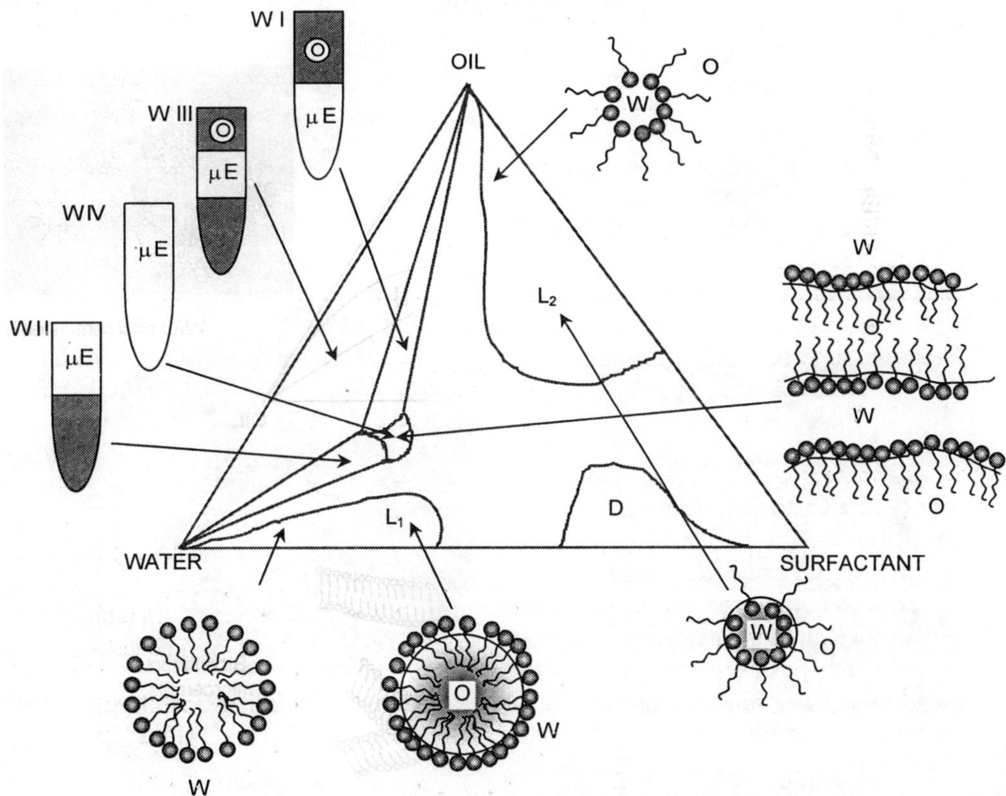

Fig. 7-4 Schematic Showing Ternary Phase Diagram of Winsor Phases (W I, W II, W III and W IV) Exists at Low Surfactant Concentration. O, Oil; W, Water; L_1, A Single Phase Region of Normal Micelles or Oil-in-Water (O/W) Microemulsion; L_2, Reverse Micelles or Water-in-Oil (W/O) Microemulsion; D, Anisotropic Lamellar Liquid Crystalline Phase; and μE Represents for Microemulsion

Table 7-3. Definitions of Some of the Common Lyotropic Phases

Phase	Basic structure
Micellar solutions (Optically isotropic)	More or less spherical, swollen, micelle containing solubilized, organic liquid
Middle phase, normal (Anisotropic)	Indefinitely long, mutually parallel rods in hexagonal array. The rods consists of more or less radially arranged amphiphiles. The hydrophiles are in contact with the surrounding continuous aqueous phase
Neat phase (Anisotropic)	Coherent double layers of amphiphilic molecules with the hydrophiles at the interfaces with intervening layers of water
Middlephase , reversed (Anisotropic)	Indefinitely long mutually parallel rods in hexagonal array. The lipophiles are arranged so that the surrounding continuous organic phase is in contact with the lipophiles .
Inverted micellar solution (Optically isotropic)	More or less spherical vertical micelles containing solubilized water

From Ekwall et al., 1975

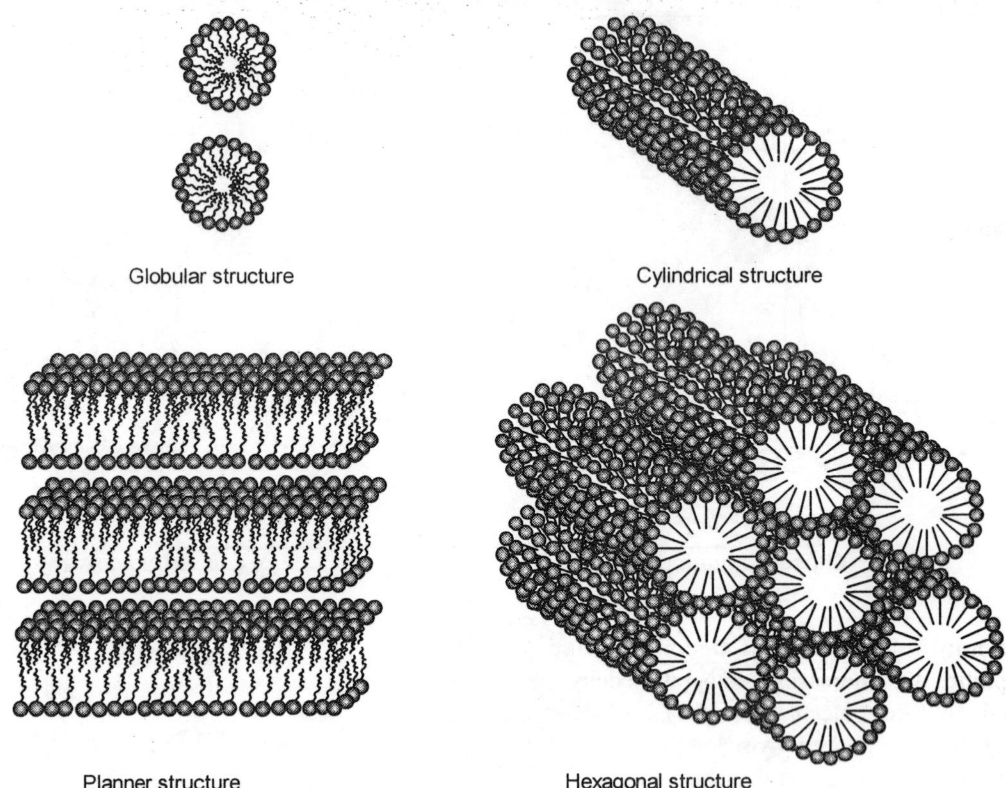

Fig. 7-5. Different Structure Formed in Oil-Water-Surfactent System Depending on Critical Packing Parameter (CPP)

water and an oil phase (Shinoda and Kunieda, 1973). The use of nonionic and ionic surfactant system makes the three-phase system to reach the maximum solubilization capacity. The change of temperature at the maximum solubilization is very sensitive for the phase behaviour. The phase behaviour becomes more temperature sensitive as the solubilization increases. Therefore, it is important to obtain the temperature-insensitive three-phase system to produce microemulsions stable against temperature change(s) in order to make it acceptable and applicable. Several attempts have been made to achieve stable microemulsions with single nonionic surfactant systems, ionic surfactant systems or mixed surfactant systems. The polyoxyethylene-type nonionic surfactants, mixed polyoxyethylene-type and sucrose-type non-ionic surfactant and mixed nonionic-ionic surfactant systems are used to get maximum desired solubilization in microemlsion systems (Kunieda and Solans, 1997).

Single Surfactant Systems

Single Nonionic Surfactant Systems

In the industrial field, the most widely used nonionic surfactants are polyoxyethylene-type nonionic surfactants. The middle-phase microemulsions are formed without the addition of cosurfactants, if the hydrophilic-lipophilic property of the nonionic surfactant is just balanced in a given water-oil system. When the weight fraction of oil in water + oil is plotted against temperature, different phases, e.g. oil-swollen miceller solution, waters-swollen reverse micellar solution phase and middle-phase microemulsion or surfactant phase appear to coexist. Figure 7-6 show the phase diagram of a water/pure homogeneous nonionic surfactant (trioxyethylene octyl ether)/ decane system as a function of temperature. The concentration of surfactant in the system is 11 %w/w.

As the temperature increases, polyoxyethylene-

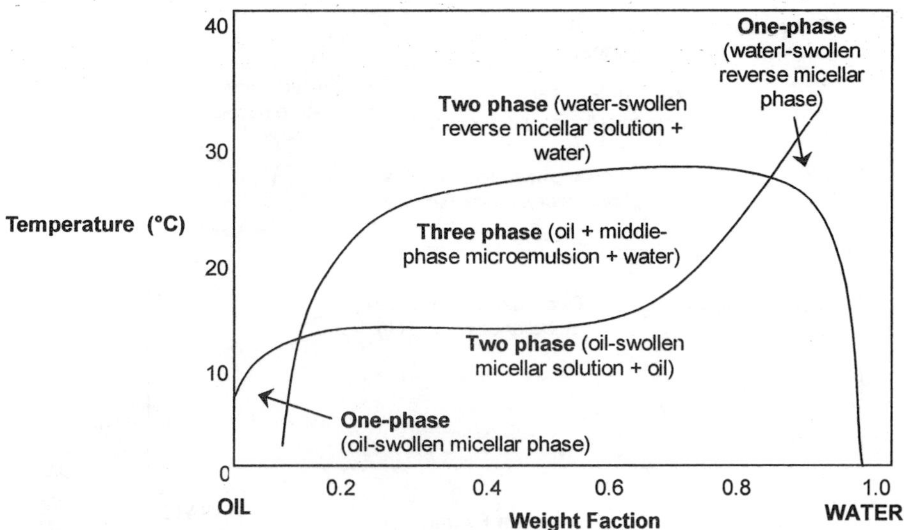

Fig. 7-6. Phase Diagram of a Water/Surfactant/Oil System as a Function of Temperature

type nonionic surfactant becomes relatively lipophilic. With increasing temperature dehydration effectively takes place as a result of conformational change in hydrophilic polyoxyethylene chains. The surfactant forms aqueous micelles and the oil-swollen aqueous micellar solution phase coexists with excess oil phase at low temperature. At high temperature, the surfactant forms a water-swollen reverse micellar solution that coexists with excess water phase. At transition temperature, the solubilization reaches its maximum and the microemulsion coexists with excess of water and oil phases. The three-phase temperature in a nonionic surfactant system is called the phase inversion temperature (PIT) in emulsion as well as the hydrophile-lipophile balance (HLB) temperature. The stability and type of emulsion are also highly dependent on temperature change. Hence, it is difficult to form temperature-insensitive stable emulsion using a single polyoxyethylene-type nonionic surfactant system.

Single Ionic Surfactant Systems

Most of the microemulsions are temperature insensitive when they are prepared in ionic surfactant systems. Three-phase microemulsions are formed in brine/double-chain ionic surfactant/oil (Kunieda and Shinoda, 1980) or brine/ionic surfactant/cosurfactant/oil systems (Kunieda et al., 1985; Winsor, 1954). Usually, for the formation of three-phase microemulsions in ionic surfactant system inorganic salts are used. Inorganic salt obviously functions to suppress the hydrophilicity of ionic surfactant, and to destroy the formation of liquid crystals. The typical three-phase behaviour of a brine/Aerosol OT/isooctane system at constant salinity and surfactant concentration is shown in Figure 7-7. The effect of temperature on this type of system is opposite to that is recorded for polyoxyethylene-type nonionic surfactant systems. At lower temperature, it forms reverse micelle in oil where as at high temperature, surfactant tends to dissolve in water. With increase in temperature the dissociation of ionic groups increases, and ionic surfactants tend to be more hydrophilic at higher temperatures at a fixed salinity. These types of systems are temperature insensitive because two critical end temperatures are well seperated yet the solubilization capacity of the system decreased.

Temperature-Insensitive Microemulsions

Three Phase Behaviour in Mixed Surfactant System

Attempts have been made to combine two surfactants whose HLBs are of opposite nature in regard to response to the temperature. When two surfactants

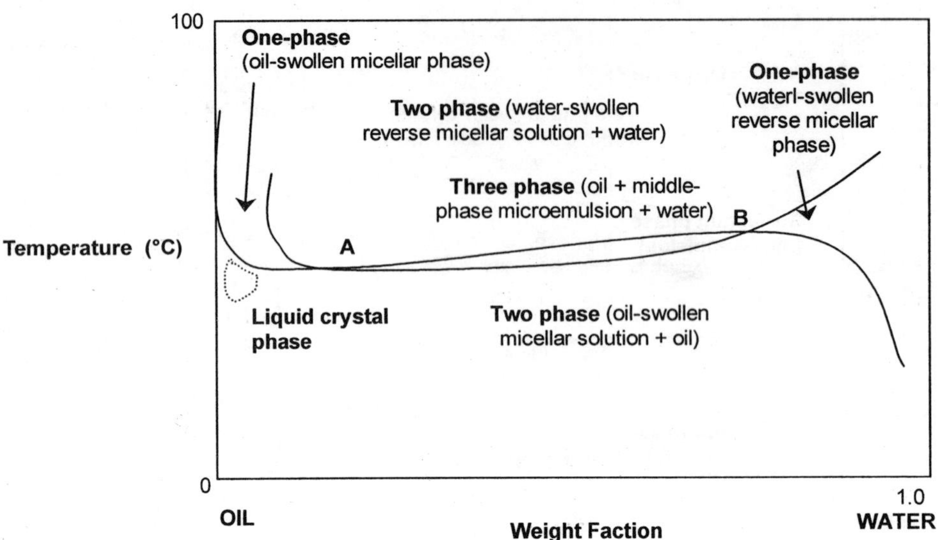

Fig. 7-7. Typical Phase Behaviour of a 0.5 wt% NaCl Aqueous/Aerosol OT/Isooctane System at Constant Salinity and Surfactant Concentration (0.2 wt.%). Points A and B are Maximum Solubilization Points in this Phase Diagram

are mixed, their distributions in aggregates or in a continuous medium are different. Figure 7-8 shows the distribution of two surfactants in three coexisting phases.

The monomeric solubility of a nonionic surfactant or cosurfactant in oil is quite higher than in aqueous phase. In the surfactant phase or middle-phase microemulsion, surfactants are distributed among the micro-water and micro-oil domains and oil-water interface (Surfactant layer). The composition of micro-water domain can be assumed as that in excess water phase of the three-phase body. Similarly, the composition of micro-oil domain as that exists in excess oil phase. If lipophilic and hydrophilic surfactants are mixed, the condition for forming the particular three-phase triangle in the midst of the three-phase body is represented by an equation;

$$W_1 = S_1^S + \frac{S_1 S_2^S - S_2 S_1^S}{1 - S_1 - S_2} R_{ow} (1/X - 1) \qquad (7\text{-}3)$$

Where W_1 is the weight fraction of lipophilic surfactant in total surfactant, R_{ow} is the weight fraction of oil in water-oil, X is weight fraction of total surfactant in the system, and S_1 and S_2 are solubilities of lipophilic and hydrophilic surfactants in excess oil phase, respectively. S_1 and S_2 can also be regarded as the surfactant concentrations in the micro-oil domain inside the microemulsion phase. S_1^S and S_2^S are the weight fractions of lipophilic and hydrophilic surfactants at water-oil interface inside the microemulsion phase. In the case of an ionic surfactant-cosurfactant mixture S_2 can be regarded as zero because ionic surfactant is practically insoluble in oil (Kunieda and Sato, 1992; Kunieda and Yamagata, 1993; Kunieda et al., 1995).

Mixtue of Polyoxyethylene-type Non-ionic Surfactants

A mixture of homologues with different lengths of polyoxyethylene chains is a commercially available polyoxyethylene-type nonionic surfactant. When a pure homogeneous nonionic surfactant system is used, the HLB temperature remains constant even if the water/oil ratio and surfactant concentration are changed. In spite of this, mixed surfactant system does not have constant HLB temperature or the three-phase body distorted in a mixed surfactant system. This distortion is caused by the difference in the distribution behaviour of each surfactant between aggregates and oil. The three-phase temperature is

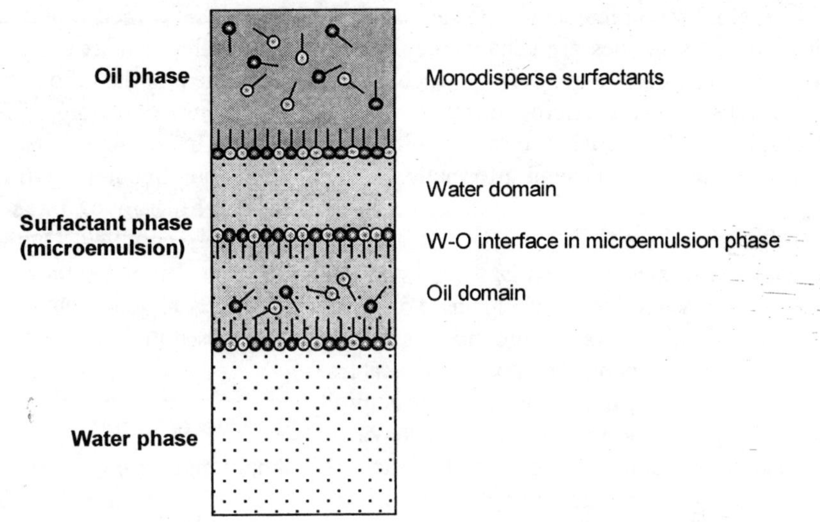

Fig. 7-8. Schematic Representation of Surfactant Distribution in Three Coexisting Phases

directly related to the mixing ratio of surfactant in aggregates or the water oil interface inside the microemulsion phase in a polyoxyethylene-type surfactant system. As the temperature increases, the the solubilities of monomers in oil of the three-phase body for lipophiic surfactants tend to decrease, whereas in the case of hydrophilic surfactant tend to increase.

Mixture of Ionic-Nonionic or Ionic-Ionic Surfactant

The weight fractions (S_1^S and S_2^S) of lipophilic and hydrophilic surfactants at the water-oil interface within the microemulsion phase, do not change with temperature in a mixed system of ionic and nonionic surfactants (Kunieda et al., 1985) because temperature has opposite effects on HLBs of ionic and polyoxyethylene-type nonionic surfactants. If the solubilities of lipophilic surfactant (S_1) and the surfactant mixing ratio at the water-oil interface inside the microemulsion (S_1^S) do not change greatly with temperature, a temperature-insensitive micro-emulsion can be obtained. In a brine/ionic surfactant/cosurfactants/oil system, if a nonionic surfactant, whose solubility in oil is low, is used a temperature-insensitive microemulsion can be obtained. For example in 1 wt.% NaCl/SDS/Aerosol OT/isooctane Aerosol OT has low solubility in oil.

Mixture of Sucrose Monoalkanoate and Polyoxyethylene-type Non-ionic Surfactants

Sucrose monoalkanoate is a strongly hydrophilic nonionic surfactant and is expected not to be highly influenced by temperature. The monomeric solubilities of sucrose monoalkanoate in both water and oil are very small and are negligible, especially when the three-phase behaviour is discussed (Kunieda et al., 1993). If more lipophilic surfactant, with HLB temperature below zero, is used, the mixing ratio may remain unchanged over a wide range of temperature and if the monomeric solubility of lipophilic surfactant kept unchanged, temperature-insensitive microemulsions can be formed. A temperature-insensitive microemulsions of large solubilization is formed in a water/sucrose alkanoate/hexanol/oil system (Pes et al., 1997).

CHARACTERIZATION OF MICROEMULSIONS

Microemulsions have been characterized using a wide variety of techniques. The characterization of microemulsions is a difficult task due to their complexity, variety of structures and components involved in these systems, as well as the limitations associated with each technique but such knowledge is essential for their successful commercial exploitation. Therefore, complementary studies using a combination of techniques are usually required to obtain a comprehensive view of the physicochemical properties and structure of microemulsions. At the macroscopic level viscosity, conductivity and dielectric methods provide useful information.

Phase Behaviour Studies

Phase behaviour studies are essential for the study of surfactant system determined by using phase diagram that provide information on the boundaries of the different phases as a function of composition variables and temperatures, and, more important, structural organization can be also inferred. Phase behaviour studies also allow comparison of the efficiency of different surfactants for a given application. In the phase behaviour studies, simple measurement and equipments are required. The boundaries of one-phase region can be assessed easily by visual observation of samples of known composition. The main drawback is long equilibrium time required for multiphase region, especially if liquid crystalline phase is involved. The phase behaviour of three-component systems at fixed temperature and pressure can be represented by a ternary phase diagram and by a triangular prism if temperature is considered as a variable (Fig. 7-9).

Other useful means and ways of representing the phase behaviour are to keep the concentration of one component or the ratio of two components constant. As the number of components increases, the number of experiments needed to define the complete phase behaviour becomes extraoridinary large and the representation of phase behaviour becomes extremely complex. One approach to characterize these multicomponent systems is by means of pseudoternary diagrams that combine more than one component in the vertices of the ternary diagram.

Scattering Techniques for Microemulsions Characterization

Small-angle X-ray scattering (SAXS), small-angle neutron scattering (SANS), and static as well as dynamic light scattering are widely applied techniques in the study of microemulsions. In the static scattering techniques, the intensity of scattered radiation I(q) is measured as a function of the scattering vector q,

$$q = (4\pi/\lambda)\ \sin\theta/2 \qquad (7\text{-}4)$$

where θ is the scattering angle and λ the wavelength of the radiation. The general expression for the scattering intensity of monodispersed spheres interacting through hard sphere repulsion is I(q) =

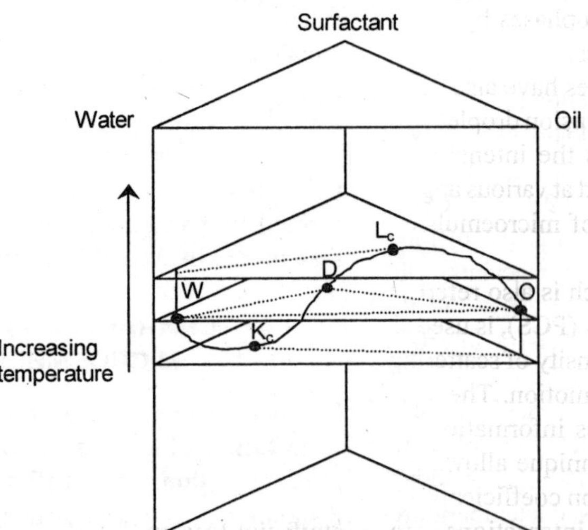

Fig. 7-9. Schematic Representation of a Three Phase Diagram when Temperature Considered as a Variable. K_c and L_c are Critical End Point. D,O and W Represent the Loci of the Phases Forming the Three Phase Triangle.

nP(q)S(q), where n is the number density of the spheres, P(q) is a form of factor, which expresses the scattering cross section of the particle, and S(q) is the structural factor, which takes into account the particle-particle interaction. P(q) and S(q) can estimated by using appropriate analytical expressions. The lower limit of size that can be measured with these techniques is about 2 nm. The upper limit is about 100 nm for SANS and SAXS and up to a few micrometers for light scattering. These methods are very valuable for obtaining quantitative informations on the size, shape and dynamics of the components. The major drawback of these technique is the dilution of the sample required for the reduction of interparticular interaction. This dilution can modify the structure and the composition of the pseudo-phases. Nevertheless, successful determinations have been carried out using a dilution technique that maintains the identity of droplets.

Small-angle X-ray scattering techniques have been used to obtain information on droplet size and shape. Using synchrotron radiation sources, in which sample-to-detector distances are bigger, significant improvements have been achieved. With synchrotron radiation more defined spectra are obtained and a wide rang of systems can be studied, including those in which the surfactant molecules are poor X-ray scatters. Small-angle neutron scattering, however, allows selective enhancement of the scattering power of different microemulsion pseudophases by using protonated or deuterated molecules.

Static light scattering techniques have also been widely used to determine microemulsion droplet size and shape. In these experiments the intensity of scattered light is generally measured at various angles and for different concentrations of microemulsion droplets.

Dynamic light scattering, which is also referred as photon correlation spectroscopy (PCS), is used to analyse the fluctuations in the intensity of scattering by the droplets due to Brownian motion. The self-correlation is measured that gives information on dynamics of the system. This technique allows the determination of z-average diffusion coefficients, D. In the absence of interpariticle interactions, the hydrodynamic radius of the particles, R_H, can be determined from the diffusion coefficient using the Stokes-Einstein equation,

$$D = kT/6\pi\eta R_H, \qquad (7\text{-}5)$$

where k is Boltzmann constant, T is the absolute temperature, and η is the viscosity of the medium.

Nuclear Magnetic Resonance Studies

The structure and dynamics of microemulsions can be studied by using nuclear magnetic resonance techniques. Self-diffusion measurements using different tracer techniques, generally radio labelling, supply information on the mobility of the components. The Fourier transform pulsed-gradient spin-echo (FT-PGSE) technique uses the magnetic gradient on the samples and it allows simultaneous and rapid determination of the self-difusion coefficients (in the range of 10^{-9} to 10^{-12} m^2s^{-1}), of many components.

Electron Microscopic Studies

The microemulsions can also be characterizated by using several electron microscopic techniques although the high lability of the samples and the possibility of artifacts, electron microscopy used to be considered a misleading technique in microemulsion studies. However, images showing clear evidence of the microstructure have been obtained. Freez-fracture electron microscopy has also been used to study microemulsion structure, however, extremely rapid cooling of the sample is required in order to maintain structure and minimize the possibility of artifacts.

Interfacial Tension, Electrical Conductivity and Viscosity Measurements

The formation and the properties of microemulsion can be studied by measuring the interfacial tension. Ultralow values of interfacial tension are correlated with phase behaviour, particularly the existence of surfactant phase or middle-phase microemulsions in equilibrium with aqueous and oil phases. Spinning-drop apparatus can be used to measure the ultralow interfacial tension. Interfacial tensions are derived form the measurement of the shape of a drop of the low-density phase, rotating it in cylindrical capillary filled with high-density phase. To determine the nature of the continuous phase and to detect phase inversion phenomena, the electrical conductivity measurements are highly useful. A sharpe increase in conductivity in certain W/O microemulsion systems was observed at low volume fractions and such behaviour was interpreted as an indication of a 'percolative behaviour' or exchange of ions between droplets before the formation of bicontinuos structures. Dielectric measurements are a powerful means of probing both structural and dynamic features of microemulsion systems.

Viscosity measurements can indicate the presence of rod-like or worm-like reverse micelle. Viscosity measurements as a function of volume fraction have been used to determine the hydrodynamic radius of droplets, as well as interactions between droplets and deviations from spherical shape by fitting the results to appropriate models (e.g. for microemulsions showing Newtonian behaviour, Einstein's equation for the relative viscosity can be used to calculate the hydrodynamic volume of the particles).

ADVANTAGES OF MICROEMULSION-BASED SYSTEMS

Microemulsions exhibit several advantages as a drug delivery system (Gasco, 1997).

1. Microemulsions are thermodynamically stable system and the stability allows self-emulsification of the system whose properties are not dependent on the process followed.
2. Microemulsions act as supersolvents of drug. They can solublize hydrophilic and lipophilic durgs including drugs that relatively insoluble in both aqueous and hydrophobilc solvents. This is due to existence of microdomains of different polarity within the same single-phase solution.
3. The dispersed phase, lipophilic or hydrophilic (oil-in-water,O/W, or water-in-oil, W/O microemulsions) can behave as a potential reservoir of lipophilic or hydrophilic drugs, respectively. The drug partitioned between dispersed and continuous phase, and when the system comes into contact with a semi-permeable membrane, the drug can be transported through the barrier. Drug release with pseudo-zero-order kinetics can be obtained, depending on the volume of the dispersed phase, the partition of the drug and the transport rate of the drug.
4. The mean diameter of droplets in microemulsions is below 0.22 μm; they can be sterilized by filtration. The small size of droplet in microemulsions, e.g. below 100 nm, yields very large interfacial area, from which the drug can quickly be released into external phase when absorption (*in vitro* or *in vivo*) takes place, maintaining the concentration in the external phase close to initial levels.
5. Same miroemulsion can carry both lipophilic and hydrophilic drugs.
6. Because of thermodynamic stability, microemulsions are easy to prepare and require no significant energy contribution during preparation. Microemulsions have low viscosity compared to other emulsions.
7. The use of microemulsion as delivery systems can improve the efficacy of a drug, allowing the total dose to be reduced and thus minimizing side effects.
8. The formation of microemulsions is reversible. They may become unstable at low or high temperature, but when the temperature returns to the stability range, the microemulsion reformed.

There are certain limitations, which are to be considered before the use of microemulsions in the field of pharmaceuticals and as drug delivery systems. The components, particularly surfactant and cosurfactant should be pharmaceutically acceptable and biocompatible.

APPLICATIONS OF MICROEMULSIONS

Microemulsions have broad area of applications some of the pharmaceutical applications are as follows;

- Oral drug delivery
- Topical drug delivery
- Ocular and pulmonary delivery
- Parenteral administration
- Perflouro microemulsions
- Microemulsions in biotechnology
- Solubilization of drugs in microemulsions

Oral Drug Delivery

The recent advances in pharmaceutical and biotechnology permit rather high amounts of peptides and proteins to be produced. Short half-life, conformational stability and biodegradability of these molecules cause considerable design difficulties in their formulation for oral administration. Microemulsions extensively studied for protection of biodegradable drugs, e.g. proteins and peptides form biological environment of peroral route.

Ritschel et al., 1990 studied the absorption of cyclosporine, a potent, neutral, cyclic endekapeptide, an immunopotent drug widely used in transplants. Cyclosporine has very poor bioavailability after oral administration. Two W/O microemulsions were administered to rat perorally and it was found that for one of them, the absolute and relative bioavailability were better than that of commercially available solutions (Fig. 7-10). A cyclosporine preparation using a W/O microemulsion containing a sorbiton ester-polyoxyethylene glycol mono ether mixture of surfactant, a low molecular weight alcohol, fatty ester and water as the vehicle for the drug was administered (Tarr and Yalkowsky, 1989). A gel-like consistency was obtained through the addition of pyrogenic silica and the microemulsions were filled and administered in hard geletin capsules. In comparison with any other preparation including i.v., the better bioavailability of the drug was recorded which was attributed to the microemulsion droplets (Ritschel et al., 1990; Ritschel et al., 1990).

The gastrointestinal absorption of three peptides (insulin, vassopressin and cyclosporine) was investigated by Ritschel, 1991 using a series of O/W microemulsion formulations. The peptides used were dissolved in the aqueous phase at a suitable pH if water-soluble (insulin, vassopressin) or otherwise added to the microemulsion (cyclosporine) and dispersed by sonication. The bioavailablity of these peptides when administered orally was not solely dependent on droplet size. Ritschel, 1991 concluded that type of lipid phase of the microemulsion, digestability of the lipid used and types of surfactant used in the formation of microemulsion also affect the systemic uptake from microemulsion on oral administration. The cyclosporin administered via hard gelatin capsules containing two O/W microemulsions (slow and fast release) and a solid micellar solution also improved the oral absorption (Drewe et al., 1992). The improved conditions for drug absorption may be related to the greater solubility of the lipophilic cyclosporine in the fast releasing microemulsion and the micellar gelified solution which probably assist instantaneous absorption and better absorption.

Topical Drug Delivery

The percuteneous route of administration has been extensively studied where the drug transport from microemulsions was recorded usually better than that from other ointment, gels and creams. A mechanism for this facilated transport is that the drugs are

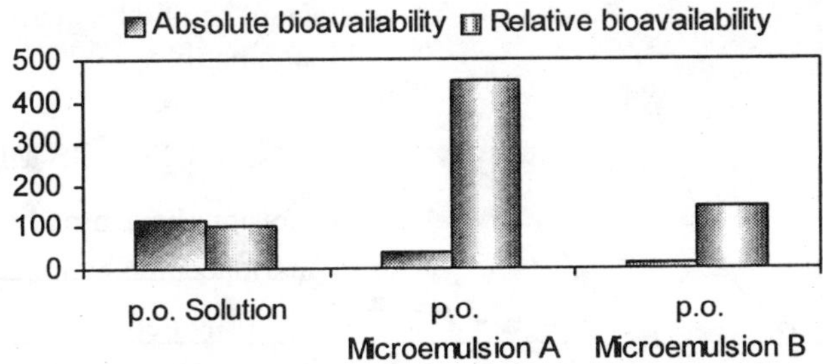

Fig. 7-10. Comparision of Absolute and Relative Bioavailability of Cyclosporine after Peroral Administration of Solution and Microemulsion Formulations. Microemulsion A : W/O Microemulsion containing a Long Chain Fatty Acid as Lipid Phase, Arlacel and Brij as Surfactant, a Low Molecular Weight Alcohol as Cosurfactant and Distilled water; Micoemulsion B : as A Except that Branched Alkyl Fatty Esters were Used as Lipid Phase.

completely dissolved in microemulsions, reaching relatively high concentrations as a consequence of the supersolvent effect of microemulsions while the dispersed phase can act as a reservoir, making it possible to maintain an almost constant concentration in the continuous phase. Thus pseudo zero-order kinetics can be achieved and some components of microemulsions *per se* can operates as enhancers.

The release of tetracycline hydrochloride form different formulations have compared by Ziegenmeyer and Fuhrer, 1980. Figure 7-11 shows the *in vitro* permeation of the drug through skin membranes versus time profile for three different formulations and results indicate that transport of the tetracycline hydrochloride is significantly better bioavailable when administered as a microemulsion. Oshborne et al., 1988 studied microemulsion consisted of AOT-octanol-water and demonstrated that the transdermal flux increased nearly six fold as the water content of the microemulsion increased from 15% to 68%. They also explained that the subsequent high water concentration serves as transport vehicle to the addenda, leading to a higher flux.

The transdermal delivery of hydrophilic drug diphenhydramine hydrochloride from a W/O microemulsion through an excised human skin has also been studied. The W/O microemulsion formulation was based on combination of Tween 80 and Span 20 with isopropyl myristate (IPM). Cholesterol and oleic acid containing two other formulations were also tested and it was found that cholesterol containing formulation increased the permeation whereas oleic acid containing formulation had no measurable effect on permanently flux (Schmalfub et al., 1997).

A combination of drug delivery strategies has been employed recently by Dalmora and Oliveira,1999. They described a formulation of an inclusion complex of the anti-inflamatory piroxicam with β-cyclodextrin in an O/W microemulsion system for topical use. Another system for topical delivery contained IPM and stabilized by cationic surfactant hexadecyltrimethylammonium bromide.

A gelatin microemulsion-based organogel (MBGs) which exploits the presence of surfactant-stabilized conducting aqueous channels has been used in the iontophoretic transdermal delivery of a model hydrophilic drug (Fig. 7-12). The MBGs were prepared using a variety of pharmaceutically acceptable surfactants and oils including Tween 80 and IPM (Kantaria et al., 1999). Novel sorbiton monosterate organogels have also been prepared from vegetable oil and IPM. Organogels are prepared at

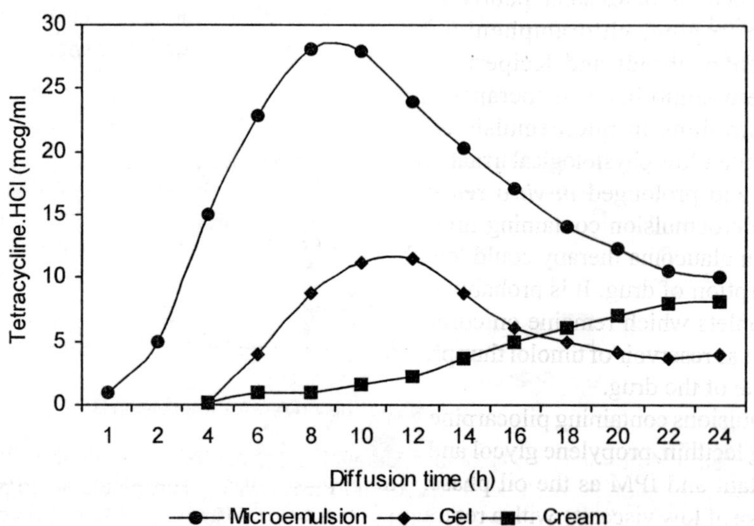

Fig. 7-11. *In vitro* Premeation of the Drug through Skin Membranes versus Time for Three Different Formulations

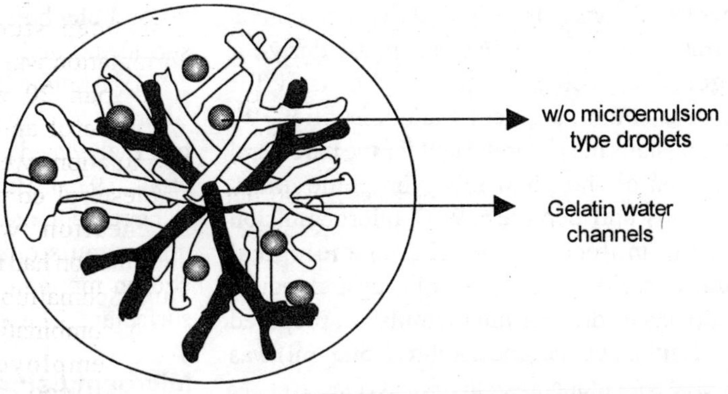

Fig. 7-12. Schematic Representation of a Gelatin Microemulsion-Based Organogel (MBGs)

elevated temperatures and then cooled, the surfactant self-assembles into inverse vesicles and then rod-shaped tubules. The organogels are opaque and thermoreversible and have been suggested as novel delivery vehicles for drugs and antigens (Murdan, et al., 1999).

Ocular and Pulmonary Delivery

For the treatment of eye diseases, drugs are essentially delivered topically. O/W microemulsions have been investigated for ocular administration, to dissolve poorly soluble drugs, to increase absorption and to attain prolong release profile. Lecithin-Tween 80 based microemulsion was developed and characterized, which dissolves some poorly soluble drugs such as atropine, chloramphenicol and indomethacin (Siebenbrodt and Keipert, 1991). These drugs were solubilized in therapeutically relevant concentrations in microemulsions. The formulation exhibited low physiological irritation and shown elevated and prolonged *in vitro* release. A lecithin based microemulsion containing timolol, a β-blocker used in glaucoma therapy could lengthen the time of absorption of drug. It is probably due to the tiny nanodroplets which remaine on cornea for some time and act as reservoir of timolol thus prolong the absrption time of the drug.

The microemulsions containing pilocarpine were formulated using lecithin, propylene glycol and PEG 200 as cosurfactant and IPM as the oil phase. The formulations were of low viscosity with a referactive index lending to ophthalmological applications (Hasse and Keipett, 1997).

The formation of a water-in-HFA propellent microemulsion stabilized by flurocarbon non-ionic surfactant and intended for pulmonary delivery has been described (Patel et al., 1998).

Solubilization of Drugs in Microemlsions

Microemulsions possess interesting physicochemical properties, i.e. transparency, low viscosity, thermodyamic stability, high solubilization power. Because of these specific properties microemulsion can be useful as a drug delivery systems. Table 7-4 show the different categories of drugs solubilized in microemulsion systems for their better therapeutic efficacy.

Parenteral Administration

In order to attain prolonged release and to administer parenterally lipophilic substances that are not soluble in water, O/W microemulsions may be used as carriers. They can be administered by intravenous, intramuscular or subcutaneous route. The potential of O/W microemulsions as a vector for flurocarbon, calcium antagonist, steroids and other lipophilic drugs has already been reported (Keipert et al., 1989). Kakutani et al., 1991 reported targeting potential of O/W microemulsions containing very lipophilic drugs to reticuloendothelial system (RES) tissue, i.e. liver and spleen. The results indicted that higher the partition coefficient of the drug,the better was the resulted targeting. For delivering the drug effectively to RES tissues, an octanol-water partition coefficient above 10^8 is required.

W/O microemulsions may be indicated for parenteral administration of hydrophilic drugs particularly for prolonged drug release and can be used for subcutaneous and intramuscular administration. W/O microemulsions may be indicated for the parenteral administration of short half-life hydrophilic drugs, small proteins and peptides. W/O microemulsion protects the molecules from harsh biological environment, prolong the release of drug and reduce the side effects of drug. A microemulsion, prepared using egg lecithin, containing insulin (0.5mg/ml) was administered subcutaneously in rabbits (Gasco et al., 1992). When the formulation compared with a solution, it was found that the half-life of insulin was 1.6 hr for the solution and reached 4.3 h for microemulsion; t_{max} values were 0.7 h for solution and 1.9 h for microemulsion.

Perfluoro Microemulsions

Fluorocarbon based microemulsions are prepared by using fluorinated surfactants. These emulsions are spontaneously formed and represent for thermodynamically stable dispersions. These emulsion systems solve long-term shelf stability problems. F-alkylated amine oxides, including XMO-10 and alcohols, were proposed by using them as surfactants and cosurfactants (Rosano and Gerbacia, 1973). Another spontaneously formed dispersion of fluorinated carbons was achieved with mixtures of two F-alkylated polyoxyethylene derivatives (Chabert et al., 1975). But these formulations were reported to be toxic in nature. Delpuech et al., 1985 obtained microemulsions with one single, appropriately chosen monodisperse F-alkylated polyoxyethylene surfactant. These systems were not biocompatible.

Microemulsions in Biotechnology

Many enzymatic and biocatalytic reactions are conducted in pure organic or aquo-organic media. Biphasic media also used for these types of reactions. The use of pure apolar media causes the denaturation of biocatalysts. The use of water-poor media is relatively advantageous. Enzymes in low water content display and have

1. Increased solubility in nonpolar reactants
2. Possibility of shifting thermodynamic equilibria in favour of condensation
3. Improvement of thermal stability of the enzymes, enabling reactions to be carried out at higher temperatures.

Table 7-4. Different Categories of Drugs are Solubilized in Different Microemulsion Systems

Category	Drug(s)	References
Antineoplasics	Doxorubicin	Gasco et al., 1988
Peptide drugs	Cyclosporin	Ritschel et al., 1990; Drewe et al., 1992
	Leutinising hormone-releasing hormone (LH-RH)	Gasco et al, 1990
Sympatholytics	Timolol	Boles et al., 1989
Local anaesthetics	Lidocaine	Carlfors et al., 1991
	Benzocaine	Delgado et al., 1995
	Tetracaine	
Steroids	Hydrocortisone	Jayakrishnan et al., 1983
	Testosterone	Malcolmson and Lawrence, 1993
	Medroxyprogesterone	
Anxiolytics	Diazepam	Trotta et al., 1991
Anti-infective drugs	Tetracycline HCl	Ziegenmeyer and Fuhrer, 1980
	Clotimazole	Garcia-Celma et al., 1994
	Ciclopiroxolamine	
Vitamins	Tocopherol	Jakobson and Sivik, 1994
	Ascorbic acid	
Anti-inflammatory drugs	Indomethcin	Farah et al., 1993
Dermatological products	Azelaic acid	Gasco et al., 1991

Many enzymes, including lipases, esterases, dehydrogenases and oxidases often function in the cells in microenvironments that are hydrophobic in nature. In biological systems many enzymes operate at the interface between hydrophobic and hydrophilic domains and these usually interfaces are stabilized by polar lipids and other natural amphiphiles. Enzymatic catalysis in microemulsions has been used for a variety of reactions, such as synthesis of esters, peptides and sugar acetals transesterification; various hydrolysis reactions and steroid transformation. The most widely used class of enzymes in microemulsion-based reactions is of lipases. The variety of proteins have been immobilized to hydrophilized solid surfaces in microemulsions (Fig. 7-13). The technique is of particular interest for solid-phase diagnostics of ELISA type.

Hatton, 1989 explored the use of W/O microemulsions (reverse micelles) for extraction of proteins and other biomolecules (Bioseparation). The procedure based on the observation that different protein molecules exhibit different affinities for properly formulated microemulsions, a property that can be used to achieve a selective separation of a protein of interest from other materials formed in an aqueous broth. Partitioning of a protein between a bulk aqueous phase and a microemulsion mainly depends on parameters related to the aqueous phase, such as pH, ionic strength and salt types as well as on the types of solvent and surfactant used in the formulation of microemulsions.

SOLID COLLOIDAL SYSTEMS PREPARED FROM MICROEMULSIONS

From W/O Microemulsions

The site-specific drug delivery can be achieved by using colloidal drug carriers. Nanoparticles prepared by emulsion polymerization, has been investigated for their potential as lisosomotropic carriers for drugs. In the preparation method, the insoluble monomers are emulsified in aqueous phase (Couvreur et al., 1982). The inner structure of nanoparticles prepared by this method are of highly porous matrix. Doxorubicin adsorbed such nanoparticles shown low toxicity. Polycyanoacrylate nanocapsules are

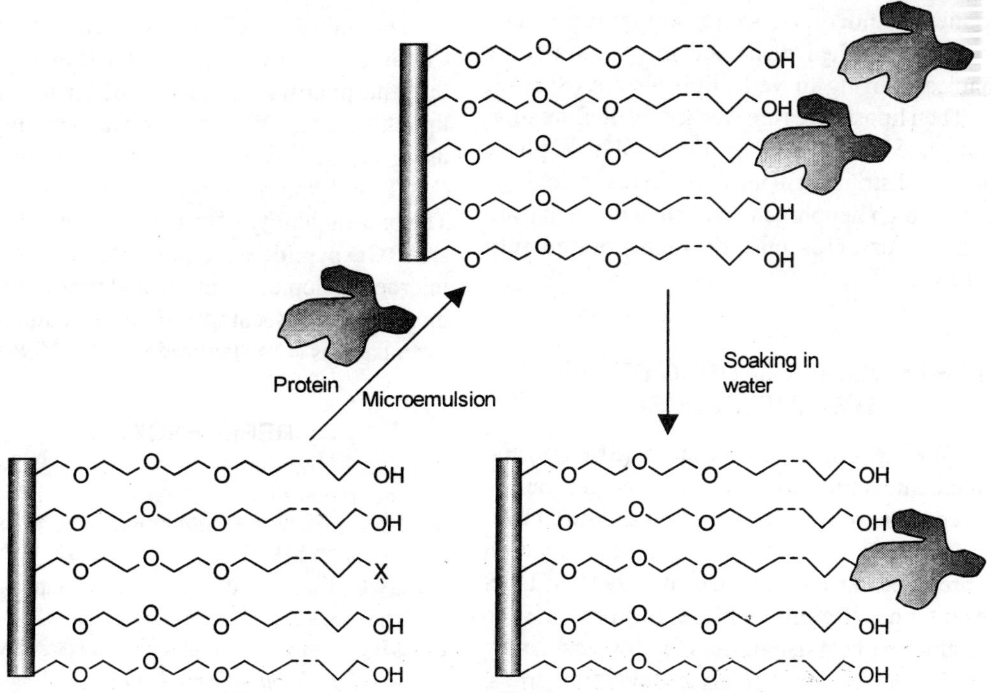

Fig. 7-13. Immobalization of Protien from a Microemulsion

prepared by dissolving the monomer alkylcyanoacrylate and a lipophilic drug in a lipidic phase. This lipidic phase then injected to an aqueous solution of a nonionic surfactant (Al-Khouri-Fallouh et al., 1986).

The polyalkylcyanoacrylate nanocapsules can prepared from W/O microemulsions (Gasco and Trotta, 1986). An *In situ* nucleophilic polymerization takes place on slow addition of the lipophilic monomer to the microemulsion and yielding colloidal nanocapsules. This reaction can also performed in waterless microemulsions, with a nuclophilic component used for the dispersed phase. A large amount of hydrophilic drug, such as doxorubicin, can be encapsulated by dissolving it in aqueous dispersed phase (Carpignano et al., 1991).

From O/W Microemulsions

Solid colloidal lipophilic systems can be prepared from warm O/W microemulsion. For the preparation of lipospheres by microemulsion, components with relatively low melting point can chosen as the oil phase, i.e. triglycerides and alkanoic acids. Warm clear systems are obtained by mixing of melted lipid components and oil at same temperature. The microemulsions then dispersed in cold water by mechanical stirring to yeild lipospheres (Speiser, 1990). Then lipospheres are washed by diafilteration and redipersed in water. Drug dissolved in oil phase is randomly distributed in the lipospheres on cooling. Drugs with high lipophilicity and other drugs that are weak bases or acids may be incorporated into lipospheres.

SELF EMULSIFYING DRUG DELIVERY SYSTEMS (SEDDS)

Self-emulsifing drug delivery systems (SEDDS) and self-microemulsifing drug delivery systems can be described as isotropic solutions of oil and surfactant, which form O/W microemulsions on mild agitation in the presence of water (Shah, et al., 1994). SEDDS represent an efficient vehicle for the *in vivo* administration of emulsions. It is for this reason they are considered for oral delivery of lipophilic drugs, provided however, that the drug has adequate solubility in oil or oil/surfactant blends. SEDDS are formulated in the absence of water by mixing an oil with a nonionic surfactant or polyglycolzed glycerides and lipid-souble drug to form an isotropic oily soulution. Upon dilution or *in vivo* administration they formed fine O/W emulsions. In order to formulate self-emulsifying O/W, four components, an oil, a blend of two surfactants and an aqueous phase (water/saline) are used. The pseudo ternary phase diagram can be the best description for these types of systems, where a constant ratio of two of the components is used and the other two are varied. For example, the mixture of the oil and oil soluble low HLB surfactant can be taken fixed and titrated with known amounts of the high HLB surfactant and water.

In order to reduce the viscosity of components, long chain glycerides, such as soyabean oil and monoolein, incorporating microemulsions are prepared at temperatures between 40 - 60 °C Monoolein is solid at room temperature, premelting at appropriate temperature is necessary before mixing with oil and other surfactant. Microemulsion incorporating medium chain glycerides can be formed spontaneously at room temperature over a wide range of compositions.

The utility of SEDDS has been investigeted by Charmen and coworkers, 1992. They demonstrated that the pharmacodynamics of an investigational lipophilic drug, WIN 54954 was greatly improved using systems based on medium chain triglycerides (MCT) and ethoxylated glyceryl trioleate (target TO). The bioavailability of calcein, a watersoluble marker and RGD peptide were shown to be increased using microemulsion concentrate and preformulated W/O microemulsions compared to the control aqueous formulations (Constantinides et al., 1996).

REFERENCES

Al-Khouri-Fallouh N., Roblot-Treupel L., Fessi H., Devissaguet J.P. and Puisiex F. (1986) *Int. J. Pharm.* **28**,125.

Auvary L., Cotton J. P., Ober R. and Taupin C. (1984) *J. phys.* **45**, 913.

Boles B., Gremmo E., Brogliatti B. and Gasco M. R. (1989) *New Trends Opthalmol.* **4**, 177.

Benita S. (1997) In: microencapsulation and industrial applications, Marcel Dekker, New york, 411.

Carlfors J., Blute I. and Shmidt V. (1991) *J. Disper. Sci. Tech.* **12**, 467.

Carpigno R., Gasco M.R. and Morel S. (1991) *Pharm. Acta Helv.* **66**, 28.

Chabert P., Foulletier L. and Lantz A., (1975) *Ger. Offen.* 2,452,513.

Charman S.A., Charman W,N., Roger M.C. Wilson T.D., Dutko T.J. and Ponton C. W. (1992) Pharm. Res. **9**, 87.

Constantinides P.P., scalart J.P., Lancaster S. Marcello , J., Marks G., Ellens H. and Smith P.L. (1994) *Pharma Res.* **11**, 1385.

Couvreur P., Roland M. and Speiser P. (1982) *U. S. Patent* 4,329,332.

Dalmora M. E. A. and Oliveira A. J. (1999) Int. J. Pharm. **184**, 157.

Delgado M. I., Solan C. and Gracia-Celma M. J. (1995) *Pharmaceutical Technology Conference* Barcelona.

Delpuech J. J., Mathis G. and Ravey J. C. (1985) *Bull. Soc. Chim. Fr.* 578.

Drewe J., Meier R., Vonderscher J., Kiss D., Posanski U., Kissel T. and Gyr K. (1992) *Br. J. Clin. Pharmacol.* **34**, 60.

Ekwall P. (1975) In: Advances in liquid crystals, brown G. H. (Ed.) Academic press, NY, 1.

Farah N., de Taddeo M., Laforet J. P. and Denis J. (1993) *AAPS Annual Meeting* Orlando, FL.

Garcia-Celma M. J., Azemar N., Pes M. A. and Solan C. (1994) *Int. J. Pharm.* **105**, 77.

Gasco M. R., Gallarate M. and Pattarino F. (1991) *Int. J. Pharm.* **69**, 193.

Gasco M. R., Morel S., Tonso E. and Viano I. (1992) *Proc. Int. Symp. Contol. Rel. Bioact. Mater.* **19**, 502.

Gasco M. R., Pattarino F. and Voltani I. (1988) *Farmaco. Ed. Prat.* **43**, 3.

Gasco M. R., Pattarino F. and Lattanzi F. (1990) *Int. J. Pharm.* **62**, 119.

Gasco M. R. and Trotta M. (1986) *Int. J.Pharm.* **29**, 267.

Hasse A. and Keipert S. (1997) *Eur. J. Pharm. Biopharm.* **43**, 179.

Hatton T. A. (1989) In: Surfactant-based Separation Processes (Surfactant series no. 33), Marcel Dekker, NewYork, 55.

Israelachvilli J. C., Mitchell D. J. and Ninham B. W. (1976) *J. Chem. Soc. Faraday Trans.* **72**, 1525.

Jakobsson M. and Sivik B. (1994) *J. Disper. Sci. Tech.* **15**, 207.

Jayakrishnan A., Kalairasi K. and Shah D. O. (1983) *J. Soc. Cosmat. Chem.* **34**, 355.

Kahlwiet M., Strey R., Haase H., Kunieda T. and Schmeling B. (1987) *J. Colloid. Interface Sci.* **118**, 436.

Kakutani T., Nishiara Y., Takahashi K., Kirano K. (1991) *Proc. Int. Symp. Contol. Rel. Bioact. Mater.* **18**, 359.

Kantaria S., Rees, G. D. and Lawrence M. J. (1999) *J. Control. Rel.* **60**, 355.

Keipert S., Siebenbrodt I., Luders F. and Bornschein M. (1989) *Pharmazie* **44**, 443.

Klang S. and Benita S. (1998) Submicron emulsions in drug delivery, Benita S. (Ed.), Hardwood Academic Publishers, India, 120.

Kunieda H. and Ishikawa N. (1985) *J. Colloid Interface Sci.* **107**, 122.

Kunieda H. and Shinoda K. (1980) *J. Colliod Interface Sci.* **75**, 601.

Kunieda H. and Solans C. (1997) In: Industrial Applications of Microemuulsions, Solans C. and Kunieda H. (Eds.), Marcel Dekker Inc., NewYork, 21.

Kunieda H. and Sato Y. (1992) In: Organized Solutions, Friberg S. E. and Lindman B. (Eds.), Marcel Dekker, New York, 67.

Kunieda H. and Yamagata M. (1993) *Langmuir* **9**, 3345.

Kunieda H., Hanno K., Yamaguchi H. and Shinoda K. (1985) *J. Colliod Interface Sci.* **107**, 129.

Kunieda H., Nakano A. and Akimaru M. (1995) *J. Colloid Interface Sci.* **170**, 78.

Kunieda H., Ushio A., Nakano A. and Miura M. (1993) *J. Colloid Interface Sci.* **159**, 37.

Lawrence M. J. and Rees G. D (2000) *Adv. Drug Deliv. Rev.* **45**, 121.

Lawrence M. J. (1994) *Eur. J. Drug Metab. Pharmacokinet.* **3**, 257.

Lovell M. W., Johnson H. W., Hui H. W., Cannon J. B., Gupta P. K. and Hsu C. C. (1994) *Int. J. Pharm.* **109**, 45.

Malcolson C. and Lawrence M. J. (1993) *J. Pharm. Pharmacol.* **45**, 141.

Murdan S., Gregoriadis G. and Florence A. T. (1999) *J. Pharm. Sc.* **88**, 608.

Oshborne D. W., Ward A. J. I. and O'Neill K. J. (1988) *Drug Dev. Ind. Pharmacy* **14**, 1203.

Patel N., Marlow M. and Lawrence M. J. (1998) In: Drug Delivery to the Lung, IX, London, The Aerosol Society, Bristol, 160.

Pes M. A., Aramaki K. and Nakamura N. (1997) *J. Colloid Interface Sci.* **191**, 34.

Rasano H. L. and Gerbacia W. E. (1973) *U.S. Patent* 3,778,381.

Ravey J. C. and Buzier M. (1984) In: Surfactants in Solutions, Mittal K. L. and Lidman B. (Eds.), Plenum, New York, 3, 1759.

Ritschel W. A. (1991) *Methods Find. Exp. Clin. Pharmacol.* **13**, 205.

Ritschel W. A., Adolph S., Ritschel G. B. and Schroeder T. (1990) *Methods Find. Exp. Clin. Pharmacol.* **12**, 127.

Ross S. and Morrison I. D. (1988) Colloidal System and Interfaces, Wiley, NewYork, 176.

Ruckenstein E. and Chi I. C. (1975) *J. Chem. Soc. Faraday Trans.* **71**, 1707.

Schulman J. H., stoekenius W. and Prince L.M. (1959) *J. Phy. Chem.* **63**, *1677.*

Schmalfub U., Neubert W. and Wohlarb W. (1997) *J. Control. Rel.* **46**, 279.

Shah N.H., Caryajal M. T., Patel C.I., Infield M.H. and Malick V. W. (1994) *Int. J. Pharm.* **106**, 15.

Shinoda K. and Kunieda H. (1973) *J. Colliod Interface Sci.* **42**, 381.

Siebenbrodt I. and Keipert S. (1991) *Pharmazie* 46, 435.

Speiser P. (1990) *Eur. Patent* O 167 825.

Tanford C. (1980) The Hydrophobic Effect, Wiley, NewYork, 52.

Tarr B. and Yalkosky S. H. (1989) *Pharm. Res.* **6**, 40.

Tibell A., Lindhom A., Sawe J., Chen G. and Norrlind B. (1995) *Pharmacol. Toxicol.* **76**, 115.

Trotta M., Gasco M. R. and Pattarino F. (1991) Proceeding of the 10th Pharmaceutical Technology Conference, Bologna, Italy, 388.

Winsor P. A. (1954) Solvent Properties of Amphiphilic Compounds, Butterworths, London, 68.

Ziegenmeyer J. and Fuhrer C. (1980) *Acta Pharm. Technol.* **26**, 273.

CHAPTER 8

Multiple Emulsions

Emulsions may be described as heterogenous systems, where one immiscible liquid is dispersed in another in the form of droplets and stabilized by a third component called emulsifying agent. These two liquids are also chemically non-reactive and form the systems that are characterized by a low thermodynamic stability. Simple emulsions are classified according to the nature of their continuous phase or dispersed phase, wherein two main classes can be identified :

- W/O system: Dispersion of droplets of aqueous phase (dispersed phase) in oil (continuous) phase.
- O/W system: Dispersion of oil droplets (dispersed phase) in aqueous (continuous) phase.

Multiple emulsion systems are novel developments in the field of emulsion technology and are more complex type of dispersed systems. Multiple emulsions are the emulsion systems in which the dispersed phase contain smaller droplets that have the same composition as the external phase. This is made possible by double emulsification hence the systems are also called as "double emulsion". These systems have been extensively studied from both academic and practical application point of view. In some disciplines certain multiple emulsions have been termed as "Liquid Membrane Systems" as the liquid film which separates the liquid phases acts as a thin semipermeable film through which solute must diffuse in order to traverse from one phase to another. The nature of liquid membrane may be hydrophilic or hydrophobic. Like simple emulsions, the multiple emulsions are also considered to be of two types :

- Oil-in-water-in-oil (O/W/O) emulsion system
- Water-in-oil-in-water (W/O/W) emulsion system

In O/W/O systems, an aqueous phase (hydrophilic) separates internal and external oil phases. In other words, O/W/O is a system in which water droplets may be surrounded in an oil phase, which in turn encloses one or more oil droplets (Fig. 8-1).

In W/O/W systems, an organic phase (hydrophobic) separates internal and external aqueous phases. In other words, W/O/W is a system in which an oil droplet may be surrounded by an aqueous phase, which in turn encloses one or several water droplets. These systems are the most studied among the multiple emulsions. The immiscible oil phase, which separates the two miscible aqueous phases is known as "liquid membrane" and acts as a diffusion barrier and semipermeable membrane for the drugs or moieties entrapped in the internal aqueous phase (Fig. 8-1).

Principles of Liquid Surfactant Membrane Emulsions

Liquid membranes (stable water-in-oil-in-water, (W/O/W) emulsions), were patented over decades ago (Li, 1960). When a W/O emulsion is dispersed in an outer aqueous phase, a three phase system is produced in which the two miscible aqueous phases are separated by an organic phase. This organic phase is called liquid membrane (Scheper, 1990) (Fig. 8-2). The organic phase is composed of a hydrocarbon solvent, emulsifiers and various additives. The composition of the organic membrane must satisfy two primary requirements. (i) It must have the ability to form a stable emulsion and (ii) it must have negligible effect on drug activity.

PREPARATION ASPECTS OF MULTIPLE EMULSION

Static aspect of Multiple Emulsion Formation

In order to specify the location of the formation region of multiple emulsions, one of the generalized phase diagram for a mixture of water-oil emulsifier proposed by Shinoda and Friberg,1986 is shown in Figure 8-3. The hydrophilic emulsifier is dissolved in water. The micellar phase of surfactant solution solubilizes a small amount of oil, while a large part of oil remains immiscible with the solution. This area can be specified by the location for providing O/W microemulsions, when one makes disruption of the interface between the two separate phases. On the other hand, a variety of the hydrophobic emulsifiers dissolved in oil phase assumable as reversed micelles solubilizes a small quantity of water. A large amount of residual water remains separated from the reversed micellar solution. This zone is featured by the area for preparing W/O microemulsions due to disruption of two-separated phase.

Some emulsifiers can neither be dissolved in water nor in oil, but they form their own continuous phase that consists of the D-phase and contains a certain amount of water and/or oil among the lamellar structure of D-phase. Such a phase can be provided

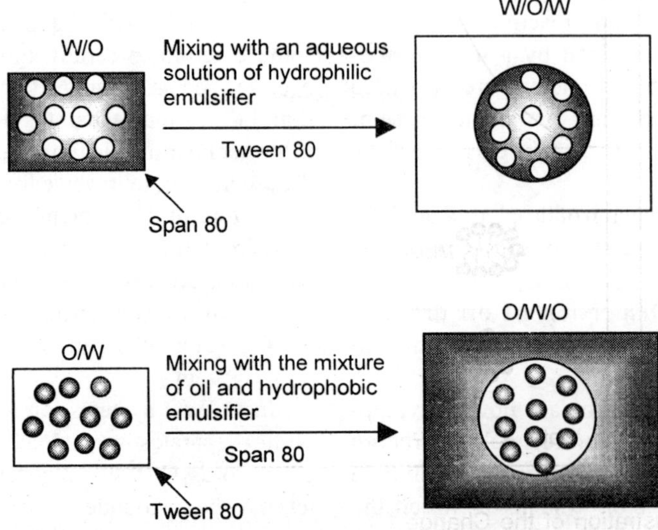

Fig. 8-1. Schematic Diagram of W/O/W and O/W/O Emulsions

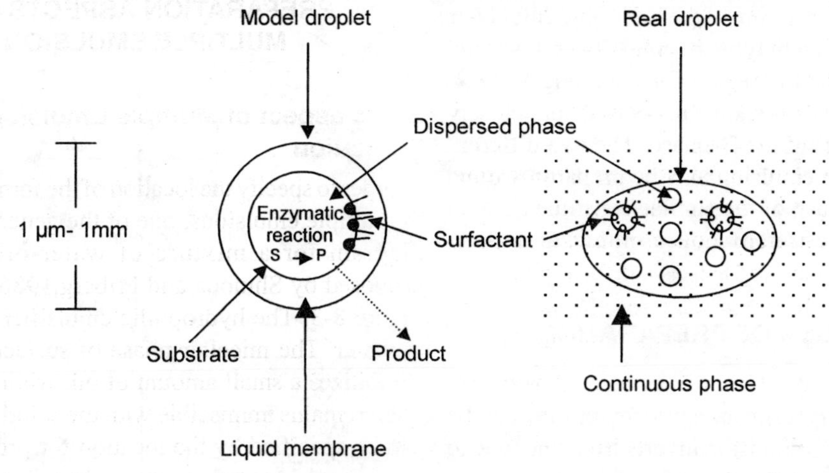

Fig. 8-2 . Principle of Liquid Membrane Emulsions

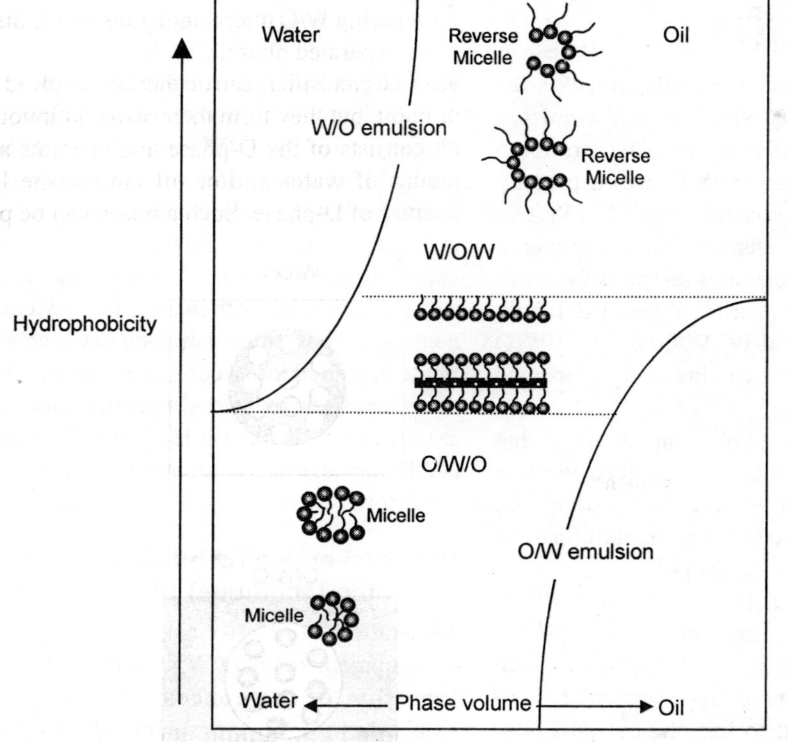

Fig. 8-3. Schematic Illustration of the Change of Solution Behaviour of Emulsifier with the Hydrophilic-Hydrophobic Balance in the Mixture of Water and Oil.

by increasing temperature of the non-ionic emulsifier or by mixing different types of emulsifiers. It should be mentioned that the region for obtaining W/O/W and O/W/O emulsions should be located very closely to the either sides of the D-phase. The two different types of multiple emulsion may be prepared around the D-phase by use of the similar constituents with judicious selection of components and their concentration levels.

METHODS OF PREPARATION

Multiple emulsion systems can be formed by the re-emulsification of a primary emulsion or they can be produced when an emulsion inverts from one type to another, for example W/O to O/W. However, in latter case the amount of internal dispersed phase created is small and such systems are probably of little use in therapeutics. Thus, for experimental studies, multiple emulsions are best prepared by re-emulsification of primary emulsion.

Two Step Emulsification (Double Emulsification)

Two step emulsification methods involve re-emulsification of primary W/O or O/W emulsion using a suitable emulsifier agent. The first step involves, obtaining an ordinary W/O or O/W primary emulsion wherein an appropriate emulsifier system is utilized. In the second step, the freshly prepared W/O or O/W primary emulsion is re-emulsified with an excess of aqueous phase or oil phase. The finally prepared emulsion could be W/O/W or O/W/O respectively. The method is schematically illustrated in Figure 8-4.

In two step emulsification it was observed that on scale of acceptability, the physicochemical characteristics of multiple emulsion systems are directly related to the ratio of the amount of Span 80 to that of a series of the hydrophilic emulsifiers existing in the entire system (Matsumoto et al., 1976; Matsumoto et al., 1977a; Matsumoto et al., 1977b). It was observed that twice or less Span 80 than Tween 80 is necessary for obtaining higher yields of O/W/O emulsions in contrast to the amount and ratio recommended for W/O/W emulsion (Kang and Matsumoto, 1988).

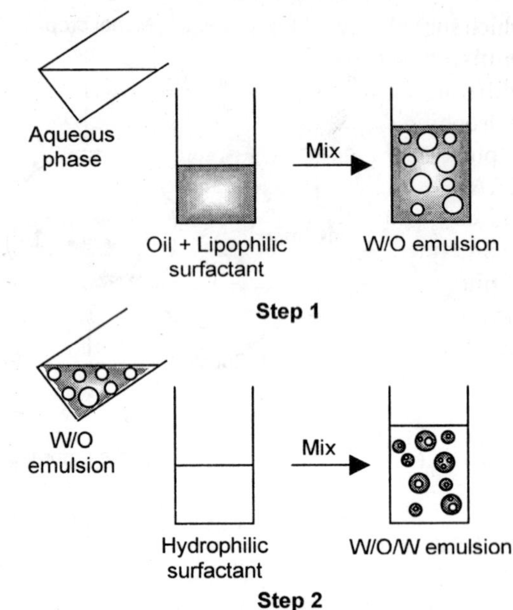

Fig. 8-4. Two-step Preparation of a W/O/W Multiple Emulsion

Recently, Okochi and Nakano, 2000 reported a modified two-step emulsification technique for the preparation of W/O/W emulsion (Fig. 8-5). This method is different from the conventional two-step technique in two points: Firstly, sonication and stirring are used to obtain fine, homogenous and stable W/O emulsion. Secondly, a continuous phase is poured into a dispersed phase for preparing W/O/W emulsion (in contrast to conventional method in which a dispersed phase is poured into a continuous phase). Moreover, the composition of internal aqueous phase-oily phase-external phase is fixed at 1:4:5, which produces most stable formulation as reported for most of W/O/W emulsions.

Phase Inversion Technique (One step Technique)

Matsumoto and co-workers first reported the development of W/O/W system during the phase inversion of the concentrated W/O emulsion (Matsumoto, 1983; Matsumoto et al., 1985a,b). An increase in volume concentration of dispersed phase may cause an increase in the phase volume ratio, which subsequently leads to the formation of multiple emulsions. The method typically involves the addition of an aqueous phase containing the hydrophilic emulsifier [Tween 80/sodium dodecyl sulphate (SDS) or Cetyl trimethyl ammonium salt (CTAB)] to an oil phase consisted of liquid paraffin and containing lipophilic emulsifier (Span 80). A well-defined volume of oil phase is placed in a vessel of pin mixer. An aqueous solution of emulsifier is then introduced successively to the oil phase in the vessel at a rate of 5 ml/min, while the pin mixer rotates steadily at 88 rpm at room temperature. When volume fraction of the aqueous solution of hydrophilic emulsifier exceeds 0.7, the continuous oil phase is substituted by the aqueous phase containing a number of the vesicular globules among the simple oil droplets, leading to phase inversion and formation of W/O/W multiple emulsion (Fig. 8-6).

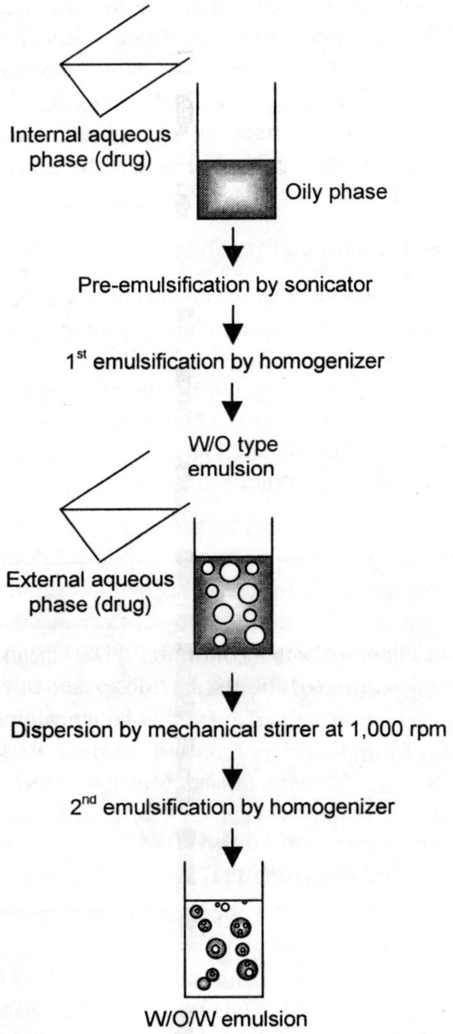

Internal aqueous phase (drug)

Oily phase

Pre-emulsification by sonicator

1st emulsification by homogenizer

W/O type emulsion

External aqueous phase (drug)

Dispersion by mechanical stirrer at 1,000 rpm

2nd emulsification by homogenizer

W/O/W emulsion

Fig. 8-5. Preparation Method of W/O/W Emulsion by a Modified Two Step Emulsification Technique

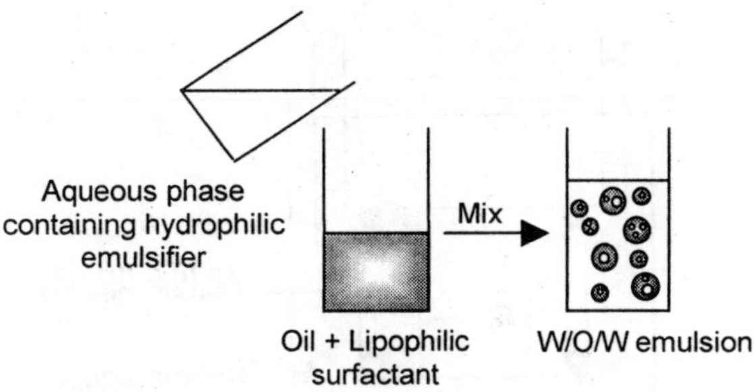

- Volume fraction of the aqueous phase should be higher than 0.7.
- Molar ratio of the hydrophobic and hydrophilic emulsifier should be optimized

Fig. 8-6. Preparation of Multiple Emulsion using Phase Inversion Technique

Membrane Emulsification Technique

Recently, a membrane emulsification procedure has been developed as a novel emulsification method (Higashi et al., 1995; 1999). Possible mechanisms involved in the membrane emulsification method are shown in Fig 8-7. In this method, a W/O emulsion (a dispersed phase) is extruded into an external aqueous phase (a continuous phase) with a constant pressure through a Porous Glass Membrane, which should have controlled and homogenous pores. The particle size of the resulting emulsion can be controlled with proper selection of Porous Glass Membrane as the droplet size depends upon the pore size of the membrane. The relation between membrane pore size and particle size of W/O/W emulsion exhibits good correlation as described by the following equation :

$$Y = 5.03\,X + 0.19 \qquad (8\text{-}1)$$

Where X is the pore size and Y is the mean

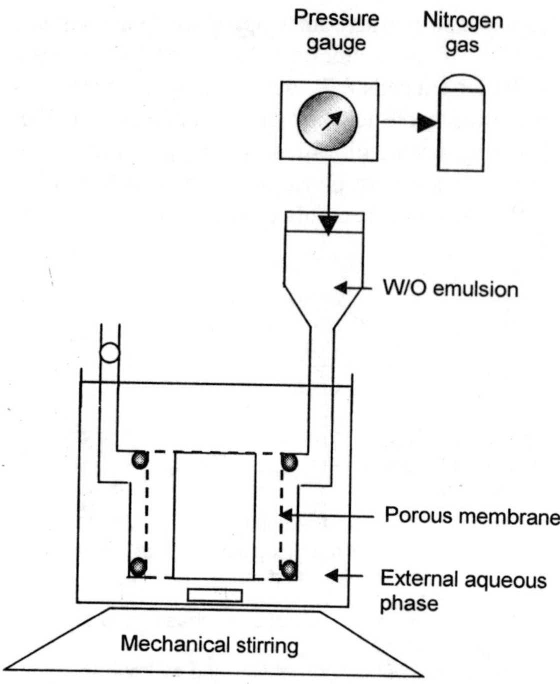

Fig. 8-7. Schematic Diagram of Apparatus used for the Multiple Emulsion Formulation using Membrane Emulsification Technique

particle size of the multiple emulsion prepared using membrane emulsification technique.

IN VITRO CHARACTERIZATION

Average Globule Size and Size Distribution

The optical microscopy method using calibrated ocular and stage micrometer can be utilized for globule size determinations of both multiple emulsion droplets as well as droplets of internal dispersed phase. Florence and Whitehill, 1982a,b used inverted phase contrast microscope and a high-speed camera. With the help of this technique, they classified multiple emulsions as coarse (>3μm diameter), fine (1-3μm diameter) and micro-multiple emulsion (<1 μm diameter). The droplet size distribution of freshly made emulsion can be measured by light scattering using a Malvern Mastersizer and surface mean droplet diameter and the specific surface area (or SSA: area per unit mass of emulsion) can also be derived. Brightfield micrographs equipped with differential interference contrast optics have been used to characterize the internal droplet of multiple emulsion. Various other techniques used to characterize colloidal carriers like Coulter counter, freeze-fracture electron microscopy and scanning electron microscopy are also used to determine average globule size and size distribution of multiple emulsions (Fig. 8-8).

Recently, NMR self-diffusion methods are adopted to multiple emulsion characterization. Using this technique, droplet size distribution for the water in the starting W/O emulsion and the water in the multiple emulsion can be evaluated. Information about the state of oil in both emulsions may also be obtained. In addition, the self-diffusion NMR technique may be used to obtain information regarding the water exchange across the oil film in the multiple emulsion.

Area of Interfaces

The average globule diameter determined can be us in the calculation of the total area of interface using the formula :

$$S = 6/d \quad (8\text{-}2)$$

S = Total area of interface (sq.cm)
D = Diameter of globules (cm)

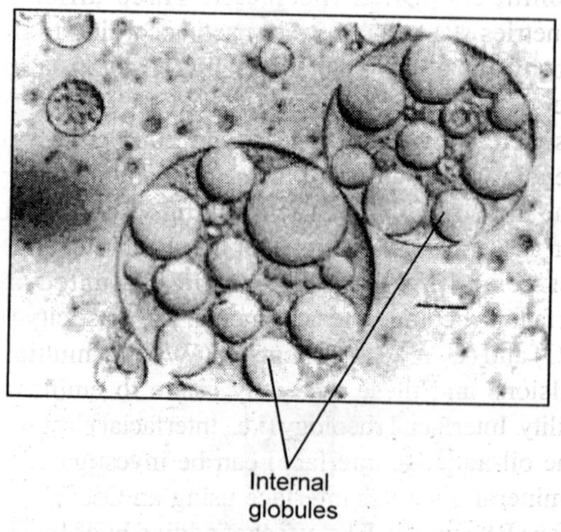

Fig. 8-8. Microphotograph of Multiple Emulsion Showing the Internal Aqueous Phase in a W/O/W Emulsion

Number of Globules

Number of globules per cubic mm can be measured using the haemocytometer cell. The emulsion is appropriately diluted, a countable number of globules are observed in each small square of the cell and counted. The globules in five groups of 16 small squares (total 80 small squares) are counted and the total number of globules in per cubic mm are calculated using the formula (Chatterjee, 1985) :

$$\text{No of globules/mm}^3 = \frac{\text{No of globules x Dilution x 4000}}{\text{No of small squares counted}} \qquad (8\text{-}3)$$

Rheological Evaluation

The rheology of multiple emulsion is an important parameter as it relates to emulsion stability and clinical performance. The viscosity and interfacial elasticity are two major parameters, which relate to product rheology. The viscosity of the multiple emulsions can be measured by Brookfield rotational viscometer. Samples are sheared for one min at 100 rpm, using an appropriate spindle and readings are taken after equilibrium of the indicator dial. Oil phase viscosity can be measured by stress viscometry using a Bohlin controlled rheometer. Three different geometries stant (5 μL) were used according to the viscosity of the samples: double-gap DG 40/50, cone-plate 4/40, and concentric cylinder C25. The shear rates were varied between 0.5 and 200 per second depending on viscosity of the sample and geometry of the measuring head. The resulting viscosity was taken as the mean viscosity over the shear rate range. Interfacial film strength can be evaluated by interfacial rheology measurements, i.e. elasticity of (W/O) and (O/W) components of (W/O/W) multiple emulsions and these data may relate to emulsion stability. Interfacial rheology (i.e., interfacial elasticity at the oil-aqueous interface) can be investigated at the mineral oil/water interface using an Oscillatory Surface Rheometer. The effect of adding hydrophilic surfactant, Tween and Spans on interfacial elasticity can also be investigated and this may provide an insight on interfacial interactions that occur at the secondary O/W interface.

Zeta Potential

The zeta potential measurements are pivotal in the designing of surface modified or ligand anchored multiple emulsion systems. The zeta potential and surface charge can be calculated using Smoluchowski's equation from the mobility and electrophoretic velocity of dispersed globules using the Zeta-potentiometer. Nakhare and Vyas, 1997 used a cylindrically bored microelectrophoresis cell equipped with platinum-iridium electrodes to measure the electrophoretic mobility of the diluted W/O/W emulsion and using the following equation, zeta potential was calculated.

$$\zeta = \frac{4\pi\eta\mu}{\varepsilon E} \times 10^3 \qquad (8\text{-}4)$$

Where,

ζ = Zeta potential (mV)

η = Viscosity of the dispersion medium (poise)

μ = Migration velocity (cm/s)

ε = Dielectric constant of the dispersion medium

E = Potential gradient (Voltage applied/ Distance between electrodes)

Percent Drug Entrapment

Percent entrapment of drug or active moiety in the multiple emulsion is generally determined using dialysis, centrifugation, filtration and conductivity measurements. However, recently an internal tracer/marker was used to evaluate the entrapment of an impermeable marker molecule contained in the inner aqueous phase of W/O/W emulsion. The unentrapped marker is calculated and the amount entrapped can be thus calculated by deducting unentrapped amount from the initially added amount. The % drug entrapment in the inner aqueous phase of W/O/W emulsion can be determined by using the dialysis method as reported by Nakhare and Vyas, 1995, 1996. The % Entrapment can be calculated using the following equation :

$$C = 100/[1\text{-}n_1 V^*/n_{10}\text{-}n_1)V_1] \qquad (8\text{-}5)$$

$$V^* = V_2 + \frac{V_d(V_1+V_2+V_0)}{V_s} \quad (8\text{-}6)$$

Where,
n_{10} = Initial concentration of drug in inner aqueous phase
n_l = Concentration of drug in dialysate
V_1, V_2 and V_0 represent the volume of inner and outer aqueous and middle oil phase respectively, and V_s and V_d represent volume of dialyzing media and dialyzed emulsion respectively.

In vitro Drug Release

The drug released from the aqueous inner phase of a W/O/W emulsion can be estimated using the conventional dialysis technique. Nakhare and Vyas, 1995 investigated the release of drug from W/O/W emulsion employing the dialysis method using cellophane tubing (Fig. 8-9). The W/O/W emulsion was placed in the dialysis bag and dialyzed against 200 ml of phosphate saline buffer (PBS, pH 7.4) at 37±1°C and a sink condition was maintained while sink contents were stirred continuously using a magnetic stirrer. Aliquots were withdrawn at different time intervals and estimated using standard procedure and the data were used to calculate cumulative drug release profile.

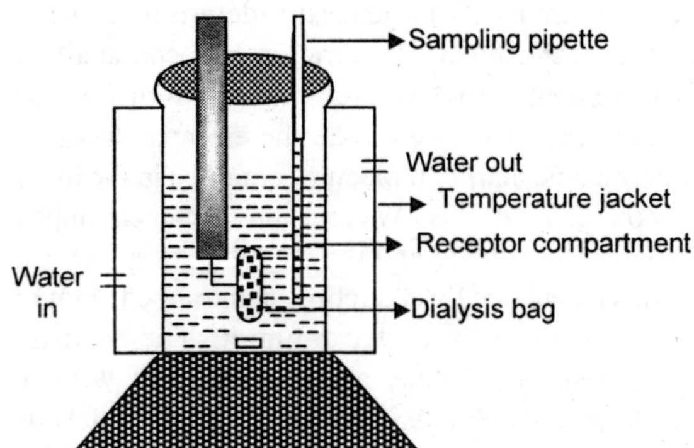

Fig. 8-9. Assembly Used for *In Vitro* Drug Release Assay

In vitro Stability Studies

Emulsion stability is determined by phase separation on storage of W/O/W emulsions. Freshly prepared multiple emulsion allowed to stand for one week at room temperature and the volume of aqueous phase separated (V_{sep}) is measured at suitable time intervals and percent phase separation is calculated using following formula (Nakhare and Vyas, 1996) :

$$B(\%) = 100\ (V_{sep}/20)/[(V_1+V_2)/\ V_1+V_2+V_0 \quad (8\text{-}7)$$

Where, V_1, V_2 and V_3 are the volumes of internal, external aqueous phase and middle oil phase respectively.

Photomicrography, difference in release of model drug and analysis of mean droplet diameters of the multiple emulsion systems as a function of time could be followed and used to study stability of W/O/W emulsions. However, to test flocculation in multiple emulsion, 5 and 100 drops of SDS (10%) are added immediately after the measurement and the emulsion is stirred gently. Then the droplet size distribution measurement is repeated and the degree of flocculation is microscopically assessed.

Nakhare and Vyas, 1996 characterized *in vitro* stability to establish the suitability of W/O/W emulsion as suitable injectable drug carrier. Osmotic fragility and turbulence shock tests were performed in addition to assess *in vitro* stability.

STABILITY OF MULTIPLE EMULSIONS

Emulsion stability is a phenomenon, which depends upon the equilibrium between water, oil and surfactant. Unfortunately, multiple emulsions are thermodynamically unstable. The possible indications of instability include :

- Leakage of the contents from the inner aqueous phase
- Expulsion of internal droplets in external phase
- Constriction or distension of the internal droplets due to osmotic gradient across the oil membrane
- Flocculation of internal aqueous phase and multiple emulsion droplets

- Disruption of oil layer on the surface of internal droplets
- Phase separation

Breakdown Pathways

Some of the breakdown pathways that may be involved in WO/W emulsion destabilization are summarized in Figure 8-10. Some breakdown pathways involve rupture of the oil layer and consequent loss of the internal aqueous drop. This results when the concentration of the primary emulsifier is depleted via transfer through the oil layer to the aqueous compartment. Partitioning effect as well as mixed micelle formation of the two surfactants (emulsifiers) may be involved, suggesting that there should be an optimum ratio of primary to secondary surfactant for greater yield of preparation with high stability (Opaware and Burgess, 1998).

Emulsifier migration is responsible for a decrease in the effective HLB of the second emulsifier. i.e. an increase in the optimal HLB is proportional to the concentration of primary emulsifier. At a fixed concentration of primary emulsifier, the HLB shift is

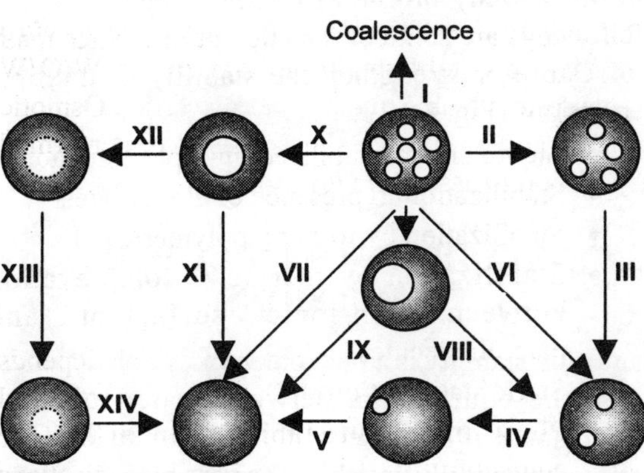

Fig. 8-10. Breakdown Process that may Occur in a W/O/W Emulsion. Pathway I, coalescence of multiple oil drops, single or multiple. Pathways II, III, IV and V, expulsion of single internal droplets. Pathways VI and VII, expulsion of more than one internal droplet. Pathways VIII and IX, coalescence of internal droplets before being expelled (X and XI). Pathways XII, XIII and XIV, shrinkage of internal droplets due to diffusion.

inversely proportional to the concentration of the secondary emulsifier. From these linear relationships it is possible to predict the optimal HLB if two emulsifier concentrations and the required HLB of the oil are known. Inversion of W/O/W emulsions to the O/W emulsion occurs if the HLB of the total emulsifiers approaches the required HLB of the oil or if the droplet size, as a result of increasing secondary emulsifier concentration, becomes too small to obtain desired internal droplet size.

Coalescence of multiple drops produces a large decrease in the oil/water interfacial area, whereas coalescence of the small internal droplets would not contribute significantly to the breakdown process. Similarly, the reduction in diameter of a multiple emulsion droplet as a result of expulsion of internal droplets by rupture of the oil membrane leads to a significant diminution of the van der Waals forces of attraction between multiple emulsion droplets (Fig. 8-11, point A). From the consideration of the free energy change on expulsion of an internal aqueous droplet emulsion that contains only a few small droplets would be expected to be more stable than the ones containing a single large droplet or many smaller droplets. The greater attraction of the internal water droplets for the continuous phase than for each other (Fig. 8-11, point C vs B) predicts that a decrease in the size of the external droplet for a given W/O primary emulsion would lead to decreased stability of the internal droplets.

Factors Affecting Stability

The factors affecting the stability of these emulsions are well identified and documented. The factors critical for stability of multiple emulsions include methods of preparation, the nature of entrapped material, particularly the effect of electrolyte, phase volume, concentration and nature of the emulsifiers and ratio of lipophilic and hydrophilic emulsifiers (Florence and Whitehill, 1982a,b).

Similarly, the rheological properties of W/O/W emulsion are remarkably affected by a number of factors (Matsumoto and Khoda, 1980). These factors depend upon the structural characteristics of the dispersed globules, such as yield of the W/O/W dispersion formation, the stability of vesicular structure of dispersed globules and the osmotic

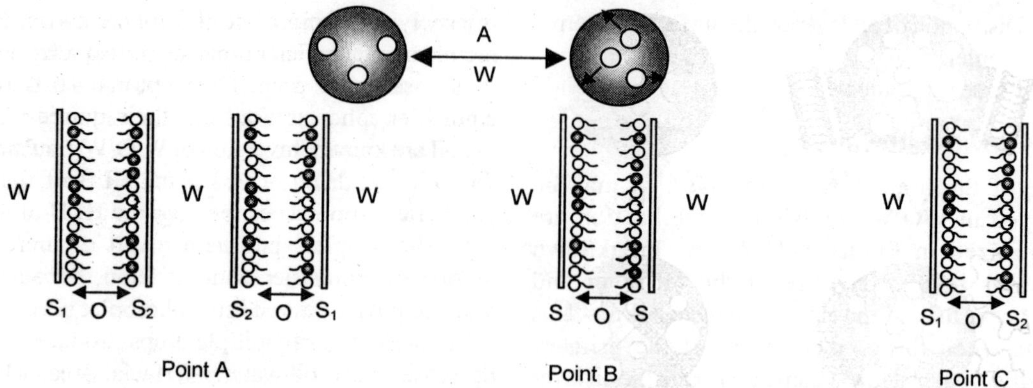

Fig. 8-11. Possible Interactions (A, B and C) Between Phases in Multiple Emulsions. Schematic Structures of Oil (O) and Water (W) Phases and Surfactant (Emulsifier) Films (S_1, S_2) Involved in the Attractive and Repulsive Interactions.

pressure gradient between the inner and outer aqueous phases of W/O/W multiple emulsion.

The changes in the bulk viscosity (Kita et al., 1978) have been measured and used as a convenient method to determine the stability of W/O/W emulsions. The viscosity of W/O/W emulsions is influenced by the osmotic pressure gradient between the aqueous compartments and the aqueous suspending fluid (Matsumoto and Khoda, 1980; Matsumoto et al., 1980).

These findings conclusively suggest that if a rupture occurs in the oil layer, the inner aqueous phase disappears instantaneously and mixes with the continuous phase. Therefore, an understanding of the exact mechanism causing instability of multiple emulsion is needed.

Essentially this goal may be reached by gaining further insights into the factors affecting the thinning process and the resultant effect on the equilibrium of liquid layer.

Methods to Stabilize Multiple Emulsions

Florence and Whitehill, 1982, 1985 suggested three methods to stabilize W/O/W emulsion as: (i) use of a high viscous oil to prevent or suppress diffusion of individual surfactant molecules, (ii) the polymerization of interfacially adsorbed surfactant molecules, and (iii) the gelation of the oily or aqueous phases of the emulsion. However, other methods like stabilization by blending (mixture) of surfactants (Opaware and Burges, 1998); by interfacial adsorption of albumin (Garti et al., 1993), acacia, gelatin or polyvinyl pyrrolidone (Omotosho, 1990, Nakhare and Vyas, 1995), colloidal microcrystalline cellulose (Oza and Frank, 1989) and poly(acrylic) acid (Cole and Whateley, 1997) are proposed. The literature is abound regarding the improvement in the stability profile of multiple emulsions. The followings are some of the attempt or studies made to restore or strengthen the stability of multiple emulsions (Fig. 8-12) :

- Liquid crystal stabilized multiple emulsion
- Stabilization in presence of electrolytes
- Stabilization by forming polymeric gel
- Stabilization by inerfacial complexation between non-ionic surfactant and macromolecules
- Steric stabilization
- Phase-inversion stabilization of W/O/W emulsion

Liquid Crystal Stabilized Multiple Emulsions

In many stable and commercially important emulsions the emulsifier, water and oil molecules contribute to regular structure of multi-molecular layers, which are known as "liquid crystal layers". These layers exist actually as a distinct phase that can exist independently after separation from the dispersion media by centrifugation. The structure of the liquid crystal layer may by determined by X-ray

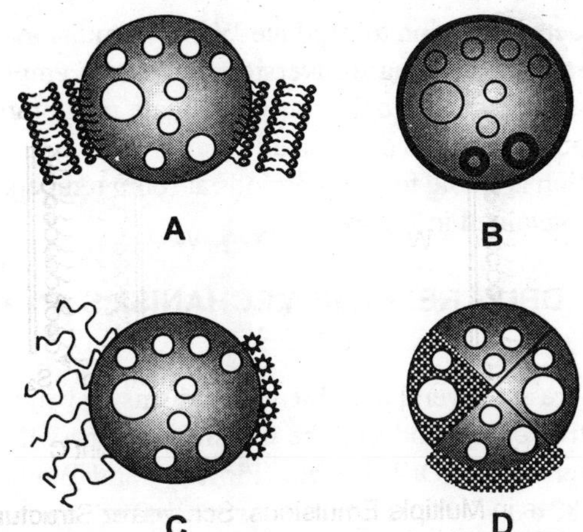

Fig. 8-12. Various Approaches to Stabilize the Liquid Membrane Systems (W/O/W Multiple Emulsion). A. Stabilization through liquid crystal formation; B. Stabilization by interfacial polymerization; C. Stabilization by adsorption of electrolyte or adsorption or covalent anchoring of polymers (steric); D. Gelation of either internal or external phase or oily core.

diffraction, optical and electron microscopy. The liquid crystal in an emulsion seems to stabilize it and several mechanisms are proposed to explain liquid crystal stabilized multiple emulsions (Friberg and Mandell, 1970; Ali and Mulley, 1978; Nakhare et al., 1994). The layers of liquid crystalline phase around the droplets act as a rheological barrier and as a result, considerably higher viscous forces are encountered, when the liquid crystalline phase is sheared. In addition, some liquid crystalline phases have a tendency to form a network similar to semisolid phase extending through the continuous phase. This network impedes the movement of the droplets and adds to the stability of emulsion.

Stabilization in Presence of Electrolytes

Matsumoto and co-workers, 1985a,b reported the use of electrolytes for obtaining a stable W/O/W emulsion. These electrolytes include ascorbic acid, acetic acid, sodium chloride and sodium citrate. The addition of lysozyme to the aqueous phase or stearylamine and oleic acid to the oil phase effectively improves the stability of the oil layer. In one of the earlier study, Matsumoto and Sherman, 1981 reported the influence of various additives, e.g. glucose, sucrose, acetic acid, citric acid, ascorbic acid, sodium chloride and sodium acetate on the stability and low grade shear viscosity of water-in-olive oil-in-water emulsion. Glucose and sucrose could increase the viscosity and as a result stability of emulsion system. Adeyeye and Price 1990 studied the effect of dextrose on internal aqueous phase formation and stability of W/O/W multiple emulsion. Microscopic study conducted on such emulsions indicated that as the dextrose concentration in internal aqueous phase increased (0-2.5%w/v), the stability recorded in terms of degree of coalescence of internal droplets and rupture rate of interfacial oily layer was increased.

Stabilization by Forming Polymeric Gel

The gelation of either internal or external phase or the oily phase (membrane) has been employed in various studies to stabilize the system. Florence and co-workers (Florence et al., 1981; Florence and Whitehill, 1982a) used two different methods to prepare stable W/O/W emulsions by forming a polymeric gel in the internal or external aqueous phase. First method is based on preparation of polyacrylamide gel/oil/water system and second method discusses the preparation of water/oil/polyacrylamide gel system. The first emulsion system has the similarities to the gelatin microspheres/oil/water system reported by Hashida et al., 1977.

Stabilization by Interfacial Complexation between Non-ionic Surfactant and Macromolecules

This mode of stabilization can be executed either through *in situ* polymerization at the interface or by interfacial interaction between a polymer and a surfactant. During the search for stable W/O/W emulsion as vehicle for sustained release preparation, numerous researchers (Law et al., 1984; Omotosho et al., 1986) have employed interfacial complexation between non-ionic surfactants and macromolecules. Another approach to obtain stable W/O/W multiple emulsion is based on the interfacial interaction between a macromolecule, e.g. albumin or polyacrylic acid (Law et al., 1986) or bovine serum albumin (Florence et al., 1985) contained in an internal aqueous phase. A lipophilic poloxamer of high molecular weight e.g. Poloxamer 331 was preferable in forming a stable W/O and the subsequent W/O/W emulsion. Similarly, hydrophilic poloxamer surfactant of high molecular weight, e.g. Poloxamer 403 was found to enhance the stability of W/O/W emulsion when used as an emulsifier.

The kinetics of swelling-breakdown of a W/O/W multiple emulsion have been studied and explored for the possible mechanisms for the lipophilic surfactant effect. Two different mechanisms were proposed and both imply the migration of the lipophilic surfactant from one simultaneously. The lipophilic surfactant could diffuse from the first to the second interface, thus rigidifying the membrane or from the oily phase to the first interface, resulting in delayed coalescence of the aqueous droplets during swelling.

Steric Stabilization

Steric stabilization can be achieved by using either adsorption or grafting of natural polymers or by using polymeric surfactants or lipid grafted polymers. The steric cloud may help prevent their instability due to environmental challenges. Iwamoto and co-workers, 1991 stabilized multiple emulsions by coating them with hydrophobized polysaccharides like cholesteroyl pullulan, mannan and amylopectin. Similar potential of Polaxamer™ or Pluronic™ coated systems can also be elucidated.

Phase-inversion Method of W/O/W Emulsion Stabilization

Hino and co-workers 2000 reported stabilization of W/O/W emulsions by means of three different methods viz., making the inner aqueous phase hypertonic, addition of chitosan in the inner phase and initiation of phase-inversion mediated through porous membrane. Making the inner aqueous phase hypertonic prevented phase separation and prolonged the release of the drug with low-partition coefficient between oil and water. Stabilization by means of chitosan was achieved after neutralizing the acetic or butyric acid with sodium hydroxide in the inner aqueous phase (pH induced gelling of chitosan). Therefore, phase separation was inhibited and the emulsion was stabilized with soft gel containing acetate and butyrate ions. Phase-inversion with a porous membrane produced W/O emulsion, which are stable on long term (shelf) storage conditions and can easily be re-dispersed in hydrophilic surfactant aqueous solution to produce W/O/W emulsion. The mechanism of phase-inversion of W/O/W emulsion by extrusion through a polycarbonate membrane to produce a physicochemically stable W/O emulsion, which is stable for long periods at room temperature is explained in Figure 8-13.

DRUG RELEASE MECHANISMS AND MODELS

There are several possible mechanisms by which the active compound may be transferred across the oil layer in a W/O/W system (Florence and Whitehill, 1982b). Various studies were based upon the intervention of these mechanisms for drug release from multiple emulsions and several models are devised simultaneously to carry out these studies. Some of the mechanisms include :

- Diffusion of unionized drug (hydrophobic species) through the oil layer
- Carrier mediated transport
- Micellar transport
- Rupture of oil membrane
- Thinning of oil membrane

Diffusion of Unionized Drug (Hydrophobic species) Through the Oil Layer (Diffusion Rate Model)

The most obvious is by diffusion of unionized drug (hydrophobic species) through the oil layer (semipermeable liquid membrane), especially in stable multiple emulsion system. Hence, the drug transport *in vitro* has been found to follow first order kinetics and obeyed Fick's law (Fig. 8-14).

$$\frac{dC_0}{dt} = \frac{-DA\,\Delta C}{dx} = \frac{-DA}{dx}(C_0 - C_i) \qquad (8\text{-}8)$$

Since $C_e = C_o/P$

$$\frac{dC_e}{dt} = \frac{P(dt)}{dC_0} = \frac{-DA}{P(dx)}\ P(C_e - Ci) \qquad (8\text{-}9)$$

Where,

C_0= Concentration of drug in the oil phase
C_i= Concentration of drug in internal aqueous phase
C_e= Concentration of drug in external aqueous phase

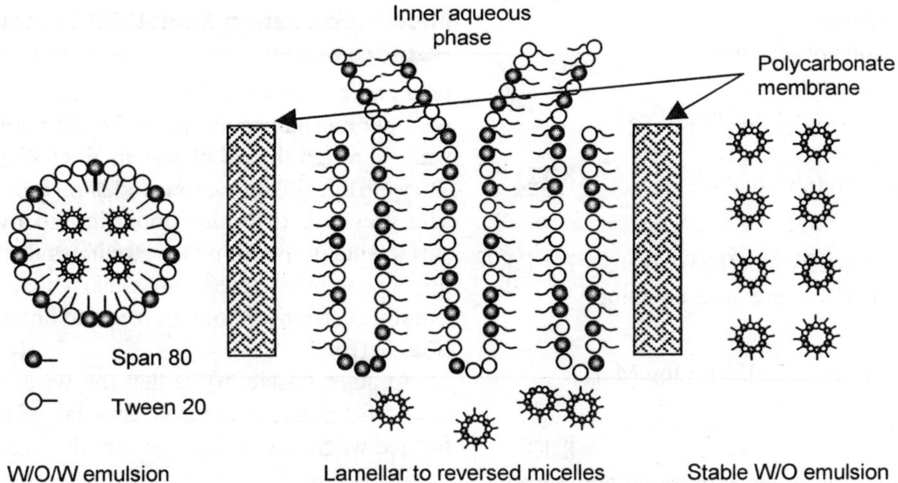

Fig. 8-13. Schematic Diagram of Phase-inversion of a W/O/W Emulsion by Extrusion through Polycarbonate Membrane to Yield Stable W/O Emulsion, which can be Reconstituted Again as W/O/W Emulsion when Required.

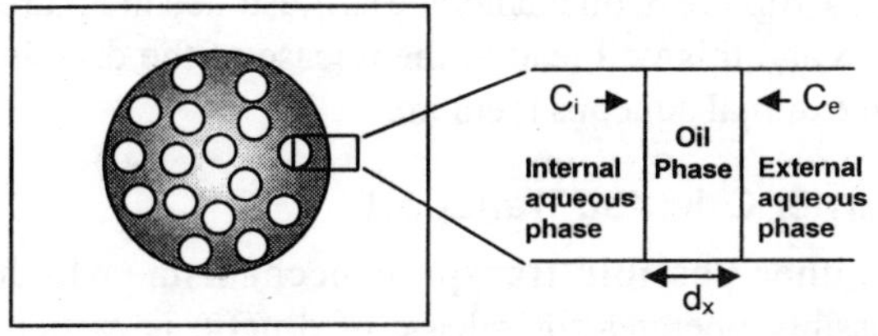

Fig. 8-14. Two-dimensional Model for Diffusion Controlled Transport of Unionized Materials from the External Aqueous Phase to the Internal Aqueous Droplets in a W/O/W System.

D= Diffusion coefficient of drug in the oil phase
dx= Diffusion layer thickness
P= Partition coefficient of drug between oil and external phase.
t= Time

When a trapping agent is used in the internal aqueous phase, the material becomes ionized and C_i turns to be negligible; equation can be written as

$$\frac{dC_e}{dt} = \frac{-DAC_e}{dx} = -KC_e \qquad (8\text{-}10)$$

The rate constant K is a function of the diffusion coefficient of the drug, the area between the external phase and the liquid membrane and membrane thickness.

Planer-sheet Model

Baker and Lonsdale,1974 have suggested the uniform planer-sheet model of multiple emulsion droplets for release mechanism. The model schematically represented in Figure 8-15.

It is generally based on the assumption that the thickness of oil phase is negligible compared to the droplet average radius (r). The area for mass transfer can be considered to be constant and a uniform planer membrane of thickness l. The equation governing the release from a slab with a non-constant source has the form :

$$M_r = \frac{M_{infinite}\{V_2 \exp[-ADK(V_1+V_2)t/\,l.V_1.V_2]+V_1\}}{V_1+V_2} \qquad (8\text{-}11)$$

Where,
M_r = Amount of drug in the internal drops at time t.
$M_{infinite}$ = Initial amount of drug
A = Surface area of multiple drops
K = Partition coefficient of solute in the oil phase
l = Thickness of the oil layer

V_1 = Internal volume
V_2 = Sink solution volume and
D = Diffusion coefficient.
Suppose $V_2 >> V_1$, equation simplifies to

$$M_r = M_{infinite} \exp(-ADKt / l.V_1) \quad (8\text{-}12)$$

The permeability coefficient (P) is given by P = DK/l and substituting (P) in previous equation.

$$\log M_r = -(AP / 2.303V_1) + \log M_{infinite} \quad (8\text{-}13)$$

This equation is first order expression and permits the evaluation of P from plots of log M_r against t.

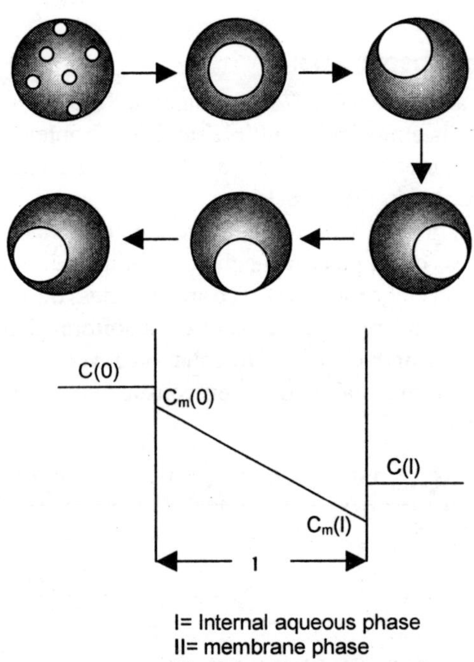

Fig. 8-15. Uniform Planer-sheet Model of Multiple Emulsion Droplets

Micelle Formation Model/ Oil Thinning or Rupture Model

Kita and co-workers, 1978 have suggested the two possible mechanisms/models for the permeation of water through the oil phases in W/O/W emulsions. They are micelle formation model/ oil rupture model. The presence of both lipophilic and hydrophilic surfactants in the oil phase facilitates the formation of water swollen inverse micelles, which may act as a mobile carrier for both ionized and unionized drug (Fig. 8-16).

Another possibility is that the water molecules may diffuse across the thin lamellae of surfactants formed where the oil layer is very thin. Experiments carried out by Kita et al., 1978 suggested that this mechanism probably comes into play when there is an osmotic pressure difference between two aqueous phases (Fig. 8-17).

Another mechanism for the drug release could be the rupture of oil membrane as illustrated in Figure 8-18 and this will lead to the release of the drug in the external aqueous medium.

Carrier Oriented Transport

Another possible transport mechanism, which possibly operates for release of drug(s) is carrier-oriented transport (Fig. 8-19). This involves either incorporation of some material into the internal aqueous phase of membrane phase, which reacts with

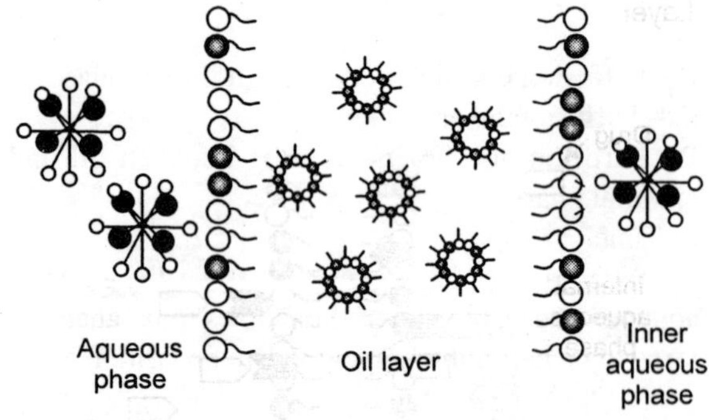

Fig. 8-16. Schematic Illusration of a Model for Micellar Transport of Water from the Outer Aqueous Phase to the Inner Aqueous Phase through the Oil Layer in W/O/W Emulsions

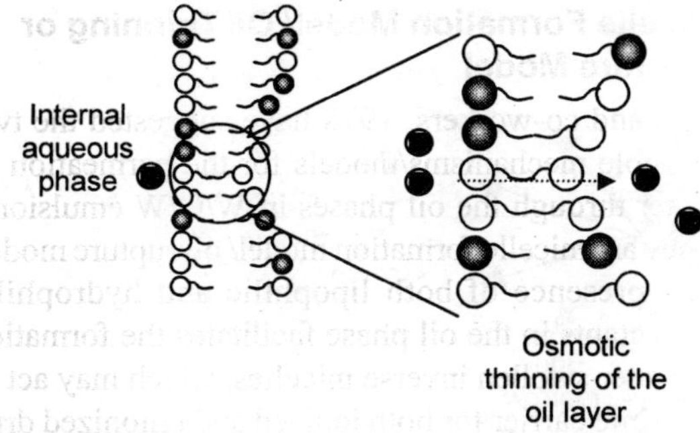

Fig. 8-17. Schematic Illustration of a Model for Water Transport through Thin Lamellae of Surfactant due to Fluctuations in the Thickness of the Oil Layer

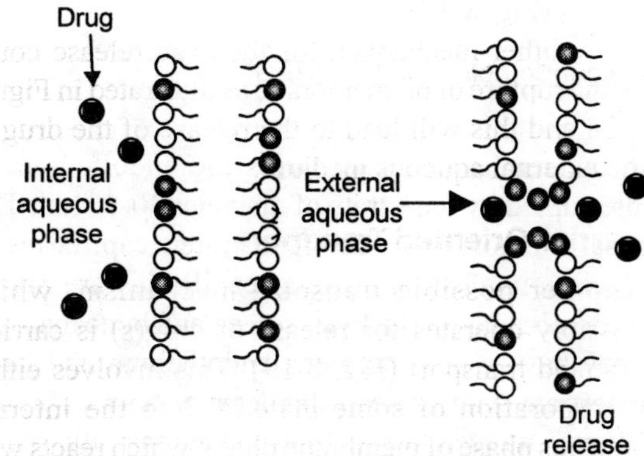

Fig. 8-18. Release of Drug on Rupturing of the Oil Layer

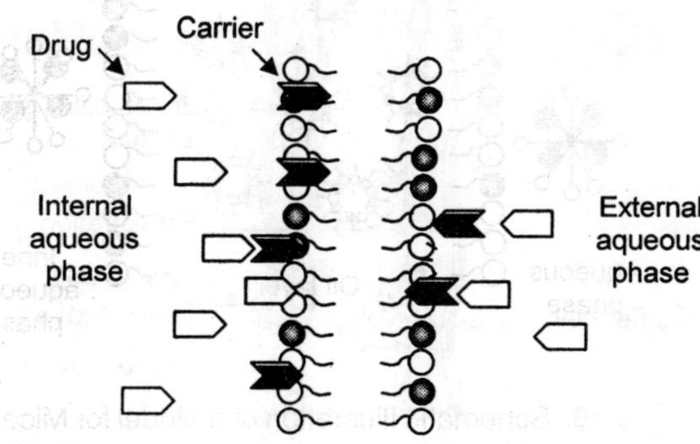

Fig. 8-19. Release Mechanism of Facilitated or Carrier Mediated Transport

the permeating compound to render it liposoluble. The carrier compounds effectively pump the permeating compound across the membrane, e.g. stearic acid facilitated diffusion of Cu^{++} ions. The mechanism is especially effective for transport of highly hydrophilic compounds (Florence and Whitehill, 1982b).

- The rapid partitioning of lipophilic molecules into oil phase and subsequently into the external medium.
- The last and probably much less important transport mechanism is solubilization of small amounts of internal phase in the membrane phase resulting into generation of diffusive passages of very small quantities of materials.

The release kinetics of the molecules across the liquid membrane systems are affected by the various factors (Florence and Whitehill, 1982a) such as :

- Internal and multiple droplet size.
- pH of internal and external aqueous phases.
- Phase volume ratios (ϕW/O and ϕW/O/W)
- Viscosity.
- Nature of entrapped material.

IN VIVO FATE OF MULTIPLE EMULSIONS

Blood, lymph, cerebrospinal fluid, synovial fluid and urine are all basically aqueous media and sustained drug delivery to these organs can be claimed if the rate of partitioning from oil into an aqueous media or dissolution of solid into aqueous media is slow and controllable. In order to reduce the diffusion of drug from an emulsion formulation. Davis and co-workers, 1987 developed a multiple W/O/W emulsion for intramuscular injection using the Iodohippuric acid as a model drug. Collings, 1971 reported that W/O/W emulsion could break down rapidly *in vivo* due to an osmotic effect. The use of isotonic system and/or the creation of thick interfacial layers or gelled systems that can withstand the osmotic stress provides systems that may have controlled drug release characteristics *in vivo* (Boyd et al., 1976). However, in all parenteral systems the most important mechanism involved is the rapid clearance of colloidal sized foreign particles from the systemic circulation by macrophages of the reticuloendothelial system (RES) (Fig. 8-20).

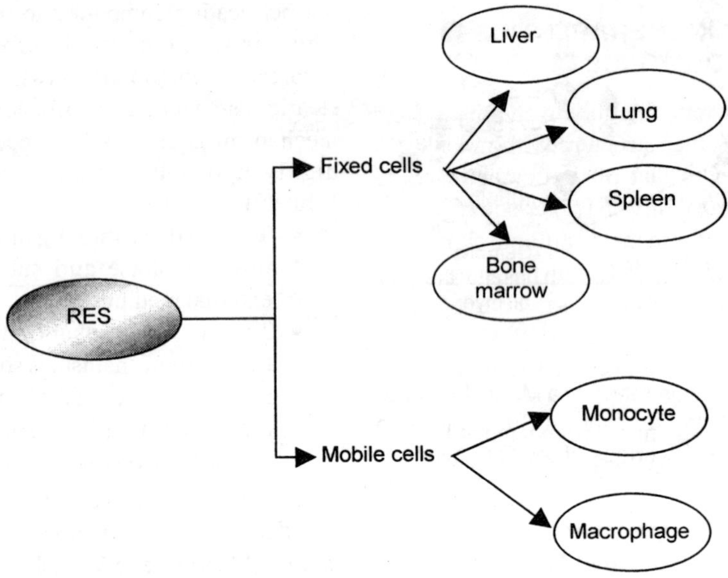

Fig. 8-20. Components of the Reticuloendothelial System (RES)

The rapid clearance of foreign particles from the circulation by macrophages lining the sinusoids in the liver, spleen and bone marrow is one of the most important non-specific host defense property. Certain serum components called "Opsonins" are effectively identified and considered to be important in the clearance of microparticles (Absolom, 1986).It is reported that enzyme entrapped in liposomes could be successfully targeted to the macrophages of RES. At the same time, it was realized that colloids previously used for radio imaging purposes could also be utilized for targeting of drugs to the RES (Moghimi and Patel, 1989). The successful delivery of different microparticles to the RES has drawn the interest on the possible mode of delivery of the microparticles to other sites in the body, such as various extra-vascular tissues. However, to date no convincing studies of specific extravascular targeting of microparticulate drug carriers has been demonstrated.

All capillaries are lined with a layer of endothelial cells set on a basement membrane (Zweitach, 1980). The three groups of capillaries have been identified (a) continuous (b) fenestrated and (c) sinusoidal. In the continuous type, the endothelial cells are connected via tight junctions to form a continuous monolayer or an uninterrupted basement membrane. In the fenestrated capillaries the endothelium is interrupted by fenestrate of diameter 30-80 nm. The basal membrane in the fenestrated capillaries is continuous. The sinusoidal capillaries are found predominantly in the liver, spleen and bone marrow. They have a discontinuous endothelium and large fenestrate with a mean diameter of about 100 nm (Wisse and De Leeuw, 1984). Diagrammatic representation and the details are shown in Figure 8-21.

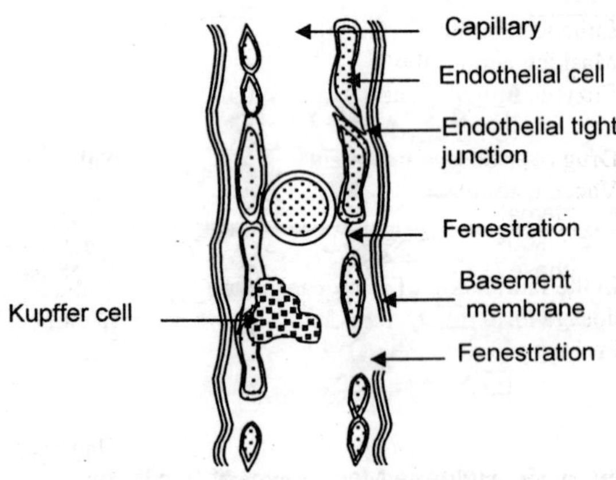

Fig. 8-21. The capillary Endothelial Barrier

APPLICATIONS IN THERAPEUTICS AND COSMTEICS

Multiple emulsion systems are finding unlimited uses because of their vesicular structure with innermost phase closely similar to that of liposomal vesicles and the selective permeability characteristic of liquid membranes. Based on these facts, multiple emulsion systems have been studied widely with respect to their practical utility, the most common is their utilization as potential drug delivery system. An O/W/O multiple emulsion may appear to be more desirable dosage form since the extra partitioning step with drug initially in the internal oil phase is expected to be the rate-limiting factor that may define the drug release characteristics.

Various prominent applications of multiple emulsions are due to the fact that biological fluids are miscible with water and a W/O/W multiple emulsion can be expected to perform essentially as a simple W/O emulsion shortly after parenteral administration. Further, the external aqueous phase would make administration much easier than W/O type emulsions (oil is an external phase), which are highly viscous and difficult to inject.

Some important applications of multiple emulsions are outlined below and summarized in Table 8-1 :

- Controlled and sustained drug delivery
- Drug targeting
- Vaccine adjuvant
- Immobilization of enzyme
- As a preparative tool for microencapsulation technology
- Food and cosmetics applications
- Absorption enhancement through gastrointestinal tract
- Miscellaneous
- As sorbent reservoir in drug overdose treatment
- Protection action
- Taste masking action

Controlled and Sustained Drug Delivery

The basic potential of multiple emulsions (both W/O/W and O/W/O) in clinical therapeutics is in the prolonged and controlled release of drugs. In both the systems drug contained in innermost phase partitions through several phases prior to release at the site of absorption and the rate of release is governed by its ability to diffuse through various phases and cross interfacial barriers. Various investigators have worked on liquid membrane system and recommended their use as a controlled release drug delivery system. Brodin et al., 1978

Table 8-1. Biomedical and Pharmaceutical Applications of Multiple Emulsions

Application(s)	Drug entrapped
Enhanced oral bioavailability	Heparin, Insulin, Griseofulvin
Masking action	Chlorpromazine HCl, Chloroquin
Enzyme immobilization	Urease, Lipase, Amylase, Pancreatic enzymes, α-Chymotrysin, L-leucine dehydrogenase
Drug over dosage treatment	Salicylates, Barbiturates, Quinine sulphate
Vaccine adjuvants	Influenza virus, Tetanus toxoid
Separation and extraction technique	Different hydrocarbons, Copper separation, purificaton of waste water and Amine extraction
In the fabrication of microcapsulated dosage form	Salbutamol sulphate, Pseudoephedrine HCl, Vitamin-B_6, Diclofenac sodium
Prolonged action	Naltrexone HCl, Pilocarpine HCl, Ephendrine HCl, Pentazocine, Xylocaine HCl, Sulphacetamide sodium, Chloroquin phosphate, Terbutaline sulphate, Haemoglobin, Nitrofurantoin, Rifampicin
In cancer therapy and drug targeting	5-Fluorouracil, Bleomycin, Methotrexate, Cysteamine, Adriamycin HCl
Other applications	Food and cosmetics

studied the potential drug delivery systems for prolonging the effect of drug with short biological half-lives. They examined *in vitro* release of Naltrexone hydrochloride and Naltrexone base from W/O/W and O/W/O systems respectively. In W/O/W system they found 70% prolongation of drug release by addition of sodium chloride or sorbitol to the internal aqueous phase.

Fukushima et al., 1983 studied *in vitro* release of cytarabine and 5-Fluorouracil (5-FU) from the W/O/W system. The release of cytarabine was prolonged while an aqueous solution of the drug released more than 90% in the first h itself, the W/O/W emulsion gave only 50% release in 12 h and less than 60% release in 24 h. Intra-arterial use of emulsions for sustained release purposes has also been explored. Lipiodol, an oily lymphographic agent, has remained selectively at a hepatic cancer site after being injected as an O/W/O emulsion into the hepatic artery (Fukushima et al., 1986).

Pandit and co-workers, 1988 prepared indomethacin containing O/W/O multiple emulsion, which when administered orally to mice, showed prolonged plasma and brain levels of the drug as compared to equivalent dose administered as free drug solution.

Mishra and Pandit, 1989 made extensive studies on both W/O/W and O/W/O multiple emulsion systems with respect to their practical utility as controlled drug delivery systems. They reported prolonged blood and tissue levels of Pentazocine after oral administration of multiple emulsion systems to mice in comparison to simple W/O and O/W emulsion and aqueous solution of Pentazocine.

Omotosho and co-workers, 1989 studied the release pattern of 5-fluorouracil (5-FU) and sodium chloride entrapped separately in internal aqueous phase of W/O/W emulsion after intramuscular administration. They found that the diffusion of the unionized species of 5-FU across the oil phase or through localized thin oil lamellae is the primary transport mechanism.

Lin and co-workers, 1992 prepared lipiodolized W/O emulsion or W/O/W multiple emulsion containing doxorubicin hydrochloride (Adriamycin HCl) with different emulsifiers and evaluated *in vitro* sustained-release behaviour, pharmacokinetic and tissue distribution function in Sprague Dawley (SD) rats. The results of dissolution studies indicate that the release of drug was significantly slow and protracted from both emulsions when HCO-60 (polyoxyethylene 60 hydrogenated castor oil) was used as an emulsifier. The results indicate that lipiodol and HCO-60 seemed to play an important role in the prolongation and selective retention of drug(s) in W/O emulsion or W/O/W multiple emulsion, *in vitro* and *in vivo*.

The *in vivo* release of four water-soluble drugs, cefadroxil, cephradine, antipyrine and 4-aminoantipyrine, from a stabilized W/O/W multiple emulsion was studied in rats (Miyakawa et al., 1993). The cefadroxil and cephradine concentrations in rat plasma following intravenous administration of their W/O/W multiple emulsions were considerably prolonged as compared to their respective aqueous solutions. However, antipyrine and 4-aminoantipyrine attained rapid systemic concentration following administration as W/O/W multiple emulsions and these plasma profiles compared well with those obtained following intravenous administration of the aqueous solutions of drugs.

Multiple W/O/W type emulsions were prepared and stabilized through interfacial complex films formation (Nakhare and Vyas, 1995; 1997). The interfacial film was formed as a result of interaction of macromolecules like gelatin, bovine serum albumin (BSA), polyvinyl alcohol (PVA) and polyacrylic acid (PAA) (each present in internal aqueous phase separately) with sorbitan monostearate (Span 60) present in the middle oil phase. The multiple emulsion containing macromolecules in their internal phase demonstrated better entrapment efficiency. Intramuscular injection drug in a W/O/W emulsion formulation provided a protracted drug plasma profile for diclofenac sodium. The C_{max} attained in case of W/O/W emulsion system with or without macromolecule (gelatin) in the inner aqueous phase was relatively lowered (750 ng/ml and 700 ng/ml) as compared against aqueous drug solution (950 ng/ml) but the overall availability was increased significantly (Fig. 8-22).

Hino and co-workers, 2000 in their study compared the *in vitro* release profile of W/O, O/W and W/O/W emulsion systems loaded with anticancer drug Famorubicin. Drug release profiles of the

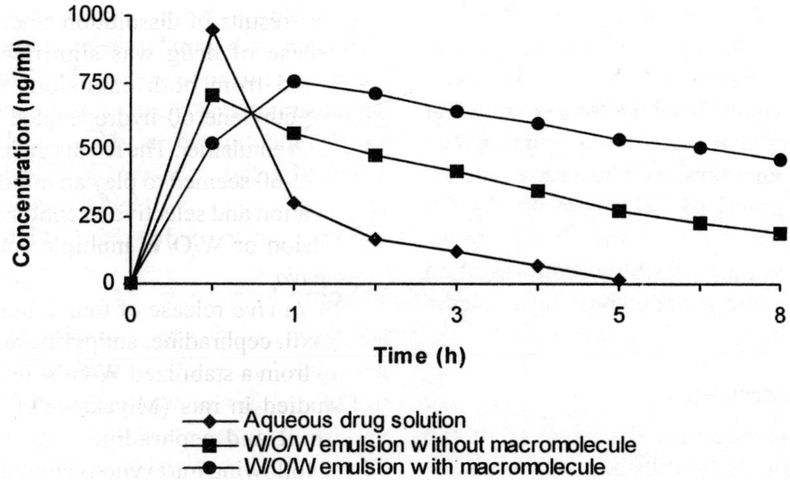

Fig. 8- 22. Plasma Concentration of Diclofenac Sodium after Intra-muscular Injection of Different Emulsion Systems

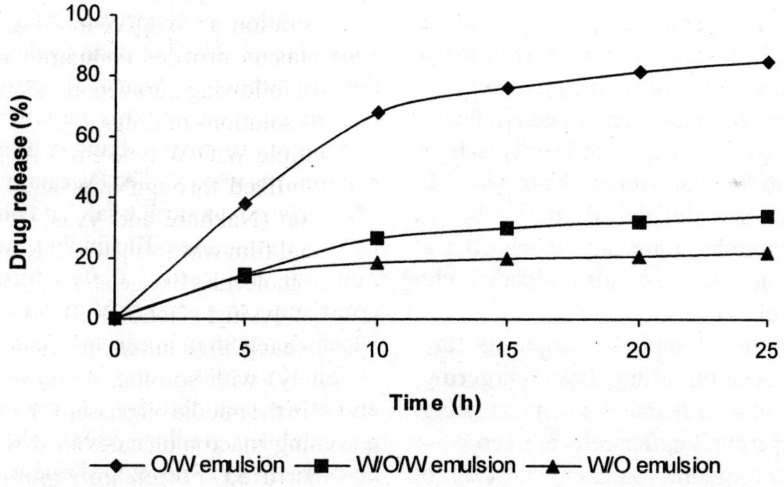

Fig. 8-23. Drug Release Profile of W/O/W, O/W and W/O Emulsion for the Anticancer Drug Famorubicin

emulsion systems are shown in Figure 8-23. The release from the W/O/W emulsion showed a sustained release pattern and was comparable to that from W/O emulsion within 7 h.

Recent research on microspheres in oil in water (S/O/W) has paved the way for the sustained and controlled delivery of bioactives. Yashioka and co-workers, 1982 prepared S/O/W systems earlier containing bleomycin and recorded improved stability with a prolonged parenteral absorption of the drug. A prolonged and sustained release albumin microspheres-in-oil-in-water emulsion (S/O/W) was prepared (Oh et al., 1998) using tegafur as a model drug. Similarly, a microsphere-in-oil emulsion was prepared by adding albumin microspheres to soybean oil containing 20% Span 80. The microsphere-in-oil emulsion was added into an aqueous solution of hydroxypropyl methylcellulose containing Pluronic

F68 to prepare an S/O/W emulsion. The t_{75} (time for 75% release of drug) of the S/O/W emulsion was recorded four-fold greater *in vitro* and the mean residence time of tegafur from the S/O/W emulsion was more than twofold *in vivo* as compared to a W/O emulsion or microsphere system. The mean residence time of 5-fluorouracil (5-FU) from an S/O/W emulsion was also greater than other dosage forms. These results suggest the possible usefulness of an S/O/W emulsion in sustained and prolonged release of drugs and bioactives.

Targeting of Bioactives

An important prerequisite for success in the application of pharmacologically active agents is site specificity. This is particularly applicable to cancer chemotherapy in which the supply of cytotoxic drugs into non-diseased tissues led to serious side effects. Multiple emulsion systems can be used as lymphotropic carriers for targeting of bioactives. The administration of lipid vehicle (O/W, W/O or W/O/W) systems intramuscularly or intraperitoneally results in emulsion droplets reaching the lymphatic system and the regional lymph nodes. This is in contrast to low molecular weight water-soluble compounds, that are delivered to the blood circulation. The targeting thus can be achieved at various levels using multiple emulsion loaded with appropriate bioactive agents :

- Organ targeting: lymphatic targeting, lung targeting, liver targeting, brain targeting, tumour and other inflammatory site targeting.
- Cellular targeting: kupffer cells of liver.
- Intracellular targeting: parenchymal cells of liver tropics.

Takahashi et al., 1973 studied the delivery of labeled 5-fluorouracil (5-FU) to regional lymph nodes following intratesticular administration. They found that the emulsion droplets reached the regional lymph nodes within 15 min and remained there for more than 7 days. Interestingly, the W/O/W system gave the highest levels within the regional lymph nodes, than other systems (aqueous solution, W/O and O/W emulsions). The same workers, 1976 used multiple emulsion system for local administration into tumours in animal and human subjects. The delivered drug (Bleomycin) was reportedly retained in tumour tissues and was slowly delivered to regional lymph node and the system was found to be virtually free of toxicity. Hashida and co-workers, 1977 and 1980 have demonstrated that ^{14}C tripalmitin labeled sesame oil and ^{131}I- iodohippuric acid (as model drug) entrapped in gelled gelatin phase of W/O emulsion could be converted into a crude Gel/O/W type emulsion which was then transported to regional lymph nodes.

Vaccine Adjuvant

Multiple emulsions have been investigated as vaccine adjuvants. Herbert, 1967 was the first to describe the use of multiple emulsion system in therapeutics as vaccine adjuvant. Standard W/O emulsion as vaccine adjuvant possess high consistency and hence difficult to inject. The re-emulsification of W/O emulsion (Herbert, 1967) to W/O/W emulsion, render them consistent enough for administration and antibody responsive than W/O system.

A multiple emulsion vaccine against *Pasteurella multocida* (P52) infection in cattle was prepared and the efficiency in terms of immunity to direct challenge, duration of this immunity for up to 1 year and the role of humoral and cell-mediated immune mechanisms were studied (Verma and Jaiswal, 1997). ME vaccine was sterile, safe and potent when tested in rabbits and calves. The findings suggested that both humoral and cell-mediated immune responses contribute to protection of animals after being vaccinated with multiple emulsion.

Similarly, Elson and co-workers, 1996 reported an oral-antigen delivery using a multiple emulsion and exhibited an enhanced oral tolerance. Tomasi and co-workers, 1997 developed a new multiple emulsion (ME) delivery system into which antigen and cholera toxins (CT) were incorporated. The purpose of the study was to evaluate whether CT would retain its mucosal adjuvanticity when sequestered within emulsion particles. ME were selectively taken up by Peyer's patches, and those containing antigen plus CT generated intestinal secretory IgA and serum IgG antibody responses in mice. Proteins incorporated in ME were protected from external acid, protease, and bile.

Lanier et al., 1999 developed high molecular weight nonionic block copolymers as vaccine adjuvants and employed these adjuvants in water-in-oil emulsion and multiple emulsion formulations with a synthetic peptide-based antigen vaccine to test their ability to prime anti-viral CD8(+) T cell responses. The results indicate that peptide vaccination using a formulation based on high molecular weight nonionic block copolymer in a simple water-in-oil or a multiple emulsion form can induce virus-specific CD8(+) T cell responses and confer enough protection to prevent the establishment of a persistent infection.

Multiple Emulsion(s) for Local Immunosuppression

A potential approach to avoid the complications of systemic immunosuppression and simultaneously enhance immunosuppressive efficacy is to deliver immunosuppressive agents locally to the site of the target organs. A water-in-oil-in-water (W/O/W) multiple emulsion has been developed for the delivery of immuno-suppressants. It has been proposed that a W/O/W emulsion of tacrolimus would possess the pharmacokinetic benefits of local immuno-suppression and evaluated the hypothesis in a rat model. The tacrolimus levels of whole blood, the liver, spleen, brain, and kidney in rats given intravenous emulsions of tacrolimus (W/O/W group) were compared with a group administered tacrolimus alone (T group). There were no significant differences between the pharmaco-kinetic parameters of W/O/W group and T group that were based on whole blood data. However, the W/O/W group had significantly decreased tacrolimus levels in the brain and kidney, and significantly increased levels in the liver and spleen compared to the T group. These data suggest that the W/O/W emulsion is applicable as an intravenous drug carrier for local immuno-suppression.

Absorption Enhancement Through Gastrointestinal Tract (GIT)

Omotosho, 1990 found increased oral absorption of griseofulvin from W/O/W emulsion in comparison to O/W emulsion and tablet dosage forms. They concluded that the administration of griseofulvin in the W/O/W emulsion may lead to the enhancement of therapeutic efficacy of the drug.

Enhanced colonic and rectal absorption of insulin reportedly occurs on administration of multiple emulsion containing eicosapentaenoic acid and docosahexaenoic acid (Suzuki et al., 1998). Histological studies revealed that the emulsion incorporating fatty acids as absorption enhancers did not induce gross morphological changes in the structure of the intestinal mucosa and facilitate the intestinal absorption of insulin without inducing any serious damage to the epithelial cells. Kajita and co-workers, 2000 evaluated the potential of Vancomycin hydrochloride (low oral bioavailability) loaded multiple emulsion incorporated with unsaturated fatty acids to improve the mucosal absorption of poorly absorbed drugs from rat intestinal loops *in situ*. The emulsion incorporating C18 unsaturated fatty acids or docosahexaenoic acid (DHA) markedly enhanced drug absorption after colonic and rectal dosing. These results indicated that W/O/W emulsions incorporating C18 unsaturated fatty acid or DHA were useful carriers for improving the absorption of poorly absorbable drugs via the intestinal tract without gross changes to tight junction function. A similar system was investigated for the increase in rectal bioavailability for insulin (Onuki et al., 2000).

Delivery of Proteins and Peptides

Multiple emulsions are unique in that a true liquid phase is maintained separate from an external aqueous phase. This may be especially important for bioactive molecules that cannot be appropriately stabilized in the solid state. In addition, the separation of aqueous phases enables highly specialized environments, conducive to protein activity (Shively, 1997). The physical instability of conventional systems remains a major factor limiting their wider application. Attempts to improve the physical stability of the aqueous dispersions through interfacial complexation and the use of microemulsions could improve the short-term stability.

To improve the stability of IgY antibody for oral administration, encapsulation of IgY in a W/O/W emulsion was attempted (Shimizu and Nakane, 1995). A stable W/O/W emulsion containing 1% IgY was prepared by using polyglyceryl condensed ricinolate (PGCR) and dextran-casein conjugate as the primary and secondary emulsifier, respectively.

However, the activity of IgY antibody, rabbit IgG, alpha-amylase, and lysozyme was reduced due to encapsulation. Molecular characterization of these proteins suggested that the rate of inactivation after encapsulation is likely to be dependent on the surface hydrophobicity and molecular stability of each protein.

Singh and co-workers, 1995 reported an insulin delivery system based on liquid surfactant membranes (W/O/W emulsion) where an organic membrane separated two aqueous phases and the internal aqueous phase contained insulin. Sesame and cottonseed oils were used as organic membranes. In order to facilitate the transportation of glucose across the organic membrane various additives such as calcium stearate, lecithin, cholesterol, hexamine, stearic acid and glyceryl tristearate were used. The additives were found to be successful carriers for the transportation of glucose to the internal aqueous phase. Similarly, viscosity enhancers, e.g. cetostearyl alcohol, in the organic phase enhanced the immobilization of insulin.

Dogru and co-workers, 2000 developed a W/O/W emulsion for oral application of Salmon calcitonin (sCT), which is a polypeptide hormone used for the treatment of osteoporosis, Paget's disease and hypercalcaemia. Oral sCT is poorly bioavailable, being susceptible to enzymatic degradation in the gastrointestinal tract. The bioavailability of sCT was recorded significantly improved in case of the multiple emulsion formulation. Incorporating sCT in the inner aqueous phase of a W/O/W emulsion appears to protect the peptide from enzymatic degradation. A protease inhibitor, aprotinin was included in the outer water phase of this system to investigate the influence of protease inhibitors on the stability of sCT. sCT was found to be yet better protected when the protease inhibitor, aprotinin, was incorporated in the outer aqueous phase.

Haemoglobin Multiple Emulsion as an Oxygen Delivery System

Multiple emulsion technology has been extended (Hb multiple emulsion) as a stable oxygen carrier system. A concentrated solution of haemoglobin (Hb) was encapsulated in the form of a Hb-in-oil-in-water (Hb/O/W) multiple emulsion (Zheng et al., 1993). Studies using mineral oil demonstrated that Hb multiple emulsions have several important characteristics that are compatible and in accordance with the blood composition that makes it a suitable blood substitute. These include: satisfactory rheological properties and good hydrodynamic stability compared to whole blood, high encapsulation concentration of Hb and high encapsulation efficiency with little met-haemoglobin generation, and satisfactory oxygen affinity and co-operative efficiency as compared to whole blood. Isovolemic exchange transfusions of Hb/O/W multiple emulsion was found to support life in rats whose hematocrit has been reduced to levels (5% or lower) and incompetent for survival at the same time without inducing any acute toxicity. The study suggests the utility of Hb/O/W as an oxygen-carrying red blood cell substitute or organ perfusion media.

Enzyme Immobilization

In recent years the main objective of the liquid surfactant membrane is to immobilize the enzyme, the latter represents for a relatively new field of biotechnology. Enzymatic conversion of water insoluble, highly lipophilic substrates, such as steroids, can be carried out in a multiple emulsion (W/O/W). The enzyme is contained in a microdroplet 'water pool', whereas the organic phase contains the substrate solution.

Hydrocarbon based liquid surfactant membranes have been used to immobilize Urease (May and Li, 1972). Immobilized enzyme retained catalytic activity and recovered by simple mechanical destruction of the liquid membrane. This technique is used in kidney diseases. Reduction and separation of nitrates and nitrites by both liquid membrane encapsulated enzyme (crude cell free extracts of *M. denitrificans*) as well as whole cell has been reported (Mohan and Li, 1974; Mohan and Li, 1975). This technique of removing nitrates and nitrites may also applied for waste water treatment.

Scheper et al. , 1984 have reported the production of L-phenyl alanine (amino acid) from the corresponding methyl ester by α-chymotrypsin immobilized in the liquid surfactant membrane. Makryalease and co-workers, 1985 also reported the reduction of L-leucine from the α-ketoisocaproate by L-leucine dehydrogenase. Iso et al., 1989 used the multiple emulsion technology for microencapsulation of lipase. The performance of the enzyme was evaluated by monitoring hydrolysis of triacetin (triglyceride of acetic acid), which is a model substrate for the enzyme.

Targeted enzyme transport is very current aspect of biotechnology. The importance of drug and enzyme targeting and numerous ways of solving the problems have been discussed in detail by Gregoriadis, 1977; Goldberg, 1983; Bruck, 1983. Furuno et al., 1987 reported microencapsulation of vitamin B_6 aqueous solution employing W/O/W emulsion technique for controlled and improved delivery.

Microencapsulation Technology using Multiple Emulsion as an Intermediate Step

Natural physiologically active compounds especially enzymes and hormones have acquired more and more importance in practical medicine. But the clinical use of these substances is still limited by number of factors such as high cost and relatively low availability of pure enzymes and hormones. The quick inactivation under physiological conditions, antigenicity, destruction of these natural physiologically active compounds under the action of endogenous proteases, natural inhibitors and difficulty of obtaining high local concentration of enzymes/hormones without increasing total administered dose, can also be cited as drawbacks for clinical applications. These problems may be resolved to a great extent by encapsulating these substances by microencapsulation using multiple emulsion technique (Iwata and McGinity, 1992; Bhatnagar et al., 1995; Pavanetto et al., 1996; Fattal et al., 1997; McGinity and O'Donnell, 1997; Leo et al., 1998; Rojas et al., 1999; Iwata et al., 1999).

Some basic techniques of microencapsulation based on multiple emulsion are described in flow charts (Fig. 8-24 and 8-25). As stated in the section of methods of stabilization of multiple emulsions that the gelation of either internal or external phase or the oily phase (membrane) results in stable emulsions. The gelation of external continuous phase is the basis of microencapsulation of bioactives by multiple emulsion technique. In case of W/O/W system

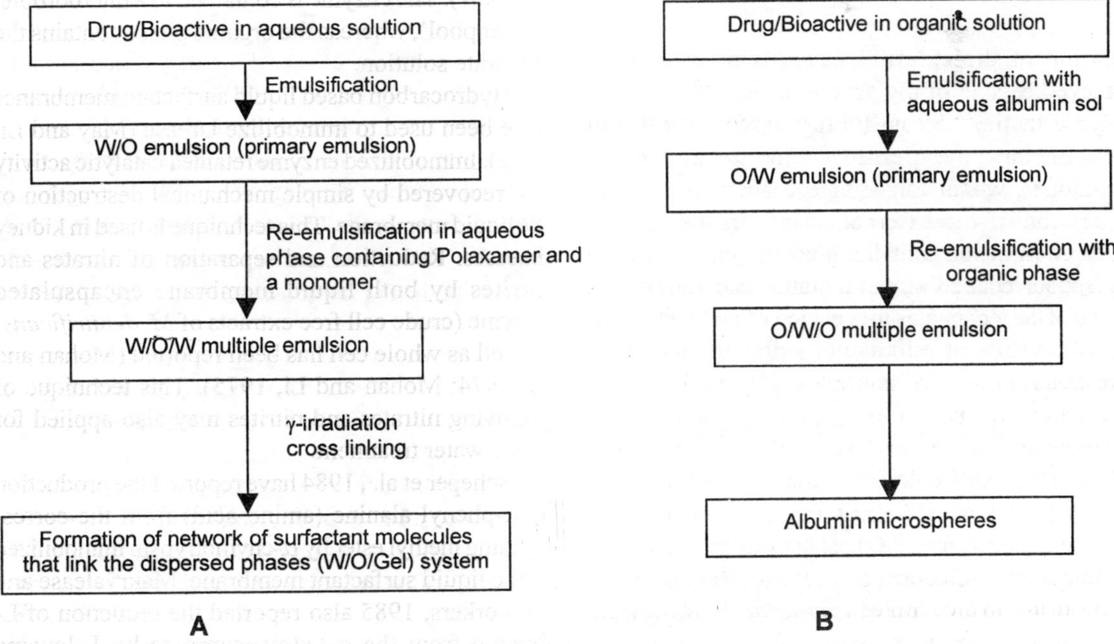

Fig. 8-24. Preparation of Microspheres using Multiple Emulsion. Gelation of External Phase in Induced either by Cross Linking (A) or by Heat Denaturation of Protein (B)

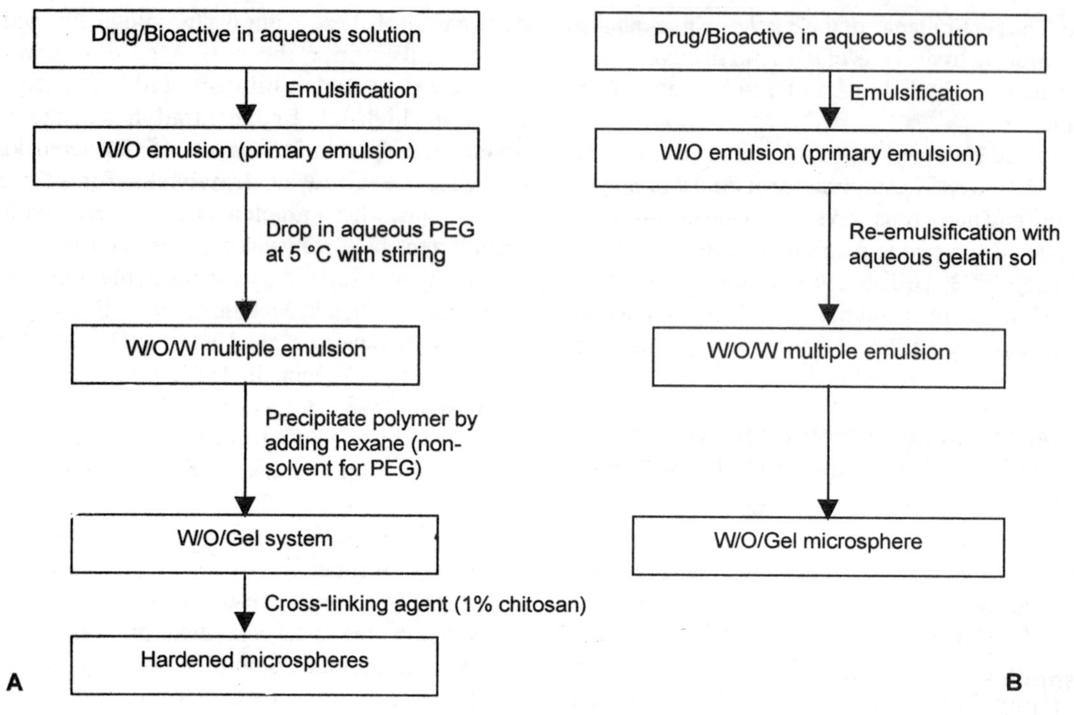

Fig. 8-25. Preparation of Microspheres using Multiple Emulsion. Gelation of external phase induced by desolvation using either non-splvent addition followed by crosslinking (A) or by salt or alcohol addition (B)

gelation of the external aqueous phase can be achieved by one of the several techniques such as polymerization, cross-linking, addition of non-solvent, salt, temperature change and other techniques, which can induce coacervation phase separation of the external phase. In the case of multiple emulsion containing volatile oil or volatile organic solvents, solvent evaporation can also be used as one of the techniques for gelation of external phase. Microcapsules of salbutamol sulphate have been prepared from W/O/W multiple emulsion containing the drug in the inner aqueous phase. The microencapsulation was executed by coacervation using gelatin and sodium chloride contained in the outer aqueous phase. Albumin microspheres were prepared (Shah et al., 1987) using a multiple emulsion technique for sulfadiazine. The drug was dissolved in the organic phase and emulsified with an aqueous phase containing the albumin. This O/W emulsion was re-emulsified with an organic phase to yield a O/W/O multiple emulsion system, where subsequent heat denaturation of the albumin yielded albumin microspheres. However, PLGA microspheres prepared using multiple emulsion and solvent evaporation/extraction method, have been the major focus of attention in recent years. Various drugs and bioactives are loaded using PLGA microspheres for example, chlorpheniramine maleate, Idoxuridine, b-lactoglobulin and somatostatin (Iwata and McGinity, 1992; Nakhre, 1996).

Recently, poly-DL-lactide-co-glycolide (PLGA) microspheres have been prepared by multiple emulsion technique as a controlled release antigen delivery system (Rojas et al., 1999). The inner aqueous phase containing the hydrophilic substances is obtained after emulsification with the immiscible organic solvent containing PLGA under stirring. This primary emulsion is stabilized with another aqueous phase containing the surfactant, poly vinyl alcohol and homogenized to get a W/O/W multiple emulsion. Subsequent solvent evaporation and extraction yielded PLGA microspheres (Fig. 8-26).

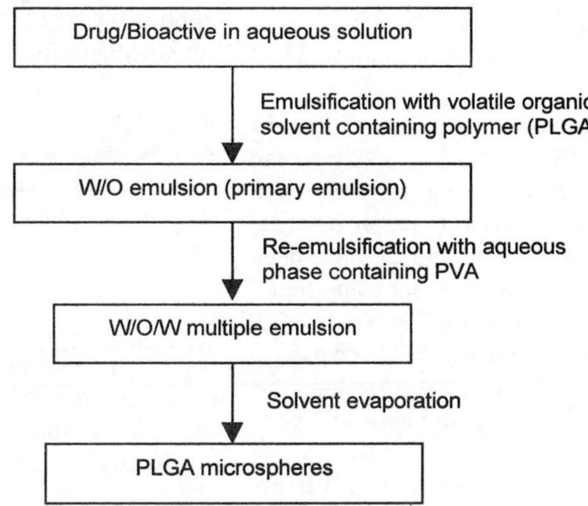

Fig. 8-26. Preparation of PLGA Microspheres using Multiple Emulsion Solvent Evaporation Technique

Cosmetics and Health Care

The basis of most cosmetics and toiletries is an emulsion of an oil-in-water, or water-in-oil, where the former is dispersed as small droplets in the other. However, more complex multiple emulsion systems are also used for moisturizing, nutritive and protective action, when applied in the form of sunscreams, hand creams, make up cleansers, shaving creams, antiperspirants and perfume preparations (Yazan et al., 1993). The use of a stable multiple phase emulsion of the $O_1/W/O_2$ type has been reported as a sun protection preparation or make-up formulation (United States Patent: 6,106,847). The O/W/O emulsion consisted of a primary oil-in-water phase consisting of a viscoplastic gel containing at least one organic UV-absorbent in the oil droplets, while the secondary oil phase (silicone oil) containing one or more inorganic UV-absorbents. The oil proportion in each phase is kept in the range from 15 to 30% by weight relative to the total weight of the emulsion. Silicone oil is preferred because it does not feel greasy, shows good spreadability on the skin and good water repellence.

W/O/W multiple emulsion prepared using non-ionic, non-ethoxylated, skin compatible emulsifiers are used for cosmetic purposes. Gallarate and co-workers, 1999 recently assessed the stability of ascorbic acid in emulsified systems for topical and cosmetic use. Chen and co-workers, 1999 reported the efficiency and protective effect of multiple emulsion (W/O/W) entrapped milk immunoglobulin G against acid (pH 2.0), alkali (pH 12.0) and proteases.

Cyclodextrin has been recently introduced to stabilize emulsions by complexation between cyclodextrins and oil at the interface of the emulsion. The cyclodextrin combines with oil plays the role of a surfactant and permits the stabilization of the emulsion . Multiple emulsions stabilized with natural cyclodextrins (i.e. without surfactants) are proposed for use in the dermo-cosmetics.

Laugel and co-workers, 2000 reported incorporation of silicones within O/W/O multiple emulsions loaded with dimethicones, as an efficient means of modulating the penetration and the distribution of drugs in the skin. The use of silicones within O/W/O multiple emulsions has been suggested to offer two principal advantages: (1) the silicones with the lowest molecular weight decrease the oily touch; (2) due to the large range of viscosity, this excipient influences the skin distribution of actives after topical application.

Miscellaneous Applications

Some of the applications of multiple emulsions are summarized as :

1. Extraction and/or separation: Liquid membrane emulsions of the W/O/W type can extract heavy metals and contaminants from the wastewater, which acts as an external phase. Metals like Cu, Ni and Zn have been extracted from wastewater plant using liquid membrane emulsion system. The system of O/W/O type on the other hand have been used to separate hydrocarbons where the aqueous phase serves as the membrane and a solvent as the external phase.
2. Treatment of drug overdose: Multiple emulsions of W/O/W types are used for the treatment of drug overdosing (Morimoto et al., 1982). A W/O/W system was designed to remove acidic drugs like barbiturates and salicylates from the gastrointestinal tract by entrapping unionized drug, permeating through the oil membrane into the inner basic phase, where it is converted to an oil insoluble anion. The extraction kinetics followed first order kinetics and the viscosity of the oil phase serve to control the influx rate.
3. Taste masking of drugs: Multiple emulsion has been employed for the taste masking of drugs like chlorpromazine HCl and chloroquine (Garti et al., 1983; Rao and Bader, 1993). By dissolving drug in the inner aqueous phase of W/O/W emulsion under conditions of good shelf stability, the formulation could be designed to release drug through the oil phase in the presence of gastric fluid.

FUTURE PERSPECTIVES

Multiple emulsions have been exploited in various diverse applications like pharmaceutics, cosmetics, food and separation techniques. Their potential pharmaceutical applications include use for red blood cell substitute; treatment of drug overdosing; immobilization of enzymes; masking the taste of drugs; enhancement of gastrointestinal absorption; and as carriers for sustained release, lymphatic uptake and transdermal drug delivery. In addition to these applications, W/O/W emulsions have been used as intermediates for the preparation of microspheres.

With the evolution of various newer techniques of preparation, stabilization and rheological characterization of these specialized emulsion systems, they can serve as potential carriers for drugs, cosmetics and pharmaceutical agents.

REFERENCES

Absolom D. R. (1986) Methods Enzymology **132**, 281.

Adeyeye C. M. and Price J. C. (1990) *Drug Dev. Ind. Pharm.* **16**, 1055.

Ali A. A. and Mulley B. A. (1978) *J. Pharm. Pharmacol.* **30**, 205.

Baker R. W. and Lonsdale H. K. (1974) In: Controlled release of biologically active agents, Tonquary A. O. and Lceoy R. E. (Eds.) Plenum Press, New York, 15.

Bhatnagar S., Nakhare S. and Vyas S. P. (1995) *J. Microencap.* **12**, 13.

Boyd J. V., Krog N. and Sherman P. (1976) The theory and practice of emulsion technology, Smith A. L. (Ed.) Academic Press, London, 123.

Brodin A. F., Kavaliunus D. R. and Frank, S. G. (1978) *Acta Pharm. Suec.* **15**, 1.

Bruck S. D. (1983) *Controlled drug delivery*, CRC press, Boca Raton, Vol. I, 187.

Chatterjee C. C. (1985) In: Human Physiology, 11th Ed., Vol. I, Medical Allied Agency, Calcutta, 174.

Chen C. C., Tu Y. Y. and Chang H. M. (1999) *J. Agric. Food Chem.* **47**, 407.

Cole M. L. and Whately T. L. (1997) *J. Control. Rel.* **49**, 51.

Collings A. J. (1971) *British Patent*, 1, 235,667.

Davis S. .S., Illum L. and Walker I. M. (1987) *Int. J. Pharm.* **38**, 133.

Dogru S. T., Calis S. and Oner F. (2000) *J. Clin. Pharm. Ther.* **25**, 435.

Elson C. O., Tomasi M., Dertzbaugh M. T., Thaggard G., Hunter R. and Weaver C. (1996) *Ann. N. Y. Acad. Sci.* **778**, 156.

Fattal E., Roques B., Puisieux F., Blanco-Prieto M. J. and Couvreur P. (1997) *Adv. Drug Deliv. Rev.* **28**, 85.

Florence A. T. and Whitehill D. (1982a) *Int. J. Pharm.*, **11**, 277.

Florence A. T. and Whitehill D. (1982b) *J. Pharm. Pharmacol.* **34**, 687.

Florence A. T. and Whitehill D. (1985) Macro- and Micro-Emulsions: Theory and Application, ACS Symposium Series, Shar D.O. (Ed.) Vol. 272, 359.

Florence A. T., Al-Saden A. A. and Whateley T. L. (1981) *Colloids and Surfaces* **2**, 49.

Florence A. T., Law T. K. and Whateley T. L. (1985) *J. Colloid Interface. Sci.* **79**, 243.

Frieberg S. and Mandell I. (1970) *J. Pharm.Sci.* **59**, 1001.

Fukushima S., Juni K. and Nakano M. (1983) *Chem. Pharm. Bull.* **31**, 4048.

Fukushima S., Nishida M., Shibuta T., Juni K., Nakano M., Uchara N., Ohkuma T., Yamishita Y. and Takahashi M. (1986) *J. Pharmacobio-Dyn.* **9**, S-18.

Furuno T., Ikeda A., Iso M., Omi S. and Yokota H. (1987) *Zairyou Gijitsu* **5**, 141.

Gallarate M., Carlotti, M. E., Trotta M. and Bovo S. (1999) *Int. J. Pharm.* **188**, 233.

Garti N., Aserin A. and Cohen Y. (1993) *J. Control. Rel.* **29**, 41.

Garti R. H., Frenkel M. and Schwartz R. (1983) *J. Disperse Sci. Technol.* **4**, 237.

Goldberg E.P. (1983) *Targeted Drugs*, John Wiley, New York, 296.

Gregoriadis G. (1977) *Nature* **265**, 407.

Hashida M., Liao M. H., Muranishi S. and Sezaki H. (1980) *Chem. Pharm. Bull.* **28**, 1659.

Hashida M., Muranishi S., Takahashi Y. and Sezaki H. (1977) *J. Pharmacokin. Biopharm.* **5**, 241.

Herbert W. J. (1967) *British Patent*, 1, 080, 994.

Higashi H., Shimizu M., Nakashima T., Iwata K., Uchiyama F., Tateno S. and Setoguchi T. (1995) *Cancer* **75**, 1245.

Higashi H., Tabata N., Kondo K. H., Maeda Y., Shimizu M. and Nakashima T. (1999) *J. Pharmacol. Exp. Ther.* **289**, 816.

Hino T., Kawashima Y. and Shimabayashi S. (2000) *Adv. Drug Deliv. Rev.* **45**, 27.

Iso M., Shirahase T., Hanamura S., Urushiyama S. and Omi S. (1989) *J. Microencaps.* **6**, 165.

Iwamoto K., Kato T., Kawahara M., Koyama N., Watanabe S., Miyake Y. and Sunamoto J. (1991) *J. Pharm. Sci.* **80**, 219.

Iwata M. and McGinity J.W. (1992) *J. Microencaps.* **9**, 201.

Iwata M., Nakamura Y. and McGinity J. W. (1999) *J. Microencaps.* **16**, 49.

Kajita M., Morishita M., Takayama K., Chiba Y., Tokiwa S. and Nagai T. (2000) *J. Pharm. Sci.* **89**, 1243.

Kang W. W. and Matsumoto S. (1988) *Int. Conf. Surface Colloid Sci.*, Kakone, Japan.

Kita Y., Matsumoto S. and Yonezawa D. (1978) *Nippon Kagaku Kaishi* **1**, 11.

Lanier J. G., Newman M. J., Lee E. M., Sette A. and Ahmed R. (1999) *Vaccine* **18**, 549.

Laugel C., Rafidison P., Potard G., Aguadisch L. and Baillet A. (2000) *J. Control. Rel.* **63**, 7.

Law T. K., Florence A. T. and Whateley T. L. (1984) *J. Pharm. Pharmacol.* **36**, 50.

Law T. K., Whateley T. L. and Florence A. T. (1986) *J. Control. Rel.* **3**, 279.

Leo E., Pecquet S., Rojas J., Couvreur P. and Fattal E. (1998) *J. Microencaps.* **15**, 421.

Li N. N. (1960) *U.S. Patent*, 3, 410.794.

Lin S. Y., Wu W. H. and Lui W. Y. (1992) *Pharmazie* **47**, 439.

Makryalease K., Scheper T., Schugent K. and Kurla M. R. (1985) *Germ. Chem. Eng.* **6**, 345.

Matsumoto S. (1983) *J. Colloid Interface*. Sci. 94, 362.

Matsumoto S. and Khoda M. (1980) *J. Colloid Interface. Sci.* **73**, 13.

Matsumoto S. and Sherman P. (1981) *J. Texture Studies* **12**, 243.

Matsumoto S., Inoue T., Khoda M. and Ikura K. (1980) *J. Colloid Interface. Sci.* **73**, 555.

Matsumoto S., Khoda M. and Murata S. (1977a) *J. Colloid Interface. Sci.* **62**, 149.

Matsumoto S., Kita Y. and Yonezawa D. (1976) *J. Colloid Interface. Sci.* **57**, 353.

Matsumoto S., Kitayama T. and Koh Y. (1985a) *J. Japan Oil Chemist's Soc.* **34**, 688.

Matsumoto S., Koh Y. and Michiura A. (1985b) *J. Disp. Sci. Tech.* **6**, 507.

Matsumoto S., Ueda Y., Kita Y. and Yonezawa D. (1977b) *Agric. Biol. Chem.* **42**, 739.

May S. W. and Li N. N. (1972) *Biochim. Biophys. Res. Commun.* **68**, 786.

McGinity J. W. and O'Donnell P. B. (1997) *Adv. Drug Deliv. Rev.* **28**, 25.

Mishra B. and Pandit J. K. (1989) *Drug Dev. Ind. Pharm.* **15**, 1217.

Miyakawa T., Zhang W., Uchida T., Kim N. S. and Goto S. (1993) *Biol. Pharm. Bull.* **16**, 268.

Moghimi S. M. and Patel H. M. (1989) *Biochim. Biophys. Acta* **984**, 379.

Mohan R. R. and Li N. N. (1974) *Biotechmol. Bioenerg.* **16**, 513.

Mohan R. R. and Li N. N. (1975) *Biotechnol. Bioeng.* **17**, 1137.

Morimoto Y., Yamaguchi Y. and Sugibayashi K. (1982) *Chem. Pharm. Bull.* **30**, 2980.

Nakhare S. (1996) Development and characterization of liquid membrane based therapeutic systems of some drugs, Ph. D. Thesis, Dr. H. S. Gour University, Sagar, India.

Nakhare S. and Vyas S. P. (1995) *J. Microencaps.* **12**, 409.

Nakhare S. and Vyas S. P. (1996) *J. Microencaps.* **13**, 281.

Nakhare S. and Vyas S. P. (1997) *Pharmazie* **52**, 224.

Nakhare S., Vyas S. P. and Jain N. K. (1994) *The Eastern Pharmacist* **8**, 65.

Oh I., Kang Y. G., Lee Y. B., Shin S. C. and Kim C. K. (1998) *Drug Dev. Ind. Pharm.* **24**, 889.

Okochi H. and Nakano M. (2000) *Adv. Drug Deliv. Rev.* **45**, 5.

Omotosho J. A. (1990) *Int. J. Pharm.* **62**, 81.

Omotosho J. A., Whateley T. L. and Florence A. T. (1989) *Biopharm. Drug Dispos.* **10**, 257.

Omotosho J. A., Whateley T. L., Law T. K. and Florence A. T. (1986) *J. Pharm. Pharmacol.* **38**, 865.

Onuki Y., Morishita M., Takayama K., Tokiwa S., Chiba Y., Isowa K. and Nagai T. (2000) *Int. J. Pharm.* **198**, 147.

Opaware F. O. and Burgess D. J. (1998) *J. Pharm. Pharmacol.* **50**, 965.

Oza K. P. and Frank S. G. (1989) *J. Dispersion Sci. Technol.* **10**, 163.

Pandit J. K., Mishra B., Krishnamurthy Y. and Mishra D. N. (1988) *Ind. J. Pharm. Sci.* **50**, 274.

Pavanetto F., Perugini P., Conti B., Modeńa T. and Genta I. (1996) *J. Microencaps.* **13**, 679.

Rao Y. M. and Bader F. (1993) *The Eastern Pharmacist*, **36**, 431.

Rojas J., Pinto-Alphandary H., Leo E., Pecquet S., Couvreur P. and Fattal E. (1999) *Int. J. Pharm.* **183**, 67.

Scheper T. (1990) *Adv. Drug Deliv. Rev.* **4**, 210.

Scheper T., Halwachs W. and Schugent K. (1984) *Chem. Eng.* **B-31**, B-37.

Shah M. V., De Gennaro M. D. and Suryakasuma H. (1987) *J. Microencaps.* **4**, 223.

Shimizu M. and Nakane Y. (1995) *Biosci. Biotechnol. Biochem.* **59**, 492.

Shinoda K. and Friberg S. (1986) Emulsion and solubilization, John Wiley and Sons, New York, 33.

Shively M. L. (1997) *Pharm. Biotechnol.* **10**, 199.

Singh S., Singh R. and Vyas S. P. (1995) *J. Microencap.* **12**, 609.

Suzuki A., Morishita M., Kajita M., Takayama K., Isowa K., Chiba Y., Tokiwa S. and Nagai T. (1998) *J. Pharm. Sci.* **87**, 1196.

Takahashi T., Mizuno M., Fujita Y., Ueda S., Nishioka B. and Majima S. (1973) *Gann.* **64**, 345.

Takahashi T., Ueda S., Kono K. and Majima S. (1976) *Cancer* **38**, 1507.

Tomasi M., Dertzbaugh M. T., Hearn T., Hunter R. L. and Elson C. O. (1997) *Eur. J. Immunol.* **27**, 2720.

Verma R. and Jaiswal T. N. (1997) *Vaccine* **15**, 1254.

Wisse E. and De Leeuw A. M. (1984) Microspheres and drug therapy: Pharmaceutical, immunological and medical aspects, Davis S. S., Illum L., Mevie J. G. and Tomlinson E. (Eds.) Elsevier, Amsterdam, 1.

Yashioka T., Ikeuchi K., Hashida M., Muranishi S. and Sezaki H. (1982) *Chem. Pharm. Bull.* **38**, 1408.

Yazan Y., Seiller M. and Puisieux F. (1993) *Boll. Chim. Farm.* **132**, 187.

Zheng S., Zheng Y., Beissinger R. L., Wasan D. T. and McCormick D. L. (1993) *Biochim. Biophys. Acta.* **1158**, 65.

Zweitach B. W. (1980) *Adv. Microcir.* **9**, 206.

CHAPTER 9

Nanoparticles

The colloidal carriers based on biodegradable and biocompatible polymeric systems have largely influenced the controlled and targeted drug delivery concepts. It was realized that the nanoparticles loaded bioactives could not only deliver drug(s) to specific organs within the body but delivery rate in addition could be controlled as being bystanders, burst, controlled, pulsatile or modulated. The possibilities and potentials further prompted the work and as a result a great deal of related information covering preparation methodologies, characterization, engineering, bio-fate and toxicology has been gathered. The understanding that relates to the biodistribution in particular has propelled and motivated the development of functionally designed nanoparticulates.

It is apparent that the polymers, the building blocks of nanoparticulate composites, belong to natural or synthetic origins. Some of them have already been exploited for their biomedical applications. Obviously, the literature is abound with concerning their safety, toxicology and biodegradation consideration.

Nanoparticles are sub-nanosized colloidal structures composed of synthetic or semi synthetic polymers. The continual quest and manoeuvering towards physical stability improvization of liposomes resulted into development of solid core nanoparticles in eighties as an alternative drug carrier. The first reported nanoparticles were based on non-biodegradable polymeric systems (polyacrylamide, polymethylmethacrylate, polystyrene etc.) (Birrenbach and Speiser, 1976; Kreuter and Speiser, 1976). The possibilities of chronic toxicity due to tissue and immunological response towards non-degradable polymeric burden, their use for systemic administration however, could not be considered. Soon the biodegradable polymers were taken up and nanoparticles based on poly(cyanoacrylate) were extensively studied (Couvreur et al., 1982; Douglas et al., 1987; Kreuter, 1991). The polymeric nanoparticles can carry drug(s) or proteinaceous substances, i.e. antigen(s). These bioactives are entrapped in the polymer matrix as particulates enmesh or solid solution or may be bound to the particle surface by physical adsorption or chemically.

The drug(s) may be added during preparation of nanoparticles or to the previously prepared nanoparticles. The term particulate is suggestively general and doesn't account for morphological and structural organization of the system. Thus they could be nanospheres, nanocapsules, nanocrystals or nanoparticulates. Nanospheres may be defined as solid core spherical particulates, which are nanometric in size. They contain drug embedded within the matrix or adsorbed on to surface; nanocapsules are vesicular system in which drug is essentially encapsulated within the central volume surrounded by an embryonic continuous polymeric sheath. In the later, drug(s) is mainly encapsulated in the solution system. The physical chemistry of these systems remains to be the same as of typical colloidal dispersions. The surface charges, dispersibility, density, hydrophobicity and hydrophilicity are some critical factors which determine the absolute stability characteristics of a system vis-a-vis its *in vivo* disposition.

Natural Hydrophilic Polymers

Among the natural macromolecules available for the manufacture of nanoparticles, proteins such as albumin, gelatin, legumin or vicilin, as well as polysaccharides like alginates or agarose have been extensively studied and characterized. These macromolecules have attracted wide interest as biomaterials due to their intrinsic biodegradability and biocompatibility. Natural hydrophilic polymers are conveniently classified as proteins and polysaccharides (Table 9-1).

The polymers of natural origin however, suffer some disadvantages including (a) batch-to-batch variation, (b) conditional biodegradability and (c) antigenicity. Parenteral administration of polymeric nanoparticles gets compromised mainly due to antigenicity. The relevant information for more systemic work to assess safety of carrier(s) based on proteins and polysaccharides are required and should be sincerely considered. Alginate based delivery systems for oral and ophthalmic administrations have been approved (Shamkhani et al., 1991). It is also reported as a homo-compatible and convincingly acceptable system for parenteral administration of bioactives. In contrast, dextran, albumin and gelatin, which are though acceptable materials for parenteral administration, manifest immunogenicity due to use of cross-linking agents, which are employed during their preparations. Chitosan on the other hand, is a homo non-compatible material and hence it should be restricted to extracorporeal uses only (Pangburn et al., 1984).

Synthetic Hydrophobic Polymers

Polymers, which are used for nanoparticle preparations are mainly those, which are conceivably employed in the preparation of microspheres. Most of them are typically hydrophobic in nature. The polymers used are either pre-polymerized or synthesized before (first group) or during the (second group) process of nanoparticle preparation (Table 9-2). The polymers from the ester class [poly (lactic acid) and poly (lactic-glycolic acid) copolymers are representative of the first group along with poly (ε–caprolactone) and already been approved for human use (Couvreur et al., 1986; Lewis, 1990; Pitt, 1990). The second group is represented by poly(alkyl-cyanoacrylates), which have received the greatest attention as polymeric nanoparticulate systems but gathered number of controversies due to the toxicity of the corresponding alkylcyanoacrylate monomer (Kattan et al., 1992). In regard to bio-degradability Couvreur and Vautier, 1991 reported that product of PACA are typically non-toxic hydrophilic oligomers, which are easily eliminated by the body through glomerular filtration.

PREPARATION TECHNIQUES OF NANOPARTICLES

The selection of the appropriate method for the preparation of nanoparticles depends on the physicochemical characteristics of the polymer and

Table 9-1. Various Proteins and Polysaccharides used for the Preparation of Nanoparticles

Proteins	Polysaccharides
Gelatin	Alginate
Albumin	Dextran
Lectins	Chitosan
Legumin	Agarose
Vicilin	Pullulan

Table 9-2. Various Synthetic Polymers used for the Preparation of Nanoparticles

Pre-polymerized	Polymerized in process
Poly (ε-caprolactone) (PECL)	Poly (isobutylcyanoacrylates) (PICA)
Poly (lactic acid) (PLA)	Poly (butylcyanoacrylates) (PBCA)
Poly (lactide-co-glycolide) (PLGA)	Polyhexylcyanoacrylate (PHCA)
Polystyrene	Poly methyl (methacrylate) (PMMA)
	Copolymer of aminoalkylmethacrylate methyl methacrylate

the drug to be loaded (Table 9-3). On the contrary, the preparation techniques largely determine the inner structure, *in vitro* release profile and the biological fate of these polymeric delivery systems (Kreuter et al., 1991). Two types of systems with different inner structures are apparently possible (Fig. 9-1) including:

- A matrix type system consisting of an entanglement of oligomer or polymer units (nanoparticles/nanospheres)
- A reservoir type of system comprised of an oily core surrounded by an embryonic polymeric shell (nanocapsules)

The drug can either be entrapped within the reservoir or the matrix or otherwise be adsorbed on the surface of these particulate systems. The polymers are strictly structured to a nanometric size range particle(s) using appropriate methodologies. These methodologies are conveniently classified as follows:

1. Amphiphilic macromolecule cross-linking
   a. Heat cross-linking
   b. Chemical cross-linking
2. Polymerization based methods
   a. Polymerization of monomers *in situ*
   b. Emulsion (micellar) polymerization
   c. Dispersion polymerization

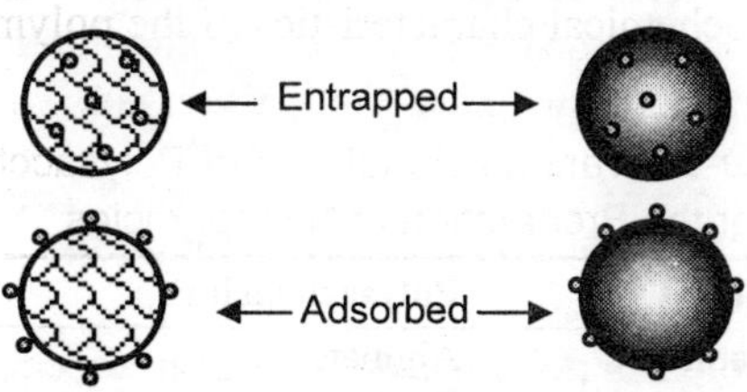

Fig. 9-1. Nanoparticles/Nanospheres and Nanocapsules With the Mode of Drug Entrapment

   d. Interfacial condensation polymerization
   e. Interfacial complexation
3. Polymer precipitation methods
   a. Solvent extraction/evaporation
   b. Solvent displacement (nanoprecipitation)
   c. Salting out

Nanoparticle(s) Preparation by Cross-Linking of Amphiphilic Macromolecules

Nanoparticles can be prepared from amphiphilic macromolecules, proteins and polysaccharides (which have affinity for aqueous and lipid solvents). The technique of their preparation involves firstly, the aggregation of amphiphile(s) followed by further stabilization either by heat denaturation (Gupta et al., 1987a,b) or chemical cross-linking (Widder et al., 1979). These processes may occur in a biphasic O/W or W/O type dispersed systems, which subdivide the amphiphile(s) prior to aggregative stabilization. It may also take place in an aqueous amphiphilic solution where on removal, extraction, or diffusion of solvent, amphiphile(s) are aggregated as tiny particulates and subsequently rigidized via chemical cross-linking. The cross-linking generally executed following dispersed phase solvent extraction, or depletion.

Cross-linking in W/O Emulsion

The cross-linking method is exhaustively used for the nano-encapsulation of drugs. The method involves the emulsification of bovine serum albumin (BSA)/ human serum albumin (HSA) or protein aqueous solution in oil using high-pressure homogenization (Kramer, 1974) or high frequency sonication (Sugibasayashi et al., 1979). The water in oil emulsion so formed is then poured into preheated oil (temperature above 100 °C). The suspension in preheated oil maintained above 100°C is held stirred

Table 9-3. Polymers used for the Preparation of Nanoparticles and Nanocapsules

Polymer use	Technique	Candidate drug
Hydrophilic		
Albumin, gelatin	Heat denaturation and cross-linking in W/O emulsion	Hydrophilic
	Desolvation and cross-linking in aqueous medium	Hydrophilic and protein affinity
Alginate, chitosan	Cross-linking in aqueous medium	Hydrophilic and protein affinity
Dextran	Polymer precipitation in an organic solvent	Hydrophilic
Hydrophobic		
Poly(alkylcyanoacrylates)	Emulsion polymerization	Hydrophilic
	Interfacial O/W polymerization	Hydrophobic
Polyesters		
Poly(lactic acid), Poly(lactide-co-glycolide), poly(ε-caprolactone)	Solvent extraction-evaporation	Hydrophilic & hydrophobic
	Solvent displacement	Soluble in polar solvent
	Salting out	Soluble in polar solvent

for a specified time in order to denature and aggregate the protein contents of aqueous pool completely and to evaporate the water (Fig. 9-2). Proteinaceous sub-nanoscopic particles are thus formed where the size of the internal phase globules mainly determines the ultimate size of particulates.

The particles are finally washed with an organic solvent to remove any adherent or adsorbed oil traces and subsequently collected by centrifugation. The crucial factors which govern the size and shape of the nanoparticles are mainly emulsification energy and temperature (used for denaturation and aggregation).

The high temperature used in the original method (Kramer, 1974) restricts the application of method to temperature-sensitive drugs. As an alternative to heat stabilization, a chemical cross-linking agent, usually glutaraldehyde, is incorporated into the system at a 3% v/v level (Nakagawa et al., 1987). Though the heat borne drawbacks are obviated, yet a need to remove residual cross-linking agent makes the method cumbersome. Further, the aggregation in process during emulsification, following emulsification or cross-linking results into variable size of nanoparticles. Gallo and associates, 1984 critically analyzed the variables, which affect the poly-dispersity of nanoparticles.

In an interesting modification, albumin containing water droplets are stabilized using cross-linking agent (Roger and Kissel, 1993). The droplets or aqueous phase is firstly emulsified in ethylcellulose solution in chloroform by homogenization followed by the addition of glutaraldehyde. The emulsion system so obtained is then stirred for several hours. The resultant nanospheres are then washed with toluene, isopropyl alcohol with water and finally freeze-dried.

Emulsion Chemical Dehydration

Chemical dehydration has been reported for producing BSA nanoparticles with a narrow size distribution. Bhargava and Aindo, 1992 suggested a simplified chemical cross-linking method. Hydroxypropyl cellulose solution in chloroform was used as a continuous phase of emulsion while a chemical dehydrating agent, i.e., 2,2, di-methyl propane, was used to translate internal aqueous phase into a solid particulate suspension. The method reportedly avoid coalescence of droplets and could produce nanoparticles of smaller size (~300 nm), probably due to sonication time required for comminution and to keep internal phase well dispersed is reduced considerably.

Phase Separation in Aqueous Medium (Desolvation)

The protein or polysaccharide from an aqueous phase can be desolvated by pH change, or change in temperature or by adding some appropriate counter ions. Cross-linking may be affected simultaneously

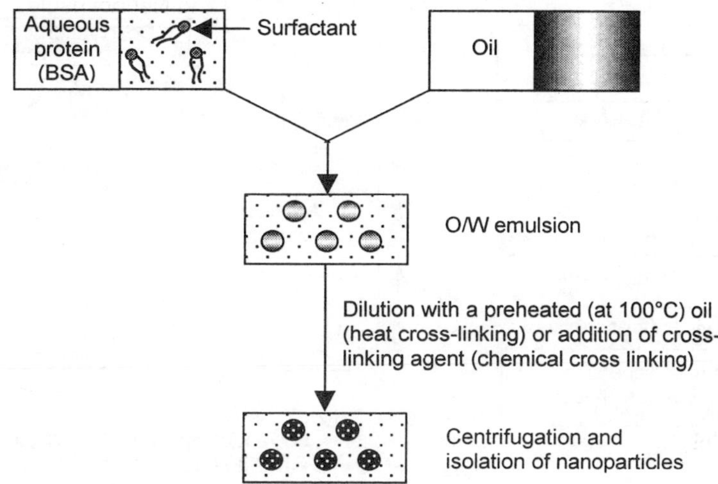

Fig. 9-2. Schematic of Macromolecular Cross-linking in a Water in Oil (W/O) Emulsion

or subsequent to the desolvation step (Marty et al., 1978; Oppenheim et al., 1982; Krause and Rohdewald, 1985; Oppenheim, 1986).

The method essentially proceeds involving three steps, i.e., protein dissolution, protein aggregation and protein deaggregation. In other words, using appropriate levels of desolvation and resolvation the aggregate size could be maintained and finally these aggregated nanoparticulates are cross-linked using glutaraldehyde.

Solvent competing agent, sodium sulphate, is mainly used as a desolvating agent while alcohol, i.e., ethanol and isopropanol are carefully added as desolvating or deaggregating agent. The addition can be optimized turbidometrically using a Nephelometer. Only desolvation may give the final product as nanospheres. Desolvation deaggregates the protein and turns the suspension colloidal and hence milky in appearance (Fig. 9-3). Both, lipophilic (Krause and Rohdewald, 1985) and hydrophilic (Oppenheim et al., 1982; Oppenheim, 1986) drugs could be entrapped in nanoparticles using this technique. Coester and co-workers, 2000 recently reported a new two step desolvation method for manufacturing gelatin nanoparticles. After the first desolvation step, the low molecular gelatin fractions present in the supernatant were removed by decanting. The high molecular weight fractions present in the sediment were redissolved and then desolvated again at pH 2.5 in the second step. Centrifugation and redispersion methods were used to purify particles so obtained.

pH Induced Aggregation

The protein phase may also be separated through pH change. The pH-induced aggregation to prepare nanoparticles has been extensively used for the preparation of nanoparticles by many workers.

Oppenheim and co-workers, 1982 successfully prepared insulin nanospheres. Insulin was firstly precipitated and then redissolved forming nanodroplets, which were hardened using glutaraldehyde. The method yielded nanoparticles of insulin itself.

Samaligy and Rohdewold, 1983 similarly prepared gelatin nanospheres. Gelatin and Tween 20 were dissolved in aqueous phase and the pH of the solution was adjusted to the optimum value. The clear solutions so obtained were heated to 40 °C followed by its quenching at 4 °C for 24 h and subsequently left at ambient temperature for 48 h. The sequential temperature treatment resulted into a colloidal dispersion of aggregated gelatin. The aggregates were finally cross-linked using glutaraldehyde as a cross-linking agent. The nanospheres thus resulted were of 200 nm average size with uniform dispersity. The optimal pH range for ideal and uniform preparation of gelatin nanospheres was 5.5-6.5. Interestingly, pH

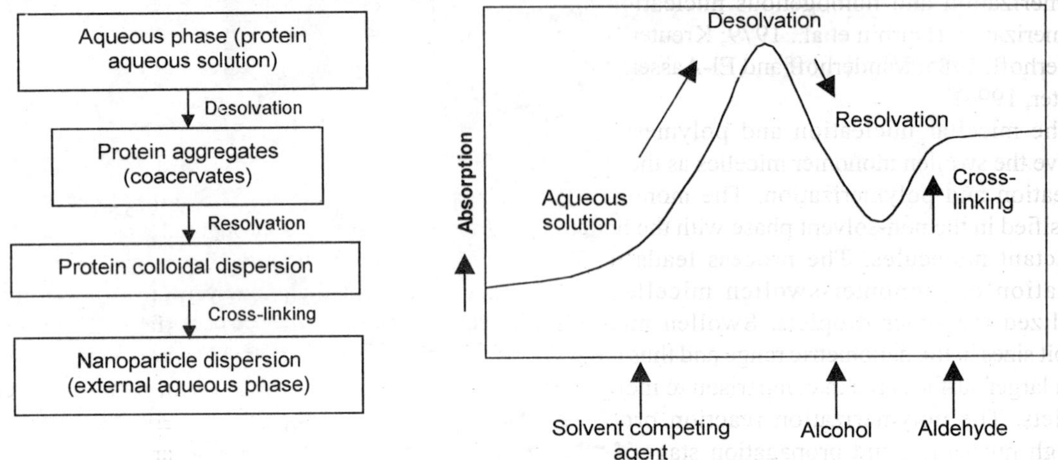

Fig. 9-3. Various Steps of Solvation and Desolvation that Leads to the Formation of Nanoparticles

value below 5.5 produced no aggregation while above 6.5 an uncontrollable aggregation led to the formation of larger nanospheres.

Counter Ion Induced Aggregation

Separation of protein phase may also occur by the presence of counter ions in the aqueous medium. The aggregation of dispersed phase (polysaccharide) can effectively be initiated by adding some appropriate counter ions. The aggregation can be propagated by adding secondary species of counter ions followed by a rigidization step. Alginate nanoparticles have recently been prepared using counter-ion induced gelation technique, where gelation was induced by Ca^{++} and continued by addition of poly (l-lysine) (Rajaonaryvony et al., 1993). Thus these nanospheres are classically based on polyelectrolyte complex. Similarly, chitosan nanospheres can be prepared by adding tripolyphosphate (highly negatively charged ions) to the medium. The size was found to be critically dependent on the concentration of both, i.e., chitosan and tri-polyphosphate ions. The residual charge on nanospheres yet remains positive suggesting negatively charged drug carrying potential of chitosan nanospheres.

Nanoparticle Preparation Using Polymerization Based Methods

The early reports on preparation of polymeric nanoparticles mainly discuss *in situ* emulsion polymerization technique. The polymers used for nanosphere preparation include poly(methylmeth acrylate), poly (acrylamide), poly (butyl cyanoacrylate), N-N'methylene-bis-acrylamide etc. (Kreuter, 1991). Two different approaches are generally adopted for the preparation of nanospheres using *in situ* polymerization technique

- Methods in which the monomer to be polymerized is emulsified in a non-solvent phase (emulsion polymerization), or
- Methods in which the monomer is dissolved in a solvent that is non-solvent for the resulting polymer (dispersion polymerization).

In emulsion polymerization method, the monomer is dissolved in an internal phase while in the case of dispersion polymerization, it is taken in the dispersed phase. It is interesting that in either of the cases, following polymerization, the polymer tends to be insoluble in internal phase or dispersed phase thus results into an ordered suspension of nanospheres.

Emulsion Polymerization

The process of emulsion polymerization can be conventional or inverse, depending upon the nature of the continuous phase in the emulsion. In the former case, the continuous phase is aqueous (O/W emulsion), whereas in the latter case it is organic (W/O emulsion). Two different mechanisms were proposed for the emulsion polymerization process and they include: micellar nucleation and polymerization and homogenous nucleation and polymerization (Durbin et al., 1979; Kreuter, 1983; Vanderhoff, 1985; Vanderhoff and El-Aasser, 1988; Kreuter, 1994).

The micellar nucleation and polymerization involve the swollen monomer micelles as the site of nucleation and polymerization. The monomer is emulsified in the non-solvent phase with the help of surfactant molecules. The process leads to the formation of monomer-swollen micelles and stabilized monomer droplets. Swollen micelles exhibit sizes in the nanometric range and thus have a much larger surface area in comparison to monomer droplets. The polymerization reaction proceeds through nucleation and propagation stage in the presence of a chemical or physical initiator. The energy provided by the initiator creates free reactive monomers in the continuous phase, which then collide with surrounding unreactive monomers and initiate the polymerization chain reaction (Fig. 9-4). Being slightly soluble in the surrounding phase, the monomer molecules reach the micelles by diffusion from the monomer droplets through the continuous phase, thus allowing the polymerization to progress within the micelles. Therefore, in this case, monomer droplets essentially act as monomer reservoirs. A second mechanism, homogenous nucleation and polymerization has been proposed, which largely applies in cases where the monomer is sufficiently soluble in the continuous outer phase (Kreuter, 1991; Kreuter, 1994). The nucleation and polymerization stages can directly occur in this phase, leading to the formation of primary chains called oligomers. In this situation, both the micelles and droplets play the role of monomer reservoirs throughout the polymer chain length. When the oligomers have reached a certain length, they precipitate and form primary particles, which are stabilized by the surfactant molecules provided by the micelles and the droplets. Depending on the bulk conditions and system stability, the end-product nanospheres are formed either by additional monomer input into the primary particles or by fusion of the primary particles (Fig. 9-5).

Poly(alkylcyanoacrylate) (PACA), a biodegradable polymer has created a great deal of interest in nanoparticulate carriers (Kreuter and Speiser, 1976; Kreuter, 1983; Chiannilkulchai et al., 1989; Couvreur and Vautier, 1991; Allemann et al., 1993a; De Verdiere et al., 1997; Soma et al., 2000a). They are essentially prepared by emulsion polymerization. Water insoluble monomer is emulsified in an external acid aqueous phase that contains a stabilizer. Monomer polymerized rapidly following anion polymerization mechanism. The polymerization rate

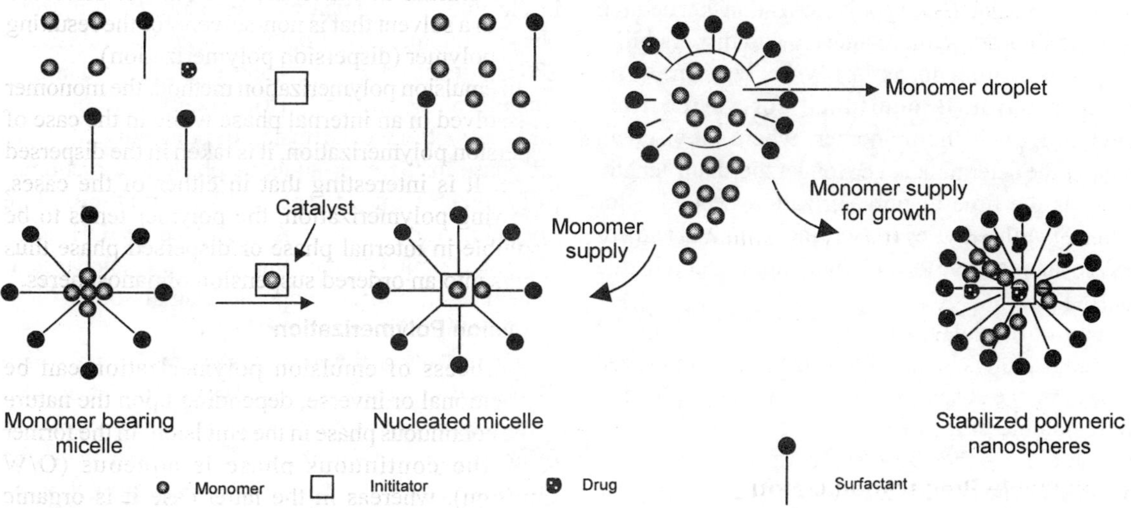

Fig. 9-4. Emulsion Polymerization (Micellar Polymerization Mechanism) for Nanoparticle Preparation
*Adopted from De Jaeghere et al., 1999

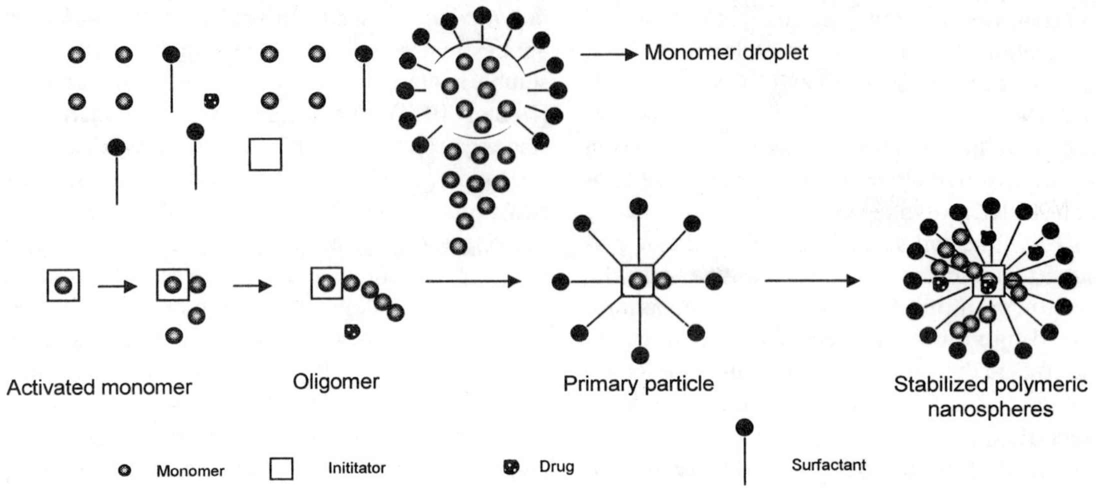

Monomer droplet
Activated monomer
Oligomer
Primary particle
Stabilized polymeric nanospheres
Monomer
Inititator
Drug
Surfactant

Fig. 9-5. Emulsion Polymerization (Homogenous Polymerization Mechanism) for Nanoparticle Preparation
*Adopted from De Jaeghere et al., 1999

is dependent on the pH of the medium. Anionic polymerization takes place in micelles after diffusion of monomer molecules through the water phase and is initiated by negatively charged compound. Thus at neutral pH the rate of polymerization being extremely fast leads to the formation of aggregates. However, at acidic pH, i.e., pH 2-4, the reaction rate remains well controlled and slow, thus producing uniform sized nanospheres of relatively high molecular weight. During polymerization the medium is stirred in order to maintain size and dispersibility of phase undergoing polymerization. The polymerization is continued for varied time depending upon the monomer, where alkyl chain length is the determinant, i.e., longer the chain length, longer is the time of polymerization needed . For instance, with ethyl cyanoacrylate it is 2 h and for hexyl cyanoacrylate the polymerization is conducted for 10-12 h.

The colloidal suspension on completion of polymerization is finally neutralized and lyophilized in the presence of some cryoprotectants, i.e., glucose. Water-soluble drugs may be associated with PACA nanoparticles either by dissolving the drug in the aqueous polymerization medium or by incubating the blank nanospheres with an aqueous solution of drug. In the former, the drug molecules are entrapped within the polymer matrix and are also adsorbed onto the surface of the nanoparticles. In the latter, the drug molecules are physically adsorbed only on the surface (Fig. 9-6).

AlKhouri-Fallouh and co-workers, 1985 discussed the polymer based nanocapsule preparation and incorporation/loading of lipophilic drug. The monomer and drug are dissolved in a mixture of polar (methanol/acetone) solvents, and oil (benzyl benzoate, coconut oil) using a lipophilic surfactant, i.e., lecithin. The oil phase is then added to an aqueous phase containing a hydrophilic surfactant. Polaxamer 188 is often used. After oil phase is dispersed into an aqueous phase, critically two processes occur at the oil-water interface. Diffusion of polar solvents from oil phase to the bulk aqueous phase and monomer polymerization at the C/W interface. The polymerization process is catalyzed by OH^- ions. Thus on completion of polymerization a nanocapsular system results where lipophilic drug dissolved in oil is incorporated in a polymeric sac.

Conversely, a dispersion system, W/O type, where dispersed aqueous phase contains the drug and stabilizer, while organic phase is typically consisted of an organic solvent (chloroform/n-hexane) and a monomer, can be used to prepare nanocapsules based upon inverse emulsification polymerization mechanism (Vauthier-Holzscherer, 1991; Gasco et al., 1991). The interfacial OH^- ions initiated

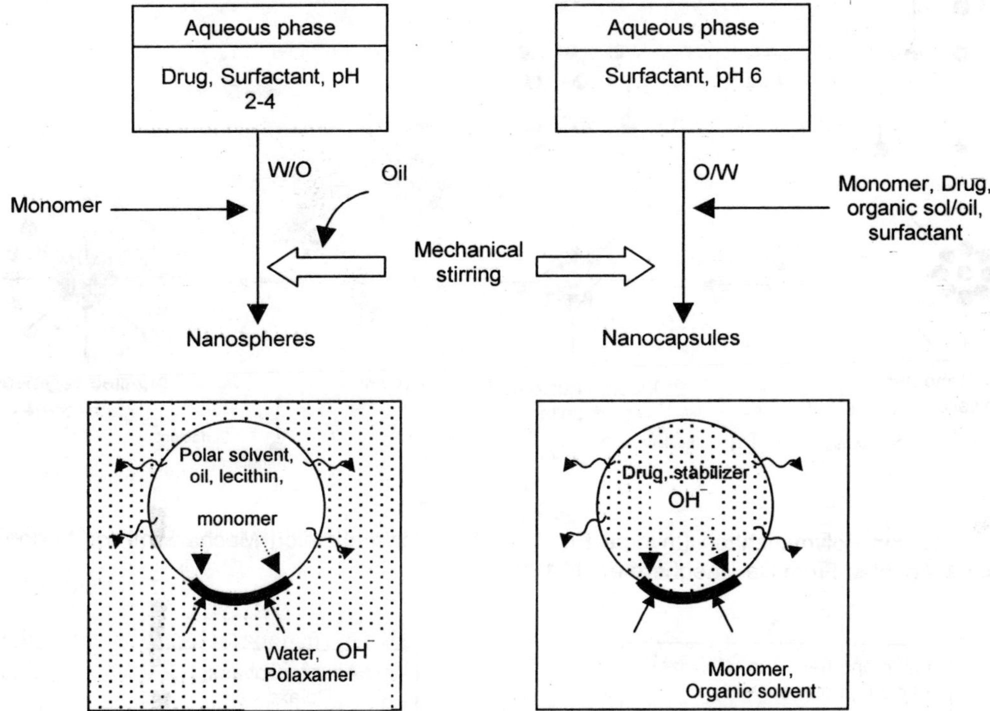

Fig. 9-6. Preparation of PACA Nanoparticles using Emulsion Polymerization Process with the Proposed Mechanisms

polymerization occurs at W/O interface enveloping aqueous phase with its drug contents in the form of nanocapsules (Fig. 9-7).

The inverse polymerization process was rapidly adopted for the preparation of biodegradable poly(alkyl cyanoacrylate) or PACA nanospheres (Gasco and Trotta, 1986; Carpignano et al., 1991) (Fig. 9-8). In these studies, the drug was dissolved in a small amount of water or hydrophilic solvent (methanol) and emulsified in an organic phase (i.e., isooctane, cyclohexane-chloroform, hexane) in the presence of large amounts of surfactants. Alkylcyanoacrylate monomers were then added directly or dissolved in an organic solvent to the preformed w/o emulsion under stirring. Hydrophilic compounds such as doxorubicin (Gasco et al., 1991), fluorescein (El-Samaligy et al., 1986) and methylene blue (Gasco and Trotta, 1986) as well as lipophilic compounds such as triamcinolone acetonide (Krause et al., 1986) were sufficiently incorporated into PACA nanoparticles prepared using this technique.

Dispersion Polymerization

The term emulsion polymerization is used when the monomer is emulsified in an immiscible (non-solvent) phase by means of surfactants. In case of dispersion polymerization however, the monomer instead of being emulsified, is dissolved in an aqueous medium which acts, as a precipitant for subsequently formed polymer. Polymerization based methods essentially involve *in situ* controlled polymerization of appropriate monomer(s) where drug may be added to monomeric phase or may be added to the formed polymeric nanoparticulates dispersion for adsorptive loading. The monomer is introduced into the dispersion medium (phase) of an emulsion or an inversed emulsion into non-solvent based polymeric solution. The polymerization is initiated by adding a catalyst and proceeds with nucleation phase followed by a growth phase (propagation). On the other hand, in the case of dispersion polymerization, the nucleation is directly induced in the aqueous monomer solution and the presence of stabilizer or

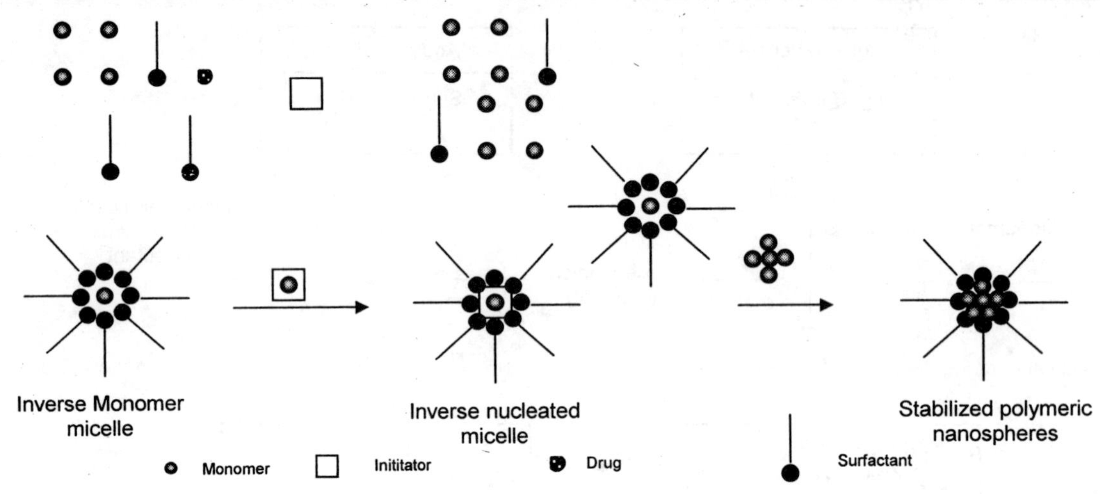

Fig. 9-7. Emulsion Polymerization (Inverse Emulsification Polymerization Mechanism) for Nanoparticle Preparation (*Adopted From De Jaeghere et al., 1999)

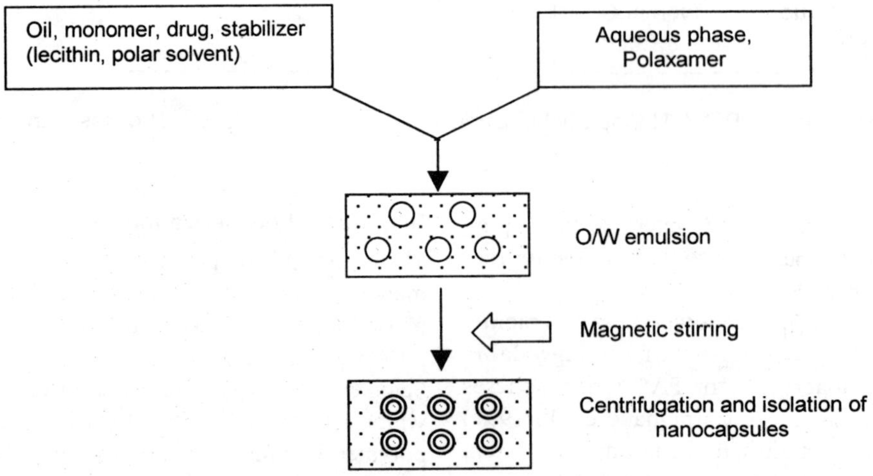

Fig. 9-8. Preparation of PACA Nanocapsules using Emulsion Polymerization Process

surfactants is not absolutely necessary for the formation of stable nanospheres (Fig. 9-9).

The method is used to prepare biodegradable polyacrylamide and polymethyl-methacrylate (PMMA) nanoparticles (Kreuter and Speiser, 1976). The acrylamide or methyl methacrylate monomer is dissolved in aqueous phase and polymerized by γ–irradiation (Kreuter and Speiser, 1976) or by chemical initiation (ammonium or potassium peroxodisulphate) combined with heating to temperature above 65 °C (Kreuter et al., 1986; Kreuter et al., 1988). The polymerization is initiated by γ–irradiation from a ^{60}Co source at elevated temperature. The redox catalyst may be used as a chemical initiator, i.e. potassium peroxodisulphate. The oligomers formed subsequently aggregate and above a certain molecular weight precipitate in the form of primary particles and propagate as

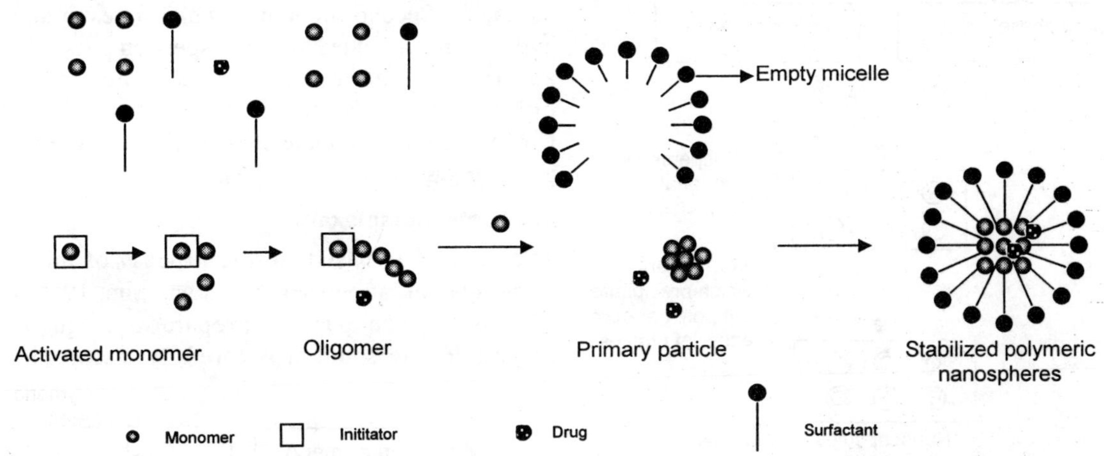

Fig. 9-9. Dispersion Polymerization Mechanism for Nanoparticle Preparation (*Adopted from De Jaeghere et al., 1999)

nanosphere which may or may not be stabilized by surfactant molecules. The monomer concentration has linear effect on the size of nanospheres where size increases with increasing monomer concentration, decreasing initiator concentration and decreasing temperature.

Being very slowly biodegradable and biocompatible, PMMA nanoparticles have been considered as optimal polymeric systems for vaccination purpose. For this application, initiation by γ–irradiation is useful for the production of PMMA nanoparticles by polymerization in the presence of antigenic material, because it operates at temperatures suitable for preservation of heat-sensitive antigenic materials, as their structure and nature remain unaffected. The antigenic materials entrapped in PMMA nanoparticles using this technique include influenza virion (Kreuter and Speiser, 1976), influenza sub unit antigen (Kreuter et al., 1988), bovine seum albumin (Kreuter et al., 1986), HIV-1 and HIV-2 antigens (Stieneker et al., 1991; Kreuter et al., 1991).

Besides PMMA nanoparticles, copolymeric methacrylic acid-based nanoparticles are also prepared by dispersion polymerization process using blends of methyl methacrylate with one or several other acrylic acid derivatives (e.g., hydroxyethyl methacrylate, methacrylic acid, ethylene glycol dimethyl acrylate, sulphopropylmethacrylate) (Bertling et al., 1989; Lukowski et al., 1992; Langer et al., 1996). These copolymer nanoparticles were developed with the intention of modifying the surface properties of the nanoparticles, namely the hydrophilicity and charge, which are important parameters governing the *in vivo* distribution of the particles.

Interfacial Polymerization

In this method, the preformed polymer phase is finally transformed to an embryonic sheath. A polymer that eventually becomes core of nanoparticle and drug molecules to be loaded are dissolved in a volatile solvent. The solution is then poured into a non-solvent for both polymer and core phase. The polymer phase is separated as a coacervate phase at O/W interface.

The resultant mixture instantaneously turns milky owing to the formation of nanocapsules (Fig. 9-10). Interfacial polymeric condensation of 2,2-bis-(4 hydroxyphenyl) propane and sebacoyl chloride is explained in Figure 9-11. The solvent is subsequently removed under vacuum. The size of nanocapsules ranges from 30-300 nm and the drug loading efficiency critically depends on drug solubility in core phase. Surfactant in small quantities can be added to stabilize the dispersion. Interfacial polymerization for the encapsulation of proteins, enzymes, antibodies

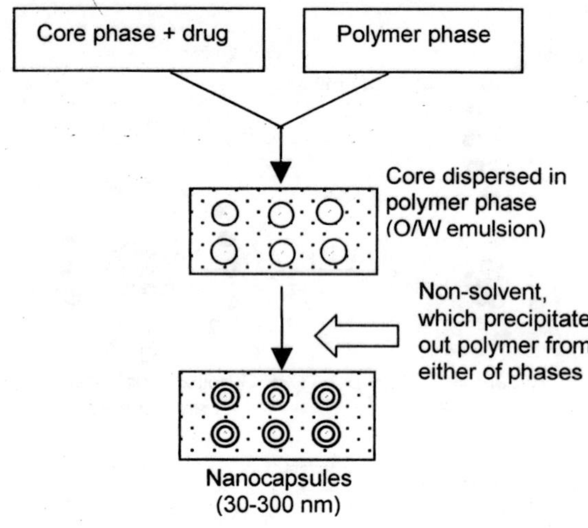

Fig. 9-10. Preparation of Nanocapsules using Interfacial Polymer Condensation

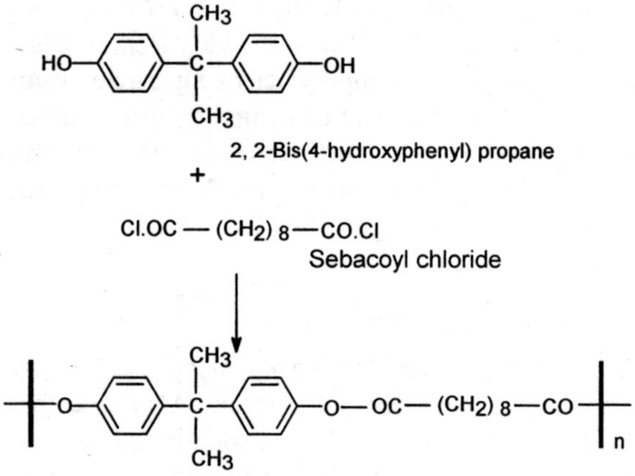

CH_3
HO–C_6H_4–C–C_6H_4–OH
CH_3
2, 2-Bis(4-hydroxyphenyl) propane
+
Cl.OC — $(CH_2)_8$ — CO.Cl
Sebacoyl chloride

$[–O–C_6H_4–C(CH_3)_2–C_6H_4–O—OC—(CH_2)_8—CO–]_n$

Fig. 9-11. Interfacial Polymerization

and cells was employed and extensively used. Such nanocapsules effectively retain protein macromolecules such as enzymes at the same time enzyme substrates and reactive products are allowed to permeate. The nanocapsules prepared by interfacial reaction of two monomers are non-immunogenic in nature. A large assortment of monomer combinations has been studied. These monomers react condensing at W/O interface. The method involves the formation of W/O microemulsion in which aqueous phase contains enzymes/protein and water soluble monomer. Second monomer, which is essentially hydrophobic, is added to bulk dispersion phase. The addition of monomer initiate condensation polymerization at the interface (Fig. 9-12). Combination of monomers could yield a variety of polymer systems (Figure 9-13).

Interfacial Complexation

The method is based on the process of microencapsulation introduced by Lin and Sun, 1969. In the case of nanoparticle preparation, aqueous polyelectrolyte solution is carefully dissolved in reverse micelles in an apolar bulk phase with the help of an appropriate surface-active agent. Subsequently, competing polyelectrolyte is added to the bulk, which allows a layer of insoluble polyelectrolyte complex to coacervate at the interface (Fig. 9-14).

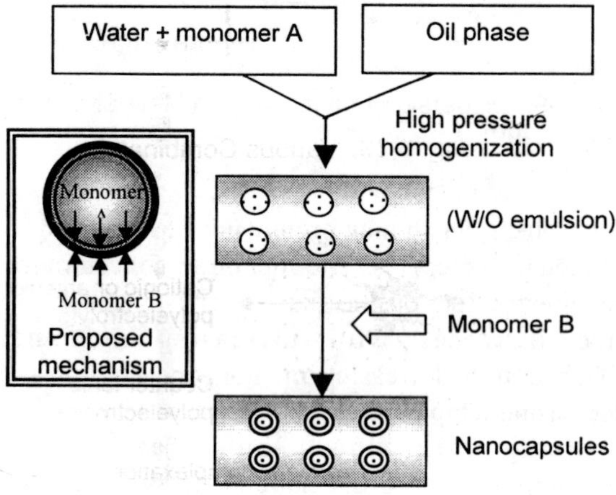

Fig. 9-12. Preparation of Nanocapsules using Interfacial Polymerization

Nanoparticle Preparation using Polymer Precipitation Methods

In these methods, the hydrophobic polymer (except dextran, mainly polyesters) and/or a hydrophobic drug is dissolved in a particular organic solvent followed by its dispersion in a continuous aqueous phase, in which the polymer is insoluble. The external phase also contains the stabilizer. Depending upon solvent miscibility techniques they are designated as solvent extraction/evaporation method (Fig. 9-15).

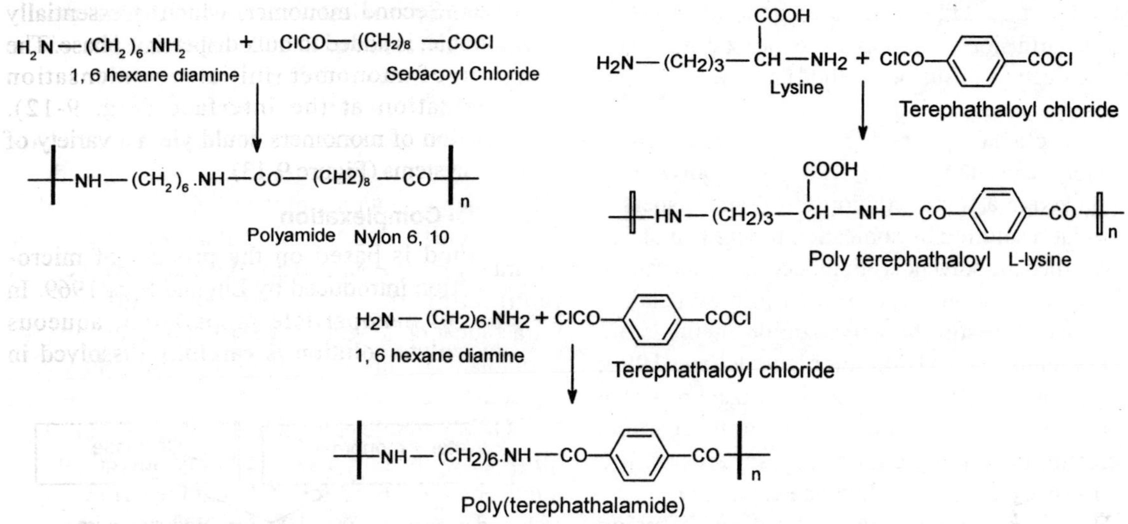

$H_2N-(CH_2)_6.NH_2$ + $ClCO-(CH_2)_8-COCl$

1, 6 hexane diamine   Sebacoyl Chloride

↓

$-[NH-(CH_2)_6.NH-CO-(CH2)_8-CO]_n-$

Polyamide Nylon 6, 10

$H_2N-(CH_2)_3-CH(COOH)-NH_2$ + $ClCO-C_6H_4-COCl$

Lysine   Terephathaloyl chloride

↓

$-[HN-(CH_2)_3-CH(COOH)-NH-CO-C_6H_4-CO]_n-$

Poly terephathaloyl L-lysine

$H_2N-(CH_2)_6.NH_2$ + $ClCO-C_6H_4-COCl$

1, 6 hexane diamine   Terephathaloyl chloride

↓

$-[NH-(CH_2)_6.NH-CO-C_6H_4-CO]_n-$

Poly(terephathalamide)

Fig. 9-13. Various Combination of Monomers with Resulatnat Polymer Systems

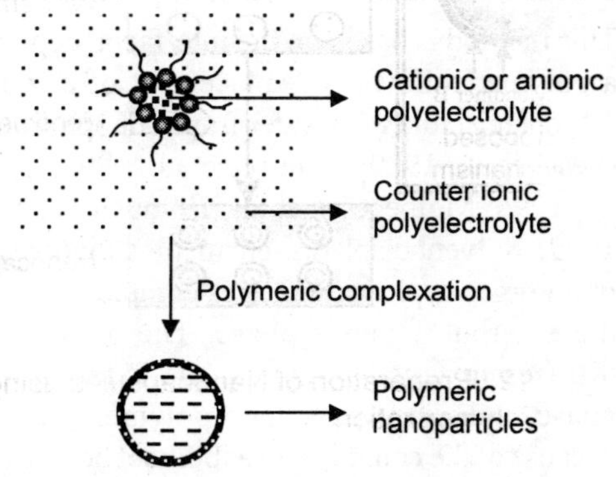

Fig. 9-14. Schematic Presentation of an Interfacial Complexation Process Between Two Competing Poly-electrolytes

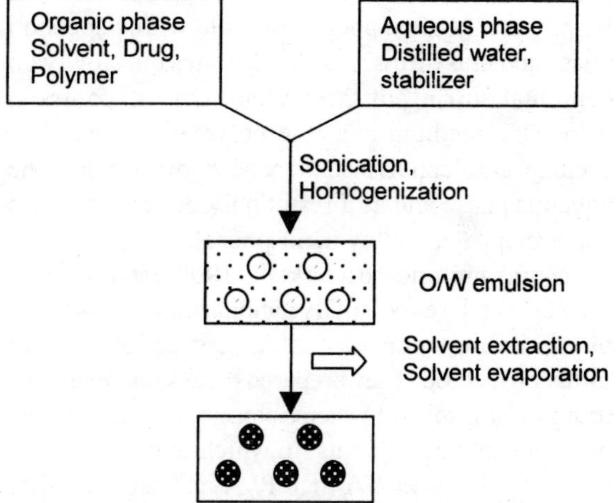

Fig. 9-15. Nanoparticle Preparation using Emulsion Solvent Evaporation Method

The polymer precipitation occurs as a consequence of the solvent extraction or evaporation, which can be brought about by:

- Increasing the solubility of the organic solvent in the external medium by adding an alcohol (i.e., isopropanol)
- By incorporating additional amount of water into the ultraemulsion (to extract or diffuse the solvent)
- By evaporation of the organic solvent at room temperature or at accelerated temperatures or by using vacuum
- Using an organic solvent that is completely soluble in the continuous aqueous phase (i.e., acetone)-nanoprecipitation

Solvent Extraction Method

This method involves the formation of a conventional O/W emulsion between a partially water miscible solvent containing the polymer and the drug, and an aqueous phase containing the stabilizer. The subsequent removal of solvent (solvent evaporation method) or the additions of water to the system so as to affect diffusion of the solvent to the external phase (emulsification diffusion method) are two variance of the solvent extraction method.

In a classic procedure to prepare PLGA nanospheres (Gumy et al., 1981), the polymer is solubilized in a solvent (chloroform) and dispersed in a gelatin solution by sonication to yield emulsion (O/W), then the solvent is eliminated by evaporation. For the evaporation purpose, apart from sonication, high speed/pressure homogenization methods are widely employed (Bodmeier and Chen, 1990; Lamprecht et al., 1999). The homogenizer breaks the initial coarse emulsion in nanodroplets (nanofluidization), yielding nanospheres with a narrow-size distribution (Julienne et al., 1992).

However, recently emulsification-diffusion method has been used on a regular basis for the solvent extraction purpose (Quintanar-Guerrero et al., 1996; 1997; 1998a. 1998b; 1999). The solvent used for polymer is often poorly miscible with dispersion phase and thus diffuses and evaporates out slowly on continual stirring of the system. On the contrary, dispersion medium miscible polymer solvent (i.e., acetone and alcohol) instantaneously diffuses into the aqueous phase and as a result polymer consolidates and precipitates as tiny nanospheres.

Murakami and co-workers, 1999 established a novel procedure for PLGA nanoparticle preparation by modifying spontaneous emulsification solvent diffusion method. They prepared PLGA nanoparticles using various solvent systems consisting of two water-miscible organic solvents, in which one solvent has more affinity to PLGA than PVA and the other has more affinity to PVA as compared to PLGA. The method has provided a good yield of nanoparticles over a wide range of composition ratios of the binary mixtures of organic solvents.

Double Emulsion Solvent Evaporation Method

Recently, emulsion solvent evaporation technique has been further modified and a double emulsion (or multiple emulsion) of water in oil in water type has been used. Following evaporation of the organic solvent(s) nanoparticles are formed which are then recovered by ultracentrifugation, washed repetitively with buffer and lyophilized (Labhasetwar et al., 1995, 1997; Song et al., 1995, 1997; Lamprecht et al., 2000) PLGA nanoparticles were prepared loaded with bovine serum albumin using double emulsion solvent evaporation method (Song et al., 1997). Owing to the high solubility of the protein in water, the double emulsion technique has been chosen as one of the appropriate methods. Figure 9-16 provides a schematic presentation of the process.

Typically, BSA and PLGA are dissolved separately in aqueous and organic phases respectively (containing the stabilizer) and subjected to ultrasonication to yield a water in oil emulsion (W_1/O emulsion). This W_1/O is further added to a PVA aqueous solution to yield the water-in-oil-in-water (W_1/O/W_2) double emulsion. The organic solvent is allowed to evaporate while being stirred first at atmosphere pressure for 16 h and then gradually at reduced pressure (from 100 mm Hg to 30 mm Hg) to yield nanoparticles (Fig. 9-16).

Solvent Displacement or Nanoprecipitation

This method is based on the interfacial deposition of a polymer following displacement of a semi-polar solvent miscible with water from a lipophilic solution (Fessi et al., 1989; Guterres et al., 1995; Chacon et al., 1996; Molpeceres et al., 1996; Govender et al., 1999). Solvent displacement method involves the use of an organic phase, which is completely soluble in the external aqueous phase. The organic solvent diffuses instantaneously to the external aqueous phase, inducing immediate polymer precipitation because of the complete miscibility of both the phases. Consequently, neither separation nor extraction of the solvent is required for the polymer precipitation. After nanoparticle preparation, the solvent is eliminated and the free-flowing nanoparticles can be obtained under reduced pressure. This method is particularly useful for drugs that are slightly soluble in water. If the drug is highly hydrophilic, it diffuses out into the external aqueous phase, whereas if the drug is highly hydrophobic, it may precipitate in the aqueous phase as nanocrystals, which further grow during storage. In the case of hydrophilic polymer, an aqueous solution of polymer is dispersed or emulsified in oil phase. The precipitation of polymer proceeds on addition of acetone. Using this technique ovalbumin loaded dextran nanospheres of ~1 μm size were prepared (Schroder and Stahl, 1984). The nanospheres were fairly stable and uniform in size.

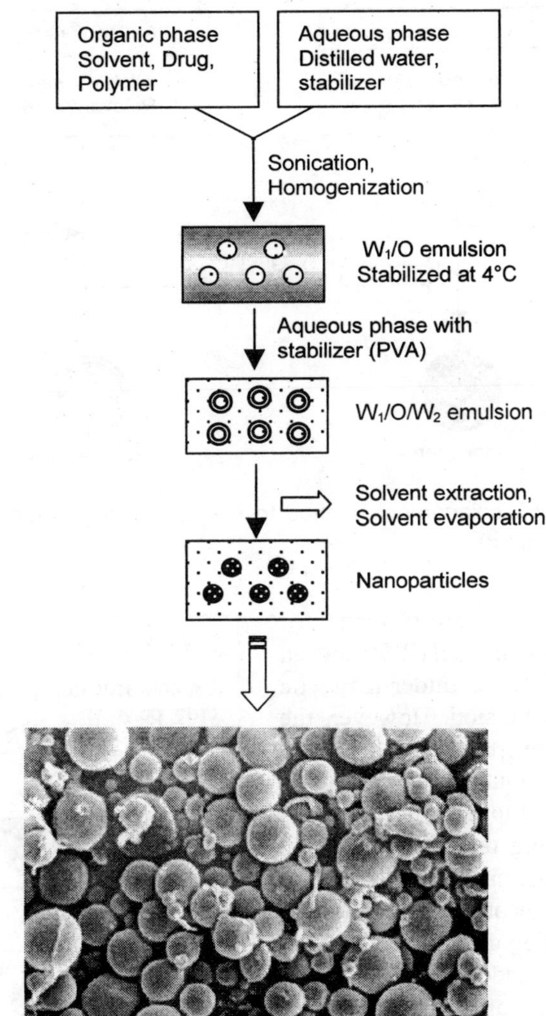

Fig. 9-16. Preparation of Nanoparticles using Double Emulsion Solvent Evaporation Method

However, the loading efficiency of lipophilic drugs, such as indomethacin (Fessi et al., 1989), metipranol (Losa et al., 1993), betaxolol (Maincent et al., 1992) in nanoparticles of PLA, PLGA and PECL has been increased using a modified solvent displacement method. In this method (Fessi et al., 1987) the drug is dissolved in a small volume of an appropriate oil and then diluted in the polar organic solvent (acetone/ethanol/methanol). When the organic solution is dispersed in the aqueous phase, the polymer precipitates around the nanodroplets, forming a reservoir system. Figure 9-17 compares the conventional (nanoparticles) and modified (nanocapsules) solvent displacement methods.

Salting Out

Salting out process is one of the most commonly adopted method used to prepare nanoparticles (Bindschaedler et al., 1990; Ibrahim et al., 1992; Allemann et al., 1992).

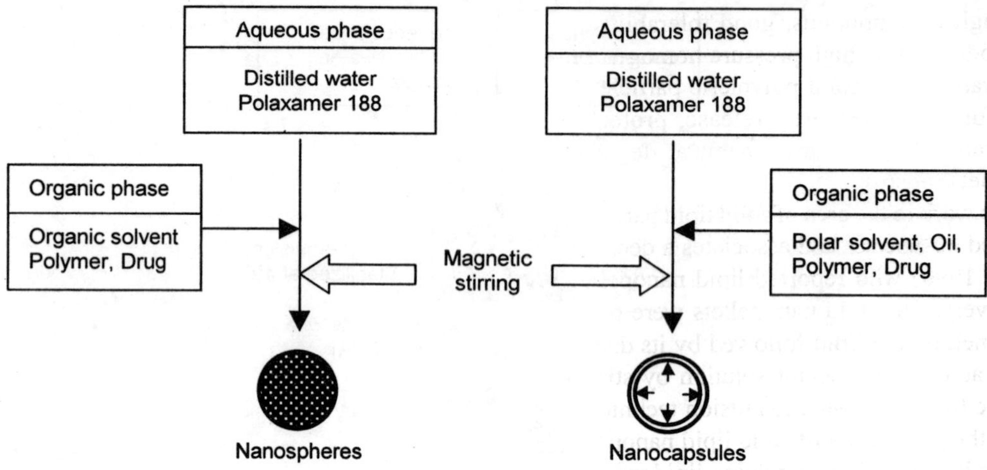

Fig. 9- 17. Use of Solvent Displacement Method to Prepare Nanoparticles (Conventional Method) and Nanocapsules (Modified Method)

The method involves the incorporation of a saturated aqueous solution of polyvinyl alcohol (PVA) into an acetone solution of the polymer under magnetic stirring to form an O/W emulsion. However, the process differs from nanoprecipitation technique as in the latter the polymeric solution (in acetone) is completely miscible with the external aqueous medium. But in the salting out technique, the miscibility of both the phases is prevented by the saturation of the external aqueous phase with PVA. The precipitation of the polymer occurs when a sufficient amount of water is added to external phase to allow complete diffusion of the acetone from internal phase into the aqueous phase. This technique is suitable for drugs and polymers that are soluble in polar solvents, such as acetone or ethanol (Fig. 9-18).

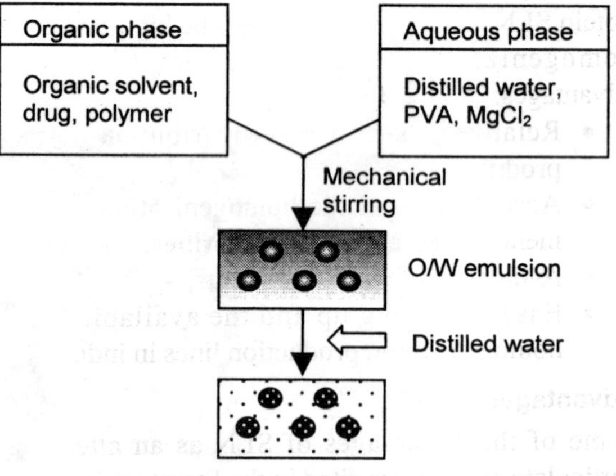

Fig. 9-18. Nanoparticle Preparation using Salting out of Polymer

NOVEL NANOPARTICULATE SYSTEMS

Solid Lipid Nanoparticles

Nanoparticles made from solid lipids are attracting major attention as novel colloidal drug carrier for intravenous applications as they have been proposed as an alternative particulate carrier system (Muller and Lucks, 1991; Muller et al., 1993; Muller and Lucks, 1996; Almeida et al., 1997; zur Muhlen et al., 1998). The solid lipid nanoparticles (SLNs) are sub-micron colloidal carriers (50-1000 nm) which are composed of physiological lipid, dispersed in water or in an aqueous surfactant solution. SLNs as colloidal drug carrier combines the advantages of polymeric nanoparticles, fat emulsions and liposomes simultaneously and avoiding some of their disadvantages.

In order to overcome the disadvantages associated with the liquid state of the oil droplets, the liquid lipid was replaced by a solid lipid, which eventually transformed into solid lipid nanoparticles (Muller et al., 1993, Muller and Lucks, 1996). The SLNs combine advantages of emulsions (composition of physiological compounds, good tolerability, large scale production by high pressure homogenization) with advantages of solid polymeric particles (solid matrix for controlled drug release, protection of incorporated drugs against chemical degradation, slower metabolism).

Basic work in the area of solid lipid particles was conducted by Speiser and associates a decade back (Speiser, 1990) who reported lipid nanopellets for oral delivery. The lipid nanopellets were produced by first melting the lipid followed by its dispersion in a hot aqueous surfactant solution by stirring or ultrasonic treatment. Microemulsion technique was used for the production of solid lipid nanoparticles. The hot microemulsion containing lipid was poured in to water leading to precipitation of nanoparticles (Gasco, 1993). Another diverse homogenization method at higher pressure for either melted or solid lipids (Muller et al., 1993) has been suggested to obtain SLN (Muller et al., 1995). The high-pressure homogenization technique offers following advantages:

- Relatively narrow size distribution of the product,
- Acceptability of the homogenization equipment by the regulatory authorities,
- Avoidance of organic solvents,
- Ease of scaling up and the availability of homogenization production lines in industry.

Advantages of SLN

Some of the advantages of SLN as an alternate particulate carriers are cited in the literature (Muller et al., 1993; Muller et al., 1995; zur Muhlen et al., 1998). Some of them are mentioned below:

- Small size and relatively narrow size distribution which provide biological opportunities for site-specific drug delivery by SLNs.
- Controlled release of active drug over a long period can be achieved.
- Protection of incorporated drug against chemical degradation.
- Possible sterilization by autoclaving or gamma irradiation.
- SLNs can be lyophilized as well as spray dried.
- No toxic metabolites are produced.
- Avoidance of organic solvents.
- Relatively cheaper and stable.
- Ease of industrial scale production by hot dispersion technique.
- Incorporation of drug can reduce distinct side effects of drug, e.g. Thrombophlebitis that is associated with i.v. injection of diazepam or etomidate.
- Surface modification can easily be accomplished and hence can be used for site - specific drug delivery system.

SLN versus other Colloidal Drug Carriers

SLN have been proven to be a better alternative carrier system than conventional O/W emulsion if a prolonged release or a protection of drug against chemical degradation is required (zur Muhlen et al., 1998). Incorporation of drug into the solid lipid matrix might surely offer a better protection than can be achieved in the oily internal phase of emulsion and liposomes. Prolonged release from emulsions does not appear to be feasible which can be achieved to a certain extent from SLN.

As compared to polymeric nanoparticles, the SLNs possess some distinctive advantages. Apart from the lower cytotoxicity, due to the absence of solvents in the production process, and a relatively low cost for the excipients the major advantage is that its large-scale production is possible by the simple process of high-pressure homogenization. Such equipment already exists in pharmaceutical industry for the production of emulsions for parenteral-nutrition and emulsions as drug carriers. While compared to liposomes the SLNs possess the advantage of offering better protection to drug against chemical degradation there is no or little access of water to the inner core of lipid particles. Depending on the nature of drug, a higher payload might be achieved. In addition, the SLNs provide more possibilities for drug release profile amelioration.

Preparation Methods of SLN

There are two well-established methods reported in literature for the production of SLN (Muller et al., 1995): homogenization of melted lipids at elevated temperature termed as hot homogenization technique and homogenization of a suspension of solid lipid at room temperature or below referred to as cold homogenization technique.

Hot Homogenization Technique

The hot homogenization technique (Fig. 9-19) can be applied to lipophilic and insoluble drugs. Even many heat sensitive drugs can be safely processed because the exposure time to high temperatures is relatively short. The technique however, does not suit for incorporation of hydrophilic drugs into SLN because of higher partition of drug in water during homogenization that results in low entrapment efficiency.

Cold Homogenization Technique

For hydrophilic drugs, the cold homogenization technique is the method of first choice. In case of too low a solubility of the hydrophilic drug in the melted lipid, surfactants can be used for solubilization of the drug (Fig. 9-20). This homogenization technique avoids and minimizes melting process of lipid and hence it is suitable for thermosensitive and thermolabile drugs. (Muller et al., 1995).

Synthetic Nanoparticles using Microemulsions as Nano-size Reactors

The techniques of microemulsions have been developed for producing nanoscale materials (Lopez-Quintela and Rivas, 1993; Lopez-Quintela et al., 1997). The microemulsion technique is based on the use of microemulsions as microreactors in order to control the growth of nanoparticles obtained. A microemulsion is defined as a thermodynamically stable dispersed system consisting of three components: two immiscible phases and a surfactant.

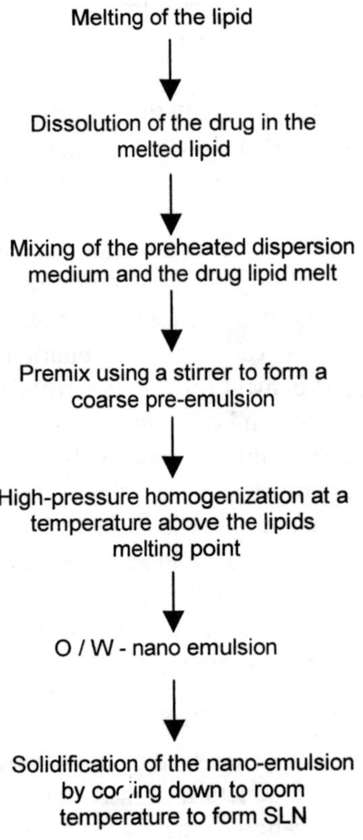

Fig. 9-19. SLN Preparation using Hot Homogenization Technique

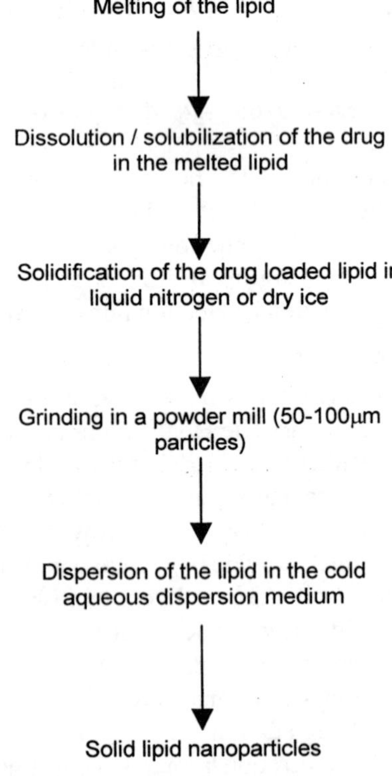

Fig. 9-20. SLN Preparation using Cold Homogenization Technique

The preparation of nano- structured systems is essentially based on mixing of two microemulsions, which contain reactants for producing desired nanoparticles. Figure 9-21 describes the process of nanoparticles formation that proceeds following mixing, interchange of reactant(s), nucleation and growth. On mixing a uniform distribution of reactant species, nanoemulsion droplets are formed. The mixing proceeds at a significantly high rate (k = 106-107 $M^{-1} S^{-1}$) and thus exchange of reactants completes within seconds. The excessively fast exchange appears to proceed through an energetic collision between two droplets in such a way that a water channel between them is generated. Following mixing a continuous exchange of contents occurs. The exchange process depends on the attractive interaction between surfactant tails and rigidity of the interface. In cases where reaction rate is extremely rapid, the rate of droplet collision determines the overall rate of reaction. Obviously, a rigid interface, by interfering with collision event, may delay the contents exchange and reaction. On the other hand, fluid interface fails in maintaining discrete dispersion of droplets and too rapid a reaction may lead to product precipitation. Conceptually, reactants A and B dissolved in two identical W/O microemulsions upon mixing, exchange the contents A and B and react forming AB complex. This precipitates within droplet environment and is stabilized by an emulgent and thus precipitate remains confined to the interior of droplets. The latter controls the process of nano-structuring and stable dispersion formation (Pillai and Shah, 1997).

In situ synthesis of a variety of nanoparticles using micro-emulsion as nanosized reactors is reported. These include *in situ* synthesis of nanoparticles of silver halides for their use in photographic emulsions (Hou and Shah, 1988; Chew et al., 1990), barium ferrite for their magnetic characteristics (Sakai et al., 1992), superconductors (Bednorz and Muller, 1986) and monodisperse particles of nickel, iron, cobalt, which have applications in heterogeneous catalysis (Nagy, 1989).

The process is (Fig. 9-21) typically represented by colloid silver halide formation, in which emulsion I contains 0.4 M aqueous solution of $AgNO_3$ as an internal phase and n-hexane as dispersion or external phase where aerosol OT (AOT) 0.15 M is used as an

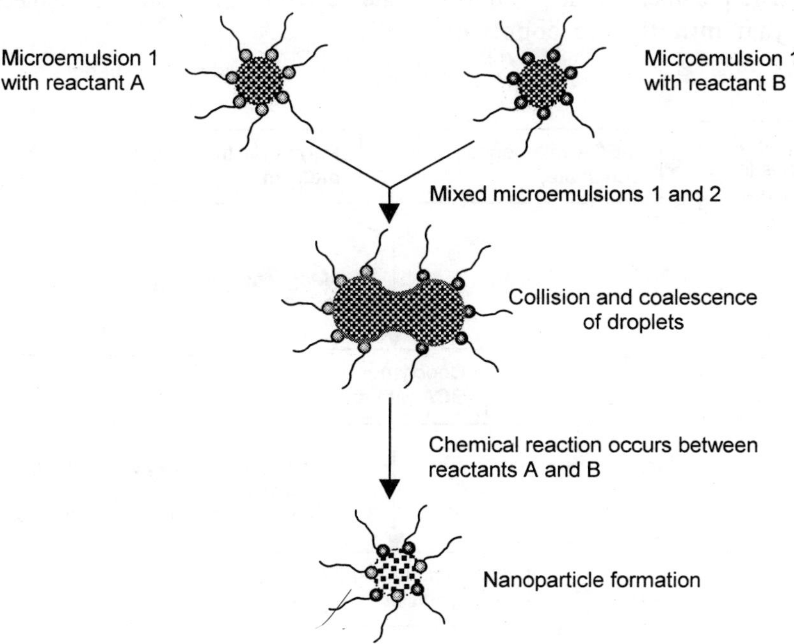

Fig. 9-21. Formation of Synthetic Nanoparticles in Microemulsion Nanoreactors

emulgent. Second emulsion contains 0.4 M NaCl in aqueous phase and other compositions remain absolutely identical. The two emulsions are then mixed under constant stirring. This leads to precipitation of AgCl as nanoscale particles. Due to reaction between the reactants following drop(s) collision, coalescence is recorded. The nanoparticles so obtained are uniform in size and spherical in shape.

Copolymerized Peptide Nanoparticles (CPP)

A novel copolymeric nanoparticulate drug delivery system, copolymerized peptide particles (CPP) has been developed as a carrier for the oral uptake of therapeutic peptides (Hillery et al., 1996). It is a drug-polymer conjugate, which forms its own nanoparticulate delivery system, in which drug moiety is covalently bound, rather physically entrapped, within the system.

By forming a copolymer delivery system using n-butylcyanoacrylate (n-BCA) as one of the monomers, the particle forming properties of the alkyl-2-cyanoacrylates could be exploited. Figure 9-22 explains the method of preparation of CPP. Various monomers can be copolymerized during the *in situ* synthesis. The polymerization reaction is manipulated so that initially the copolymer precipitated out of the reaction. After decantation of the aqueous phase, the precipitated co-polymer is dried, dissolved in DMF and subsequently recovered as nanoparticles, by the addition of "particle forming" polymerization medium. Particles of size range ~100 nm can be prepared using the technique. Thus, the process involves the copolymerization of a peptide derivative with other monomers, formulated so that the copolymer forms its own particulate delivery system.

Hydrogel Nanoparticles

Hydrogel nanoparticles are formed in water by self-assemblage and self-aggregation of natural polymer amphiphiles such as hydrophobized polysaccharides, like cholesteroyl pullulan, cholesteroyl mannan and cholesteroyl dextran (Akiyoshi and Sunamoto, 1992; Ohki et al., 1994; Akiyoshi et al., 1995, Nishikawa et al., 1996). Cholesterol bearing polysaccharides (CHP) self-aggregate to form a mono-disperse and stable hydrogel nanoparticles, in which the domains of the associated cholesterol groups of cholesteroyl polysaccharides provide cross-linking points in a non-covalent manner (Fig. 9-23). The size and density of hydrogel nanoparticles can be controlled by changing the degree of substitution of cholesterol groups of CHP.

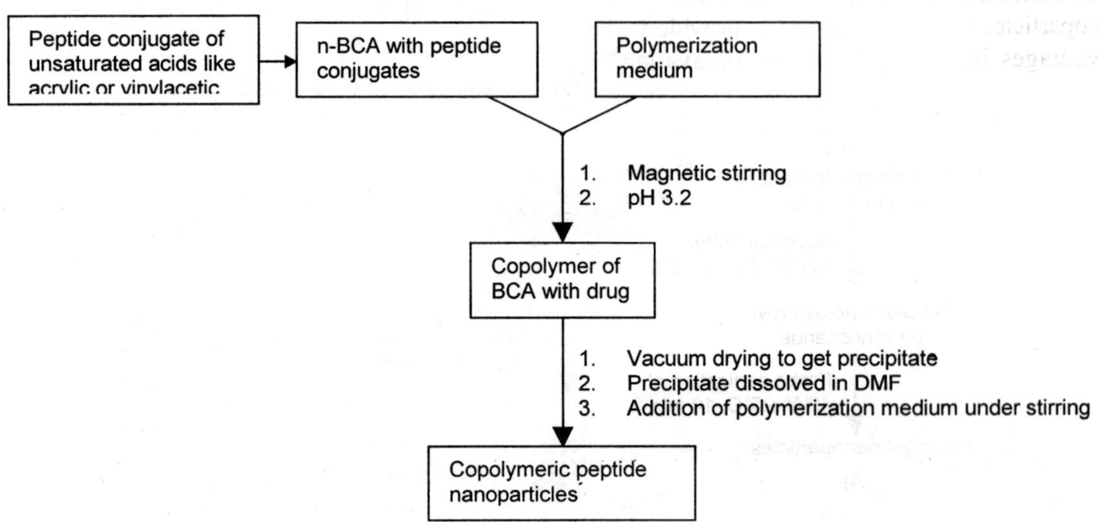

Fig. 9-22. Preparation Steps of Copolymeric Peptide Nanoparticles

Nanocrystals and Nanosuspension

Recent investigations in drug delivery research have directed towards overcoming drug solubility problems of poorly soluble drugs. Typical problems encountered with poorly soluble drugs are low bioavailability and erratic absorption (oral administration) and problems of preparing parenteral dosage forms.

Nanocrystals (NanoSystems, Elan) and nanosuspensions are two recently introduced aspects to the drug delivery research. The basic theme is to convert micronized drug powders (i.e., drug microparticles) to drug nanoparticles. To produce Nanocrystals, the drug powder is dispersed in a surfactant solution and the obtained suspension undergoes a pearl milling process for hours up to several days. To produce Nanosuspension (SkyePharm PLC; Drug Delivery Service, GmbH, Germany) the drug powder is dispersed in an aqueous surfactant solution by high speed stirring. The obtained macro-suspension is passed through a high-speed homogenizer leading to the formation of nanosuspension of the poorly water-soluble drug (Fig. 9-24).

Muller and co-workers, 2001 in a recent review have discussed mucoadhesive nanosuspension for oral delivery and surface-modified drug nanoparticles for site-specific delivery to brain. The oral administration of drugs in the form of drug nanoparticles has been reported to provide various advantages including, improved bioavailability, improved dose proportionality, reduced fed/fast variability, reduced inter-subject variability and enhanced absorption rate (Muller et al., 2001). These workers suggested that drug nanoparticles offer potential for targeting to the mucosa of the gastrointestinal tract after oral administration, and to the cells of the mononuclear phagocytic system (MPS) to treat infections of MPS.

DRUG LOADING AND *IN VITRO* RELEASE PROCESS

Lipophilic or poorly water-soluble drugs are often incorporated in a nanocapsule or nanoparticles using hydrophobic polymers. In encapsulation procedure inner phase which constitutes reservoir of system (oil + organic solvent) contains drug(s), with an emulsion stabilizer at an appropriate level in aqueous dispersion phase. The solubility of drug at large governs the selection of organic solvent in the case of nanocapsular system (Ammoury et al., 1990). Depending on drug hydrophobicity, it may require highly apolar solvents like chloroform or methylene chloride, hence an additional cumbersome step for their removal. Solvent extraction evaporation or interfacial polymerization methods can successfully be used. Since the procedures proceed via diffusion followed by solvent evaporation, this may lead to nanoprecipitation of drug in dispersion phase, which often grows into crystals during storage. The release of incorporated drug depends on partitioning behaviour between capsular reservoir and dispersion

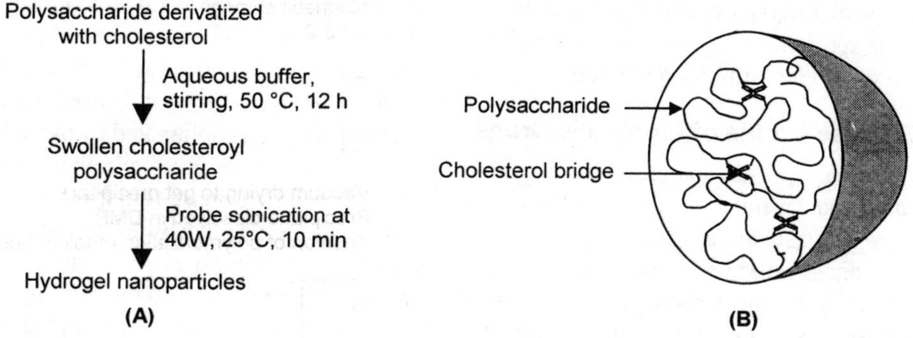

Fig. 9-23. Hydrogel Nanoparticles Prepared using Cholesteroyl Polysaccharides (A) and Diagram of Hydrogel Nanoparticle (B)

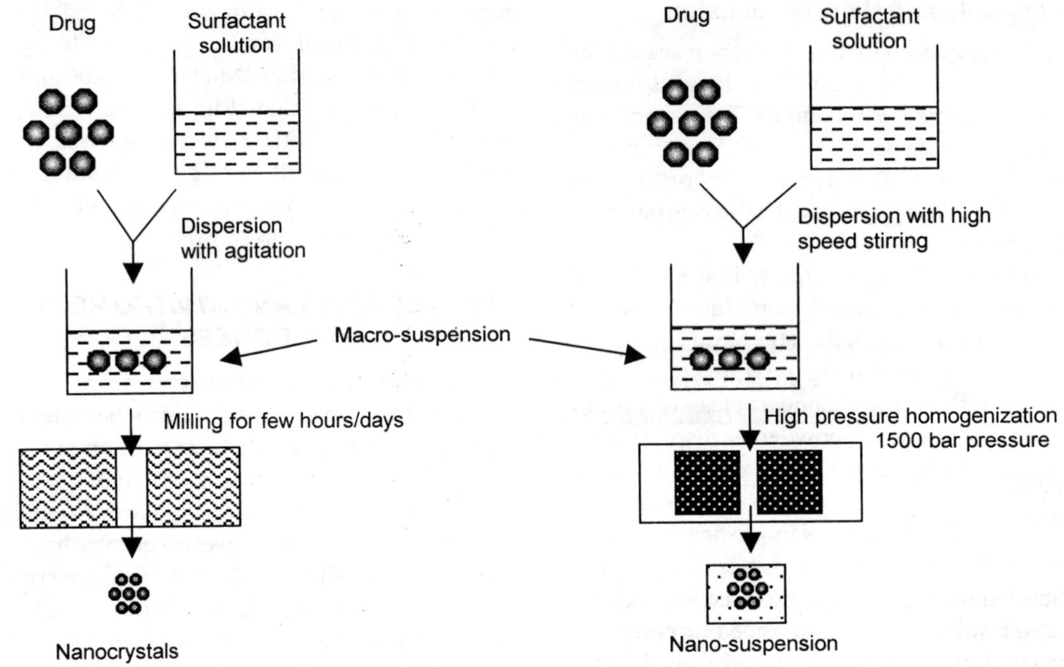

Fig. 9-24. Presentation of Nanocrystals and Nanosuspension

phase sink and so the retention of loaded drug by the carrier system.

In the case of hydrophilic drugs, however, the aqueous phase contains the bioactives, which are embedded in a polymeric cross-linked matrix. Obviously, drug-polymer affinity and interaction may be the critical factors that determine and regulate drug payload or percent drug incorporation and drug release (Henry-Micheland et al., 1987). The encapsulation of drug(s) in hydrophilic polymers requires some appropriate organic solvent depending on the procedural and formulation factors.

In vitro Release Profile of Lipophilic Drugs

The *in vitro* release profile changes with the nature of loaded drug and depending on the type of polymer. The *in vitro* release behaviour of a lipophilic compound from a polymeric colloidal system is largely affected by its inner structure. It is ascertained that the release pattern of drugs from nanocapsules (reservoir system) is dominated by the drug partition from the colloidal suspension to the external sink solution and thus in turn depends upon drug solubility in the oily core and external receptor medium. This behaviour has been documented with various drugs, such as indomethacin (Ammoury et al., 1990), metipranol (Losa et al., 1993), betaxolol (Maincent et al., 1992) and cyclosporine (Bonduelle et al., 1992; Sanchez and Alonso, 1995).

Consequently, these nanocapsular systems should not be considered as controlled release delivery systems though the release continues for several hours. Probably, the main function of the polymer coat is to avoid the coalescence of the oily droplets. On the other hand, the *in vitro* release characteristics of the lipophilic compounds from the nanoparticles (matrix system) is dominated by the polymer erosion and in most of the cases a biphasic release pattern results. The first phase (burst release) is due to the release of the drug adsorbed on the particle surface, and the second phase is due to drug diffusion out of the polymer matrices and the erosion of the polymer matrix. Figure 9-25 demonstrates the *in vitro* release profile of cyclosporin A from PLGA microspheres and nanospheres and indicates that the initial phase of release on the first day relates to the size of the

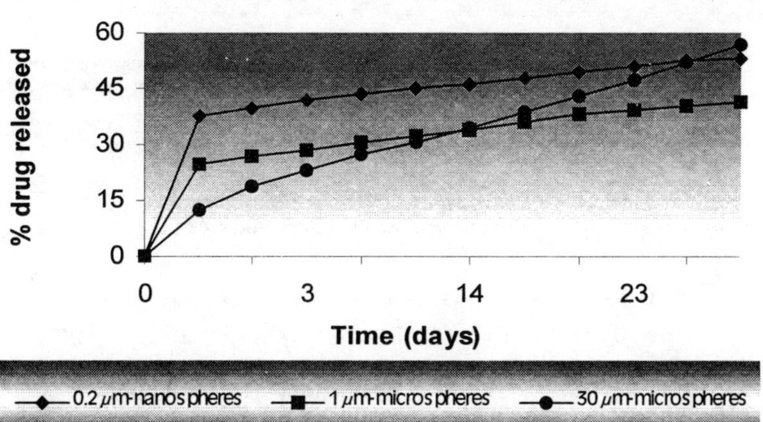

Fig. 9-25. *In Vitro* Release Profile of Cyclosporine From PLGA Micro- and Nanospheres Prepared by Solvent Evaporation Techniques

particulates whereas the second phase is suggestively affected by the degradation/erosion rate profile of the polymer (Sanchez and Alonso, 1995).

In vitro Release Profile of Hydrophilic Drugs

A different release pattern is observed when the hydrophilic molecules are incorporated during the nanoparticle preparation (Oppenheim, 1986; Henry-Micheland et al., 1987; Allemann et al., 1993b; Rajaonaryvony et al., 1993). In those cases, when the loading is carried out in an aqueous environment (monomer polymerization, protein desolvation, carbohydrates cross-linking) the drug is dissolved in the aqueous medium, and its entrapment in nanoparticles is very much dependent upon drug-polymer affinity. However, in cases where the loading requires the use of organic solvent (PLA, PLGA or PECL nanoparticles prepared from polymer precipitation), the drug loading efficiency depends on the formulation conditions.

A hydrophilic compound can be adsorbed onto preformed nanospheres or entrapped within a polymer matrix composed of natural macromolecules or synthetic polymers. Generally in the first case, the release of hydrophilic drugs from polymeric nanoparticles occurs relatively fast (1-2 days) and the release rate reflects the affinity of the drug for the polymer (Fig. 9-26). In the second case however, the polymer degradation rate and inner structure (porosity, degree of cross-linkage) of nanoparticle in combination may influence the drug release process.

PHARMACEUTICAL ASPECTS OF NANOPARTICLES

From a pharmaceutical point of view nanoparticles prepared using the above mentioned methods should be free from potentially toxic impurities, should be easy to store and administer and should be sterile if parenteral use is advocated. Accordingly three important process parameters are performed before releasing them for clinical trails. (Allemann et al., 1993a, Langer et al., 1994, Rolland et al., 1986).

- Purification
- Freeze drying
- Sterilization

Purification of Nanoparticles

Nanoparticles are prepared using a diverse range of methods, which may yield toxic impurities in the nanoparticle suspension including organic solvents, residual monomers, polymerization initiators, electrolytes, stabilizers and large polymer aggregates. The most commonly reported methods used for purification are gel filtration (Langer et al., 1994), dialysis (Rolland et al., 1986) and ultra-centrifugation (Allemann et al., 1993a). However, these methods

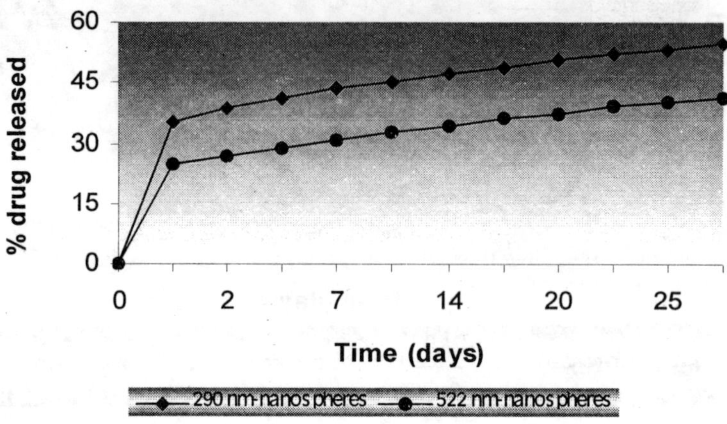

Fig. 9-26. *In Vitro* Release Profile of BSA From PLGA Nanospheres Prepared by Solvent Extraction Technique

are not entirely satisfactory as they are restricted to the laboratory scale and they are incapable of eliminating molecules with high molecular weight (Table 9-4).

A new methodology, known as "cross-flow filtration method" has been used and suggested for the purification of nanoparticles and the method can be scaled up from an industrial standpoint (Allemann et al., 1993b). In this method, the nanoparticles suspension is filtered through membranes, with the direction of fluid being tangential to the surface of the membrane. In contrast to the perpendicular filtration modes, the clogging of the filters is therefore avoided (Fig. 9-27). Depending upon the type of membrane used either micro-filtration or ultra-filtration can be performed. The suspension is subjected to several filtration cycles, while the filtrate, containing components smaller than the pores of the membrane as well as soluble impurities, is discarded. This leads to the concentration of the suspension. This is followed by addition of purified water at the same filtration rate, allowing the circulation volume to remain constant (diafiltration). This method is not only simple to perform but it also allows the fast purification of large amounts of nanoparticles with no alteration in their size.

Table 9-4. Methods Adopted for the Purification of Nanoparticles*

Purification method	Schematic principle	Remarks
Gel filtration		High molecular weight substances and impurities are difficult to remove
Dialysis		High molecular weight impurities are difficult to remove; Time consuming process; Scaling up is difficult
Ultra-centrifugation		Aggregation of particles; Time consuming process; Scaling up difficult

*Adopted from De Jaeghere et al., 1999

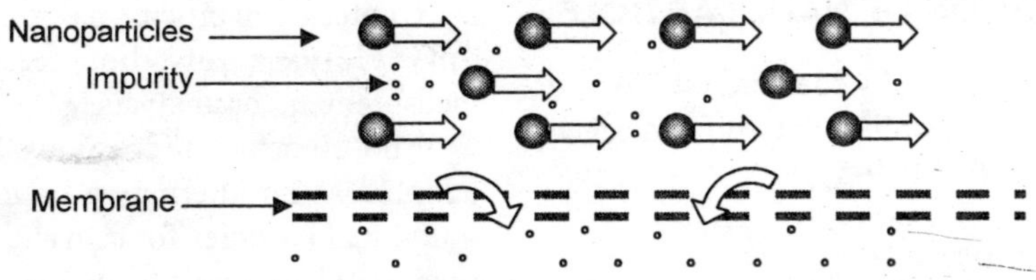

Nanoparticles
Impurity
Membrane

Fig. 9-27. Cross-flow Filtration Technique used for the Purification of Nanoparticles After Preparation (*Adopted from De Jaeghere et al., 1999)

Freeze Drying of Nanoparticles

This technique involves the freezing of the nanoparticle suspension and subsequent sublimation of its water content under reduced pressure to get a freeflowing powered material (Auvillain et al., 1989). Following advantages are cited for the freeze drying of nanoparticles:

- Prevention from degradation and/or solubilization of the polymer
- Prevention from drug leakage, drug desorption, and/or drug degradation
- Easy to handle and store and helps in long term preservation/conservation of nanoparticles
- Readily dispersible in water without modifications in their physicochemical properties

Nevertheless, some problems occur during freeze drying process. In some cases, full redispersion of the system may de difficult to achieve. For example, nanocapsules composed of an oily core surrounded by a tiny polymeric wall tend to aggregate during the freeze drying process (Auvillain et al., 1989). Similarly, nanospheres also tend to aggregate (Sommerfeld et al., 1997) during lyophilization process. These problems can be circumvented by desiccating these systems in the presence of an appropriate lyoprotective agent such as mono- or di-saccharides (e.g., trehalose, glucose, sucrose) (De Jaeghere et al., 1999). It is commonly suggested that during freeze drying sugars may interact with the solute of interest through hydrogen binding. As a result, the solute might be maintained in a "pseudo-hydrated" state during the dehydrating step of freeze drying, and would therefore be protected from damage caused during dehydration and subsequent rehydration. Such a protective interaction is made possible by the ability of sugars to remain amorphous during freeze drying. However, the addition of sugar may change the isotonicity of the nanoparticle dispersion, which should be maintained or adjusted accordingly.

Sterilization of Nanoparticles

Nanoparticles intended for parenteral use should be sterilized to be pyrogen free before they are allowed for administration to animal models or to human use. Some of the well established methods of sterilization for other delivery systems like filtration through 0.22 μm membrane filter do not always work for nanoparticles because microorganisms and nanoparticles may be larger in size (0.25-1.0 μm). However, sterilization in case of nanoparticles is best achieved by using aseptic technique throughout their preparation and processing and formulation and/or by subsequent sterilizing treatments like autoclaving or γ–irradiation (Allemann et al., 1993b; Alonso, 1996).

Processing under aseptic conditions is not completely safe and a terminal sterilization step is required to ensure the microbiological safety of the final product. The choice of the terminal sterilization process however, depends upon the physical stability of the system. Autoclaving and γ–irradiation were shown to have an impact on the physicochemical properties of the particles with a resultant modification in the particle size, stability and drug release characteristics as reported by Masson et al., 1997. It is deduced from these considerations that the sterilization of nanoparticles is a critical step that should be systematically investigated during formulation development stage.

CHARACTERIZATION OF NANOPARTICLES

The nanoparticles are generally characterized for size, density, electrophoretic mobility, angle of contact and specific surface area (Table 9-5).

Size and Morphology

The particle size is one of the most important parameters of nanoparticles. Particle size and sizing of sub-optical particulates is a different procedure, as it involves not only procedural variability, but some of the surface associated properties may even change during sizing procedure. Two main techniques are being used to determine the particle size distribution of nanoparticles and include photon correlation spectroscopy (PCS) and electron microscopy (EM) (Douglas et al., 1987; Kreuter, 1983; Kreuter, 1991; Fusai et al., 1997). The latter includes scanning electron microscopy (SEM), transmission electron microscopy (TEM) and freeze-fracture techniques. The size evaluation of nanoparticle dispersion demonstrates better results with freeze-fracturing microscopy and photon correlation spectroscopy as quantitative methods. The freeze-fracturing with poly(methyl methacrylate) is confronted with and interrupted by in process particles aggregation which only yields a few discrete particles for size measurement or analysis.

The electron microscopy however, could be adopted as an alternative option, which measures individual particles for size and its distribution. It is relatively less time consuming. Additionally, freeze fracturing of particles allows for morphological determination of inner structure of particles. In combination with freeze fracture procedures, TEM permits differentiation among nanocapsules, nanoparticles and emulsion droplets. Similarly, scanning electron microscopy is much less time consuming. However, since particles are based on organic and non-conductive material, they require gold coating. The thickness of gold coat may vary from 30-50 nm. Thus determined size should be denoted as gold-coated particle size rather than a particle size (Fig. 9-28).

Atomic force microscopy (AFM) is an advanced nanoscopic technique that has been applied for the characterization of PLA nanospheres (Gref et al., 1994; Quintanar-Guerrero et al., 1998b) and solid lipid nanoparticles (zur Muhlen et al., 1996). The AFM images can be obtained in an aqueous medium

Table 9-5. Different Parameters and Characterization Methods for Nanoparticles

Parameter	Characterization method (s)
Particle size and size distribution	Photon correlation spectroscopy (PCS)
	Laser defractometry
	Transmission electron microscopy
	Scanning electron microscopy
	Atomic force microscopy
	Mercury porositometry
Charge determination	Laser Doppler Anemometry
	Zeta potentiometer
Surface hydrophobicity	Water contact angle measurements
	Rose bengal (dye) binding
	Hydrophobic interaction chromatography
	X-ray photoelectron spectroscopy
Chemical analysis of surface	Static secondary ion mass spectrometry
	Sorptometer
Carrier-drug interaction	Differential scanning calorimetry
Nanoparticle dispersion stability	Critical flocculation temperature (CFT)
Release profile	*In vitro* release characteristics under physiologic and sink conditions
Drug stability	Bioassay of drug extracted from nanoparticles
	Chemical analysis of drug

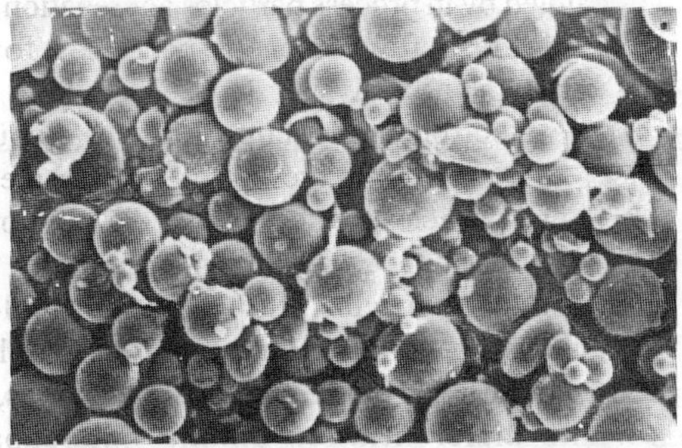

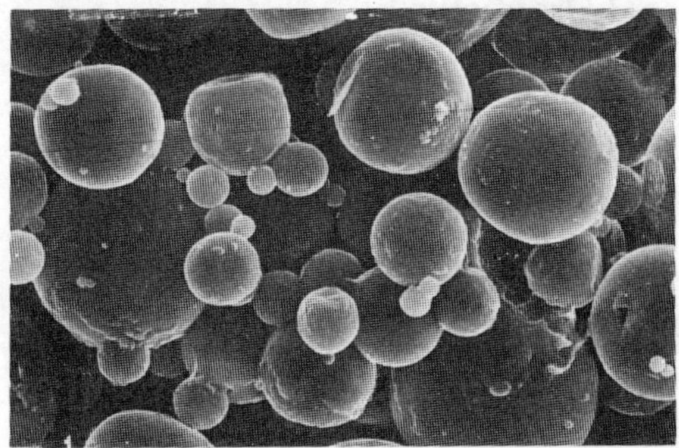

Fig. 9-28. Scanning Electron Microscope Photograph of Gold-coated Nanoparticles

and for this reason it is an effective means for the investigation of nanoparticle behaviour in biological environment.

Mercury porositometry is equally suitable technique for the sizing of nano-particulates (Kreuter, 1983). The freeze-dried nanoparticles are filled in a dilatometer under vacuum and then measured with the help of a mercury pressure porositometer. The method largely measures particulate agglomerates as mercury fails to penetrate to a greater extent within the primary particles.

Specific Surface

The specific surface area of freeze-dried nanoparticles is generally determined with the help of Sorptometer (Kreuter, 1983). The equation given below can be used in the calculation of specific surface area.

$$A = 6 / \partial . d \qquad (9\text{-}1)$$

Where A is the specific surface area, ∂ is the density and d, is the diameter of the particle.

In most of the cases, the measured and calculated specific surface areas fairly compare while in some cases the residual surfactant could affect deviation in measured values. The surfactant coating apparently reduces the specific surface area.

Surface Charge and Electrophoretic Mobility

The nature and intensity of the surface charge of nanoparticles is very important as it determines their interaction with the biological environment as well as their electrostatic interaction with bioactive compounds. The surface charge of colloidal particles in general and nanoparticles in particular can be determined by measuring the particle velocity in an electric field. Laser light scattering technique, i.e. Laser Doppler Anemometry or Velocimetry, has become available as fast and high-resolution technique for the determination of nanoparticle velocities (Sestier et al., 1998).

The surface charge of colloidal particles could also be measured as electrophoretic mobility. The charge composition critically decides the bio-distribution of drug carrying nanoparticles. Generally, the electrophoretic mobility of nanoparticles is determined in phosphate saline buffer (PBS, pH 7.4) and human serum.

The aggregated bands of nanoparticles are visualized distinctively. It is important that free drug adherent or solubilized in aqueous phase and residual surfactant should be removed before electrophoretic mobility is determined. Repeated washing using centrifugation however, may lead to aggregation. Nevertheless, the aggregated nanoparticles suit best for electrophoretic mobility determination as they contribute to a well visible band.

Phosphate saline buffer (pH 7.4) relatively reduces the absolute charge value due to ionic interaction of buffer components with the charged surface of nanoparticles. The zeta potential can be obtained by measuring the electrophoretic mobility applying the Helmholtz-Smoluchowski equation (Hunter, 1983).

Surface Hydrophobicity

The surface hydrophobicity of nanoparticles has an important influence on the interaction of colloidal particles with the biological environment (e.g. protein adsorption and cell adhesion). The hydrophobicity and hydrophilicity collectively determine the bio-fate of nanoparticles and their contents. Hydrophobicity regulates the extent and type of hydrophobic interactions of nanoparticulates with blood components. Several methods, including hydrophobic interaction chromatography, two-phase partition, adsorption of hydrophobic fluorescent or radiolabeled probes, and contact angle measurements have been adopted to evaluate surface hydrophobicity (Carstensen et al., 1991). The measurement of angle of contact suggests about the hydrophobicity or hydrophilicity of the nanoparticles. The water contact angle is measured only on plain surface hence nanoparticles are compressed as tablet/pellet. To study the effect of blood components on resultant *in vivo* hydrophilicity or hydrophobicity the particles are first incubated with blood serum, then centrifuged and lyophilized. The dried nanoparticles are then compressed and angle of contact with water (water contact angle) is determined. The serum components decrease the contact angle by 20°. This suggests that blood components are adsorbed strongly and affect subsequent wettability characteristics of the nanoparticles. Recently, several sophisticated methods of surface chemistry analysis have been used. For example, X-ray photoelectron spectroscopy (XPS) permits the identification of specific chemical groups on the surface of nanoparticles (Scholes et al., 1999).

Density

In addition to surface scanning electron microscopy, transmission electron microscopy following freeze fracturing could successfully be used in morphological investigation of nanoparticles. The interiors are continuous or some structural imperfections exist that provide an indication about the density distribution across the matrix. Some polymeric nanoparticles specially polycyanoacrylate and poly(methyl methacrylate) seem to have porous interior and they also exhibit more irregular and rough surface. The density of nanoparticles is determined with helium or air using a gas Pycnometer (Kreuter, 1983). The value obtained with air and with helium may differ noticeably from each other. The difference is much more pronounced due to specific surface area and porosity of the structure.

Molecular Weight Measurements of Nanoparticles

Molecular weight of the polymer and its distribution in the matrix can be evaluated by gel permeation chromatography (GPC) using a refractive index detector (van Snick et al., 1985). Sukuma and co-workers, 1997 determined the number average and weight average molecular weight of macromolecules on the polystyrene nanoparticles having surface grafted hydrophilic polymeric chains and correlated these parameters with a good water dispersibility of the system. Using gel permeation chromatography, it was shown that PACA nanoparticles are built by an entanglement of numerous small oligomeric subunits rather than by the rolling up of one or a few long polymer chains (Soma et al., 2000a,b).

Nanoparticle Recovery and Drug Incorporation Efficiency

The nanoparticle recovery, which is also referred to as nanoparticle yield in the literature (Govender et al, 1999) can be calculated using the following equation.

$$\text{Nanoparticle Recovery (\%)} = \frac{\text{Conc of drug in nanoparticles}}{\text{Conc of nanoparticles recovered}} \times 100 \qquad (9\text{-}2)$$

Drug incorporation efficiency has been expressed both as drug content (% w/w), which is also referred as drug loading in the literature (Govender et al., 1999) and drug entrapment (%), represented by following equations:

$$\text{Drug content (\% w/w)} = \frac{\text{Conc of drug in nanoparticles}}{\text{Conc of nanoparticles recovered}} \times 100 \qquad (9\text{-}3)$$

In Vitro Release

In vitro release profile can be determined using standard dialysis, diffusion cell or recently introduced modified ultrafiltration technique (Kreuter, 1983; Kreuter, 1991; Magenheim et al, 1993).

In vitro drug release from the nanoparticles can be evaluated in phosphate buffer utilizing double chamber diffusion cells on a shaker stand. A Millipore hydrophilic low-protein binding membrane is placed between the two chambers. The donor chamber is filled with nanoparticulate suspension and the receptor chamber with plain buffer. The receptor compartment is assayed at different time intervals for the released drug using standard procedures.

Magenheim and co-workers, 1993 used a modified ultrafiltration technique to determine *in vitro* release behaviour of the nanoparticles. The nanoparticle suspension is added directly into a stirred ultrafiltration cell-containing buffer. At different time intervals aliquots of the dissolution medium are filtered through the ultrafiltration membrane using less than 2 bar positive nitrogen pressure and assayed for the released drug using standard procedures.

IN VIVO FATE AND BIODISTRIBUTION OF NANOPARTICLES

Following intravenous administration, the colloidal carriers first come into contact with plasma/serum proteins before they reach target cells. Most notably, the interaction of the colloidal carriers with the phagocytes often requires some serum components and then subsequently interaction with complement receptors, Fc receptors and sugar/lectin receptors on the macrophage, lymphocytes or other cells. Soluble carriers can be pinocytosed via Fc or lectin receptors. A number of other receptors are expressed on different cell types which negotiate the transportation of various endogenous ligands or colloidal carriers appended with their synthetic mimics (Vyas and Sihorkar, 2000; Vyas et al., 2001). Normally, intravenous injections of colloidal carriers follow their interactions with at least two distinct groups of plasma proteins. It is now recognized that phagocytosis of particulates by elements of RES (liver, spleen, bone marrow) and specially with reference to liver (Kupffer cells) is regulated by the presence and balance between two groups of serum components: opsonins that promote phagocytosis, and dysopsonins, that suppress the process (Absolom, 1986; Moghimi & Patel, 1989; Moghimi & Patel, 1998). The so-called opsonins adsorb on to the surface of the colloidal carriers and render particles recognizable and more "palatable" to the RES (Fig. 9-29). Thus they mediate their endocytosis by the fixed macrophages of the RES and circulating monocytes.

Immunoglobulins and components of complement systems (particularly C3 and C5) are known as classical opsonin molecules, while fibronectin, C-reactive protein and tuftsin are also known to enhance recognition of various particulates by different macrophages. Immunoglobulin IgA and secretory IgA are the best known dysopsonins (Absolom, 1986). The mode of dysopsonins is not

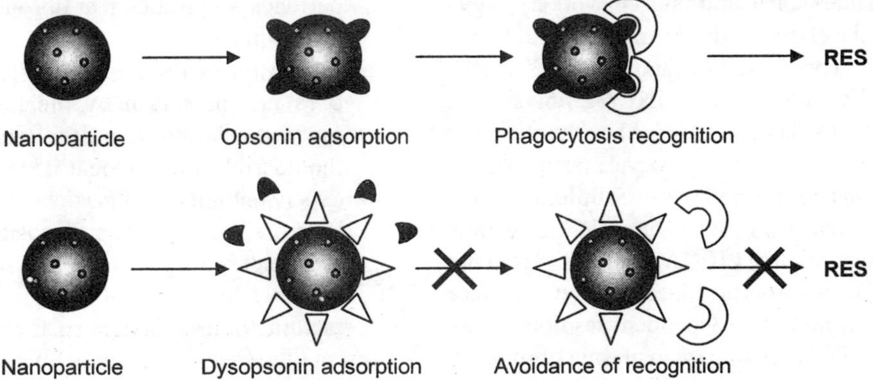

Fig. 9-29. *In Vivo* Fate of Nanoparticles after Adsorption of Serum Components

well documented however their hydrophilicity could be assumed to be responsible for their action. Recently, efforts are being waged to "disguise" the recognition of particulates by RES and enable nanoparticles escape RES capture.

The central dogma in the opsonin driven phagocytosis (opsono-phagocytosis) is the higher protein adsorbability of hydrophobic relative to hydrophilic surfaces. The same has been related to the enhanced uptake of more hydrophobic particles by phagocytosis *in vitro* and rapid removal of hydrophobic particles *in vivo*. Essentially, the macrophages located in the reticuloendothelial systems play a crucial role in opsonin mediated phagocytosis of the injected particulate systems. Polystyrene particles as small as 60 nm showed higher clearance rates from circulation (Illum et al., 1987). Similarly, short circulation half lives were observed irrespective of the compositions of the injected micro-particulate systems of albumin, poly(lactic acid), poly(lactide-co-glycolide), poly(cyanoacrylate) or polyacryl starch (Stolnik et al., 1995). Therefore, using these systems, it is only possible to target drugs to RES-rich organs. Wide ranges of serum components, which are expressed on either at the metastatic states or as a result of changes in circadian rhythm of the different target sites, are thought to play key roles in determining the *in vivo* fate of the particulate systems. Polystyrene particles (PS) (60 nm in diameter) and colloidal gold particles (17 nm in diameter) were found to be opsonized by fibronectins but the adsorption was allegedly prevented after the coating of the particles with polaxamine-908 (Moghimi et al., 1993). In another study, Fernandez-Urrusuno and co-workers, 1996 investigated the effect of administration of polymeric nanoparticles of polyisobutylcyanoacrylate (PIBCA), polyisohexyl-cyanoacrylate (PIHCA), polystyrene (PS) and poly(D,L lactic acid) (PLA) on the clearance activity of the mononuclear phagocyte system in mice. The study was performed with colloidal carbon particles by measuring the serum clearance rate. Single administration of PIBCA and PIHCA (but not PLA and PS) nanoparticles reduced carbon-clearance in both a time- and dose-dependent fashion. These results coupled with a decrease in plasma fibronectin levels resulting from nanoparticulate systems indicate the possible implication of fibronectin in the removal of colloidal particles from the circulation. Recently, Ogawara and co-workers, 1999 demonstrated that serum components play an important role in the hepatic disposition of polystyrene particles and the complement C3b and fibronectins are involved as serum opsonins. In a very unique set of studies they tried to identify the entity of several serum opsonins and dysopsonins responsible for the hepatic uptake of polystyrene particles of 50 nm and 500 nm. The results of their studies are summarized below:

1. Pretreatment of liver by trypsin significantly suppressed the serum dependent hepatic uptake of both types of particles (50 nm and 500 nm), suggesting that serum components involved in opsonization are proteinaceous in nature.
2. Pretreatment with anti-CD3 antibody of serum reduced the promotive effect of serum on the hepatic uptake of 500-nm particles (whereas it was already established that serum in the perfusate inhibited and promoted the hepatic disposition of 50-nm and 500-nm particles at 37°C, respectively). This suggested that complement factor C3b is involved.
3. Hepatic disposition of both particles at 4°C was reduced on addition of serum in the perfusate. These results could be ascribed to the reduction of the surface hydrophilicity due to the adsorption of serum proteins onto the surface of particles and to resultant decrease in non-specific disposition to the liver.
4. Pretreatment of the serum with anti-fibronectin antibody resulted in a significant reduction in the hepatic disposition of 500-nm sized particles, suggesting that fibronectin works as an opsonin.
5. Inhibition of the hepatic disposition in the presence of serum by the addition of N-acetylgalactosamine into the perfusate, suggest the possible involvement of lectin in serum-dependent uptake of particles.
6. Potentiation of hepatic disposition in plasma as compared against serum, suggesting the possible involvement of blood-coagulation factors, such as fibrinogen as an opsonin.

From these results, serum is inferred to function both as the opsonin to enhance the hepatic uptake of particles and as an inhibitor by reducing non-specific interaction between particles serum components (a possible dysopsonic effect). In a very interesting study, Luck and co-workers, 1999 analyzed the mechanisms for C3 binding to the particle surface and subsequent inactivation by cleavage using two-dimensional electrophoresis (2-DE). It could be demonstrated that 2-DE analysis provides the possibility to distinguish between adsorption and covalent attachment of C3 to particulate surfaces. The findings suggest that covalent binding of the C3 component C3b to the particles' surface caused complement activation. The authors stated that the influence of the incubation medium on the *in vitro* protein adsorption of particulate drug carriers has to be considered when a correlation between the protein adsorption pattern and the *in vivc* behaviour of the particles is to be correlated

SURFACE ENGINEERING OF NANOPARTICLES

Nanoparticles are surface engineered for various purposes. On the basis of the reports in the literature, they are classified as:

- Steric stabilized (stealth) nanoparticles
- Bio-mimetic nanoparticles
- Antibody coated nanoparticles
- Magnetically guided nanoparticles
- Bioadhesive nanoparticles

Steric Stabilized (stealth) Nanoparticles

The concept of surface modification of particulate carriers to control or deter them from opsonization process and the specific and non-specific interactions with serum components, have been appreciated with a number of materials. These materials upon coating or grafting to nanoparticle surface could impart a stealth behaviour to them (Torchilin and Trubetskoy, 1995; Araujo et al., 1999).

Materials Used for Steric Stabilization

Unlike liposomes, where monosialo-gangliosides impart stealth behaviour, similar approaches failed in the case of particulate systems to increase circulation half-life (Allen, 1994). A similar approach has been applied to poly(isobutyl cyanoacrylate) nanoparticles where orosomucoid, a sialic acid rich glycoprotein, was used (Olivier et al., 1996). However, *in vitro* results showed that the adsorbed orosomucoid layer can be sorbed/replaced with serum proteins and it is unlikely that this system would demonstrate acceptable long-circulatory *in vivo* behaviour. There are many biocompatible hydrophilic macromolecules and polymers, which in principle may form the hydrophilic, hydrated steric barrier on the particle surface. However, the effect of gelatin coating on poly(lactide)/poly(glycolide) nanospheres on their *in vitro* phagocytosis illustrates that any hydrophilic layer does not necessarily have the anti-phagocytic effect (Tabata and Ikada, 1989). Gelatin encourages fibronectin, a serum component that provides particle recognition for opsono-phagocytosis. Another hydrophilic polymer, dextran, also failed to prevent accumulation of coated poly(butyl cyanoacrylate) nanoparticles in the RES-rich organs after intravenous administration in rabbits (Douglas et al., 1986).

However, polyethylene oxide (PEO) has been the most successful synthetic material used to modify the interactions of particulate systems with serum components and has been either grafted as homo-polymer or copolymer with amphipathic materials (Harper et al., 1991). The research in last decade however, has been focused on poly(ethylene glycol) and its copolymers with poly(ethylene oxide). A range of amphipathic PEO/PEG copolymers with poly(propylene oxide)/poly(propylene glycol) (PPO/PPG)) has been preferentially used to modify the surface of model polystyrene carriers rather than PEO/PEG homopolymers (Torchilin and Trubetskoy, 1995). This rationale is based on the experience in colloidal science where amphipathic copolymers have been shown to provide effective steric stabilization. Various amphipathic PEO/PEG and PPO/PPG copolymers of different compositions and molecular weights are commercially available as Polaxamers™ and Polaxamines™ (BASF, Wyandote, USA) (also known as Pluronics™ and Tetronics™, Fluca, Switzerland).

Polaxamers have ABA block structure with central PPO/PPG block and two terminal PEO/PEG blocks (PEO/PEG-PPO/PPG-PEO/PEG), whereas Polaxamines are tetra-functional block copolymers with four PEO-PPO or PEG-PPG blocks joined together by a central ethylene diamine bridge [(PEO-PPO)$_2$-x-(PPO-PEO)$_2$] or [(PEG-PPG)$_2$-x-(PPG-PEG)$_2$]. Other commercially available poly(ethylene oxide)-containing surfactants have also been tested including a range of poly(ethylene oxide) sorbitan mono-ester (Polysorbates 20, 40 and 80) for the surface modification of poly(methyl methacrylate) nanoparticles (Muller et al., 1992) (Fig. 9-30).

Mechanism of Steric Stabilization and/or Long Circulation

Illum and Davis, 1983, 1984, 1986 and Illum et al., 1987 in their pioneer work on sterically stabilized systems highlighted the effects of coating on the particulate systems with various Polaxamers and Polaxamines. It was observed that in contrast to uncoated material, which targets the liver, Polaxamer 407 coated nanoparticles target the bone marrow, and Polaxamine 908 coating retains the materials in the circulation (Illum et al., 1987). These results raised concerns over the single dominant factor involvement in the stealth systems, and concerted efforts are being waged since then to resolve and establish various parameters and mechanisms (Torchilin and Trubetskoy, 1995). In recent years, the mechanisms and factors influencing the stealth and long circulatory behaviour of hydrophilic polymers have been discussed in great detail.

The effect of polymer coated particulate systems on protein adsorption has been attributed to several factors including those related to particles and polymers or a combinations of the both. These include the surface hydrophobicity, degree of hydrophilicity conferred by the polymer cap, particle size, particle charge, nature of particle surface, biodegradability and non-biodegradability of the system. The efforts are being made to correlate these factors with *in vivo* interactions with biological systems. Among the various mechanisms, which possibly play their parts in imparting the stealth behaviour to the particulate systems are:

1. Increased hydrophilicity provided by the hydrophilic chains of the polymers
2. Decreased interactions with serum components and activity of dysopsonins in serum
3. Flexible versus rigid polymers
4. Contact angle between the phagocytic cells and the particle surface
5. The presence of hydrophobicity on the coating surface

Increased hydrophilicity was earlier thought as the sole reason for the stealth behaviour of the polymer coated particulate systems. As demonstrated in the case of polystyrene nanoparticles, the more hydrophobic PPG blocks adsorbed on the polystyrene surface, and more hydrophilic PEG blocks stick out of the surface and form a protective coating/barrier (Illum and Davis, 1984) (Fig. 9-31).

These hydrophilic regions on the polymer backbone retard the attack of serum components through various mechanisms. The effects of polyethylene blocks on protein adsorption have been attributed to several factors involving, among others, the unique solution properties and molecular conformations of PEG in aqueous solutions (Illum et al., 1987). PEG produces a surface that is in liquid-like state with the polymer chains exhibiting considerable flexibility and mobility. The high

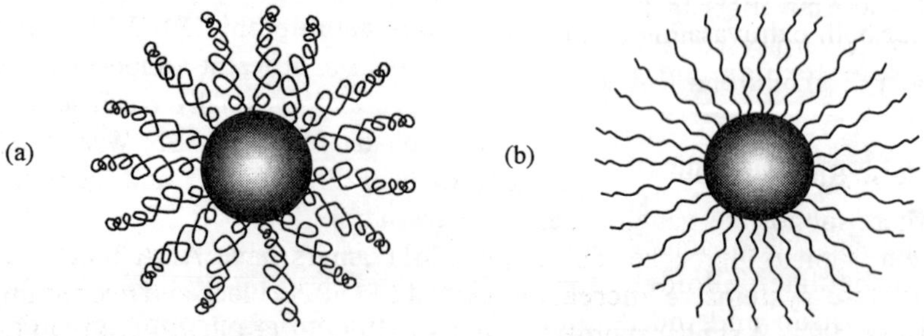

Fig. 9-30. Scheme Illustrating Stealth (Long Circulating) Nanoparticles. (A) Nanoparticles Coated with Polaxamers/Polaxamines. (B) Nanoparticles Coated with Grafted PEO.

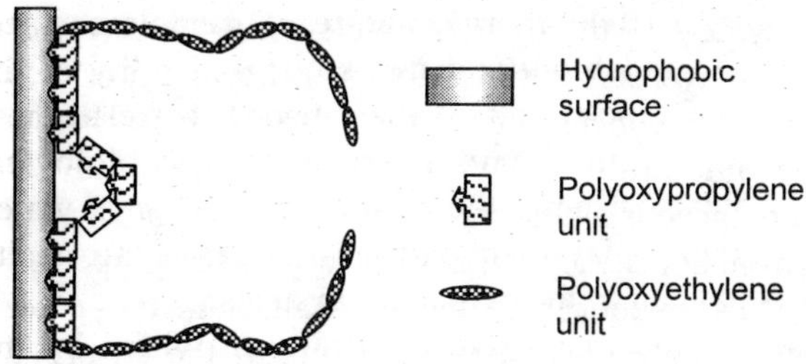

Fig. 9-31. Schematic Representation of the Mechanism of Adsorption of Block Copolymers to the Surface of a Hydrophobic Particle

mobility of PEG chains has been proposed to repel approaching serum proteins from the surface because the protein does not have sufficient contact time with the mobile phase to adsorb. Due to the transient, flexible and rapidly changing structure of PEG, the immune system may also encounter hindrance in modeling opsonic serum immunoglobulin around it. The protective layer of PEG is considered as a "cloud" of possible chain conformations, with a density high enough to prevent the interactions with the surface of the particles (Tan et al., 1993; Torchilin and Trubetskoy, 1995). These facts instruct that only, if a polymer chain possesses both hydrophilicity and flexible properties (to enable a high number of possible chain conformations), it can serve as an effective coating barrier for particulate systems against opsonization. Interestingly, PEG and other polymers provide significant clearance prolongation of clearance when they are present not only in the form of dense particle coating, but also in the form of a relatively loose brush as well. Hydrophilic brush like interfaces assemblages of non-reactive and non-immunogenic polymer chains proved to be effective in the prolongation of both extravasating and non-extravasating macromolecular and colloidal candidates.

Mathematical Models for Mechanistic of Steric Stabilization

Proteins of the serum and that of immune origin adsorb on to the particulate/colloidal carriers immediately after injection and the resultant opsonization imparts them preferred orientation that favours phagocytic uptake especially by macrophages of the reticuloendothelial system. The molecular origin of these interactions is mostly long range electrostatic, Vander Waals and short-range hydrophobic interactions of colloidal/particulate surface with the macromolecules in the serum (Jeon et al., 1991; Blunk et al., 1993; Gref et al., 1995). While electrostatic and hydrophobic interactions can be minimized by the selective manipulation of the materials of construction, for example in the case of bilayered vesicles, the use of neutral lipids and mechanically strong bilayers could minimize these interactions. However, Vander Waals interactions need the coating of these surfaces with some components which mechanically and spatially hinder its interactions with the serum components. Gref and co-workers, 1995 studied the conditions that lead to repulsion of serum component from hydrophobic plane surfaces to which some hydrophilic steric molecules are tagged.

A mathematical model has been proposed (Jeon et al., 1991; Jeon and Andrade, 1991) that accounts and explains four types of interactions between a serum component (usually a protein) and a hydrophobic substrate (Fig. 9-32). The best conditions for repulsion of serum components are offered by long PEG chain length (L) and high surface density. These workers have calculated the distance between the anchorage to the substrate of two terminally attached PEG chains (D) and reported that the value of D may vary for the smaller and larger

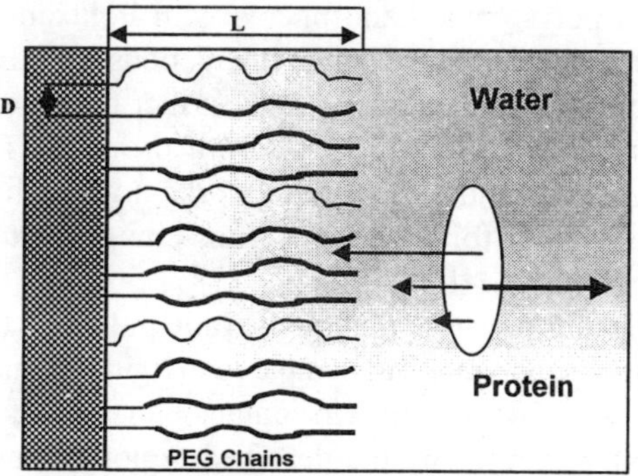

Fig. 9-32. Interactions of Protein and Hydrophobic Substrate with Attached PEG Chains. Adopted From Eon and co-workers, 1991, with Modifications

proteins from serum. It was further suggested that the reductions in the adsorption of certain serum components (dysopsonins) prevent the recognition and uptake of the particulate systems by the macrophages; the competition between these two mechanisms is believed to be the decisive in controlling the particulate uptake by the macrophages. Moghimi and coworkers, 1993 confirmed the role of dysopsonization in the particulate systems similar to that demonstrated in stealth liposomes by Patel, 1992. These workers (Moghimi et al., 1993) coated the surfaces of colloidal gold particles (17 nm in diameter) and polystyrene nanospheres (60 nm in diameter) with Polaxamine 908. The colloidal gold particles demonstrated fibronectin dominant opsonization and accumulated in Kupffer cells when treated in autologous plasma. In contrast, coating of gold particles with Polaxamine 908 prior to plasma opsonization prevented the adsorption of fibronectin onto their surface. Simultaneously, Kupffer cells failed to recognize Polaxamine 908 coated gold particles before and after opsonization. Unlike Kupffer cells, liver endothelial cells endocytosed Polaxamine 908-coated gold particles prior to opsonization but failed to recognize them after the opsonization process. Moghimi et al., 1993 explained this activity as an indication of the presence of dysopsonic activity in plasma/serum. This dysopsonic activity was further elaborated using polystyrene latex nanospheres, where the uptake of such particles by phagocytes is known to be independent of opsonization. The coating of ^{111}In-labeled polystyrene nanospheres with Polaxamine 908 dramatically reduced their interactions with liver sinusoidal cells. The uptake was further reduced in the presence of autologous serum proteins. The dysopsonin identified by these workers was a heat stable (60 °C for 15 min) serum component of molecular mass >100 KDa.

It is thus apparent that the flexible polymers (all hydrophilic polymers) as compared to rigid polymers are adsorbed with regions in contact with the surface (trains), separated by the detached regions (loops) with polymer projects away from the surface (tails) (Norde, 1984; Norde, 1992). These tailed portions provide hydrophilicity to the coated particulate system (Fig. 9-33). The adsorption of hydrophilic polymers to the hydrophobic surfaces is a typical monolayer adsorption. However, beyond a critical polymer concentration, the adsorption isotherms become multiple. While these polymers do not spontaneously desorb, when come in contact with serum fluids, they can be displaced by serum species. Displacement can be due to the attachment of other macromolecules when segments of the adsorbed polymer detach. Another priori for the RES-avoiding effects of these flexible polymers relates to the contact angle between the phagocytic cells and the particle surface.

Van Oss et al., 1975 showed that the addition of complement and antiserum to non-phagocytosed bacteria resulted in phagocytosis (using human neutrophils). In line with their work the phagocytosis was traced as surface phenomenon, it was noted that the contact angles of saline on the bacteria were all below 18°, until the complement and anti-serum was added. After the addition of these plasma components, the contact angles were raised significantly. The workers claimed that the difference in contact angle between the phagocytic cells and the bacterial cells were critical and determine whether phagocytosis will occur or not. The treatment of the bacterial cells by the body can be expected to be analogous to a typically colloidal drug delivery system and thus substantiates their relevance in targeted drug delivery. Contact angle method was utilized to investigate the affinity of the hydrophilic polymers for model carrier materials. They used Polaxamines and Polaxamers, as well as other surfactants (Polysorbates and Sorbitan fatty acids)

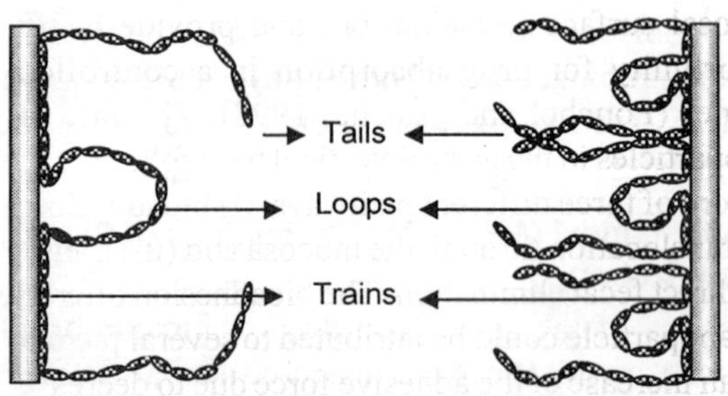

Fig. 9-33. Schematic Adsorption of a Flexible Polymer to a Solid Surface, showing Multiple Contact Points. Adopted From Norde, 1992, with Modification

for the adsorption on the model hydrophobic surface of poly(methyl methacrylate) (Muller and Wallis, 1993). With the help of parameters like advancing angles, receding angles and contact angle hysteresis effect, these workers concluded that polymers and surfactants having a strong interaction with the solid, should have a low receding angle (high hysteresis).

The hysteresis is the difference between the advancing and the receding angle, and can be a measure of chemical heterogeneity of the solid surface, and an indication of the surface roughness. This parameter suggests that the strength of surfactant adsorption largely determines whether opsonizing serum proteins gain an access to the surface (as well as steric stabilization). The need for a strong interaction between the hydrophobe of the polymer and the solid surface has been demonstrated by the fact that Polaxamers do not prevent opsonization of biodegradable drug carriers (Carstensen et al., 1991). This is because certain carrier particles are not sufficiently hydrophobic to provide a driving force for Polaxamer adsorption. It was further demonstrated that the nature of adsorption or anchoring of the hydrophobe to the polymer surface is critical in determining the conformation of the polymer, and eventually the surface nature of the adsorbed polymer (Ceh et al., 1997).

Nanoparticles for Bioadhesion

The oral route is the most preferred route for drug administration. However, numerous drugs remain poorly available when administered by this route. In order to circumvent this problem, it has been proposed to associate drugs to polymeric bioadhesive nanoparticulate systems because they adhere to mucosal surface (bioadhesion) and provide better opportunity for drug absorption in a controlled manner (Ponchel and Irache, 1998). The fate of nanoparticles in the gastrointestinal tract follows one or more of three different pathways: (i) bioadhesion, (ii) translocation through the mucosa and (iii) transit and direct fecal elimination. The bioadhesion offered by nanoparticle could be attributed to several factors like an increase of the adhesive force due to decrease in size (nanoscopic), or a prolongation of the gastrointestinal transit time. Bioadhesion can be achieved by building up either non-specific interactions with the mucosal surface, which are mediated through physicochemical properties of the particles and the surfaces, or specific interactions when a ligand (i.e., lectin) attached to the particle is used for the recognition and attachment to a specific site at the mucosal surface (Fig. 9-34).

The specific interactions between three lectin-latex conjugates and different structures of rat intestinal mucosa have been studied *ex vivo*. These systems were prepared by covalent coupling of different ligands, i.e., tomato lectin (TL), asparagus pea lectin (AL), mycoplasma gallisepticum lectin (ML), and bovine serum albumin (BSA) as control, to poly(styrene) latex nanospheres (Irache et al., 1996). Photomicrographs with fluorescent lattices have confirmed the specificity of the ML- and AL-latex conjugates for the Peyer's patches region and of the TL-latex conjugates for the mucus gel. The usefulness of a surface-conjugated, bioadhesive molecule, tomato lectin, to augment and facilitate intestinal uptake of orally administered inert nanoparticles was demonstrated by Hussain and co-workers, 1997. The application of tomato lectin as a bioadhesive ligand has been demonstrated to enhance subsequent intestinal transcytosis of colloidal particulates to which it is bound.

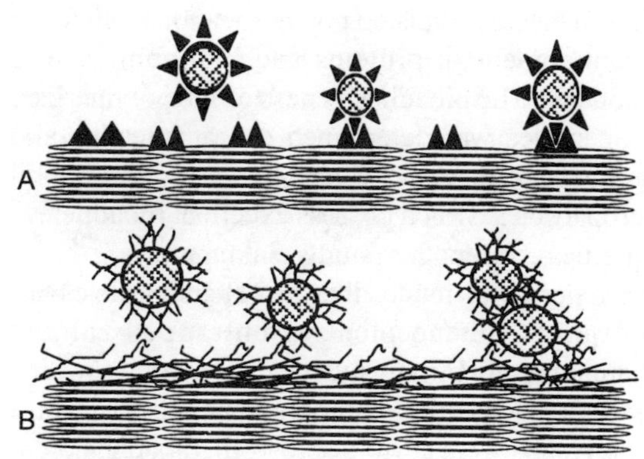

Fig. 9-34. Mechanistic Approaches for the Delivery of Drugs/Peptides by Bioadhesive Nanoparticles to Gastric Mucosa . A. Signifies high affinity binding of ligand (lectin) anchored nanoparticles and B. Signifies non-specific binding using surface properties

Ulex europaeus lectin-gliadin nanoparticle conjugates (UE-GNP) were also evaluated for their *in vitro* bioadhesive properties (Ezpeleta et al., 1999). The mucin adhesion activity of these conjugates tested with bovine submaxillary gland mucin (BSM) and the level of mucin binding was always much greater with UE-GNP compared to control (gliadin nanoparticles). However, the presence of 50 μmol fucose, which is the reported specific sugar for *U. europaeus* lectin, specifically inhibited the activity of these conjugates. These results showed that the activity and specificity of *U. europaeus* lectin was preserved after covalent coupling to these biodegradable carriers.

Recently, bioadhesive potential of *Dolichos biflorus* lectin (DBA)-gliadin nanoparticles was evaluated by Arangoa and associates, 2000. The bioadhesive activity of nanoparticles and DBA conjugates was determined in small and large rat intestinal mucosa. The higher level of interaction with the mucosa was proposed due to gliadin composition. In fact, gliadin is rich in neutral and lipophilic residues. As suggested by these scientists, neutral amino acids can promote hydrogen-bonding interactions with the mucosa, while the lipophilic components can interact with the biological tissue through hydrophobic interactions.

However, Kriwt and co-workers, 1998 prepared bioadhesive poly(acrylic acid) nanoparticles prepared using an inverse emulsion polymerization method for the entrapment of proteins and hydrophilic drug candidates. The bioadhesiveness of the polymerized nanoparticles was determined on rat intestine and found to be comparable with reference (polycarbophil microparticles, which possess excellent bioadhesive properties). In another study, Sakuma et al., 1997, 1999 reported the mucoadhesion of nanoparticles and absorption enhancement of entrapped salmon calcitonin (sCT) by polystyrene nanoparticles, which possess surface grafted hydrophilic polymeric chains. These results were attributed to both, bioadhesion of nanoparticles to GI mucosa and an increase in the stability of entrapped sCT in GI tract. Findings obtained using *in situ* intestinal perfusion technique indicated that the strength of mucoadhesion depends on the structure of the hydrophilic polymer chains on the polystyrene nanoparticle surface.

Bio-mimetic Nanoparticles

The coating of nanoparticles with endogenous serum components may circumvent their uptake through mononuclear phagocytic system (MPS). These bio-mimetic particles mimic the biological environment and disguise their recognition from RES components. The rationale for using albumin and complement components as bio-mimetic ligands has been proposed by some workers (Verrecchia et al., 1995; Olivier et al., 1996). Albumin is the main protein present in the blood (40 g/l), whereas complement moieties are among the most important opsonins involved in clearance mechanisms. Sialic acids may also serve as a bio-mimetic ligand to prevent the drug carrier from being recognized by RES, by imitating the sialylated surface. Human orosomucoid, a sialic acid rich serum glycoprotein, has been recently used to coat PACA nanoparticles (Olivier et al., 1996). However, the bio-mimetic coatings were found to provide iadequate protection against opsonin adsorption and RES uptake, presumably due to rapid desorption of these ligands, which turns out to be insufficient in negotiating stealthing effect.

Magnetic Nanoparticles

The concept of magnetically modulated drug delivery and strategies has emerged and exploited, which include nanoparticle based systems as well. These strategies mainly rely upon reversal of passive bioprocessing, through minimizing nanoparticles uptake by the RES and by enhancing their access to extra-vascular sites, particularly to tumours. Nanoparticles are rendered magnetic by incorporating Fe_3O_4 particles (10-20 nm) simultaneously with the drug during the preparation stage. The magnetic nanoparticles are then injected through the artery supplying the tumour tissue and guided externally with the help of an external magnet in order to target the nanoparticulate carrier and contents. This technique has been investigated with albumin nanoparticles but the production of poly-glutaraldehyde, PACA and PMMA magnetic nanoparticles is also reported (Allemann et al., 1993a; Kreuter, 1994).

Vyas and Malaiya, 1988, 1989 studied the *in vivo* magnet responsiveness and kinetics of distribution of indomethacin entrapped in magnetic poly (methyl methacrylate) nanoparticles on a rat tail model and periodically monitored drug concentration in various visceral organs after intraarterial and intravenous administration (Fig. 9-35). Up to 60 min post injection time 60-fold higher concentrations could be achieved in tail target segment which resulted in considerably reduced drug concentration in other organs like liver and spleen. Magnetic nanoparticle of indomethacin demonstrated selective targeting under magnetic field of 8000 Oe strength. Following normal administration (no magnetic field applied) the drug concentration was higher in the liver and spleen where endocytosis and phagocytosis could occur.

Super-paramagnetic iron oxide nanoparticles have been used by Guimaraes and co-workers, 1994 for MR lymphography as pathologic basis for contrast enhancement. After i.v. injection of super-paramagnetic nanoparticles, a decrease in signal intensity indicates active uptake of particles by macrophages, whereas an increase in signal intensity indicates altered capillary permeability to the tumour. These findings in rats may prove to be clinically useful for differentiating benign from malignant enlarged lymph nodes.

Moore and co-workers, 2000 investigated the accumulation and cellular uptake of long-circulating dextran-coated iron oxide (LCDIO) particles in malignant neoplasms *in vivo*. LCDIO was preferentially localized in tumour cells (49.0%±4.6) but was also taken up by macrophages in tumours (21.0%± 3.1) and by endothelial cells in the areas of active angiogenesis (where actively new blood capillaries are developed).

Nanoparticles Coated with Antibodies

The anchoring of target specific antibodies to the nanoparticle surface may facilitate their delivery to specific sites. Selectivity in drug targeting can, in theory, be achieved by the attachment of monoclonal antibody as a site-directing device. *In vitro* and *in vivo* studies with nanoparticles coated with monoclonal antibodies have been carried out (Douglas et al., 1987). Monoclonal antibodies can be fixed on nanoparticles by direct adsorption or via a spacer molecule (protein A) or by covalent linkage (e.g., carbodiimide, cyanogen bromide and glutaraldehyde reaction) (Illum et al., 1984). In this way, antibodies are bound to the particles via their Fc part and therefore projecting the antigen specific binding sites (Fab') for the target specificity. This technique has been applied to a wide variety of nanoparticles including PACA, polymethyl-methacrylate and albumin (Illum et al., 1984; Rolland et al., 1987; Breton et al., 1996). These studies however reflected the specificity of these immunonanoparticles to bind specifically tumour cells *in vitro*. Nevertheless, such systems failed to record a significant accumulation of the carriers in targeted tumours *in vivo*. This could be explained due to a probable competitive displacement of the

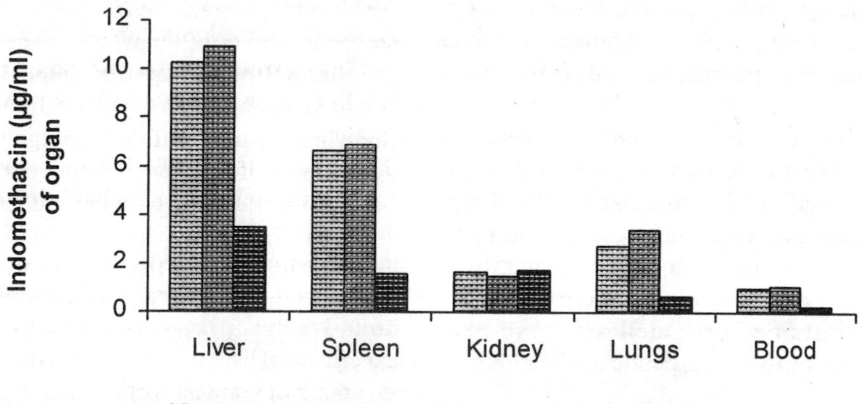

Fig. 9-35. *In Vivo* Organ Distribution of Indomethacin Loaded PMMA Plain and Magentic Nanoparticles after Intravenous Administration (*Adopted From Vyas And Malaiya, 1989)

antibodies (in case they are adsorbed) by blood components, secondary coating of opsonin components and/or insufficient access to the target site. Tumour-specific monoclonal antibodies conjugated to super-paramagnetic monocrystalline iron oxide nanoparticles (MION) could be used to yield specific diagnoses with the use of MR imaging. Tiefenauer and co-workers, 1996 evaluated magnetite nanoparticles as a tumour contrast agent in MRI. Magnetite nanoparticles, coated by three different artificial polypeptides, were conjugated to an antibody specific to the carcinoembryonic antigen (CEA). To protect the particles from fast blood elimination, the surfaces were modified using various sugars, polyethyleneglycol, albumin, and sialoproteins, respectively. The protective effect was determined by using a specific *in vitro* test and by analyzing the biodistribution of the nanoparticles in nude mice grafted with CEA-tumours. The tumour accumulation was slightly improved by coating the nanoparticle surface using sialoprotein glycophorin B. However, coating long circulatory and sterically stabilized nanoparticles with site-specific antibodies or lectins remains to be explored.

THERAPEUTIC APPLICATIONS OF NANOPARTICLES

Nanoparticles with different compositions and characteristics have been formulated and investigated for various therapeutic applications (Table 9-6). Several different types of biodegradable polymers including biopolymers (e.g. gelatin, albumin, casein, polysaccharide, lectin etc.) and synthetic polymers (polycaprolactone, polyesters, polyanhydrides, polycyanoacrylates) with various drug release characteristics ranging from several hours to several months have been used to formulate sustained release nanoparticles. It is the submicron size of this delivery system, which makes it more efficient in certain drug therapy applications, such as in intracellular localization of therapeutic agents. These systems, in addition to sustained drug delivery have been investigated for various therapeutic applications.

Intracellular Targeting

The treatment of infections caused by obligate and facultative intracellular microorganism is difficult because most of the available antibiotics have following limitations:

- Poor intracellular diffusion or reduced activity at the acidic pH of the phagosomes and lysosomes (Moghimi and Patel, 1989).
- Most intracellular infections are difficult to eradicate because bacteria inside phagosomes are protected from antibiotics (Horwitz, 1982).
- Multi drug resistance due to the functional P-glycoprotein pumps (Kartner et al., 1985).

The nature of antibiotics also determines their fate *in vivo*. Thus antibiotics with basic character (aminoglycosides) lead to lysosomal overloading whereas they display a reduced activity in acidic environment (Tulkens and Trouet, 1978). Conversely, acidic antibiotics (β–lactams) do not diffuse through the lysosomal membrane because of their ionic character at neutral extracellular or cytoplasmic pH (Trouet and Tulkens, 1981). Finally, certain antibiotics, which permeate the cell more rapidly and to a larger extent (clindamycin) are poorly, retained in the cell (Johnson et al., 1980) as they efflux out fast.

The need for antibiotics with greater intracellular efficacy led to the development of endocytosable drug carriers including nanoparticles, which mimic the entry path of the bacteria by penetrating the cells into phagosomes and lysosomes (Fig. 9-36). Nanoparticles and mostly all non polymer-coated particles following intravenous administration rapidly accumulate in liver and spleen (MPS rich organs) which are the main organs of reticuloendothelial system associated infections (Table 9-7).

The effectiveness of ampicillin loaded polyhexylcyanoacrylate (PIHCA) nanoparticles was first tested on experimental salmonellosis in mice (Fattal et al., 1989; 1991). A total dose of 0.8 mg of ampicillin bound to nanoparticles suppressed all mortality compared to three doses of 32 mg each of the free drug required to suppress mortality. The antimicrobial efficiency of PIHCA nanoparticle bound ampicillin was confirmed *in vivo* in experimental listerosis in athymic nude mice, a model involving a chronic infection of both liver and spleen macrophages (Youssef et al., 1988). The therapeutic index of ampicillin for liver bacterial counts rise at least 20-fold after its linkage to PIHCA nanoparticles.

Table 9-6. Various Therapeutic Applications of Nanoparticles/Nanocapsules

Application	Material	Purpose
Cancer therapy	Poly (alkylcyanoacrylate) nanoparticles with anticancer agents, oligonucleotides	Targeting, reduced toxicity, enhanced uptake of antitumour agents, improved *in vitro* and *in vivo* stability
Intracellular targeting	Poly (alkylcyanoacrylate) Polyester nanoparticles with anti-parasitic or antiviral agents	Target reticuloendothelial systems for intracellular infections
Prolonged systemic circulation	Polyesters with adsorbed polyethylene glycols or pluronics or derivatized polyesters	Prolong systemic drug effect, avoid uptake by the reticuloendothelial system
Vaccine adjuvant	Poly (methylmethacrylate) nanoparticles with vaccines (oral and intramuscular immunization)	Enhances immune response, alternate acceptable adjuvant
Peroral absorption	Poly (methylmethacrylate) nanoparticles with proteins and therapeutic agents	Enhanced bioavailability, protection from gastrointestinal enzymes
Ocular delivery	Poly (alkylcyanoacrylate) nanoparticles with steroids, anti-inflammatory agents, anti-bacterial agents for glucoma	Improved retention of drug/reduced wash out
DNA delivery	DNA-gelatin nanoparticles, DNA-chitosan nanoparticles, PDNA- poly(DL-lactide-co-glycolide) nanoparticle	Enhanced delivery and significantly higher expression levels
Oligonucleotide delivery	Alginate nanoparticles, poly (D,L) lactic acid nanoparticles	Enhanced delivery of oligonucleotide
Other applications	Poly (alkylcyanoacrylate) nanoparticles with peptides	Crosses blood-brain barrier
	Poly (alkylcyanoacrylate) nanoparticles for transdermal application	Improved absorption and permeation
	Nanoparticles with adsorbed enzymes	Enzyme immunoassays
	Nanoparticles with radioactive or contrast agents	Radio-imaging
	Copolymerized peptide nanoparticles of n-butyl cyanoacrylate and activated peptides	Oral delivery of peptides

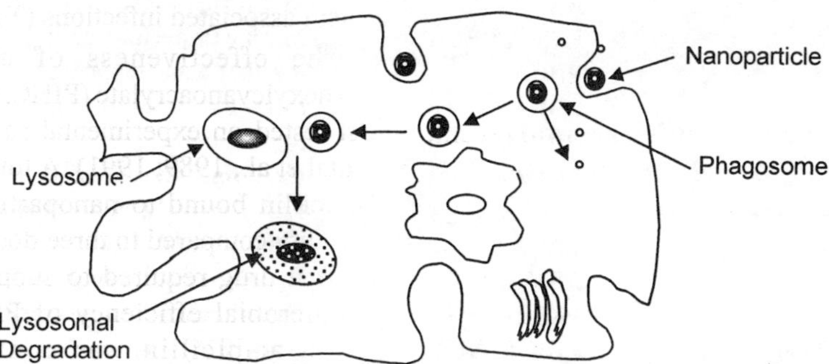

Fig. 9-36. Schematic Presentation of Possible Localization of Nanoparticle in Infected Cell. Nanoparticles loaded with drug enter through phagocytosis and form phagosomes, phagolysosome and then liberate the drug in the lysosomes.

Table 9-7. Various Intracellular Bacterial and Parasitic Infections where Nanoparticle Loaded Antibiotics could Potentially be Used

Leishmaniasis
Salmonellosis
Trypanosis
Listerosis
Malaria

They have also been used as carriers of primaquine to treat intracellular parasites of the RES, such as *Leishmania donovani* in intracellular leishmaniasis (Gaspard et al., 1992a,b). This leads to a reduction in the acute toxicity due to nonspecific accumulation or distribution of the therapeutic agents. Surprisingly, it was observed that the carrier on its own (unloaded) exhibited a significant anti-leishmanial activity. This was proposed due to the phagocytosis of PIHCA nanoparticles leading to the induction of a respiratory burst (and associated oxygen radicals and intermediates). The effect was more pronounced in infected than in non-infected macrophages.

In a study to treat intracellular infection using antibiotics, nanoparticle-bound ampicillin has been demonstrated to have a 20-fold higher therapeutic index in liver compared to free drug (Pinto-Alphandary et al., 1994) and the strategy was effective in the treatment of salmonellosis in mice. Venier-Julienne and co-workers (Venier-Julienne and Benoit, 1992; Venier-Julienne et al., 1992) tested the anti-leishmanial activity of unloaded and amphotericin B loaded PLGA nanoparticles on cultured macrophages. They also reported an anti-leishmanial activity of unloaded PLGA nanoparticles and attributed it to an indirect effect mediated through macrophage activation.

Recently, Gonalez-Martin and co-workers, 2000a, 2000b evaluated nifurtimox and allopurinol loaded polyethyl-cyanoacrylate nanoparticles as potential lysosomotropic carrier for the trypanocidal activity against *Trypanosoma cruzi*, which is responsible for Chagas' disease. Various approaches of macrophage targeting through nanoparticles as drug delivery systems are summarized in Table 9-8.

It is desirable in certain physiologic conditions that on i.v. administration the colloidal particles should evade and avoid rapid recognition and uptake by the RES and achieve prolonged systemic circulation. These applications include a prolonged systemic drug delivery, use as an imaging agent, or for site specific localization of nanoparticles other than the liver and spleen. This can be achieved by using following methods:

- Nanoparticles can be prepared by using derivatized polymers, which orient projecting their hydrophilic segment exposed to aqueous

Table 9-8. Approaches of Macrophage Targeting using Nanoparticles*

Bioactive	Polymers	Target site
^{3}H dactinomycin	PBCA	Murine peritoneal macrophage
^{3}H vinblastin	PMCA/PECA	Murine tissue macrophage
^{3}H dactinomycin	PBCA	Rat tissue macrophages
5-Fluorouracil	PBCA	Murine resident macrophages
Doxorubicin	PIHCA	Murine hepatic metastases
Ampicillin	PHCA	Experimental salmonellosis
Ampicillin	PIHCA	Experimental listeriosis in mice
Dehydroemetine	PACA	Experimental leishmaniasis in mice
Primaquine	PIHCA	Experimental leishmaniasis in mice
Amphotericin B	PMMA	Experimental leishmaniasis in mice
Antisense oligonucleotide oligo(thymidinate)	PIBCA/PIHCA	Anti-HIV

Abbreviations: PBCA polybutyl cyanoacrylate; PMCA polymethyl cyanoacrylate; PECA polyethyl cyanoacrylate; PIHCA polyisohexyl cyanoacrylate; PHCA polyhexyl cyanoacrylate; PACA polyalkyl cyanoacrylate; PMMAPolymethyl methacrylate; PIBCA polyisobutyl cyanoacrylate

*Adopted from Vyas et al., 2001

bulk while hydrophobic segment(s) are shielded, thus the resultant surface tends to be hydrophilic and evade recognition from RES (Gref et al., 1995).

- Surface modification of the preformed nanoparticles with different block copolymers (Pluronics™/Polaxamers™) or polyethylene glycols, which produce several fold higher systemic circulation time compared to unmodified nanoparticles following i.v. administration (Torchilin and Trubetskoy, 1995).

Nanoparticles in Chemotherapy

The most promising application of nanoparticles is their possible use as carriers for antitumour agents (Couvreur et al., 1990; Kreuter, 1991). Enhanced endocytic activity and leaky vasculature of the tumour favours accumulation of intravenously administered nanoparticles. However, to facilitate and optimize drug targeting to tumour tissues, the "stealth" behaviour using polyoxyethylene could contribute to excessive extravasation. Stealth nanoparticles are prepared by coating them with soluble polyoxyethylene, or by using dialykyl polyoxyethylene and phospholipids. The accumulation of non-stealth (conventional) nanoparticles in RES may also be exploited for cancer chemotherapy.

Chemoembolization

One of the approach, chemoembolization, makes use of the biodegradable particles administration to the liver tumours using a catheter that passes directly into an artery of the tumour (Fig. 9-37).

The accumulation of non-stealth mitomycin-C microparticles within the Kupffer cells (liver) has been used to target hepatic neoplasm indirectly (Natsume et al., 1990). This is executed by providing a depot of drug for killing nearby neoplastic tissues, as the particles (non-stealth) are not actually taken up by the neoplastic tissue. Similar targeting strategies using trans-catheter chemoembolization has been reported for cisplatin (Li et al., 1994), doxorubicin (Cay et al., 1996), taxol (Wang et al., 1996), rifampicin (Kassab et al., 1997) and 5-fluorouracil (Denkbas et al., 1999).

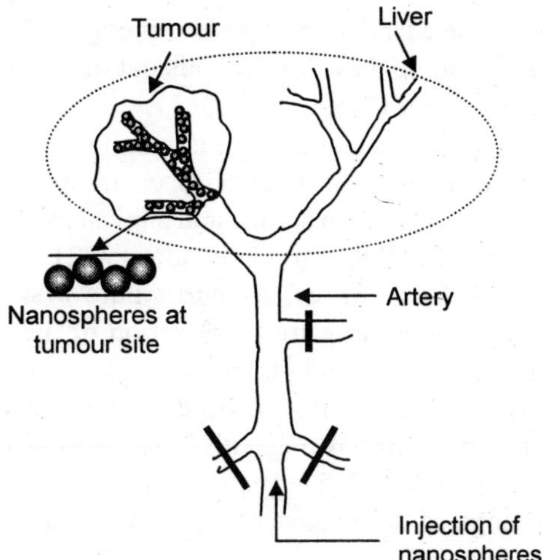

Fig. 9-37. Infusion of Albumin Particles for Chemo-embolization into Liver (Adopted From Natsume et al., 1990)

Several studies are reported for prolonged drug retention in tumours, reduction in tumour growth, and prolonged survival of tumour bearing animals using nanoparticle loaded antitumour agents compared to free drug.

Avoidance of Multi-drug Resistance

Multi-drug resistance is the main cause of the failure of chemotherapeutic agents (Endicott and Ling, 1989). This can severely affect the effectiveness of some types of chemotherapy. It is often associated with the over-expression of a cell membrane glycoprotein of 170 KDa molecular weight (Kartner et al., 1985. The glycoprotein (P-glycoprotein) is a membrane spanning ATPase and located in the plasma membrane. This multi-drug resistance transporter could act as an efflux pump and reject positively charged amphipathic drugs from the cells as shown for bacterial transport proteins. Over-expression of P-glycoprotein in tumour cells can lead to a marked decrease in drug sensitivity. Thus multi-drug resistance is associated with a low intracellular accumulation of these drugs. This is more pronounced with drugs which enter the cell by passive diffusion through the lipid bilayer, for example, doxorubicin (an anticancer drug). Upon entering the cell, these drugs bind to P-glycoprotein, which forms transmembrane channels and uses the energy of ATP hydrolysis to pump these compounds out of the cell (Kartenr and Ling, 1989).

Nanoparticle loaded drugs has resulted in the effective treatment of a number of chemotherapy refractory cancers both in animal and clinical models (Kubiak et al., 1989; Cuvier et al., 1992). The lysosomal localization of the particulate system protects the loaded drug from the action of the P-glycoprotein, thus avoiding immediate contact with P-glycoprotein transporter located at the plasma membrane (Fig. 9-38). Along with cell sensitization, nanoparticulate drug delivery may help overcome a broader range of drug resistance due to favourable pharmacokinetics.

Cuvier et al., 1992 demonstrated an enhanced cellular accumulation of doxorubicin following the administration of polyisohexylcyanoacrylate nanoparticle-bound doxorubicin (as compared to free drug) in a multi-drug resistant tumour cell line.

Delivery of Anticancer Drugs

The polyalkylcyanoacrylate nanoparticles have been studied in recent years as a possible means of targeting drugs to specific sites in the body, with particular emphasis to cancer chemotherapy. The small colloidal carriers are biodegradable and drug substances can be incorporated normally by a process of surface adsorption. Some of the anticancer drugs that are either entrapped or adsorbed onto polyalkylcyanoacrylate nanoparticles are doxorubicin associated with polyisohexylcyanoacrylate nanoparticles (Chiannilkulchai et al., 1989), mitoxantrone in polybutylcyanoacrylate nanoparticles (Beck et al., 1993), aclacinomycin A in polyisobutylcyanoacrylate nanoparticle (Jiang and Liao, 1995), granulocyte-colony stimulating factor (G-CSF) in polyalkylcyanoacrylate nanoparticles (Gibaud et al., 1998), acyclovir in polybutylcyanoacrylate nanoparticles (Zhang et al., 1998) and doxorubicin in polyalkylcyanoacrylate nanoparticles (Soma et al., 2000b).

However, other biodegradable polymers like poly(lactide-co-glycolide) and polyvinylpyrrolidone are also investigated for drug delivery in cancer therapy. These include dexamethasone in poly-(lactide-co-glycolide) nanoparticle (Chacon et al., 1996) and Taxol in polyvinylpyrrolidone nanoparticles (Sharma et al., 1996).

Adjuvant Effect for Vaccines

An adjuvant effect of the nanoparticles with either matrix entrapped or surface adsorbed vaccine has been demonstrated in several studies on subcutaneous or oral administration. The adjuvant effect of nanoparticles could be ascribed to the sustained release of the entrapped antigen or improved uptake and subsequent processing of the nanoparticle bound antigen by the immune system of the body. Kreuter and co-workers observed that polymethyl-

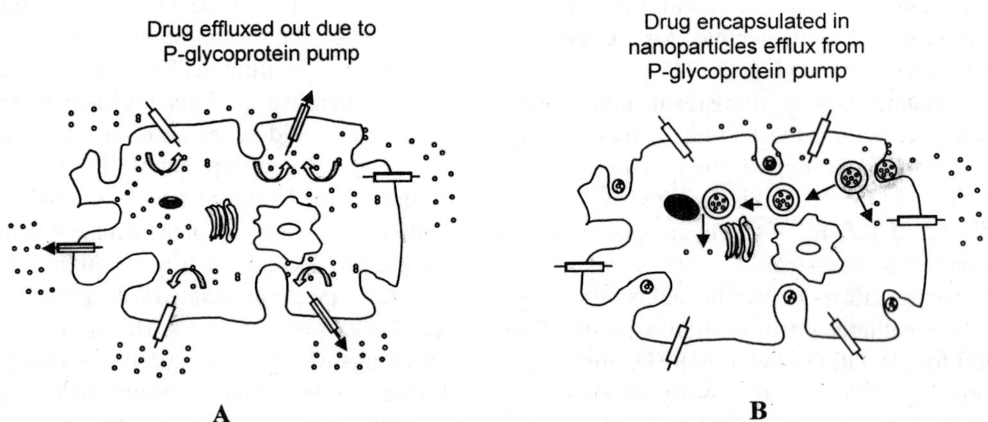

Fig. 9-38. Schematic Diagram of Proposed Drug Trafficking into Multi-Drug Resistant Cell of Free Drug (A) and of Drug Associated With Nanoparticles (B). Adopted from Cuvier et al., 1992, with modifications

methacrylate nanoparticles containing the influenza antigen induced significant antibody response and protected mice against a challenge with mouse-adapted influenza virus to a greater extent than the antigen alone or an alum preparation of the antigen (Kreuter and Haenzel, 1978; Kreuter et al., 1986; 1988; Kreuter, 1991). These workers further demonstrated that a decrease in particle size and an increase in hydrophobicity of the nanoparticles increased the adjuvant effect. These nanoparticles were biodegradable after subcutaneous or intramuscular injection. Stieneker and co-workers, 1991 found 10- to 100-fold higher IgG titre, when polymethylmethacrylate nanoparticles were used as adjuvants for HIV-2 whole virus vaccine in mice and showed excellent adjuvanticity as compared to aluminum hydroxide or an aqueous control solution.

Oral delivery of antigens with nanoparticles may be an elegant means of producing an increased IgA antibody response. Orally administered nanoparticle associated antigens are protected from the gastric enzymes and acidic pH and are subsequently taken up by the gut associated lymphoid tissue. Biodegradable poly(butyl-2-cyanoacrylate)particles have been shown to enhance the secretory immune response after their oral administration in association with ovalbumin (O'Hagan et al., 1989). Pappo et al., 1991 reported polystyrene nanoparticles conjugated to the anti-M cell monoclonal antibody 5B11 to target Peyer's patch M cells. Desai and co-workers, 1995 found that nanoparticles formulated with poly (lactic-co-glycolic acid) co-polymer (PLGA) (~100 nm diameter) have several fold higher uptake by the Peyer's patch tissue compared to larger size nanoparticles in a rat *in situ* intestinal loop model and these systems hold promise for mucosal vaccination.

Nanoparticles for Peroral Administration of Proteins and Peptides

Proteins and peptides are increasingly seen as therapeutic drugs. As they are quite susceptible to proteolytic degradation, and therefore lead to problems of physicochemical and bio-stability coupled with their short biological half-life and inability to pass most of the biological barriers. For protein/peptide delivery, nanoparticles offer an attractive possibility. Nanoparticles have been employed as peroral drug carriers with the following objectives:

1. Improvement of the bioavailability of drugs with poor absorption characteristics
2. Delivery of vaccine antigens to the gut-associated lymphoid tissue (GALT)
3. Controlled or sustained release of the drug
4. Reduction of the gastrointestinal mucosa irritation caused by drugs
5. Assurance of the stability of drugs in the gastrointestinal tract.

The majority of studies however, deal with the stability aspects of the nanoparticle associated peptides against challenges from the luminal proteases in the gastrointestinal tract. Polyalkyl-cyanoacrylate nanoparticles and nanocapsules were developed as peptide carriers for insulin (Damage et al., 1990; Michel et al., 1991) and Growth Hormone Releasing Factor (Grangier et al., 1991; Gautier et al., 1992). PACA nanoparticles were also proposed as possible drug delivery system for cyclosporin A, a cyclic oligopeptide having a specific immuno-suppressive activity (Bonduelle et al., 1992). Efforts are directed on delivery of proteins and peptides, especially using biodegradable nanoparticles (PLA/PLG nanoparticles). Nanoparticles of PLGA loaded with amphotericin B, another cyclic peptide (Venier-Julienne et al., 1992) have been reported for site specific delivery with better therapeutic index and low incidences of toxic manifestations.

Insulin encapsulated into nanoparticulate systems when administered orally was found to induce hypoglycaemic effects for several days in fasted and fed diabetic rabbits. Encapsulation protects insulin against proteolytic enzymes. In addition, nanoparticles are known to cross the gut lumen by paracellular pathway and enter the blood circulation, thus demonstrating a systemic drug effect. This strategy is under investigation for an oral administration of other proteins and peptides, and receptor mediated transport through gut wall using glycoprotein and glycopeptide conjugated nanoparticles (Kukan et al., 1989; Scherer et al., 1993; Desai et al., 1995; Florence et al., 1995). Thus nanoparticle-bound peptides can be used for the sustained oral delivery and also to improve the absorption and bioavailability. The mechanism of the absorption enhancement of peptide and protein drugs by nanoparticles has been investigated (Sakuma et al., 1997). These workers examined the mechanism of enhancement of Salmon calcitonin (sCT) by poly-(N-isopropylacrylamide) nanoparticles and proved that the absorption enhancement results mainly from both mucoadhesion of nanoparticles in the GI tract and an increase in the stability of sCT against degradation by digestive enzymes as demonstrated in Figure 9-39. Recently, copolymerized peptide particles (CPP) have been developed as carriers for oral uptake of therapeutic peptides. Hillery and co-workers, 1996 reported *in vitro* stability of CPP of leutinizing hormone releasing hormone (LHRH) when incubated in luminal contents, mucosal scrapings and serum and recorded significant *in vitro* intestinal transport of associated hormone (LHRH) using the Caco-2 cell lines.

Nanoparticles for Intra-arterial Applications

Nanoparticles possess several advantages as a carrier system for the intra-arterial localization of therapeutic agents. These advantages include their subcellular size, targeted surface, good suspensibility and uniform dispersity for catheter-based therapy, and an easy penetration into the arterial wall without causing trauma. Nanoparticles could prove to be an effective dosage form for an intra-arterial localization of therapeutic agents for preventing restenosis (Fig. 9-40). Restenosis may be defined as the process of re-obstruction of an artery following interventional procedures such as angioplasty, atherectomy, or stenting and forms the major limitations of these well-established therapies. Nanoparticles are putative drug carriers for the treatment of restenosis as they localize the therapeutic agents at the site of artery injury rather than systemic administration (Labhasetwar et al., 1995; Song et al., 1997). These workers demonstrated that local delivery of drugs like dexamethasone, heparin and U-86983 (an anti-proliferative agent) was facilitated and high regional concentration could be built with prolonged retention in lower doses with reduced systemic toxicity. These systems are also promised as carriers for genes in restenosis and other gene therapy applications (Guzman et al., 1996).

Nanoparticles for Ocular Delivery

The most applications of drug-loaded ophthalmic delivery systems are for glaucoma therapy, especially cholinergic agonists like pilocarpine. The short elimination half life of aqueous eye drops (due probably to lachrymal drainage) can be extended from a very short time (1-3 min) to prolonged time (15-20 min) using nanoparticles, which have biodegradable properties. These include, polyalkylcyanoacrylate nanoparticles (Li et al., 1986; Losa et al., 1991), poly-ε-carolactone (Marchal-Heussler et al., 1992), polyester nanoparticles (Marchal-Heussler et al., 1992), albumin nanoparticles (Zimmer et al., 1995). In addition, it has been demonstrated that nanoparticles adhere to the inflammed tissue in a more quantitative manner as compared to the healthy tissue, thus these could also be used for targeting of anti-inflammatory drugs to inflammed eyes. Various advantages are proposed for the polyalkylcyano-acrylate nanoparticles specially PHCA nanoparticles including their biodegradability, tissue adhesion and

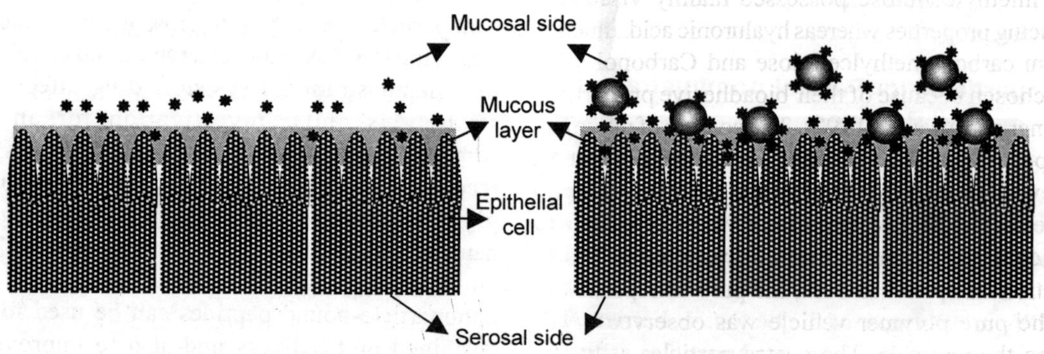

Fig. 9-39. Enhanced Oral Delivery of Nanoparticle Associated Protein and Peptidal Drugs via Mucoadhesion

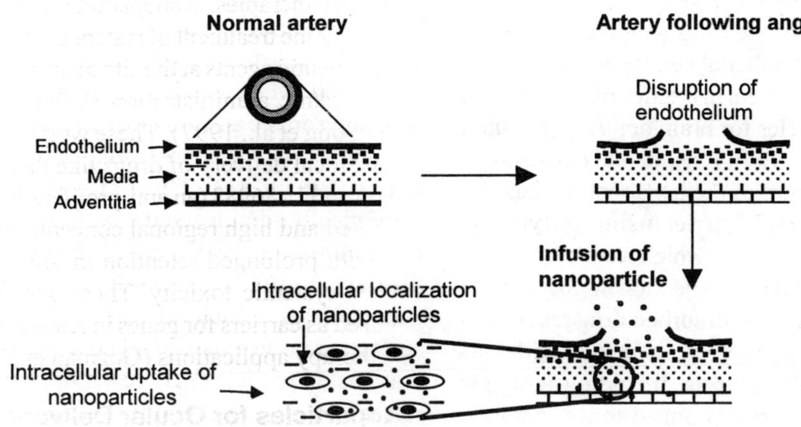

Fig. 9-40. Intra-arterial Delivery of Nanoparticles for Restenosis

increased elimination half-life of their drainage coupled with a slow clearance. It was found that pilocarpine and betaxolol loaded polyalkylcyano-acrylate nanoparticles could prolong and maintain the reduced the intraocular pressure in rabbits for more than 9 h (Diepold et al., 1989; Marchal-Heussler et al., 1990). Zimmer and co-workers, 1994a, 1994b used pilocarpine loaded polybutyl cyanoacrylate nanoparticles for ocular delivery. A better pilocarpine pharmacokinetics as well as pharmacodynamic response in terms of intraocular pressure (IOP) lowering effect and enhanced mitosis, was established. A possibility to increase the efficacy of pilocarpine-loaded nanoparticles is the classic approach of coating them with bioadhesive or viscous polymers (Zimmer et al., 1995). The poymers methylcellulose, polyvinylalcohol and hydroxy-propylmethylcellulose possessed mainly viscosity enhancing properties whereas hyaluronic acid, mucin, sodium carboxymethylcellulose and Carbopol 941 were chosen because of their bioadhesive properties (Zimmer and Kreuter, 1997). The coating of albumin nanoparticles with viscosity imparting polymers however, failed in bringing an additive effect. However, with the bioadhesive polymers an additional improvement in mitotic response and IOP reduction compared to both, the pure nanoparticles and the pure polymer vehicle was observed after coating the particles. The coated particles seem to adhere to conjuctival mucin thus prolonging the residence time of the drug-loaded particles in the precorneal area.

Nanoparticles for Brain Delivery

The blood-brain barrier represents one of the hurdles for drugs including antibiotics, antineoplastic agents and a variety of neuroleptic drugs. One of the possibilities suggested to overcome this barrier is drug delivery to the brain using nanoparticles. Drugs that have successfully been used for brain targeting using nanoparticles include the hexapeptide dalargin, the dipeptide kyotropin, loperamide, tubocurarine and doxorubicin. A number of prospects are accounted for the enhanced delivery of drugs to the brain using nanoparticles:

1. Higher concentration gradient at the blood brain barrier that may enhance the transport across the endothelial cell layer and hence increased retention in the brain.
2. Solubilization of endothelial cell membrane lipids by surfactant action of nanoparticles leading to membrane fluidization and enhanced drug permeability to BBB.
3. Loosening of tight junctions between endothelial cells and increased permeability of drug or drug-nanoparticle conjugates through these channels.
4. Endocytosis of nanoparticles by the endothelial cells followed by the release of the drug intra-cellularly.

5. Transcyotosis of the drug bound nanoparticle through the endothelial cell layer.

Kreuter and co-workers in a series of studies have advocated nanoparticles for brain delivery (Kreuter, 1994; Kreuter et al., 1995). Kreuter and co-workers, 1995 reported transport of the hexapeptide dalargin across the blood-brain barrier using poly(butyl cyanoacrylate) nanoparticles, which were coated with polysorbate 80. Intravenous injection of polysorbate 80 coated nanoparticles with sorbed drug resulted in significant analgesic effect in mice model as compared against all controls, including a simple mixture of the three components (drugs, nanoparticles, and surfactant) mixed directly before i.v. injection. Fluorescent and electron microscopic studies indicated that the passage of the particle-bound drug occurred by phagocytic uptake of the polysorbate 80-coated nanoparticles by the brain blood vessel endothelial cells.

Some neuropeptides are also delivered across blood-brain barrier using nanoparticle technology. Leu-enkephalin dalargin and the Met-enkephalin kyotorphin are neuropeptides that normally do not cross the blood-brain barrier (BBB) when given systemically. To transport these neuropeptides across the BBB they were adsorbed onto the surface of poly(butylcyanoacrylate) nanoparticles, which were coated with polysorbate 80 (Schroeder et al., 1998). In a recent study, Gulyaev and co-workers, 1999 investigated the delivery of anticancer drugs into the brain using polysorbate 80 coated nanoparticles. High brain concentrations of doxorubicin (>6 μg/g) were achieved with the nanoparticles coated with polysorbate 80, whereas with controls (plain drug, drug with polysorbate and drug loaded plain nanoparticle), the brain concentrations were below the detection limits (Fig. 9-41). The brain concentration of systemically administered doxorubicin was found to be enhanced over 60-fold by binding to biodegradable poly(butyl cyanoacrylate) nanoparticles, which are coated with the nonionic surfactant polysorbate 80. These workers proposed that coated particles may reach the brain intact and release the drug after endocytosis by the brain blood vessel endothelial cells. The polysorbate 80 used as the coating agent could inhibit the P-glycoprotein efflux pump and thus could increase the brain delivery of the drug.

Nanoparticle(s) for DNA Delivery

Nanoparticles have been recently used as a delivery vehicle for the transfection of plasmid DNA and to improve their stability in the bio-environment. Truong-Le and co-workers, 1998 developed a novel system for gene delivery based on the use of DNA-gelatin nanoparticles (nanospheres) formed by salt-induced complex coacervation of gelatin and plasmid DNA. Nanosphere-DNA incubated in bovine serum was more resistant to nuclease digestion compared to naked DNA (Fig. 9-42). Various bioactive agents could be encapsulated in the nanospheres through ionic interaction with the matrix components,

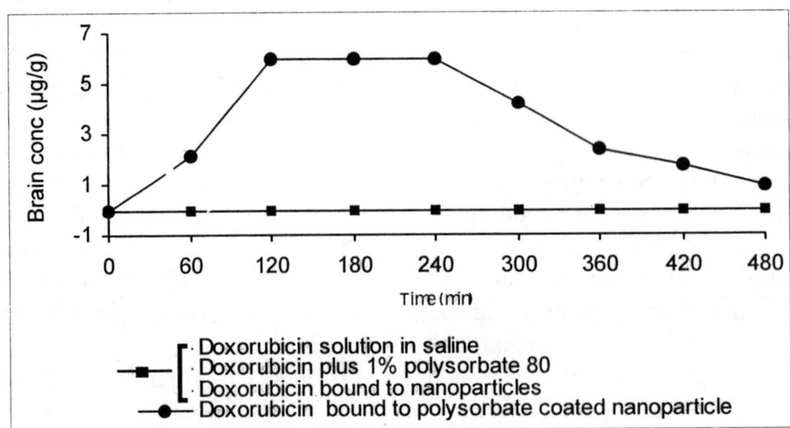

Fig. 9-41. Doxorubicin Brain Concentration after Intravenous Injection of Polysorbate Coated Nanoparticles

physical entrapment, or covalent conjugation. Truong-Le and associates, 1999 further developed DNA-gelatin nanoparticle system contain-ing chloroquine and calcium. The targeting ligand, transferrin, was covalently bound to the gelatin, as a gene delivery vehicle. Optimum cell transfection by nanosphere-DNA required the presence of calcium and nanospheres containing transferrin.

Janes and co-workers, 2001 reported chitosan-DNA hybrid colloidal systems either as chitosan-DNA complex or as chitosan-DNA nanosphere and reported comparatively better gene expression. Oral administration of DNA nanoparticles synthesized by complexing plasmid DNA with chitosan, a natural biocompatible polysaccharide, resulted in transduced gene expression in the intestinal epithelium (Roy et al., 1999). Mice receiving nanoparticles containing a dominant peanut allergen gene (pCMVArah2) produced secretory IgA and serum IgG2a. Compared with non-immunized mice or mice treated with 'naked' DNA, mice immunized with nanoparticles showed a substantial reduction in allergen-induced anaphylaxis associated with reduced levels of IgE, plasma histamine and vascular leakage.

Kneuer and co-workers, 2000a, 2000b synthesized silica nanoparticles (SiNP) with covalently linked cationic surface modifications. The study demonstra-ted the ability of silica nanoparticles to electro-statically bind, condense and protect plasmid DNA. These particles might be utilized as DNA carriers for gene delivery. The ability of colloidal silica particles with covalently attached cationic surface modifications to transfect plasmid DNA *in vitro* is investigated and the complex was given the name nanoplex.

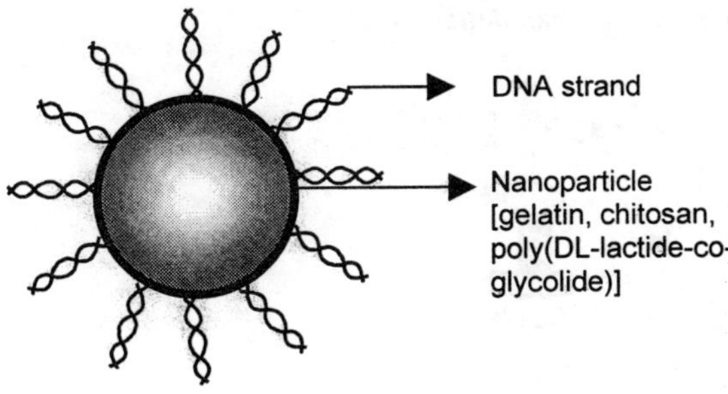

Fig. 9-42. DNA-Nanoparticle Conjugates used for Transfection of Plasmid DNA and to Improve their Stability in Bioenvironment

Biodegradable and biocompatible poly(DL-lactide-co-glycolide) polymer was used to enacapsulate pDNA (alkaline phosphatase, AP, a reporter gene) in submicron size particles (Cohen et al., 2000). Gene expression mediated by the nanoparticles (NP) was evaluated *in vitro* and *in vivo* and compared with cationic-liposome delivery. Nano size range (600 nm) pDNA-loaded in poly(DL-lactide-co-glycolide) polymer particles with high encapsulation efficiency (70%) exhibited sustained release of pDNA over a month. The entrapped plasmid maintained its structural and functional integrity. *In vitro* transfection by pDNA-NP resulted in significantly higher expression levels in comparison to naked pDNA.

Nanoparticle for Oligonucleotide Delivery

Antisense therapeutic agents bind to DNA or RNA sequences, blocking the synthesis of cellular proteins with unparalleled specificity. Transcription and translation are the two processes with which the agents interfere. There are three major classes of antisense agents: antisense sequences, commonly called antisense oligonucleotides; antigene sequences; and ribozymes (Putnam, 1996). Antisense sequences are derivatives of nucleic acids that hybridize cytosolic messenger RNA (mRNA) sense strands through hydrogen bonding to complementary nucleic acid bases. Antigene sequences hybridize double-stranded DNA in the nucleus, forming triple helixes. Ribozymes, rather than inhibiting protein synthesis simply by binding to a single targeted mRNA, combine enzymatic processes with the specificity of antisense base pairing, creating a molecule that can incapacitate multiple targeted mRNAs. Antisense oligonucleotides (ODNs) are being investigated *in vitro* and *in vivo* for evaluating their possible use in treating human immunodeficiency virus infection, hepatitis B virus infection, Herpes Simplex Virus infection, papillomavirus infection, cancer, restenosis, rheumatoid arthritis, and allergic disorders. A major goal in developing methods of delivering antisense agents is to reduce their susceptibility to nucleases while retaining their ability to bind to targeted sites. Carrier systems designed to protect the antisense structure and improve passage through the cell membrane include liposomes, water-soluble polymers, and nanoparticles (Fig. 9-43).

Due to their hydrophilic and polyanionic character, ODNs poorly combine with polymeric systems, however, three main strategies have been put forward recently for binding of ODN and nanoparticles (Fig. 9-44):

1. ODNs may covalently link to hydrophobic anchor allowing insertion with polymer surface (A)
2. Cationic polymers coated particles will interact with the negatively charged ODN molecules (B)
3. Loading of ODN can be achieved using a specialized naoparticulate system, nanosponge, which uses diffusion/reptation process for the loading of ODNs (C)

Oligonucleotides adsorbed onto polyalkylcyanoacrylate nanoparticles have been demonstrated to enhance stability against nucleases and more ideal cellular disposition.

Positively charged nanoparticles prepared from diethylaminoethyl (DEAE)-dextran and polyhexylcyanoacrylate (PHCA) were evaluated as carriers for ODNs (Zobel et al., 1997). Oligonucleotides adsorbed to the surface of the nanoparticles remained protected against degradation by the endonuclease DNase I and under *in vitro* cell culture conditions, whereas unprotected ODNs were totally digested under these conditions. Fattal and co-workers, 1998 studied oligonucleotides associated biodegradable polyalkylcyanoacrylate nanoparticles through the formation of ion pairs between the negatively charged oligonucleotides and hydrophobic cations. Oligonucleotides bound to these nanoparticles were protected from nuclease attack in cell culture media and their cellular uptake was increased as a result of the capture of nanoparticles by an endocytotic/phagocytotic pathway. Berton and co-workers, 1999 investigated nanoparticles (NP) of poly (D,L) lactic acid for the intracellular delivery of oligonucleotides and reported their intracellular compartmentalization. Aynie and co-workers, 1999 designed a new antisense oligonucleotide (ON) carrier system based on "sponge-like" alginate nanoparticles and investigated

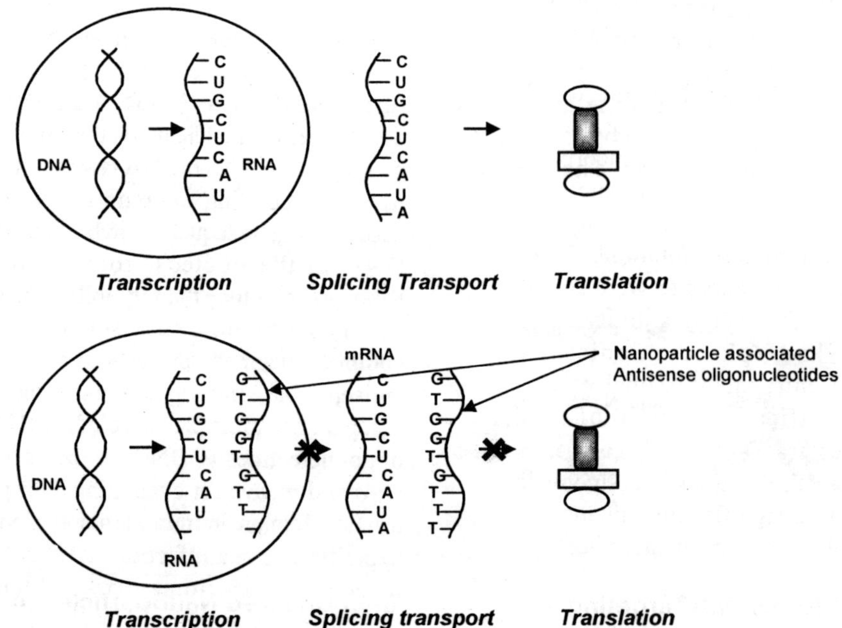

Fig. 9-43. Protection of Antisense Structure and Improve Passage through the Cell Membrane when Associated with Nanoparticles

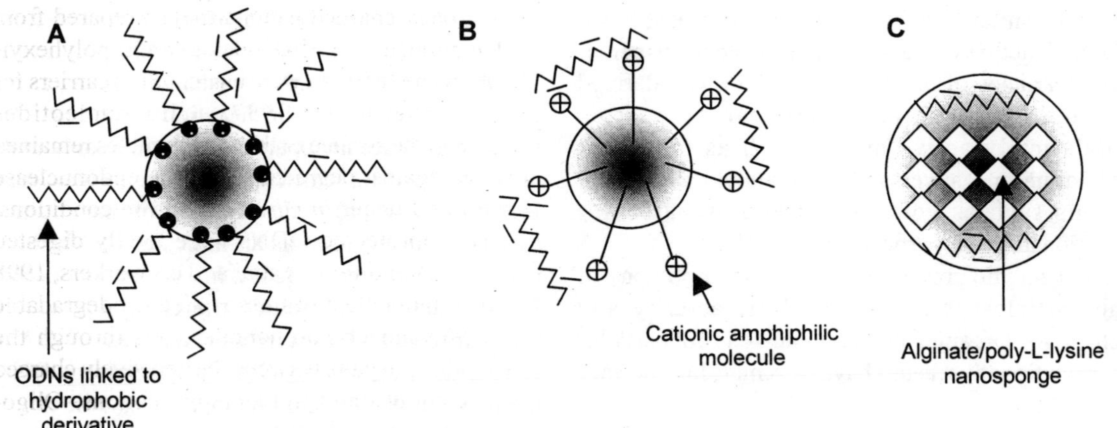

Fig. 9-44. Different Mechanisms by which ODN can be Associated with Nanoparticles

its ability to protect ON from degradation in the presence of serum. This new alginate-based system was found to be able to protect [^{33}P]-radiolabeled ON from degradation in bovine serum medium and exhibited modified biodistribution in the lungs, liver and spleen after intravenous administration into mice. Such nanosponges are promising carriers for specific delivery of ON to lungs, liver, and spleen. Recent studies suggested that lipophilic polymethylmethacrylate (PMMA) homopolymer nanoparticles show a negative surface charge and, therefore, are not suitable for the adsorption of anionic oligonucleotides. However, if the surface charge is changed to positive values by the incorporation of basic monomers, the resultant cationic copolymer (aminoalkylmethacrylate methylmethacrylate copolymer) nanoparticles containing 30% (w/w) methylaminoethyl-methacrylate were found to be optimal in regard to biocompatibility and carrier properties for hydrophilic anionic antisense oligonucleotide entrapment (Zobel et al., 1999; 2000). A significant portion of adsorbed oligonucleotides was protected from enzymatic degradation. The cellular uptake of oligonucleotides into Vero cells was significantly enhanced by this methylaminoethyl-methacrylate derivative.

Nanoparticles for Lymph Targeting

The major purpose of lymph targeting is to provide an effective anticancer chemotherapy to prevent the metastasis of tumour cells by accumulating the drug in the regional lymph node via subcutaneous administration. The objective of lymph node targeting also involve the localization of diagnostic agent to the regional lymph node for the lymphatic vessel visualization before surgery and also the improvement of peroral bioavailability of macromolecular drugs like polypeptides and proteins, which are absorbed via Peyer's patches in the intestine. A wide range of studies are carried out to date for the lymphatic targeting using nanoparticle as drug carriers:

1. Polyalkylcyanoacrylate nanoparticles bearing anticancer drugs (Couvreur et al., 1990) for tumour of peritoneal cavity
2. Polyisobutylcyanoacrylate nanoparticles loaded with insulin for peroral peptide delivery through Peyer's patches (Damge et al., 1990)
3. Poly(lactide-co-glycolide) nanoparticles for the lymphatic delivery of diagnostic agents (Hawley et al., 1997)
4. Magnetite-dextran nanoparticles as a contrast agent in magnetic resonance imaging (Chouly et al., 1996)
5. Polyalkylcyanoacrylate nanocapsules bearing marker (ASA) for lymphatic delivery (Nishioka and Yoshino, 2001).

Functionalized Nanoparticles: A New Dimension in Innovative Research

Functionalized nanoparticles can be prepared from catalytically active and non-catalytically active metals with or without additional surface active groups. These functionalized systems are mono-disperse-sized particles of uniform shape with well-defined surface compositions. Nanoparticles from catalytically active metals such as platinum, palladium and silver and non-catalytically active metals such as gold, have been prepared for functionalization purposes (Fig. 9-45).

In catalytic process, the size and morphology of the particles determine catalytic activity and selectivity. Organically functionalized nanoparticles of catalytic active metals have extremely high surface

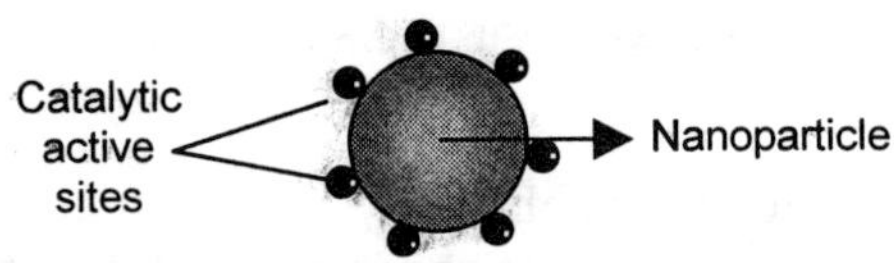

Fig. 9-45 Functionalized Nanoparticles With Multiple Catalytic (or Non-catalytic) Active Binding Sites

area (a large number of catalytic active sites per particle) and unique size-dependent chemical behaviour. This enables their application in a variety of homogenous and heterogenous catalytic processes from petroleum cracking to polymer synthesis, biopolymer templating, biomolecular lithography and fabricating nanoelectronic devices. Gold nanoparticles (non-catalytically active) are often employed as size-markers for measuring the dimensions of biological structures. Several applications are proposed for functionalized nanoparticles and include:

- Biomedical and medical applications of surface modified functionalized nanoparticles (specific cell labeling, specific cell preparation, affinity chromatography, cell growth, diagnostics)
- Specific hemo-perfusion (specific removal from whole blood of toxic materials such as antigens, antibodies, immuno-complexes and heavy metal ions)
- Synthesis, characterization and biological use of functionalized thin film coatings (self-assembled monolayer and multilayer coatings on substrates)
- Enzyme immobilization
- Controlled release polymeric systems

Recently, Mirkin and co-workers, 1996, 2000a, 2000b demonstrated DNA-based gold nanoparticle assembly approach for the detection of specific DNA sequences. Since nanoparticles assemble only in the presence of a complementary DNA strand, the change in the material properties induced by nanoparticle assembly can be used as an indicator of whether a particular sequence is present in a sample or not (Fig. 9-46). Such ploys include the changing optical, mechanical and electric properties of DNA-functionalized nanoparticles, for example, on DNA-mediated assembly, gold nanoparticles will change from red to blue, and this change can be correlated to the presence of a DNA target.

Mirkin and co-workers, 2000a,b have further extended the nanoparticle assembly strategy to analyze combinatorial DNA arrays (or "gene chips"). DNA-functionalized gold nanoparticles assemble onto a sensor surface only in the presence of a complementary ligand. In case a patterned sensor surface of multiple DNA strands is used, the technique can detect different DNA sequences simultaneously.

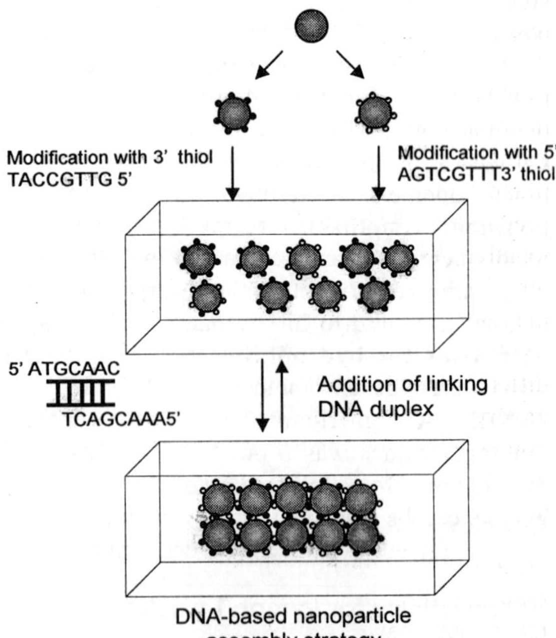

Fig. 9-46. DNA-based Nanoparticle Assembly Strategy

Recently, polymeric nanoparticles were functionalized with surface associated amino acids and used in extraction or purification purposes. Darkow et al., 1999 reported functionalized nanoparticles for endotoxin binding and subsequent removal from pure water, dialysis fluids, plasma or blood. Nanoparticles consisting of a polystyrene core and a polyglycidyl methacrylate shell were prepared by a two-step emulsion polymerization. Particles were found to be monodisperse with a mean diameter of about 85 nm. Parent particles were modified with a number of different ligands including diamines of increasing chain length, amino acids and corresponding amines and higher molecular weight ligands like polymyxin B. The modified particles were tested for their endotoxin (ET) binding capacity in water and physiological sodium chloride solution with the Limulus amebocyte lysate (LAL) assay. It was found that the ET binding properties of the different ligands depend both on the ability of the ligand to form Coulomb- and Vander Waals-interactions with the ET molecule influenced by the nature of the suspension medium. Therefore, the choice of ligands for particle modification has to consider minutely the conditions under which ET is to be removed, e.g. removal from pure water, dialysis fluids, plasma or blood. Mullaney and co-workers, 1999 investigated plasma protein adsorption on functionalized nanoparticles for their application in apheresis. Particles with specific ligands for the adsorption of plasma proteins can be used in therapeutic or preparative apheresis. Nanoparticles were functionalized with aliphatic diamines of increasing chain length; with the amino acids lysine, tryptophan, histidine, and their corresponding amines; and with tryptophan and histidine spaced with diamines of different length (Mullaney et al., 1999). However, nanoparticles functionalized with aliphatic diamines bound significantly higher amounts of fibrinogen than all other ligands.

Conclusions

Nanoparticles containing contrast agents or gamma-emitters such as radioactive iodine, indium or technetium have been used as imaging agents in tumour localization and also for imaging of other body compartments (Guo et al., 1992). Other applications of nanoparticles include solid phase for enzyme immunoassays, and sustained intramuscular depot injection of proteins, peptides and other therapeutic agents (Nilsson, 1989). In addition, nanoparticles have been used as a drug carrier in transdermal formulations to enhance absorption of therapeutic agents (de Vringer and de Ronde, 1995). With the advent of novel nanoparticulate systems like co-polymerized peptide particles, synthetic nanoemulsions, aquasomes, dendrimers and others, the nanoparticulate technology seems to dominate the field of drug delivery and drug targeting in future.

REFERENCES

Absolom D. R. (1986) *Methods Enzymol.* **132**, 281.

Akiyoshi K. and Sunamoto S. (1992) *J. Surfactants Sci. Ser.* **44**, 289.

Akiyoshi K., Nishikawa T., Shichibe S. and Sunamoto J. (1995) *Chem. Lett.* 707.

Al Khouri Fallouh N., Roblot-Treupel L., Fessi H., Devissaguet J. P. and Puisieux F. (1985) *Int. J. Pharm.* **28**, 125.

Allemann E., Gurny R. and Doelker E. (1992) *Int. J. Pharm.* **87**, 247.

Allemann E., Gurny R. and Doelker E. (1993a) *Eur. J. Pharmcol. Biopharm.* **39**, 173.

Allemann E., Leroux J. C., Gurny R. and Doelker E. (1993b) *Pharm. Res.* **10**, 1732.

Allen T. M. (1994) *Adv. Drug Deliv. Rev.* **13**, 285.

Almeida A. J., Runge S. and Muller R. H. (1997) *Int. J. Pharm.* **149**, 255.

Alonso M. J. (1996) In: Microparticulate systems for the delivery of proteins and vaccines, Cohen S. and Bernstein H. (Eds.), Marcel Dekker, New York, 203.

Ammoury N., Fessi H., Devissaget J. P., Puisieux F. and Benita S. (1990) *J. Pharm. Sci.* **79**, 763.

Arangoa M. A., Ponchel G., Orecchioni A. M., Renedo M. J., Duchene D. and Irache J. M. (2000) *Eur. J. Pharm. Sci.* **11**, 333.

Araujo L., Lobenberg R. and Kreuter J. (1999) *J. Drug Target.* **6**, 373.

Auvillain M., Cave G., Fessi H. and Devissaguet J. P. (1989) *STP Pharm. Sci.* **5**, 738.

Aynie I., Vauthier C., Chacun H., Fattal E. and Couvreur P. (1999) *Antisense Nucleic Acid Drug Dev.* **9**, 301.

Beck P., Kreuter J., Reszka R. and Fichtner I. (1993) *J. Microencap.* **10**, 101.

Bednorz J. and Muller A. (1986) *Z. Phys.* **B64**, 189.

Bertling W. M., Gareis M., Paspaleeva V., Zimer A., Kreuter J., Numberg E. and Harrer P. (1989) *Biotechnol. Appl. Biochem.* **13**, 390.

Berton M., Allemann E., Stein C. A. and Gurny R. (1999) *Eur. J. Pharm. Sci.* **9**, 163.

Bhargava K. and Aindo H. Y. (1992) *Pharm. Res.* **9**, 776.

Bindschaedler C., Gurny R. and Doelker E. (1990) *US Patent* 4,968,350.

Birrenbach G. and Speiser R. (1976) *J. Pharm. Sci.* **65**, 1763.

Blunk T., Hochstrasser D. F., Sanchez J. C., Muller B. W. and Muller R. H. (1993) *Electrophoresis* **14**, 1382.

Bodmeier R. and Chen H. (1990) *J. Control. Rel.* **12**, 223.

Bonduelle S., Foucher C., Leroux J. C., Chouinard F., Cadieux C. and Linaerts V. (1992) *J. Microenacap.* **9**, 173.

Breton P. (1996) *Eur. J. Pharm. Biopharm.* **43**, 95.

Carpignano R., Gasco M. R. and Morel S. (1991) *Pharm. Acta helv.* **66**, 28.

Carstensen H., Muller B. W. and Muller R. H. (1991) *Int. J. Pharm.* **67**, 29.

Cay O., Kruskal J., Thomas P. (1996) *J Vasc Interv Radiol.* **7**, 409.

Chacon M., Berges L., Molpeceres J. Aberturas M. R. and Guzman M. (1996) *Int. J. pharm.* **141**, 81.

Chew C. H., Gan L. M. and Shah D. O. (1990) *J. Dispers. Sci. Technol.* **11**, 593.

Chiannilkulchai N., Driouich Z., Benoit J.P., Parodi A. L. and Couvreur P. (1989) *Sel. Cancer Ther.* **5**, 1.

Chouly C., Pouliquen D., Lucet I., Jeune J. J. and Jallet P. (1996) *J. Microencaps.* **13**, 245.

Coester C. J., Langer K., Briesen H. V. and Kreuter J. (2000) *J. Microencap.* **17**, 187.

Cohen H., Levy R. J., Gao J., Fishbein I., Kousaev V., Sosnowski S., Slomkowski S. and Golomb G. (2000) *Gene Ther.* **7**, 1896.

Couvreur P. and Vauthier C. (1991) *J. Control. Rel.* **17**, 187.

Couvreur P., Grislain L., Linaerts V., Brasseur P., Guiot P. and Biernacki A. (1986) In:Biodegradable polymeric nanoparticles as drug carriers for anti-tumour agents, Polymeric nanoparticles as drug carriers for antitumour agents, Guiot P. and Couvreur P. (Eds.), CRC Press, Boca Raton, FL, 27.

Couvreur P., Kante B., Grislain L., Roland M. and Speiser P. (1982) *J. Pharm. Sci.* **71**, 790.

Couvreur P., Roblot-Treupel L., Poupon M. F., Brasseur F. and Puisieux F. (1990) *Adv. Drug Deliv. Rev.* **5**, 209.

Cuvier C., Roblot-Treupel L., Millot J. M., Lizard G., Chevillard S., Manfait M., Couvreur P. and Poupon M. F. (1992) *Biochem. Pharmacol.* **44**, 509.

Damage C., Michel C., Aprahamiam M., Couvreur P. and Devissaguet J. P. (1990) *J. Control. Rel.* **13**, 233.

Darkow R., Groth T., Albrecht W., Lutzow K. and Paul D. (1999) *Biomaterials* **20**, 1277.

De Jaeghere F., Alleman E., Leroux J. C., Stevels W., Feijen J., Doelker E. and Gumy R. (1999) *Pharm. Res.* **16**, 859.

De Jaeghere F., Doelker E., and Gumy R. (1999) In: Encyclopedia of controlled drug delivery, Mathiowitz, E. (Ed.), Vol. II, John Wiley and Sons, New York, 641.

De Verdiere C., Dubernet C., Nemati F., Soma E., Appel M., Ferte J., Bernard S., Puisieux F. and Couvreur P. (1997) *Br. J. Cancer* **76**, 198.

De Vringer T. and De Ronde H. (1995) *J. Pharm. Sci.* **84**, 466.

Denkbas E. B., Seyyal M. and Piskin E. (1999) *J Microencapsul.* **16**, 741.

Desai M., Labhasetwar V., Song S., Qu X., Amidon G. and Levy R. (1995) *Pharm. Res.* **12**, S233.

Diepold R., Kreuter J., Himber J., Gury R., Lee V. H. I., Robinson J. R., Seattone M. F. and Schnaudingel, O. F. (1989) *Archieve Clin. Exp. Opthalmol.* **227**, 188.

Douglas S. J., Davis S. S. and Illum L. (1986) *Int. J. Pharm.* **34**, 145.

Douglas S. J., Davis S. S. and Illum L. (1987) *CRC Crit Rev. Ther Drug Carr. Syst.* **3**, 233.

Durbin D. P., El-Aasser M. S., Poehlein G. W. and Vanderhoff J. W. (1979) *J. Appl. Polym. Sci.* **24**, 703.

El-Samaligy M. S., Rohdewald P. and Mahmoud H.A. (1986) *J. Pharm. Pharmacol.* **38**, 216.

Endicott J. A. and Ling V. (1989) *Annu. Rev. Biochem.* **58**, 137.

Ezpeleta I., Arangoa M. A., Irache J. M., Stainmesse S., Chabenat C., Popineau Y. and Orecchioni A. M. (1999) *Int. J. Pharm.* **191**, 25.

Fattal E., Vauthier C., Aynie I., Nakada Y., Lambert G., Malvy C. and Couvreur P. (1998) *J. Control. Rel.* **53**, 137.

Fattal F., Rojas J., Roblot-Troupel L., Andremont A. and Couvreur P. (1991) *J. Microencap.* **8**, 29.

Fattal F., Youssef M., Couvreur P. and Andremont A. (1989) *Antimicrob. Agents Chemother.* **33**, 1540.

Fernandez-Urrusuno F. R., Fattal E., Rodrigues J. M., Jr., Feger J., Bedossa P. and Couvreur, P. (1996) *J. Biomed. Mater. Res.* **31**, 401.

Fessi H., Puisieux F. and Devissaguet J. P. (1987) *European Patent* 274 961.

Fessi H., Puisieux F., Devissaguet J. P., Ammoury N. and Benita S. (1989) *Int. J. Pharm.* **55**, R1.

Florence A. T., Hillery A. M., Hussain N. and Jani P. U. (1995) *J. Drug Target.* **3**, 65.

Fusai T., Boulard Y., Durand R., Paul M., Bories C., Rivollet D., Astier A., Houin R. and Deniau M. (1997) *Parasite* **4**, 133.

Gallo J. M., Hung C. T. and Perrier D. G. (1984) *Int. J. Pharm.* **22**, 63.

Gasco M. R. (1993) *European Patent Application*, 9 111 3152.2.

Gasco M. R. and Trotta M. (1986) *Int. J. Pharm*. 29, 267.

Gasco, M. R. Morel S. and Viano I. (1991) *Pharm. Acta helv*. **66**, 47.

Gaspard R., Opperdoes F. R., Preat V. And Roland M. (1992a) *Annals Of Tropical Medicine And Parasitology* **86**, 41.

Gaspard R., Preat V., Opperdoes F. R.and Roland M. (1992b) *Pharm. Res*. **9**, 782.

Gautier J. C., Grangier J. I., Barbier A., Dupoint P., Dussossoy D., Pastor G. and Couvreur P. (1992) *J. Control. Rel*. **20**, 67.

Gibaud S., Rousseau C., Weingarten C., Favier R., Douay L., Andreux J. P. and Couvreur P. (1998) *J. Control. Rel*. **52**, 131.

Gonalez-Martin G., Figueroa C., Merino I. and Osuna A. (2000a) *Eur. J. Pharm. Biopharm*. **49**, 137.

Gonalez-Martin G., Merino I., Rodriguez-Cabezas M. N., Torres M., Nunez R. and Osuna A. (2000b) *J. Pharm. Pharmacol*. **50**, 29.

Govender T., Stolnik S., Garnett M. C., Illlum L. and Davis S. S. (1999) *J. Control. Rel*. **57**, 171.

Grangier J. I., Puygrenier M., Gautier J. C. and Couvreur P. (1991) *J. Control. Rel*. **15**, 3.

Gref R., Domb A., Quellec P., Blunk T., Muller R. H., Verbavatz J. M. and Langer R. (1995) *Adv. Drug Deliv. Rev*. **16**, 215.

Gref R., Minimitake Y., Perrachia M. T., Trubetskoy V., Torchilin V. and Langer R. (1994) *Science* **263**, 1600.

Guimaraes R., Clement O., Bittoun J., Carnot F. and Frija G. (1994) *Am. J. Roentgenol*. **162**, 201.

Guzman L., Labhasetwar V., Song C., Jang Y., Lincoff M. A., Levy R. J. and Topol E. J. (1996) *Circulation* **92**, I-292.

Gulyaev A. E., Gelperina S. E., Skidan I. N., Antropov A. S., Kivman G. Y. and Kreuter J. (1999) *Pharm. Res*. **16**, 1564.

Gumy R., Peppas N. A., Harrington D. D. and Banker G. S. (1981) *Drug Dev. Ind. Pharm*. **7**, 1.

Guo C. Y., Shankar R. R., Abe S., Ye Z., Thomas R. N. and Kuo J. E. (1992) *Anal. Biochem*. **207**, 241.

Gupta P. K., Gallo J. M., Hung C. T. and Perrier D. G. (1987a) *Drug Dev Ind. Pharm*. **13**, 1471.

Gupta P.K., Hung, C.T., Lam, F.C. and Perrier, D.G. (1987b) *Int. J. Pharm*. **43**, 167.

Guterres S. S., Fessi H., Barrat G., Devissaguest J. P. and Puisiex F. (1995) *Int. J. Pharm*. **113**, 57.

Harper G. R., Davies M. C., Davis S. S., Tadors Th. F., Taylor D. C., Irving M. P. and Waters J. A. (1991) *Biomaterials* **12**, 695.

Hawley A. E., Illum L., Davis S. S. (1997) *Pharm. Res*. **14**, 657.

Henry-Micheland M. J., Alonso M. J., Andermout A., Sazueres J. and Couvreur P. (1987) *Int. J. Pharm*. **35**, 121.

Hillery A. M., Toth I., Shaw A. J. and Florence A. T. (1996) *J. Control. Rel*. **41**, 271.

Horwitz M. A. (1982) *Rev. Infect. Dist*. **4**, 104.

Hou M. J. and Shah D. O. (1988) In: Interfacial phenomenon in biotechnology and materials processing, Attia Y. A., Moudgil B. M. and Chander S. (Eds.), Elsevier, Amsterdam, 443.

Hunter R.J. (1983) In: Zeta potential in colloidal sciences: principle and applications, Academic Press, London.

Hussain N., Jani P. U. and Florence A. T. (1997) *Pharm. Res*. **14**, 613.

Ibrahim H., Bindschaedler C., Doelker E., Buri P. and Gurny R. (1992) *Int. J. Pharm*. **87**, 239.

Illum L. and Davis S. S. (1983) *J. Pharm. Sci*. **72**, 1086.

Illum L. and Davis S. S. (1984) *FEBS Lett*. **167**, 79.

Illum L. and Davis S. S. (1986) *Int. J. Pharm*. **29**, 53.

Illum L., Davis S. S., Muller R. H., Mak E. and West P. (1987) *Life Sci*. **40**, 367.

Illum L., Jones P. D. E., Baldwin R. W. and Davis S. S. (1984) In: Microspheres And Drug Therapy: Pharmaceutical, Immunological And Medical Aspects Davis S. S., Illum L., Mcvie J. G. and Tomlinson E. (Eds.) Elsevier, Amsterdam, 353.

Irache J. M., Durrer C., Duchene D. and Ponchel G. (1996) *Pharm. Res*. **13**, 1716.

Jeon S. I. and Andrade J. D. (1991) *J. Colloid Interf. Sci*. **142**, 159.

Jiang X. and Liao G. (1995) *Hua. His. I. Ko. Ta. Hsueh. Hsueh. Pao*. **26**, 163.

Johnson J. D., Hand W. L., Francis J. B., King-Thompson N. and Corwin R. W. (1980) *J. Lab. Clinic. Pract*. **95**, 429.

Julienne M. C., Alonso M. J., Gomez J. L. and Benoit J. P. (1992) *Drug Dev. Ind. Pharm*. **18**, 1063.

Kartner N. and Ling V. (1989) *Scientific American* 44, 25.

Kartner N., Evernden-Porelle D., Bradley G. and Ling V. (1985) *Nature* **316**, 820.

Kassab A. C., Xu K., Denkbas E. B., Dou Y., Zhao S. and Piskin E. (1997) *J Biomater Sci Polym*. **8**, 947.

Kattan J., Droz J. P., Couvreur P., Marino J. P., Bouton-Laroze A., Rougier P., Brauls P., Vranks H., Grognet J., Morge X. and Sancho H. (1992) *Invest. New Drugs* **10**, 191.

Kneuer C., Sameti M., Bakowsky U., Schiestel T., Schirra H., Schmidt H. and Lehr C. M. (2000a) *Bioconjug. Chem*. **11**, 926.

Kneuer C., Sameti M., Haltner E. G., Schiestel T., Schirra H., Schmidt H. and Lehr C.M. (2000b) *Int. J. Pharm*. **196**, 257.

Kramer P. A. (1974) *J. Pharm. Sci*. **63**, 1647.

Krause H. J. and Rohdewald P. (1985) *Pharm. Res.* **5**, 239.

Krause H. J., Schwarz A. and Rohdewald P. (1986) *Drug Dev. Ind. Pharm.* **12**, 527.

Kreuter J. (1983) *Int. J. Pharm.* **14**, 43.

Kreuter J. (1991) *J. Control. Rel.* **16**, 169.

Kreuter J. (1994) *Eur. J. Drug Metab. Pharmacokinet.* **19**, 253.

Kreuter J. And Haenzel I. (1978) *Infect. Immun.* **19**, 667.

Kreuter J. and Speiser P. (1976) *J. Pharm. Sci.* **65**, 1624.

Kreuter J. Alyautdin R. N., Kharkevich D. A. and Ivanov A. A. (1995) *Brain Res.* **674**, 171.

Kreuter J., Berg U., Liehl E., Soiva M. and Speiser P. P. (1986) *Vaccine* **4**, 125.

Kreuter J. (1994) In: Colloidal drug delivery systems, Kreuter J. (Ed.), Marcel Dekker, New York, 219.

Kreuter J., Liehl E., Berg U., Soiva M. and Speiser P. P. (1988) *Vaccine* **6**, 253.

Kreuter J., Stieneker F. and Lower J. (1991) *Poc. Int. Symp. Controlled Release Bioact. Mater.* **18**, 277.

Kriwet B., Walter E. and Kissel T. (1998) *J. Control. Rel.* **56**, 149.

Kubiak C., Manil L., Clausse B. and Couvreur P. (1989) *Biomaterials* **10**, 553.

Kukan M., Bezek S., Koprda V., Labsky J., Kalal J., Bauerova K. And Trnovec T. (1989) *Pharmazie* **44**, 309.

Labhasetwar V., Song C. and Levy R. J. (1997) *Adv. Drug Deliv. Rev.* **24**, 63.

Labhasetwar V., Song C. X., Humphery W. R., Shebuski R. J. and Levy R. J. (1995) *Proc. Int. Symp. Control. Release Bioact. Mater.* **22**, 182.

Lamprecht A., Ubrich N., Hombreiro Perez M., Lehr C., Hoffman M. and Maincent P. (1999) *Int. J. Pharm.* **184**, 97.

Lamprecht A., Ubrich N., Hombreiro Perez M., Lehr C., Hoffman M. and Maincent P. (2000) *Int. J. Pharm.* **196**, 177.

Langer K. (1996) *Int. J. Pharm.* **137**, 67.

Langer K., Seegmullaer E., Zimmer A. and Kreuter J. (1994) *Int. J. Pharm.* **110**, 21.

Lewis D. H. (1990) In: Controlled release of bioactive agents from lactide/glycolide polymers, Biodegradable polymers as drug carrier systems. Chasin M. and Langer R. (Eds.) Marcel Dekker, New York, 1.

Li C., Yang D. J., Nikiforow S., Tansey W., Kuang L. R., Wright K. C. and Wallace S. (1994) *Pharm. Res.* **11**, 1792.

Li V. H., Wood R. W., Kreuter J., Harmia T. and Robinson J. R. (1986) *J. Microencap.* **3**, 213.

Lopez-Quintela M. A. and Rivas J. (1993) *J. Colloid. Interface Sci.* **158**, 446.

Lopez-Quintela M. A., Quiben-Solla J. and Rivas J. (1997) In: Use of microemulsions in the production of nano-structured materials, Industrial applications of micro-emulsion. Solans C. and Kunieda H. (Eds.), Macel Dekker Inc., New York, 248.

Losa C., Calvo P., Castro E., Villa J. J. and Alonso M. J. (1991) *J. Pharm. Pharmacol.* **43**, 548.

Losa C., Marchal-Heussler L., Orallo F., Vila Jato J. L. and Alonso M. J. (1993) *Pharm. Res.* **10**, 80.

Luck M., Schroder W., Paulke B. R., Blunk T. and Muller R. H. (1999) *Biomaterials* **20**, 2063.

Lukowski G., Muller R. H., Muller B. W. and Dittgen M. (1992) *Int. J. Pharm.* **84**, 23.

Magenheim B., Levy M. Y. and Benita S. (1993) *Int. J. Pharm.* **94**, 115.

Maincent P., Marchal-Heussler L., Sirbat D., Thouvenot P., Hoffman M. and Vallet J. A. (1992) *Proc. Int. Symp. Controlled Release Bioact. Mater.* **18**, 226.

Malaiya A. and Vyas S. P. (1988) *J. Microencaps.* **5**, 243.

Marchal-Heussler L., Fessi H., Devissaguet J. P., Hoffman M. and Maincent P. (1992) *S.T.P. Pharm. Science* **2**, 98.

Marchal-Heussler L., Maincent P., Hoffman M., Spittler J. and Couvreur P. (1990) *Int. J. Pharm.* **58**, 115.

Marty J. J., Oppenheim R. C. and Speiser P. (1978) *Pharm Acta Helv* **53**, 17.

Masson V., Maurin F., Fessi H. and Devissaguet J. P. (1997) *Biomaterials* **18**, 327.

Michel C., Aprahamiam M., Defontaine L., Couvreur P. and Damage C. (1991) *J. Pharm. Pharmacol.* **43**, 1.

Mirkin C. A. (2000a) *MRS Bulletin.* **25**, 43.

Mirkin C. A. (2000b) *Inorg. Chem.* **39**, 2258.

Mirkin C. A., Mucic R. C., Letsinger R. L., Storhoff J. J. (1996) *Nature* **382**, 607.

Moghimi S. M. and Patel H. M. (1989) *Biochim. Biophys. Acta.* **984**, 379.

Moghimi S. M. and Patel H. M., (1998) *Adv. Drug Deliv. Rev.* **32**, 45.

Moghimi S. M., Muir I. S., Illum L., Davis S. S. and Kolb-Bachofen V. (1993) *Biochim. Biophys. Acta* **1179**, 157.

Molpeceres J., Guzman M., Aberturas M. R., Chacon M. and Berges L. (1996) *J. Pharm. Sci.* **85**, 206.

Moore A., Marecos E., Bogdanov A. Jr. and Weissleder R. (2000) *Radiology* **214**, 568.

Mullaney M., Groth T., Darkow R., Hesse R., Albrecht W., Paul D. and Von Sengbusch G. (1999) *Artif. Organs* **23**, 87.

Muller R. H. and Lucks J. S. (1991) *German Patent Application* P41 31 562.6.

Muller R. H. and Lucks J. S. (1996) *European Patent* 0 605 497 B1.

Muller R. H. and Wallis K. H. (1993) *Int. J. Pharm.* **89**, 25.

Muller R. H., Jacobes C. and Kayser O. (2001) *Adv. Drug Deliv. Rev.* **47**, 3.

Muller R. H., Mehnert W., Lucks J. S., Schwarz C., Zur Muhlen A., Weyhers H., Freitas C. and Ruhl D. (1995) *Eur. J. Pharm. Biopharm.* **41**, 62.

Muller R. H., Schwarz C., Mehnert W. and Lucks J. S. (1993) *Proc. Int. Symp. Controlled Release Bioact. Mater.* **20**, 480.

Muller R. H., Wallis K. H., Troster S. D. and Kreuter J. (1992) *J. Control. Rel.* **20**, 237.

Murakami H., Kobayashi M., Takeuchi H. and Kawashima Y. (1999) *Int. J. Pharm.* **187**, 143.

Nagy J. B. (1989) *Colloids Surfaces* **35**, 201.

Nakagawa Y., Takayama K., Ueda H., Machida Y. and Nagai T. (1987) *Drug Des Deliv.* **2**, 99.

Natsume H., Sugibayashi K., Juni K., Morimoto Y., Shibata T. and Fujimoto S. (1990) *Int. J. Pharm.* **58**, 79.

Nilsson K. G. (1989) *J. immunol. Methods* **122**, 273.

Nishikawa T., Akiyoshi K. and Sunamoto J. (1996) *J. Am. Chem. Soc.* **118**, 6110.

Nishioka Y. and Yoshino H. (2001) *Adv. Drug Deliv. Rev.* **47**, 55.

Norde W. (1984) In: Physicochemical aspects of the behaviour of biological components at the solid/liquid interface, microspheres and drug therapy: pharmaceutical, immunological and medical aspects. Davis S. S., Illum L., Mcvie J. G. and Tomlinson E. (Eds.) Elsevier, Amsterdam, 39.

Norde W. (1992) *J. Dispersion Sci. Technol.* **13**, 363.

O'Hagan D. T., Palin K. and Davis K. K. (1989) *Vaccine* 7, 213.

Ogawara K., Yoshida M., Kubo J., Mnishikawa M., Takakura Y., Hashida M., Higaki K. and Kimura T. (1999) *J. Control. Rel.* **61**, 241.

Ohki A., Naka K., Ito O. and Maeda S. (1994) *Chem. Lett.* 1065.

Olivier J. C. (1996) *J. Control. Rel.* **40**, 157.

Oppenheim R. C. (1986) In: Nanoparticulate drug delivery systems based on gelatin and albumin, Polymeric nanoparticles as drug carriers for antitumour agents. Guiot P. and Couvreur P. (Eds.), CRC Press, Boca Raton, FL, 27.

Oppenheim R. C., Stewart N. F., Gordon L. and Patel H. M. (1982) *Drug Dev. Ind. Phar.* **8**, 531.

Pangburn S. H., Trecony P. V. and Heller J. (1984) In:Partially deacetylated chitin: its use in self-regulated drug delivery system, Chitin, Chitosan and related enzymes Louis J.P. (Ed.) Academic Press, New York, 3.

Pappo J., Ermak L. H. and Steger H. J. (1991) *Immunol.* **73**, 277.

Patel H. M. (1992) *Crit. Rev. Ther. Drug Carr. Syst.* **9**, 39.

Pillai V. and Shah D. O. (1997) In: Microemulsions as nanosize reactors for the synthesis of nanoparticles of advanced materials, Industrial applications of microemulsions. Solans C. and Kunieda H. (Eds.) Macel Dekker Inc., New York, 227.

Pinto-Alphandary H., Balland O., Laurent M., Andermont A., Puisieux F. and Couvreur P. (1994) *Pharm. Res.* **11**, 38.

Pitt C. G. (1990) In: Poly (ε−carolactone) and its copolymers, Biodegradable polymers as drug carrier systems Chasin M. and Langer R. (Eds.) Marcel Dekker, New York, 71.

Ponchel G. and Irache J. (1998) *Adv. Drug Deliv. Rev.* **34**, 191.

Putnam D. A. (1996) *Am. J. Health Syst. Pharm.* **53**, 151.

Quintanar-Guerrero D., Allemann E., Fessi H. and Doelker E. (1999) *Int. J. Pharm.* **188**, 155.

Quintanar-Guerrero D., Allemann E. and Doelker E. and Fessi H., (1997) *Colloid Polym. Sci.* **275**, 640.

Quintanar-Guerrero D., Allemann E., Doelker E. and Fessi H. (1998b) *Pharm. Res.* **15**, 1056.

Quintanar-Guerrero D., Fessi H., Allemann E. and Doelker E. (1996) *Int. J. Pharm.* **143**, 133.

Quintanar-Guerrero D., Ganem-Quintanar A., Fessi H., Allemann E. and Doelker E. (1998a) *J. Microencap.* **15**, 107.

Rajaonaryvony M. J., Vauthier C., Couarraze G., Puisieux F. and Couvreur P. (1993) *J. Pharm. Sci.* **82**, 912.

Roger M. and Kissel T. (1993) *Eur. J. Pharmacol. Biopharm.* **39**, 8.

Rolland A., Bourel D., Genetet B. and Le Verge R. (1987) *Int. J. Pharm.* **39**, 173.

Rolland A., Collet B., Le Verge R. and Toujas L. (1989) *J. Pharm. Sci.* **78**, 481.

Rolland A., Gibassier D., Sado P. and Le Verge R. (1986) *J. Pharm. Belg.* **41**, 94.

Roy K., Mao H. Q., Huang S. K. and Leong K. W. (1999) *Nat. Med.* **5**, 387.

Sakai H., Hanawa K. and Aoyagi K. (1992) *IEEE Trans. Magn. MAG.* **28**, 3355.

Sakuma S., Sudo R., Suzuki N., Kikuchi H., Akashi M. and Hayashi M. (1999) *Int. J. Pharm.* **177**, 161.

Sakuma S., Suzuki N., Kikuchi H., Hiwatari K., Arikawa K., Kishida A. and Akashi M. (1997) *Int. J. Pharm.* **158**, 69.

Samaligy M. S. and Rohdewald P. (1983) *J. Pharm. Pharmacol.* **35**, 537.

Sanchez A. and Alonso M. J. (1995) *Eur. J. Pharmacol. Biopharm.* **41**, 31.

Scherer D., Mooren F. C., Kinne R. K. and Kreuter J. (1993) *J. Drug Target.* **1**, 21.

Scholes P. D., Coombes A. G., Illum L., Davis S. S., Watts J. F., Ustariz C., Vert M. and Davies, M. C. (1999) *J. Control. Rel.* **59**, 261.

Schroder U. and Sthal A. (1984) *J. Immunol. Methods* **70**, 127.

Schroeder U., Sommerfeld P., Ulrich S. and Sabel B. A. (1998) *J. Pharm. Sci.* **87**, 1305.

Sestier, C., Da-Silva, M.F., Sabolovic, D., Roger, J. and Pons, J.N. (1998) *Electrophoresis* **19**, 1220.

Shamkhani A., Bhakoo M., Metzger A. T. and Duncan R. (1991) *Proc. Control. Rel. Bioact. Mat.* Amsterdam, 213.

Sharma D., Chelvi T. P., Kaur J., Chakravorty K., De T. K., Maitra A. and Ralhan R. (1996) *Oncol. Res.* **8**, 281.

Soma C.E., Dubernet C., Barratt G., Benita S. and Couvreur P. (2000b) *J. Control. Rel.* **68**, 283.

Soma C. E., Dubernet C., Bentolia D., Benita S. and Couvreur P. (2000a) *Biomaterials* **21**, 1.

Sommerfeld P., Schroeder U. and Sabel B. A. (1997) *Int. J. Pharm.* **155**, 201.

Song C. X., Labhasetwar V., Gujman L., Topol E. and Levy R. J. (1995) *Proc. Int. Symp. Control. Release Bioact. Mater.* **22**, 444.

Song C. X., Labhasetwar V., Murphy H., Qu X., Humphery W. R., Shebuski R. J. and Levy R. J. (1997) *J. Control. Rel.* **43**, 197.

Speiser P. (1990) *European Patent* EP 0 167 825.

Stieneker F., Kreuter J. and Lower J. (1991) *AIDS* **5**, 431.

Storhoff J. J. and Mirkin C. A. (1999) *Chem. Rev.* **99**, 1849.

Sugibasayashi K., Morimotot Y., Nada T., Kato Y., Hasegawa A. and Arita T. (1979) *Chem. Pharm. Bull.*, **27**, 204.

Sukuma S., Suzuki N., Kikuchi H., Hiwatari K., Arikawa K., Kishida A. and Akashi M. (1997) *Int. J. pharm.* **149**, 93.

Tabata Y. and Ikada Y. (1989) *Pharm. Res.* **6**, 296.

Tan J., Butterfield D., Voycheck C., Caldwell K. and Li J. (1993) *Biomaterials* **14**, 823.

Tiefenauer L. X. Tschirky A., Kuhne G. and Andres R. Y. (1996) *Magn. Reson. Imaging* **14**, 391.

Torchilin V. P. and Trubetskoy V. S. (1995) *Adv. Drug Deliv. Rev.* **16**, 141.

Trouet A. and Tulkens P. (1981) In: The future of antibiotherapy and antibiotic research. Ninet L., Bost P. E., Bouanchaud D. H. and Florent J. (Eds.), Elsevier, Amsterdam, 179.

Truong-Le V. L., August J. T. and Leong K. W. (1998) *Hum. Gene Ther.* **9**, 1709.

Truong-Le V. L. Walsh S. M. Schweibert E., Mao H. Q. Guggino W. B., August J. T. and Leong, K. W. (1999) *Arch. Biochem. Biophys.* **361**, 47.

Tulkens P. and Trouet A. (1978) *Biochem. Pharmacol.* **27**, 415.

Van Oss C. J., Gillman C. F. and Neumann A. W. (1975) In:Phagocytic engulfment and cell adhesiveness as cellular surface phenomena, Marcel Dekker, New York.

Van Snick L., Couvreur P., Vrancks H., Lenarets V. and Ronald M. (1985) *Pharm. Res.* **1**, 36.

Vanderhoff J. W. (1985) *J. Polym. Sci. Polym. Symp.* **72**, 161.

Vanderhoff J. W. and El-Aasser M. S. (1988) In: Pharmaceutical dosage forms: Dispersed systems, Marcel Dekker, New York, 93.

Vauthier-Holzscherer C. (1991) *S.T.P. Pharm. Sci.* 1, 109.

Venier-Julienne M. C. and Benoit J. P. (1992) *Proc. Int. Conf. Pharm. Tech.* **2**, 301.

Venier-Julienne M. C., Vouldoukis I., Monjour L. and Benoit J. P. (1992) *Proc. Int. Conf. Pharm. Tech.* **5**, 4249.

Verrecchia T., Spenlehauer G. and Bazile D. V. (1995) *J. Control. Rel.* **36**, 49.

Vyas S. P. and Malaiya A. (1989) *J. Microencaps.* **6**, 493.

Vyas S. P. and Sihorkar V. (2000) *Adv. Drug Deliv. Rev.* **43**, 101.

Vyas S. P., Singh A. and Sihorkar V. (2001) *Crit. Rev. Ther. Drug Carr. Syst.* **18**, 1.

Wang Y. M., Sato H., Adachi I., Horikoshi I. (1996) *Chem Pharm Bull (Tokyo)* **44**, 1935.

Widder K., Flouret G. and Senyei A. (1979) *J. Pharm. Sci.* **68**, 79.

Youssef M., Fattal F., Alonso M. J., Roblot-Troupel L., Sauzieres J., Tandrade C., Omnes A., Couvreur P. and Andremont A. (1988) *Antimicrob. Agents Chemother.* **32**, 1204.

Zhang Q., Liao G. and Yin H. (1998) *Hua. His. I. Ko. Ta. Hsueh. Hsueh. Pao.* **26**, 172.

Zimmer A. and Kreuter J. (1997) *Adv. Drug Deliv. Rev.* **16**, 61.

Zimmer A., Mutschler E., Lambrecht G., Mayer D. and Kreuter J. (1994a) *Pharm. Res.* **11**, 1435.

Zimmer A., Saettone M. F., Zerbe H. and Kreuter J. (1995) *J. Control. Rel.* **33**, 31.

Zimmer, A., Zerbe, H. and Kreuter, J. (1994b) *J. Control. Rel.* **32**, 57-70.

Zobel H. P., Junghans M., Maienschein V., Werner D., Gilbert M., Zimmermann H., Noe C., Kreuter J. and Zimmer A. (2000) *Eur. J. Pharm. Biopharm.* **49**, 203.

Zobel H. P., Kreuter J., Werner D., Noe C. R., Kumel G. and Zimmer A. (1997) *Antisense Nucleic Acid Drug Dev.* **7**, 483.

Zobel H. P., Stieneker F., Atmaca-Abdel Aziz S., Gilbert M., Werner D., Noe C., Kreuter J. and Zimmer A. (1999) *Eur. J. Pharm. Biopharm.* **48**, 1.

Zur Muhlen A., Schwarz C. and Mehnert W. (1998) *Eur. J. Pharm. Biopharm.* **45**, 149.

Zur Muhlen A., Zur Muhlen E., Niehus H. and Mehnert W. (1996) *Pharm. Res.* **13**, 1411.

CHAPTER 10

Resealed Erythrocytes

Amongst various carriers explored for target oriented drug delivery, vesicular, microparticulate and cellular carriers meet several criteria rendering them useful in clinical applications. Among these carriers, the most important are the one that at least mimic body's intrinsic components and avoid provoking an immune response on intravenous administration. Various cellular carriers proposed are: (a) lymphocytes, (b) leukocytes, (c) platelets, (d) granulocytes, and (e) erythrocytes. Out of all these carriers, erythrocytes have been the most extensively investigated and found to possess great potential in novel drug delivery (Ihler et al., 1973; Zimmermann and Beckers, 1978, Deloach et al., 1989; Juliano, 1980; Vyas and Jain, 1994; Magnani et al., 1998).

DRUG CARRYING POTENTIAL OF ERYTHROCYTES

Red blood cells (RBC, erythrocytes) were discovered in 1658. The developing RBC has the capacity to synthesize haemoglobin, however, adult RBCs do not have this capacity and serve as carriers for haemoglobin. The prime function of these RBCs is to transport gases for respiratory processes. The carrier potential of these cells was first realized in early 1970. The use of cells as drug delivery systems requires that drug (or enzymes) which are normally unable to permeate the membrane, should be made to traverse the membrane without causing any irreversible changes in the membrane structure and permeability. Furthermore, the cells must be able to release the entrapped drug in a controlled manner upon reaching the desired target. The first stage in the processing of drug entrapment requires a reversible and transient permeability change in the membrane, which can be achieved by various physical and chemical means. Once loaded, these cells can be used either for carrying the drug to desired site or they themselves may function as circulating bioreactor. Erythrocytes have been proposed and recently utilized as carriers for a wide range of bioactive components including drugs, enzymes, pesticides, DNA molecules and others. Their capability for prevention of premature degradation or inactivation, slow release profile of loaded drug(s), targeting potential to reticuloendothelial system (RES) and serving as circulatory biovectors for enzymes make them versatile carriers in modern pharmaceutical research and development. However, they are difficult to engineer for a non-RES target, but recent innovations based on biophysically modulated devices may render them suitable for targeting to organs other than RES (Juliano, 1980; DeLoach et al, 1991; Vyas and Jain, 1994; Magnani et al., 1998).

The desirable properties, which substantiate the suitability of red blood cells (erythrocytes) (Fig. 10- 1) as drug carriers are :

- Biodegradability.
- Circulate throughout the circulatory system.
- Large quantities of material can be encapsulated within small volume of cells.
- Can be utilized for organ targeting within RES.
- A wide variety of bioactive agents can be encapsulated within them.
- Erythrocytes are biocompatible provided that compatible cells are used in patients there is no possibility of triggered immunological response.

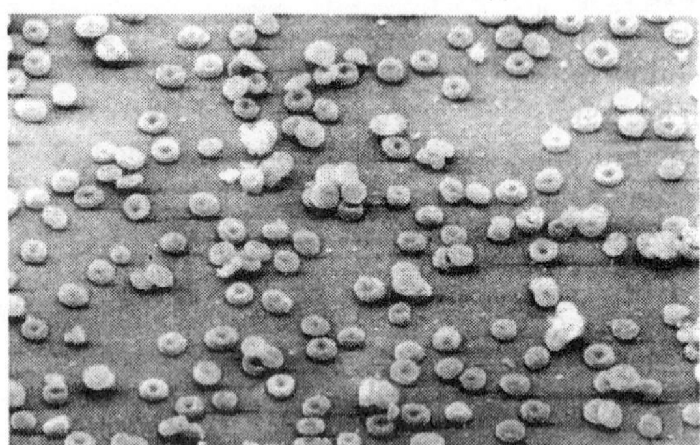

Fig. 10-1. Scanning Electron Microscope (SEM) Photograph of Drug Loaded Resealed Erythrocytes

BASIC FEATURES OF ERYTHROCYTES

Composition of Erythrocytes

The blood contains about 55% of fluid portion (plasma) and nearly 45% of corpuscles or formed elements. The fluid portion contains a large number of organic and inorganic substances in solution, which may be diffusible (electrolytes, anabolic and catabolic substances formed during metabolism) and non-diffusible (proteins) (Chatterjee, 1995). The formed element or cellular portion of the blood consists of erythrocytes (red blood cells), leukocytes (white blood cells) and thrombocytes (platelets). The plasma constituents help in maintaining the isotonicity and the morphology of the red blood cells. Manipulation in plasma compositions *ex vivo* could be used to design various delivery systems. Normal blood cells have extensile, elastic, biconcave and non-nucleated configuration with a diameter ranging from 6-9 μ with a mean diameter of 7.5 μ. The thickness is nearly 1 μ in the center with an increased thickness (~2μ) near the periphery. They have a life span of about 100-120 days. The erythrocytes being non-nucleated do not have the machinery to synthesize new carbohydrates, proteins and lipids and replace them with plasma components to rebuild its membrane constituents. Erythrocytes have a solid content of about 35% (rest 65% being water) most of which is haemoglobin which remains tightly bound to the stroma of the cell membrane.

Haemoglobin is determined spectrophotometrically at 540 nm, either directly or after the conversion of haemoglobin to cyanomethyl-haemoglobin using Drabkin's reagent. Most of the remaining solid is represented by proteins and lipids, which form the stroma or framework which concentrate on the cell surface as limiting membrane (cell wall). The phosphate content (50-100 mg/100 gm) of the erythrocytes is higher than that found in the plasma, most of which is organic in nature, i.e., triphosphate, hexosephosphate, ATP and traces of NAD and NADP. The lipid content of the erythrocytes essentially includes cholesterol, lecithin and cephaelins.

Electrolyte Composition of Erythrocytes

The electrolyte composition of the erythrocytes is although qualitatively similar to that of plasma however, quantitatively it differs from that of plasma.

The concentration of K^+ and Na^+ differ in that the former is more in erythrocytes and the later in plasma. The osmotic pressure of the interior of the erythrocytes is equal to that of plasma and termed as isotonic (normally equivalent to the osmotic pressure of 0.9% NaCl, commonly known as normal or physiological saline). Changes in the osmotic pressure of the medium surrounding the red blood cells (either *in vivo* or *in vitro*) change and manipulate the morphology and tonicity of the cells. If the medium is hypotonic water diffuses into the cells and they get swelled and eventually loose all their haemoglobin content and may burst. On the other hand, if the medium is hypertonic, (i.e., one having a higher osmotic pressure than 0.9% NaCl) they will shrink and become irregular (crenated) in appearance. However, 0.9% saline solution lack necessary ions for the functionality of the cells. Balanced ion solutions like Ringer's, Ringer-Loche and Tyrode's solution, which are not only isotonic but also contain ions in proper quantity, are used in erythrocyte related experiments.

The flexibility of red blood cells (erythrocytes, RBC) retains its shape and morphology when placed in isotonic saline after being challenged with altered tonicity environments (Fig. 10-2). These properties lend them suitable carriers for drugs and enzymes.

Haematocrit Value and Erythrocyte Sedimentation Rate

The blood volume in normal individuals is about 7% (for male) and ~6.5% (female) of body weight respectively. The haematocrit is the percent volume occupied by the cells and is determined by simple centrifugation of the blood. When blood, in the presence of some anticoagulant is centrifuged the cells settle down to the bottom of the tube, while the plasma rises up to the top. Normally the cells constitute about 45% (for males) and 41% (for females) of the total volume. This is referred to as normal haematocrit or in modern terminology as volume of packed red cells (VPRC). Expressed in International units, the normal VPRC for males is 0.45 litres per litre (l/l), and for females, it is about 0.41 l/l (Chatterjee, 1995).

The erythrocytes are often characterized in terms of haematocrit value, i.e., the fraction of erythrocyte portion to total blood. It is expressed as the volume ratio of packed cell to total volume of the blood. The haematocrit value is a parameter that indicates both the number and size of the erythrocytes. The erythrocytes are also characterized by erythrocyte sedimentation rate (ESR). When the blood is mixed with an anticoagulant and kept for sometime, the erythrocytes form aggregates and settle down under the force of gravity alone, the rate at which this settling occurs is known as erythrocyte sedimentation rate. The volume of clear plasma above the sedimenting erythrocyte at the end of 1 h determines the erythrocyte sedimentation rate.

SOURCE, FRACTIONATION AND ISOLATION OF ERYTHROCYTES

Different mammalian erythrocytes have been exploited for drug loading, resealing and subsequent use in drug and enzyme delivery. Majority of them is constructed of red blood cells of mice, cattle, pigs, dogs, sheep, goats, monkeys, chicken, rats and rabbits. Usually to isolate erythrocytes, blood is collected into heparinized tubes by venipuncture. EDTA or heparin can be used as an anticoagulant (Bailleul et al., 1990). Whole blood from horse, sheep, goat, dog and rabbit is easily collected through venipuncture. However, with mice, either the orbital sinus or the heart is used as a collection site. The differences in encapsulation efficiencies of

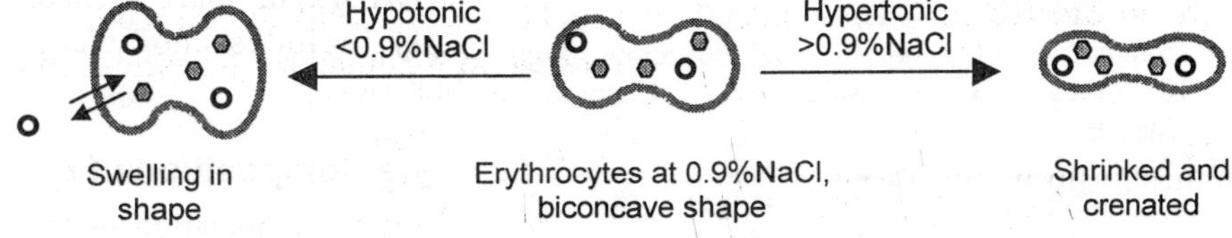

Fig. 10-2. Various Shapes and Morphology of Erythrocytes Under Different Osmotic Environments

erythrocytes isolated from the aged and fresh blood could be cited as reasons behind using fresh whole animal blood for the isolation of erythrocytes for drug delivery purpose. Fresh whole blood in this sense is defined as any blood collected and immediately chilled to 4 °C and stored for not more than 2 days. Red blood cells are harvested and washed by centrifugation. Two major differences in all procedures documented so far are the use of different centrifugal (g) force and the composition of the washing buffer. A 10-15 mmol phosphate buffer having a pH of 7.0-7.4 containing 144 mmol NaCl, 5 mmol $MgCl_2$ and 10 mM glucose is adequate for most species (Dale, 1987). With mouse RBCs, centrifugation at 100-500 g results in cells appearing normal by their morphological characteristics. Table 10-1 provides a comparative account of various conditions and centrifugal force used for isolation of erythrocytes and their use in the drug delivery studies (DeLoach, 1987).

Erythrocytes for the purpose of drug delivery studies could be isolated from the blood of any source as described previously using a well established protocol by Jain and Vyas, 1994. After recovering the blood from cardiac puncture and admixing with heparin, it is centrifuged at 2000 g for 5 min at 4±1 °C. This helps in separation of plasma and buffy coat. Packed erythrocytes so obtained are washed with buffer solution (NaCl, 140 mmol/l; KCl, 16 mmol; $MgCl_2$, 4 mmol; $CaCl_2$, 2 mmol; and Tris, 5 mmol, pH 7.4). The erythrocytes recovered after proper washing periods are adjusted with buffer solutions at different haematocrit values as desired in the study. These erythrocytes are often stored in acid-citrate-dextrose buffer at 4 °C upto 48 h prior to use.

METHODS OF DRUG LOADING

In general, the potential use of erythrocytes depends on their ability to encapsulate exogenous enzymes or other substance into erythrocytes. Mostly hypotonic lysis of cells in a solution containing the drug/enzyme to be entrapped followed by restoration of tonicity to reseal them serves as a loading procedure. But other techniques such as electrical breakdown, endocytosis, chemical perturbation of membrane and lipid-erythrocyte fusion have also been utilized. These methods can be classified as described in Figure 10-3.

Hypotonic Haemolysis and Isotonic Resealing Methods

This method is based upon hypotonic lysis of cells in a solution containing the drug/enzyme to be entrapped followed by restoration of tonicity to reseal them (Fig. 10-4). Four variations of the procedure have been described (Table 10-2) based upon modes, by which hypotonicity is produced. The ghost populations so obtained are heterogenous (Ihler et al., 1973; DeLoach et al., 1979; Juliano, 1980; DeLoach, 1986). Three types of ghosts can be distinguished: type I ghosts which reseal immediately after haemolysis; type II ghosts which reseal after

Table 10-1. Various Conditions and Centrifugal Force Used for the Isolation of Erythrocytes

Species	Washing buffer	Centrifugal force (g)
Mouse	10 mmol KH_2PO_4/Na_2HPO_4, pH 7.0; 5 mmol adenosine; 5mmol $MgCl_2$; 10 mmol glucose	100-500
Human	154 mmol NaCl or 10 mmol KH_2PO_4/Na_2HPO_4, pH 7.0; 2mmol $MgCl_2$; 10 mmol glucose	<500
Rabbit	10 mmol KH_2PO_4/Na_2HPO_4, pH 7.0	500-1000
Dog	15 mmol KH_2PO_4/Na_2HPO_4, pH 7.0; 5mmol $MgCl_2$; 10 mmol glucose	500-1000
Cow	10-15 mmol KH_2PO_4/Na_2HPO_4, pH 7.0; 2mmol $MgCl_2$; 10 mmol glucose	1000
Goat	10 mmol KH_2PO_4/Na_2HPO_4, pH 7.0	500-1000
Horse	10 mmol KH_2PO_4/Na_2HPO_4, pH 7.0; 2mmol $MgCl_2$; 10 mmol glucose	1000
Pig	10 mmol KH_2PO_4/Na_2HPO_4, pH 7.0	500-1000
Sheep	10 mmol KH_2PO_4/Na_2HPO_4, pH 7.0, 5mmol $MgCl_2$	500-1000

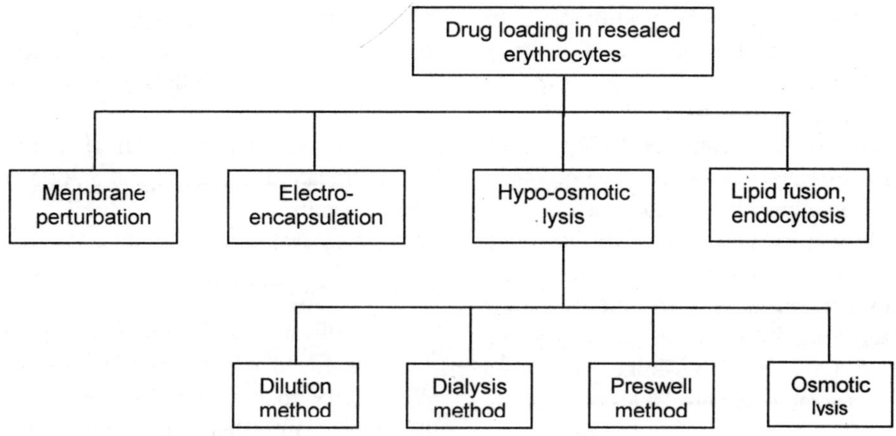

Fig. 10-3. Various Methods of Preparations of Resealed Erytrhocytes

Table 10-2. Comparison of Various Hypoosmotic Lysis Methods

Method	% Loading	Advantages	Disadvantages
Dilution method	1-8%	Fastest and simplest especially for low molecular weight drugs	Entrapment efficiency is very less (1-8%).
Dialysis	30-45%	Better *in vivo* survival of erythrocytes; better structural integrity of membrane due to lesser ionic load	Time consuming; heterogeneous size distribution of resealed erythrocytes
Preswell dilution	20-70%	Good retention of cytoplasm constituents and good survival *in vivo*.	-
Isotonic osmotic lysis	-	Better *in vivo* surveillance	Impermeable only to large molecules, process is time consuming

reversal of haemolysis by addition of alkali ions; and type III ghosts which remain leaky under different experimental conditions. The ratio of three fractions depends on temperature at which haemolysis is affected and on time interval between haemolysis and restoration of tonicity.

Erythrocytes have an exceptional capability for reversible shape changes with or without accompanying volume changes and for reversible deformation under distension (stress). Increase in volume initially leads to conversion of normal biconcave discocytes (normal erythrocytes) to spherocytes. This is because they do not have superfluous membrane or internal membranes and no capacity to synthesize additional plasma membranes, the surface area is inevitably fixed. Thus the cells becomes spheres as they accommodate additional volume with a fixed surface area. However, these swollen erythrocytes have little capacity to resist volume greater than 50-75% of the initial volume and when placed in solutions less than about 150mOsm/kg (corresponding to about 0.4% w/v NaCl), the membrane ruptures, permitting escape of the cellular components.

The principle of using erythrocytes as drug carriers resides in the fact that these ruptured membranes can be resealed by raising the salt concentration to its original (isotonic) levels and upon incubation, the resealed erythrocytes resume their normal biconcave shape and recover their normal impermeability to both macromolecules and ions. Erythrocytes are resealed on addition of sufficient

1.54 M KCl, which restores isotonicity. In experiments where preservation of energy metabolism within the cells is desirable; magnesium salts, glucose and adenosine are included during resealing to attain final concentrations of 4 mM, 10 mM and 2 mM respectively (Ihler and Tsang, 1987). These cells are then allowed to incubate at 37 °C for 30-60 min followed by washing of the resealed erythrocytes with isotonic buffer generally three times to remove unentrapped components. These erythrocytes serve as drug carriers which can be surface modified, i.e. either cross-linked or grafted with antibodies to achieve various levles of targeting (Fig. 10-4)

Loading by "Red Cell Loader"

Magnani and coworkers, 1998 developed a novel method for the entrapment of non-diffusible drugs into human erythrocytes. The equipment designed for this method was termed as "red cell loader". The method requires as little as 50 ml of blood. By using a new apparatus, it is possible to entrap a variety of biological compounds into erythrocytes in as little time as 2 h at room temperature under blood banking conditions. The method is based on two sequential and controlled hypotonic dilutions of washed red blood cells followed by concentration with a haemofilter. Subsequent isotonic resealing of

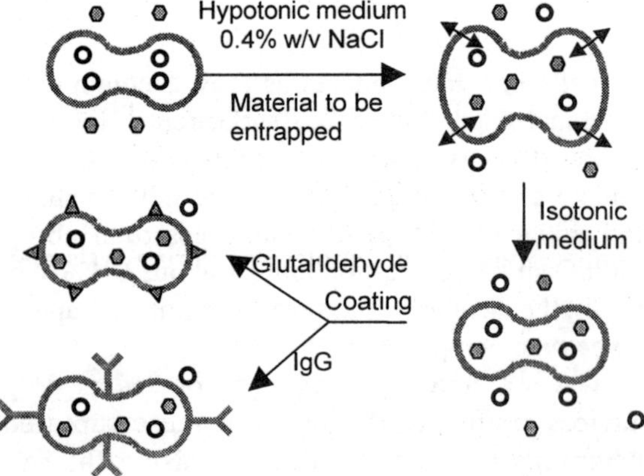

Fig. 10-4. Schematic of Hypotonic Haemolysis and Isotonic Resealing Method of Loading Erythrocytes with Drugs or Enzymes and Haemoglobin is Equilibrated in the Process

erythrocytes allow a 35-50% cell recovery and approximate 30% entrapment of added drug. The resulting processed erythrocytes possess a normal survival *in vivo* and can further be modified using chemical cross-linking by using the same apparatus. The modifications are largely incorporated to increase their recognition by tissue macrophages to perform as drug targeting system.

Dilutional Haemolysis

Population of erythrocytes when exposed to hypotonic saline solution (0.4% NaCl), swells until it reaches a critical value of volume or pressure where membrane ruptures and becomes permeable to macromolecules and ions, therefore permitting the escape of cellular components (Ihler et al., 1973; Ihler and Tsang, 1987). One volume of washed erythrocytes could be treated with 2-20 volumes of materials to be loaded in a hypotonic buffer at 0°C or 5 min. Further incubation at 25 °C in an isotonic solution (0.9% NaCl) reseal them again. In general, the method is rapid and simplest especially for low molecular weight drugs, however the entrapment efficiency remains to be low (1-8%).

Preswell Dilutional Haemolysis

The technique is based upon initial controlled swelling of erythrocytes without lysis by placing them in slightly hypotonic solution followed by centrifugation at low 'g' to take them up to point of lysis (Humphreys et al., 1981; Ihler and Tsang, 1987). Finally, the addition of small volume of drug solution to attain drug loaded resealed erythrocytes (Fig. 10-5). Rechsteiner, 1975 initially utilized the technique, which was further modified by Pitt and co-workers, 1983. Haemolysis and resealing is implemented in three steps :

- First, one volume of washed cells is suspended in five volumes of slightly hypotonic buffer (0.6% w/v NaCl). Under these conditions, only a small percentage of cells lysed and constitute the most fragile population of the erythrocytes. However, the remaining cells, though remain intact but contain an increased cell volume averaging about 150% of the normal cell volume.
- Second, after incubation at 0 °C for 5 min, the cells were recovered by gentle centrifugation.

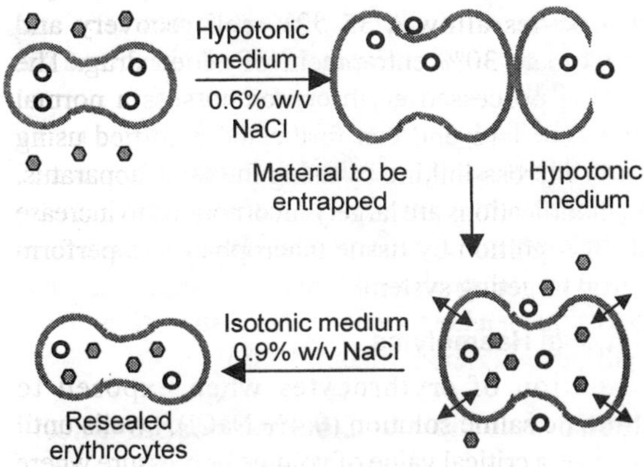

Fig. 10-5. Schematic of Preswell Dilutional Haemolysis and Isotonic Resealing Method of Loading Erythrocytes with Drugs or Enzymes and Haemoglobin is Equilibrated in the Process.

- Third, the swelling procedure is further extended by addition of a volume of hypotonic buffer equal to one half the volume of the swollen cells to effect lysis of the cells. This hypotonic buffer medium also contains the material to be loaded and the cells are allowed to remain lysed for 10 min at 0°C. This is followed by restoration of tonicity and resealing of the membrane.

The gentle swelling of cells results in good retention of cytoplasmic constituents thus a good survival ensues *in vivo*. The encapsulation efficiency by this technique has been reported to be as much as 72% by Field and co-workers, 1989.

Isotonic Osmotic Lysis

In order to avoid the potential disadvantages associated with hypotonic haemolysis, efforts were made to prepare resealed erythrocytes under isotonic (and/or isoionic) conditions. Haemolysis in isotonic solutions can be achieved both by chemical and physical means. If erythrocytes are incubated in solutions of a substance with high transerythrocytic membrane permeability (i.e., small reflection coefficient as defined by the thermodynamics of irreversible processes) the solute will diffuse into the cells due to inwardly directed chemical potential gradient. This will be followed by water uptake until osmotic equilibrium is restored. Various methods are based on this mechanism including :

- Conventional (classical) haemolysis in isotonic urea solutions (Davson and Danielli, 1970)
- Polyethylene induced haemolysis (Billah et al., 1976)
- Ammonium chloride induced haemolysis

The technique of polyethylene glycol induced haemolysis technique is based upon producing transient permeability in the erythrocyte membrane using propylene glycol and this establishes equilibrium within the environment with resultant diffusion of the drugs/bioactives. Incubation of the treated cells under isotonic condition can then reseal the equilibrated erythrocytes by diluting with a glycol free buffer medium (Billah et al., 1977). However ghost cells, obtained from glycol-induced haemolysis seem to be impermeable only to large molecules of dextran and have limited applications as carriers. Ghost cells obtained by NH_4Cl induced haemolysis on the other hand, exhibit properties very similar to normal cells with respect to their permeability to sulphate, monosaccharide, meso-erythitol, sucrose and L-lactate (small molecules). However, even in these methods that exploit isotonic solutions, it is generally impossible to rule out changes in the membrane structure and composition due to the presence of the membrane lytic substances.

Dialysis

The major limitation of dilution procedure, is low entrapment efficiency. It can be overcome by carrying out lysis and resealing within a dialysis tube (DeLoach and Ihler, 1977; Dale et al., 1977; Dale, 1987). Several methods for dialysis based loading of erythrocytes are reported but all take advantage of the common principle that the semipermeable dialysis membrane maximizes the intracellular:extracellular volume ratio for macromolecules during lysis and resealing, but also allows for free flow of small ions, responsible for lysis and resealing of the erythrocytes. It is this intracellular:extracellular volume ratio during the time that the erythrocyte membrane tends to be permeable that determines the % entrapment of bioactives. It considerably reduces the extracellular solution volume that equilibrates with intracellular spaces of erythrocytes during lysis (Fig. 10-6). Haemolysis and resealing is implemented in three steps :

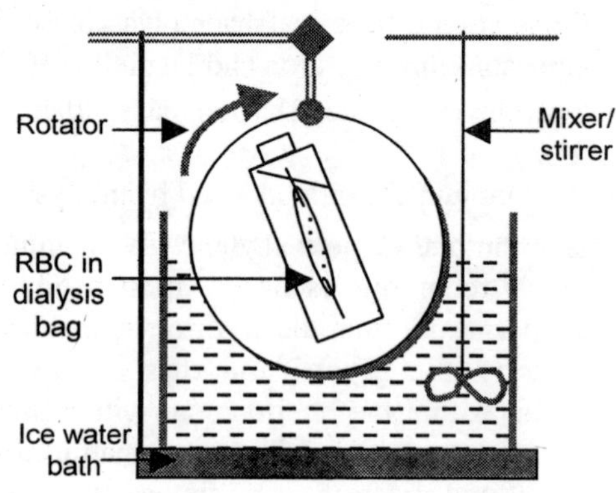

Fig. 10-6. Schematic Presentation of Erythrocyte Dialyzer Apparatus for Entrapping Proteins into Erythrocytes Using Dialysis Method.

- First, washed erythrocytes (haematocrit 85-95%) are mixed with phosphate buffered saline (0.15 M NaCl, 5 mM sodium phosphate, pH 7.4) containing the drug/protein to be entrapped. The volume of buffer used is optimized to a lower haematocrit value of red cells ~ not less than 80% (for example, 7 ml of erythrocyte solution with a haematocrit of 90% needs to be diluted with 0.875 ml of buffer to yield a haematocrit of 80%). This erythrocyte/drug (or protein) mixture is then placed in a dialysis bag.
- The dialysis bag is inflated with an air bubble and sealed in such a way that the erythrocyte suspension occupies no more than 75% of the internal volume. This bubble is critical for the procedure, in that during lysis and resealing, it traverses through the length of the dialysis tubing and serves to blend the contents of the dialysis bag.
- The sealed dialysis bag is then placed in a bottle (or any similar device) containing at least 200 ml of lysis buffer (0.1% w/v NaCl, 0°C) and placed on a mechanical rotator for 2 h at 4°C.
- After the initial lysis at 0°C, the dialysis bag is transferred to a bottle containing at least 200 ml of resealing buffer at room temperature for 30 min.

These dialysis methods considerably improve the drug incorporation efficiencies with high haematocrit values of the resealed cells. The entrapment efficiency increases to 30-45% (Ihler, 1983). This method was successfully utilized for encapsulation of ^{125}I albumin (Ihler and Tsang, 1987). For better *in vivo* survival of erythrocytes the method is most suitable as it imparts structural integrity to membrane presumably due to lesser ionic load and related in process stresses. However, the method is time consuming and does not results in a homogenous size distribution of host erythrocytes (Zimmermann, 1985).

Electro-insertion or Electro-encapsulation

Kinsota and Tsong, 1977, 1978 have suggested the use of transient electrolysis to generate desirable membrane permeability for drug loading into red blood cells. The erythrocyte membrane could be opened by dielectric breakdown and subsequently the pores can be resealed by incubation at 37°C in an osmotically balanced medium. The method is based on creating electrically induced permeability changes at high membrane potential differences. Electric-breakdown is evident when the membrane is polarized for microseconds using varied voltage values. The components can be entrapped when an electric pulse of greater than a threshold voltage of 2 kV/cm is applied for 20μ sec (Teissie et al., 1982). The potential difference across the membrane is built up either directly by inter- and intracellular electrodes or indirectly by applying internal electric field to the cells. The electromechanical compression of the membrane after breakdown leads to formation of pores. The extent of pore formation depends upon the electric field strength, pulse duration and ionic strength of the suspending medium (Tsong, 1987). Once the membrane is perforated, regardless of the size of the pores, ions rapidly distribute between the extra-and intracellular space to attain Donnan equilibrium, however the membrane still remain impermeable to its cytoplasmic macromolecules. The cell membrane eventually lyses because of the colloidal osmotic pressure of its macromolecular contents. In the case of red blood cells, the colloidal osmotic pressure of haemoglobin is about 30 mOsm. This pressure drives water and ion influx as a result leads to swelling of the cells. The membrane is ruptured when the cell volume reaches 155% of its original volume. Thus, cell lysis is a secondary effect of electric modification of the membrane. Since the cell lysis is due to the colloidal osmotic swelling, the rational to prevent lysis is to balance the colloidal osmotic pressure of cellular (or cytoplasmic) macromolecules. This can be affected by the addition of large molecules (like tetrasaccharide stachyose or protein such as bovine serum albumin) and ribonuclease. This helps to counteract the colloidal osmotic swelling of electrically perforated erythrocytes (Fig. 10-7). Thus, the cells do not swell even after their membranes are perforated with small pores. Under these osmotically balanced conditions pores stay open at 4 °C for a few days. If drugs of small molecular weight are added at this point, they permeate into the red blood cells. A suitable procedure could subsequently be used to reseal these pores. Various bioactives like, methotrexate (Zimmerman and Beckers, 1978), isoniazid (Mitchell et al., 1991) and human glycophorin (Mouneimne et al., 1994) have been entrapped using this method. Electrohaemolysis and resealing is implemented in three steps :

1. Washed erythrocytes (haematocrit 10-20%) are suspended in a pulsation medium (mixture of isotonic saline, 150 mM, and isoosmotic sucrose solution, 300 mM) and kept at 4 °C.
2. 0.15 ml of erythrocyte suspension (10-20% haematocrit in a pulsation medium) is transferred to a high voltage pulsation device equipped with a single electric pulse of 2.2 kV/cm (above the threshold value) for a duration of 20 μsec (at 25 °C). However, to make an osmotically balanced loading, macromolecules like saccharides or proteins are added to the erythrocyte suspension, which could subsequently be treated with a 3.7 kV/cm, 20 μsec electric pulse in a medium composed of a 3:7 mixture of isotonic NaCl and isoosmotic sucrose. The cell suspension is transferred to a pre-cooled tube and kept at 4 °C.
3. Resealing of electrically perforated erythrocyte membrane is then affected by incubation at 37 °C in an osmotically balanced medium (Fig. 10-8).

Excellent *in vivo* performance has been reported and normal haemoglobin properties were retained. The technique can also be used to insert proteins into erythrocyte membranes. Mangal and Kaur , 1991 reported that drug loaded erythrocytes prepared by electro-encapsulation method can give a sustained release of entrapped drug. Since the method causes no to negligible membranolytic or deleterious effects, the erythrocytes are not intercepted and sequestered by RES. Thus, they are allowed to remain in circulation and during the course control the release of contents. However, the method is time-consuming and the cost factor is the major disadvantage as compared against preswell and dilution methods.

Loading by Electric Cell Fusion

In this method, the molecules are first loaded into erythrocyte ghosts. These ghosts are then caused to adhere to target cells. Electric pulses are applied to induce fusion of ghost with target cells with subsequent release of the encapsulated molecule. This loading can be exemplified with the loading of cell specific monoclonal antibody to erythrocyte ghosts (Lo et al., 1984; Tsong, 1987). An antibody against

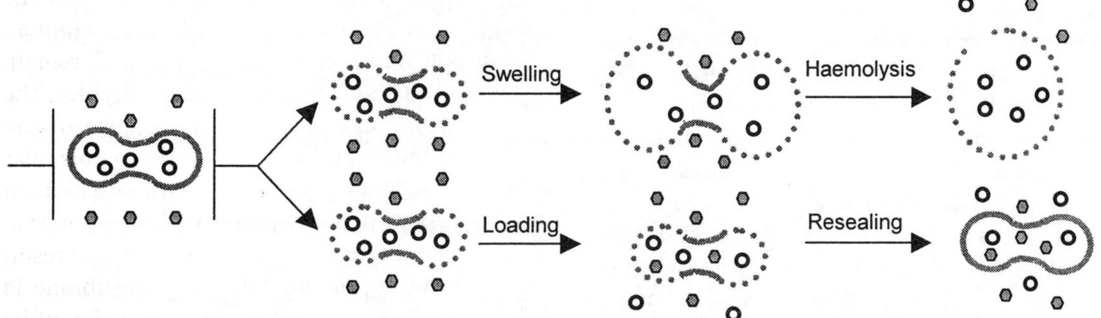

Fig. 10-7. Schematic Presentation of Electro-encapsulation, Where Osmotic Haemolysis of Electrically Perforated Red Cells Causes Loading with Subsequent Resealing of Pores (Adopted from Tsong, 1987)

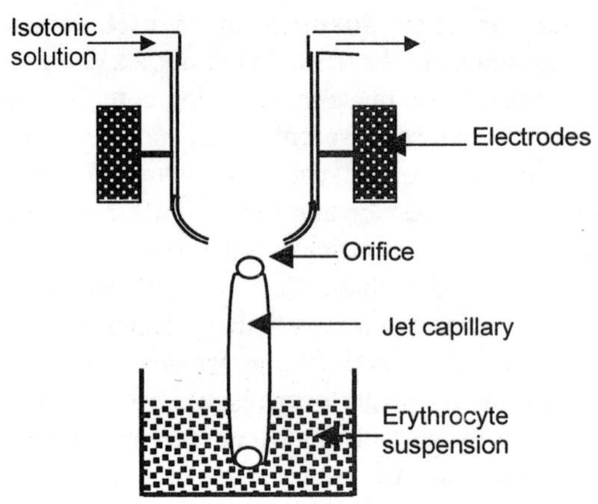

Fig. 10-8. A Schematic Diagram of the System Used to Produce Ghost Cells by Electric Breakdown. (Adopted from Ihler and Tsang, 1987 with minor modifications)

a specific surface protein of the target cells can be chemically cross-linked to drug loaded ghosts. The antibody will direct these ghosts to target cell for adhesion. Electric cell fusion then allows injection of these drugs into the target cells.

Entrapment by Endocytosis

Schrier and co-workers, 1975 described drug entrapment in erythrocyte ghosts by endocytosis. The vesicle membrane separates the endocytosed substance from the cytoplasm, which may shelter drugs prone to inactivation in erythrocytes or alternatively protect the erythrocytes from drug. The resulting erythrocytes contain vacuoles and probably have different *in vivo* survival characteristics from resealed cells, prepared using other methods. The swollen ghosts so prepared exhibit larger (>0.5 μ diameter) endocytic vacuoles. The drug substances are trapped in these endocytic vacuoles (Fig. 10-9). Drug induced endocytosis is quite common and a variety of amphiphilic cations/drugs produce first stomatocytosis and then, mostly at the advancing lip of the stoma, inside-out endocytic vacuole formation. Several classes of drugs as reported by Schrier, 1987 can produce this phenomenon of visible invagination. The best studied are primaquine and related 8-aminoquinolines, vinblastine, chlorpromazine and other cationic phenothiazines, hydrocortisone,

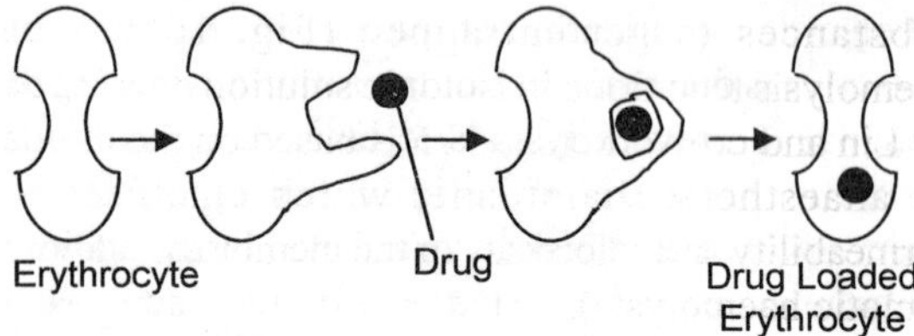

Fig. 10-9. Erythrocyte Endocytosis Produced by Cations and Trapping of Molecules in the Invagination or Inside Out Endocytic Vacuoles.

propranolol, tetracaine and vitamin A (Schrier et al., 1975; Tsang et al., 1982; Schrier, 1987; DeLoach et al., 1991).

Entrapment by endocytosis categorically involves three steps :

- First, one volume of washed packed erythrocytes is added with nine volumes of buffer containing ATP, $MgCl_2$ and $CaCl_2$ to yield final concentrations of 2.5 mM, 2.5 mM and 1 mM, respectively and incubated for 2 min at room temperature.
- Resealing of erythrocyte membrane by the addition of NaCl to 154 mM, followed by incubation for 2 min at 37°C. These resealed cells are washed in 5 mM imidazole-glycylglycine buffer, pH 7.4, containing 154 mM NaCl.
- Third, entrapment of the material by allowing endocytosis following incubation of washed resealed cells with buffer containing the material to be entrapped for 30 min at 37 °C.

The intracellular vesicles could be induced in erythrocytes containing small molecules, drugs or viruses derived from external medium. This also provides an alternative means for loading erythrocytes and allow for successful encapsulation of DNA or particles as large as bacteria which are difficult to be entrapped using the hypotonic haemolysis methods.

Loading by Chemical Perturbation of Membrane (Drug Mediated Loading)

This method is based upon the observation that the permeability of the erythrocytic membrane is increased, when it is exposed to some chemical agents. This allows the low molecular weight substances to get entrapped (Fig. 10-10). A haemolysis technique in isotonic solution developed by Lin and co-workers, 1975 is based on the use of an anaesthetic, halothane, which changes the permeability and selectivity of the membrane (colloid osmotic haemolysis).

Amphotericin B, a polyene antifungal antibiotic, damages microorganism by increasing permeability of their membranes to metabolites and ions. Kitao and Hattori, 1980 utilized this feature for the entrapment of daunomycin in human and mouse erythrocytes. The *in vivo* survival of loaded erythrocytes by this technique however was found to be poor. Due to residual membrane defects they are sequestered from circulation by RES predominant organs.

Loading by Lipid Fusion

Lipid vesicles containing drug can be directly fused with human erythrocytes leading to exchange of lipid entrapped drug. Nicolau and Gresonele, 1979 used this technique for loading of inositol hexaphosphate into resealed erythrocytes for the increased oxygen carrying capacity. The method, however gives very low encapsulation efficiency (1%).

IN VITRO CHARACTERIZATION

Resealed erythrocytes after loading are characterized for following parameters. These *in vitro* characterizations are pivotal to ensure their *in vivo* performance and therapeutic benefits. Table 10-3 records various parameters often used with their

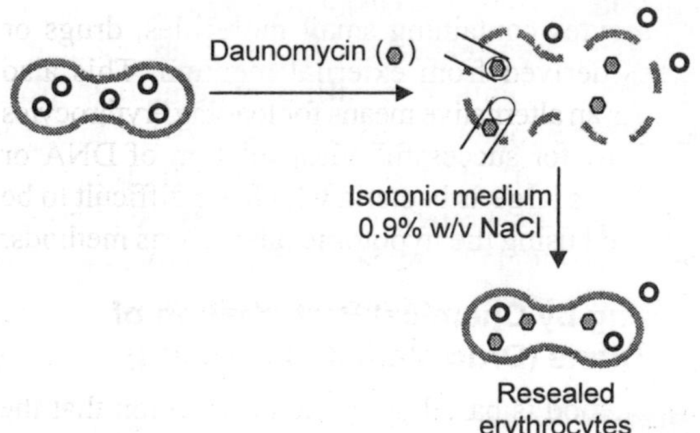

Fig. 10-10. Schematic of Loading by Chemical Perturbation of Membrane (Drug Mediated Loading)

preferred mode of investigations. Some of the routine characterization parameters used to evaluate resealed erythrocytes are described in brief.

Drug Content

Packed loaded erythrocytes (0.5 ml) are first deproteinized with acetonitrile (2.0 ml) and subjected to centrifugation at 2500 rpm for 10 min. The clear supernatant is analyzed for the drug content using specified estimation methodology for entrapped drug (Vyas and Jain, 1994). In case, the resealed erythrocytes are loaded with magnetite to make them magnoresponsive (Jain and Vyas, 1994), a horse shoe magnet (1200 G) is placed adjacent to the base of the centrifuge tube in order to retain the entrapped magnetite. The magnetite concentration in drug loaded erythrocytes could be determined using atomic absorption spectroscopy or some other appropriate procedures (Jain and Vyas, 1994).

In vitro Drug and Haemoglobin Release

Normal and loaded erythrocytes are incubated at 37±2°C in phosphate buffer saline (pH 7.4) at 50% haematocrit in a metabolic rotating wheel incubator bath. Periodically, the samples are withdrawn with the help of a hypodermic syringe fitted with a 0.8 μ Spectropore membrane filter. The samples are then deproteinized with acetonitirle and can be estimated for the amount of drug released. Percent haemoglobin can similarly be calculated at various time intervals at 540 nm spectrophotometrically (Vyas and Jain, 1994). The cumulative % release profile as function of time can be calculated. Percent haemolysis can also be determined by comparing the absorbance of supernatant with the absorbance obtained after complete hydrolysis of same number of cells in distilled water (Jain and Vyas, 1994). Laser light scattering may also be used to evaluate haemoglobin content of individual resealed erythrocytes (Green, 1985).

Another parameter, which evaluates the haemoglobin disposition after the resealing, is the mean corpuscular haemoglobin. It is the mean concentration of haemoglobin per 100 ml of cells, and is an index, which is independent of the size of the red cell and therefore, it is a true expression of their haemoglobin content. It is expressed as :

Table 10-3. Erythrocyte Characterization with Their Quality Control Assays

Characterization parameters	Analytical methods/Instrumentation
Physical characterization	
Shape and surface morphology	Transmission electron microscopy, scanning electron microscopy, phase-contrast optical microscopy
Vesicle size and size distribution	Transmission electron microscopy, optical microscopy
Drug release	Diffusion cell/ dialysis
% Encapsulation [(Amount encapsulated/ amount added to RBC) ×100]	Deproteinization (using methanol or acetonitrile) of cell membrane and assay for released drug or radio-labeled markers
Electrical surface potential and surface pH	Zeta potential measurements and pH sensitive probes
Cell related characterization	
% Haemoglobin content/volume	Deproteinization (using methanol or acetonitrile) of cell membrane and assay for Hb; Laser light scattering for cell volume
Mean corpuscular haemoglobin [Haemoglobin (g/100 ml) ×10/erythrocyte count (per cu mm)]	Laser light scattering
Percent cell recovery (Number of intact cells per cubic mm)	Haematological analyzer; Neubeur's chamber
Osmotic fragility	Stepwise incubation with isotonic to hypotonic saline solutions and estimation of drug and Hb
Osmotic shock	Dilution with distilled water and estimation of drug and Hb
Turbulent shock	Passing cell suspension through a 23 gauge needle hypodermic needle (10 ml/min) and estimation of residual drug and Hb
Erythrocyte sedimentation rate	ESR apparatus
Biological characterization	
Sterility	Aerobic or anaerobic cultures
Pyrogenicity	Rabbit fever response test or LAL test
Animal toxicity	

$$\text{Mean corpuscular haemoglobin} = \frac{[\text{Haemoglobin (g/100 ml)} \times 10}{\text{Erythrocyte count (per mm}^3)} \quad (10\text{-}1)$$

Osmotic Fragility

It is the parameter, which simulates and mimics the bio-environmental conditions that are encountered on *in vivo* administration, *in vitro* handling and the effect of loaded contents on the survival rates of the erythrocytes. When red blood cells are exposed to solutions of varying tonicities their shape changes (swell in hypotonic and shrink in hypertonic environments) due to osmotic imbalance (Sprandel and Zollner, 1985). To evaluate the effects of varying tonicities, drug loaded erythrocytes are incubated with saline solutions of different tonicities (from isotonic to hypotonic, i.e., 0.9 %w/v to 0.1% w/v) at 37±2 °C for 10 min. The suspension after centrifugation at 30 g for 15 min is assayed for drug and/or haemoglobin release, which should be in the acceptable range for a system to be therapeutically effective.

Osmotic Shock

Osmotic shock describes a sudden (and not tapering) exposure of drug loaded erythrocytes to an environment, which is far from isotonic to evaluate the ability of resealed erythrocytes to withstand the stress and maintain their integrity as well as appearance (Ingrosso et al., 1997). Incubating the resealed erythrocytes (1 ml, 10-50% haematocrit) with distilled water (5 ml) for 15 min followed by centrifugation at 3000 rpm for 15 min, may cause the release of haemoglobin to varying degrees, which could be estimated spectrophotometrically.

Turbulence Shock

The parameter indicates the effects of shear force and pressure by which resealed erythrocytes formulations are injected, on the integrity of the loaded cells. Loaded erythrocytes (10% haematocrit, 5 ml) are passed through a 23-gauge hypodermic needle at a flow rate of 10 ml/min (Vyas and Jain, 1994). After every pass, aliquote of the suspension is withdrawn and centrifuged at 300 G for 15 min, and haemoglobin content, leached out are estimated spectrophotometrically. Resealing of the erythrocytes make them sensitive towards turbulence or mechanical agitation and hence an estimation of turbulence shock study provides their expected performance *in vivo*.

Morphology and Percent Cellular Recovery

Phase-contrast optical microscopy, transmission electron microscopy and scanning electron microscopy are the microscopic methods used to evaluate the shape, size and the surface features of the loaded erythrocytes. Percent cell recovery (after loading) can be determined by assessing the number of intact erythrocytes remaining per cubic mm with the help of a haemocytometer.

DIFFERENT FORMS OF DRUG LOADED RED BLOOD CELLS

Normally, more than 80% of the erythrocyte ghosts loaded with drugs or enzymes appear as biconcave disks (discocytes) when they are observed under electron microscope. Less than 20% cells show abnormal morphology (Fig. 10-11). The rest appear as stomatocytes or spherocytes or echinocytes, cells with different infoldins and other abnormal or destroyed forms (Sprandel et al., 1981; 1987). This is due to osmotic balance, which the cells experience when they are exposed during hypotonic drug loading conditions (swell in hypotonic and shrink in hypertonic environments).

On swelling, the cells get converted from diskocytes to spherocytes (sphere shaped structures) and thus get compromised with a lower ratio of surface features (surface area to surface volume). Further increase in hypotonicity may lead to the formation of echinocytes and cells with different infoldings and other damaged forms.

Erythrocytes on haemolysis and washing with large volumes of hypotonic medium, loose nearly all their haemoglobin and on resealing the resultant cells appear as pale or transparent in appearance and are referred to as "Erythrocytes ghosts" or "White resealable erythrocytes ghosts" (Schrier, 1987). However, these ghosts contain 5-10% of their original haemoglobin (as a major cytosolic component), they can not be resealed if they are depleted of all cytosolic components through multiple washing steps. This can be overcome by using gel filtration method for producing ghosts (Schrier, 1987). If haemolysis is allowed to take place under flow conditions, where the relative velocity of the membrane is greater than that of the adjacent medium, then the cytosolic materials continue to diffuse into a medium free of haemolyzate. Diffusion can continue until no

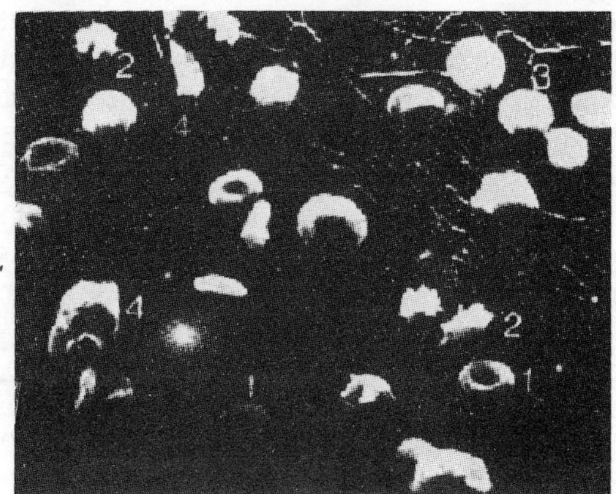

Fig. 10-11 Scanning Electron Microscopy of Different Forms of Red Blood Cells Observed After Loading of Erythrocytes. 1. Discocytes, 2. Spherocytes, 3. Echinocytes, and 4. Some Irregular Infoldings

cytosolic material is present on either side of the membrane. With the proper adjustment of pH to allow maximum desorption of protein from the membrane and, in addition, to allow maximal resealing, a resealable ghost membrane is formed. However, the composition of the cytosol may be restored by the addition of a concentrated stock solution and subsequently, the membrane is resealed by incubation at an elevated temperature. These ghost cells though have little or no capacity for survival *in vivo*, but are useful for the delivery of substances to lysosomes of erythrophagocytic cells. The resealed ghosts have been used frequently to study various transport pathways found in the erythrocyte membrane including the anion-exchange system, sodium pump, and the calcium-activated potassium channel. However more recently, these are used as a vehicle for drug delivery and enzyme therapy.

SHELF AND STORAGE STABILITY OF RESEALED ERYTHROCYTE

Storage of resealed erythrocytes places a major challenge in their practical utility as drug delivery system. Lewis and Alpar, 1984 have reported that encapsulated product and carrier both exhibit satisfactory self-stability when stored in Hank's balanced salt solution (HBSS) at 4 °C for 2 weeks. Similar results were obtained by suspending cells in oxygenated HBSS containing 1% soft bloom gelatin. The cells were recovered after liquefying the gel by placing the tubes in water bath at 37 °C followed by centrifugation. Under clinical conditions standard blood bags may be used for both, encapsulation and storage. The procedure would be to use Group 'O' (universal donor) cells and by using preswell or dialysis technique, batches of preparation could be prepared in adequate amounts and stored as normal erythrocytes, which are used in transfusion (Lewis and Alpar, 1984). Another method utilized for storage has been the cryopreservation of erythrocytes in liquid nitrogen temperatures (Brearly et al., 1988; 1990).

IN VIVO SURVIVAL AND IMMUNOLOGICAL CONSEQUENCES

Erythrocytes loaded using hypotonic haemolysis followed by isotonic resealing; dialysis and electro-encapsulation methods appear to sustain normally in the circulation. A bimodal type of survival kinetics is observed: a rapid loss of cells during first 24 h followed by much slower loss afterwards (Vyas and Jain, 1994). The early loss possibly accounts for removal of nearly 15% of total cell population, this represents the cells that are severely damaged during drug loading procedures. The second phase has a half-life of the orders of weeks for different mammalian erythrocytes. The erythrocyte carriers constructed of red blood cells of mice, cattle, pigs, dogs, sheep, goats and monkeys exhibit comparable circulation profile when compared with unloaded normal erythrocytes. On the other hand, resealed erythrocytes prepared from red blood cells of chicken, rats and rabbits exhibit relatively poor circulation profile as compared against unloaded normal erythrocytes. These inter-subject and inter-species variations from different sources require a judicial analysis and use of the source before experiment protocol is designed.

There are three general modes of efflux of loaded contents from resealed erythrocytes: phagocytosis, diffusion or specific transport mechanisms once placed *in vivo*. RBCs are normally removed from circulation by the process of phagocytosis (Bratosin et al., 1997). Phagocytosis occurs within the reticuloendothelial system (RES). The degree of cross-linking determines whether liver or spleen will preferentially remove the cells. Similarly, carrier erythrocytes following heat treatment, sulphydryl treatment, or antibody cross-linking are quickly removed from the circulation by phagocytic cells located mainly in liver and spleen. Eichler and co-workers, 1986a; 1986b; 1986c investigated *in vivo* survival and reported the potential of erythrocytes in formulating a prolonged and slow release drug carrier system.

It is observed that erythrocyte carriers constructed of autologous sources do not elicit immunological consequences. However, it is customary to realize that during loading process, some antigenic impurities may get entrapped resulting in immunological manifestations. Nevertheless, different studies (Thorpe et al., 1974, 1977; Bax et al., 1999) indicate that autologous sources do not generally contribute to undesirable immune responses.

INFLUENCE OF MEMBRANOLYTIC AND MEMBRANOTROPIC SUBSTRATES

Certain substances influence the geometric balance of normal biconcave discocytes and in turn influence the functioning of erythrocytes in circulation. The parameters affected include normal metabolism, deformability, viscosity and morphology and surface characteristics. These substances which are either utilized in cases of drug loading or chemical cross-linking to render a specific surface property to the resealed erythrocytes can be categorized as follows :

- Membrane active substrates
- Membrane lytic substrates

Ions including sodium, phosphate and magnesium are important and are used in the resealing and annealing medium of loading procedures. These help in keeping a proper balance and osmolarity of the resealing solution and the resultant carriers function optimally in circulation.

Even substrates like glucose and adenosine are required to keep the tonicity of the red blood cells maintained in the resealing solutions. Both calcium ions and oleic acid are membrane active and affect shape of the erythrocytes but has no extracellular effects (Ihler et al., 1973). With an enhanced intracellular concentration of calcium ions, carrier erythrocytes undergo a shape change from discocytes to stomatocytes and finally to spherocytes, however the ghost erythrocytes often convert from discocytes to echinocytes (Sprandel et al., 1981). On the other hand, oleic acid transforms biconcave discocytes into the echinocytes and its effects are both intracellular and extracellular. Moreover, to operate at extracellular level at least 10-fold higher concentration is required. These membrane-modulating effects could serve as physiological models in haematology and in studying membrane behaviour (Sprandel et al., 1987).

On the other hand, some drugs like daunomycin, amphotericin B and primaquine affect the erythrocytes in different way altogether. Amphotericin B, a polyene antifungal antibiotic, damages microorganism by increasing permeability of their membranes to metabolites and ions.

Kitao and Hattori, 1980 utilized this feature for the entrapment of daunomycin in human and mouse erythrocytes. Several classes of drugs as reported by Schrier, 1987 can produce the phenomenon of endocytic invagination. The best studied are primaquine and related analogues of 8-amino-quinolines, vinblastine, chlorpromazine as well as other cationic phenothiazines, hydrocortisone, propranolol, tetracaine and vitamin A.

BIOMEDICAL APPLICATIONS OF RESEALED ERYTHROCYTES

Resealed erythrocytes have found a large number of possible applications in various fields of human and veterinary medicine (Table 10-4) (Bailleul et al., 1990; Gneushev and Gneusheva, 1996; Magnani et al., 1998).

Erythrocytes as Drug/Enzyme Carriers

Erythrocytes could be used as circulating carrier to disseminate bioactive agents over a prolonged period of time in circulation or selectively to liver, spleen and lymph nodes.

Erythrocytes as Carriers for Enzymes

Resealed erythrocytes serve as an ideal carrier for enzymes in the treatment of inherited metabolic diseases. The entrapment of catalase, urease, uricase, invertase, arginase, asparaginase, β-glucuronidase, β-fructouronidase, and β-galactosidase in erythrocytes using hypotonic lysis method has proved that erythrocytes could operate as enzyme carriers (Ihler et al., 1973; Thorpe et al., 1974; Bailleul et al., 1990; DeLoach, 1991). Lizano and co-workers, 1998 reported alcohol dehydrogenase and acetaldehyde dehydrogenase encapsulated into human erythrocytes and used *in vivo* for complete metabolization of ethanol. Sanz and co-workers, 1999 loaded enzyme, glutamate dehydrogenase (GDH) encapsulated in erythrocytes can be used as a potential carrier system for the *in vivo* removal of high levels of ammonia from blood.

Erythrocytes as Carriers for Drugs

Various bioactive agents encapsulated in erythrocytes are developed for the slow and sustained release in circulation to allow effective treatment of parasitic diseases. Resealed erythrocytes serve as an ideal carrier for antineoplastic agents like bleomycin, adriamycin, actinomycin-D, or cytosine arabinoside

TABLE 10-4. Various Applications of Resealed Erythrocytes

Application	Drug/enzyme/macromolecules	References
Enzyme deficiency, replacement therapy	β-galactosidase, β-fructo-furonodase; Urease, Glucose-6-phosphate dehydrogenase; Corticol-2-phosphate; Adenylosuccinate lyase	Ihler et al., 1973; Ihler et al., 1975; Pitt *et al.*, 1983
Thrombolytic Activity	Brinase, Aspirin, Heparin	Flynn *et al.*, 1994; Orekhova *et al.*, 1990; Eichler *et al.*, 1986b
Iron overload	Desferroxamine	Green, 1985
Chemotherapy	Rubomycin, Methotrexate, L-Asparaginase, Doxorubicin, Daunomycin, Cytosine arabinoside, Adriamycin	Kitao and Hattori, 1980; DeLoach, 1982; Benatti *et al.*, 1989
Immuno-therapy	Human recombinant Interleukin-2	DeLoach *et al.*, 1991; Kirch *et al.*, 1994
Circulating carriers	Albumin, Prednisolone, Salbutamol, Tyrosine kinase, Phosphotriesterase	Pitt *et al.*, 1983,
Circulating bioreactor	Arginase, Uricase, Luciferase, Acetaldehyde dehydrogenase	Adriaenssenents *et al.*, 1976; Magnani *et al.*, 1992; Vitvitsky, 1992
Targeting to RES	Pentamidine, Mycotoxin, Imidocarb dipropionate, Homidium bromide, Ricin A chain	DeLoach *et al.*, 1988; DeLoach *et al.*, 1981
Targeting to sites other than RES	Daunomycin, Methotrexate, Diclofenac sodium	Kitao *et al.*, 1978; Flynn *et al.*, 1994; Jain and Vyas, 1994; Vyas and Jain, 1994

in erythrocyte ghosts (Tonetti et al., 1990). DeLoach et al., 1991 used erythrocytes as carrier prolongation bio-life and circulation half-life of cytosine arabinoside. Various antimicrobial drugs like trypanocidal and babesicides, antibiotics and vitamins and steroids have been encapsulated in resealed erythrocytes (reviewed in Magnani et al., 1998).

Erythrocytes as Carriers for Proteins and Macromolecules

Zolla and co-workers, 1991 reported red blood cells as carriers for delivering of proteins. Bird et al., 1983 proposed erythrocytes as carrier for insulin for its sustained release. They have examined a number of low molecular weight compounds for their suitability as inhibitor of insulin degrading system found in erythrocytes. DeLoach and co-workers, 1988 reported the delivery of highly toxic molecules like mycotoxins specifically to liver macrophages by encapsulating in erythrocytes. Garin and co-workers, 1996 reported that carrier RBC-preparations may serve as a cellular sustained delivery system for *in vivo* administration of recombinant human erythropoietin (rHuEpo). Red blood cells coated with recombinant interleukin-2 (rIL-2) are reported by Moyes and co-workers, 1996 to provide a slow and sustained delivery so as to allow low and non-toxic concentrations of IL-2 in the circulation.

Drug Targeting

A drug delivery should ideally be site-specific and target oriented in order to exhibit maximal therapeutic index and minimum side and toxic effects. It has been observed that osmotically loaded erythrocytes can act as drug carriers in systemic circulation, whereas chemically surface modified erythrocytes are targeted to organs of the mononuclear phagocytic system/ reticuloendothelial system (MPS/RES) because of changes incorporated in the membrane that are recognized by macrophage cells (Alvarez et al., 1996). However, recently approaches are employed to target these cellular carriers to sites other than MPS/ RES.

Drug Targeting to RES Organs

The damaged erythrocytes are quickly removed from circulation by phagocytic Kupffer cells located in liver and spleen. Though, resealed erythrocytes have been proposed for passive auto-vectorization to MPS/

RES system where modified surface characteristics lend them the selectivity and specificity towards target cells (mainly liver and spleen). Previous investigation has shown that osmotically loaded erythrocytes can act as drug carriers in systemic circulation, whereas chemically modified erythrocytes can be targeted to organs of the mononuclear phagocytic system because of changes introduced in the membrane that are recognized by macrophage cells (Fig. 10-12). Various approaches for modifying the circulatory and tissue uptake parameters of resealed erythrocytes to make them site specific and target oriented are adopted and are described below.

Surface Modification with Antibodies

Circulatory half-life is shortened on coating resealed erythrocytes with antibodies. Lightly coated (modified) resealed erythrocytes cause a reduction of the half-life from 27 days to several minutes and the majority of the erythrocytes are sequestered by the spleen macrophages. On the other hand, heavily modified cells cause a similar reduction in circulating half-life while in this case, the majority of the erythrocytes are sequestered by liver macrophages, and as a result accommodated in these organs.

Surface Modification with Glutaraldehyde

Lightly damaged or modified erythrocytes are sequestered by spleen similar to normal senescent erythrocytes, whereas liver sequesters/recognizes heavily modified erythrocytes. Since, the liver is perfused 7 times greater than the spleen, the severely damaged cells are predominantly localized to the liver Kupffer cells.

Surface Modification-involving Carbohydrates

Enzymatically modified cell surface carbohydrates of erythrocytes exhibit a different biodistribution as compared to their plain version. Sialidase, an enzyme that removes sialic acid from external glycoproteins and glycolipids, causes a significant reduction in the circulatory half life of the erythrocytes, and make them prone to macrophage uptake especially in liver and spleen (Franco et al., 1981).

Surface Modification with Sulphydryls

The external sulphydryls of erythrocytes can be oxidized to varying degrees and the thus circulatory half-life of the cells can be manipulated from a normal value of 27 days to several minutes (8 min).

Surface Chemical Cross-linking

Cross-linking of loaded erythrocytes increases delivery of encapsulated substance to macrophages. The delivery of ^{125}I-labelled carbonic anhydrase (^{125}I-CA) carried by mouse erythrocytes, either loaded, or loaded and cross-linked with bis(sulphosuccinimidyl) suberate (BS3) and 3,3'-dithiobis-(sulphosuccinimidyl propionate), into homologous peritoneal macrophages was reported by Alvarez et al., 1998. The hypotonically loaded mouse erythrocytes showed a weak recognition by macrophages, similar to native erythrocytes. CA loaded in erythrocytes is thus delivered to a limited extent into macrophages. Neither the number of recognized loaded ^{51}Cr-labelled erythrocytes nor the amount of delivered ^{125}I-CA is affected by the presence of serum components or IgG. In contrast, cross-linking these loaded erythrocytes results in a greater phagocytosis by macrophages as assessed by microscopic observations, producing a markedly increased amount of targeted enzyme. The amount of CA delivered into macrophages, after BS3 cross-linker treatment of erythrocytes, is dependent on the presence of serum components in the incubation

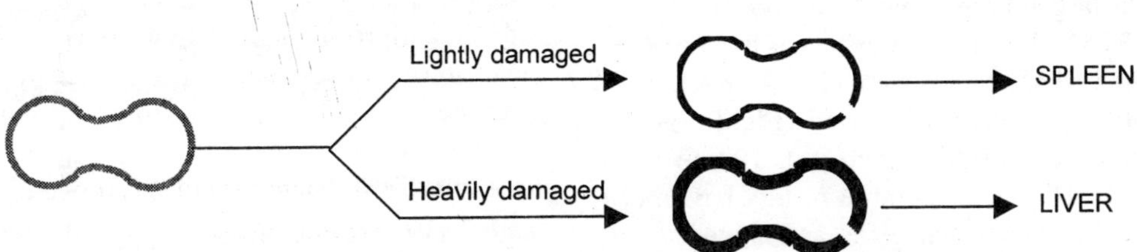

Fig. 10-12 Schematic Presentation of the Bio-fate of Chemically Modified Erythrocytes. Lightly modified or senescent erythrocytes are taken up by spleen, whereas liver captures heavily modified erythrocytes.

medium. Thus these cross-linking treatments improve the capacity of loaded mouse erythrocytes to deliver significant amounts of targeted enzyme to macrophage cells, and thus increase the therapeutic potential of carrier erythrocytes.

Drug Targeting to Liver

Enzyme Deficiency/Replacement Therapy

Enzymes can be injected into blood stream to replace the missing or deficient enzyme in a metabolic disorder. Lysosomal storage disorders (such as Gaucher's disease), hyperargininaemia, hyperuricaemia, hyperphenylalaninaemia, and kidney failure are some examples of metabolic disorders that can be treated by enzyme(s) based therapy. Exogenous enzyme therapy is complicated by the short half-life of enzymes in blood stream, allergic reactions and occasional toxicity against normal tissues.

As a strategy to eliminate or minimize the problems of immunological nature and toxicity, encapsulated enzyme administration has been employed. The entrapment of enzymes in erythrocytes using hypotonic haemolysis methods has enabled erythrocytes to be used as enzyme carriers in either enzyme deficiency therapy or in enzyme replacement therapy. The disease caused due to accumulation of glucocerebroside in liver and spleen can be combated as reported by DeLoach and Ihler, 1977 by the use of glucocerebrosidase encapsulated in erythrocytes. The Resealed erythrocytes have been used (Ihler et al., 1979) for replacement of enzyme in lysosomes. α-glucuronidase, α-galactosidase and α-glucosidase were encapsulated in erythrocytes for lysosomal disorder.

Treatment of Liver Tumours

Anticancer agents encapsulated in erythrocytes can be used for targeting to hepatic carcinomas (Lynch et al., 1985). Various agents as bleomycin, adriamycin, carboplatin, gentamycin, L-asparaginase and methotrexate have been tried (Eichler et al., 1986a; Bennati et al., 1989; Lynch et al., 1985; Tonetti et al., 1992). Highly favourable results have been obtained using methotrexate as anticancer agent. Bennati et al., 1989 have proposed adriamycin loaded glutaraldehyde treated erythrocytes as a promising system against liver tumour. Erythrocyte membrane-bound daunorubicin has also been used as a delivery system in anticancer treatment.

Gaudreault et al., 1989 proposed drug encapsulation in erythrocytes to extend its biological lifetime. Molecules encapsulated this way are protected against rapid cellular metabolism and body elimination.

Unfortunately, drugs such as daunorubicin cannot be efficiently entrapped in erythrocytes since they diffuse rapidly from the cells. In order to overcome this problem, Gaudreault and co-workers, 1989 covalently linked daunorubicin to erythrocyte membranes (ghosts) using two different types of linking arms: glutaraldehyde and cis-aconitic acid. Both ghost-daunorubicin conjugates were tested *in vitro* on mouse leukaemia cells (P388D1) and on human osteosarcoma cells (CRL-1427). Results showed a better cytotoxic activity for ghost-glutaraldehyde-daunorubicin conjugate than for ghost-cis-aconityl-daunorubicin conjugate. Both conjugates were also tested *in vivo* on CDF1 mice bearing P388D1 cells. T/C% of 161 and 103 were observed with ghost-glutaraldehyde-daunorubicin and ghost-cis-aconityl-daunorubicin conjugate respectively at 6.0 mg/kg dose. Compared to free drug, the increase in survival time could be explained by a slow release of daunomycin in the circulation from the erythrocyte membranes, leading to a more complete absorption by cancer cells.

Tonetti and co-workers, 1992 encapsulated antineoplastic drug, carboplatin, in resealed erythrocytes as a therapeutic strategy for increasing the drug concentration in specific organs, notably liver. Analysis of the intra-erythrocytic metabolism of carboplatin showed that, in spite of its relatively high stability in aqueous solutions, in haemolysates and in the loaded erythrocytes a significant percentage of drug is rapidly converted to other species that still retain an antiproliferative activity *in vitro*. This fast conversion could be extensively inhibited by previous conversion of oxyhaemoglobin to methaeamoglobin or carbomonoxyhaemoglobin, suggesting an important role of haem iron in this process.

Treatment of Parasitic Diseases

The ability of resealed erythrocytes to selectively accumulate within the RES rich organs make them versatile drug carriers for the delivery of antiparasitic agents. This is further beneficial as they behave as circulating bioreactor and hence can be engineered to release the encapsulated drug in the RES organs. Parasitic diseases in which the parasite resides in RES system have been effectively treated with resealed erythrocytes. Pentamidine, primaquine phosphate and metronidazole have been successfully utilized for treatment of leishmaniasis, malaria and extraintestinal amoebiasis on experimental laboratory models.

Removal of RES Iron Overload

In iron overload resulting from repeated blood transfusion, RES cells are the primary and the major sites of iron accumulation. Iron-chelating drug (e.g., desferrioxamine) has been entrapped by Green, 1985, in erythrocytes, for promoting excretion of iron that is present as intracellular ferritin and haemosiderin deposit. The drug forms soluble chelates and depletes the depot.

Removal of Toxic Agents

Cannon and co-workers, 1994 reported antagonism of cyanide intoxication with murine carrier erythrocytes containing bovine rhodanese and sodium thiosulphate. Murine carrier erythrocytes containing bovine rhodanese and sodium thiosulphate are being explored as a new approach to antagonize the lethal effects of potassium cyanide in mice. Prior studies indicated that these carrier erythrocytes persist in the vascular system for the comparable length of time as normal erythrocytes and can enhance metabolism of cyanide to thiocyanate. The studies demonstrate the ability of these carrier red blood cells containing rhodanese and thiosulphate to antagonize the lethal effects of cyanide either alone or in various combinations with sodium nitrite and/or sodium thiosulphate. Potency ratios are compared in groups of mice treated with sodium nitrite, sodium thiosulphate, and carrier erythrocytes containing rhodanese and sodium thiosulphate either alone or in various combinations prior to the administration of potassium cyanide. These results indicate that the administration of carrier erythrocytes containing rhodanese and thiosulphate alone can provide significant protection against the lethal effects of cyanide. These carrier erythrocytes potentiate the antidote effect of sodium thiosulphate alone or the combination of sodium nitrite and sodium thiosulphate. The mechanisms of cyanide antagonism by these carrier erythrocytes and their broader conceptual significance to the antagonism of other chemical toxicants are discussed.

A relatively new approach was employed to antagonize organophosphorus intoxication by using resealed carrier erythrocytes containing a recombinant phosphotriesterase (Pei and co-workers, 1994). This enzyme has been reported to hydrolyze many organophosphorus compounds, including paraoxon, a potent cholinesterase inhibitor. Paraoxon is rapidly hydrolyzed by this enzyme to p-nitrophenol and diethylphosphate. Incorporation of phosphotriesterase within resealed murine erythrocytes was accomplished by hypotonic dialysis. The properties of this enzyme within these resealed erythrocytes were investigated. Addition of paraoxon to reaction mixtures containing these resealed erythrocytes loaded with phosphotriesterase resulted in the rapid hydrolysis of paraoxon. Hydrolysis of paraoxon did not occur when these carrier erythrocytes contained no phosphotriesterase. These *in vitro* studies suggest that carrier erythrocytes may be developed as an effective approach for the prophylactic and therapeutic antagonism of organophosphorus intoxication.

Targeting to sites other than RES-rich Organs

Resealed erythrocytes have the ability to deliver a drug or enzyme to the macrophage-rich organs, this is, unfortunately the premium limitation of this delivery system. Kitao and co-workers , 1978 reported the use of lectin (wheat germ agglutinin) to target daunomycin loaded erythrocytes to tumour cells. Organ targeting other than RES have been tried recently with resealed erythrocytes. Some of the representative approaches (Fig 10-13) are discussed in brief.

Magnet-responsive Erythrocyte Ghosts

Magnetic erythrocytes have been reported as an intelligent version for site-specific biophysically modulated targeting strategy. Zimmermann and Beckers, 1978 proposed that the encapsulation of small paramagnetic particles into erythrocytes might allow their localization to a particular location under the influence of external magnetic field. Recently, the loading of ferrofluids (colloidal suspension of magnetite, Fe_3O_4, Ferrofluidics Corp., New Hampshire) in erythrocytes has been reported in a study by Sprandel *et al.*, 1987. These ferromagnetic micro molecules upon entrapment in erythrocyte ghosts can be directed to deliver the entrapped drug under the influence of externally applied magnetic fields. Vyas and Jain, 1994 entrapped anti-inflammatory drugs, Diclofenac sodium and Ibuprofen into magnoresponsive erythrocytes and recorded improved stability and shelf life of the preparation in regard to drug and magnetite retention by reducing the cytotoxic effects of magnetite (Fig 10-13). These workers have devised an instrument to assess the *in vivo* magnetic responsiveness of drug loaded magnetic erythrocytes . The *in vivo* target specificity and selectivity of the drug loaded magnoresponsive erythrocytes was evaluated by assessing drug content at target site and other cutaneous and subcutaneous parts.

Photosensitized Erythrocytes

Photosensitized erythrocytes have been studied by Flynn and co-workers , 1994 as a photo-triggered carrier/delivery system for methotrexate in tumour therapy. Erythrocytes were loaded with methotrexate and photosensitized by subsequent exposure to a haematoporphyrin derivative. Following their accumulation at the site these were photoirradiated for effective photodynamic effect. Thus a combination of chemotherapy and photodynamic therapy could be a useful modality in the treatment of tumours of body located at site other than RES predominant organs.

Antibody Anchored Erythrocytes (Immunoerythrocytes)

Antibody coating of resealed drug carrier erythrocytes may be useful for drug targeting to the RES (Eichler et al., 1986b). Chiarantini et al., 1995 reported *in vitro* targeting of erythrocytes to cytotoxic T-cells by coupling of Thy-1.2 monoclonal antibody. Mouse erythrocytes were coupled with an anti-Thy-1.2 monoclonal antibody by two methods. Chromic chloride coupling of antibody was preferred to biotinylation. The morphology, osmotic fragility, and the haematological values of treated cells were normal and compared well with those of control erythrocytes. Antibody-coupled erythrocytes were incubated with cytotoxic T-lymphocytes (CTL) *in vitro* at a 20:1 ratio. Approximately 60-70% of the CTL formed rosettes. The cell mixture was subjected to gradient centrifugation and separated into four fractions.

The rosettes were clearly identified only in the treated group containing anti-Thy-1.2-coupled erythrocytes. No rosettes were found when a specific monoclonal antibody was coupled to erythrocytes. Examination by scanning and transmission electron microscopy revealed CTL with 4-5 erythrocytes attached to them but did not show any evidence of membrane fusion. Rosettes of CTL incubated *in vitro* proliferated as CTL alone and maintained their dependency on interleukin-2. Targeting of erythrocyte carriers to lymphocytes offers the potential for delivery of molecules directly to the target cell.

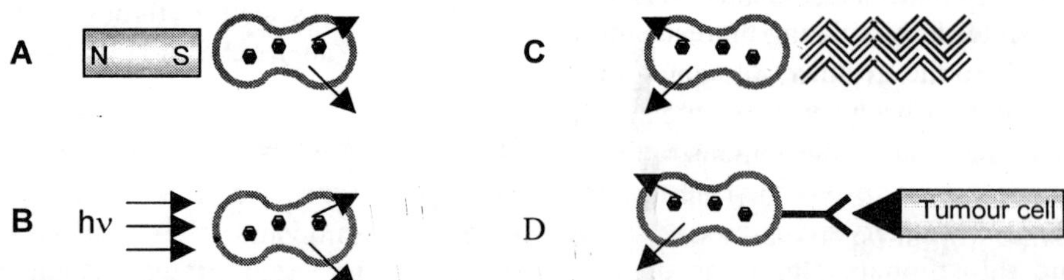

Fig. 10-13. Various Delivery Strategies Adopted to Avoid RES Uptake and Confer Targetability to Carrier Erythrocytes. (A) Targeting Using Paramagnetic Particles Loaded Inside the Erythrocytes. (B). Targeting Using Photosensitive Elements Loaded Within Erythrocytes Irradiated to Release the Drug Within the Target Vicinity. (C). Targeting Using Ultrasound Waves and (D). Targeting Using Target Specific Immunoglobulin (Antibody) Attached to Erythrocytes

Ultrasound Mediated Delivery of Erythrocytes loaded drug(s)

Price et al., 1998 reported the delivery of colloidal particles and red blood cells to tissue through microvessel ruptures created by targeted microbubble destruction with ultrasound. The application of ultrasound to thin-shelled microbubbles flowing through small microvessels (<7 μ in diameter) produces vessel wall ruptures *in vivo*. The endothelial barrier limits many intravascular drug and gene delivery vehicles. These workers hypothesized that this phenomenon could be used to deliver drug-bearing vehicles to tissue. Intravascular fluorescent red blood cells were delivered to the interstitium of rat skeletal muscle through microvessel ruptures created by insonifying microbubbles *in vivo*. Microvessel ruptures caused by insonification of microbubbles *in vivo* provided a non-invasive means for delivering engineered red blood cells across the endothelial lining of barrier(s) to the target tissue.

Erythrocytes as Circulating Bioreactors

Erythrocytes have been realized as carriers for enzymes to serve as circulating bioreactors. Sometimes it is desirable to decrease the level of circulating metabolites that can enter erythrocytes. The immobilization of enzymes, which catalyze these reactions, can be used as bioreactor. It is the perm-selectivity of the erythrocyte membrane, which allows it to act as a portal for enzyme allowing selective action on excessive pool of substrate and thus lowering down their blood levels. Adriaenssens and co-workers , 1976 demonstrated the efficacy of arginase loaded erythrocytes in reducing plasma arginine levels by 40% within 2 h of infusion into a patient with hyperargininaemia. Magnani et al., 1997 proposed erythrocytes as circulating bioreactors of blood acetaldehyde in the treatment of alcoholism. Erythrocytes have also been used as circulating bioreactors for the controlled delivery of antiviral drugs.

Delivery of Antiviral Agents

Several reports are available in the literature for the antiviral agents encapsulated in the resealed erythrocytes for effective delivery and targeting (Magnani et al., 1997). Because of the rapid plasma elimination and toxicity of the most commonly used drugs, daily multiple-drug therapies must often be continued throughout life, frequently causing major side effects and, as a consequence, poor patient compliance. Therefore, alternative strategies that reduce the toxicity of the drugs and allow prolonged application intervals are needed. Since most of the antiviral drugs are either nucleotides or nucleoside analogues, their entrapment and exit through membrane needs due consideration. Both purine and pyrimidine nucleosides are transported extremely rapidly by facilitated diffusion. Nucleotides however, are not transported across the membrane and thus remain entrapped causing a prolonged release profile. Release of nucleotides from erythrocytes thus requires a conversion of nucleotides to purine or pyrimidine bases (Fig. 10-14). This inter-conversion of non-transportable form of the drug to transportable form of drug can be brought about in two different ways :

- Normal erythrocyte enzymes can take part in the inter-conversion as in the case of ara CTP (arabinoside cytosine triphosphate), where phosphatase present in the erythrocyte removes phosphates from ara CTP.
- Non erythrocyte enzymes could be conjugated or entrapped in the erythrocytes to perform inter-conversion as in the case of pyridoxine and pyridoxal, which are transported through facilitated diffusion. Once transported they can be phosphorylated and inter-converted.

Thus, erythrocytes loaded with antiviral drugs may act "*in vitro*" as bioreactors ensuring sustained and potentially useful release of these drugs. Human immunodeficiency virus (HIV) and associated herpes virus (HSVs) (in HIV-1-immunocompromised patients) are distributed worldwide and are among the most frequent causes of viral infections. Hence, therapeutic strategies able to inhibit HSV-1 and HIV-1 replication are needed. Until now, the most common therapies against HSV-1 and HIV-1 infectivity have been based on the administration of nucleoside analogues; however, to be active, these antiviral drugs must be converted into their triphosphorylated derivatives by viral and/or cellular kinases. At the cellular level, the main problems involved in the use of such drugs are their limited phosphorylation in some cells (e.g., antiretroviral drugs in macrophages)

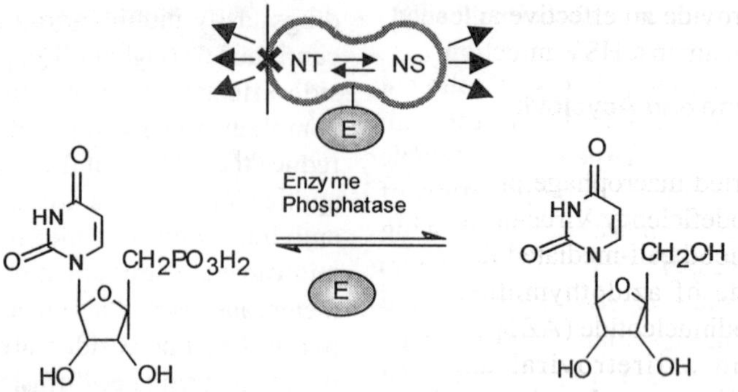

Fig. 10-14. The Interconversion of Nucleotides to Purine and Pyrimidine Bases and Thence Facilitated Diffusion to the Environment. Since Nucleotides Themselves are Impermeable to Erythrocyte Membrane, thus They Form a Circulating Bioreactor, Which can be Controlled by Intracellular Enzyme System or Exogenously Provided or Erythrocyte Anchored Enzyme System

and the cytotoxic side effects of nucleoside analogue triphosphates. To overcome these limitations, some of the strategies, which are adopted for the delivery of antiviral drugs are summarized in the following section

Delivery of Azidothymidine Derivative

Benatti and co-workers , 1996 reported Azidothymidine homodinucleotide-loaded erythrocytes and bioreactors for slow delivery of the antiretroviral drug azidothymidine. A new Azidothymidine derivative, di-(thymidine-3'- azido-2',3'-dideoxy-D-riboside)-5'-5'-p1-p2-pyrophosphate (AZTp2AZT), was encapsulated in human erythrocytes using hypotonic shock-isotonic resealing and reannealing method. Like, erythrocyte lysates supplemented with 1 mM ATP, intact red cells too were found to convert AZTp2AZT into 3'-Azido-3'-deoxythymidine which was then released linearly in plasma.

Delivery of Deoxycytidine Derivatives

Magnani and co-workers , 1997 reported targeting of antiviral nucleotide analogues encapsulated into erythrocytes to macrophages. Macrophages are important target cells for human immunodeficiency virus type 1 (HIV-1) infection. These workers developed a drug targeting system for the selective delivery of phosphorylated nucleoside analogues to these phagocytosing cells. They encapsulated phosphorylated drugs into autologous erythrocytes and on the subsequent selective modification of their membranes, macrophage recognition and phagocytosis was recorded. Targeted delivery of phosphorylated nucleoside analogues to human, feline, and murine macrophages inhibits the infectivity of HIV-1, feline immunodeficiency virus, and LP-BM5 viruses more efficiently than the administration of the corresponding nucleoside analogues. *In vivo* administration of 2',3'-dideoxycytidine 5'-triphosphate (ddCTP) encapsulated into autologous erythrocytes to LP-BM5-infected mice was found to reduce infectivity and disease progression. Furthermore, the simultaneous administration of AZT or ddC produced additive antiviral effects.

Delivery of Recombinant HSV-1 Glycoprotein B

Chiarantini *et al.*, 1995 reported red blood cells as delivery system for recombinant HSV-1 glycoprotein B. The immunotherapeutic potential of autologous red blood cells (RBC) coupled to the secretory form of Herpes Simplex Virus type 1 (HSV-1) glycoprotein B (gB1s) was examined with a mouse model of HSV-1 infection. Mice immunized with RBC coupled gB1s were protected against lethal and latent HSV-1 infection, and developed an anti-HSV antibody response, as measured by ELISA and HSV-1 neutralization assays, similar or higher than that elicited by the same antigen in Freund's complete adjuvant. This suggested that autologous RBC coupled to gB1s may provide an effective and safe method of immunization against HSV infection.

Delivery of Azathioprene and Acyclovir Derivatives

Rossi et al., 1998 reported macrophage protection against Human Immunodeficiency Virus or Herpes Simplex Virus by red blood cell-mediated delivery of a heterodinucleotide of azidothymidine and acyclovir. A new heterodinucleotide (AZTp2ACV) consisting of both an antiretroviral and an antiherpetic drug, bound by a pyrophosphate bridge, was designed and synthesized. The impermeant AZTp2ACV was encapsulated into autologous erythrocytes modified to increase their recognition and phagocytosis by human macrophages. Once inside the macrophages, metabolic activation of the drug occurred. The addition of AZTp2ACV-loaded erythrocytes to human macrophages provided effective and almost complete *in vitro* protection from HIV-1 and HSV-1 replications, respectively.

Delivery of Fludarabine Phosphate

2-Fluoro-ara-AMP (fludarabine phosphate) is a purine analogue with antineoplastic activity in lymphoproliferative malignancies. Fraternale and co-workers, 1996 encapsulated fludarabine phosphate in human erythrocytes and found that it is slowly released as fludarabine for more than four days. Encapsulated fludarabine phosphate does not affect erythrocyte metabolism and is rapidly converted by erythrocyte enzymes to pharmacologically active fludarabine.

Delivery of Ethambutol Derivative

Since erythrocytes (RBCs) can behave as bioreactors able to convert impermeant prodrugs to membrane-releasable active drugs, new compounds consisting of both an antiretroviral and an antimicrobial drug were designed and synthesized. Rossi et al., 1999 reported that heterodimer-loaded erythrocytes act as bioreactors for slow delivery of the antiviral drug azidothymidine and the antimycobacterial drug ethambutol (AZTpEMB, AZTpEMBpAZT and AZTp2EMB). Among these, only AZTp2EMB was hydrolyzed by erythrocyte enzymes and could be encapsulated inside RBCs. Moreover, when AZTp2EMB-loaded erythrocytes were incubated for 6 days in the presence of human macrophages infected with *Mycobacterium avium* (*M. avium*) a marked bactericidal effect (>1 log) was observed.

Macrophage Activation

Gautam and co-workers, 1987 used resealed erythrocytes as delivery system for biological response modifiers to generate macrophage-mediated tumouricidal activity. C-reactive protein associated with red cell ghosts inhibited established lung metastasis of T241 fibrosarcoma in the experimental mice.

Glucocorticoids are a widely used class of anti-inflammatory and immunosuppressive drugs, but their therapeutic use is limited by endocrine and metabolic side effects that they produce when given systemically. Since cells of the monocyte/macrophage lineage play an important role in the pathogenesis of several auto-immune and inflammatory diseases, dexamethasone, a potent glucocorticoid analogue, was encapsulated in erythrocytes and selectively delivered to macrophages. In addition, lipopolysaccharide (LPS) stimulation of dexamethasone-targeted macrophages results in the suppression of TNF-alpha secretion. Crinelli et al., 2000 demonstrated that the administration of dexamethasone to macrophages by means of opsonized red blood cells allows efficient interference with NF-kB activation. Furthermore, NF-kB inactivation correlated with down regulation of TNF-alpha mRNA expression, demonstrating that suppression of TNF-alpha production in dexamethasone-targeted cells occurs at the transcriptional level.

Thrombolytic Therapy

Entrapment of anti-thrombolytic agents in resealed erythrocytes has been proved effective. Eichler and co-workers , 1986a,c reported heparin entrapped resealed erythrocytes as useful modality in the prevention of thromboembolism because heparin is suggested to be released during retraction of fresh thrombi. Several other compounds are reported to be encapsulated in red blood cells for local prevention of thrombus and include aspirin (Orekhova et al., 1990) and Brinase (Flynn et al., 1994). Orekhova and co-workers, 1990 loaded erythrocytes with aspirin and ferromagnetic colloids and guided the loaded cells with externally modulated magnetic fields to program the release of aspirin to the retraction site.

Delivery of Interleukins

In order to circumvent the toxicity associated with high-dose interleukin 2 (IL 2) administration and its rapid clearance from the circulation, a carrier system for IL 2 is needed.

Kirch et al., 1994 evaluated the effect of targeted erythrocytes coated with recombinant human interleukin 2 (rIL-2) on T-lymphocyte proliferation *in vitro*. Mouse red blood cells (RBC) were incubated with rIL-2 in protein-free media. Of the added cytokine, about 20% was bound to the cells. RBC were covalently coupled to specific monoclonal antibody (mAb) towards the lymphocyte cell-surface marker Thyl.2, coated with rIL-2, subsequently exposed to the target CTL cells, then evaluated for CTL/RBC rosette formation. The attachment of mAb to the RBCs surface did not markedly change the succeeding rIL-2 adsorption, and the bound rIL 2 did not impair antigen recognition by the mAb.

In another report Moyes and coworkers, 1996 reported enhanced biological activity of human recombinant interleukin 2 (IL-2) coupled to mouse red blood cells as evaluated using the mouse Meth A sarcoma model.

Red blood cells (RBCs) coated with recombinant interleukin 2 (rIL-2) provide a means of delivering IL-2 into the system in a continuous low-dose manner which, in turn, maintains a low, potentially non-toxic, IL-2 concentration. Moreover, the RBC-rIL-2 vehicle is able to induce tumouricidal cytotoxicity with very low rIL-2 concentrations (about 10,000 i.u. of rIL-2/mouse).

Oxygen Deficiency Therapy

Resealed erythrocytes are also used in cases of oxygen deficiency where an improved oxygen supply is required as in the following cases :

- High altitude conditions (where partial pressure of oxygen is low).
- Small number of alveoli (where lung exchange surface is low).
- Increased resistance to oxygen diffusion in the lungs.
- Reduction in oxygen transport capacity.
- Mutation or chemical modification (where oxygen affinity of the haemoglobin is increased.
- Liver mediated detoxification processes (where an increased oxygen supply is a requirement).
- Increased radiosensitivity of radiation sensitive tumours.

In these cases, resealed erythrocytes can be used to improve the oxygen releasing capacity of the native erythrocytes. The underlying problem with normal erythrocytes is that 95% of the haemoglobin is normally saturated with oxygen in the lungs whereas under physiological conditions in the peripheral blood stream only about 25% of the oxygenated haemoglobin become deoxygenated. Thus the major fraction of the oxygen bound to haemoglobin is recirculated with the venous blood to the lungs. The use of this bound fraction has been suggested for the therapy of oxygen deficiency. This is possible when oxygen release is facilitated and increased in the capillary system and its affinity towards haemoglobin is reduced. This can be achieved by the enhancement of the 2,3-diphosphoglycerate (DPG) level or its substitute in the erythrocytes.

Inositol hexaphosphate (IHP, phytic acid) loaded into erythrocytes (performed by lipid-vesicle fusion) binds irreversibly to the haemoglobin and reduces its oxygen binding thus releasing the same in the capillaries. Erythrocyte entrapped IHP has a long life because no hydrolytic enzymes that have specificity for IHP is present in the normal erythrocytes.

A technique is described for opening the membrane of a red blood cell by electroporation in a manner, which permits free exchange of the native haemoglobin with exogenous haemoglobin in the surrounding medium (Fischer and Yabuki, 1998). After resealing the RBC's demonstrate near normal size and haemoglobin content and retain an effective methaemoglobin reduction system.

This method can be used to introduce natural or genetically engineered haemoglobins with altered oxygen-binding characteristics, which should be useful to treat tissue hypoxia from a variety of causes.

Resealed Erythrocytes in Cell Biological Applications

Microinjection of Macromolecules into Cultured cells using erythrocyte ghosts

Biological functions of the macromolecules like DNA, RNA and proteins are exploited for various cell biological applications. Hence various methods are used to introduce these macromolecules into cultured cells ("microinjection"). These include calcium phosphate or DEAE-dextran-mediated transfection, direct microinjection with microcapillaries, protoplast fusion, polybrene, electroporation, virus receptors, liposomes and resealed erythrocytes (red blood cells) or erythrocyte ghosts.

All these methods differ in their way of presentation of exogenous macromolecules into the cytoplasm. They can be efficiently presented using either Sendai virus (haemagglutinating virus of Japan, HVJ) or PEG-mediated fusion, and then the macromolecules are transferred efficiently from cytoplasm to the nucleus for their expression.

The technique involves loading of macromolecules into the erythrocyte ghosts using hypotonic haemolysis method. This is followed by fusion of erythrocyte ghosts with HVJ positive cell lines. When cells without HVJ receptors, such as lymphocytes are used as targets, polyethylene glycol (PEG) can be used. However, the fusion efficiency with PEG is lower as compared to that achieved using HVJ as fusion agent.

Erythrocyte ghost-cell fusion method mediated by HVJ is relatively easier, and has the special advantage that it can be used for microinjection into many cells at the same time. Furusawa and co-workers, 1974 first demonstrated the ability of erythrocyte ghost-cell fusion using fluorescein isothiocyanate (FITC) as a marker. Schlegel and Rechsteiner, 1978 also reported erythrocyte-mediated microinjection method. However in a series of studies, Yoneda and Kaneda, 1993 reported quantitative evaluation of the role of erythrocyte ghosts for the microinjection of the macromolecules using FITC-BSA as a fluorescent marker.

This method has certain advantages and disadvantages as listed below :

Advantages

- It can be employed for quantitative injection of material into cells.
- It does not require any special apparatus and/ or technique.
- Simultaneous introduction of materials into a large number of cells is possible.
- It permits introduction of materials into cells in suspension culture.
- The damage to the cells is minimal.

Disadvantages

- Co-introduction of the erythrocyte membranes, viral envelopes, viral RNA and residual haemoglobin may have unpredicted effects on the cells.
- A comparatively larger amount of test material is desired than that for the microcapillary method.
- Direct injection into the cell nucleus is not feasible.

Cell Biological Applications

The technique has been used in several cell biological applications :

1. Yamaizumi and co-workers , 1978(a,b) demonstrated that fragment A of diphtheria toxin (which on entering the cytoplasm inhibits peptide chain elongation in translation and causing cell death) can be introduced into target cells by the erythrocyte ghost-cell fusion (microinjection).
2. Yamaizumi et al., 1979 examined the feasibility of using antibody that can function in a cell The studies using antibody against diphtheria toxin fragment indicated that the antigen-antibody reaction occurs in a living cell (*in vivo*) as effectively as in a cell free system (*in vitro*). More than 50% of the initial activity of the anti-fragment A antibody was found to remain intact even after incubation of the cells containing the antibody at 37°C for 20 h. This indicates that the antibody against fragment A retains its function equally well *in vitro* and *in vivo*.
3. Various workers (Yamaizumi et al., 1978a,b, Sugawa et al., 1985; Tsuneoka et al., 1986; Yoneda, 1993) have demonstrated the

mechanistic of protein import into the nucleus (the mechanism of microinjection) using erythrocyte ghost-fusion method. These workers have used different nuclear proteins including: ^{125}I labeled nonhistone chromosomal protein (Yamaizumi et al., 1978), nucleo-plasmin-IgG conjugate (Sugawa et al., 1985), nonhistone chromosomal protein high mobility group-1 (HMG-1) and monoclonal antibody conjugate (Tsuneoka et al., 1986) and simian virus 40 large T-antigen (Yoneda, 1993). Thus by using synthetic peptides containing the nuclear location signal sequence, desired nonnuclear proteins, such as anti-target antibody, can be introduced into the nucleus by injecting them into the cytoplasm by the erythrocyte ghost-cell fusion method.

As shown in Figure 10-15, a synthetic peptide has been used containing the nuclear location signal of SV 40 large T antigen (T-peptide). In a parallel step (A) bovine serum albumin (BSA) is treated with the synthetic peptide (T-peptide) to make the conjugate. The conjugate T-BSA, in which BSA is chemically cross-linked with T-peptides, is completed (B). During dialysis against hypotonic PBS, T-BSA enters erythrocyte ghosts through transient holes in their membranes (C). During dialysis against isotonic PBS, the ruptured erythrocyte membrane is resealed and T-BSA is trapped in the ghost (D). Ghost containing T-BSA are mixed with target cells and HVJ at 4°C, resulting in agglutination (E). During incubation at 37°C for 30 min, the ghosts and target cells fuse and T-BSA trapped in the ghosts enters the cytoplasm of the cells (F). After incubation at 37°C for 1-2 h, T-BSA migrates into the nucleus (G). Molecules of the erythrocyte membrane and target cells are then intermixed.

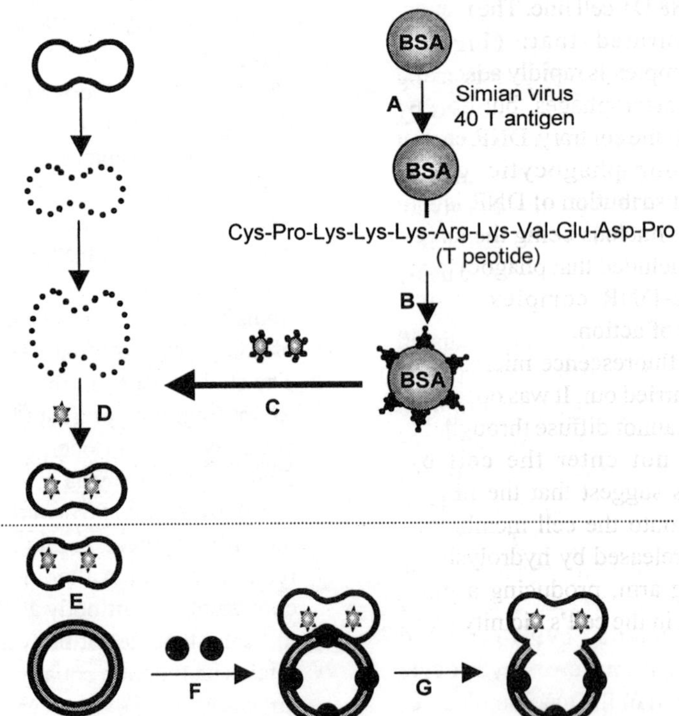

Fig. 10-15. The Steps involved in an Experiment on the Nuclear Transport Mechanism (Adopted from Yoneda, 1993, with modification)

NOVEL SYSTEMS

Nanoerythrosomes

An erythrocyte based new drug carrier, named nanoerythrosome has been developed which is prepared by extrusion of erythrocyte ghosts to produce small vesicles having an average diameter of 100 nm (Moorjani et al., 1996; Lejeune et al., 1997). Daunorubicin (DNR) was covalently conjugated to the nEryt (nEryt-DNR) using glutaraldehyde as homobifunctional linking arm. This led to a complex that is more active than free DNR both *in vitro* and *in vivo*. Daunorubicin (DNR) conjugated to these nanoerythrosomes has a higher antineoplastic index than the free drug. Moreover, since nanoerythrosomes are particles, phagocytosis may be involved in their mechanism of potentiation. Lejeune and co-workers, 1997 in their independent studies have compared the mechanism of penetration between free DNR and conjugate DNR linked to nanoerythrosomes, on cells presenting high phagocytic activity, macrophages, and cells lacking phagocytic activity, the P388 D1 cell line. The results of their study demonstrated that: (1) The nanoerythrosome-DNR complex is rapidly adsorbed and phagocytosed by the macrophages, but not by the P388 D1 cell line. (2) On the contrary, DNR enters both phagocytic and non-phagocytic cells. Furthermore, the cellular distribution of DNR is the same in both cell lines, the nucleus being the target organelle. The workers concluded that phagocytosis of the nanoerythrosome-DNR complex is not involved in its mechanism of action.

Further studies using fluorescence microscopy and cellular-uptake were carried out. It was observed that nEryt-DNR complex cannot diffuse through the cell membrane and do not enter the cell by endocytosis. These results suggest that the nEryt-DNR is rapidly absorbed onto the cell membrane. Free DNR is then slowly released by hydrolysis of the glutaraldehyde-linking arm, producing a high concentration of free DNR in the cell's vicinity over a long period of time.

Erythrosomes

Erythrosomes are specially engineered vesicular systems in which chemically cross-linked human erythrocyte cytoskeletons are used as a support upon which a lipid bilayer is coated. This can be achieved by a modified procedure normally adopted for reverse phase evaporation. Erythrosomes are proposed as useful encapsulation systems for drug delivery particularly for macromolecular drugs (Cuppoletti et al., 1981; Jung, 1987; Vyas and Dxit, 1999).

FUTURE PERSPECTIVES

The concept of employing erythrocytes as drug or bioactive carrier still needs further optimization . A large amount of valuable work is needed so as to utilize the potentials of erythrocytes in passive as well as active targeting of drugs. Diseases like cancer could surely find its cure. Genetic engineering aspects can be coupled to give a newer dimension to the existing cellular drug carrier concept.

REFERENCES

Adriaenseen K., Karcher D., Lonwenthal A. and Terheggen-H. G. (1976) *Clin. Chem.* **22**, 323.

Ahn Y. S., Byrness J. J., Harrington W. J., Cayer M. L., Smith D. S. Brunskill D. E. and Pall L. M. (1978) *N. Engl. J. Med.* **298**, 1101.

Alvarez F. J., Herraez A., Murciano J. C., Jordan J. A., Diez J. C. and Tejedor M. C. (1996) *J. Biochem.* **120**, 286.

Alvarez F. J., Jordan J. A., Calleja P., Lotero L. A., Olmos G., Diez J. C. and Tejedor M. C. (1998) *Biotechnol. Appl. Biochem.* **27**, 139.

Bailleul C., Kravtzoff R., Chestier N., Laguerre M., Chassaigne M. and Ropars C. (1990) *Biomed. Biochim. Acta.* **49**, S344.

Baker R. F. and Gills N. R. (1969) *Blood* **33**, 170.

Bax B. E. Bain M. D., Talbot P. J., Parker-Williams E. J. and Chalmers R. A. (1999) *Clin. Sci.* **96**, 171.

Benatti U., Giovine M., Damonte G., Gasparini A., Scarfi S., De Flora A., Fraternale A., Rossi L. and Magnani M. (1996) *Biochem. Biophys. Res. Commun.* **220**, 20.

Benatti U., Zocchi E., Tonetti M., Guida L., Polvani C. and De Flora A. (1989) *Pharmacol. Res.* **21**, S2, 27.

Bentler E., Dale G. L. Guinto E., Kuhl W. (1977) *Proc. Natl. Acad Sc. U SA.* **74**, 4620.

Berman J. D. and Aikawa M. (1984) *Am. J. Trop. Med. Hyg.* **33**, 1112.

Billah M. M., Finen J. B., Colfman R. and Michell R. H. (1976) *Biochim. Biophys. Acta* **433**, 54.

Billah M. M., Finen J. B., Colfman R. and Michell R. H. (1977) *Biochim. Biophys. Acta* **465**, 515.

Bird J., Bast R. and Lewis D.A. (1983) *J. Pharm. Pharmacol.* **35**, 246.

Bratosin D., Mazurier J., Slomianny C., Aminoff D. and Montreuil J. (1997) *Cytometry* **30**, 269.

Brearly C. A., Hodges N. A. and Olliff C. J. (1990) *J. Pharm. Pharmacol.* **42**, 297.

Brearly C. A., Lloyd A. W., Hodges N. A. and Olliff C. J. (1988) *Biochem. Soc. Trans.* **16**, 354.

Cannon E. P., Leung P., Hawkins A., Petrikovics I., DeLoach J. and Way J. L. (1994) *J. Toxicol. Environ. Health* **41**, 267.

Chatterjee C. C. (1995) Human Physiology, 3rd Ed., National Book Centre, Calcutta.

Chiarantini L., Rossi L., Fraternale A. and Magnani M. (1995) *Mol. Cell Biochem.* **144**, 53.

Crinelli R., Antonelli A., Bianchi M., Gentilini L., Scaramucci S. and Magnani M. (2000) *Blood Cells Mol. Dis.* **26**, 211.

Cuppoletti J., Mayhew E., Zobel C. R. and Jung C. Y. (1981) *Proc. Natl. Acad. Sci. USA* **78**, 2786.

Dale G. L. (1987) Methods in Enzymology 149, Academic Press, New York, 229.

Dale G. L. Villocorte D. G. and Gentler G. (1977) *Biochem. Med.* **18**, 220.

Dale G. L., Khul W. and Bentler E. (1979) *Proc. Natl. Acad. Sci. U.S.A* **76**, 473.

Davson H. and Danielli J. F. (1970) Dannen Conn. Hanfer Publishing Company, 80.

DeFlora A, Zocchi E., Guida L., Polvani C. and Benatti U. (1988) *Proc. Natl. Acad. Sci. U.S.A.* **31**, 45.

DeFlora, A., Banatti, U., Guida L. and Zoechi E. (1989) *Proc. Natl. Acad. Sci., U.S.A.* **83**, 7029.

DeLoach J. and lhler G. (1977) *Biochim. Biophys. Acta.* **496**, 136.

DeLoach J. R. (1982) *J. Appl. Biochem.* **4**, 533.

DeLoach J. R. (1985) *Res. Exp. Med.* **185**, 345.

DeLoach J. R. (1986) *Med. Res. Rev.* **6**, 487.

DeLoach J. R. (1987) Methods in Enzymology 149, Academic Press, New York, 235.

DeLoach J. R. Peters S., Pinkard O., Glew R. and lhler G. (1977) *Biochim. Biophys. Acta* **496**, 507.

DeLoach J. R. (1983) *J. Appl. Biochem.* **5**, 149.

DeLoach J. R., Andrews K. and Naqi A. (1988) *Biotechnol. Appl. Biochem.* **10**, 154.

DeLoach J. R., Barton C. (1981) *Am. J. Vet. Res.* **42**, 1971.

DeLoach J. R., Droleskey R. E. and Andrews K. (1991) *Biotechnol. Appl. Biochem.* **13**, 72.

DeLoach J. R., Tanger C. H. and Barton C. (1983) *Res. Exp. Med.* **183**, 167.

DeLoach J. R., Wagner G. G. and Corrier D. E. (1989) *J. Control. Rel.* **9**, 243.

DeLoach J. R., Wagner G. G., Craig T. M. (1981) *J. Appl. Biochem.* **3**, 254.

Ehrlich P. (1956) Collected papers of Paul Ehrlich: Immunology and Cancer Research, Pergamon Press, London, Vol. II, 352.

Eichler H. G. Rameis H., Bauer K., Kon A., Gasic S. and Bacher S. (1986a) *Eur. J. Clin. Ivest.* **16**, 39.

Eichler H. G., Gasic S., Bauer K., Korn A. and Bacher S. (1986b) *Clin. Pharmacol. Ther.* **40**, 300.

Eichler H. G., Schneider W., Raberger G., Bacher S. and Pabinger I. (1986c) *Res. Exp. Med.* **186**, 407.

Field W. N., Gamble C. M., Lewis D. A. (1989) *Int. J. Pharm.* **512**, 175.

Fischer J. J. and Yabuki H. (1998) *Artif. Cells Blood Substit. Immobil. Biotechnol.* **26**, 377.

Flynn G., McHale L. and McHale A. P. (1994) *Cancer Lett.* **82**, 225.

Franco M., Nordt F. J., Corfield A. P. and Schauer R. (1981) *Acta Biol. Med. Ger.* **40**, 409.

Fraternale A., Rossi L. and Magnani M. (1996) *Biochim. Biophys. Acta* **1291**, 149.

Furusawa M., Nishimura T., Yamaizumi M. and Okada Y. (1974) *Nature* **249**, 449.

Garin M.I., Lopez R. M., Sanz S., Pinilla M. and Luque J. (1996) *Pharm. Res.* **13**, 869.

Gaudreault R. C., Bellemare B. and Lacroix J. (1989) *Anticancer Res.* **9**, 1201.

Gautam S., Barna B., Chiang T. Pettay J. and Deodhar S. (1987) *J. Biol. Response Mod.* **6**, 346.

Gneushev E. T. and Gneusheva I. A. (1996) *Eksp. Klin. Farmakol.* **59**, 71.

Green R. (1985) *Bibl. Haematol.* **51**, 25.

Green R., Laman J. and Curran D. (1980) *Lancet* **2**, 327.

Humphreys J., Edlind T. and Ihler G. (1981) *J. Appl. Biochem.* **3**, 199.

Ihler G., Lantzy A., Purpura J. and Glew R.H. (1975) *J. Clin. Invest.* **56**, 595.

Ihler G. M. (1983) *Pharmacol. Therap.* **20**, 151.

Ihler G. M. and Tsang H. C. W. (1987) Methods in Enzymology 149, Academic Press, New York, 221.

Ihler G. M., Glew R. H. and Schnure F. W. (1973) *Proc. Natl. Acad. Sci. USA* **70**, 2663.

Ingrosso D., Cotticelli M. G., D'Angelo S., Buro M. D., Zappia V. and Galletti P. (1997) *Eur. J. Biochem.* **244**, 918.

Jain S. K. and Vyas S. P. (1994) *J. Microencaps.* **11**, 141.

Jausel-Husken S. and Deuticke B. (1981) *J. Memb. Biol.* **63**, 61.

Juliano R. L. (1980) Drug Delivery Systems, Oxford University Press, New York, 9.

Jung C. Y. (1987) Methods in Enzymology 149, Academic Press, New York, 217.

Kinosita K. and Tsong T. Y. (1977) *Nature* **268**, 438.

Kinosita K. and Tsong T. Y. (1978) *Nature* **272**, 258.

Kirch H. J., Moyes R. B., Chiarantini L. and DeLoach J. R. (1994) *Biotechnol. Appl. Biochem*. **19**, 331.

Kitao T. and Hattori K. (1980) *Cancer Res*. **40**, 351.

Kitao T., Hattori K. and Takeshita M. (1978) *Experimentia* **341**, 94.

Kruse C. A. Mierau G. W. and James G. T. (1989) *Biotechnol. Appl. Biochem.* **11**, 571.

Lejeune A., Poyet P., Gaudreault R. C. and Gicquaud C. (1997) *Anticancer Res.* **17**, 3599.

Lewis D. A. and Alpar O. H. (1984) *Int. J. Pharm.* **22**, 137.

Lhler G. M., Glew R. H. and Schnare F. W. (1973) *Proc. Natl. Acad. Sci. U.S.A.* **70**, 2663.

Lo M. M. S., Tsong T.Y., Conard M. K., Strittmatter S. M., Hester L. D. and Snyder S. H. (1984) *Nature* **310**, 792.

Lynch H. E., Sartiano, G.P. and Ghaffar, A. (1980) *Am. J. Hematolol.*, **9**, 249.

Lynch, W. E., Sartiano G. P., Rosenblum S. L., Calkins J. H. and Ramsey C. B. (1985) *Bibl. Haematol.* **51**, 42.

Magnani M., Laguerre M., Rossi L., Bianci M., Ninfali P., Mangani F. and Roppars C. (1989) *Alcoholism Clin. Exp. Res.* **13**, 849.

Magnani M., Rossi L., Fraternale A., Casabianca A., Brandi G., Benatti U. and De Flora A. (1997) *J. Leukoc. Biol*. **62**, 133.

Magnani M., Rossi L., D'ascenzo M., Panzani I., Bigi L. and Zanella A. (1998) *Biotechnol. Appl. Biochem.* **28**, 1.

Mangal P. C. and Kaur A. (1991) *Ind. J. Biochem. Biophys.* **28**, 219.

Mishra K. P. and Singh B. B. (1984) *Ind. J. Exp. Biol*. **19**, 320.

Mitchell D. H., James G. T. and Kruse C. A. (1991) *Biotechnol. Appl. Biochem.* **12**, 264.

Moorjani M., Lejeune A., Gicquaud C., Lacroix J., Poyet P. and Gaudreault R. C. (1996) *Anticancer Res.* **16**, 2831.

Moyes R. B., Kirch H. and DeLoach J. R. (1996) *Biotechnol. Appl. Biochem*. **23**, 29.

Nicolau C. and Gresonele K. (1979) *Naturewissenschaftern* **66**, 563.

Orekhova N. M., Akchurin R. S., Belyaev A. A., Smirnov M. D., Ragimov S. E. and Orekhov A. N. (1990) *Thromb. Res.* **57**, 611.

Pitt E., Johnson C. M., Lewis D. A., Jenner D. A. and Offord R. E. (1983) *Biochem. Pharmacol.* **32**, 3359.

Price R. J., Skyba D. M., Kaul S. and Skalak T. C. (1998) *Circulation* **98**, 1264.

Rechsteiner M. C. (1978) *Natl. Cancer Inst. Monogr.* **48**, 57.

Rechsteiner M. C. (1975) *Exp. Cell. Res.* **93**, 487.

Rossi L., Brandi G., Schiavano G. F., Scarfi S., Millo E., Damonte G., Benatti U., De Flora A and Magnani M. (1999) *AIDS Res. Hum. Retroviruses* **15**, 345.

Rossi R., Barra D., Bellelli A., Boumis G., Canofeni S., Di Simplicio P., Lusini L., Pascarella S. and Amiconi G. (1998) *J. Biol. Chem*. **273**, 19198.

Sanz S., Lizano C., Luque J. and Pinilla M. (1999) *Life Sci.* **65**, 2781.

Schlegel R. A. and Rechsteiner M. C. (1975) *Cell* **5**, 371.

Schrier S. L. (1987) Methods in Enzymology 149, Academic Press, New York, 260.

Schrier S. L., Bensch K. G., Johnson M. and Janga L. (1975) *J. Clin. Invest.* **56**, 8.

Segal A. W. (1979) In: Drug Carriers in Biology and Medicine, Gregoriadis G. (Ed.), Academic Press, New York, 155.

Serandel U., Franz D. J. and Horston W. (1987) Methods in Enzymology 149, Academic Press, New York, 301.

Sprandel U. and Zollner N. (1985) *Res. Exp. Med.* **185**, 77.

Sprandel U., Franz D. J. and Horston W. (1987) *Methods in Enzymology* **149**, 301.

Sprandel U., Hubbard A. R. and Chalmers R. A. (1981) *Clin. Sci.* **59**, 7.

Sugawa H., Uchida T., Yoneda Y., Ishiura M. and Okada Y. (1985) *Exp. Cell Res.* **159**, 410.

Talwar N. and Jain N.K. (1992) *Drug Dev. Ind. Pharm*. **18**, 128.

Teissie J., Knutson V. P., Song, T. Y. and Lane M. D. (1982) *Science* **216**, 537.

Thorpe S. R., Fiddler M. B. and Desnik R. J. (1977) *Pediatr. Res.* **9**, 918.

Thorpe S. R., Fiddler M. R. and Desnik R. J. (1974) *Biochem. Biophys. Res. Comm.* **61**, 1464.

Tonetti M., Astroff B., Satterfield W., De Flora A., Benatti U. and DeLoach J. R. (1990). *Biotechnol. Appl. Biochem.* **12**, 621.

Tonetti M., Gasparini A., Giovine M., Bini D., Mazzucotelli A., De Paz F., Benatti U. and De Flora A. (1992) *Biotechnol. Appl. Biochem.* **15**, 267.

Tsang H. C., Mollenhauer H. and Ihler G. (1982) *J. Appl. Biochem.* **4**, 418.

Tsong T. Y. (1987) Methods in Enzymology 149, Academic Press, New York, 248.

Tsuneoka M., Imamoto N. S. and Uchida T. (1986) *J. Biol. Chem.* **261**, 1829.

Tyrell D. A. and Rymen B. E. (1976) *Biochem. Soc. Trans.* **4**, 677.

Vyas S. P. and Dixit V. K. (1999) Pharmaceutical Biotechnology, CBS publishers, New Delhi, 656.

Vyas S. P. and Jain S. K. (1994) *J. Microencaps.* **11**, 19.

Yamaizumi M., Mekada E., Uchida T. and Okada Y. (1978b) *Cell* **15**, 245.

Yamaizumi M., Uchida T., Mekada E. and Okada Y. (1979) *Cell* **18**, 1009.

Yamaizumi M., Uchida T., Okada Y. and Furusawa M. (1978) *Cell* **13**, 227.

Yoneda Y. (1993) *Methods Enzymol.* **221**, 306.

Zimmermann U. and Beckers F. (1978) *Planta.* **138**, 173.

Zimmermann U. and Riemann F. (1976) *Biochem. Biophys. Acta* **436**, 460.

Zimmermann U. (1985) In: Targeted Drug, Goldberg E. P. (Ed.), 2, 153.

Zimmermann U., Pilwat G. and Esser B. (1978) *J. Clin. Chem. Clin. Biochem.* **16**, 135.

Zolla L., Lupidi G., Marcheggiani M., Falcioni G. and Brunori M. (1991) *Ann. Ist Super Sanita* **27**, 97.

CHAPTER 11

Microspheres

- Introduction
- Material(s) used
- Prerequisites for ideal microparticulate carriers
- General methods of preparation
- Loading of drug
- Drug release kinetics
- Polymeric microspheres
- Fate of microspheres in body
- Characterization
- Applications
- Future perspective
- References

The concept of drug delivery has been revolutionized. The strides have been made to lend patient derive maximum benefits of a drug. The drug should be delivered to specific target sites at a rate and concentration that permit optimal therapeutic efficacy while reducing side effects to minimum. Another aspect to be considered in drug delivery is patient compliance during the drug therapy.

The concept of the advanced drug delivery systems especially those offering a sustained and controlled action of drug to desired area of effect, attained great appeal for nearly half a century. However, prior to advent of improved alternate methods, drug delivery systems were considered only as a means of getting the drug into the patient's body. Actual practice of controlled release began with advent of timed release coating to the pills or solid drug particles in order to mask their unacceptable taste or make them more palatable.

Between 1940s and 1960s, the concept of chemical microencapsulation technology began as an alternative means of delivering drugs. In continued quest for the more refined systems, in 1980s polymer/membrane technology came to be known at forefront. Further, the process of targeting and site specific delivery with absolute accuracy can be achieved by attaching bioactive molecule to liposomes, bioerodible polymer, implants, monoclonal antibodies and various particulate carriers (e.g., nanoparticles and microspheres, etc.). The micro-particulate delivery systems are considered and accepted as a reliable means to deliver the drug to the target site with specificity, if modified, and to maintain the desired concentration at the site of interest without untoward effect(s).

The term microcapsule, is defined as a spherical particle with size varying from 50 nm to 2 mm, containing a core substance. Microspheres are, in strict sense, spherical empty particles. However, the terms microcapsules and microspheres are often used synonymously. In addition, some related terms are used as well. For example, essentially "microbeads" and "beads" are used alternatively. Spheres and spherical particles are also used for a large size and rigid morphology. The microsphere are characteristically free flowing powders consisting of proteins or synthetic polymers, which are biodegradable in nature, and ideally having a particle size less than 200 μm. Solid biodegradable microspheres incorporating a drug dispersed or dissolved throughout particle matrix have the potential for the controlled release of drug. These carriers received much attention not only for prolonged release but also for the targeting of the anticancer drugs to the tumour. (Widder et al., 1979).

MATERIAL(S) USED

A number of different substances both biodegradable as well as non-biodegradable have been investigated for the preparation of microspheres. These materials include the polymers of natural and synthetic origin and also modified natural substances. Synthetic polymers employed as carrier materials are methyl methacrylate (Kreuter et al., 1983), acrolein (Margel and Wiesel 1984), lactide, glycolide and their copolymers (Wakiyama et al., 1981, bod, et al., 1984a), ethylene vinylacetate copolymer (Stefan et al., 1984), polyanhydrides, etc. The natural polymers used for the purpose are albumin (Sugibayashi et al., 1979, Lee et al, 1981), gelatin (Yoshioaka et al, 1981, 1982), starch (Russel 1983, Lindberg et al., 1984), collagen and carrageenan, etc. Some of the polymers used in the preparation of the microspheres are classified and listed in the Table 11-1.

PREREQUISITES FOR IDEAL MICROPARTICULATE CARRIERS

The material utilized for the preparation of microparticulates should ideally fulfil the following prerequisites:

- Longer duration of action
- Control of content release
- Increase of therapeutic efficiency
- Protection of drug
- Reduction of toxicity
- Biocompatibility
- Sterilizability
- Relative stability
- Water solubility or dispersability
- Bioresorbability

Table 11-1. Classification of Polymers

SYNTHETIC POLYMERS

Non-biodegradable

- PMMA
- Acrolein
- Glycidyl methacrylate
- Epoxy polymers

Biodegradable

- Lactides and glycolides and their copolymers
- Polyalkyl cyano acrylates
- Polyanhydrides

NATURAL MATERIALS

Proteins

- Albumins
- Gelatin
- Collagen

Carbohydrates

- Starch
- Agarose
- Carrageenan
- Chitosan

Chemically modified carbohydrates

- DEAE cellulose
- Poly(acryl)dextran
- Poly(acryl)starch

- Targetability
- Polyvalent

GENERAL METHODS OF PREPARATION

The microspheres can be prepared by using any of the several techniques discussed in the following sections, (Rajeev jain 2000) but the choice of the technique mainly depends on the nature of the polymer used, the drug, the intended use and the duration of therapy. Moreover, the method of preparation and its choice are equivocally determined by some formulation and technology related factors as mentioned below:

1. The particle size requirement.
2. The drug or the protein should not be adversely affected by the process.
3. Reproducibility of the release profile and the method.
4. No stability problem.
5. There should be no toxic product(s) associated with the final product.

Synthetic polymers are now materials of choice for the controlled release as well as targeted micro particulate carriers. The initial work was carried out on the non-biodegradable polymers but later on, the interest has been shifted to the biodegradable polymers. Different types of methods are employed for the preparation of the microspheres. These include *in situ* polymerization, solvent evaporation, coacervation phase separation, spray drying and spray congealing, etc.

Single Emulsion Technique

The microparticulate carriers of natural polymers, i.e. those of proteins and carbohydrates are prepared by single emulsion technique (Fig. 11-1). The natural polymers are dissolved or dispersed in aqueous medium followed by dispersion in the non-aqueous medium e.g., oil. In the second step of preparation, cross linking of the dispersed globule is carried out. The cross-linking can be achieved either by means of heat or by using the chemical cross linkers. The chemical cross-linking agents used include glutaraldehyde, formaldehyde, terephthaloyl chloride, diacid chloride, etc. Cross-linking by heat is affected by adding the dispersion to previously heated oil. Heat denaturation is however, not suitable for the thermolabile drugs while the chemical cross-linking suffers disadvantage of excessive exposure of active ingredient to chemicals if added at the time of preparation.

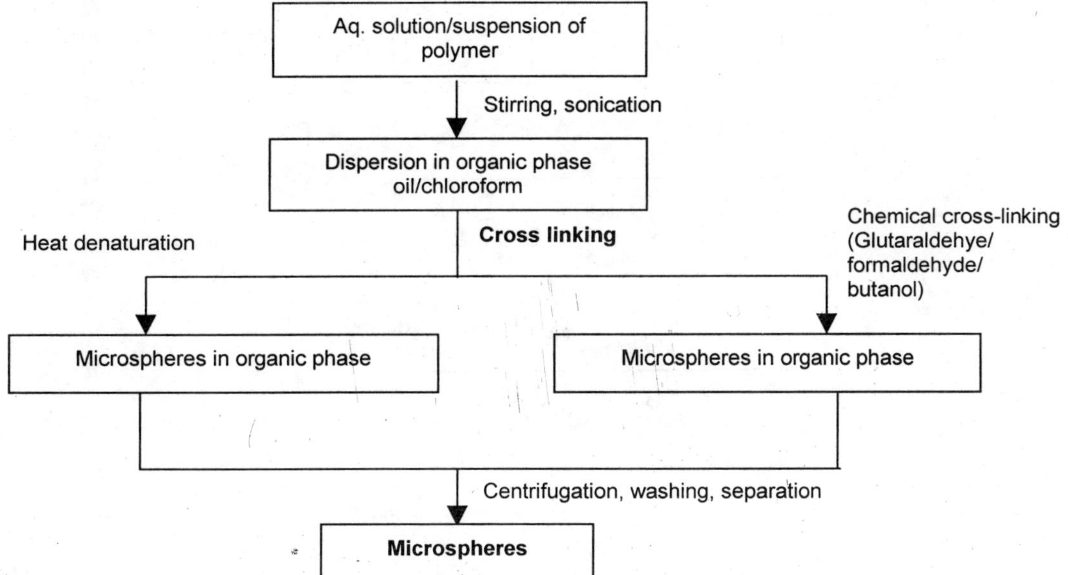

Fig. 11-1. Schematic Representation of Simple Emulsion Based Method of Microspheres Preparation

Double Emulsion Techniques

Briefly, double emulsion method of microspheres preparation involves the formation of the multiple emulsions or the double emulsion of type w/o/w (Fig. 11-2) and is best suited to the water-soluble drugs, peptides, proteins and the vaccines. This method can be used with both the natural as well as the synthetic polymers. The aqueous protein solution is dispersed in a lipophilic organic continuous phase. This protein solution may contain the active constituents. The continuous phase is generally consisted of the polymer solution that eventually encapsulates of the protein contained in dispersed aqueous phase. The primary emulsion is then subjected to the homogenization or the sonication before addition to the aqueous solution of the poly vinyl alcohol (PVA). This results in the formation of a double emulsion. The emulsion is then subjected to solvent removal either by solvent evaporation or by solvent extraction process. The solvent evaporation is carried out by maintaining emulsion at reduced pressure or by stirring the emulsion so that the organic phase evaporates out. In the latter case, the emulsion is added to the large quantity of water (with or without surfactant) into which organic phase diffuses out. The solid microspheres are subsequently obtained by filtration and washing. A number of hydrophilic drugs like leutinizing hormone releasing hormone(LH-RH) agonist, vaccines, protein/ peptides and conventional molecules are successfully incorporated in to the microspheres using the method of double emulsion solvent evaporation/extraction.

Polymerization Techniques

The polymerization techniques conventionally used for the preparation of the microspheres are mainly classified as:

I. Normal polymerization
II. Interfacial polymerization

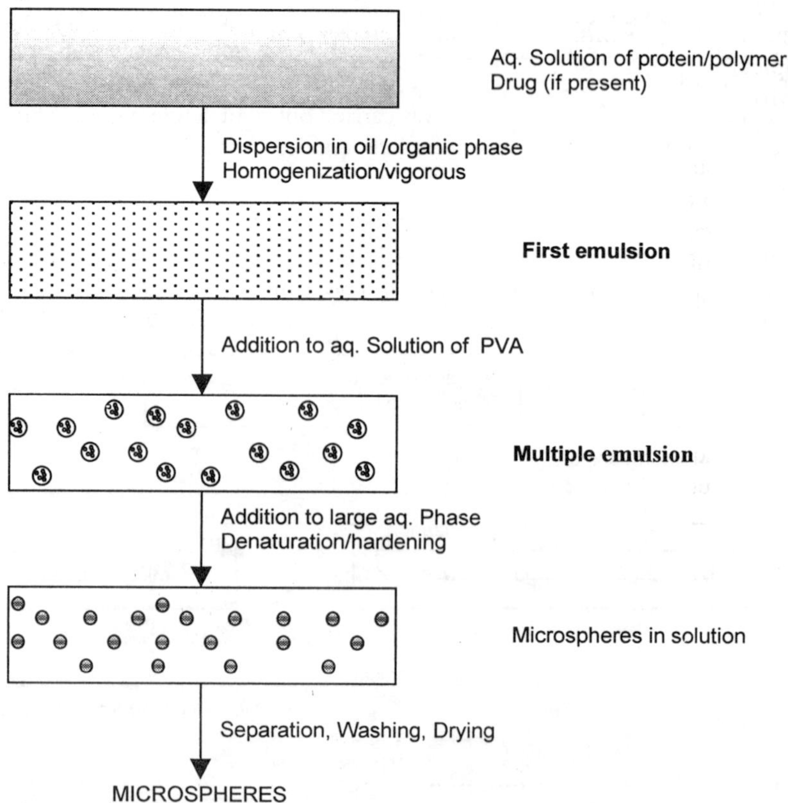

Fig. 11-2. Schematic Representation of Double Emulsion Method of Microspheres Preparation

Normal Polymerization

The two processes are carried out in a liquid phase. Normal polymerization proceeds and carried out using different techniques as bulk, suspension precipitation, emulsion and miceller polymerization processes.

In bulk polymerization, a monomer or a mixture of monomer along with the initiator is usually heated to initiate the polymerization and carry out the process. The catalyst or the initiator is added to the reaction mixture to facilitate or accelerate the rate of the reaction. The polymer so obtained may be moulded or fragmented as microspheres. For loading of drug, adsorptive drug loading or adding drug during the process of polymerization may be opted. The scheme of the bulk polymerization is represented in the Figure 11-3.

The suspension polymerization, which is also referred to as the bead or pearl polymerization is carried out by heating the monomer or mixture of monomers with active principles (drugs) as droplets dispersion in a continuous aqueous phase. The droplets may also contain an initiator and other additives. The scheme for the suspension polymerization is given in Figure 11-4.

The emulsion polymerization, however, (Fig. 11-5) differs from the suspension polymerization as due to presence of the initiator in the aqueous phase, which later on diffuses to the surface of the micelles or the emulsion globules (Fig. 11-6). The bulk polymeri-zation has an advantage of formation of the pure polymer, but it also suffers a disadvantage, as it is very difficult to dissipate the heat of reaction, which can adversely affect the thermolabile active ingredients. On the other hand the suspension and emulsion polymerization can be carried out at lower temperature, since continuous external phase is normally water through which heat can easily dissipate. The two processes also lead to the formation of the higher molecular weight polymer at relatively faster rate. The major disadvantage of suspension and emulsion polymerization is, association of polymer with the unreacted monomer and other additives.

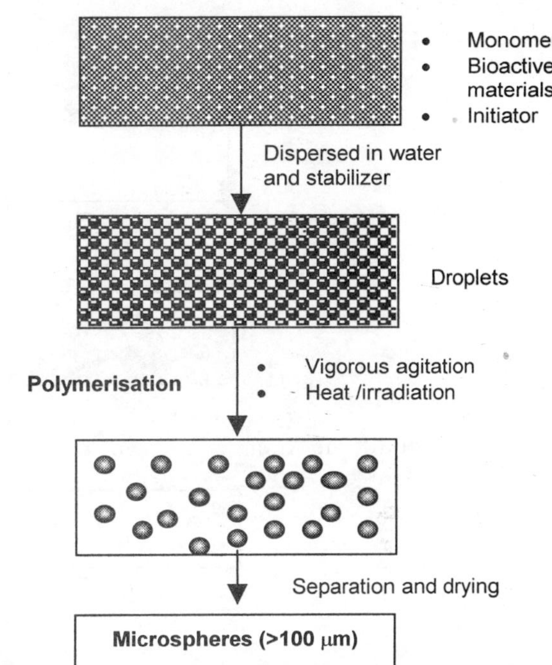

Fig. 11-4. Schematic Representation of Suspension Polymerization for Microspheres Formation

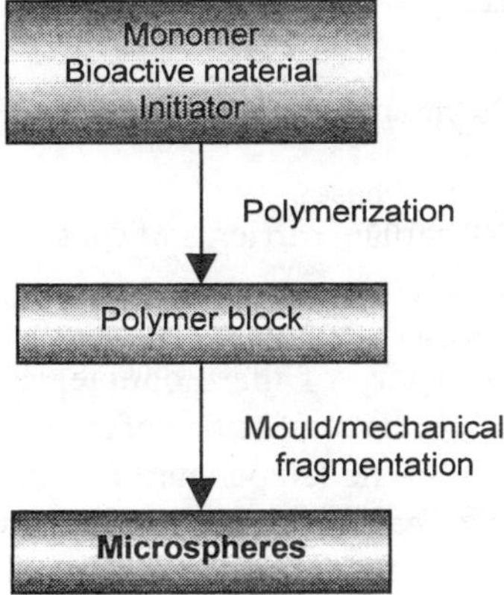

Fig. 11-3. Schematic for Bulk Polymerization

Interfacial Polymerization

Interfacial polymerization essentially proceeds involving reaction of various monomers at the interface between the two immiscible liquid phases to form a film of polymer that essentially envelops the dispersed phase. In this technique two reacting monomers are employed; one of which is dissolved in the continuous phase while the other being

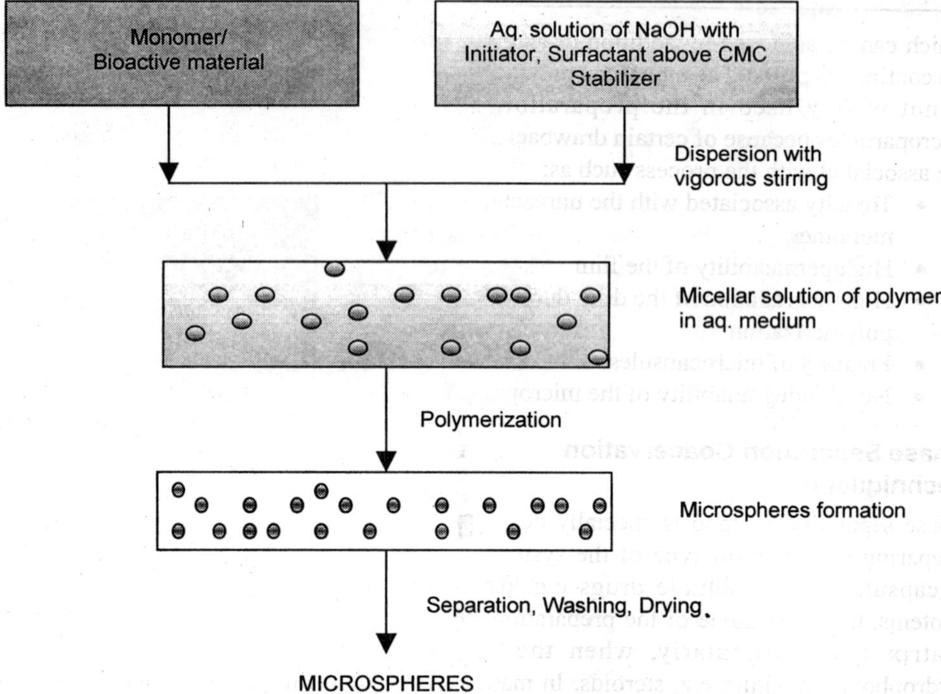

Fig. 11-5. Schematic Representation of Emulsion Polymerization

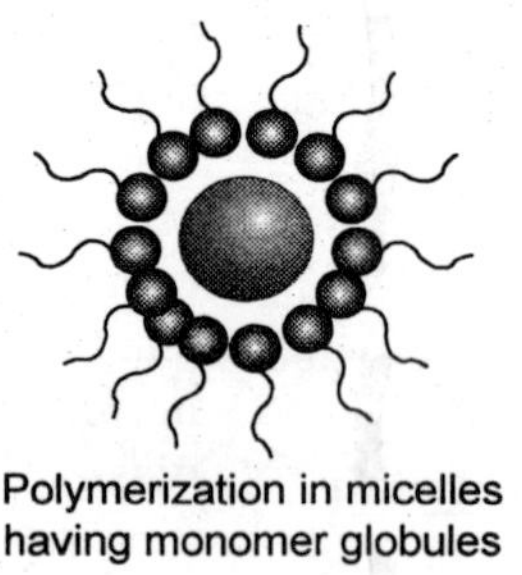

Polymerization in micelles having monomer globules

Fig. 11-6. Micelles as a Site of Polymerization

dispersed in the continuous phase. The continuous phase is generally aqueous in nature throughout which the second monomer is emulsified. The monomers present in either phases diffuse rapidly and polymerize rapidly at the interface. Two conditions arise depending upon the solubility of formed polymer in the emulsion droplet. If the polymer is soluble in the droplet it will lead to the formation of the monolithic type of the carrier on the other hand if the polymer is insoluble in the monomer droplet, the formed carrier is of capsular (reservoir) type.

The degree of polymerization can be controlled by the reactivity of the monomer chosen, their concentration, the composition of the vehicle of either phases and by the temperature of the system. The particle size can be controlled by controlling the droplets or globules size of the disperse phase. The polymerization reaction can be controlled by maintaining the concentration of the monomers, which can be achieved by addition of an excess of the continuous phase. The interfacial polymerization is not widely used in the preparation of the microparticles because of certain drawbacks, which are associated with the process such as:

- Toxicity associated with the unreacted monomer
- High permeability of the film
- High degradation of the drug during the polymerization
- Fragility of microcapsules
- Non-biodegradability of the microparticles

Phase Separation Coacervation Technique(s)

Phase separation method is specially designed for preparing the reservoir type of the system, i.e. to encapsulate water soluble drugs e.g. peptides, proteins, however, some of the preparations are of matrix type particularly, when the drug is hydrophobic in nature e.g. steroids. In matrix type device, the drug or the protein is soluble in the polymer phase. The process is based on the principle of decreasing the solubility of the polymer in the organic phase to affect the formation of the polymer rich phase called the coacervates. The coacervation can be brought about by addition of the third component to the system which results in the formation of the two phases, one rich in the polymer, while the other one, i.e. supernatant, depleted of the polymer. There are various means and methods, which are effectively employed for coacervate phase separation. The method choice is largely dependent upon the polymer and set of conditions. The method are based on salt addition non-solvent addition, addition of the incompatible polymer or change in pH.

In this technique, (Fig. 11-7) the polymer is first dissolved in a suitable solvent and then drug is dispersed by making its aqueous solution, if hydrophilic or dissolved in the polymer solution itself, if hydrophobic. Phase separation is then accomplished by changing the solution conditions by using any of the method mentioned above. The process is carried out under continuous stirring to control the size of the microparticles. The process

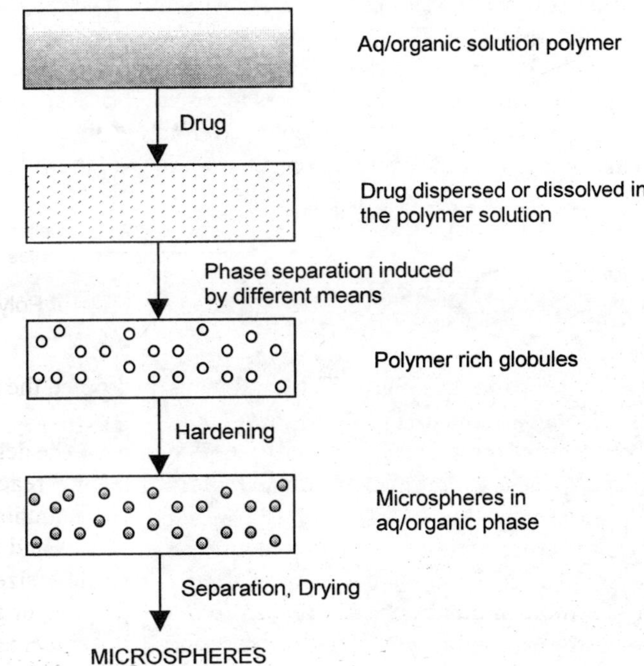

Fig. 11-7. Schematic Representation of Microspheres Formation by Phase Separation Method

variables are very important since the rate of achieving the coacervate determines the distribution of the polymer film, the particle size and agglomeration of the formed particles. The agglomeration must be avoided by stirring the suspension using a suitable speed stirrer since as the process of microspheres formation begins the formed polymerize globules start to stick and form the agglomerates. Therefore, the process variable are critical as they control the kinetic of the formed particles since there is no defined state of equilibrium attainment.

Spray Drying and Spray Congealing

Spray drying and spray congealing methods are based on the drying of the mist of the polymer and drug in the air. Depending upon the removal of the solvent or the cooling of the solution, the two processes are named spray drying and the spray congealing respectively. The polymer is first dissolved in a suitable volatile organic solvent such as dichloromethane, acetone, etc. The drug in the solid form is then dispersed in the polymer solution under high-speed homogenization. This dispersion is then atomized in a stream of hot air. The atomization leads to the formation of the small droplets or the fine mist from which the solvent evaporates instantaneously leading the formation of the microspheres in a size range 1-100 μm. Microparticles are separated from the hot air by means of the cyclone separator while the traces of solvent are removed by vacuum drying. One of the major advantages of the process is feasibility of operation under aseptic conditions. The two processes are rapid, requiring single stage operation, suitable for both batch and bulk manufacturing. These techniques have been used to encapsulate a large number of the drugs. The spray drying process is used to encapsulate various penicillins. Thiamine mononitrate (Koff, 1963) and sulpha ethylthiadizole (John and Becker, 1968; Cushimano and Becker, 1968) are encapsulated in a mixture of mono- and diglycerides of stearic and palmitic acid using spray congealing. The rate of solvent removal by evaporation strongly influences the characteristics of the formed microspheres and it depends on the temperature, pressure, and the solubility parameter of the polymer, the solvent and the dispersion media. Very rapid solvent evaporation, however leads to the formation of porous microparticles (Photomicrograph 11-1).

Solvent Extraction

Solvent extraction method used for the preparation of microparticles, involves removal of the organic phase by extraction of the organic solvent. The method involves water miscible organic solvents such as isopropanol. Organic phase is removed by extraction with water. This process decreases the hardening time for the microspheres. One variation of the process involves direct addition of the drug or

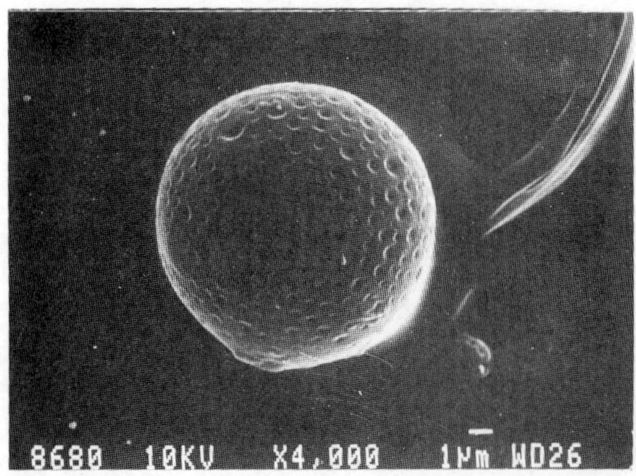

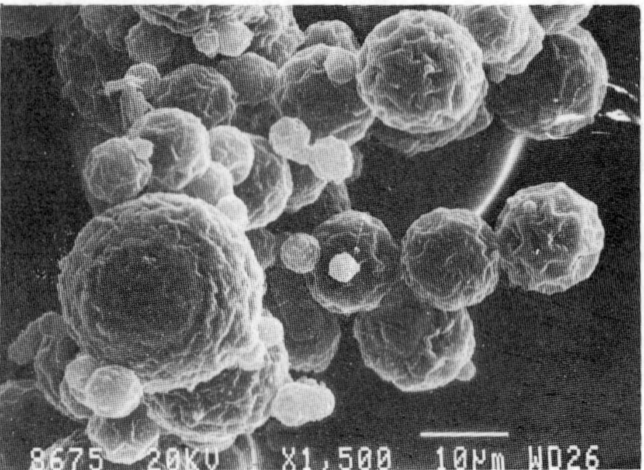

Photomicrograph 11-1. Porous Microspheres Photomicrograph

protein to polymer organic solution. The rate of solvent removal by extraction method depends on the temperature of water, ratio of emulsion volume to the water and the solubility profile of the polymer.

LOADING OF DRUG

The active components are loaded over the microspheres principally using two methods, i.e. during the preparation of the microsphere or after the formation of the microspheres by incubating them with the drug/protein. The active component can be loaded by means of the physical entrapment, chemical linkage and surface adsorption. The entrapment largely depends on the method of preparation and nature of the drug or polymer (monomer, if used). Maximum loading can be achieved by incorporating the drug during the time of preparation but it may get affected by many other process variables such as method of preparation, presence of additives (e.g. cross-linking agent, surfactant stabilizers, etc.) heat of polymerization, agitation intensity, etc. Percent incorporation in pre-formed microspheres is relatively less but the major advantage of the loading method being there no effect of process variables. The loading is carried out in pre-formed microspheres by incubating them with high concentration of the drug in a suitable solvent. The drug in these microspheres is loaded via penetration or diffusion of the drug through the pores in the microspheres as well as adsorption on their surface. The solvent is then removed, leaving drug-loaded microsphere. The drugs and protein can also be incorporated by physical or chemical linkage. The adsorption of the drugs/proteins depends on the nature of the polymers (Kipling, 1965). The Freundlich model is applied to determine the adsorption of the drugs. The Freundlich equation is

$$\frac{X}{M} = KC^{P}_{eq} \qquad (11\text{-}1)$$

Where K is a constant related to the capacity of the adsorbent for the adsorbate and P is a constant related to the affinity of the adsorbent for the adsorbate. Although this equation was first employed empirically, it can be derived with the assumption of a continuously varying heat of adsorption. The Freundlich model unfortunately predicts both infinite adsorption at infinite concentration and an infinite heat of adsorption at zero coverage.

DRUG RELEASE KINETICS

Release of the active constituent is an important consideration in case of microspheres. Many theoretically possible mechanisms may be considered for the release of drug from the microparticulates.

1. Liberation due to polymer erosion or degradation,
2. Self diffusion through the pore,
3. Release from the surface of the polymer,
4. Pulsed delivery initiated by the application of an oscillating or sonic field.

In most of the cases, a combination of more than one mechanism for drug of release may operate so the distinction amongst the mechanisms is not always trivial. The release profile from the microspheres depends on the nature of the polymer used in the preparation as well as on the nature of the active drug. The release of drug from both biodegradable as well as non-biodegradable microsphere(s) is influenced by structure or micro-morphology of the carrier and the properties of the polymer itself. The drugs could be released through the microspheres by any of the three methods, first is the osmotically driven burst mechanism, second pore diffusion mechanism and third by erosion or the degradation of the polymer. In osmotically driven burst mechanism, water diffuses into the core through biodegradable or non-biodegradable coating, creating sufficient pressure that ruptures the membrane. The burst effect is mainly controlled by three factors the macromolecule/polymer ratio, particle size of the dispersed macromolecule and the particle size of the microspheres. The pore diffusion method is named so because as penetrating waterfront continue to diffuse towards the core. The dispersed protein/drug dissolve creating a water filled pore network through which the active principle diffuses out in a controlled manner. In case of the biodegradable polymers, the release is controlled by both the erosion as well as diffusion process. The polymer erosion, i.e. loss of polymer is accompanied by accumulation of the monomer in the release medium. The erosion of the polymer begins with the changes in the microstructure of the carrier as water penetrates within it leading to the plasticization of the matrix. This plasticization of the matrix finally leads to the cleavage of the hydrolytic bonds. The cleavage of the bond is also facilitated by the presence of the enzyme (lysozymes) in the surroundings. The erosion of the polymer may be either surfacial or it may be bulk leading to the rapid release of the drug/active components. The rate and extent of water uptake therefore determines release profile of the system and depends on type of the polymer, porosity of the polymer matrix, protein drug loading, etc.

Factors affecting the release of the drug from the particulate system in relation to drug, microspheres and bioenvironment (Tomlinson, 1983):

- Drug
  - Position in microspheres
  - Molecular weight
  - Physicochemical properties
  - Concentration
  - Interaction with matrix
- Microspheres
  - Type and amount of the matrix polymer
  - Size and density of the microspheres
  - Extent of cross linking, denaturation or -polymerization
  - Adjuvants
- Environment
  - pH
  - Polarity
  - Presence of enzyme

Drug release from the non-biodegradable type of polymers can be understood by considering the geometry of the carrier. The geometry of the carrier, i.e. whether it is reservoir type where the drug is present as a core, or matrix type in which drug is dispersed throughout the carrier, governs overall release profile of the drug or active ingredients.

Reservoir Type System

Release from the reservoir type system with rate controlling membrane proceeds by first penetration of the water through the membrane followed by dissolution of the drug in the penetrating dissolution fluid. The dissolved drug after partitioning through the membrane diffuses across the stagnant diffusion layer. The release is essentially governed by the Fick's first law of diffusion as

$$J = -D(dc/dx) \qquad (11\text{-}2)$$

Where, J is flux per unit area, D is diffusion coefficient, and dc/dx is concentration gradient.

Diffusion across the membrane determines the effectiveness of the carrier system. The cumulative amount of drug that is released through the unit area, 'Q_t' at any time 't' is given by equation;

$$Q_t = \frac{C_s K D_m D_d t}{K D_m l_m + D_d l_d} \qquad (11\text{-}3)$$

Where, C_s represents saturation solubility of drug in dispersion medium, D_m is diffusion coefficient of drug in membrane of thickness l_m, D_d is diffusion coefficient of drug in static diffusion layer of thickness l_d, K is Partition coefficient of drug between membrane and reservoir compartments.

The release rate from the carriers can be modified by changing both the composition and the thickness of the polymeric membrane.

Matrix Type System

Release profile of the drug from the matrix type of the device critically depends on the state of drug whether it is dissolved or dispersed in the polymer matrix. In the case of the drug dissolved in the polymeric matrix, amount of drug, and the nature of the polymer (whether hydrophobic or hydrophilic) affect the release profile.

In case of drug dissolved in the polymeric matrix, the amount of drug appearing in the receptor phase at time 't' is approximated by two separate equations. The first equation determines the initial 60 percent of the drug release while the second shows the release profile at later stage.

$$\frac{dM_t}{dt} = 2M_x \ (D/\pi \ l^2 t)^{1/2} \qquad (11\text{-}4)$$

$$\frac{dM_t}{dt} = \frac{8\,D\,M_x}{l^2} \exp \frac{\pi^2 Dt}{l^2} \qquad (11\text{-}5)$$

where l is thickness of polymer slab, D is diffusion coefficient, M_x is the total amount of drug present in the matrix and M_t is the amount of drug released in time t. When the drug is dispersed throughout the polymer matrix then the release profile follows Higuchi's equation

$$\frac{dM_t}{dt} = \frac{A}{2} \frac{(2\,D\,C_s\,C_o)^{1/2}}{t} \qquad (11\text{-}6)$$

Where, A is area of matrix, C_s is solubility of the drug in the matrix and C_o represents total concentration in the matrix.

Taking porosity (ε) and tortuosity (τ) of the matrix into the consideration the above equation can be rewritten as

$$\frac{dM_t}{dt} = \left[\frac{\varepsilon}{\tau} D_m\,(2C_o - \varepsilon\ C_s)C_s t\right]^{1/2} \qquad (11\text{-}7)$$

POLYMERIC MICROSPHERES

Albumin Microspheres

The albumin is a widely distributed natural protein. The particulate or the colloidal form of albumin is considered as the potential carrier of drug/proteins for either their site-specific localization or their local application into anatomical discrete sites. Much of earlier use of serum albumin microspheres was limited to the diagnostic purpose as the microsphere of different size range locate themselves differentially at selected sites to facilitate the imaging. Now because of selected uptake of protein carrier by tumour cells, the microspheres of albumin are being widely used for the targeted drug delivery to the tumour cells. The preparation of the albumin microparticles is easy and particles of size range 15 nm to 150 μm diameter are easy to prepare. There are numerous methods available for preparation of the albumin microspheres, which involve the drug incorporation either during the preparation or after the formation of the particles as the conditions may be. On the basis of changes in process variables at the time of preparation the degradation time (Table 11-2) and diameter of microspheres (Table 11-3) can be varied. Albumin microparticle are mainly prepared by emulsion polymerization, using either heat denaturation of the particles at elevated temperature (100-180 °C) or chemical cross-linking. The albumin microspheres can also be prepared by denaturation of the protein aerosol in gas medium (Przyborowski et al., 1982) or an aerosol step followed by denaturation in oil (Millar et al., 1982).

The microspheres prepared by above methods are hydrophobic in nature, and therefore small amount of surface-active agent is needed to disperse them in parenteral preparation. Hydrophobic microspheres are rapidly cleared from the body. The hydrophilic microspheres are considered to be good carriers as they can carry large amounts of drug. Microspheres with increased hydrophilicity are advantageous because (i) they may exhibit enhanced surface physical and chemical properties *in vivo* (ii) they do not require surfactants currently needed to prepare aqueous dispersions which may influence tissue interaction, drug release, and activity (iii) hydrophilicity facilitates aqueous chemical modification (iv) high concentration of drug can be incorporated after preparation. In order to make the albumin microspheres to be hydrophilic a method was proposed by Longo et al., 1982. In this method the albumin droplets are stabilized using a high molecular weight polymer solution followed be cross-linking with glutaraldehyde introduced through organic phase, e.g. toluene. This in turn produces high cross-linking density at or near the surface accompanied by high concentration of mono reacted aldehyde (Fig. 11-8). This process increases the anionic character and leads to incorporation of greater hydrophilicity. The drug release from albumin microspheres depends on the degree of cross-linking. The surface free aldehyde and carboxyl groups (latter formed by

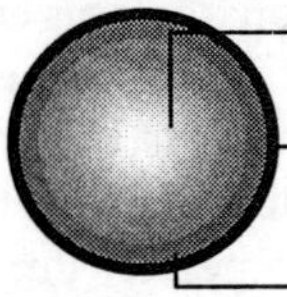

Low cross linking density

Reactive surface with CHO, COO⁻

High cross linking density

Fig. 11-8. Surface Cross-Linked Functional Microspheres

oxidation) can be used for further surface and bulk chemical modification. The reactive CHO groups are readily quenched or capped with compounds containing primary amino groups such as aminoalcohols or aminoacids (e.g. Glycine). Glycine conjugation leads to an increased anionic character and hence hydrophilicity.

The albumin microspheres were evaluated for the targeting potential of the chemotherapeutic agents. Albumin microspheres loaded with anticancer drug such as mitomycin C were found to be more effective than the drug alone. Burger et al., 1985 observed that cisplatin-loaded microspheres are 10 times more potent in targeting the drug to the patient with hypervascular liver carcinoma. Albumin microspheres can also be targeted to the various organ and cell lines and they are found to decrease the toxicity of the incorporated drugs. Intravenous injection can provide efficient targeting of albumin microspheres either to the lung or to the liver. Their ultimate location will depend on the size range of the microspheres. Microspheres of particle size range 15-30 μm or larger will pass through the heart and deposited in the capillary bed of lung with 99% efficiency. The microspheres of 1-3 μm sizes will pass into reticuloendothelial system where they deposit with 90% efficiency in the liver. Microspheres with particle size less then 1 μm, when injected intravenously, lead to about 80-90% deposition in lung, about 5-8% in spleen and about 1-2% in bone marrow. The release of drug from heat stabilized albumin microsphere is frequently biphasic in character. This biphasic profile is dependent to some degree on the water solubility of the entrapped drug. Highly water-soluble drug exhibits very noticeable biphasic release characteristics. Relatively water insoluble drugs such as steroids, which diffuse relatively slowly from the matrix, exhibit less pronounced biphasic release properties. The concentration of drug incorporated in the microspheres also plays a major role in governing the biphasic character of the drug release.

Gelatin Microspheres

Gelatin is proteinacious biodegradable polymer obtained from the partial hydrolysis of the collagen derived from the skin, connective tissues and bones of animals. The acid treated collagen is called type A and the alkali treated is referred to as type B gelatin. Gelatin microspheres are extensively studied because

Table 11-2. Effect of Cross-Linking Temperature on Albumin Microspheres Degradation

Cross linking temperature (°C)	50% solubilization time
135	24hr
160	84hr
170	4days
190	30 days

Table 11-3. Effect of Process Variable on the Diameter of Albumin Microspheres (Burger et al., 1985)

Process variables	Effect on diameter
Increased oil amount	Increase
Decreased oil viscosity	Increase
Increase protein amount	Increase
Increase aqueous phase	Increase
Increasing stirring speed	Decrease
Surfactant addition	No effect

they are prone to strong opsonization (Ikada and Tabata, 1986). Figure 11-9 represents minor details of macrophage morphology which on activation of macrophage explicitly translated into multifold protruded membrane as pseudopods. Thus, gelatin microspheres of suitable size range can be used as an efficient carrier system capable of delivering the drug or biological response modifiers such as interferon to the phagocytes (macrophages). Sustained release was obtained with the glutaraldehyde cross-linked microsphere while zero order release in case of the ethyl cellulose coated microspheres. Gelatin microspheres are reported to be taken up by some of the tumour cells, which do not take albumin (Oppenheim and Stewart, 1979).

Gelatin microspheres is prepared by cross linking gelatin in water in oil emulsion with glutaraldehyde. Opsonic gelatin microsphere are also prepared by similar method by dispersing gelatin having IFN-α A/D in oil followed by cross-linking with glutaraldehyde (Tabata and Ikada, 1989). The shape of the microspheres prepared by this method is spherical and size of the microspheres can be reduced to average diameter of about 1.5 μm by sonicating the emulsion. This size is suitable for macrophagic phagocytosis (Tabata and Ikada, 1988). The size and the surface characteristics of gelatin microspheres have great influence on the macrophage uptake (North, 1970; Cohn, 1970; Griffin et al., 1975; Stossel, 1975; Van Oss, 1975). Gelatin microspheres are found to be more opsonic than immunoglobulins and fibronectin, which are serum opsonic proteins (Ikada and Tabata, 1986; Tabata and Ikada, 1990). The gelatin microspheres have affinity towards the proteins so in presence of the serum, the microspheres may get coated by the serum proteins leading to an increased opsonization.

The gelatin microspheres being susceptible for the macrophage recognition, can be used as carrier for the antigens. The antigens from microspheres are released within the macrophages upon their degradation leading to enhanced production of antigen specific antibodies. Thus, gelatin microspheres can be used as immunoadjuvants (Kreuter et al., 1986a, 1986b; Tabata et al., 1995).

A number of different drugs have been studied for their targeting using gelatin based microparticulate carriers, such as sulphanilamide (Tanaka et al., 1963) for GIT; bleomycin (Nakamoto et al., 1975; Hashida et al., 1979) for lymph; mitomycin C (Yoshioka et al., 1981) for liver and joints and daunorubicin and fluorouracil (Oppenheim, 1981; Elsamaligy and Rohdewald, 1981) for liver tumours etc.

Starch Microspheres

Starch is one of the most abundant biodegradable polymers that belongs to carbohydrate class. It consists of the principle glucopyranose unit, which undergoes hydrolysis to yield D-glucose. Starch being a polysaccharide, consists of larger number of the

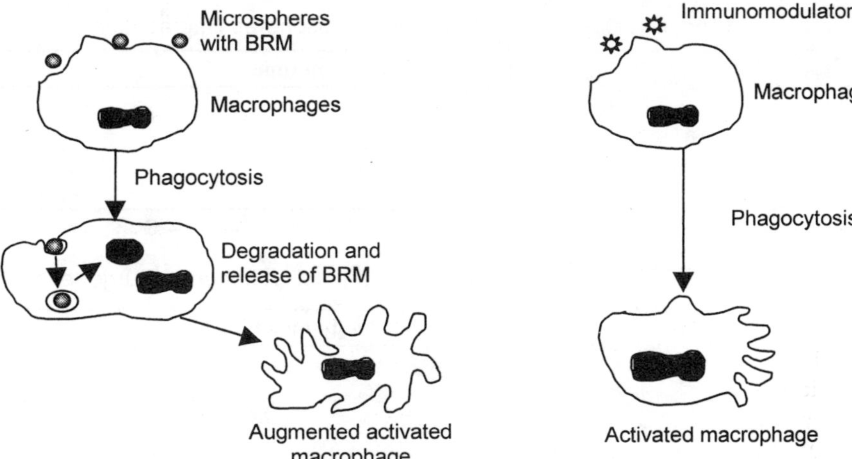

Fig. 11-9. Opsonization of Macrophages by Gelatin Microspheres

free hydroxyl groups. By means of these free hydroxyl groups a large number of the active ingredients can be incorporated within as well as active on surface of microspheres. The starch microspheres when introduced into the body cavity undergo potential swelling, leading to the development of mucoadhesive character. Therefore, they are not cleared rapidly from the body cavity. Intranasally administered insulin starch microspheres are cleared slowly and offer a delivery mode for protein and small molecules (Bjork and Edman, 1988).

Dextran Microspheres

Dextran, a carbohydrate is used to prepare hydrogel type of biodegradable and biocompatible systems. It can be chemically modified that provide higher percentage of drug or proteins incorporation. Simple method of incorporating aldehydes group to dextran is by oxidation using sodium iodate (Fig. 11-10). Protein loaded dextran microspheres are prepared by water in water emulsion technique (Fig. 11-11). In this method an aqueous solution of the methacrylated dextran is emulsified in aqueous solution of polyethylene glycol (PEG). The dispersed methacrylated phase is then cross-linked by using radical polymerization of the dextran bound methacrylate groups. This leads to the formation of the dexran microspheres with hydrogel character. The method is based on the phenomenon that phase separation occurs in aqueous solution of the dextran and polyethylene glycol (PEG) (Stenkes et al., 1998; Franssen and Hennink, 1998). The microspheres were rendered biodegradable by co entrapment of the dextranase. By using water and water emulsion technology it is possible to encapsulate IgG with very high entrapment or loading efficiency (more than 88%) (Franssen et al., 1999).

The release from the hydrogel matrix is dependent on the diffusion of the protein through the hydrogel matrix, if the protein diameter is smaller than the pore size of the matrix, it results in typical first order release. When the protein diameter is larger than the pore diameter, the release tends to be dependent on degradation rate of the gel. The rate of degradation of dextran microspheres depends entirely on the

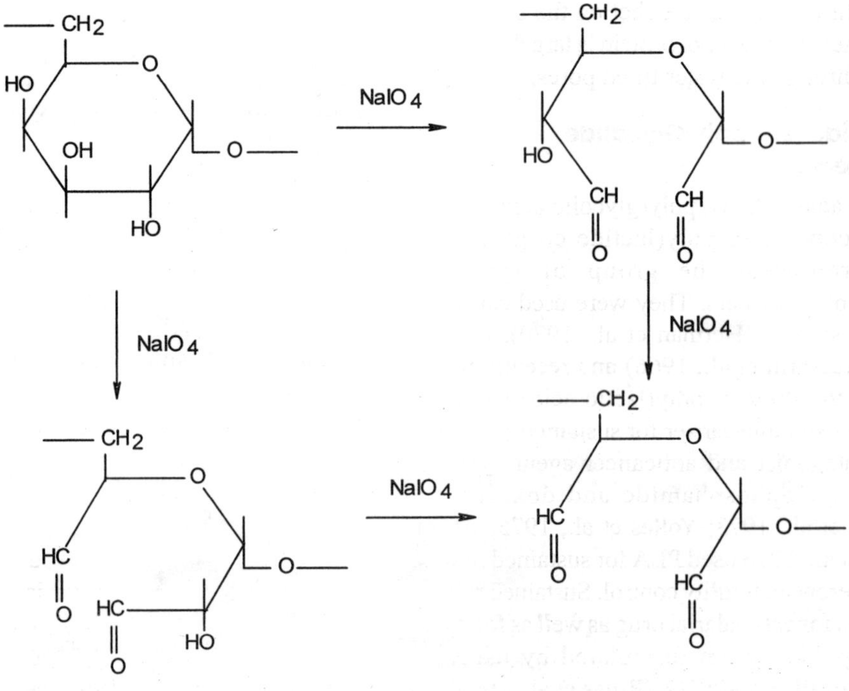

Fig. 11-10. Method for Aldehyde Incorporation in Dextran

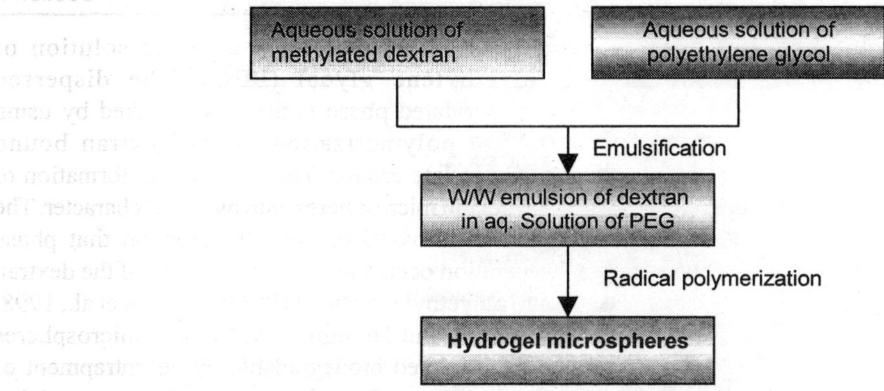

Fig. 11-11. Schematic Representation of Dextran Hydrogel Microspheres Preparation

degree of substitution of the dextran and the amount of dextranase enzyme incorporated. The optimization of the water content reduces the episodes of burst effect to less than 10%. Similarly, incorporation of dextranase helps in tailoring the release rate of the microspheres. A linear relationship between the amount of the dextranase and the initial degradation is generally recorded.

The major advantage of dextran water in water emulsion technique is that no organic solvent is used, which might have adverse effect on the stability of drug or protein and second, protein is largely allowed to release through the water filled pores.

Poly Lactide and poly Glycolide Microspheres

Poly(lactic acid) (PLA), poly(glycolic acid) (PGA) and their copolymer poly(lactide co glycolide) (PLGA) represent the group of synthetic biodegradable polymers. They were used earlier as absorbable sutures (Herman et al., 1970), implant material (Kulkarni et al., 1966) and recently as the carrier for the drug. L poly(lactic acid) has been reported as a suitable carrier for sustained release of narcotic antagonist and anticancer agents such as cisplatin, cyclophosphamide and doxorubicin (Woodland et al., 1973; Yolles et al., 1975, 1978). Anderson et al., 1976 used PLA for sustained release of norethisterone in fertility control. Sustained release preparations for antimalarial drug as well as for many other drugs have been formulated by using of copolymer of PLA and PGA (Rojas et al., 1999).

Microspheres from the PLA, PGA or PLGA may be prepared by any of the microparticles preparation techniques like single emulsion technique, double emulsion technique, phase separation coacervation, spray drying, etc. The PLGA microsphere are successfully prepared by double emulsion technique and phase separation methods. The phase separation method produces agglomerated microsphere in case of large scale production while the double emulsion method requires a lengthy and cumbersome procedure and it is difficult to incorporate the hydrophilic drugs (Jalil and Nixon, 1990; Takada et al., 1995). In contrast to these, spray drying method is fast and by controlling the different process variable desired type of microspheres can be obtained (Bodmeir and McGnity, 1987).

Double walled microsphere (Fig. 11-12) in size range 4-22 μm can be obtained in order to protect antigen (e.g. hepatitis) from the harmful effects of solvent. The method involves prior production of core microparticles by mixing hepatitis B antigen with hydroxy propyl cellulose (HPC) followed by spray drying (Lee et al., 1996). These core microparticle are then suspended in the PLGA/ ethyl acetate solution and spray dried to yield double walled microspheres.

To improve patient acceptance and to overcome drawbacks of traditional methods as (i) requirement of reconstitution before administration in the body cavity; (ii) presence of residual solvent and (iii) hazard of using organic solvents. A novel implant system has been developed, which after administration (in

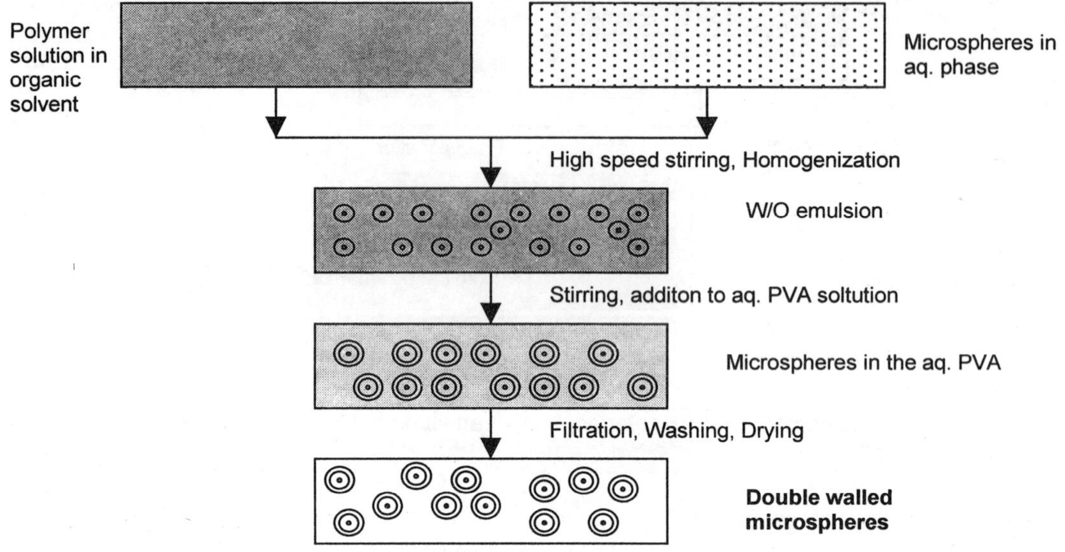

Fig. 11-12. Preparation of Double Walled Microspheres

liquid form) solidifies *in situ* (Shively et al., 1995; Shah et al., 1993). This method is reported by a number of scientists to deliver a number of antigen and variety of therapeutic classes. Figure 11-13 represents the method of preparation of these novel microspheres.

After injection, protein release occurs from biodegradable microspheres, as the protein diffuses from the interior of the microsphere through pores more void is created by polymer degradation or dissolution of encapsulated solids. The duration of release, which can range from days to months, is determined by polymer molecular weight, lactide:glycolide ratio, and the presence of hydrophobic end-groups. Excipients, such as zinc salts, can be included to stabilize the protein.

Polyanhydride Microspheres

Polyanhydrides are biodegradable and biocompatible polymers. They were first prepared using aromatic monomers (Bucher and Slade, 1990). The first aliphatic polyanhydride was prepared as a raw material for the textile purposes. In 1980's the polyanhydrides were rediscovered as they can be used for the erosion controlled devices in the area of drug delivery (Rosen et al., 1983). The polyanhydride can be manufactured with desired features (such as crystallinity, controlled degradation rate, degree of cross-linking, water uptake, etc.) by employing different monomers (Fig. 11-14) and controlling the polymerization process variables.

Polyanhydride microspheres can be prepared by solvent evaporation, solvent extraction, hot melt technique and spray drying techniques. For the hot melt encapsulation procedure, polyanhydrides were melted, and drug was dispersed in the melted polymer. This suspension was then transformed into microspheres by addition to or of a non-solvent such as silicone or olive oil, at 5 °C above the melting point of the polymer. The spheres solidified on subsequent cooling and were washed with petroleum ether. The temperature of the preparation is a limiting step of the method. Apart from these the double walled polyanhydride microspheres having two different polymer layers can be prepared using one of the two methods. The first method is based on the partial or complete insolubility of one polymer into other. The cosolution of the two polymers is then added to poly vinyl alcohol (PVA) aqueous solution followed by evaporation of the solvent. On evaporation of the solvent, the polymers separates from each other and finally give rise to core of one polymer while the coat of the other (Pekarek et al., 1994). The second method (Fig. 11-12) is based on

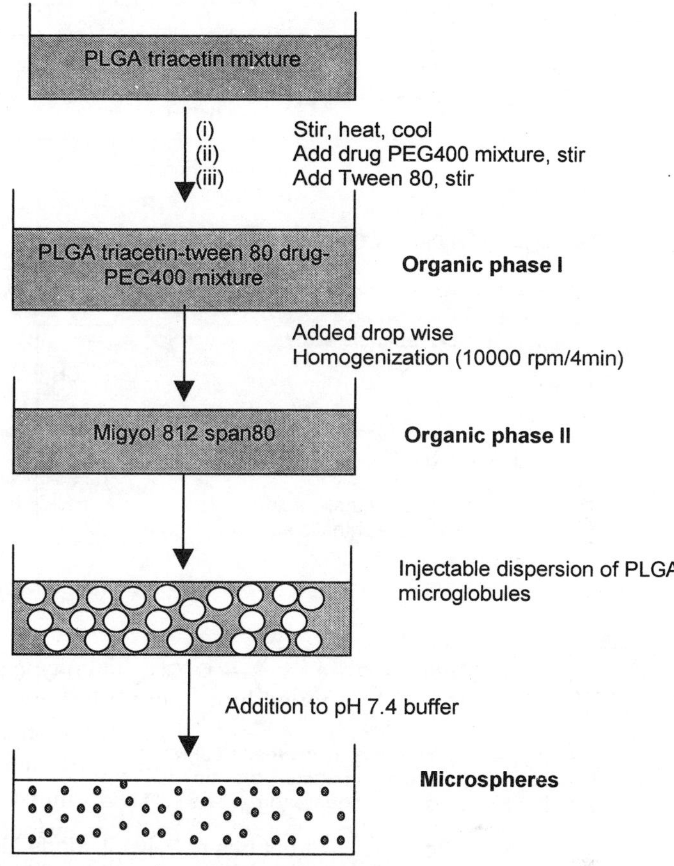

Fig. 11-13. Schematic for Novel PLA/PLGA Microspheres Formulation

the modified double emulsion technique. In this method the microspheres in aqueous phase are dispersed in a polymer solution in organic phase to form w/o emulsion. This is then added to the aqueous PVA solution to form the double walled microspheres instantaneously (Gopferich et al., 1994).

Polyanhydride microspheres of average particle size range 40 μm have been investigated to extend the precorneal residence time for ocular delivery (Albertson et al., 1993). Poly(adipic anhydride) was used to encapsulate timolol maleate for ocular delivery. Similarly, insulin loaded microspheres of p-carboxy propane were studied for use as release rate modifier (Mathiowitz and Langer, 1987).

Polyphosphazene Microspheres

Polyphosphazene polymers have a long chain backbone of alternating nitrogen and phosphorus atom with two side group attached to each phosphorus atom (Fig. 11-15). Polyphosphazene polymers form highly swollen ionotropic gel in the presence of the multivalent ions in aqueous media, such as calcium. Because of this property the polyphosphazene microspheres can be prepared under very mild conditions of low temperature and in absence of the organic solvent (Allcock and Kwon, 1989; Cohen et al., 1990). The microspheres are prepared by using a droplet apparatus, which produces spherical gel particle of size range 0.5-1.5 μm. In this method a 2.5% w/v phosphazene solution is added in the form of the droplets to a 7.5% w/v aqueous solution of calcium chloride. The microspheres (1-10 μm) have been used to target Peyer's Patch M cells and sub epithelial macrophages (Payne et al., 1995a, 1995b). The method describes

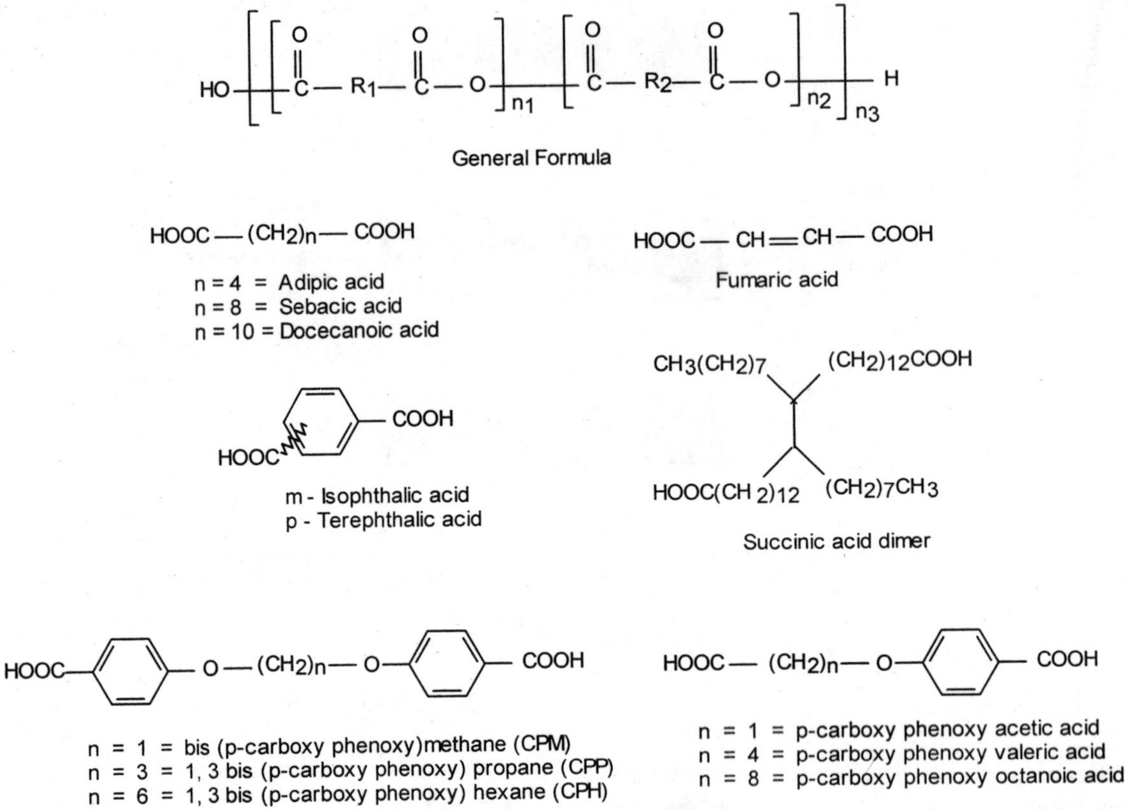

General Formula

$HOOC-(CH_2)_n-COOH$

n = 4 = Adipic acid
n = 8 = Sebacic acid
n = 10 = Docecanoic acid

$HOOC-CH{=}CH-COOH$

Fumaric acid

m - Isophthalic acid
p - Terephthalic acid

Succinic acid dimer

n = 1 = bis (p-carboxy phenoxy)methane (CPM)
n = 3 = 1, 3 bis (p-carboxy phenoxy) propane (CPP)
n = 6 = 1, 3 bis (p-carboxy phenoxy) hexane (CPH)

n = 1 = p-carboxy phenoxy acetic acid
n = 4 = p-carboxy phenoxy valeric acid
n = 8 = p-carboxy phenoxy octanoic acid

Fig. 11-14. Structures of Polyanhydride Monomers

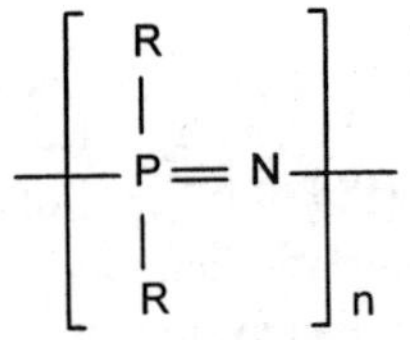

Fig. 11-15. General Formula for Polyphosphazene Polymer

the preparation of microspheres, where polyphosphazene polymer solution at pressure (40 Psi) is sprayed through an ultrasonic spray nozzle, which produces a spray cloud having the microdroplets of the polymer solution. This cloud when collide with the calcium chloride solution, instantaneously gels to form the microspheres (Fig. 11-16). The nature of the substrate and the gelation condition determine the encapsulation efficiency and the bioavailability and bioactivity of the substrate. Using this method the entrapment of ß-galactosidase enzyme was reported to be about 80%. Hydroma cells were encapsulated up to 30% with recorded viability of about 70%. The polyphosphazene microspheres are sensitive to the ionic environment of the surroundings. They can be stabilized by coating with positively charged polyelectrolytes such as poly(L-lysine) (Andrianov et al., 1993). The hydrophobicity of the polyphosphazene can be manipulated by subsequent reaction of PLA surface with the polycation solution. The formation of the inter polymer complex at the surface and within provides stability to the microspheres in saline solution (Tsuchida and Abe, 1986; Kabanov and Zezin, 1982).

Chitosan Microspheres

Recently, natural polymers such as polysaccharides and proteins have received much attention in the pharmaceutical field owing to their good

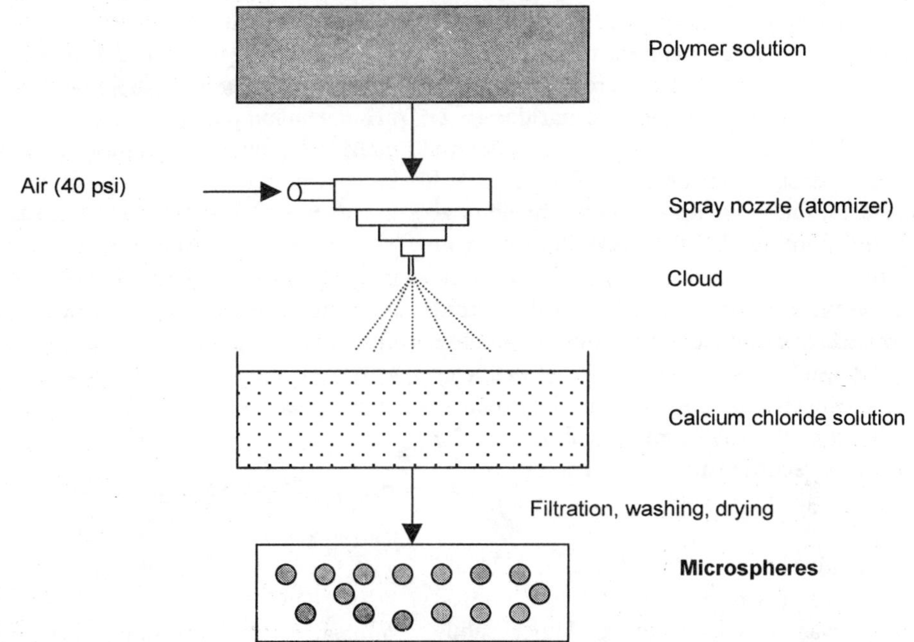

Fig. 11-16. Schematic **Representing** the Formation of Polyphosphazene

biocompatibility and biodegradability. Among polysaccharides, chitosan, the deacetylated product of chitin, is one of the most useful natural polymers from the viewpoint of possible exploitation of natural resources. Chitosan is insoluble at neutral and alkaline pH values, but forms salts with inorganic and organic acids such as hydrochloric acid. Upon dissolution, the amine groups of chitosan get protonated and the resultant polymer becomes positively charged. Since chitosan exhibits net positive charge, it has been recently introduced in the market as an aid for weight loss and as cholesterol-lowering agent. The mechanism behind chitosan may be its effect on lipid transport in the gut, where the positively charged chitosan can bind to the free fatty acids and bile salt components and hence disrupts overall lipid absorption (Ravi kumar, 2000).

The effect of chitosan has been considered mainly because of its positive charge; however, the adsorption process could also be the result of other forces that might exist between molecules, such as hydrogen bonding or Vander Waal's forces. These interactions might have a strong impact on the absorption and bioavailability of pharmaceutical compounds, especially drugs that are potent and have low water solubility.

Yao et al., 1995 highlighted the preparation and properties of microcapsules and microspheres of chitosan. Due to attractive properties and wider applications of chitosan-based microcapsules and microspheres, they are used as a carrier for the applications in controlled drug release. Moreover, microcapsules and microspheres have an edge over other forms in regard to their handling and administration.

Polysaccharides or Lipid Crosslinked Chitosan Microspheres

Ohya and Takei, 1993 studied 5-fluorouracil (5-FU) and its amino derivatives, loaded cross linked chitosan microspheres coated with polysaccharide or lipid for controlled and targeted drug delivery. The microspheres were prepared with an inverse emulsion of 5-FU or its salt solution with chitosan contained in aqueous phase while toluene containing span 80 served as dispersion phase. Chitosan was cross-linked with Schiff's salt formation on addition of glutaraldehyde toluene solution. At the same time, the amino derivatives of 5-FU were immobilized, obviously resulting in an increase in drug content within the microspheres. The microspheres were further coated with anionic polysaccharides (e.g. carboxymethylchitin) through a polyion complexation reaction. In the case of lipid coated microsphere, the microspheres along with dipalmitoyl phosphatidyl choline (DPPC) were dispersed in chloroform. After evaporation of the solvent, microspheres were obtained coated with DPPC lipid multilayers, which exhibited a transition temperature of a liquid crystal phase at 41.4 °C. The diameter range of microspheres was 250-300 nm with a narrow size distribution. Improvement in stability of the dispersion was recorded following coating of the microspheres with anionic polysaccharide or a lipid multilayer.

A comparative study on the release of 5-FU and its derivatives from polysaccharide coated microspheres was carried out in physiological saline at 37 °C. Data indicated that the 5-FU-release rate decreased in the order: free-5-FU > carboxymethyl type 5-FU > ester type 5-FU. The results revealed that the coating imposed the effective barriers to 5-FU release. The lipid mutilayers with a homogeneous composition generally show a transition of gel-liquid crystal. When the temperature raises to 42 °C, i.e. above the phase transition temperature (41.4 °C), the amount of 5-FU released is increased. In contrast the amount of drug delivered decreased at 37 °C or at temperature below the transition temperature. Due to the improved recognition function of polysaccharide chains for animal cell membranes, it is reasonable to develop targeted delivery systems using polysaccharide for coating of the microspheres.

Chitosan/gelatin polymers based microspheres are reported for controlled release of cimetidine. The drug loaded microspheres were prepared by dissolving chitosan, gelatin (1:1 by weight) and cimetidine in 5% acetic acid. A certain amount of Tween-80 and liquid paraffin at a water to oil ratio of 1:10 was added to the chitosan/gelatin mixture under agitation at 650 rpm at 30 °C. A suitable amount of 25% w/v aqueous glutaraldehyde solution was added to the inverse emulsion and maintained for 2 h. Finally, the liquid paraffin was vaporized under vacuum to obtain microspheres. The drug release studies were performed in 0.1N hydrochloric acid solution (pH 1.0) and potassium dihydrogen phosphate buffer (pH 7.8, ionic strength 0.1 m/L). A pH dependent pulsed-release behaviour of the HPN matrix was observed. Moreover, the release rate can be controlled via the composition of the HPN and the degree of deacetylation of chitosan. Gohel et al., 1994 reported the preparation of chitosan microspheres containing diclofenac sodium by co-acervation phase separation method. Chitosan and glutaraldehyde were used as coating material and crosslinking agent respectively. Moreover, the microspheres were found to be stable at 45 °C for 30 days.

Carrageenan Microsphere

Carrageenan is an anionic polymer of hemisulphate galactose and 3-4 anhydrogalactose residue alternately linked by α 1-3 and ß1-4 glycosidic linkage. Hemisulphate ester groups impart negative charge to the polymer. Based on the sulphate groups esterification pattern, the polymer is graded as the L, κ, and δ. L-carrageenan has been proved to be a better candidate for the preparation of the microspheres using aqueous microencapsulation process that avoids the use of the organic solvents, which may alter the biological properties. Patil and Speaker, 2000 uses carrageenan for the formulation of model protein horseradish peroxide in the water based microsphers delivery system. Patil and Speaker, 1997 have described the method for carrageenan microspheres preparation (Fig. 11-17). They pumped mixture of 0.6 mM L-carrageenan (9 ml) and 1 mg/ml horseradish peroxide at the flow rate of the 1 ml/min through a 76 μm orifice to produce a continuous jet. Against the side of the capillary, sonic pulsing was applied to produce uniform droplets. The formed droplets were allowed to fall into a magnetically stirred amine solution (15 ml). To establish the correct concentration of the amine the concentration of amine is varied and tested for stable microspheres. Prepared microspheres were separated by the centrifugation (10000 g) and washed twice with 10 ml distilled water.

Alginate Microspheres

Many of the present controlled release devices in their preparation involve harsh and hazardous chemicals

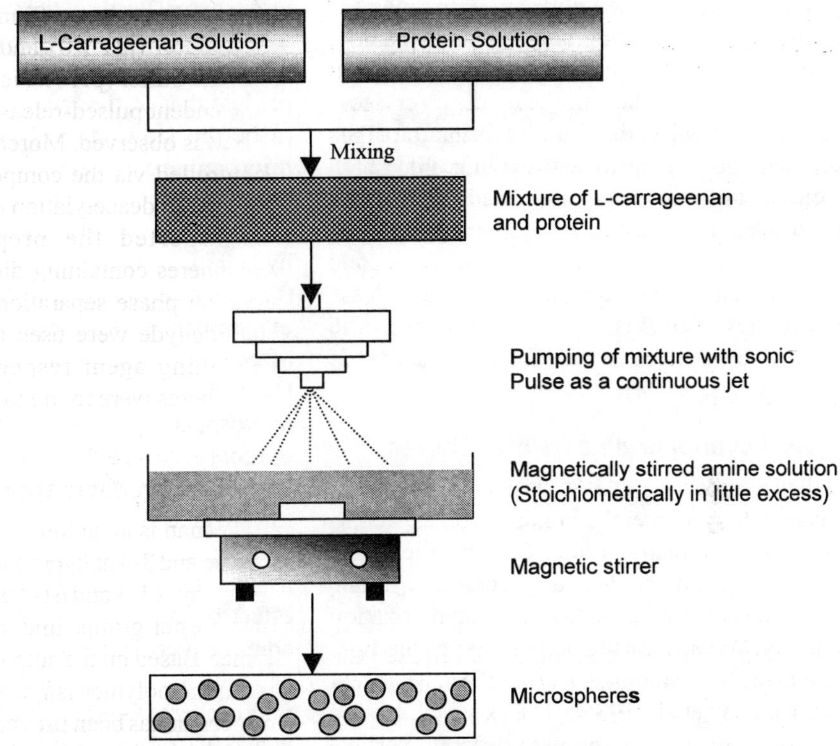

Fig. 11-17. Schematic for Carrageenan preparation

such as organic solvents or extreme conditions such as high temperature, which can adversely affect the drug or the proteins. Alginate microspheres are suggested for such sensitive drugs. Sodium alginate (NaAlg), a water soluble salt of alginic acid, is a natural polysaccharide extracted from marine brown algae. It contains two uronic acids, ß-D-mannuronic acid (M) and α-L-glucouronic acid (G), and it is composed of homopolymeric blocks MM or GG, and blocks with an alternating sequence (MG blocks). NaAlg has been used as a matrix for entrapment of drugs and macromolecules. Some of the applications of NaAlg relate to its particular property: it can form hydrophilic gels by interaction with bivalent metal ions. Since alginate gel can easily be formed by this ionic interaction in aqueous medium, gel beads are commonly obtained by dropping solutions of sodium alginate into solutions of calcium chloride. Many grades of sodium alginate are available and are selected depending upon the purpose, e.g. high L-glucouronic acid content gives high gel strength. Most of the alginic acids consist of the homopolymeric block of the D-mannuronic acid and L-glucouronic acid. Enzymatic degradation using a poly (L-glucouronate) lyase to leave the poly mannuronic blocks intact, has shown that these blocks have a uniform chain length of 24 residues (Mumper et al., 1994; Kim and Lee, 1992; Kikuchi et al., 1996; Yotsuyanagi et al., 1991).

The alginate microspheres are usually prepared by suspending the protein in sodium alginate solution and spraying this solution into 1.3%w/v buffered (HEPES Buffer) calcium chloride to form cross linked microcapsules. Poor formation of the capsule occurs due to strong protein alginate interaction. As a result, diffusion technique is employed for the incorporation of the drug and proteins. In this technique the plain alginate microsphere are produced using the previous technique. Protein is then subsequently loaded by allowing its stepwise diffusion from solution of increasing concentration. The drug loaded capsules are coated with a final layer of polycation. In all, three polycation coatings are used, i.e. two prior loading and one after loading. The first coating influences the size, integrity, and loading capacity of the microcapsule. Very low concentration of polycation leads to formation of the capsule with poor integrity and loading while high concentration prevents the loading of the microcapsules. The first coat also influences duration of the drug release, size and burst effect. The second coat too influences the drug loading and the release characteristics. The final coat however, has little effect on the drug release profile (Timida et al., 1993; Rubio and Ghaly, 1994).

Poly(alkyl cyanoacrylate) Microspheres

Poly(alkyl cyanoacrylate), PAC, is potential colloidal drug carrier for parenteral administration as well as through other alternative routes (ophthalmic, oral). The microspheres of the PAC are prepared by simple polymerization techniques. Several polymerization systems can be used for the preparation of the PAC microspheres (Couvreur and Aurby, 1984; Maincent , 1982; Douglas et al., 1985a; 1986), which lead to the microspheres production with different particle size ranges. The general method of preparation of PAC microspheres involves addition of the monomer (1% v/v) to the rapidly stirred aqueous phase. The pH of the system is critical in deciding the polymerization rate of the alkyl cyanoacrylate monomers. The pH of the system is normally adjusted to 2-4 for optimum polymerization rate. pH more than 4 leads to very rapid polymerization while in case of pH less than 2, the rate of the polymerization tends to be too slow. In body polyalkyl cyanoacrylate microspheres degrade by reverse Knovenagel reaction (Leonard et al., 1966) resulting in the production of alkyl 2-cyanoacrylate and formaldehyde (Fig. 11-18). The rate of degradation varies with the ester chain length and pH of the media. The choice of the monomer and the polymerization condition also affect the degradation rate of the microspheres (Douglas et al., 1985b). Poly cyano-acrylate microspheres loaded with anticancerous agents are extensively studied for the purpose of tumour targeting. PAC microspheres have natural affinity towards the tumours and they also possess inherent anti tumour activity. These are found to have higher tumour uptake. The studies indicate that anti tumour effect of cytotoxic drugs increases when they are administered contained in the PAC microspheres. Monoclonal antibodies may be used to target PAC microspheres (Kreuter and Hartmen, 1983; Brasseur et al. 1980). Monoclonal antibodies can be attached to the microspheres either via spacer group or by simple adsorption. These particles are specifically taken by the tumour cells. The PAC microspheres are also used for the targeting of the liver diseases. The tissue toxicity of PAC microspheres decreases

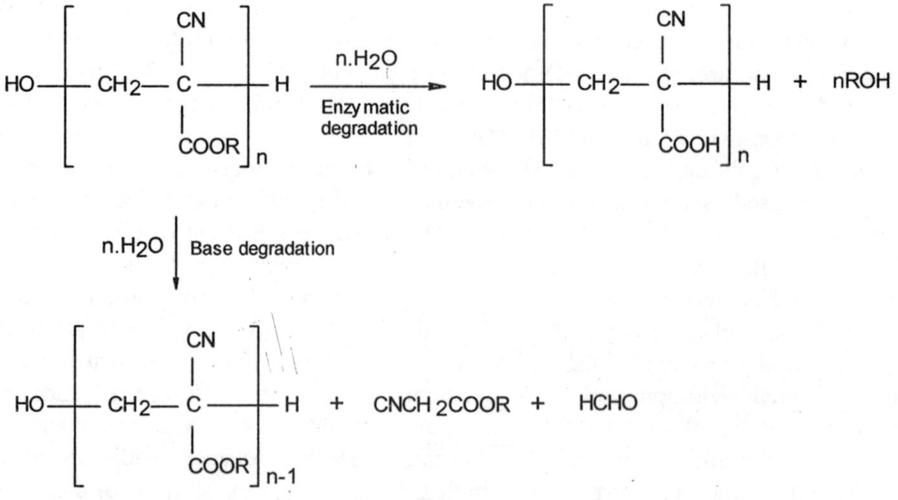

$$HO-\left[CH_2-\underset{COOR}{\overset{CN}{C}}\right]_n-H \xrightarrow[\text{Enzymatic degradation}]{n.H_2O} HO-\left[CH_2-\underset{COOH}{\overset{CN}{C}}\right]_n-H + nROH$$

$$\Big\downarrow \; n.H_2O \quad \text{Base degradation}$$

$$HO-\left[CH_2-\underset{COOR}{\overset{CN}{C}}\right]_{n-1}-H + CNCH_2COOR + HCHO$$

Fig. 11-18. Degradation Pathways of Poly(alkyl cyanoacrylate) Microspheres

with decrease in the rate of degradation and it increases in a homologous series. Polymethyl cyanoacrylate was found to be more toxic in the series because of rapid degradation of the polymer. LD_{50} value for the isobutyl and butyl microsphere was found to be 196 mg and 230 mg/kg following the intravenous injection, which shows an increase in toxicity within the homologous series (Kante et al., 1982). The rate of administration also determines the toxicity of the polymer (Avila, 1983).

Polyacrolein Microspheres

Poly acrolein microspheres are functional type of the microspheres. These microspheres do not require any activation step since the surfacial free aldehyde groups over the poly acrolein can react with amine group of the protein to form Schiff's base. Poly acrolein microspheres remain active for more than a month when stored at 4 °C. The hydrophilicity can be generated by copolymerizing the acrolein monomer with monomers such as hydroxy ethyl methacrylate, styrene or methyl methacrylate (Rembaum 1983; Rembaum and Dreyer, 1980). The poly acrolein microspheres are prepared by alkaline polymerization of acrolein monomer (Fig. 11-19) or by copolymerization of acrolein monomer with other monomers. Acrolein microspheres can be prepared by simple radiation polymerization using Cobalt 60. Acrolein molecules have two functionality one is carboxyl while other is vinyl. Studies have shown that acrolein polymerizes through its vinyl groups. The resultant polymer exists in equilibrium with the acetal isomer (Fig. 11-20). Poly acrolein microspheres were successfully prepared by aqueous polymerization of acrolein in the presence of an appropriate surfactant under alkaline condition (Fig. 11-21). Agarose poly acrolein micro beads can be prepared by encapsulating poly acrolein microspheres in agarose gel matrix. The cross linking is affected using divinyl sulphone. This system acts as an efficient immunoadsorbent.

FATE OF MICROSPHERES IN BODY

Microparticulate carrier systems can be administered through different routes such as intravenous, ocular, intra muscular, intra arterial, oral, etc. Each route has its own biological significance, limitation and pharmaceutical feasibility. The microparticles are intended to be administered through different routes to achieve desired activity of either sustained action or targeting or both. Through different routes different mechanisms of uptake, transport and fate of translocated particles have been proposed.

Biodegradable microparticulate carriers are of interest for oral delivery of drugs to improve the bioavailability (Maincent et al., 1986), to enhance drug absorption (Couvreur et al., 1979, 1984, Illum

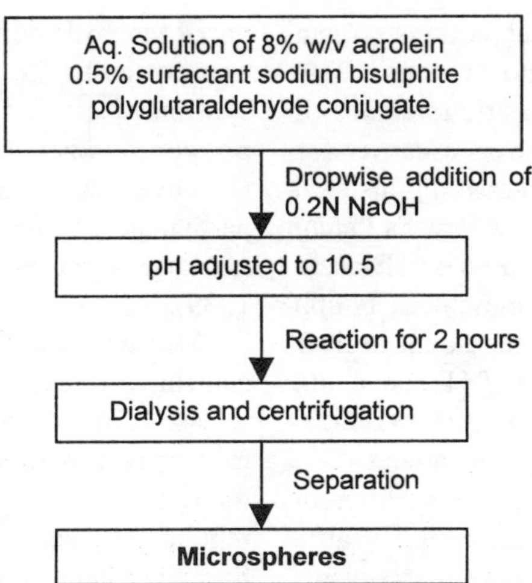

Fig. 11-19. Schematic Representation of Polyacrolein Microspheres Preparation

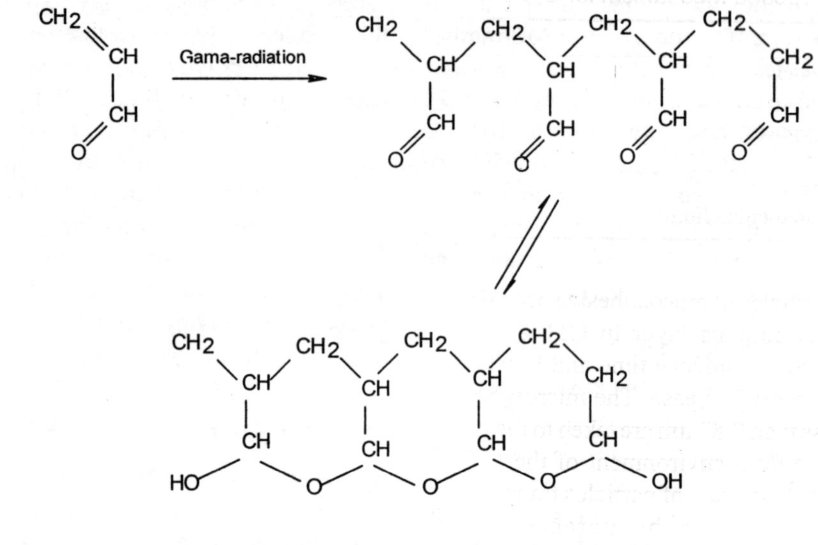

Fig. 11-20. Radiation Polymerization of Polyacrolein

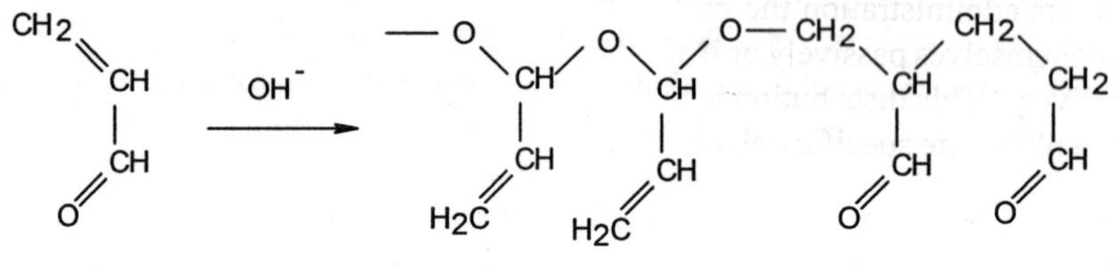

Fig. 11-21. Base Catalysed Polymerization in Polyacrolein

et al., 1987, Kreuter 1983), to target particular organ and reduced toxicity (Kramer and burstein 1976; Marty et al., 1978), to improve gastric tolerance of gastric irritant to the stomach and as a carrier for antigen. The polystyrene microspheres administered orally are reported to be taken up by Peyer's Patch. They are subsequently translocated to discrete anatomical compartments such as mesenteric lymph vessels, lymph nodes and to a lesser extent in liver and spleen (Sanders and Ashworth 1961, Jani et al., 1990). The particulate matters gain entry into follicle associated epithelium through Peyer's Patches.

After the uptake of the particulate carrier via different mechanism their fate becomes important (Table 11-4) (O'Hagan, 1990). Some uptake mechanisms avoid the lysosomal system of the enterocytes. The particles following uptake by enterocytes are transported to the mesenteric lymph, followed by systemic circulation and are subsequently phagocytosized by the Kupffer cells of liver. However, after uptake by enterocytes, some particulate carriers may be taken up into vacuoles and discharged back into gut lumen (Alpar et al., 1989).

Microspheres can also be designed for the controlled release to the gastrointestinal tract. The release of the drug content depends on the size of microparticles and the drug content within microspheres. The release of the drug could be regulated by selecting an appropriate hydrophilic / lipophilic balance of the matrix such as in case of matrix of polyglycerol esters of fatty acid (Ebel,

Table 11-4. Proposed Mechanism for Uptake of Particulate

Site	Size range	Fate
Enterocyte/Endocyte	<220 nm	RES uptake
Paracellular uptake	100-200 nm	Unknown
Intestinal macrophage	1 μm	MLN
Persorption	5-150μm	Blood & Excretory fluids
Peyer's Patches	20 nm-10μm	PP and MLN
Follicle associated epithelium	< 750 nm	MLN.

1990). Microparticles of mucoadhesive polymers get attached to the mucous layer in GIT and hence prolong the gastric residence time and functionally offer a sustained drug release. The microspheres of particle size less than 0.87 μm are taken to the general circulation. The fluid environment of the GIT can affect the number and rate of particles translocation.

Microspheres given by parenteral route (intravenous) distribute themselves according to their size range. The microparticulate carriers are rapidly cleared from the circulation mainly by means of reticuloendothelial system (Fig. 11-22).

After intravenous administration the particulate carriers distribute themselves passively or if suitably designed, then actively. This distribution is referred to as passive mode of the site specific delivery of the microparticulates.

CHARACTERIZATION

The characterization of the microparticulate carrier is an important phenomenon, which helps to design a suitable carrier for the proteins, drug or antigen delivery. The microspheres have different microstructures, which depend on their method of preparation and conditions during preparation (Schugens et al 1994). These microstructures determine the release and the stability of the carrier. A number of other parameters are generally evaluated for the characterization of microspheres.

Particle Size and Shape

The most widely used procedures to visualize microparticles are conventional light microscopy (LM) and scanning electron microscopy (SEM). Both techniques can be used to determine the shape and outer structure of the microparticles. Nevertheless, they have certain limitations when used for the analysis of the internal structure of such particles. Particle size and its distribution are determined by light microscopy, scanning electron microscopy, electron microscopy etc. Light microscopy provides a control over coating parameters in case of double walled microspheres. The microsphere structures can be visualized before and after coating and the change can be measured microscopically.

The scanning electron microscopy (SEM) provides higher resolution in contrast to the light microscopy (Mathews and Nixon, 1974). SEM allows investigations of the microspheres surfaces and after particles are cross-sectioned, it can also be used for the investigation of double walled systems.

Confocal laser scanning microscopy (CLSM) is applied as a nondestructive visualization technique for microparticles. Moreover, CLSM allows visualization and characterization of structures not only on the surface, but also inside the particles, provided the material is sufficiently transparent and can be fluorescently labeled. By collecting several coplanar cross sections, a three-dimensional reconstruction of the inspected objects is possible. CLSM has already been used in the evaluation and characterization of solid pharmaceutical formulations, including determination of the release kinetics of the entrapped drugs and examination of the swelling of microparticles by using fluorescein-containing aqueous media. Furthermore, microparticles were visualized in order to depict the dispersion of the entrapped phase and polymer structures on the surface.

Confocal fluorescence microscopy is used for the structure characterization of multiple walled microspheres. The core and the coating polymers are stained with two different dyes and they show two different absorption spectra. Using proper filters the two spectra can be separated and analyzed for

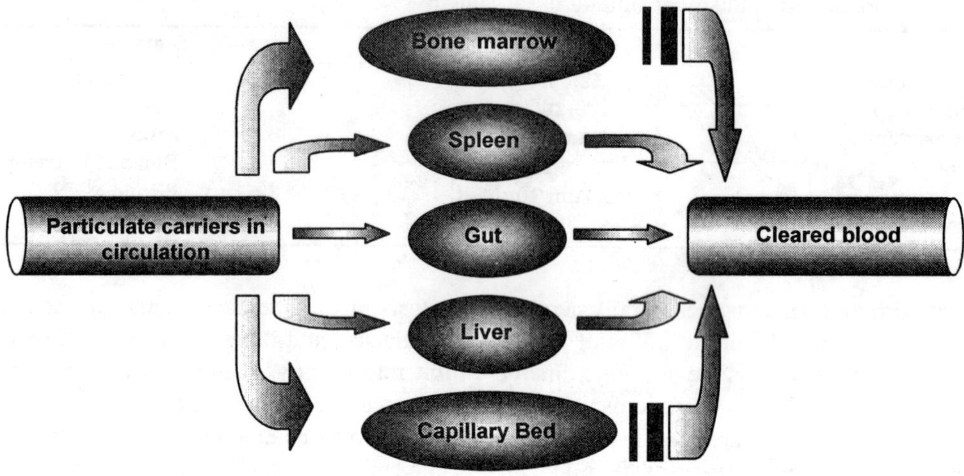

Fig. 11–22. RES Systems for Microparticulate Clearance

the core and coating polymer (Lamprecht et al., 2000). Laser light scattering and multisize coulter counter are other instrumental methods, which can be used for the characterization of size, shape and morphology of the microspheres.

Electron Spectroscopy for Chemical Analysis

The surface chemistry of the microspheres can be determined using the electron spectroscopy for chemical analysis (ESCA). ESCA provides a means for the determination of the atomic composition of the surface. The spectra obtained using ESCA can be used to determine the surfacial degradation of the biodegradable microspheres.

Attenuated Total Reflectance Fourier Transform-Infrared Spectroscopy

FTIR is used to determine the degradation of the polymeric matrix of the carrier system. The surface of the microspheres is investigated measuring alternated total reflectance (ATR) (Fig. 11-23). The IR beam passing through the ATR cell reflected many times through the sample to provide IR spectra mainly of surface material. The ATR-FTIR provides information about the surface composition of the microspheres depending upon manufacturing procedure and conditions.

Density Determination

The density of the microspheres can be measured by using a multivolume pychnometer. Accurately weighed sample in a cup is placed into the multivolume pychnometer. Helium is introduced at a constant pressure in the chamber and allowed to expand. This expansion results in a decrease in pressure within the chamber. Two consecutive readings of reduction in pressure at different initial pressure are noted. From two pressure readings the volume and hence the density of the microsphere carrier is determined.

Isoelectric Point

The microelectrophoresis is an apparatus used to measure the electrophoretic mobility of microspheres from which the isoelectric point can be determined. The mean velocity at different pH values ranging from 3-10 is calculated by measuring the time of particle movement over a distance of 1 mm. Using these data the electrical mobility of the particle can be determined. The electrophoretic mobility can be related to surface contained charge, ionisable behaviour or ion absorption nature of the microspheres.

Surface Carboxylic Acid Residue

The surface carboxylic acid residue is measured by using radioactive glycine. The radioactive glycine

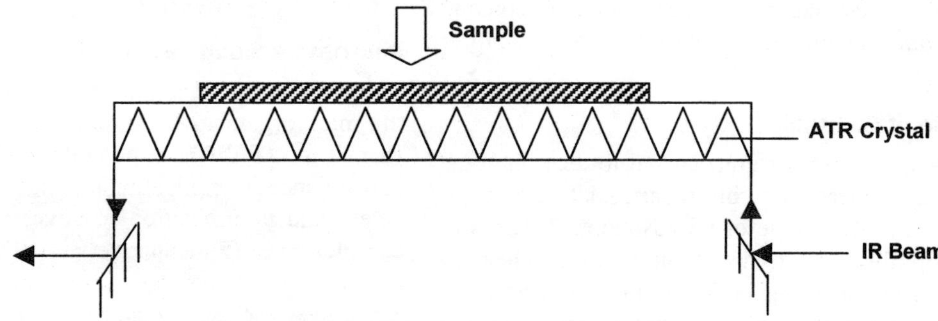

Fig. 11-23. Attenuated Total Reflectance Spectroscopy

conjugate is prepared by reaction of ^{14}C-glycine ethyl ester hydrochloride with the microspheres. The glycine residue is linked using a water soluble condensing agent 1-ethyl-3 (3-dimethyl amino propyl) carbidiimide (EDAC). The radioactivity of the conjugate is then measured using liquid scintillation counter. Thus the carboxylic acid residue can be compared and correlated. The free carboxylic acid residue can be measured for hydrophobic or hydrophilic or any other derivatized type of the microspheres.

Surface Amino Acid Residue

Surface associated amino acid residue is determined by the radioactive ^{14}C - acetic acid conjugate. The carboxylic acid residue is measured through the liquid scintillation counter and hence the amino acid residue can be determined indirectly. EDAC is used to condense the amino group and the ^{14}C-acetic acid carboxylic acid residue. The method used for determining the free amino or the free carboxylic acid residues are based on indirect estimation, by measuring the radioactivity of the ^{14}C having acetic acid or the glycine conjugate. The accuracy of the method however, depends on the time allowed for conjugation of the radioactive moiety and the reactivity of free functional group (MacAdams et al., 1997).

Capture Efficiency

The capture efficiency of the microspheres or the percent entrapment can be determined by allowing washed microspheres to lyse. The lysate is then subjected to the determination of active constituents as per monograph requirement. The percent encapsulation efficiency is calculated using following equation:

$$\% \text{ Entrapment} = \frac{\text{Actual content}}{\text{Theoretical content}} \times 100$$

Release Studies

Release studies for microspheres in phosphate saline buffer of pH 7.4, are carried out using rotating paddle apparatus or by using dialysis method. In case of the paddle apparatus the sample is agitated at 100 rpm. The samples are taken at specific time intervals and are replaced by same amount of saline. The active ingredient in the sample withdrawn is analysed as per the monograph requirement and release profile is determined using the plot of amount released as a function of time. The release profile of the drugs or proteins generally depends on the method of formulation, formulation conditions (process variable), and more importantly on the nature of the polymer used for the preparation. Degradation profile of the polymer is another important parameter, which determines, whether the release is sustained, prolonged or burst type. Dialysis is another method used to study the release of the drugs/proteins from the microspheres. The method involves the use of the assembly shown in the Fig. 11-24. The microspheres are kept in a dialysing bag or tube with membrane, while the dialysing media is continuously stirred and samples of dialysate are taken. The withdrawn samples are estimated for drug content. Each time the volume is replaced using fresh buffer solution.

Angle of Contact

The angle of contact is measured to determine the wetting property of a microparticulate carrier. It determines the nature of microspheres in terms of hydrophilicity or hydrophobicity. This thermodynamic property is specific to solid and affected by the presence of the adsorbed component. The angle of contact is measured at the solid/air/water interface. The method for the determination of the angle of contact is given by Nutt who proposed that the particle floating at interface is subjected to number of forces such as gravitational, Archimedean thrust, etc. These forces affect the angle of contact. The advancing and receding angle of contact are measured by placing a droplet in a circular cell mounted above objective of inverted microscope. Contact angle is measured at 20 °C within a minute of deposition of microspheres.

APPLICATIONS

Microspheres in Vaccine Delivery

The prerequisite of a vaccine is protection against the microorganism or its toxic product. An ideal vaccine must fulfil the requirement of efficacy, safety, convenience in application and cost. The aspect of safety and minimization of adverse reaction is a complex issue (Fudenberg et al., 1978). The aspect of safety and the degree of production of antibody responses are closely related to mode of application. Biodegradable delivery systems for vaccines that are given by parenteral route may overcome the shortcoming of the conventional vaccines (Capron et al., 1994; Edelman, 1993; Drews, 1984; Spier, 1993). The interest in parenteral (subcutaneous, intra muscular, intradermal) carrier lies since they offer specific advantages including:

1. Improved antigenicity by adjuvant action,
2. Modulation of antigen release,
3. Stabilization of antigen.

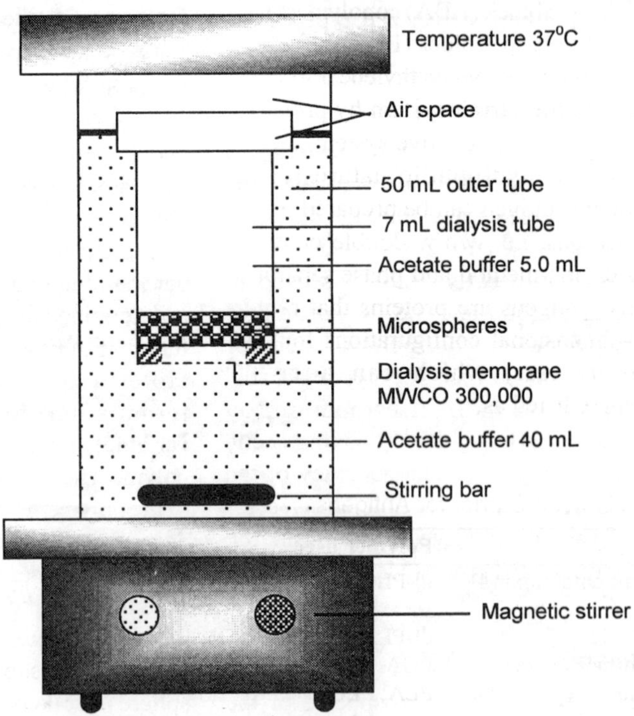

Fig. 11-24 Dialysis Assembly

Polymers for Vaccine Delivery System

Biodegradable polymers belong to a class of choice for the delivery of the vaccine since they do not require surgical removal. Apart from biodegradation kinetics, the mode and rate of presentation of antigen, toxicity, tissue compatibility as well as antigen stability are properties that are critically considered for the selection of the appropriate polymer and method of preparation. Thermoplastic polyesters of poly (lactic acid), poly (glycolic acid) and their copolymers poly (lactides co glycolides) (PLGA) are studied extensively as the carrier for many antigens (Table 11-5).

Stability

Antigen polymer compatibility is a major barrier encountered in the design of a suitable carrier because it may lead to the stability problem. The polymer compatibility can be increased by coencapsulating buffer salts and stabilizers for proteins which are thought to increase the antigen stability by modifying the internal pH of microspheres and accelerating swelling. The use of triblock (ABA) copolymers (Fig. 11-25) having hydrophilic A block (PLA or PLAGA) and hydrophilic B block (Polyoxyethylene, PEO) also provide stability to the carrier system by providing more gentle and an accommodative system

Microspheres of hydrophilic nature for the delivery of proteins/antigen can be prepared by any of the three methods, i.e. w/o/w double emulsion method, spray drying method and phase separation method. Mostly, antigens are proteins that require specific three-dimensional configurations for their activity. The factors, which can alter the conformations, are listed as,

- Polymer
- Moisture
- Lyophilization
- pH
- Shearing
- Temperature
- Rotation
- Hydrophilic/hydrophobic surface
- Salt
- Organic solvent

Antigen Release

The release of antigens from the microspheres is influenced by the structure, micro-morphology, nature and type of the biodegradable polymer. The antigen release from microspheres can be of different types viz., burst mechanism, pore diffusion mechanism, erosion or combination of them. The basic mechanisms of release are presented schematically in Figure 11-26 and the release profile in Figure 11-27.

Microparticles with core of antigen may release antigen by osmotically driven burst effect. The burst release mechanism is a result of influx of water through the coat, into the core causing increase in intra matrix pressure. This increased pressure results in rupturing of the wall of microspheres and hence release of antigens. The burst effect can be avoided by using the balance of protein-polymer ratio, the particle size of dispersed phase and the particle size of microspheres. In pore diffusion method, the pores are created as a result of the movement of water front towards the core of microparticles. The dispersed particles are dissolved in water and diffuse out through the pores or the channels created by water (Brown et al., 1983; Langer, 1980; Siegel and Langer,

Table 11-5. Polymeric Carrier for Antigens

Antigen	Polymer used	Method of preparation	Reference
Staphylococcus enterotoxin B	dl-PLGA	Solvent evaporation	Hora et al., 1990 Eldridge et al., 1991
Diphtheria toxoid	dl-PLA	W/O/W emulsion	Singh et al., 1991
Hepatitis B surface antigen	PGA	Phase separation suspension	Nellore et al., 1992
Tetanus toxoid	PLA, PLGA	Emulsion	Esparza and Kissel 1992 Alonoso et al., 1992
Bovine serum albumin	PLA	Adsorption	Almeida et al., 1993

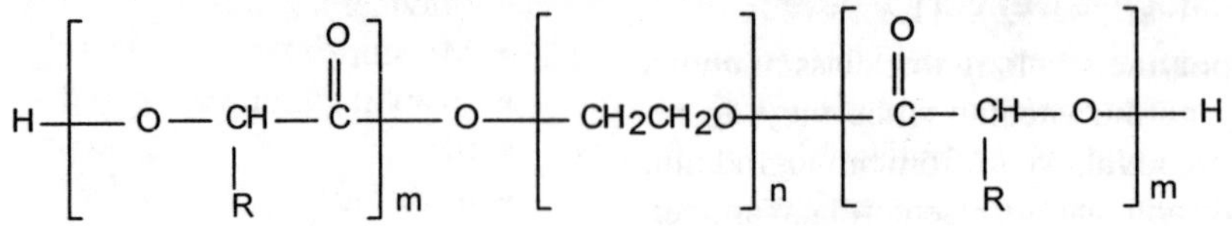

$$H\left[O-\underset{\mid \atop R}{CH}-\overset{O \atop \|}{C}\right]_m O\left[CH_2CH_2O\right]_n\left[\overset{O \atop \|}{C}-\underset{\mid \atop R}{CH}-O\right]_m H$$

A = PLA/PLGA
B = PEO
ABA - Triblock copolymer

Fig. 11-25. ABA Triblock Polymer of PLA/PLGA

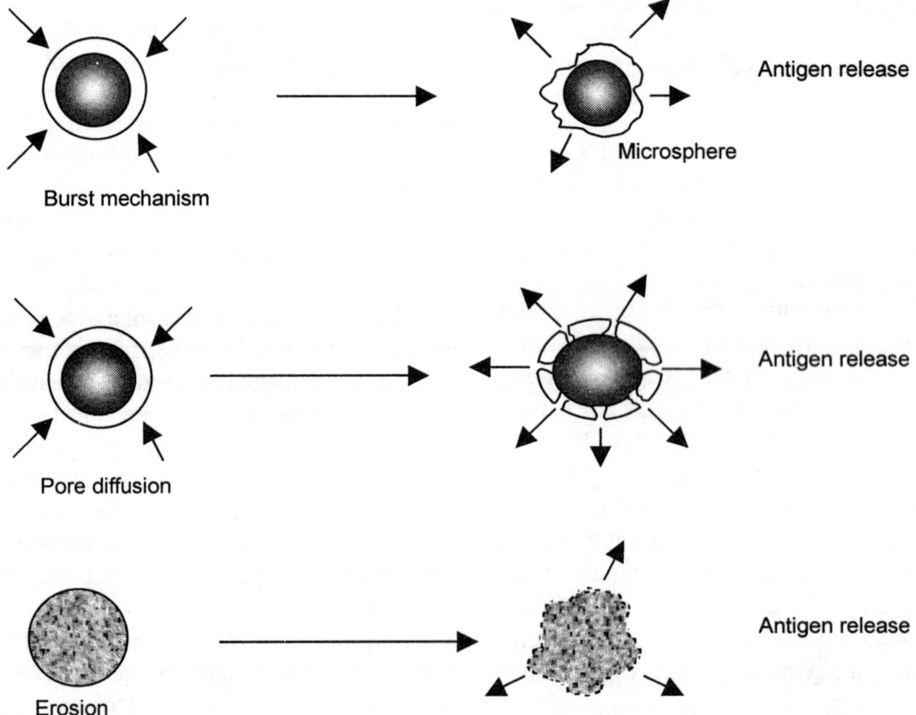

Fig. 11-26. Schematic Showing the Mechanism of Release of Antigens from Microspheres

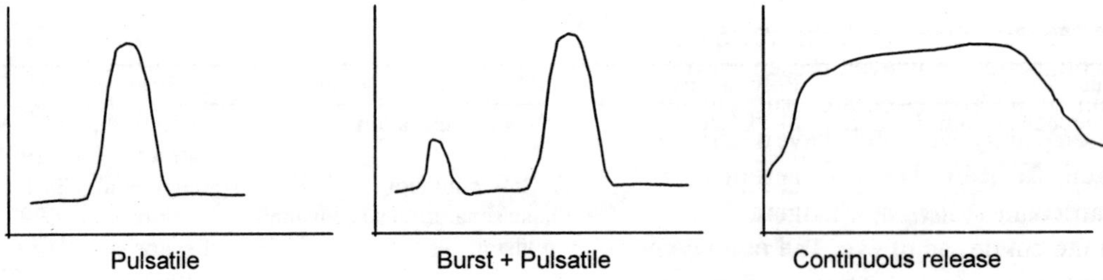

Fig. 11-27. Release Profiles by Different Mechanisms

1984; Bodmer et al., 1992). The third and an important mechanism is erosion. The erosion is catalyzed by pH and presence of enzymes. The rate of degradation or catalysis of hydrophilic bonds determines the release pattern of the antigen from a matrix.

Microspheres and Immune System

The interaction of the microspheres with macrophages (Fig. 11-28) depends upon the particle size. Microspheres of particle size less than 10 μm are directly taken up by the antigen presenting cells. The microparticles with particle size range greater than 10 μm first undergo degradation or release of antigens, which are then phagocytosized by antigen presenting cells (Anderson, 1994). The antigen presenting cells are responsible for the activation of B and T cells and hence immunological consequences (Stites and Terr, 1991; Roitte et al., 1991). A number of antigens are under investigation as shown in Table 11-5 for their efficient delivery through microspheres.

Targeting Using Microparticulate Carriers

The concept of targeting, i.e. site specific drug delivery is a well established dogma, which is gaining full attention. The therapeutic efficacy of the drug relies on its access and specific interaction with its candidate receptors.

The ability to leave the blood pool in reproducible, efficient and specific manner is centre to drug action mediated by use of a carrier system. Placement of the particles in discrete anatomical compartment leads to their retention either because of the physical properties of the environment or biophysical interaction of the particles with the cellular content of the target tissue.

Ocular

The eye and the cornea are easily accessible targets. The washout effect, however, presents difficulties in retention of microparticulate drug carrier in the corneal sac. Gurny et al., 1985 have described a novel approach to increase the retention of the microparticulate system by changing them to the gel form in the cul de sac of eye. The rapid conversion of the particulate suspension to gel form reportedly leads to their longer retention in the eye.

Intranasal

The intranasal route is exploited for the delivery of the peptides and proteins. The conventional dosage form are rapidly cleared from the nasal mucosa. Bioadhesive gels have been proposed to increase the retention of the insulin and calcitonin. The bioadhesive microspheres are used as the alternative to the gel dosage formulations. In comparison to the gel dosage form the bioadhesive microspheres have greater control over the surface character and the release pattern. Various improvised therapeutic applications of microspheres in intranasal delivery are widely reported and discussed.

Oral

Oral route is one of the most preferred and convenient routes for administration of the drug. Thus, a number of the controlled release systems have been developed for oral administration. Single unit system has disadvantage of being removed with the chyme. Thus, their gastrointestinal transit time is determined by the frequency of the stomach emptying and casual localization in the vicinity of pylorus. In comparison to single unit systems, multiple unit system has marked advantages as it spreads over a large area and avoids the exposure of high concentration of drug to the mucosa. The risk of dose dumping is considerably minimized (Akiyama et al., 1993). The drug release is affected by the size of the microspheres as well as the drug content. The smaller size particles and high drug loaded particles show faster release. The faster release from microspheres with high drug content is due to the formation of pores as the drug dissolution proceeds.

Oral route is also suggested for the delivery of the soluble antigens. This as viable alternative can be considered due to the ability of the particles of definite size range to gain access to the Payer's patches. The particulate carriers are effective for delivery of both the entrapped and adsorbed antigen (Eldridge et. al.,1990, O'Hagen et al., 1989a, O'Hagen et al., 1989b).

Many drug substances are characterized by poor solubility in aqueous media and thus they pose problems in formulation intended specially for oral administration. Inspite of promising potentials demonstrated *in vitro*, the development of such

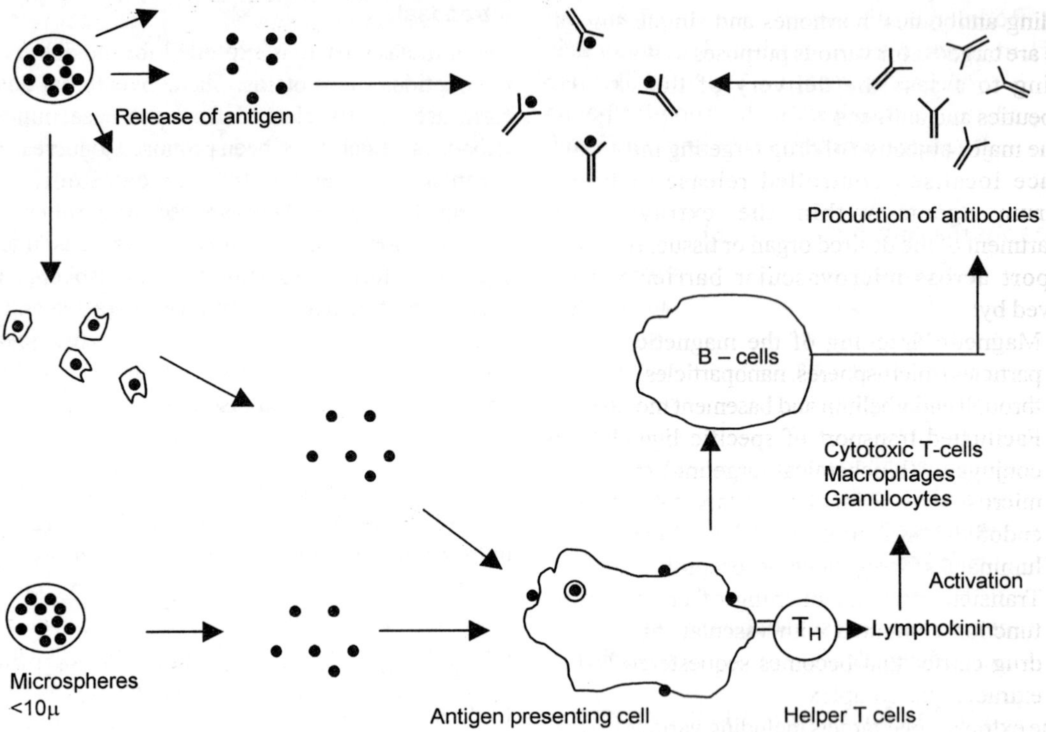

Fig. 11–28. Antigenic Microspheres Interacting with Macrophages

substances is often prematurely halted as a consequence of their inadequate oral bioavailability. Beside the use of cosolvents or absorption enhancers, incorporation in carrier systems has been proposed as an alternative way to render poorly water-soluble drugs better administrable through oral route. pH-sensitive microparticles are particles composed of polymers having a pH-dependent solubility. While remaining stable at a low pH environment such as in the stomach, these particles are expected to allow an improved enteric drug delivery. The incorporation of anti-infective agents of poor aqueous solubility into pH-sensitive microparticles provides an efficient means for oral delivery.

There is preferential size dependent deposition of microparticles or nanoparticles in the inflamed tissue in inflammatory bowel disease after oral administration. Such targeted delivery of an entrapped drug reduces side effects. In the inflamed colonic tissue, an increased adherence of particles is observed. This probably results from an increased attachment to the thicker mucus layer at the inflamed regions and an accumulation inside the ulcerated colonic tissue. A size dependency of the deposition is observed. For 10 μm particles only fair deposition was observed, 1 μm particles showed higher binding. The highest deposition in inflamed tissue was shown by 0.1 μm particles. Moreover, attached particles showed a prolonged residence time in the inflamed regions for up to five days. The size dependent deposition of particles in the inflamed tissue may allow designing of carrier systems for the site-specific treatment of inflammatory bowel disease.

The introduction of the drug in the systemic circulation along with the microparticles provides a means to target either to the vasculature or to the extravascular compartments, accessible via capillary endothelium. The intravascular targets are mononuclear phagocytic system, diagnostic imaging, and the blood cells that may be recognised by ligands including antibodies, hormones and simple sugars. These are targeted for various purposes as diagnostic imaging to assess the delivery of the chemotherapeutics and antigens.

The major objective of drug targeting must be to produce localised controlled release of broad spectrum agents within the extravascular compartment of the desired organ or tissue. Efficient transport across microvascular barrier can be achieved by:

1. Magnetic dragging of the magnetic microparticles (microspheres, nanoparticles) directly through endothelium and basement membrane.
2. Facilitated transport of specific ligand drug conjugates (biochemical targeting) or coated microspheres (bioadhesive targeting) across endothelium as a result of ligand binding to luminal surface antigen or receptors.
3. Transient regional opening of endothelium function combined with vascular infusion of drug carrier that becomes sequestered in the extracellular complex.

The extravascular targets including various tissues and organs utilize carriers especially for selective drug delivery, i.e. tumour sites.

Magnetic Microspheres

Targeting of drug under controlled, burst or modulated release using biophysical approaches is a new way to achieve site specific drug delivery. These approaches utilize a wide range of modalities as hyperthermia, arterial perfusion, arterial chemoembolization, intra cavity injection and use of extra corporeal magnetic field. In developing different approaches to target, it is instructive to observe how the body localizes its own biopharmaceuticals in the desired tissues.

Magnetic monitoring has the advantage of being efficient in allowing high local concentration of therapeutic agents. A variety of magnetically responsive carriers have been proposed for chemotherapeutic agents. These include magnetite containing matrices (microspheres or nanoparticles of the starch, albumin, ethyl cellulose, etc.), ethyl oleate based emulsion and natural cells such as erythrocyte ghosts. Magnetic targeting is one of the most efficient methods developed for targeting of active agents. Up to 60% of injected dose can be targeted and released to the selected non-endothelial organs. Multiple body regions can be accessed using magnetic microspheres but this must be accomplished sequentially. In order to avoid toxicity due to focal overdosing a magnet with constant gradient may effectively be used.

Magnetic microspheres are prepared by mixing water soluble drugs (for lipophilic drugs, along with the dispersing agents) and 10 nm magnetite (Fe_3O_4) particles in an aqueous solvent of matrix material. This mixture is then emulsified in the oil. Ultrasonication or shearing is done to produce particle of suitable size range. The matrix is then stabilized by chemical cross linking or heating. Magnetic microspheres are administered via intraarterial or intravenous injection. Intraarterial injection is given to achieve high systemic targeting while intravenous administration helps in achieving high pulmonary targeting or medium systemic targeting. Magnetic microspheres in response to extra corporeal magnetic field get captured in small arterioles and capillaries of magnetic target organ.

Magnetic targeting is based on the force exerted by external magnetic field over the magnetically susceptible microspheres. The equation determining force can be given as

$$F = M \nabla H \qquad (11\text{-}8)$$

where,

F = force on particles
M = magnetic moment of particles
∇H = magnetic field gradients

The monitoring of the carrier localization is an important part of magnetic targeting that avoids the normal tissue injury. Magnetic shielding is desirable to restrict the capture of the magnetic microspheres to the desired tissue and avoid adjacent tissue localization. The tissue carrier localization monitoring is also important in order to determine the free tissue level of drug at various times after targeting. Solid tumours are first targeted using the adriamycin loaded magnetic microspheres. In rat tail model the tumour undergoes complete remission in 75% of animal at a dose of 0.5 mg/kg. In a second study microspheres, targeted vindesin sulphate produce total remission of the tumours in 85% of rats at both 0.25 and 0.5 mg/kg dose levels. A number of different drugs are under trials for the targeting via magnetic microspheres. Amphotericin B is targeted for pulmonary aspergillosis using magnetic microspheres. Interleukin-2 is also targeted to stimulate the anti tumour response of the macrophages using magnetic microspheres.

Monoclonal Antibodies Mediated Microspheres Targeting-Immunomicrospheres:

Monoclonal antibodies mediated targeting is a method used to achieve selective targeting to the specific sites. Monoclonal antibodies are extremely specific molecules. This extreme specificity of the monoclonal antibodies (Mabs) can be utilized to target microspheres loaded bioactive molecules to selected sites. Mabs can be directly attached to the microspheres by means of covalent coupling. The free aldehyde groups, amino groups, or hydroxyl groups on the surface of the microspheres can be linked to the antibodies. Microspheres from different material (e.g. bovine serum albumin and poly acrolein) and prepared using different methods, carry different functional groups, which help in the coupling of the antibodies. The Mabs can be attached to the microspheres by any of the following methods:

1. Non specific adsorption
2. Specific adsorption
3. Direct coupling
4. Coupling via reagents

Mabs can be adsorbed non specifically on to the surface of the hydrophobic microspheres by physical adsorption, which renders them more hydrophilic. Hydrophilic microspheres are more suitable for the cell targeting. Monoclonal antibodies form immunomicrospheres on coupling with the microspheres. Immunomicrospheres are formed non-specifically by Vander Waals - London forces (Van Oss and Singer, 1966; Van Oss et al., 1975). Mabs can be adsorbed on the surface of poly hexyl cyanoacrylate microparticles by simple incubation of microspheres with an excess of antibodies at 4 °C in phosphate buffer saline (Illum et. al., 1983)

Specific adsorption can be conducted by means of the ligands, which interact directly with intact or modified antibodies. proteins A-from *Staphylococcus aureus* and avidin biotin are two specific ligands that are used for specific adsorption purpose. *Staphylococcus aureus* protein A binds with Fc portion of the antibodies of sub class IgG (Widder et al., 1981; Kandzia et al., 1981; Couvreur and Aurby 1984). Mabs can be adsorbed by briefly incubating with microspheres carrying protein A at 37 °C. Protein A can be incorporated within the microsphere at the time of preparation of the microspheres along with the matrix material. Protein A is used for linking monoclonal antibodies against HLA-BW6 type of carcinoma to human/bovine serum albumin microspheres. Biotinylated monoclonal antibodies similarly can be linked to poly methacrylate microspheres bearing acetylated avidin (Fig. 11-29). Specific adsorption occurs because of natural affinity of some of the natural molecules to their counterparts, e.g. avidin for biotin.

Direct coupling is achieved through free functional groups present on the surface of the microspheres. The functional microspheres undergo direct coupling, e.g. polyacrolein microspheres have free functional carboxyl groups, which help them to couple with the monoclonal antibodies. Rembaum et al., 1978 described that polyglutaraldehyde coated microspheres have relatively long chains extending from surface to the surrounding aqueous medium (Fig. 11-30). These chains are capable of reacting with several protein molecules including Mabs (Fig. 11-31).

Coupling of microspheres with monoclonal antibodies can also be achieved by means of the reagents when microspheres of choice do not contain functional groups or carry functional groups, which are not capable of coupling. Different methods depending upon the reagent used include

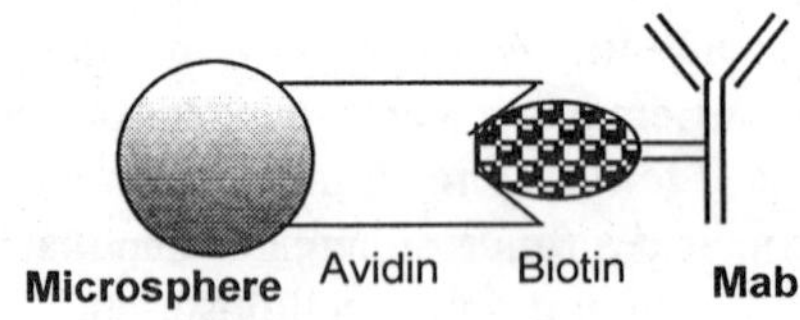

Fig. 11-29. Schematic Showing Microsphere Avidin Biotin Mab Complex

carbodiimide method (Goodfriend et al., 1964), cyanogen bromide method (Axen et al., 1967), glutaraldehyde method (Richard and Knowles, 1968), EEDQ method (Sunderam, 1974), Woodward's reagent K (WRK) method (Patel et al., 1967), SPDP method (Barbet et al., 1981), Dextran bridge method (Arnon and Sela 1982), etc. (Fig. 11-32).

Chemoembolization

Chemoembolization is an endovascular therapy, which involves the selective arterial embolization of a tumour together with simultaneous or subsequent local delivery of the chemotherapeutic agent.

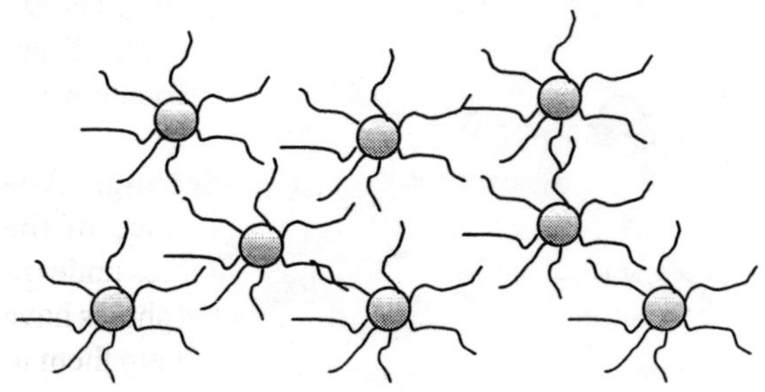

Fig. 11-30. Poly Glutaraldehyde Coated Microspheres

Chemoembolization is an extension of traditional percutaneous embolization techniques. With chemoembolization, investigators embolize tumours with microparticles soaked with chemotherapeutic agents. The theoretical advantage is that such embolizations will not only provide vascular occlusion but will bring about sustained therapeutic levels of chemotherapeutics in the areas of tumour. Generalized ischemia so created would reduce the ability of the cell to relieve itself from the toxicity of chemotherapy. In a human Sk hepatoma and colon carcinoma cell cultures, hypoxia increased the uptake of daunomycin. Despite widespread usage of such chemoembolization, no randomized study to date has demonstrated that the theoretical advantage of adding chemotherapy could be translated into a clinical advantage. Indeed, even in HCC where embolization is most often used, the randomized trials to date have not demonstrated an advantage of chemo-embolization. Degradable starch microspheres injected intra-arterially are trapped in an extra-capillary network (Fig. 11-33) formed in liver metastases. Drug dissolved in the microspheres suspension gets retained in the blood vessels of the target organ as long as the blood flow remains blocked and then gradually releases the chemotherapeutic agents, resulting in a longer duration of tumour

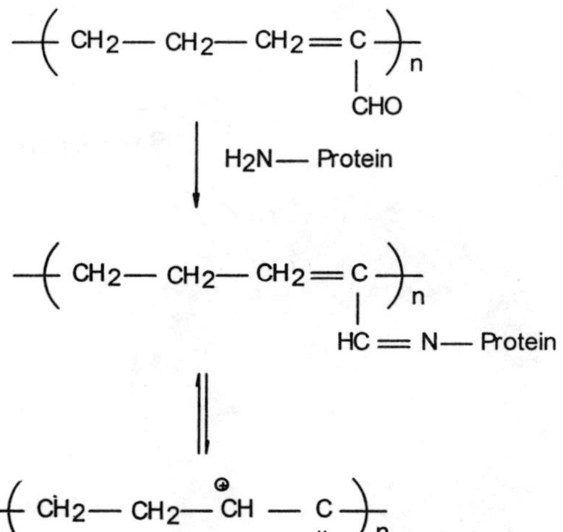

$$-\!\!\left(CH_2-CH_2-CH_2=\underset{\displaystyle CHO}{\underset{|}{C}}\right)_{\!n}\!\!-$$

$$\Big\downarrow \; H_2N-\text{Protein}$$

$$-\!\!\left(CH_2-CH_2-CH_2=\underset{\displaystyle HC=N-\text{Protein}}{\underset{|}{C}}\right)_{\!n}\!\!-$$

$$\Updownarrow$$

$$-\!\!\left(\dot{C}H_2-CH_2-\overset{\oplus}{CH}-\underset{\displaystyle HC-\underset{\ominus}{N}-\text{Protein}}{\underset{\|}{C}}\right)_{\!n}\!\!-$$

Fig .11-31. Poly Gluteraldehyde Mediated Coupling of Mabs (Proteins) to Microspheres

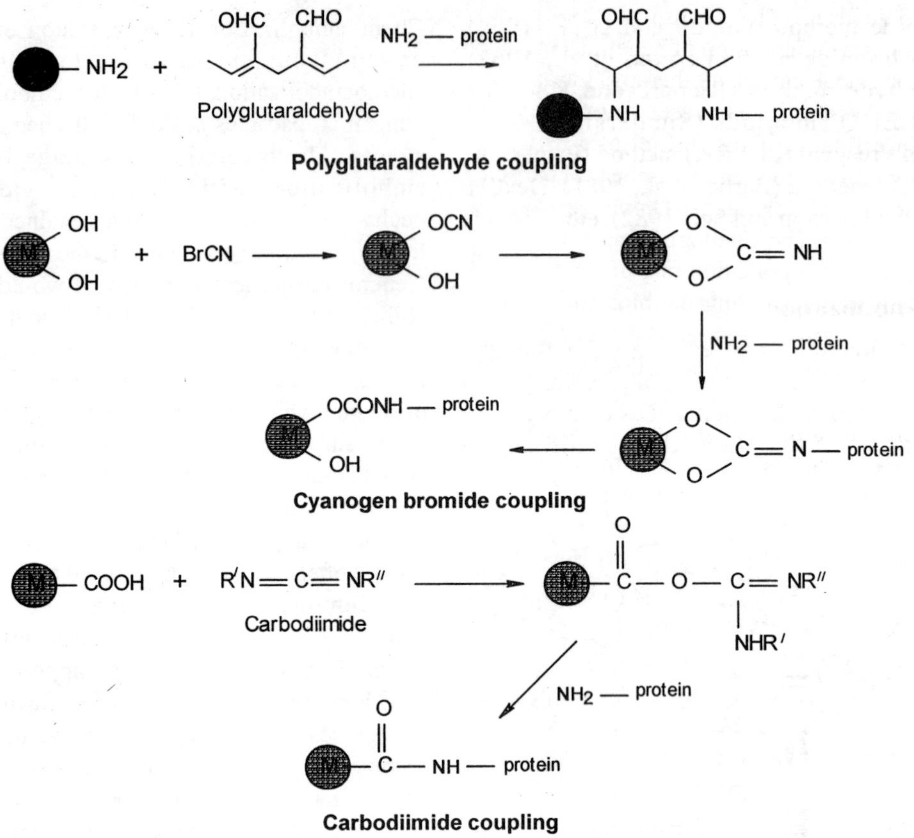

M—NH_2 + Polyglutaraldehyde (OHC, CHO) $\xrightarrow{NH_2\text{—protein}}$ M—NH … NH—protein

Polyglutaraldehyde coupling

M(OH)(OH) + BrCN ⟶ M(OCN)(OH) ⟶ M(O)(O)C═NH $\xrightarrow{NH_2\text{—protein}}$ M(O)(O)C═N—protein ⟶ M(OCONH—protein)(OH)

Cyanogen bromide coupling

M—COOH + R′N═C═NR″ (Carbodiimide) ⟶ M—C(═O)—O—C(═NR″)—NHR′ $\xrightarrow{NH_2\text{—protein}}$ M—C(═O)—NH—protein

Carbodiimide coupling

Fig. 11-32. Coupling of Antibodies with Microspheres via Ligands

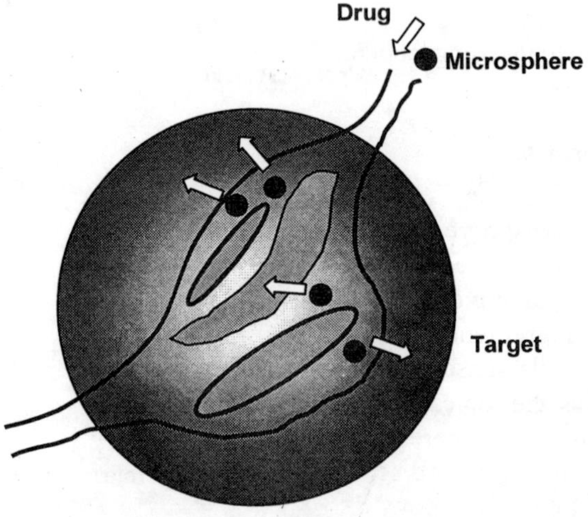

Fig. 11-33. Chemoembolization as a Method of Targeting

exposure to the drug. The technique of chemo-embolization is a combination of beneficial effect of embolization and local chemotherapy. Intraarterial injection of the microspheres increases the therapeutic efficacy of the antimitotic drugs by causing temporary embolization. Spherical particles are most useful in achieving distal homogeneous and effective embolism. The kinetics of drug release from the emboli and biodegradation rate of drug carriers are important in determining the bioavailability of the drug in the restricted area. The biodegradable microspheres of starch, PLA or PLGA may be used for the purpose of achieving the occlusion. The microspheres of size >40 μm are injected intra arterially, which causes blockade of the arteriole at the tumour sites. This blockade of the arterioles and the capillary bed may be beneficial in two ways, first it increases the time of absorption of drugs at the tumour site and second, due to blockade of feeder vessels it causes ischemia and hence leads to the tumour regression (Kassab et al., 1997).

Imaging

The microspheres have been extensively studied and used for the targeting purposes. Various cells, cell lines, tissues and organs can be imaged using radiolabelled microspheres. The particle size range of microspheres is an important factor in determining the imaging of particular sites. The particles injected intravenously apart from the portal vein will become entrapped in the capillary bed of the lungs. This phenomenon is exploited for the scintiographic imaging of the tumour masses in lungs using labelled human serum albumin microspheres.

Microsponges: Topical porous microspheres

Microsponges are porous microspheres having myriad of interconnected voids of particle size range 5-300 μm. These microsponges having capacity to entrap wide range of active ingredients such as emollients, fragrances, essential oils, sunscreens and anti-infectives, etc. are used as the topical carrier system. Further, these porous microspheres with active ingredients can be incorporated in to formulations such as creams, lotions and powders. Microsponges consists of non collapsible structures with porous surface through which active ingredients are released in a controlled manner (Nachts and Martin, 1990). Depending upon the size, the total pore length may range up to 10 ft and pore volume up to 1 ml/g. The porous microspheres are prepared by suspension polymerization method in a liquid-liquid system. In their preparation, the monomers are first dissolved along with active ingredients in a suitable solvent. The solution of monomer is then dispersed in the aqueous phase, which consists of additives (surfactants, suspending agent, etc. to aid in formation of suspension). The polymerization is then initiated by adding catalyst or by increasing temperature or irradiation. The various steps in the preparation of microsponge are summarized as:

- Selection of monomer or combination of monomers
- Formation of chain of monomers as polymerization begins
- Formation of ladders as a result of cross linking between chains of monomers
- Folding of monomer ladders to form spherical particles (microspheres)
- Agglomeration of microspheres, which gives rise to formation of bunches of microspheres
- Binding of bunches to form microsponges.

The polymerization process leads to formation of reservoir type of system which opens at the surface through pores. In some cases the active substances are not capable of forming pores at the surface. In these cases an inert liquid immiscible with water but completely miscible with monomer is used during polymerization to form pore network. After polymerization the liquid is removed leaving the porous microspheres, i.e. microsponges. The functional substances are then incorporated by impregnating them within preformed microsponge. Sometimes solvent may be used for faster and efficient incorporation of the active substances. The microsponges act as the topical carriers for variety of functional substances, e.g. anti acne, anti inflammatory, anti pruritics, anti fungal, rubefacients, etc.

Surface Modified Microspheres

The objective of drug therapy using carriers is the selective delivery of drug to specific sites in the body. The phagocytosis of colloidal carriers, rapid clearance and passive distribution are common disadvantages of particulate systems. The change in the biophysical behaviour of the particles helps to avoid the difficulties in targeting. Different approaches have been utilized to change the surface properties of carriers to protect them against phagocytic clearance and to alter their body distribution pattern. The adsorption of the poloxamer on the surface of the polystyrene, polyester or poly methylmethacrylate microspheres renders them more hydrophilic and hence decreases their MPS uptake. Protein microspheres covalently modified by PEG derivatives show decreased immunogenecity and clearance. Among the most studied surface modifiers are (Torchilin and Trubetskov, 1996):

1. Antibodies and their fragments.
2. Proteins.
3. Mono-, Oligo-, and polysaccharides.
4. Chelating compounds (EDTA, DTPA or Desferroxamine).
5. Synthetic soluble polymers.

The surface of the albumin microspheres can be modified by covalent attachment of polyoxy (C1-4) alkyene chain having terminal ether groups. The polyoxyethylene moiety may react with surface amino or carboxyl residues by condensation with an appropriate functional group in the presence of condensing agent, e.g. 1,1-carbonyldiimidazole and N-(3-dimethyl amino propyl)-N'-ethyl carbodiimide hydrochloride (EDAC). The surface modified albumin microspheres having terminally linked galactose moiety are used for the liver targeting of antitumour 5-flurouracil. Such modifications are provided to the surface of the microspheres in order to achieve the targeting to the discrete organs and to avoid rapid clearance from the body.

FUTURE PERSPECTIVES

With the availability of various biodegradable and bio-inspired polymers it shall be now possible to design microsphere systems for protracted drug release, organ imaging, effective immunization and in the development of bio-implantable, bio-reactors, bio-chips, bio-sensors and tissue surrogates prosthesis. Furthermore, in future by combining various other strategies, microspheres will find the central place in novel drug delivery, particularly in diseased cell sorting, diagnostics, gene and genetic materials, safe, targeted and effective *in vivo* delivery, which may have its implications in gene therapy, genetic customization and supplements as miniature versions of diseased organ and tissues in the body.

REFERENCES

Akiyama Y., Yoshioka M., Horibe H., Hirai S., Kitamori N. and Toguchi H. (1993) *J. Control. Rel.* **26**, 1.

Albertson A C., Carlfors J. and Sturesson C. (1993) *J. Appl. Polym. Sci.* **62**, 695.

Allcock H. R. and Kwon S. (1989) *Macromolecul* **22**, 75.

Almeida A. J., Alpar H. O. and Brown M. R. W. (1993) *Proc. Int. Symp. Control. Rel. Bioact. Mater.* **20**, 390.

Alonso M. J., Cohen S., Park T. W., Gupta R. K., Siber G. R. and Langer R. (1992) *Proc. Int. Symp. Controlled Release Bioact. Mater.* **19**, 120.

Alpar H. O., Field W. N., Hyde R. and Lewis D. A. (1989) *J. Pharm. Pharmcol.* **41**, 194.

Anderson J. M. (1994) *Eur. J. Pharmcol. Biopharm.* **10**, 1.

Anderson L. C., Wise D. L. and Howes J. F. (1976) *Contraception* **13**, 375.

Andrianov A. K., Cohen S., Visscher K. B., Payne L. G., Allcock H. R. and Langer R. (1993) *J. Cont. Rel.* **27**, 69.

Arnon R. and Sela M. (1982) *Immunology Rev.* **62**, 5.

Avila J. L. (1983) *Interscienci*a. **8**, 405.

Axen R., Porath J. and Ernback S. (1967) *Nature* **214**, 1302.

Barbet J., Machy P. and Laserman L. D. (1981) *J. Supramol. Struct. Cell Biochem.* **16**, 243.

Benita S., Benoit J. P., Puisieux F. and Thies C. (1984a) *J Pharm Sci.* **73**, 1721.

Benita S., Fickat R., benoit J. P., Bonnemain B., Samaille J. P. and Madoule P. (1984b) *J. Microencapsul.* **1**, 317.

Bjork J. and Edman P. (1988) *Int. J. Pharm.* **47**, 233.

Bodmeier R. and McGinity J. (1987) *J Microencapsul.* **4**, 279.

Bodmer D., Kissel T. and Traechslin E. (1992) *J. Controlled Release.* **21**, 129.

Brasseur F., Couvreur P., Kante B., Deckers-Passau L., Roland M., Deckers C. and Speiser P. (1980) *Eur. J. Cancer.* **16**, 1441.

Brown R., Wei C. L. and Langer R. (1983) *J. Pharm. Sci.*

72, 1181.

Bucher J. E. and Slade W. C. (1990) *J. Am. Chem. Soc.* **31**, 1319.

Burger J. J., Tomlinson E., Mudler E. M. A. and McVie J. G. (1985) *Int. J. Pharm.* **23**, 333.

Capron A. C., Locht C. and Fracchia G. N. (1994) *Vaccine.* **12**, 667.

Cohen S., Bano M. C., Visscher K. B., Chaw M., Allcock H. R., and Langer R. (1990) *J. Am. Chem. Soc.* **112**, 7832.

Cohn Z. A. (1970) In:Mononuclear phagocytes., Van R. (Ed.) Blackwell Scientific, Oxford. 121.

Couvreur P. and Aurby J. (1984) In: Topics in Pharmaceutical Sciences, Breimer D. D. (Ed.) Vol II Elsevier Biomedical Press, Amsterdam, 305.

Couvreur P., Kante B., Roland M. and Speiser P. (1979) *J. Pharm. Scs.* **68**, 1521.

Couvreur P., Lenaerts V., Leyh D., Guiot P. and Roland M. (1984) In: Microspheres and drug therapy. Pharmaceuticals, immunologicals and medical aspects. Davis S. S., Illum L., McVie J. G. and Tomlinson E. (Eds.) Elsevier Science publishers, Amsterdam, 103.

Cushimano A. G. and Becker C. H, (1968) *J. Pharm. Sci.* **57**, 1104.

Douglas S. J., Illum L. and Davis S. S. (1985a) *J. Colloid Interface.* **103**,154.

Douglas S J., Illum L. and Davis S S. (1986) *J. Control. Rel.* **15**, 315.

Douglas S. J., Illum L. and Holding S. R. (1985b) *Br. Polym. J.* **17**, 339.

Drews J. (1984) *Immunostimulantien, Klin. Wochenschr.* **62**, 254.

Ebel J. P. (1990) *Pharm Res.* **7**, 848.

Edelman R. (1993) *Vaccine* **11**, 1361.

Eldridge J. H., Hammond C. J., Meulbroek J. A., Staas J. K., Gilley R. M. and Tice T. R. (1990) *J. Control. Rel.* **11**, 205.

Eldridge J H., Staas J K., Meulbrock J A., McGee J P. Tice T R. and Gilley R M. (1991) *Mol. Immunol.* **28**, 287.

El-Samaligy M. S. and Rohdewald P. (1981) *Pharm Act. Helv.* **57**, 201.

Esparza I. and Kissel T. (1992) *Vaccine* **10**, 714.

Franssen O. and Hennink W. E. (1998) *Int. J. Pharm.* **168**, 1.

Franssen O., Stenekes R. J. H. and Hennink W. E. (1999) *J. Cont. Rel.* **59**, 219.

Fudenberg H. H., Stites D. P., Caldwel J. L. and Wells J. V. (1978) In: Basic and clinical immunology, 2 ed., Lange Medical, Los Altos CA.

Gohel M. C., Sheth M. N., Patel M. M., Jani G. K., and Patel H., (1994) *Indian J Pharm Sci.* **56** ,210.

Goodfriend T. L., Levine L. and Fasman G. D. (1964) *Science* **144**, 1344.

Gopferich A., Alonso M. J. and langer R. (1994) *Pharm Res.* **11**, 1568.

Griffin F. M., Griffin J. A., leider J. E. and Silverstein S. C. (1975) *J. Exp. Med.* **142**, 1263.

Gurny R., Boyle T. and Ibrahim H. (1985) *J. Control. Rel.* **2**, 353.

Hashida M., Muranishi S., Sezaki H., Tangigawa Nsotomura K. and Hikasa Y. (1979) *Int. J. Pharm.* **2**, 145.

Hermann J. B., Kelly R. J. and Higgins G. A. (1970) *Arch. Surg.* **100**, 486.

Hora M. S., Rana R. K., Nunberg J. H., Tice T. R., Gilley R. M. and Hudson M. E. (1990) *Pharm. Res.* **7**, 1190.

Ikada Y. and Tabata Y. (1982) *J. Bioact. Compt. Polym.* **1**, 31.

Illum L., Davis S. S., Muller R. H., Mak E. and West P. (1987) *Life Sci.* **40**, 367.

Illum L., Jones P. D. E., kreuter J., Baldwin R. W. and Davis S. S. (1983) *Int. J. Pharm.* **17**, 65.

Jalil R. and Nixon J. R. (1990) *J. Microecapsulation* **7**, 297.

Jani P., Halbert G. W., Langridge J. and Florence A. T. (1990) *J. Pharm. Pharmacol.* **42**, 821.

John P. M. and Becker C. H. (1968) *J. Pharm. Sci.* **57**, 584.

Kabanov and Zezin A. B. (1982) *Sol. Sci. Rev. Sec Bio Chem. Rev.* **4**, 207.

Kandjia J., Anderson M. J. D. and Muller-Ruchholtz W. (1981) *J. Cancer Res. Clin. Oncol.* **101**, 165.

Kante B., Couvreur P., Dubois-Krack G., De Meester C., GuoitP., Roland M., Mercier M. and Speiser P. (1982) *J. Pharm. Sci.* **71**, 786.

Kassab A.C., Xu K., Denkbas E. B., Dou Y., Zhao S. and Piskin E. (1997) *J. Biomat. Sci.: Polymer Edition*, Vol. 8, 12, 947.

Kikuchi A., Kawabuchi M., Sugihara M., Sakurai Y. and Okano T. (1996) *Proceed Intern Symp Control Rel Bioact Mater.* **23**, 737.

Kim C. K. and Lee E. J. (1992) *Int J Pharm.* **79**, 11.

Kipling J. J. (1965) In: Adsorption from Solutions of Non-electrolytes, Academic Press Inc., London, 1.

Koff *US Patent* (March 2 1963) 3,080,292 .

Kramer P. A. and Burnstein T. (1976) *Life Sci.* **19**, 515.

Kreuter J. and Hartmann H R. (1983) *Oncology*. **40**, 363.

Kreuter J. (1983) *Int. J. Pharm.* **14**, 43.

Kreuter J., Berg U., Leihl E., Soliva M. and Speiser P. P. (1986a) *Vaccine* **4**, 125.

Kreuter J., Berg U., Leihl E., Soliva M. and Speiser P. P. (1986b) *Vaccine* **4**, 253.

Kreuter J., Nefzger M., Liehl E., Czok R. and Voges R. (1983) *J. pharm. Sci.* **72**, 1146.

Kulkarni R. K., Pani K. C. Neuman C. and Leonard F. (1966) *Arch. Surg.* **93**, 893.

Lamprecht A., Schäfer U. F. and Lehr Ç. M. (2000) *Eur J Pharm Biopharm*. **49**, 1.

Langer R. (1980) *Chem. Eng. Commun.* **6**, 1.

Lee T. K., Sokoloksi T. D. and Royer G. P. (1981) *Science* **213**, 233.

Lee H. K., Park J. H. and Kowan K. C. (1996) *Proc. Int. Symp. Control. Rel. Bioact. Mater*. **23**, 333.

Leonard F., Kulkarni R. K., Brandes G., Nelson J. and Cameron J J. (1966) *J. Appl. Polym. Sci.* **10**, 259.

Lindberg B., LoteK. and Teder H. (1984) In: Microsphere and Drug Therapy, Davis S. S., Illum L., McVie J. G. and Tomlinson E. (Eds.), Elsevier science, 153.

Longo W. E., Iwata H., Lindheimer T. A. and Goldberg E. P. (1982) *J. Pharm. Sci.* **71**, 1323.

MacAdam A. B., Shafi J. B., James S. L., Marriott C. and Martin G. P. (1997) *Int. J. Pharma.* **151**, 47.

Maincent P., Verge R. L., Sado P. A., Couvreur P. and Devissaguet J. P. (1986) *J. Pharm. Sci.* **75**, 955.

Maincent P. (1982) *PhD Thesis* university of Paris-Sud.

Margel S. and Wiesel E. (1984) *J. Polym. Sci.* **22**, 145.

Marty J. J., Oppenheim R. C. and Speiser P. P. (1978) *Pharm. Acta. Helv*. **53**, 17.

Mathews B. R. and Nixon J. R. (1974) *J Pharm Pharmacol.* **26**, 383.

Mathiowitz E. and Langer R. (1987) *J. Cont. Rel.* **5**, 13.

Millar A. M., McMillan L., Hannan W. J., Emmett P. C. and Aitken R. J. (1982) *Int. J. Appl. Radiat. Isot.* **33**, 1423.

Mumper R. J., Hoffman A. S., Poulakkainen P. A., Bouchard L. S. and Gombotz W. R. (1994) *J. Control. Rel.* **30**, 241.

Nachts S. and Martin K. (1990) In: The microsponges a novel topical programmable delivery formulation, Marcel Dekker Inc., New York, 299

Nakamoto Y., Hashida M., Muranishi N. and Sezaki H. (1975) *Chem. Pharm. Bull.* **23**, 3125.

Nellore R. V., Pande P. G., Young D. and Bhagat H. R. (1992) *J. Parent. Sci. Tech.* **46**, 176.

North R. J. (1970) *Semin. Hematol.* **7**, 161.

O'Hagen D. T., Palin K. and Davis S. S. (1989a) *Vaccine* **7**, 213.

O'Hagen D. T., Palin K. Davis S. S., Artursson P. and Sjoholm I. (1989b) *Vaccine* **7**, 421.

O'Hagen D. T. (1990) *Adv. Drug Del. Rev.* **5**, 265.

Ohya Y. and Takei T. (1993) *Chem Ind (Jpn.)* **46**, 798.

Oppenheim R. C. (1981) *Int. J. Pharm.* **8**, 217.

Oppenheim R. C. and Stewart N. F. (1979) *Drug. Dev. Ind. Pharm.* **5**, 563.

Patel R. P., Lopiekes D. V., Brown S. P. and Price S. (1967) *Biopolymers* **5**, 577.

Patil R. T. and Speaker T. J. (1997) *J. Micrencapsul.* **14**, 169.

Patil R. T. and Speaker T. J. (2000) *J. Pharm. Sci.* **89**, 9.

Payne L. G, Jenkins S. A., Andrianov A. K, Langer R. and Roberts B. E. (1995a) Adv. Mucosal immunology, Mestecky J. et al., (Eds.) Plennum press, New York, 475.

Payne L. G., Jenkins S. A., Andrianov A. K. and Roberts B. E. (1995b) In: Vaccine design, Powell M. F. and Neuman M. J. (Eds.) Plennum press, New York, 473.

Pekarek K. J., Jacob J. S. and Mathiowitz E. (1994) *Nature* **367**, 258.

Przyborowski M., Lacknik E., Wiza J. and Lieinska I. (1982) *Eur. J. Nucl. Med.* **7**, 71.

R. Won (sept 1 1987)*US Patent* 4 690, 825 .

Rajeev A. Jain (2000) *Biomaterial* **21**, 2475.

Ravi kumar M. N. V. (2000) *J. Pharmaceu. Sci.* **3**, 234.

Rembaum A. and Dreyer W. J. (1980) *Science* **208**, 364.

Rembaum A. (1983) *US Patent* 4,413,070.

Rembaum A., Margel S. and Levy J. (1978) *J. Immunol. Methods* **24**, 239.

Richards F. M. and Knowles J. R. (1968) *J. Mol. Bio*. **37**, 231.

Roitt I. M., Brostoff J. and Male D. K. (1991) *Kurzes Lehrbuch der Immunologie.* George Thieme Verlag. Stuttgart.

Rojas J., Pinto-Alphandary H., Leo E., Pecquet S., Couvreur P., Gulik A. and Fattal E. (1999) *Pharm Res.* **16**, 255.

Rosen H. B., Chang J., Wnek G. E., Linhardt R. J. and Langer R. (1983) *Biomaterisls* **4**, 131.

Rubio M. R. and Ghaly E. S. (1994) *Drug Dev Ind Pharm* . **20**, 1239.

Russel G. F. (1983) *Pharm. Int*. **4**, 260.

Sanders E. and Ashworth C. T. (1961) *Exp. Cell Res*. **22**, 137.

Schugens C., Laruelle N., Nihant N., Grandfils C., Jerome R. and Teyssie P. (1994) *J. Control. Rel.* **32**, 161.

Stefon M., Brown L. R. and Langer R. S. (1984) *J. pharm. Sci.* **73**, 1859.

Shah N. H., Railkar A. S., Chen F. C., Tarantino R., Kumar S., Murjani M., Palmer D., Infeld M. H. and Malick A. W. (1993) *J. Control Rel.* **27**, 139.

Shilvey M. L., Coonts B. A., Renner W. D., Southhard H. and Benett A. T. (1995) *J. Control Rel.* **33**, 237.

Siegel R. A. and Langer R. (1984) *Pharm. Res.* **1**, 1.

Singh M., Singh A. and Talwar G. P. (1991) *Pharm. Res.* **8**, 958.

Spier R. E. (1993) Vaccine **11**, 1450.

Stenekes R. J. H., Franssen O., Van Bommel E. M. G., Crommelin D. J. A. and Hennink W. E. (1998) *Pharm. Res.* **15**, 555.

Stites D. P. and Terr A. I. *Basic and Clinical immunology*, 2nd ed. Appleton and Lange, Norwalk CT.1991.

Stossel T. P. (1975) *Semin hematol.* **12**, 83.

Sugibayashi K., Akimoto M., Moromoto Y., Nadai T. and Kato Y. (1979) *Pharmacobiodyn.* **23**, 50.

Sunderam P. V. (1974) *Biochem Biophys. Res. Commun.* **61**, 717.

Tabata Y. and Ikada Y. (1988) *Biomaterials* **9**, 356.

Tabata Y. and Ikada Y. (1989) *Pharm. Res.* **6**, 422.

Tabata Y. and Ikada Y. (1990) *Adv. Poly. Sci.* **94**, 107.

Tabata Y., Nakaoka R. and Ikada Y. (1995) *Vaccine* **13**, 653.

Takada S., Uda Y., Toguchi H. and Ogawa Y. (1995) *J. Pharm. Sci. Technol.* **49**, 180.

Tanake N., Takino S. and Utsumi I. (1963) *J. Pharm. Sci.* **52,** 664.

Timida H., Mizuo C., Nakamura C. and Kiryu S. (1993) *Chem. Pharm Bull.* **41**, 1475.

Tomlinson E. (1983) *Int. J. Pharm. Tech. Prod. Mfr.* **4**, 49.

Torchilin V. P. and Trubetskoy V. S. (1996) In: Microparticulate systems for the delivery of proteins and vaccines, Cohen S. and Bernstein H. (Eds.) Marcel Dekker Inc. New York, 243.

Tsuchida E. and Abe K. (1986) In: Polyelectrolyte complexes: Development in ionic polymers-2, Prosser H. J. and Wilson A D. (Eds.) Elsevier Applied Science, New York. 191.

Van Oss C. F. and Singer J. H. (1966) *J. Reticuloendothel. Soc.* **3**, 29.

Van Oss C. F., Gilman C. F. and Neumann A. W. (1975) In: Phagocytic engulfment and cell adhesiveness, Marcel Dekker , New York.

Van Oss C. J. (1975) Phagocytic Engulfment and cell adhesiveness, Marcel Dekker, NewYork.

Wakiyama N., Juni K. and Nakano M. (1981) *Chem. Pharm. Bull.* **29**, 3363.

Widder K. J., Sanyei A. E., Ovadia H. and Paterson P. Y. (1981) *J. Pharm Sci.* **70**, 387.

Widder K. J., Senyei A. E., Ovadia H. and Paterson P. Y. (1979) *Clin. Immuno. Immunopathol.* **14**, 395.

Woodland J. H. R., Yolles S., Blake D. A., Helrich M. and Meyer F. J. (1973) *J. Med. Chem.* **16**, 897.

Yao K. D., Peng T., Yu J. J., Xu M. X. and Goosen M. F. A. (1995) *J M S-Rev Macromol Chem Phys,* C35, 155.

Yolles S., Leafe T. D. and Meyer F. (1975) *J. Pharm. Sci.* **64**, 115.

Yolles S., Morton J. F. and Rosenberg B. (1978) *Acta. Pharm. Sci.* **15**, 382.

Yoshioka T., Hashida M., Muranishi S. and Sezaki H. (1981) *Int. J. Pharm.* **8**, 131.

Yoshioka T., Ikeuchi K., Hashida M., Muranishi S. and Sezaki H. (1982) *Chem. Pharm. Bulle.* **30**, 1408.

Yotsuyanagi T., Yoshioka I., Segi N. and Ikada K. (1991) *Chem. Pharm Bull.* **39**,1072.

CHAPTER 12

Magnetically Modulated Drug Delivery

In recent years, polymeric controlled drug delivery systems have evolved as one of the most attractive areas in drug delivery research. The drug release is controlled by the properties of the polymer-drug system and to some extent environmental factors such as pH, enzymes and inter-patient variance.

Despite the several advantages offered by controlled drug release, one important problem pertinent to the entire field is that all the systems so far developed give release rates that either are constant or decrease with time. Augmented delivery on demand could be beneficial in a number of situations like, delivery of insulin for patients with diabetes mellitus, antiarrhythmics for patients with heart disorders and nitrates for patients with angina pectoris. Augmented delivery on demand is also required in selective β-adrenergic blockade, birth control and general hormone replacement, immunization, cancer chemotherapy and long term immunosuppression. This "augmented delivery on demand" can be achieved by the systems, which are associated with external or feed back control such as magnetic control (Tyle, 1988). For drug targeting, various carrier systems have been exploited including liposomes, microspheres, nanoparticles, antibodies, cellular carriers and macromolecules. The difficulty of targeting drugs *in vivo* using these carrier systems is that the body contains not one, but three major tubes: the vascular, extracellular and intracellular compart-ments. Reticuloendothelial organs exhibit micro-vascular barriers that severely restrict the extravasation of drug carriers above 3-5 nm in molecular diameter. This means that many potential carriers of sufficient molecular size to encode receptor-binding information are excluded from the extravascular compartments of normal target organs other than liver, lung, spleen, bone marrow, and kidney. Diseased regions of the organs exhibit variable breakdown of microvascular barriers. For example, in experimental tumour whose vascular filtration properties have been sized using fluoresceinated dextrans, moderate permeabilities are reported for 1,50,000 dalton species and lower permeabilities for upto 30,00,000 dalton species. Even with partial breakdown, the largest soluble molecules (e.g., drug DNA complexes), molecular microaggregates (of 3-100 nm) and the smallest particles (≥50 nm in diameter) experience lesional accumulation rates that are generally too slow to complete with faster rates of active hepatic/RES clearance. This highlights the major challenges facing drug targeting *in vivo*, namely, the initial biodistribution of drug carrier and bioengineering problems that must be addressed before the possibilities of cell-receptor binding and cell uptake can be meaningfully explored (Ranny and Huffaker, 1987).

An alternative to the above systems has been to magnetize the carriers so that these particles can be retained at or guided to the target site by the application of an external magnetic field of appropriate strength (Widder et al., 1978). Retention of magnetic carrier at target site will delay reticuloendothelial clearance, facilitate extravasation and thus prolong the systemic action of drug (Fig. 12-1). Magnetic fields are believed to be harmless to biological systems and adaptable to any part of the body. Upto 60% of an injected dose can be deposited and released in a controlled manner in selected non-reticuloendothelial organs. Magnetic targeting has several advantages, which include :

- Therapeutic responses in target organs at only one tenth of the free drug dose.
- Controlled drug release within target tissues for intervals of 30 min to 30 h, as desired.
- Avoidance of acute drug toxicity directed against endothelium and normal parenchymal cells.
- Adaptable to any part of the body.

However, this novel approach suffers from certain disadvantages also as given below :

- Magnetic targeting is an expensive, technical approach and requires specialized manufacture and quality control system.
- It needs specialized magnet for targeting, advanced techniques for monitoring, and trained personnel to perform procedures.
- Magnets must have relatively constant gradients, in order to avoid focal over-dosing with toxic drugs.
- A large fraction (40-60%) of the magnetite, which is entrapped in carriers, is deposited permanently in target tissues.

Due to these limitations magnetic drug targeting is likely to be approved only for very severe diseases that are refractory to other approaches. Such targeting is limited to specialized centers; and to antitumour, antifungal, transplantation, and CNS acting agents that are highly toxic or labile (Ranny and Huffaker, 1987).

This chapter describes magnetically modulated drug carriers and drug delivery devices. In these systems, the release rate of substances from carriers and polymeric matrices can be repeatedly modulated at desired rate, by magnetic control.

HISTORY OF MAGNETIC GUIDANCE

The earliest use of magnet for selective delivery of clinical agents involved treatment of arterial thrombosis by angiography and intravascular localization of carbonyl iron with guidance of catheters. Continuous efforts by researchers established that microparticles of carbonyl iron (1-3 μm) are retained at selected intravascular sites in the presence of arterial flow, under the influence of strong magnetic fields. Little amount of iron remained at the site for 7 days suggesting migration of some of the particles to the arterial walls and tissues. Initially drugs were grafted on to the surface of magnetite particles, but it suffers from certain drawbacks like very low loading capacity for clinically acceptable limits of dosing with magnetite and irreversible particle aggregation under the exposure of magnetic fields, which ultimately causes embolization of large blood vessels and non-homogeneous particle distribution in capillary bed. Coating of ferromagnetic materials with albumin and other charged polymers however, circumvent the aggregation problem by making it reversible. This led to the introduction of a new approach involving albumin emulsification for preparation of small particles, which encapsulate ferromagnetic material.

MAGNETICALLY MODULATED MICROCARRIERS

Magnetic microcarriers are supramolecular particles that are small enough to circulate through capillaries

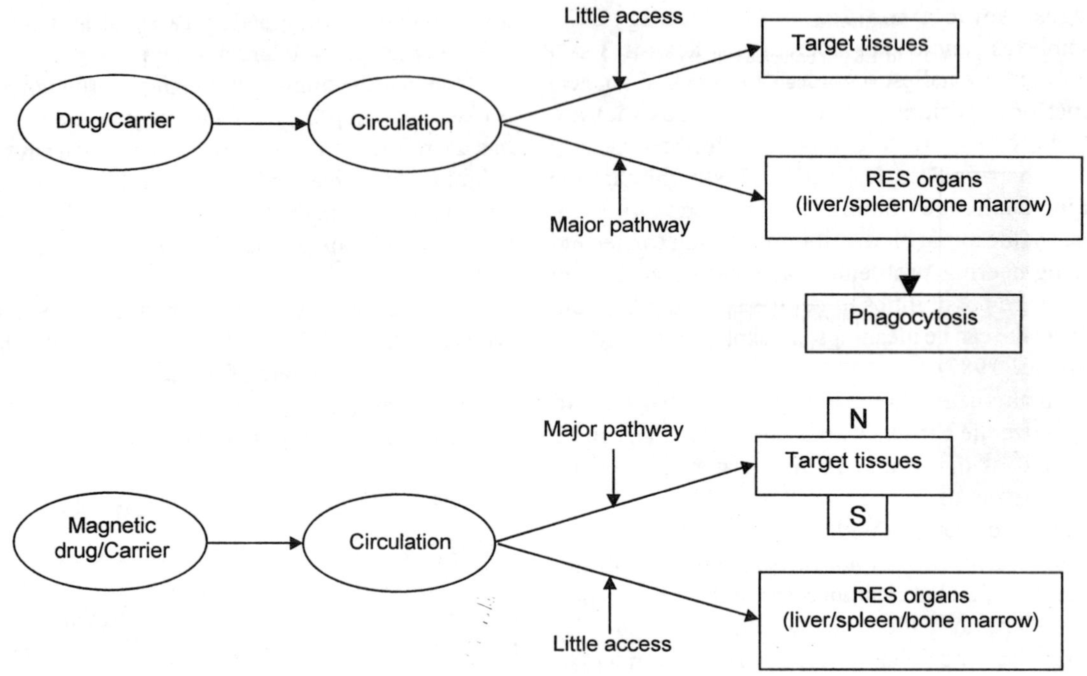

Fig. 12-1. Principle of Magnetic Drug Targeting

without producing embolic occlusion (<4 μm), but are sufficiently susceptible (ferromagnetic) to become captured in microvessels and dragged in to the adjacent tissues by magnetic fields of 0.5-0.8 tesla (T). These microcarriers include microspheres, liposomes, cells, nanoparticles, etc.

Magnetic Microspheres

The use of magnetic force for the site-specific drug delivery by using albumin microspheres containing magnetite appears to be a promising strategy. Significant improvements in response can be incorporated and obtained with the magnetic albumin microspheres delivery system compared with conventional and nonmagnetic microspheres drug regimens. In the presence of a suitable magnetic field, the microspheres are internalized by the endothelial cells of the target tissue in healthy as well as tumour bearing animals (Fig. 12-2) (Widder et al., 1978).

A labeled marker contained in magnetic microspheres was significantly fixed at a part of the rat-tail where a magnetic field was applied after injection into the tail artery (Senyei et al., 1981). The localization of magnetic microspheres in the head and hind leg, besides the tail, after arterial infusion was achieved by the use of a powerful samarium-cobalt permanent magnet. Injected foreign particles are known to be mainly taken up by the reticuloendothelial system (RES) in the liver and spleen in normal circumstances. The uptake in these organs was suppressed by applying a magnetic field at other parts of the body (Ovadia et al., 1983).

The magnetically carried microspheres and liposomes were employed to selectively transport the curare like drugs (pyrocurine, diadonium) to the muscles of one of the limbs of the cat. The use of magnetic microspheres produced no changes in systemic arterial blood pressure, local blood flow, EEG or ECG. The method also diminished the respiratory depression produced by the curare like substances when they are routinely used for body muscle relaxation (Kharkevich et al., 1985 and 1989).

New magnetic microsphere carriers that localize drugs by both biochemical and physical means have been designed (Fig. 12-3). The microspheres, prepared from the polysaccharide, chitosan, are

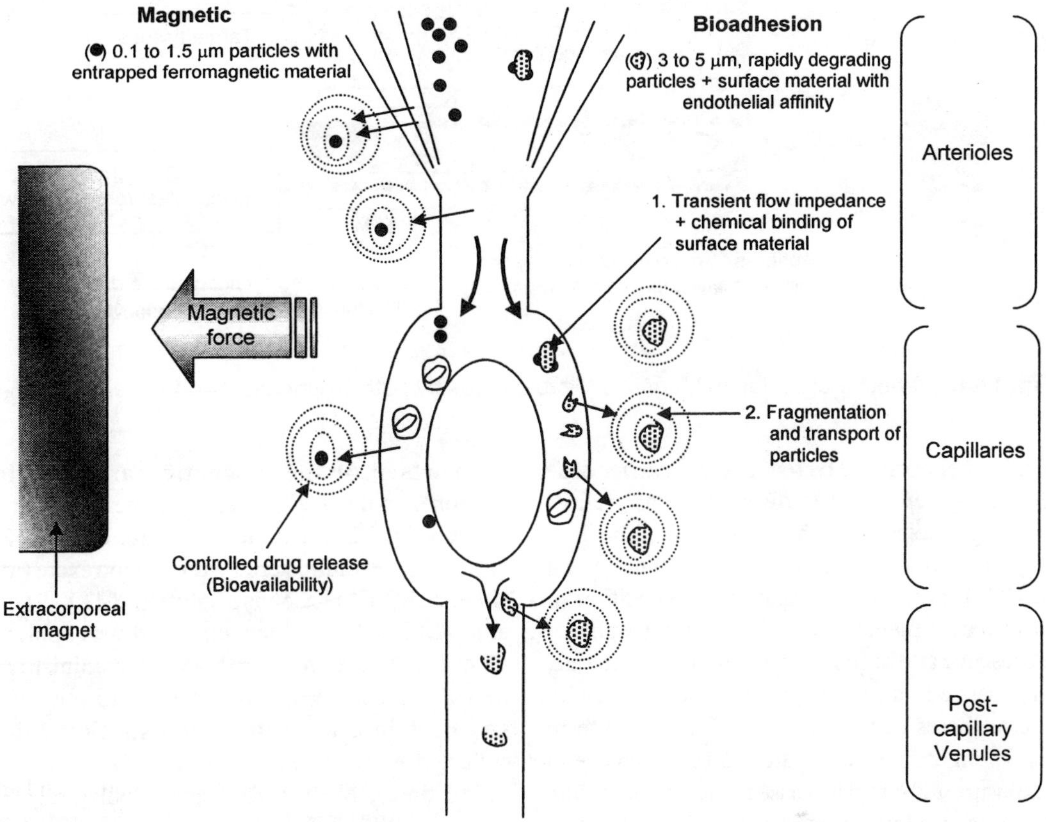

Magnetic
(●) 0.1 to 1.5 μm particles with entrapped ferromagnetic material

Bioadhesion
(◌) 3 to 5 μm, rapidly degrading particles + surface material with endothelial affinity

Arterioles

1. Transient flow impedance + chemical binding of surface material

Magnetic force

2. Fragmentation and transport of particles

Capillaries

Controlled drug release (Bioavailability)

Extracorporeal magnet

Post-capillary Venules

Fig. 12-2. Methods of Microsphere Targeting

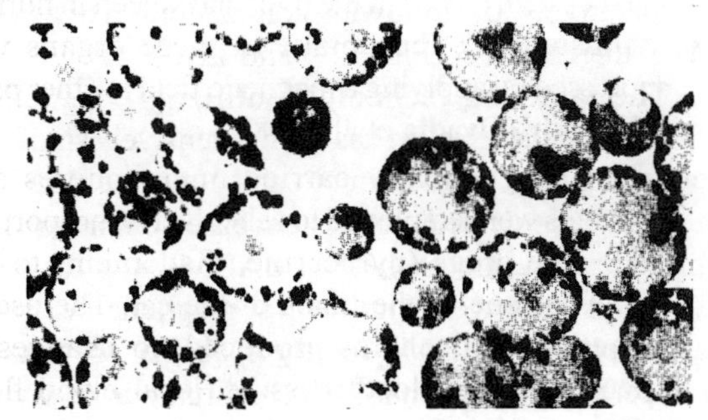

Fig. 12-3. TEM of Albumin Microspheres containing Entrapped Magnetite and Adriamycin

designed to bind to anionic glycosaminoglycan receptors on the surface of capillary endothelial cells. Formation of complexes between the microspheres and heparin has been demonstrated, where heparin served as a model glycosaminoglycan (Fig. 12-4) (Gallo and Hassan, 1988). The disposition of adriamycin following its intra-arterial administration in rats as a solution or magnetic albumin microsphere dispersion has been studied. It was demonstrated that the magnetic albumin microspheres altered the tissue distribution of adriamycin in rats. Administration of drug containing magnetic microspheres was shown to increase the relative drug exposure to both tail target segment and liver (Gallo et al., 1989).

The effect of carrier dose on the multiple tissue disposition of doxorubicin hydrochloride administered via magnetic albumin microspheres in rats was determined. Again the rat tail was used as a target organ and two groups of animals were administered 2.0 or 0.04 mg/kg of microspheres entrapped drug via the ventral caudal artery, and the preidentified tail target site was exposed to a 8000-G magnetic field

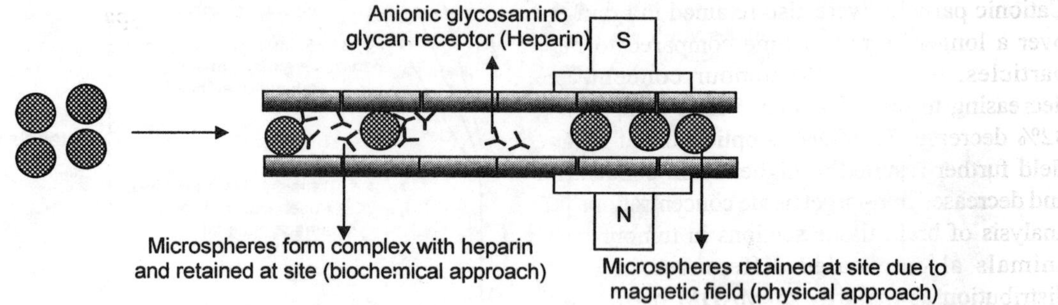

Fig. 12-4. Targeting of Chitosan Magnetic Microspheres by both Biochemical and Physical Means

for 30 min after dosing. The reduction in carrier dose was found to increase drug distribution as well as the targeting efficiency for the target tissue. The drug delivery to heart and liver was reduced (Gupta and Hung, 1989). Studies of comparative disposition of adriamycin bearing magnetic albumin microspheres in the presence and absence of magnetic field in rats, was also carried out. In presence of magnetic field, the microspheres demonstrated 16 fold increase in the maximum drug concentration, 6 fold increase in drug exposure and 6 fold increase in the drug targeting efficiency to rats tail target segment. Drug delivery to the most of the non-target tissues, including heart and liver, was substantially reduced. The results quantitatively suggested that the efficacy of magnetic albumin microspheres in the targeted delivery of incorporated therapeutic agent is predominantly due to the magnetic effects, and not entirely due to the characteristics of the microcarrier system.

Various *in vitro* parameters and *in vivo* efficacy of non-magnetic and magnetic albumin-globulin mix microspheres of mefenamic acid were studied (Lalla and Ahuja, 1991). The distribution of ^{99m}Tc labeled magnetic gelatin microspheres in rabbits was studied (Wu et al., 1993). When magnet was used, the radioactivity in the head (target site) was 15 times more than that when magnet was not used. At the same time, the radioactivity in the lung was recorded to be 5 times less than when magnet was not used.

A novel magnetic microsphere-methotrexate (MM-MTX) drug delivery system was developed and evaluated in rats bearing rat glioma-2 (RG-2) tumour (Devineni et al., 1995). Methotrexate was linked to the surface of the magnetic particles via an aminohexanol linker that released free drug following hydrolysis. Male Fischer 344 rats bearing RG-2 tumour were administered with methotrexate (MTX) either as MM-MTX or as a solution (MTX-S) over 5 min. A 6000 Gauss magnetic field was applied for 15 min from the end of MM-MTX administrations. Serial sacrifices were conducted at 15 min, 30 min and 45 min after drug administrations, organs collected and analyzed for total MTX by a radioassay. At all times, MTX right brain (ipsilateral), brain tumour, and left brain concentrations were approximately 3.5 to 5 fold greater in the MM-MTX treated group compared to the MTX-S treated group. MTX concentrations in all other organs were comparatively low following administration of MM-MTX than MTX-S (Fig. 12-5 and 12-6).

The targeting technology utilizing magnetic microparticulate system has been extensively studied for cancer therapy (Morimoto and Natsume, 1998). A novel cationic delivery system based on magnetic aminodextran microspheres (MADM) was formulated and compared with neutral magnetic dextran microspheres (MDM) for their ability to target intracerebral rat glioma-2 (RG-2) tumour *in vivo*. Overall, the administration of cationic MADM and neutral MDM particles in normal animals resulted in low brain tissue concentrations with the concomitant highest concentrations observed in lung and spleen. In contrast, studies in brain tumour bearing animals resulted in cationic MADM particles being concentrated in brain tumour at a level significantly higher than neutral MDM particles.

Cationic particles were also retained in brain tissue over a longer period of time compared to neutral particles, with MADM tumour concentrations decreasing to only 4% after 6 h as compared to a 32% decrease for MDM. Application of magnetic field further resulted in higher brain concentration and decreased non-target tissue concentrations. TEM analysis of brain tissue sections in tumour bearing animals also revealed differences in particle distribution as majority of MADM particles were observed in the interstitial space while MDM particles found trapped in the vasculature (Fig. 12-7).

Magnetite (Fe_3O_4)

Magnetite is known as the magnetic oxide of iron and is a combination of the two oxides, FeO and Fe_2O_3. It is also referred to as ferrous ferrite. It shows magnetic property just like pure iron. It is in the form of fine particles and has been used for various applica-

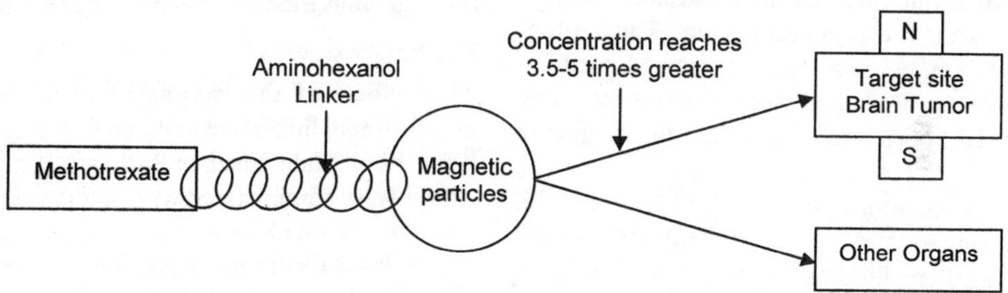

Fig. 12-5. Schematic Representation of Targeting of Magnetic Particles Conjugated with Drug Molecule

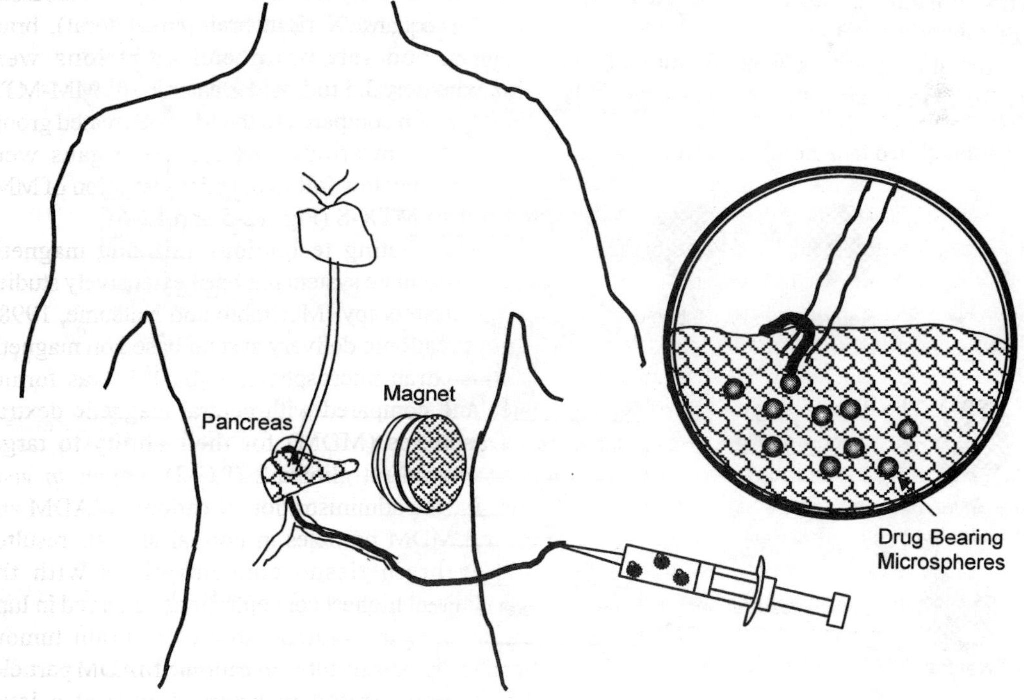

Fig. 12-6. Magnetic Targeting of Antitumour Microspheres to Pancreas

tions *in vivo*, in transmission radiography, as contrast gastrointestinal agent, in inducing clotting in arteriovenous malformation, as a tracer of blood flow and in radionuclide angiography. Iron particles of 50-200 Å in diameter could pass through even the smallest capillaries in the body, when properly conditioned (Freeman et al., 1960).

Studies have confirmed that iron particles could be magnetically controlled in the vasculature of experimental animals (Meyers et al., 1963). The iron particles could be held in place or localized by a magnetic field but when the field is removed, they disappear from the roentgenogram. The mutual attractive forces between two aggregated particles were apparently weakened when the non-magnetic film is casted in order to encapsulate the magnetite particles.

Further a magnoresponsive fluid is available, which is commercially known as ferrofluids (Cobalt-ferrite) from Ferrofluidics Corp. U.S.A. and has a varying size distribution. These normally contain anionic surface active agents for the purpose of stabilization which have haemolytic properties. These haemolytic substances can be removed by the addition of Amberlite MB_2.

Conventional magnetite is generally not a good candidate for magnetizing the carriers especially liposomes because it is insoluble in both aqueous and organic solvents. Moreover, it has got relatively high toxicity as represented by its LD_{50} (mouse, i.v. dose) of 300-600 mg/kg. So a novel magnetic material dextran-magnetite conjugate (DM) was proposed (Hasegawa and Hokkoku, 1978). DM is a submicron complex consisting of magnetic iron oxide core surrounded by dextran chains. It disperses uniformly in aqueous phase and its toxicity was also found to be very low (LD_{50} 2000 to 6000 mg/Kg) in comparison to conventional magnetite.

Magnet Design

The force exerted by a gradient magnetic field is an important parameter that governs in magnetic targeting of microcarriers. The relationship of magnetic force to field gradient and magnetic moment of particles is expressed by following equation :

$$F = M \nabla H \qquad (12\text{-}1)$$

Where; F is force on particles; M is magnetic moment of particles after saturation magnetism; ∇H is magnetic field gradient

This equation explains that spheres with increased magnetic moments will experience forces sufficient for extravascular migration at proportionately lower

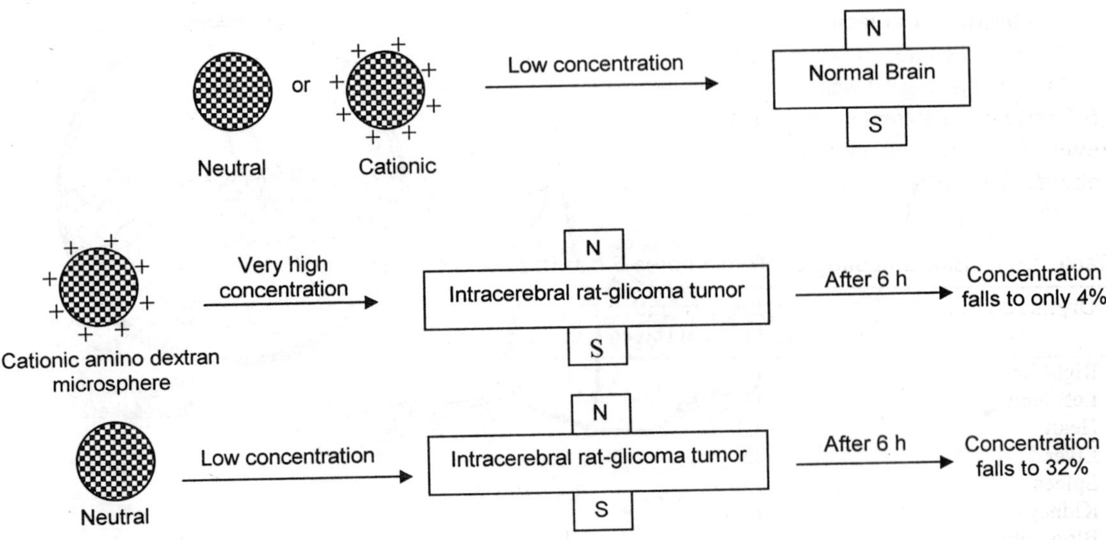

Fig. 12-7. Working Principle of Novel Cationic Delivery System Composed of Magnetic Amino Dextran Microspheres

field gradients. The magnetic moments of microsphere magnetite can be increased in three ways,

1. By magnetizing the spheres to saturation levels prior to vascular targeting
2. By clustering magnetite at the centre of each sphere to produce larger macrodomains
3. By substituting one of the newer ferromagnetic materials that has higher susceptibility than Fe_3O_4.

The acute and chronic toxicities of several new magnetic alloys must be assessed before using them in delivery devices.

Biodistribution and Tissue Concentration of Microspheres

By injecting microspheres in a physiological solution containing 0.1 % (w/v) Tween 80 or a viscosity enhancing agent, such as 50 % (w/v) dextran, aggregation in target vessels can be minimized. For spheres smaller than 3 μm, initial (5-30 min) biodistribution is a function of,

1. The dose relative to the capacity of target capillaries
2. The degree to which the magnetic field overlaps microvessels supplied by the injection vessel
3. The extent of venous shunting before microspheres reach the field
4. The flow rates in target vessels.

In a study, large doses of trace-labeled spheres (6.6 mg/kg, sufficient to produce effective tissue levels of f-met-leu-phe peptide) were infused intravenously in to rats over a 3 min interval, allowed to travel at native flow rates in to the central venous system through the right heart in to both lungs, and captured by an 0.55 T magnetic field (gradient of 0.01 T/mm), which enveloped the right thorax and the middle half of the left thorax (Ranney, 1985). The results are presented in Table 12-1. The splenic and renal concentrations of spheres in the later study were slightly higher because there was greater vascular shunting due to incomplete magnetic envelopment of the left lung.

Carrier Localization

Injury to normal regions of target circulation can be prevented by infusing washed microspheres of appropriate size at moderate rates, however blood flow rate and tissue perfusion are additionally critical. Monitoring the mass of microspheres that becomes localized in a given mass of tissue is also important. Studies for targeting involving trace labeled microspheres provide the basis for modification in drug regimen. Gamma dosimetry and gamma camera imaging provide means to quantify carrier localization with a resolution of 0.5 to 1 cm (Bartlett et al., 1984; Schlafke-Stelson and Watson, 1986). Advanced techniques, like high frequency ultrasound or magnetic resonance (MR) are used to evaluate targeting at submillimeter levels. These two techniques are successfully utilized to assess microspheres distribution in critical anatomical subregions of the target site. Therefore, these techniques are capable of detecting small group of untreated tumour cells or microorganisms that might be missed by lower resolution positron emission topography (PET) and gamma isotopic techniques.

Table 12-1. Biodistribution of Microspheres 5 min Post Injection (Ranney, 1985)

Organs and blood	Biodistribution of microspheres (as % of injected dose)	Tissue concentration of microspheres μg/g wet weight)
Right lung	15.9	195
Left lung	11.2	135
Heart	3.3	67
Liver	45	37
Spleen	7.6	27
Kidneys	11.3	24
Blood plasma	3.4	3
Circulating white blood cells	<0.1	<0.004
	Total dose recovered - 97.8%	

Drug Release

Classical methods frequently fail to monitor drug, due to reduction in circulating free drug levels by a factor exceeding 100 when magnetic targeting is used (Ranney, 1985). Even the blood levels monitored by some feasible methods do not give results when correlated with tissue levels. Estimates of free tissue drug can be made at different intervals from the simultaneous interpretation of results obtained from carrier localization studies in tissue and drug release profile *in vitro*. This method is crude and ignores some factors that influence drug release from carrier *in vivo* viz., enzymatic digestion of microspheres accelerated drug release and retrodiffusion of the drug back to microvessels enhances drug clearance. The accurate and precise results can be obtained by measuring the drug levels of the target site *per se* using magnetic resonance methods.

Tissue Levels

Determination of naturally occurring ^{31}P metabolites and ^{13}C labeled metabolic precursors by magnetic resonance spectroscopy provides a means to monitor tissue responses to localized drugs. Treatment of human melanomas grown in nude mice with diphtheria toxin has shown an acute and reversible decrease in spectral peaks of high-energy phosphates (ATP and phosphocreatine). A more prolonged (24 h) decrease has been recorded at the pH of inorganic phosphates, however this change is reversible but recovery is slow and corresponds in time to resultant major tissue damages.

Another approach to tissue monitoring using MR technique involves acute broadening of spectral peaks observed in rat organs that were excised and studied shortly after the induction of acute inflammation. Peaks broadening reflects, shortened tissue T2 relaxation times and are due to long-lived free radicals generated in inflamed tissues. Treatment with antiinflammatory agents leads to reversal of spectral change.

Biomodulators

Biological response modifiers (BRMs) alter host, tumour as well as microbial responses in four ways,

1. Augmentation of host effector mechanisms directed against tumour cells or microorganisms.
2. Decrease in host response that interferes with tumour resistance by a quantitative increase in endogenous effector resistance by an increase in endogenous effector molecules or redirecting their sites and duration of action.
3. Augmentation of tumour sensitivity to host cells by redifferentiating tumour cells.
4. Increase in host tolerance of conventional cancer treatment.

There are basically two types of agents; indirect and direct (Heberman, 1985). Indirect agents include white cell chemoattractant/activator peptides, interleukins (1 to 4) and immunomodulators such as the interferons (α, β and γ). Indirect BRMs seem to act by enhancing the responses of monocytes, neutrophils, macrophages, B and T lymphocytes and natural killer cells. Direct acting BRMs are the final lymphocyte effector molecules. These are exemplified by antibodies, lymphotoxin and tumour necrosis factor (TNF, also called as Cachetin). A potential advantage with these molecules is that they do not have an upper limit to their pharmacological actions.

Chemoattractant Microspheres

Neutrophil chemoattractant, f-met-leu-phe was the first selected biomodulator for magnetic targeting (Ranney, 1985) due to its lethal property when administered freely in the circulation at a concentration exceeding 2×10^{-7}M. It requires a site specific and local delivery to modulate inflammation and is a small, bacterially derived peptide, stable during microspheres preparation. It can be entrapped successfully in microparticles. f-met-leu-phe microspheres have been used either in disease modeling or clinical therapy. In pulmonary medicine these delivery systems are used as (1) an experimental method to test new agents that prevent neutrophil degradation of lung elastin in smokers, (2) a means of studying the contribution of acute alveolar damage to acute type respiratory distress syndrome and (3) as an adjuvant method in treating invasive pulmonary aspergillosis suffering patients.

Magnetic Neutrophils

In certain clinical conditions, where patient sera contains chemotactic factor inactivators (Ward, 1984) and neutrophils directed inhibitors of chemotaxis

(Chopp et al., 1985), an indirect approach of targeting white cells by chemoattraction fails. These disorders include chronic lymphocytic leukemia, alcoholic cirrhosis, Crohn's disease, hemodialysis, sarcoidosis and Hodgkin's disease. Even though failure of chemotaxis is not observed in all patients, such conditions are life threatening. Therefore, a means of making neutrophil ingest magnetite base system ought to be developed, so that the sites of severe infection can be selectively approached for therapy (Ranney and Huffaker, 1987).

Interleukin 2 Microspheres

Interleukin 2 (IL-2) is an important immuno-modulator with a molecular weight 15,000. It is chemically a glycoprotein made by activated T-lymphocytes that enhance cellular immune response to infection and certain tumours (Lotze et al., 1986). IL-2 activates certain cell types like T-helper cells, cytotoxic T-lymphocytes, natural killer cells and possibly macrophages. It is an appropriate molecule for drug delivery systems due to its attractive properties. It is stable, active in mice and human being and is available in large quantities as a product of genetic engineering. Studies revealed that high doses of IL-2 lead to regression of pulmonary and hepatic metastasis in several murine tumours (Rosenberg et al., 1985). IL-2 has also been found effective against disseminated human melanomas and renal cell carcinomas, which are generally non-responsive to conventional therapy.

Magnetic Nanoparticles

Immunospecific ferromagnetic iron-dextran reagents for the labeling and magnetic separation of cells were studied (Molday and Mackenzie, 1982). Ferro-magnetic iron-dextran nanoparticles were prepared by reacting a mixture of ferrous chloride and ferric chloride with dextran polymers under alkaline conditions. The particles of average size range (30-40 nm) showed little non-specific binding to cells and had a magnetic moment. Protein A from *Staphylococcus aureus* was covalantly linked to periodate oxidized ferromagnetic iron-dextran particles. These conjugates were used to indirectly label antigen sites on human red blood cells and thymocytes for visualization by scanning and transmission electron microscopy. Cells labeled with these immunospecific ferromagnetic particles were quantitatively retained by a simple permanent magnet and could be separated from unlabeled cells. Possibilities of these novel reagents in the separation of cells, cell membranes and receptors in drug targeting have been discussed (Fig. 12-8).

Magnetic carbohydrate nanoparticles have been proposed for use in affinity cell separation. Magnetically responsive nanoparticles were prepared from enzymatically hydrolyzed starch and magnetite. Two different monoclonal antibodies were covalantly coupled to the particles. Using these magnetic nanoparticles (average size range 100-300 nm) coupled with monoclonal mouse anti-rat Ig kappa light chain antibody, a very high depletion of surface Ig positive cells (mostly B-cells) from one million rat peripheral blood mononuclear cells could be achieved. The separation efficiency of this technique was evaluated by flow cytofluorometric analysis and the technique has been reported to permit the detection of a small number of surface Ig positive cells among 10,000 negative cells (Schroder et al., 1986).

Indomethacin bearing magnetic nanoparticles of polymethylmethacrylate, were prepared by the emulsion polymerization technique (Vyas and Malaiya, 1989). The controlled growth of ferric hydroxide particles in the presence of non-ionic surfactant was affected to obtain nano-sized particles and these were subsequently heated to obtain magnetite. The effect of various parameters, i.e. monomer concentration and magnetite concentration, as well as the stirring rate was studied to characterize the particle size and its distribution. The factors, which affect the total drug payload were also assessed. The *in vivo* magnet responsiveness and kinetics of distribution of these magnetic and plain nanoparticles were characterized and reported. Up to 60 min post injection time, 60-fold higher drug concentration in target tail segment was recorded which resulted in considerably reduced drug concentration in other organs as evinced by data from control rats. Following normal administration (without magnetic field) drug concentration was higher in liver and spleen, where endocytosis and phagocytosis takes place (Fig. 12-9). Tumour-specific

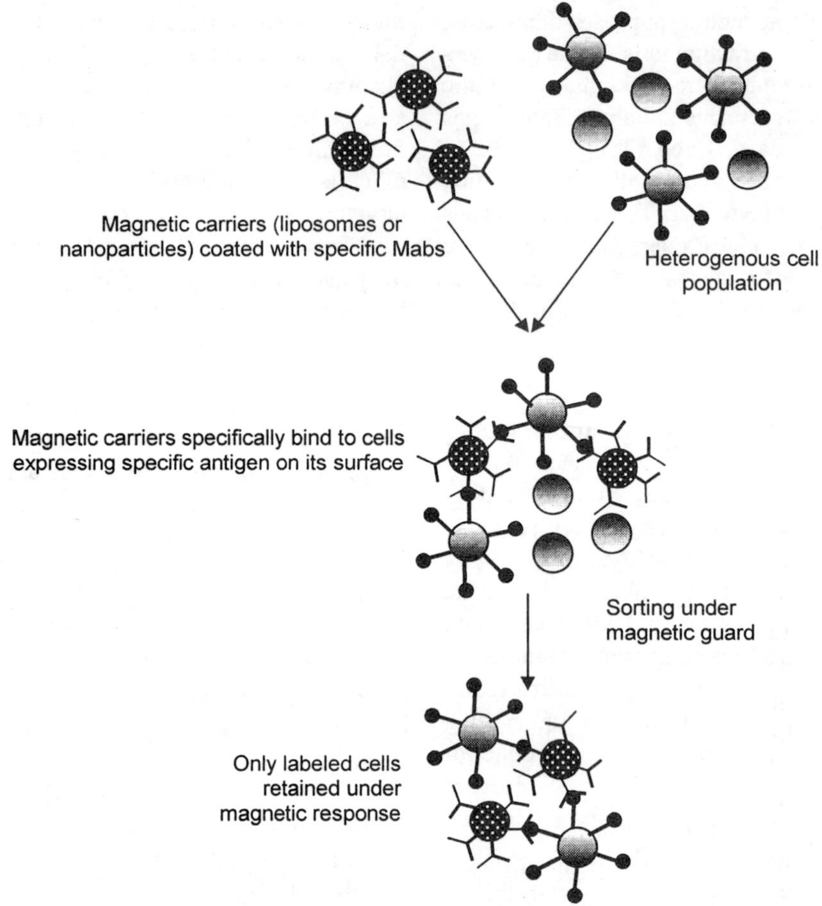

Fig. 12-8. Principle of Cellular Sorting using Magnetic Carriers

superparamagnetic particles (SMP) were prepared and characterized. Particles of uniform size (9.6 ± 0.8 nm) were prepared from an alkaline solution of ferric and ferrous ions and isolated by differential centrifugation. The resulting nanoparticles suspension was stabilized in buffer using a polypeptide coat to which a monoclonal antibody, specific to carcinoembryonic antigen (CEA), was covalantly attached at the hinge region. The resulting anti-CEA SMP antibody had a hydrodynamic radius of less than 50 nm with specific binding affinity to CEA *in vitro*. The visualization of epitopes, present on a cell surface in very low density as expected for tumour antigens or receptors may be achieved. Furthermore, the polypeptide coat chosen provided an ideal platform for the attachment of biological modifiers needed for the reduction of the antigenicity and blood clearance rate of anti-CEA SMP (Tiefenauer et al., 1993).

Superparamagnetic iron oxide particles represent a new class of contrast agents that increase the detectability of hepatic and splenic tumour by magnetic resonance imaging (MRI). The main steps of the biodegradation and metabolism of the magnetite-dextran nanoparticles in rats were investigated (Okon et al., 1994). The radioactive tracer data and histochemistry features showed that the iron oxide cores were accumulated into the Kupffer cells and the macrophages of the splenic marginal zone. With time, the number of the granules was decreased whereas the fine iron granules appeared in the cytoplasm. Immunopositive staining

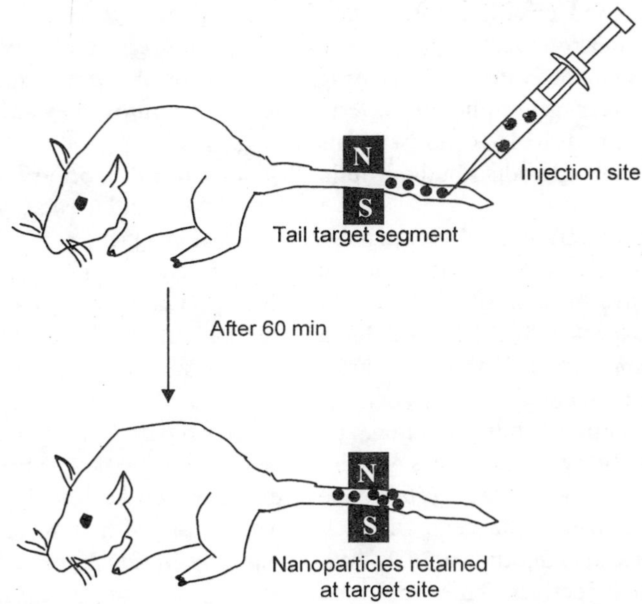

Fig. 12-9. Schematic Representation of retaining of Magnetic Nanoparticles at Rat Tail Target Segment

for ferritin was markedly increased in the liver hepatocytes as observed for 3 days after injection. The splenic marginal zone macrophages stained prominantly14 days after injection. The data pointed to the early biodegradation of the magnetite-dextran nanoparticles and they thus appear as an interesting biodegradable new contrast agent first devoted to MRI of liver and spleen diseases that could be further extended to heart, kidneys, and other organs. *In vivo* evaluation of magnetite nanoparticles for use as a tumour contrast agent in MRI has been carried out and discussed by Tiefenauer et al., 1996. Magnetite nanoparticles, coated by three different artificial polypeptides, were conjugated to an antibody specific to the carcinoembryonic antigen (CEA) (Fig. 12-10). To protect the particles from fast blood elimination, the coats were modified by various sugars, polyethylene glycol, albumin, and sialoproteins, respectively and their biodistribution in nude mice grafted with CEA-tumour was determined. A

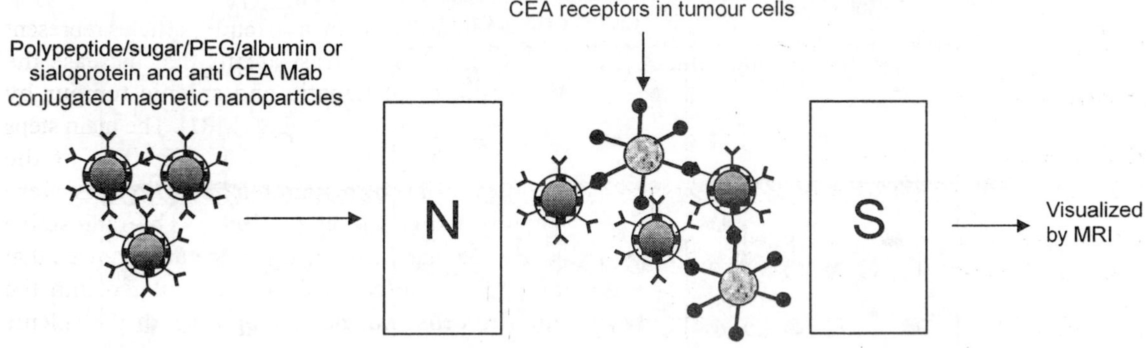

Fig. 12-10. Schematic Presentation of use of Magnetic Nanoparticles as Tumour Contrast agent

prolongation of the blood circulation time and decreased rates of elimination were recorded. The tumour accumulation was slightly improved by using the specific sialoprotein glycophorin B. The usefulness of nanoparticles as image contrast agents is probably limited by their microdistribution within the tumour tissue.

Blood brain barrier (BBB) permeability to magnetic dextran nanoparticles (MD_3) after osmotic disruption in rats was investigated. After intravenous mannitol infusion, as expected, the BBB breakdown was immediate and temporary as judged by soluble molecule diffusion. MD_3 nanoparticles crossed the BBB 12 h after intravenous mannitol injection, at a time when brain permeability for molecules or small particles returns to normal. Magnetite crystals were found in cytoplasmic vesicles of glial cells. On MRI, signal intensity decreased after injection of MD_3, even 12 h after mannitol injection. This could be particularly useful in the study of focal pathological lesions accompanied by BBB permeability modifications. In such conditions, super paramagnetic particles based contrast agents could be caught by the BBB, allowing the observations of impaired BBB areas without detectable cellular lesions (Fig. 12-11) (Roussean et al., 1997).

Surface modification of superparamagnetic nanoparticles (Ferrofluid) with particle electrophoresis and their application in specific targeting of cells was studied. Colloidal aqueous suspension of superparamagnetic nanoparticles (diameter 9 nm) was covalently coupled with lectins, enzymes or antibodies, applying specific thiol chemistry. Changes in particle electrophoretic mobility (PEM) were shown to correlate well with the amount of ligand fixed on the particles, as proved by its biological activity (Sestier et al., 1998).

Colloidal iron oxide nanoparticles were synthesized and used as MRI contrast agent. These superparamagnetic particles were constituted of solid cores (diameter of 5-15 nm) generally coated by a thick polysaccharide layer (hydrodynamic radius of 30-100 nm), and formulated by direct coprecipitation of iron salts in the presence of polymeric material (Babes et al., 1999).

Similarly, magnetic nanoparticles were incorporated in new hybrid network based on tetrafunctionalized heteropolyanions and polyacrylamide, which resulted in a magnetic hybrid hydrogel with super absorption properties. The magnetic properties of the nanoparticles which enable their mobility inside the network, were estimated and their release during the swelling of the hydrogel was monitored (Mayer et al., 1999).

The use of magnetic nanospheres for the well directed delivery of radionuclides to a tumour after the intravenous administration of the biodegradable colloidal suspension is well documented and proposed (Schutt et al., 1999).

A novel magnetic drug carrier based on carboxymethyl dextran magnetic nanoparticles (CMD MNPs) was prepared (Shi et al., 2000). Adriamycin (ADR) was coupled with two types of carriers; neutral dextran MNPs and anionic CMD MNPs, by

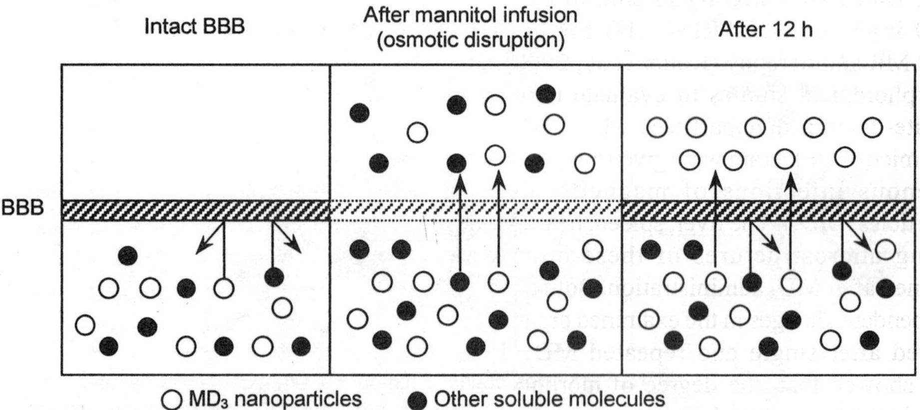

Fig. 12-11. Blood Brain Barrier Permeability to Magnetic Dextran Nanoparticles

periodated oxidation. The physico-chemical characteristics and the magnetic guidance effects *in vitro* and *in vivo* of ADR-CMD MNPs were studied. The distribution profiles of liver and spleen revealed that on conjugation with neutral dextran MNPs, excessive accumulation resulted in liver and spleen after intravenous administration. On the other hand, conjugation with CMD MNPs gave a markedly lower concentration in these organs, which indicated less uptake of ADR-CMD conjugate MNPs by RES. It is therefore, considered advantageous for delivering loaded drug to sites other than the RES.

A cell labeling approach using short HIV-Tat peptides was developed to derivatize magnetic nanoparticles for *in vivo* tracking and recovery of progenitor cells. The particles were efficiently internalized into hematopoietic and neutral progenitor cells in quantity upto 10-30 pg of iron per cell. Iron incorporation did not affect viability, differentiation, or proliferation of CD34+ cells. Following intra-venous injection into immuno-deficient mice, 4% of magnetized CD34+ cells homed in to the bone marrow and discrete single cells could be detected by magnetic resonance (MR) imaging in tissue samples. In addition, magnetically labeled cells homed to bone narrow could be recovered by using a magnetic separation columns. Localization and retrieval of cell populations *in vivo* enable detailed analysis of specific stem cell and organ interactions critical for advancing the therapeutic use of stem cells (Lewin et al., 2000).

Monocrystalline iron oxide containing nanoparticles were prepared with an oxidized starch coating, which are currently in clinical trials (NC 100150 injection; CLARISCAN) for positive-contrast MR angiography (Keller et al., 2000).

Morphological studies to evaluate toxicity of magnetite-dextran nanoparticles were performed. Female mice of OFI strain were given single repeated intravenous injections of magnetite-dextran nanoparticles (MD_3). The liver, spleen, heart, kidney and lung microstructures of these mice were determined after MD_3 administration. Both dose and time dependent changes in the examined organs were compared after single and repeated MD_3 doses. Results showed that, the degree of morphological changes in the liver and spleen appeared to be rather low even after a single MD_3 dose that exceeds approximately 200 times a dose necessary for diagnostic MRI (Okon et al., 2000).

Magnetic Liposomes

The magnetic liposomes have been used in cellular sorting successfully. Liposomes bearing anti-fibronectin antibodies and associated with ferromagnetic particles bound firmly to the surface of mouse embryo fibroblasts. Upon binding magnetoliposomes, the cells could be sorted under influence of a magnetic field (Margolis et al., 1983). The feasibility of magnetic liposomes as a targeting device for drugs was explored. They incorporated ultrafine magnetite particles within vesicles composed of egg-PC and tocopherol using film hydration method. The liposomes were targeted to Yoshida sarcoma implanted in a footpad of rats. A very small amount of the liposomes, but significantly more than the control, was found trapped at the tumour tissue (Kiwada et al., 1986).

The magnetoliposomes were biophysically characterized and the potentialities of magneto-liposomes in symmetric and asymmetric phospholipid transfer processes were explored. They presented classical binding characteristics and thermal behaviour of cytochrome-C oxidase bearing magnetic liposomes (Cuyper and Joniau, 1988 and 1992). The preparation, physicochemical properties of magnetoliposomes, and their possible use as a targeting carrier have also been described (Ishii et al., 1990). Human peripheral blood mononuclear cells (PBMCs) were incubated with large unilamellar vesicles containing encapsulated dextran-magnetite particles (DPM). This resulted in an efficient incorporation of DMP within cells. Electron microscopy revealed the presence of DMP in cells mainly in phagosomes and secondary lysosomes. The fraction of DMP containing PBMCs could be enriched by magnetic cell separation. The major population of the DMP containing cells were identified to be monocytes. The labeling of these cells was used in studies of selective MR imaging of *in vivo* cells migration in a variety of immunologically compromised tissue states, e.g. tumour transplantations and abscesses (Fig. 12-12) (Bulte et al., 1993).

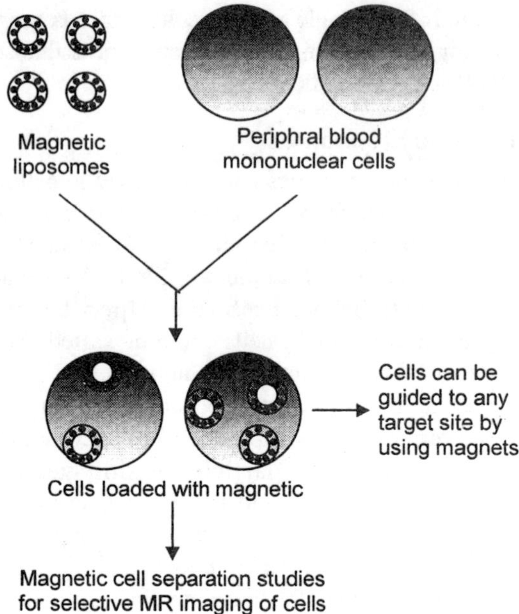

Fig. 12-12. Incorporation of Dextran-Magnetic Particles within PBM cells and their Monitoring

A procedure for increased iron oxide incorporation in liposomes without liposomal aggregation or fusion was developed (Bogdanov et al.,1994). It essentially employs dextran stabilized iron oxide nanoparticles (MION) encapsulated in REV's by transient binding of oxidized dextran with amine groups of aminophospholipids with the formation of covalent Schiff's bonds. Phosphatidyl ethanolamine (PE) containing lipids in organic phase were combined with oxidized MION during the preparation of water/ lipid emulsion, which resulted in an increased entrapment of colloids in REVs. In REV's, the iron oxide/dextran is attached to internal monolayer of the bilayer and may be detached by altering the pH. This detachment was supposed to be a result of the stability of the Schiff's bond at acidic pH values. These highly super paramagnetic liposomes were termed as ferrosomes, in which remaining amine groups were used either for grafting targeting ligands or for acylation.

The liposomal constructs based on DPPC/DSPC (dipalmitoyl/distearoyl PC) with optimum molar ratio of cholesterol (to optimize phase transformation above the physiological temperature) and dextran magnetite (incorporated to endow them with thermosensitivity and magnetic responsiveness), were successfully developed. Based on the discussed principle, a DPPC based liposomal surface modified by Me-PEG-PE has been reported for the selective doxorubicin chemotherapy (Viroonchatapan et al., 1998).

Magnetofluorescent liposomes for increased sensitivity of immunofluorescence were suggested. LUV's loaded with carboxyfluorescein and small magnetic particles, were prepared by membrane extrusion and magnetic filtration. The magneto-liposomes proved to be useful for improvement of sensitivity of detection and physical separation at large or to quantitate the biodistribution or to sort phagocytic cells at low levels. The high affinity IL-2 receptor CD25 is expressed in low density on a significant fraction of resting B and T lymphocytes in human peripheral blood, as can be shown exclusively by magnetofluorescent liposomes (Scheffold et al., 1995).

The possibility of dextran magnetite (DM) incorporated thermosensitive liposomes, namely thermosensitive magnetoliposomes (TMs), as a physically modulated temperature responsive system, was studied (Masuko et al., 1995). The temperature of TMs suspensions and cancer tumour injected with TMs suspensions was elevated up to 42°C by electromagnetic induced heating at a frequency of 500 KHz under both *in vitro* and *in vivo* conditions. The temperature rise obtained at various concentrations of TMs suggested that approximately 15 mg Fe/cm^3 tumour volume was adequate as a therapeutic dose of TMs for efficient selective hyperthermia. Their possibility for magnetic drug targeting was further investigated (Viroonchatapan et al., 1995). Due to water-soluble property of DM, higher content, i.e. 490 mg per mmols of DPPC were successfully incorporated in calcein bearing REV's. A novel on-line flow apparatus was engineered to assess the magnetic responsiveness of TMs, whereas calcein release was a measure of thermosensitivity in response to hyperthermia. Virooenchatapan and co-workers, 1996 have reported dextran-magnetite as a promising strategy in targeting of thermosensitive magnetoliposomes to mouse livers in *in situ* on-line perfusion system (Fig. 12-13). The group established an efficient targeting of thermosensitive magnetoliposomes in RES blocked livers with a targeting advantage index (TAI) of 1.6-3.1 (compared to TAI in normal liver of 1.1-1.4) revealing a critical role of RES uptake in the physically modulated systems. The release of 5-Fluorouracil (5-FU) from TMs was assessed (Viroonchatapan et al., 1998). TMs was injected into the tumour mass of B16-BL6 melanoma in mice and subsequently the tumour temperature was raised by using a 500 KHz electromagnetic field. The temperature of TMs selectively in the tumour was effectively elevated to 42°C and maintained at this temperature, overcoming the 'cooling effect' of blood flow and surrounding tissues. The analysis of release kinetics of 5-FU allowed the estimated prediction of intra-tumour drug concentrations during electromagnetic field exposure under various conditions.

Antibody coated magnetoliposomes for hyperthermia treatment of cancer were prepared by coating phospholipid on to magnetic particles (Shinkai et al., 1995). The magnetoliposomes were coated with hydrazide pullulan to stabilize the phospholipid capsules and provide a site selective anchor for the immobilization of antibodies. By this method, 90-180 molecules of a monoclonal antibody were immobilized on to a magnetoliposome. When the antibody-conjugated magnetoliposomes were incubated with cancer cells, they were adsorbed on to the cell surface and taken up by the cells about 12 times more effectively than the control after 4 h. The heating properties of the magnetoliposomes were also assessed and found to vary with the size of the core contained magnetite (Fig. 12-14).

Positively charged vesicles with encapsulated magnetite, named as magnetite cationic liposomes (MCLs), were developed as a means to generate intracellular hyperthermia (Shinkai et al., 1996). Affinity of the MCLs to glioma cells was estimated to be 10 times higher than that of magnetic neutral liposomes due to the electrostatic interaction based on the positive charge of the MCLs. In an *in vitro* study, heat generation of the MCLs was studied using agar phantoms and small pellets of rat glioma cells.

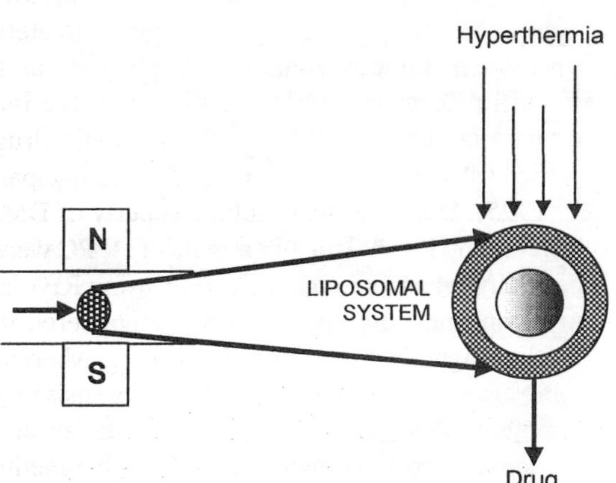

Fig. 12-13. Dextran Magnetite Based Thermosensitive Magnetoliposomes

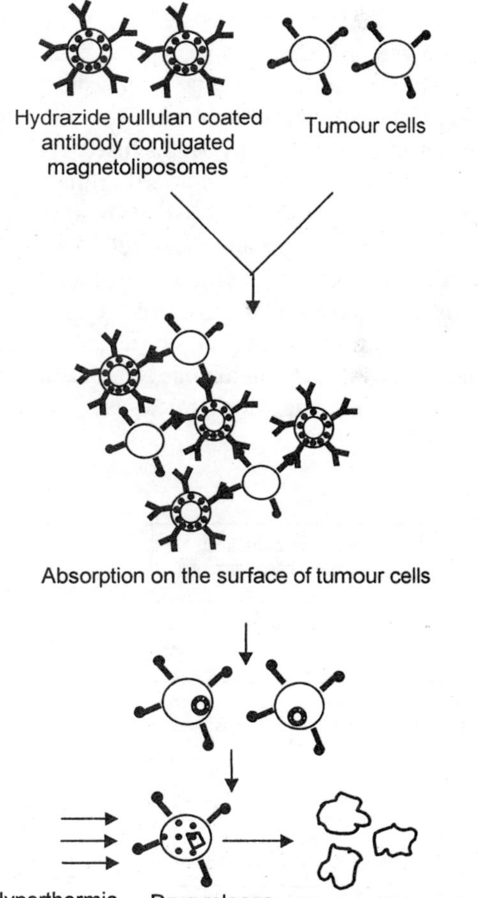

Fig. 12-14. Hyperthermia Treatment of Cancer using Antibody coated Magnetic Liposomes

When a high-frequency magnetic field, 118 KHz, 384 Oe was applied to glioma cells in the presence of MCLs, the glioma cells pellet of 80 μl (5.4 nm in diameter) got heated to over 43°C and all the cells died on 40 min irradiation owing to the hyperthermic effect. On the basis of these *in vitro* results the same group of scientists further studied MCLs for hyperthermic treatment of solid tumour in *ex vivo* (Yanase et al., 1997) and *in vivo* studies (Yanase et al., 1998). Complete tumour regression was recorded in 87.5% of the rats treated with MCLs and subjected to irradiation for 30 min (three times) by an alternating magnetic field (118 KHz, 384 Oe). Furthermore, the treated rats showed no severe side effects. In addition to killing the tumour cells by heat, a host immune response was also induced (Yanase et al., 1998). Cellular pellets consisted of T-9 rat glioma cells into which MCLs was incorporated in a petri dish, were implanted subcutaneously in the left femoral region of female F344 rats. The cell pellets were heated to over 43°C by MCLs (used as heating mediators for intracellular hyperthermia) in the magnetic field (384 Oe, 118 MHz) by applying 3 cycles of 60 min. Almost all glioma cells were found to be killed. To examine the induction of antitumour immunity, rats were re-challenged with T-9 cells after a 3-month period and it was observed that after transient growth phase, all tumour cells disappeared. Furthermore, immunocytochemical assay revealed that the host immune response induced by the hyperthermia treatment was mediated by both CD8+ T and CD4+ cells with a marked augmentation of tumour-selective cytotoxic T-lymphocyte activity.

Three different types of liposomes containing superparamagnetic iron oxide particles (SPIOs) as a contrast agent were tested by magnetic resonance imaging (MRI) for intratumour enrichment (Pauser et al., 1997). The liposomes encapsulated SPIOs were investigated for comparison with AMI-227, dextran coated SPIOs in two different dosage using the CC531 adenocarcinoma in the liver of WAG/RIJ rats as a model. Reduction of the relative signal intensity (SI) in the tumour in T2-weighted MR images was assumed as a measure of the liposomes enrichment in the tumour or adjacent tissue. The samples were also tested at dosages with isomolar iron content and at dosage producing the same MR relaxivity.

Magnetically responsive polymerized liposomes as potential oral delivery vehicles were prepared to protect complex molecules such as proteins or peptides (e.g., vaccines) from the harsh gastrointestinal environment and targeting them to the Peyer's patches (Fig. 12-15) (Chen and Langer, 1997). The intestinal transit of liposomes is relatively fast in mice (1-2 h for small intestine). During this time, liposomes are continuously pushed downward by intestinal flow as well as intestinal motions. As a result, most liposomes fail to have sufficient time to reach the

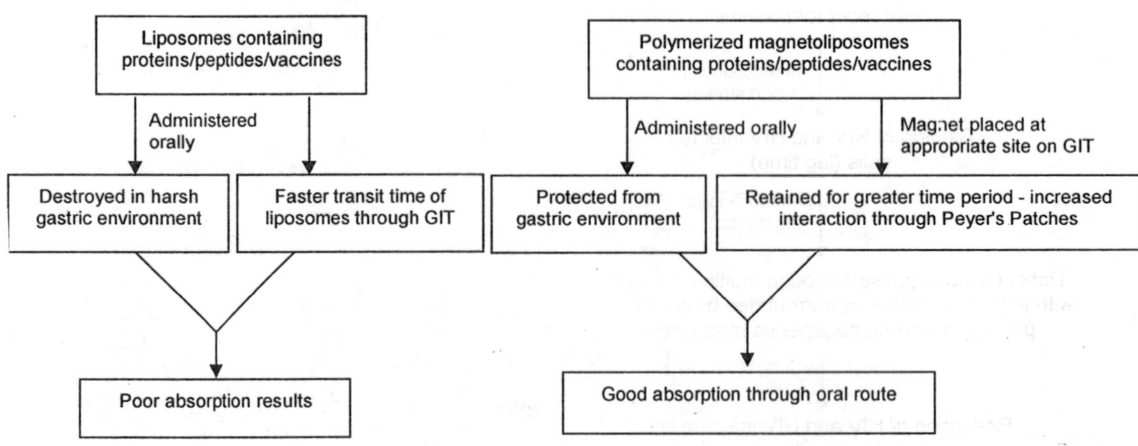

Fig. 12-15. Possibility of Polymerized Magnetoliposomes as a Possible Oral Delivery Vehicle

Peyer's patches before they are swept further down. In order to slow down the liposomes transit so as to retain them in the intestine for a prolonged period of time, magnetically responsive liposomes were prepared. These liposomes were localized at desired areas by exposing them to an external magnetic field. *In vivo* absorption of the Fe_3O_4 containing liposomes was examined in mice. After liposomes administration, the mice were given access to food and water for 40 min before they were restrained and exposed to the magnetic field. In this way, when the external magnetic field was applied, the majority of the liposomes were localized within the intestine instead of the stomach as measured by the amount of radioactivity retained in various tissue samples.

A simple method for the treatment of AIDS was proposed by introducing magnetoliposomes coupled with HIV receptor proteins that could be effective treatment modules against HIV virus (Fig. 12-16) (Babincova and Machova, 1998). After a time lag, needed for binding of HIV and HIV-infected cells to magnetoliposomes, the arteriovenous shunt, as used with dialysis patient could be inserted and the patient's blood is passed through multiple tubes filled with stainless steel wool, each of which was surrounded by a coil producing a strong non-homogeneous magnetic field, which resulted in a substantial reduction of HIV and HIV-infected cells in the infected body by their selective retention and subsequent removal.

The relaxation enhancement and biodistribution of conventional vs long-circulating magnetoliposomes as a new contrast agent for MR imaging of bone marrow was evaluated. Magnetoliposomes with (ML-PEG) and without (ML) incorporation of PEG 2000 were prepared. PEGylation selectively enhanced the T2 relaxivity of magnetoliposomes by 10% to 15%. The formulations were administered intravenously into Sprague-Dawley rats at 100 pmol Fe/kg. PEGylation increased blood half-life. MR imaging revealed their pronounced uptake in bone marrow, including the iliac bone, femur, tibia, and upper and lower vertebrae. The bone marrow uptake of ML-PEG was comparable to that of ML, with both reaching a plateau within 30 min following injection. Fast spin-echo T2 imaging was found to provide optimal contrast enhancement and allowed a clear depiction of red-yellow marrow conversion due to normal aging, while the use of magnetoliposomes provided an added benefit of therapeutic drug or gene delivery (Bulte et al., 1999).

Due to the magnetite particles, which are strong microwave absorbers, magnetoliposomes could be heated to higher temperatures, which may subsequently lead to a leakage of encapsulated drug. Influence of static magnetic field on liposomes in

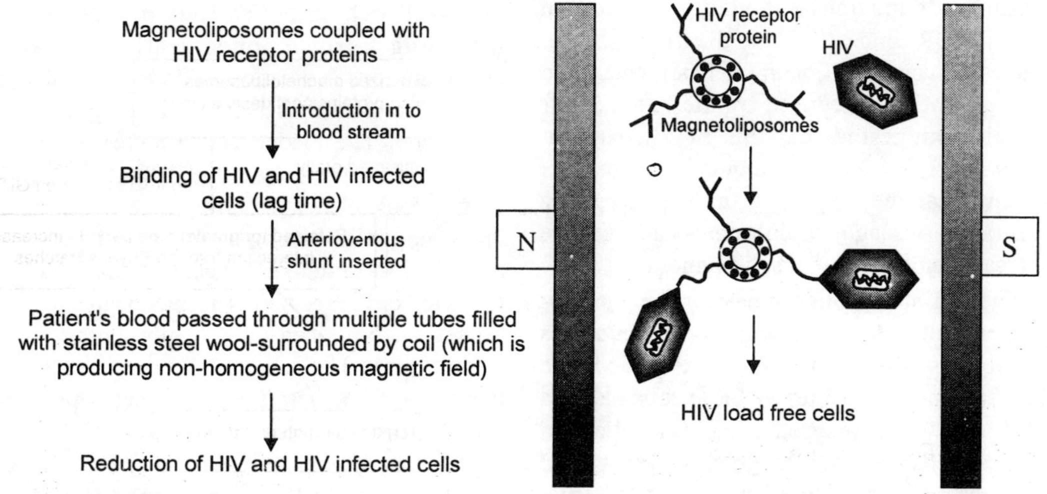

Fig. 12-16. Schematic Representation of HIV Treatment by Magnetoliposomes

the blood stream was analyzed (Babincova et al., 2000). Human serum albumin labeled with technetium 99m together with magnetite particles were further encapsulated into phosphatidyl choline/ cholesterol liposomes. For *in vivo* targeting a SmCo permanent magnet with intensity approximately 0.35 T was attached near the right kidney. Difference between the relative radioactivity in the magnetically targeted right kidney (25.92 ± 5.84%) and non-targeted left kidney (0.93 ± 0.05%) was sufficiently high for relevant clinical applications.

Magnetic liposomes designed to act as anticancer drug carriers, could be effectively delivered to solid tumour via intravenous route (Kubo et al., 2000). Magnetic liposomes with incorporated adriamycin (magnetic ADR lipsomes) were prepared by reverse-phase evaporation technique and an *in vivo* study was carried out to assess the magnetic targeting of these liposomes osteosarcoma site. Syrian male hamsters inoculated with osteosarcoma, Os 515, in the right hind limb were studied 7 days after inoculation. After the hamsters had received an intravenous administration of either magnetic ADR liposomes or ADR solution (corresponding to 5 mg ADR/kg), the ADR concentrations in plasma, tumour, liver, lung, heart and kidney were determined at designated time intervals. Administration of magnetic ADR liposomes under magnetic force (0.4 T) produced an approximately 4 fold higher ADR concentration in the tumour than did administration of ADR solution. The former administration modality induced an increase in ADR concentration in the liver and lung and decreased concentration in the heart, compared with concentrations produced by the latter. Their results also suggested that this new treatment approach which involved a combination of magnet implantation at the target site and intravenous administration of magnetic liposomes can improve the clinical chemotherapy of solid tumour.

Engineered magnetoliposomes for their preferential presentation to circulating blood monocytes and neutrophils (phagocytic cells) were studied. The uptake of magnetoliposomes by these cells resulted in both drug as well as magnetite content localization within these cells and due to magnetite content these cells become magnetic which respond to an external magnetic field. Due to the chemotaxis and diapedesis properties of these cells, they migrate towards inflammatory sites and their migration (natural phenomenon of these cells) could be supplied by placing the magnet at the inflammatory site. By utilizing this carrier-cellular co-ordinated targeting approach, the author targeted the bioactives to brain tissues (Jain, 2000). The strategy is schematically presented in Figure 12-17.

Magnetic Resealed Erythrocytes

Local thrombosis in animal arteries was prevented by means of magnetic targeting of aspirin loaded red cells (Fig. 12-18). Thrombosis was induced in 18 dogs and 16 rabbits arteries by surgically inverting a vascular wall flap into its lumen. A completely occluding red thrombus was developed inside the vessel after 4 to 5 h in 80% of cases. SmCo5 magnet was secured externally to one of the arteries. The constant magnetic field produced by the magnet had no influence on the clot formation. Autologous red cells loaded with ferromagnetic colloid compound and aspirin were administered intravenously, and completely aborted arteriothrombosis on magnet application side with no deterioratory effect on clot formation in the control artery was recorded (Orekhova et al., 1990).

Magnetically responsive ibuprofen-loaded erythrocytes were prepared and characterized *in vitro* (Vyas and Jain, 1994). The erythrocytes were loaded with ibuprofen and magnetite (ferrofluids) using the preswell technique. Various process variables including drug concentration, magnetite concentration, sonication of ferrofluids that could affect the loading of drug and magnetite were optimized. The loaded erythrocytes were characterized for *in vitro* drug efflux, haemoglobin release, morphology, osmotic fragility, turbulence shock, *in vitro* magnetic responsiveness and percent cell recovery. In optimum concentrations, erythrocytes could tolerate ibuprofen as no appreciable detrimental effects were noticed on cell morphology, osmotic fragility and turbulence shock, when compared with normal erythrocytes. The drug release profile from the cellular system was observed to follow approximately zero-order kinetics. The loaded cells effectively responded to an external magnetic field of 8.0 KOe. In the continuous study, diclofenac

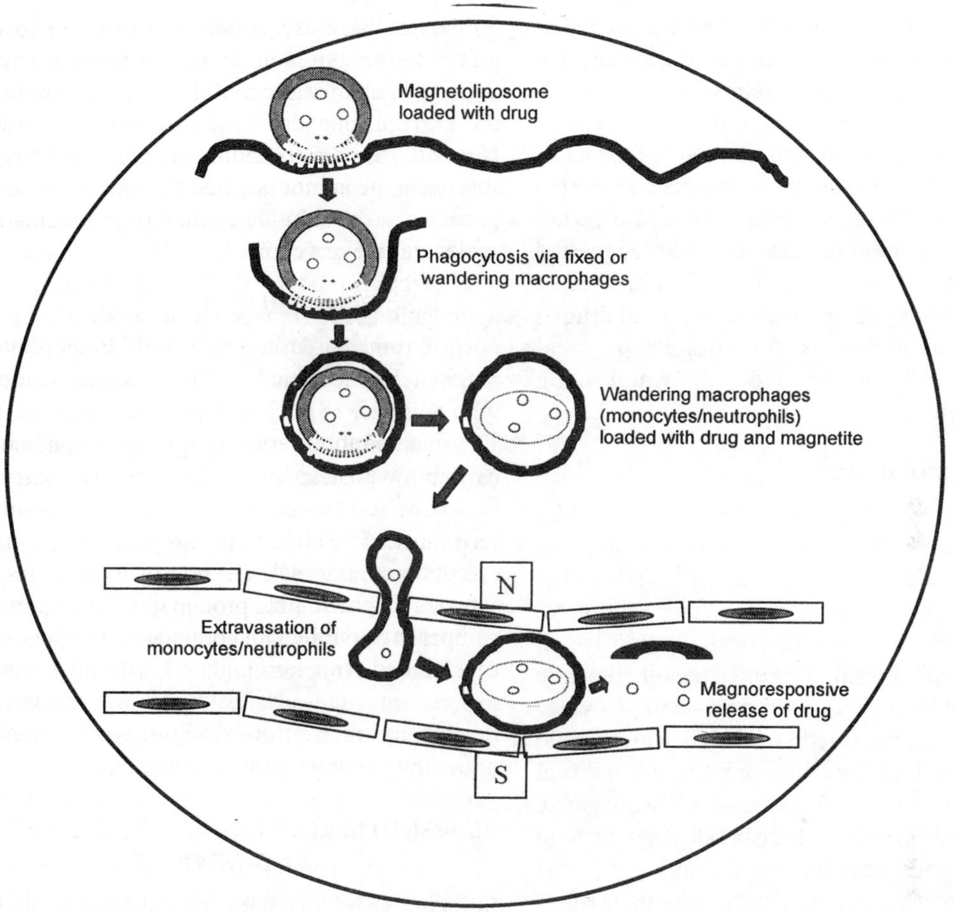

Fig. 12-17. Carrier-Celluar Co-ordiated Targeting Strategy

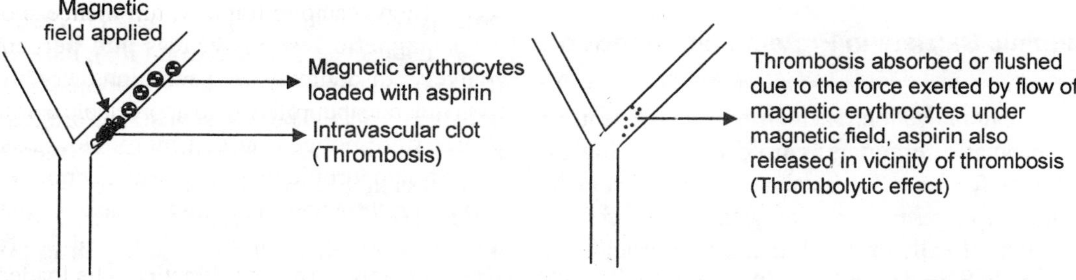

Fig. 12-18. Prevention of Arterial Thrombosis by Aspirin loaded Magnetic Resealed Erythrocytes

sodium-bearing magnetic erythrocytes were prepared using a preswell technique and characterized for various *in vitro* parameters. (Jain and Vyas, 1994). The drug-loaded magnetic erythrocytes responded effectively for an external magnetic field of 8.0 KOe. In the unpublished studies these co-workers targeted these drug loaded magnetic erythrocytes into the tail target segment of the albino rats. The study suggested the potentiality of diclofenac sodium-loaded magnetic erythrocytes, for active delivery of drug to painful inflammed joints, for possible physical modulation of carrier and contained drug biodistribution.

Magnetic Emulsions

Besides magnetically modulated systems, like microcapsules/microspheres, magnetic emulsions have been also tried as drug carrier for chemotherapeutic agents (Akimoto and Morimoto, 1983). The emulsion is a magnetically responsive oil in water type of emulsion bearing chemotherapeutic agent 1-(2-chloroethyl)-3-(trans-4-methyl cyclohexyl)-1-nitrosourea (methyl-CCNU) which could selectively be localized by applying an external magnetic field to a specific target site. The magnetic emulsion consists of ethyl oleate based magnetic fluid as the dispersed phase and casein solution as the continuous phase. The anticancer agent, methyl-CCNU, was trapped in the oily dispersed phase. The emulsion showed high retention by a magnetic field *in vitro*. After i. v. injection in the rat, the magnetic emulsion was mainly localized in the lungs by application of an electromagnet over the chest. Therefore, magnetic emulsions appear to have potential in conferring site specificity to certain chemotherapeutic agents.

Magnetic Carriers in Protein Immobilization

Magnetic materials were suggested as carriers for protein immobilization. Their property to concentrate near magnetic terminals is used in technological processes for selective catalyst removal from the reaction mixture, in immunological studies for the separation of cells to which magnetic particles are specifically bound modified with antibodies against cell surface components, in experiments for the drug targeting *in vivo* into appropriate tissues under guidance of an external magnetic field. A number of methods are available to obtain porous magnetic carriers, containing immobilized matter not only on the surface, but also in the volume of a particle. Normally, these preparations are obtained by granule formation from the suspension of ferromagnetic particles in the solution or melt of appropriate high molecular weight compound. The drawbacks of the above mentioned methods include pronounced aggregation of ferromagnetic particles, which do not permit the use of concentrated suspensions of magnetic particles and lead to formation of product with a variety of sizes and magnetic properties.

An attempt was made to synthesize the magnetic carrier for protein immobilization. The method is based on commercial adsorptional fixation of ferromagnetic particles in the pores of the carrier (Torchilin et al., 1985). The properties of the magnetic sephadex as carrier for protein immobilization were compared by parallel immobilization on both carriers of α-chymotrypsin and ^{131}I albumin. *In vivo* experiments suggest the ability of magnetic sephadex to concentrate in a desired region of the circulation under the action of external magnetic field.

MAGNETICALLY MODULATED SYSTEMS AND DEVICES

In recent years, magnetically modulated polymeric controlled drug delivery systems that deliver the drugs at increased rate on demand have been developed (Edelman et al., 1985; Hsich et al., 1981). These systems consist of a polymeric matrix where in drug powder is dispersed. The polymeric matrix is generally composed of ethylene vinyl acetate copolymer (EVAc) with some magnetic beads. The beads used are either magnetic steel beads composed principally of iron (79%), chromium (17%), carbon (1%), manganese (1%), silicon (1%), molybdenum (0.75%) and phosphorous (0.04%) or small samarium cobalt magnets. These systems are formulated by adding approximately 50 % of drug-polymer mixture to a glass mould, which is cooled to – 80°C using dry ice (Fig. 12-19), then the magnetic particles are added followed by the remaining drug-polymer mixture (Edelman et al., 1985). For the *in vitro* experiments, the magnetic tablets are placed in glass vials.

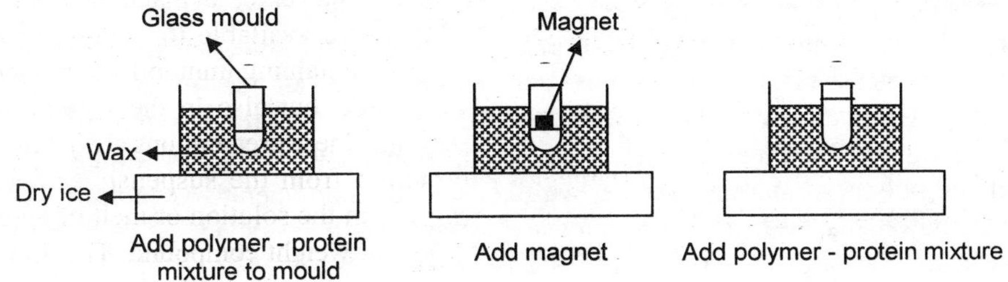

Fig. 12-19. Procedure for Preparation of Magnetically Controlled Release Polymers

An oscillating external magnetic field, which is generated by a device that rotates the permanent magnets below the vials, controls release rates. For *in vivo* studies, small plastic cages containing animals are placed on the tabletop (Fig. 12-20).

The systems can release up to 30 times more drug when exposed to the magnetic field, and release rates return to normal when the magnetic field is removed. Furthermore, these systems do not cause inflammation *in vivo*. This was confirmed by lack of edema, cellular infiltrate, or neovascularization as concluded by gross and histological examination of tissues in rabbits. (Hsich and Langer, 1983).

System Parameters

The important factors that control the release rate of magnetic polymeric devices are magnetic field characteristics and the mechanical properties of the polymer matrix. In a study, the amplitude of the magnetic field was varied by increasing the difference between the external and embedded magnet's strength. The results concluded that the extent of release enhancement increases as the field amplitude increases. In another study, the magnetic orientation has been studied using samples containing a single 1100 G magnet. In half of the cases, the magnet was placed perpendicular to the applied field while in the other half it was oriented parallel to the field. The mean release rate enhancement was 2.1 times in the parallel cases and 12.4 times in the perpendicular cases. The rotational torque caused the difference between the two. When placed in parallel, the magnet rotates in an attempt to align its pole vector with the field and therefore the displacement remains smaller. The extent of magnetic force enhancement is also

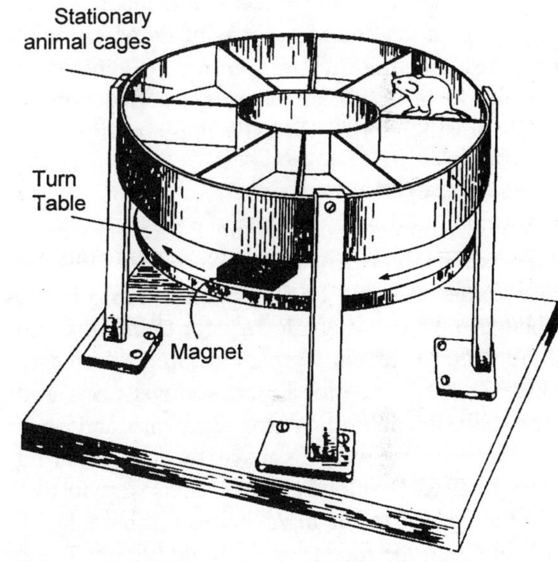

Fig. 12-20. Schematic Diagram of Device used to Generate an Oscillating Magnetic Field

affected by the mechanical properties of the polymeric matrix (Kost et al., 1986). For example, changes in the vinyl acetate content of the polymer can alter the modules of elasticity of the polymeric matrix.

Mechanism

The release of macromolecules from EVAc systems without magnetic beads, suggest that molecules with molecular weight greater than 300 can not permeate the polymer. The direct incorporation of macromolecules in the polymer-macromolecule using cast procedure caused a tortuous and complex series of pores formation within the matrix (Siegal and Langer, 1984). The release rates are determined by factors affecting permeation of water in to the polymer and drug out of these pores. Video recordings of the polymeric matrix surface, with magnetic beads, showed that the beads actually move within the matrix in response to the external magnetic field and as a result displace adjacent material containing polymer and drug with it, "squeezing" out the dissolved drug through the pores (McCarthy et al., 1984). A model for the enhanced release suggested that the major effect originates from the alternate compression and expansion deformation of the pores, causing the fluid within to generate a pulsatile flow, which alone (no net convection) is able to greatly improve diffusive mass transfer.

In vivo Experiments

In a study, implants containing EVAc embedded magnets and bovine zinc insulin were used for the *in vivo* experiments. The implants are placed subcutaneously in diabetic rats for 2 months and blood glucose levels were monitored (Kost and Langer, 1984). The blood glucose level decreased due to diffusion of insulin from the polymer and when the diabetic rats were exposed to an oscillating magnetic field, the blood glucose levels were further lowered from 50 to 200 mg/dl below this basal level, depending on the magnetic field conditions. These results were confirmed by radioimmunoassay (RIA).

Magnetically Modulated, Implantable, Hemispheric Drug Delivery Device

Polymeric drug delivery devices associated with a magnetically operated or triggered mechanism can improve the release rates of macromolecules from the polymeric controlled drug delivery devices. A zero order drug release profile could be achieved by using a hemisphere shaped geometry design (Heich and Langer, 1983). By adopting this approach, a subdermally implantable, magnetic modulated hemispheric drug delivery device has been developed. It contains a doughnut shaped magnet at the center of a biocompatible polymer matrix, the latter contains a homogeneous dispersion of a macromolecular drug at a high drug:polymer ratio, to form a hemi-spheric magnetic pellet. This pellet is then coated with a pure polymer (ethyl vinyl acetate copolymer or silicone elastomers) on all sides, except the cavity at the center of the flat surface, to permit the release of macromolecular drug only through the cavity.

Under non-operative condition, the hemispheric magnetic delivery device can release macromolecular drug at a controlled basal rate, following a diffusion mechanism. However, when external magnetic field is applied, it tends to release the drug at higher rate under the activation (Fig. 12-21).

Magnetic Systems in Contraceptive Drug Delivery

In these magnetically controlled systems, the drug and small magnetic beads are uniformly dispersed within a polymer material. On exposure to aqueous media, the drug is released in a diffusion controlled fashion. Moreover, the rate can be increased or modulated on application of an oscillating external magnetic field (Robinson and Lee, 1987). These systems may be useful when drug delivery is designed responsive to the changes in steroid secretion during the menstrual cycle (Fig. 12-22).

Magnetically Programmable Infusion Pumps

Magnetic technology is widely used for external programming of cardiac pacemakers. The same principle was adopted to an implantable infusion pump. The development of such pumps to a prototype stage, the newer method of radiofrequency (rf) signaling could improve the magnetic approach because of greater programming flexibility and bi-directional transmission capability. In rf-programmable pump, the receiver is initially switched to a programmable mode by a permanent magnet located in the extracorporeal programming head (Vogelzang, 1984). When the magnetic field and a recognizable rf pulse sequence are applied simultaneously, the re-programming occurs.

Some of the experimental applications of programmable pumps are :

1. Continuous, time-pulsed or circadian infusion of antitumour agents into systemic and portal veins
2. Control of pain in cancer patients by intrathecal

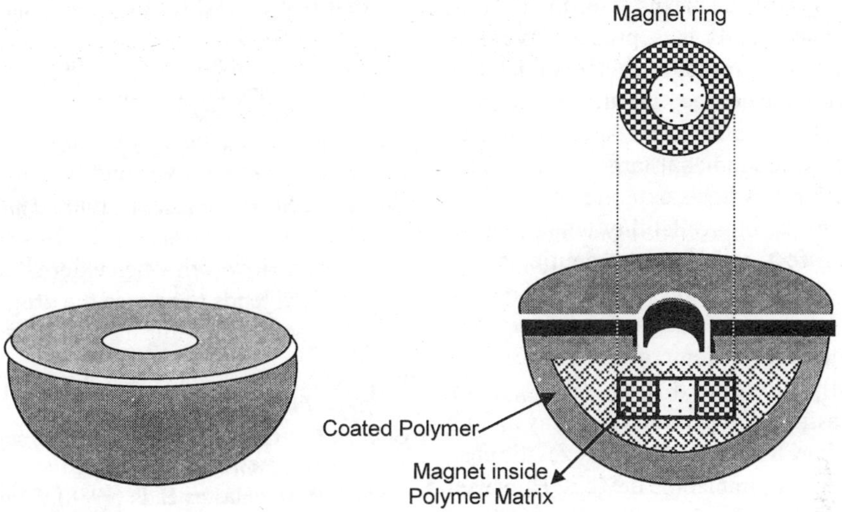

Fig. 12-21. Diagrammatic Illustration of a Magnetism-activated Drug Delivery Device (Hemispheric Magnetic Pellets)

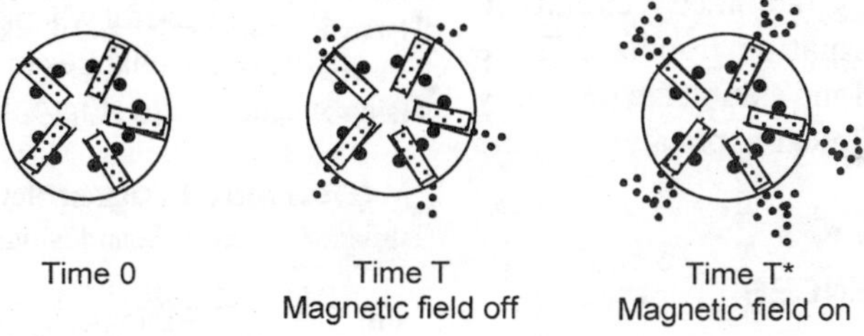

Fig. 12-22. Magnetically Controlled Contraceptive Delivery

or epidural infusion of morphine (Penn et al., 1984; Hrushesky, 1985)

3. Treatment of motor specificity in multiple sclerosis with intraspinal infusion of baclofen (a GABA binder).

The advantages of programmable pumps over polymeric implants are :

1. Drug output can be increased to compensate for biological tolerance to pain medications.
2. Catheter tips can be inserted in to very small spaces or vessels where polymer slabs and even injectable microspheres will not fit.
3. Pump reservoirs require infrequent filling, only once every 2-6 weeks depending on drug stability (Vogelzang et al., 1985).
4. The pumps are designed to run for up to 2 years on their original batteries.

The disadvantages however include :

1. Requirement for drug stability in solution at 37°C
2. Relatively high expense
3. Bulkiness of the central pump unit
4. Failure rate of up to 12 %
5. Occasional plugging of the outflow catheter
6. Minor difficulty in accessing the injection port.

CONCLUSION

Magnetics seems to serve as a common function of opening a new vista of a multi-barrier or multi-step drug delivery. It has been established that magnetic drug targeting is an efficient means of localizing toxic or labile pharmaceuticals in a preselective site. Magnetic targeting is a process of choice for delivery of about 45-60% of the new peptide and recombinant proteins at a level of 25-50% localization of injected dose in non-reticuloendothelial target tissues. This means of targeting has been exploited to achieve adequate drug levels, bioavailability enhancement, localizing the effect of biopharmaceuticals and avoidance of toxic manifestations. Magnetic targeting also offers advantages of magnetic capture and retention to endothelium of microvasculature.

Magnetically modulated drug release from implants, successfully compensate any decay in drug release against time. Moreover, it minimizes the cost, size and complexity of implanted devices. However, utility of such implants has been compromised due to irreproducibility of magnetic modulation and necessity of surgery to replace such implants after complete drug release. Externally programmable infusion pumps, need magnetic modulation only to a limited extent for activating radiometry circuits to allow bi-directional information transfer. These pumps are potentially useful and exhibit the flexibility required in the complex clinical applications of the forthcoming future.

REFERENCES

Akimoto M. and Morimoto Y. (1983) *Biomaterials* **4**, 49.

Babes L., Denizot B., Tanguy G., Le Jeune J. J. and Jallet P. (1999) *J. Colloid Interface Sci.* **212**, 474.

Babincova M., Altanerova V., Lampert M., Altaner C., Machova E., Sramka M. and Babinec P. (2000) *Z Naturforsch [C]* **55**, 278.

Babincova M. and Machova E. (1998) *Z Naturforsch [C]* **53**, 935.

Bartlett J. M., Richardson R. C., Elliott G. S., Blevins W. E., Janus W., Hale J. R. and Silver R. L. (1984) In: Microspheres and Drug Therapy: Pharmaceutical Immunological and Medical Aspects, Davis S. S., Illum L., McVie J. G. and Tomlinson E. (Eds.), Elsevier, Amsterdam, 413.

Bogdanov A. A. Jr., Martin C., Weissleder R. and Brady T. J. (1994) *Biochim. Biophys. Acta* **1193**, 212.

Bulte J. W., Cuyper de Y., Despres D. and Frank T. A. (1999) *J. Magn. Reson. Imaging* **9**, 329.

Bulte J. W., Ma L. D., Magin R. L., Kamman R. L., Hultstaert C. E., Go K. G. and de Leij L. (1993) *Magn. Reson. Med.* **29**, 32.

Chen H. and Langer R. (1997) *Pharm. Res.* **14**, 537.

Chopp M., Helporn J. A., Ewing J. R. and Welch K. M. (1985) *Magn. Resonance Imaging* **3**, 399.

Cuyper De M. and Joniau M. (1992) *Biotechnol. Appl. Biochem.* **16**, 201.

Cuyper De M. and Joniau M. (1988) *Eur. Biophys. J.* **15**, 311.

Devineni D., Klein-Szanto A. and Gallo J. M. (1995) *J. Neurooncol.* **24**, 143.

Edelman E., Kost J., Bobek H. and Langer R. (1985) *J. Biomed. Meter. Res.* **19**, 67.

Freeman M. W., Arnott A. and Watson J. H. I. (1960) *J. Appl. Phys.* **31**, 4045.

Gallo J. M., Gupta P. K., Hung C. T. and Perrier D. G. (1989) *J. Pharm. Sci.* **78**, 190.

Gallo J. M. and Hassan E. E. (1988) *Pharm. Res.* 5, 300.

Gupta P. K. and Hung C. T. (1989) *J. Pharm. Sci.* **78**, 745.

Hasegawa M. and Hokkoku S. (1978) *U.S. patent* 18,101,435.

Heberman R. B. (1985) *Cancer Tract. Rep.* **69**, 1169.

Hrushesky W. J. M. (1985) *Science* **228**, 73.

Hsich R., Langer R. and Folkman J. (1981) *Proc. Natl. Acad. Sci. USA* **78**, 1863.

Hsich R. and Langer R. (1983) In: Controlled Release of Bioactive Materials, Mansdorff Z. and Roseman J. J. (Eds.) Marcel Dekkar, New York, 121.

Ishii F., Takamura A. and Ishigami Y. (1990) *J. Dispersion Sci. Technol.* **11**, 581.

Jain. S. (2000) Biologically Modulated Carrier-Cellular Co-ordinated Site Specific Delivery System-Development and Characterization, M.Pharm Thesis, Dr. H.S.Gour University, Sagar. M.P. India.

Jain S. K. and Vyas S. P. (1994) *J. Microencapsul.* **11**, 141.

Keller K. E., Fujii D. K., Gunther W. H., Briley-Saebo K., Bjornerud A., Spiller M. and Koenig S. H. (2000) *J. Magn. Reson. Imaging* **11**, 488.

Kost J. and Langer R. (1984) *Trends. Biotechnol.* **2**, 47.

Kost J., Noecker R., Kunica E. and Langer R. (1986) *J. Biomed. Mater. Res.* **19**, 935.

Kharkevich D. A., Aliautdin R. N., Kasparov S. A., Nemirovskii A. I. and Tankovich N. I. (1985) *Farmakol Toksilol.* **48**, 32.

Kharkevich D. A., Aliautdin R. N. and Filippov V. I. (1989) *J. Pharm. Pharmcol.* **41**, 286.

Kiwada H., Sato J., Yamada S. and Kato Y. (1986) *Chem. Pharm. Bull.* **34**, 4253.

Kubo T., Sugita T., Shimose S., Nitta Y., Ikuta Y. and Murakami T. (2000) *Int. J. Oncol.* **17**, 309.

Lalla J. K. and Ahuja P. L. (1991) *J. Microencapsul.* **8**, 37.

Lewin M., Carlesso N., Tung C. H., Tang S. W., Cory D., Scadden D. T. and Weissleder R. (2000) *Nat. Biotechnol.* **18**, 410.

Lotze M. T., Chang A. E., Seipp C. A., Simpson C., Vetto J. T. and Rosenberg S. A. (1986) *JAMA* **286**, 3117.

Margolis L. B., Namiot V. A. and Kljkin L. M. (1983) *Biochim. Biophys. Acta* **735**, 193.

Masuko Y., Tazawa K., Viroon Chatapan E., Takemon S., Shimizu T., Fujimaki M., Nagae H., Sato H. and Horikoshi I. (1995) *Biol. Pharm. Bull.* **18**, 1802.

Mayer C. R., Cabuil V., Lalot T. and Thouvenot R. (1999) *Angen. Chem. Int. Ed. Engl.* **38**, 3672.

McCarthy M., Soong D. and Edelman E. (1984) *J. Cont. Rel.* **1**, 143.

Meyers P. H., Cronic F. and Nice C. M. (1963) *Amer. J. Radiol.* **90**, 1068.

Molday R. S. and Mackenzie D. (1982) *J. Immunol. Methods* **52**, 353.

Morimoto Y. and Natsume H. (1998) *Nippon Rinsho* **56**, 649.

Okon E., Pouliquen D., Okon P., Kovaleva Z. W., Stepanova T. P., Lavit S. G., Kudriavtsev B. N. and Jallet P. (1994) *Lab. Invest.* **71**, 895.

Okon I. E., Pulikan D., Pereverzer A. E., Kudriavtsev B. N. and Zhale P. (2000) *Tsitologiia* **42**, 358.

Orekhova N. M., Akchurin R. S., Belyaev A. A., Smirnor M. D., Ragimov S. E. and Orekhov A. N. (1990) *Thromb. Res.* **57**, 611.

Ovadia H., Paterson P. Y. and Hale J. R. (1983) *Isr. J. Med. Sci.* **19**, 631.

Pauser S., Reszka R., Wagner S., Wolf K. J., Buhr H. J. and Berger G. (1997) *Anticancer Drug Des.* **12**, 125.

Penn R. D., Paice J. A., Gottschulk W. and Ivankovich A. D. (1984) *J. Neurosurg.* **61**, 302.

Ranny D. F. (1985) *Science* **227**, 182.

Ranny D. F. and Huffaker H. H. (1987) In: Biological Approaches to the Controlled Delivery of Drugs, Juliano R. L. (Ed.), The New York Academy of Sciences, New York, 104.

Robinson R. J. and Lee V. H. (1987) Controlled Drug Delivery : Fundamentals and Applications, 2nd Edition, Marcel Dekkar Inc., New York, 504.

Roussean V., Denizot B., Pouliquen D., Jallet P. and Jeune Le J. J. (1997) *MAGMA* **5**, 213.

Rosenberg S. A., Mule J. J., Spiess P. J., Reichert C. M. and Schwartz S. L. (1985) *J. Exp. Med.* **161**, 1169.

Scheffold A., Mittenyi S. and Radbruch A. (1995) *Immunotechnology* **2**, 127.

Schlafke-Stelson A. T. and Watson E. E. (1986) Proceedings of the Fourth International Radio-pharmaceutical Dosimetry Symposium, Oak Ridge, TN, 1.

Schroder U., Segren S., Gemmetors C., Hedlund G., Jansson B., Sjogren H. O. and Borrebaeck C. A. (1986) *J. Immunol. Methods* **93**, 45.

Schutt W., Gruttner C., Teller J., Westphal F., Hafeli U., Paulke B., Goetz P. and Finck W. (1999) ***Artif. Organs*** **23**, 98.

Senyei A. E., Reich S. D., Gonezy C. and Widder K. J. (1981) *J.Pharm. Sci.* **70**, 389.

Sestier C., Da-Silva M. F., Sabolovic D., Roger J. and Pons J. N. (1998) *Electrophoresis* **19**, 1220.

Shi K., Li C. and He B. (2000) *Sheng Wu Yi Xue Gong Cheng Xue Za Zhi* **17**, 21.

Shinkai M., Suzuki M., Iijima S. and Kobayashi T. (1995) *Biotechnol. Appl. Biochem.* **21**, 125.

Shinkai M., Yanase M., Honda H., Wakabayashi T., Yoshida J. and Kobayashi T. (1996) *Jpn. J. Cancer Res.* **87**, 1179.

Siegal R. and Langer. (1984) *Pharm. Res.* **1**, 2.

Tiefenauer L. X., Kuhne G. and Andres R. Y. (1993) *Bioconjug. Chem.* **4**, 347.

Teifenauer L. X., Tschirky A., Kuhne G. and Andres R. Y. (1996) *Magn. Reson. Imaging* **14**, 391.

Torchilin V. P., Papisov M. L. and Smirnov V. N. (1985) *J. Biomed. Mater. Res.* **19**, 461.

Tyle P. (1988) Drug Delivery Devices : Fundamentals and Applications, Marcel Dekkar Inc., New York, 326.

Viroonchatapan E., Sato H., Ueno M., Adachi I., Murata J., Saiki I., Tazawa K. and Horikoshi I. (1998) *J. Drug Target.* **5**, 379.

Viroonchatapan E., Sato H., Ueno M. Adachi I., Tazawa K. and Horikoshi I. (1996) *Life Sci.* **58**, 2251.

Viroonchatapan E., Ueno M., Sato H., Adachi I., Nagae H., Tazawa K. and Horikoshi I. (1995) *Pharm. Res.* **12**, 1176.

Widder K. J., Senyei A. E. and Scarpelli D. G. (1978) *Proc. Soc. Exp. Biol. Med.* **58**, 141.

Wu C. B., Zhao Y. L. and He S. M. (1993) *Yao Xue Xue Bao* **28**, 464.

Ward P. A. (1984) *Am. J. Pathol.* **77**, 520.

Vogelzang N. J. (1984) *J. Clin. Oncol.* **2**, 1289.

Vogelzang N. J., Ruane M. and De Meester K. (1985) *J. Clin. Oncol.* **3**, 407.

Vyas S. P. and Jain S. K. (1994) *J. Microencapsul.* **2**, 19.

Vyas S. P. and Malaiya A. (1989) *J. Microencapsul.* **6**, 493.

Yanase M., Shinkai M., Honda H., Wakabayashi T., Yoshida J. and Kobayashi T. (1997) *Jpn. J. Cancer Res.* **88**, 630.

Yanase M., Shinkai M., Honda H., Wakabayashi T., Yoshida J. and Kobayashi T. (1998) *Jpn. J. Cander Res.* **89**, 463.

SECTION III

SITE-SPECIFIC DRUG DELIVERY

CHAPTER 13

Drug Delivery to Brain

The advances in our understanding makes us aware of mechanisms involved in pharmacodynamic activity of neuroactive agents, physiopathology and etiology of neurogenerative disorders, impediments and limitations to effective therapeutics. The drug accessibility to the central nervous system (CNS) is mainly limited by the blood-brain-barrier(BBB). In the treatment of diseases or conditions that result from the lack of simple hormones and peptides, the administration of these compounds in a controlled fashion could provide effective management of diseases and therapy. Conditions such as diabetic neuropathy, amylotropic lateral sclerosis (ALS) and Huntington's disease and Parkisonism's disease may be treated with better pharmacodynamic effects using targeted drug strategies. Brain related diseases of diversed etiology are the major causes of debilitation, agony and death. Various brain disorders are summarized in Table 13-1(Greig et al., 1990). The management of brain related diseases with present available therapeutic systems is very difficult, as insufficient amount of drug reaches to the brain, due to highly lypophilic nature of blood-brain-barrier (BBB). Drug delivery to the brain requires advances in both, drug delivery technologies and drug discovery. Due to the presence of the blood-brain-barrier only small, lipid soluble drugs in the circulation are delivered to the brain cells. Therefore, practical strategies are required for mediating drug transport across blood-brain-barrier. New strategies for selective delivery to the brain arise from investigation that critically reveals the physiological mechanisms involved with the solute transport across the blood-brain-barrier(McComb et al,1994; Cancilla et al., 1993).

Recent transbarrier transport kinetics, metabolic, cellular and molecular studies have given a major impetus to the better understanding as to how the BBB functions, and what advantages from these bio-processes can possibly be availed for therapeutic selective brain targeting. It has been demonstrated that several classes of metabolic substrates, neuroactives and regulatory peptides, plasma derived- proteins, and various groups of centrally

Table 14-1. Diseases Related to Brain and Their Etiology

Brain Disorders	Etiology/Disease	Currently used drugs
Meningitis		
1. Acute	*E.coli*	Penicillins
	Haemophilus influenzae	Cephalosporins
	Neisseria meningitidis	Vancomycin (Penicillin resistant strains)
	Streptococcus pneumoniae	
2. Chronic meningitis	*Tuberculous meningitis*	Rifampicin
	Tubercle bacillus	Isoniazid
	Cryptococcal meningits	
Encephalitis		
1. Bacterial	Type A encephalitis	Wide spectrum antibiotics
2. Viral	Type B encephalitis	
	Herpes zoster	Acyclovir
	Herpes simplex	Viderabine
Degenerative diseases		
1. Cerebral cortex	Alzheimer's	
2. Basal ganglia and brain stem	Pick's	
	Huntington's	
	Parkinson's	DOPA
Tumours	Glioblastoma	Nitrosourea
		Carmustin
		BNCU
		Methotrexate
		Interferon-α
AIDS (abscess in brain)	HIV	Azidothymidine(AZT)

active pharmacotherapeutics are able to utilize specialized 'shuttle' services at the BBB. The current concept of a BBB states that the microvascular endothelium in coordination with astrocytes, pericytes and possibly microglia, regulates and facilitates the homeostasis of the neural milieu, rather than impeding solute exchanges between blood and brain.

THE FLUID-BRAIN BARRIERS

The fluid-brain barriers are group of cells that inhibit the ready passage of non-lipid-soluble molecules between the environment external to the CNS (i.e., air, blood) and the CNS milieu (Boardwell, 1992). These fluid-brain barriers include

1. The blood-brain barrier (BBB) associated with capillary, venule, and arteriole nonfenestrated endothelia of cerebral blood vessels;
2. The bloodcerebrospinal fluid (CSF) barrier associated with epithelia of the choroid plexus and other circumventricular organs (e.g., median eminence, area postrema);
3. The nose-brain barrier associated with epithelia of the nasal mucosa; and
4. The arachnoid mater-CSF barrier.

Each of the barriers is believed to be attributed to circumferential belts of intercellular tight junctional complexes that preclude the extracellular movement of non-lipid-soluble micromolecules and macromolecules bidirectionally between the external environment and the CNS. The characteristics of these barriers are summarized in Table 13-2.

Cell Biology and Anatomy of BBB

The cell biology of the BBB reveals about the close proximity and paracrine type of interactions between

Table 13-2. Characteristics of Blood Brain Barrier (Compiled from Boardwell, 1992)

Cell types

Blood-brain barrier

Nonfenestrated endothelia
Circumferential belts of tight junctional complexes
Secondary lysosomes containing acid hydrolases
Extralysosomal hydrolytic enzymes (e.g., monoamine oxidase)

Blood-CSF barrier

Choroid plexus epithelium
Circumferential belts of tight junctional complexes
Secondary lysosomes containing acid hydrolases
Arachnoid mater
Circumferential belts of tight junctional complexes

Phagocytes

Circumventricular organ/subarachnoid macrophages
Perivascular cells: pericytes, microglia, macrophages
Supraependymal macrophages, Kolmer cells

Polarity of the BBB

The endothelium is polarized with regard to demonstrable internalization or recycling of its cell surface membrane and endocytosis of non-lipid-soluble macromolecules. These events occur from the blood side but not from the brain side of the endothelium.

Blood-brain barrier vs. brain-blood barrier

BBB is not absolute, whereas its counterpart-the brain-blood barrier-may be. Potential adsorptive and receptor-mediated transcytoses of macromolecules through the barrier is from blood to brain but not from brain to blood; hence, transcytosis through the endothelium appears to be vectorial.

Blood-CSF barrier is not polarized

Internalization of cell surface membrane associated with fluid-phase and adsorptive endocytoses is circumferential in epithelial cells of the choroid plexus and median eminence .
Adsorptive transcytosis through these epithelial cells is bidirectional.

cerebral endothelial cells, pericytes, astrocytes, microglia, and neurons. Figure 13-1 illustrates the anatomic relationship between different cells involved with the functionality of the BBB complex. Anatomically the BBB is a continuous zipper-like tight junctioned endothelial cellular layer. The microvascular endothelium shares a common basement membrane with astrocytes and pericytes. Astrocytes send their foot processes to invest more than 90% of endothelial capillaries, while in the capillaries the ratio between pericytes and endothelial cells is approximately 1:2. Neuronal endings may directly innervate the endothelium, while microglia is located in the vicinity of pericytes (Cancilla et al., 1993; Herman, 1993).

The endothelial layer needs to be viewed as two separate membranes, one on the inside of the vessels (luminal) and other to the outside (abluminal), separated by 300 to 500 nm thick layer of cytoplasm. The surface area of cerebral capillary endothelium is about 100 cm^2 per gram of brain tissue. In a adult human brain the total surface area of microvasculature is estimated to be nearly 12 m^2, the total length of capillaries equals 650 km, with a 6μm diameter of capillary lumen, and the capillaries are well separated apart by a distance 40μm. The endothelial cells express numerous functional proteins that are generally involved with various transports, receptor-signal transduction and cell-mediated mechanisms, which effectively operate for normal functioning of the brain. It appears that different regulatory molecules, mostly peptides, are involved in the control of BBB related transport mechanisms. They may be secreted by astrocytes

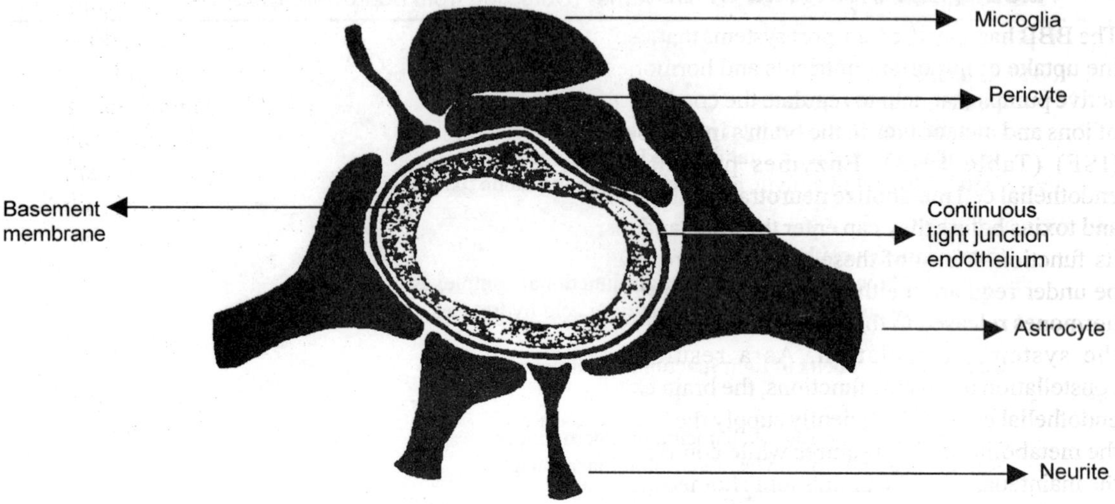

Fig. 13-1. Schematic Representation of Cell Biology of Blood Brain Barrier

and to some extent possibly by some neural endings, active in a typical paracrine fashion on the abluminal side of the BBB, and/or alternatively may originate from circulating blood acting on the luminal side of the BBB.

The tight-junctions exclude paracellular pathway for solute movement through the BBB and the virtual absence of pinocytosis across brain capillary endothelium, ablates transcellular bulk flow of circulating solute through the BBB. Under these conditions solute may gain an access to brain interestitium via only one or two pathways i.e., lipid mediated transport or catalyzed transport. Further, the lipid-mediated transport is restricted to small molecules. It is generally related to the lipid solubility of the molecule. Catalyzed transport system involves carrier mediated or receptor mediated process (Pardridge, 1993; Brightman, 1977).

Collectively, these characteristics impart the BBB a very selective and dynamic filtering interface that effectively excludes most water soluble substances, including peptides and proteins, from entering the central nervous system (CNS) through blood. Exceptions include relatively lipophilic substances and some CNS required nutrients (e.g. glucose, amino acids, choline, etc.) for which specific, saturable BBB transport systems exist. Therapeutic applications of blood borne substances directed to the CNS are therefore dependent on the delivery strategies, which overcome permeability limitations, imposed by BBB. During the past decade, a number of central nervous system (CNS) activating peptide drugs have been discovered. Although these neuro-peptides have many uses as neuro-pharmaceuticals, the clinical application has yet to be completely realized. One of the most crucial problems encountered in the development of CNS acting peptide drugs is to increase the cerebral availability of the peptide drug after administration.

Evidence exists suggesting that biologically significant amounts of some peptides (eg. leu-enkephalin, peptide T-like peptides, tyr-MIF-1, vassopressin; delta-sleep-inducing peptide) may cross the BBB by either passive transmembrane diffusion or through saturable carrier mechanisms. While evidences for peptide penetration of the BBB are accumulative, the biochemical nature of the processes permitting transmembrane passage of peptides still remains poorly defined. Realization of the potential therapeutic utility of peptides and proteins necessitates for more precise knowledge of the mechanisms by which peptides may permeate across the barrier membrane.

MULTIPLE FUNCTIONS OF BBB

The BBB has specific transport systems that facilitate the uptake of important nutrients and hormones and active pumps that help to regulate the concentrations of ions and metabolites in the brain's interstitial fluid (ISF) (Table 13-3). Enzymes present in the endothelial cell metabolize neurotransmitters, drugs, and toxins before they can enter the brain and disrupt its function. Many of these properties are likely to be under regulation either of neurotransmitters and hormones released in the brain or of those present in the systemic circulation. As a result of this constellation of diverse functions, the brain capillary endothelial cells ISF efficiently supply the brain with the metabolites that it requires while contributing to the maintenance of the brain's ionic homeostasis and protecting it from circulating toxins (Betz, 1992).

The BBB as an Active Pump

BBB transport systems not operate equally well in both the blood-to-brain and brain-to-blood directions. The transport of potassium is asymmetric. Potassium is transported out of the brain by a saturable transport system that can be inhibited by ouabain, whereas the flux of potassium from blood to brain is low and not inhibited by ouabain. This is due to the presence of the active pump Na,K-ATPase on the abluminal but not the luminal side of the brain capillary endothelial cell (Betz , 1992) (Fig. 13-2).

Similarly, the distribution of ion transporters in fluid-transporting epithelial cells present in the choroid plexus are asymmetry and this cellular polarity forms the basis for their ability to actively secrete ions and water. Other features that the brain capillary endothelium has in common with a typical epithelium include the presence of continuous tight junctions, a transcellular electrical resistance of approximately 2,000 cm^2 , a low hydraulic conductivity and a high mitochondrial content, which is believed to be related to a high capacity for active transport. Since the brain capillary shares so many structural features in common with epithelia, it has been proposed that it functions like an epithelium as well. If the BBB does indeed secrete fluid, this could be the explanation for the 10 to 30 percent of CSF that is produced from extrachoroidal sources; and it could account for the bulk flow of fluid through the brain's interstitial space. In addition to the presence of Na,K-ATPase on one side, fluid-secreting epithelial cells contain other sodium transporters on

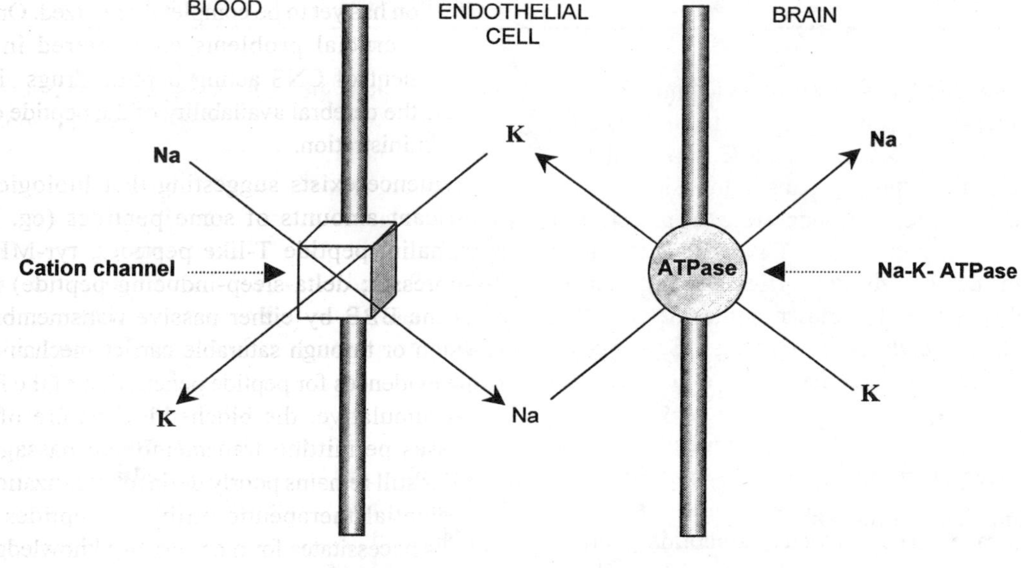

Fig. 13-2. The BBB as an Active Pump (Betz, 1992)

Table 13-3. Different Transport Systems that Operate from Blood to Brain at BBB (Bentz, 1992)

Transport System	Typical Substrate
Metabolites	
Hexose	Glucose
Large neutral amino acid	Phenylalanine
Basic amino acid	Lysine
Acidic amino acid	Glutamate
Monocarboxylic acid	Lactate
Amine	Choline
Purine	Adenine
Nucleoside	Adenosine
Saturated fatty acid	Octanoate
Micronutrients	
Thiamine	Thramine
Pantothenic acid	Pantothenic acid
Biotin	Biotin
Vitamin B6	Pyridoxal
Riboflavin	Riboflavin
Niacinamide	Niacinamide
Carnitine	Carnitine
Lnositol	Myo-inositol
Electrolytes	
Sodium-chloride cotransport	Sodium chloride
Cation channel	Sodium, potassium
Heavy metal	Lead
Hormones	
Thyroid hormone	T3
Vasopressin	Arginine vasopressin
Insulin	Insulin
Other Peptides	
Transferrin	Transferrin
Enkephalins	Leu-enkephalin

the opposite side that allow sodium to enter the cell. Using intracarotid bolus injections to study single-pass sodium uptake, Betz, 1983 reported two saturable sodium entry systems in the BBB. One is inhibited by furosemide, suggesting the presence of a Na-Cl cotransport system. The other is inhibited by amiloride. but its properties are not clearly identical to either the known amiloride-sensitive sodium channel or the Na/H exchanger. Specifically, Betz, 1983 reported that the brain capillary sodium channel is highly sensitive to inhibition by amiloride as IS the sodium channel in tight epithelia, but it is nonselective since amiloride also inhibits brain rubidium uptake. Recent studies confirm that brain sodium uptake can be inhibited by amiloride (Murphy and Johanson, 1989) and that brain capillary endothelial cells contain an amiloride-sensitive cation channel that is permeable to both sodium and potassium (Vigne et al., 1989). Active transport of ions across the brain capillary endothelium may play a role not only in fluid secretion but also in regulation of the potassium concentration of the brain's interstitial fluid (ISF). The potassium concentration of the CSF and ISF is held remarkably constant at approximately 3 mM despite acute or chronic changes in plasma potassium between 1.6 and 7 mM (Bradbury and Stulcova 1970). The low permeability of the BBB to potassium in the blood-to-brain direction contributes to this potassium homeostasis. However, potassium efflux, mediated by Na,K-ATPase located on the abluminal side of the brain capillary endothelial cell and the apical side of the choroid plexus epithelial cell (Ernst et al., 1986), also plays a major role (Bradbury and Stulcova, 1970;

Betz, 1986). Given that the total influx of potassium across the BBB is 10 times greater than across the blood-CSF barrier, the brain capillary is probably more important than the choroid plexus in brain potassium homeostasis. Astrocytic glial cells also are believed to play an important role in maintaining potassium homeostasis in brain. This specialized glial cell has a large potassium conductance in its end-feet that allows it to quickly take up potassium from the surrounding fluid (Newman, 1986). Localized uptake in an area where potassium is high is accompanied by the dumping of potassium in another area where its concentration is low. This type of spatial buffering of potassium is believed to be important for the second-to-second regulation of localized ISF potassium concentration but it cannot by itself account for long-term global regulation of ISF potassium. For this, the brain capillary endothelial cell probably plays the primary role. One reason the brain capillary endothelial cell is so closely invested with glial foot processes may be to permit astrocytes and endothelial cells to work together to maintain potassium homeostasis. The presence of other asymmetrically distributed transporters in the brain capillary endothelial cell (Table 13-4) can be deduced by differences in transport rates in the blood-to-brain and brain-to-blood directions as explained above. Another approach is to study uptake by isolated brain capillaries *in vitro*. Since these structures have their abluminal membranes exposed to the incubation medium, transporters that are present on this side of the cell can be studied easily. Thus, those substances that are taken up by isolated capillaries, but that do not appreciably enter the brain from the blood, probably have transporters on the abluminal but not the luminal membrane of the endothelial cell. This approach has been used to demonstrate an asymmetry of A-system and ASC-system transporters for small neutral amino acids as well as transporters for taurine and monoamines (Betz and Goldstein, 1978; Tayarani et al., 1987a). However, one must be aware that the isolated brain capillaries contain other cells, such as pericytes, that also might be transport sites.

Finally, the presence of active transport out of the brain can be deduced by using transport inhibitors. When a substance is present under steady-state conditions at a lower concentration in the brain's ISF than in blood and a transport inhibitor increases the brain concentration, then the presence of an active efflux system can be deduced. This approach has been used to demonstrate active BBB efflux systems for iodide prostaglandins (Bito et al., 1976).

The BBB as a Metabolic Barrier

The BBB is formed by a cell layer with different properties of the membranes on either side. These cells also have an intracellular cytoplasm and organelles containing specific enzymes that play an important role in BBB function. The rat brain capillary endothelial cells are richly endowed in enzymes involved with neurotransmitter synthesis (e.g., aromatic amino acid decarboxylase) and degradation (e.g., monoamine oxidase [MAO]) (Hardebo and Owman, 1980). Since neuro-transmitter precursors such as L-3,4- dihydroxy-phenylalanine (L-dopa) can enter the endothelial cell from the blood via the L-system for large neutral amino acid transport, the subsequent intraendothelial metabolism provides an effective mechanism for preventing neurotransmitters from moving beyond the endothelial cell and into the brain. Neurotransmitter degrading enzymes present in the endothelial cells also may play a role in inactivating neurotransmitters released during neuronal activity since transport systems for uptake of catecholamines by the endothelial cell appear to be present on the abluminal membrane. Brain capillary endothelial cells contain many enzymes in addition to those involved with neurotransmitter metabolism (Mrsulja and Djuricic, 1981). Besides the enzymes involved in energy metabolism, these cells also contain acid hydrolases typically found in lysosomes and aminopeptidase (Baranczyk-Kuzma and Audus, 1987). Similar to other endothelial cells, they contain angiotensin-converting enzyme (Gimbrone et al., 1979) xanthine oxidase (Betz ,1985), and enzymes that protect cells from peroxidatrve damage such as superoxide dismutase, catalase, and glutathione peroxidase (Tayarani et al., 1987b).

MAO present in brain capillaries may serve to provide protection of the brain from circulating toxins. Brain capillary endothelial cells are well equipped to handle circulating drugs and toxins since

Table 13-4. Asymmetrically Distributed BBB Transport Systems (Betz, 1992)

Transport System	Typical Substrate	Probable Location
Na,K-ATPase	Potassium	Abluminal
Sodium-chloride cotransport	Sodium chloride	Luminal
Cation channel	Sodium, potassium	Luminal
Sodium-hydrogen exchanger	Sodium, hydrogen	Abluminal
A-system for neutral amino adds	Glycine	Abluminal
ASC-system for neutral amino acids	Cysteine	Abluminal
B-amino acid	Taurine	Abluminal
Monoamine	Dopamine	Abluminal
Organic anion	p-Aminohippurate	Abluminal
Inorganic anion	Iodide	Abluminal
Prostaglandin	pGF20	Abluminal

they contain drug-metabolizing enzyme systems such as cytochrome P-450-linked monooxygenases, epoxide hydrolase, NADPH:cytochrome P-450 reductase, and 1-napthol UDP-glucuronosyl transferase, which are typically found in the liver. They also contain a multidrug transport protein, P170 (Thiebaut et al., 1989).

Regulation of BBB Function

The brain capillary endothelial cells contain many neurotransmitter- and hormone-binding sites, as listed below in Table 13-5.

These receptors have been detected either by directly studying binding of radiolabeled ligands to the isolated capillaries or by observing changes in intracellular second messengers following exposure to agonists. The β-adrenergic receptors appear to be in some way involved with regulation of ion transport since ablation of adrenergic input to the cerebral microvasculature by lesioning the locus ceruleus leads to up-regulation of ß-adrenergic receptors on the endothelial cells (Kalaria et al., 1989) and a down-regulation of their Na,K-ATPase activity (Harik, 1986). Atrial natriuretic peptide (ANP) receptors also may play a role in ion transport regulation because ANP inhibits the amiloride-sensitive cation channel (Doczi et al., 1990; lbaragi et al. 1989). Finally, some receptors (e.g., those for insulin, transferrin, and vasopressin) may play a role in receptor-mediated transcytosis rather than regulating endothelial cell function. The endothelial cells also must contain other, as yet unidentified, receptors that allow them to respond to modulators present in brain and probably released by the astrocytes. Glial cells may be an important source of such signals since astrocytes or astrocyte-conditioned medium induce morphological and functional changes in brain capillary endothelial cells in tissue culture.

LIMITATIONS IN BRAIN UPTAKE OF DRUGS

A number of drug peptide, biological response modifiers and monoclonal antibodies and fragments are presently available which have been proven to be of valuable in inhibiting a variety of malignant infectious diseases, and rectification of neuro-transmitter and enzyme imbalance in tissue culture systems. However, their *in vivo* therapeutic efficacy is frequently compromized by their inability to reach and maintain active concentration at the diseased site located in brain.

There are few more cases where inadequate pharmacokinetics can limit drug therapy when a disease is located within the central nervous system. This problem is commonly encountered in patients with acute cerebral bacterial or viral infections, as well as with neurogenerative diseases, such as Parkinson's, Hunttington's or Tay-Sach disease. However, the most extreme cases are encountered by neuroncologist in treating patients with brain tumours (Greig, 1987).

TRANSPORT THROGH BBB

Circulating molecules use a number of different mechanisms available at the BBB for their transport

Table 13-5. Neurotransmitter and Hormone Binding Sites at Brain Capillary Endothelial Cells (Betz, 1992)

ß-Adrenergic	Insulin
Adrenergic	Transferrin
Dopamine	Vasoactive intestinal peptide
Histamine	Parathyroid hormone
Adenosine	Atrial natriuretic peptide
Muscarinic cholinergic	Vasopressin
Prostaglandin	Angiotensin II
Leukotriene C4	Bradykinin

across the barrier as shown in Fig. 13-3 (McComb et al., 1994). Non-lipid-soluble micromolecules and macromolecules from the periphery are capable of circumventing the fluid-brain barriers by intracellular routes related to three separate and distinct endocytic processes. The three endocytic processes from the least to the most specific are fluid- or bulk-phase endocytosis, adsorptive endocytosis, and receptor-mediated endocytosis (Table 13-6). All three processes involve the internalization of the external molecule in association with cell surface membrane. Adsorptive endocytosis concerns molecules such as lectins (e.g., wheat germ agglutinin [WGA]) that bind to carbohydrate moieties on the cell surface and positively charged (&ionized) molecules that bind to negatively charged cell surface components. Receptor-mediated endocytosis is identified with the binding of a ligand (e.g., insulin, transferrin) to a cell surface receptor specific for that ligand; the binding then triggers the internalization of the receptor-ligand complex (Dautry-Varsat and Lodish, 1984).

Various blood brain barrier transport mechanisms include lipid mediated transport of many small highly lipophilic drugs; carrier mediated transport for hydrophilic nutrients and their analogues; plasma-protein mediated transport of acidic drugs, peptides and highly lipophilic drugs; carrier-receptor, and/or absorptive mediated transcytosis of peptides including proteins; and bulk flow transcytosis, i.e. pinocytosis and tubulocanalicular transport irrespective of the molecular size i.e., minimal under normal physiologic conditions, but may become significant under certain varied pathologic circumstances (Banks et al, 1991).

Transport mechanisms operating at the BBB for peptides and proteins can be classified into the following categories (Table 13-7)

- Transport via carrier mediated systems
- Receptor mediated transcytosis (RMT)
- Absorptive mediated transcytosis (AMT).

Carrier Mediated Transport system

Several peptide transport systems (PTS) present at the BBB. These systems seen to be restricted to transportation of a limited number of structurally related peptides. Peptides transported from blood to brain via PTS include Tyr-Pro-Leu-Gly-amide, methionine, enkephalin, orginine and vassopressin. The permeability coefficient for peptide transport from blood to the brain via PTS usually ranges between 1 to 10 ml/min/g brain, which is about 10 fold faster than could be predicted from their lipid solubilities. Transport from brain to blood is also mediated by PTS for Tyr-Pro-Leu-Gly-amide, methionine, enkephaliln, orginine, vassopressin, oxytocin, LHRH and somatostatin, with half lives in the range of 10 - 50 min (Farnk and Pardridge,1987; Pardridge et al., 1987; Duffy et al., 1988).

Such characteristics of bidirectional transport from blood to brain and from brain to blood may explain why most peptides have low and variable rates of entry into the brain. If we can inhibit relevant transport system, then a substantial accumulation of some peptides in the CNS may be generated which could be of great therapeutic significance. On other hand; enhancement of peptide transport from brain to blood by some means might be a useful way to minimize CNS drug accumulation related side effects of peripherally active peptides (Killer and Borchardt, 1988; Miller and Borchardt, 1991).

Receptor Mediated Transcytosis (RMT)

Peptides such as insulin, transferrin, insulin like growth factor (IGF) I and IGF II exhibit high affinity

Table 13-6. Different Endocytic Processes (Broadwell, 1992)

Types	Examples	Specificity	Organelles
Fluid phase	HRP, ferritin	Nonspecific	Vesicles, endosomes, lysosomes
Adsorptive phase	WGA, rein, Cationized probes	Specific oligosaccharides	Vesicles, endosomes, golgi complex
Receptor-mediated	Insulin, transferrin	Specific receptors	Vesicles, endosomes, lysosomes, golgi complex

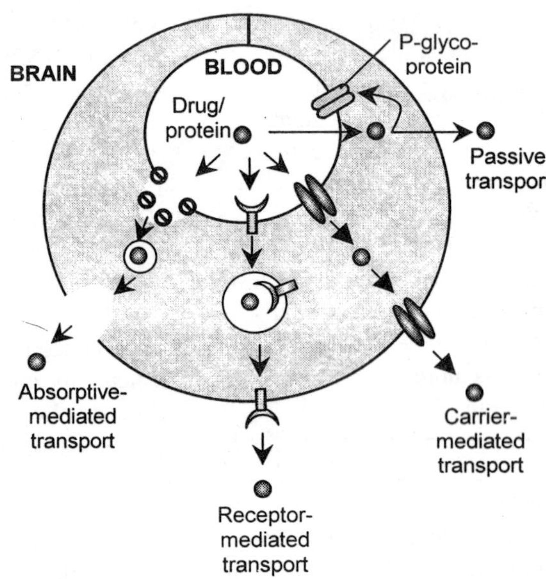

Fig. 13-3. Transport Mechanisms of Drugs Across the Blood Brain Barrier

to receptors expressed on the brain capillaries. These receptors mediate the transcytosis of insulin, transferrin and IGF through the BBB involving three successive steps:

1. Receptor mediated endocytosis at the luminal or blood side of BBB.
2. Movement of the ligand receptor complex through the endothelial cytoplasm.
3. Receptor mediated exocytosis of the ligand into the brain interstitial fluid at the antiluminal or brain side of the BBB.

Following the binding of ligand to its affinity receptor the process of endocytosis is intiated. Transferrin affinity to BBB receptor is usually high with a dissociation constant (KD) of about 5 nM. It has the maximum binding capacity (a measure of the total number of binding sites) on the endothelium of about 0.10 pmol/mg protein for transferrin has been reported. Recent work using primary cultured monolayers of bovine BCEC suggest that transferrin is internalized through BCEC expressed on the apical side and is recycled, predominantly intact to the apical side to the cells. Unlike transferrin, insulin undergoes a time dependent degradation upon internalization by BCEC monolayer.

Similar pathways would apply for receptor-mediated transcytosis through epithelia of the blood-CSF barrier. Immunohistochemistry has demonstrated that endothelia possessing the receptor for ferrotransferrin (f-TRF; MW 35,000) are restricted to cerebral vessels (Jefferies et al., 1984). Receptor recognition of f-TRF may promote the transport and

Table 13-7. Different Transport Mechanisms for Drug/Peptides at BBB

Transport mechanism	Peptide/drug
Receptor-mediated transcytosis	$sA\beta_{1-40}$-Apolipoprotein J Apolipoprotein J Arginine vasopressin $sA\beta_{1-40}$(Soluble amyloid) Insulin
Absorptive -mediated transcytosis	Cationized IgG Cationized BSA Cationized BSA-D-(ala^2)-β- endorphin IgG(native, species homologous)
Carries-mediated transport at the luminal side	Leucine enkephalin Delta sleep inducing peptide
Non-transport Process (e.g. endocytosis, absorption, metabolism)	Apolipoprotein E3 Apolipoprotein E Apolipoprotein E4 $sA\beta_{1-40}$apolipoprotein E3 $sA\beta_{1-40}$apolipoprotein E D-(ala^2)β-endorphin β-endorphin Inter polar molecules Sucrose DextranMannitol
Non-specific transport	Cyclosporin A Thyrotropin releasing hormone

delivery of transferrin and iron from plasma into brain. At 1 hour postinjection, reaction product for f-TRF-HRP is observed within endothelial endocytic vesicles, tubules, spherical endosomes, and dense bodies and within the perivascular clefts and perivascular phagocytes. Subarachnoid macrophages, the circumventricular organs, and Golgi saccules in BBB endothelia are not associated with reaction product. Infrequently, reaction product loads a presumptive "exocytic vesicle" or pit positioned at the abluminal plasmalemma. The entire f-TRF-HRP conjugate reportedly undergoes receptor-mediated transcytosis through the BBB. The stated specificity of the endothelial transferring (TRF) receptor in brain, in combination with blood-borne TRF may be an ideal vehicle for ferrying substances across the barrier.

The receptor mediated transcytosis of f-TRF-HRP through cerebral endothelia differs from that in other cell types. In the hepatocyte, for example, the f-TRF associated with the cell surface f-TRF receptor is internalized and directed to endosomes, wherein iron is dissociated from the transferrin peptide and transferred to the iron-storing protein ferritin and the iron-free apotransferrin remains bound to its membrane receptor and is recycled with it to the cell surface (Dautry-Varsat and Lodish, 1983). The iron-free apotransferrin is released to bind additional iron when the receptor-apotransferrin complex encounters the neutral pH of the extracellular medium. Broadwell and colleagues hypothesize that the fate of f-TRF in the endosome of BBB endothelia is dissociation of the ligand from its receptor, which is recycled to the luminal surface; f-TRF is anticipated to be transferred to a vesicle of endosome origin for export and exocytosis at the abluminal front (Broadwell, 1989). Iron would dissociate from the TRF once exocytosis into the perivascular space commences. Perivascular phagocytes could endocytose the free TRF.

There are evidences that some viruses express antigens that have affinity for various receptor or absorptive mediated mechanism associated with the BBB, while the expression of specific adhesion molecules on both the leukocytes and brain endothelial cells are required for the cellular interactions to occur.

Absorptive Mediated Transcytosis(AMT)

Absorptive mediated transcytosis(AMT) through BBB is functionally similar to RMT, except that initial triggering of the endocytotic event starts at the luminal side of the BBB membrane. The examples of peptides that penetrate the BBB via AMT include polycationic proteins such as cationized albumin, cationized IgG, histone, avidin and recombinant CD4 (Kumargi et al., 1987; Triguero et al., 1989; Pardridge and Boado, 1981; Pardridge et al., 1992).

Lectins and cationized molecules are not specific for cells, those located within the CNS as well as those situated peripherally. WGA (wheat germ agglutinin) (MW 36,000) conjugated to HRP (horse reddish peroxidase) is transported via adsorptive transcytosis through the blood-brain barriers, specifically cerebral endothelia and choroid epithelia (Balin and Broadwell, 1988; Broadwell, 1989; Broadwell et al., 1988). Cationized serum proteins can also transported via adsorptive transcytosis through BBB endothelia (Triguero et al., 1989). Lectins and cationized molecules, therefore, may represent excellent vehicles for brain delivery of molecules normally excluded entry by the fluid-brain barriers. Subsequently, the innermost saccule of the Golgi complex also labels with reaction product for WGA-HRP. The signals for transcytosis of WGA-HRP through BBB endothelia are

1. Sequestration of reaction product for blood-borne WGA-HRP within the inner Golgi saccule of cerebral endothelia;
2. Reaction product filling the perivascular clefts;
3. WGA-HRP reaction product in the innermost Golgi saccule of perivascular phagocytes; and
4. WGA-HRP occupying extracellular clefts and processes in the neuropil beyond the basal lamina surrounding the perivascular phagocytes and endothelia (Broadwell et al., 1988).

WGA-HRP labeling of the Golgi complex may be a consequence of overwhelming accumulation of the cellular endosomal compartment by the internalization of cell surface membrane tagged with the lectin conjugate. The endosome compartment is the common nexus among fluid-phase, adsorptive, and receptor-mediated endocytic processes; it represents a clearing center and first intracellular stop in the endocytic pathway for internalized cell surface membrane associated with lectin, the ligand-receptor complex, and fluid-phase molecules (Dautry-Varsat and Lodish, 1984). The endosome serve and dissociates internalized membrane from the attached lectin/ligand so that the membrane can be recycled to the cell surface, leaving the lectin/ligand within the endosome.

In fluid-phase endocytosis, internalized cell surface membrane recycles from endosomes to the plasmalemma after endocytic vesicles have deposited their contents in endosomes. Broadwell and colleagues (Balin and Broadwell 1988) speculated that, when individual endosomes accumulate the endocytic membrane associated with WGA-HRP, the "normal" intracellular endocytic pathway may be perturbed. As a consequence, internalized membrane with attached lectin may be diverted to the inner Golgi saccule wherein a bucket of specific enzymes contributes to the processing of membrane macromolecules, such as the addition or replacement of sialic acid (Bennett et al., 1981) to which WGA binds on the cell surface. Membrane and WGA-HRP recycled through the inner Golgi saccule are packaged for export to other organelles (e.g., endosomes, secondary lysosomes, and plasmalemma) as well as for exocytosis. WGA-HRP delivered into the lateral cerebral ventricle is endocytosed avidly by choroid epithelia at the microvillus face of the cells and transcytosed through the epithelia within 10 minutes for binding to fenestrated endothelia located at the opposite pole of the epithelia. This transcytosis occurs in advance of WGAHRP labeling of the innermost Golgi saccule and is assumed to utilize the endosome compartment as an intermediary in the transcytotic pathway (Balin and Broadwell, 1988). The binding of blood-borne WGA-HRP to luminal and abluminal surfaces of fenestrated endothelia supplying the choroids plexus is so prominent that extracellular availability of the lectin for adsorptive endocytosis by choroid epithelia appears rather compromised (Balin and Broadwell, 1988). Figure 13-4 shows the possible membrane trafficking within choroid epithelia.

Although the physiological relevance of absorptive mediated endocytosis/absorptive mediated transcytosis at the BBB has not been clarified, yet the systems demonstrated promising pathways for the delivery of several kinds of basic peptides to the brain. One of the advantages of utilizing this system is that it operates independent of primary structure and molecular size of peptide(s), hence not restricted to specific peptide(s).

FACTORS AFFECTING DRUG PERMEATION THROUGH BBB

The factors that govern the permeation of a drug across the normal BBB and determine its time dependent concentration within the brain following its systemic administration have been examined by a number of investigators (Greig, 1987; Bardbury, 1979; Davson, 1972; Rapoport, 1976). The factors identified include the followings.

- The time dependent plasma concentration profile of the compound, this is related to its distribution and elimination process.
- The binding of agent to plasma constituents and tissue, and binding off rates from them (plasma clearance).
- The permeability of the BBB to the agent.
- Local cerebral blood flow.

The cerebral availability of peptide/drugs depends on the route of administration. Intracerebral, intraventricular or intracarotid arterial administration provides high concentrations in CSF and diffusion of the peptide drug from CSF through interstitial fluid (ISF) is significantly limited. Factors which affect the pharmacokinetics of a peptide drug after systemic administration include:

- Elimination from the systemic circulation (e.g. hepatic uptake, enzymetic metabolism in the blood and liver, and renal excretion);
- Plasma protein binding;
- Transport at the BBB;
- Enzymatic stability in the brain ISF and
- Diffusion in the brain ISF.

In order to improve the pharmacokinetic characteristics of peptide drugs, it is necessary to understand the concerted biochemical mechanisms operative effecting aforementioned distribution processes. These distribution processes could be studied by chemically modifying native peptides and synthesizing analogue peptides, as has been accomplished in the case of synthetic antibiotics (e.g. β- lactam antibiotics that are di-ol-tri-peptide drugs).

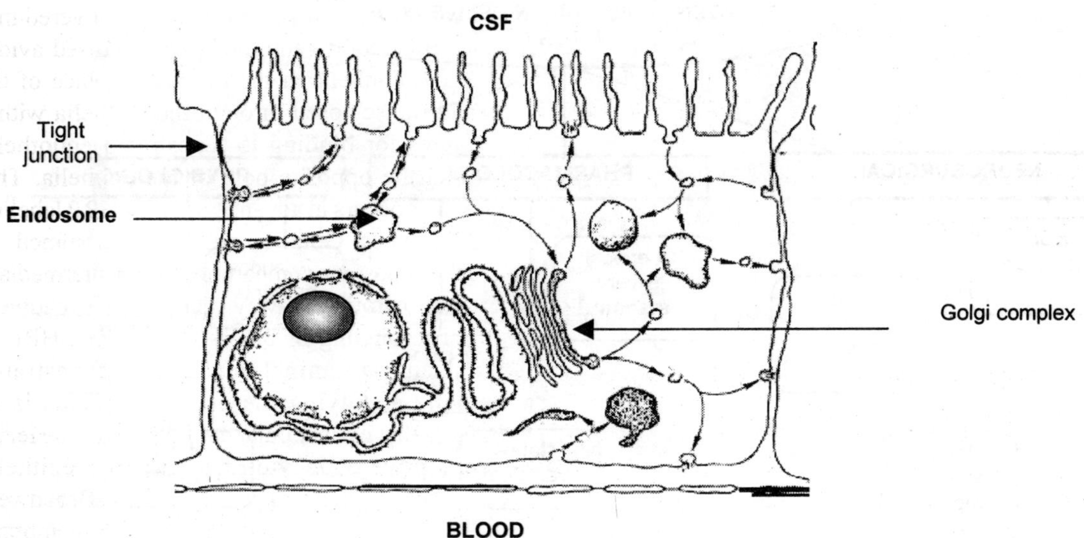

Fig. 13-4. The Possible Membrane Trafficking within Choroid Epithelia (Boardwell, 1992)

BRAIN DRUG DELIVERY STRATEGIES

It is obvious that BBB could be overcome using some active drug carrying system(s) based on novel strategies capable of utilizing bio-events judiously without disturbing their intrinsic characteristics. Some of the strategies appreciated, designed and evaluated for selective brain drug delivery (Fig. 13-5) are broadly classified as:

- Neurosurgical based or invasive;
- Physiologic based strategies;
- Pharmacologic based.

Neurosurgical or Invasive Strategies

Neurosurgical-based strategies include BBB disruption, intraventricular drug infusion, and intracerebral implants.

Hyperosmolar BBB Disruption

Rapoport and coworker (Rapoport, 1970; Rapoport et al., 1972) reported that the BBB might be modified to be more permeable by applying hypertonic solutions on either side of the vascular wall and thereby osmotically shrinking vascular endothelial cells. They investigated the effects of hypertonic solutions, applied topically (extravascularly) for 10 minutes to the arachnoid surface of the rabbit brain, on the permeabilities of pial arterioles and venules to intravascular Evans blue-albumin. Minimal (threshold) concentrations were determined for various electrolytes and nonelectrolytes for increasing the permeability of the pial vessels to this tracer. When Evans blue was administered intravenously, 30 minutes later a threshold concentration of a particular test solution was applied to the brain surface for 10 minutes, the absence or presence of its extravasation demonstrated for reversibly of osmotic BBB opening (Neuwelt and Rapoport, 1984; Warnke et al., 1987; Baba et al., 1991; Pardridge, 1991). An inverse relation between threshold con-centration and octanol:water partition coefficient was demonstrated for reversibly acting agents, that is, those agents less lipid-soluble than ethylene glycol (octanol:water partition coefficient 0.012) This relation was interpreted to indicate that osmotic BBB opening was mediated by shrinkage of cerebro-vascular endothelial cells, stressing and thereby widening interendothelial tight junctions. This suggested mechanism subsequently was confirmed, using electron microscopy and an electron dense tracer (horseradish peroxidase or ionic lanthanum) following intracarotid infusion of hypertonic urea or arabinose in animals (Rapoport,

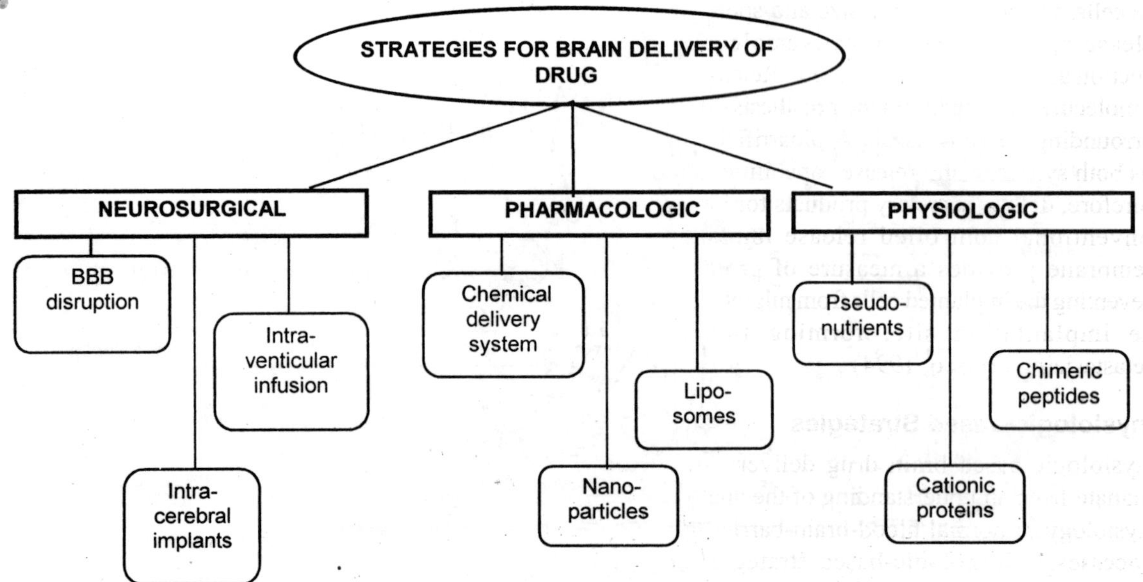

Fig. 13-5. Various Strategies for Brain Delivery of Drugs (Modified from Pardridge, 1996)

1992). The hyperosmolar challenge has been found to opens up the BBB in normal brain relatively more than that in the tumour brain. Recently, biochemical forms of BBB disruption have been demonstrated to preferentially open the BBB of tumour bearing brain rather than normal, if vasoactive compound (e.g. Leukotrienes) is administered via carotid artery.

Intraventricular Drug Infusion

Another strategy which could be employed to reach the brain via neurosurgical means is seemingly intraventricular drug infusion is an ideal source for distributing drug to the surface of the brain, however it poorly delivers drug to brain parenchyma.

Intracerebral Implants

A recently explored alternative relies upon an implantable, bioartificial prosthesis composed of a neurosecretory cell core surrounded by a semi-permeable membrane. This type of implant is similar to controlled release systems in that it allows for site-specific delivery to affected brain areas, but differs in regard to living cells incorporated within the structure. The cells are kept alive by allowing passive exchange of nutrients and waste products with surrounding extracellular fluid through pores in the encapsulating membrane.

The rationale behind the approach is based on the cells, which both synthesize and spontaneously release appropriate neuroactivemolecules may function as a 'Biological Sustained - Release System' as molecules released from the prosthesis diffuse into surrounding nervous tissue. A bioartificial implant has both synthetic and release capabilities and may, therefore, deliver secretary products for longer than conventional controlled release implants. The membrane provides a measure of protection by preventing the implanted cells from migrating beyond the implantation site, forming tumours or metastasizing (Tresco, 1994).

Physiologic-based Strategies

Physiologic-based brain drug delivery strategies emanate from an understanding of the anatomy and physiology of normal blood-brain-barrier transport processes. Physiologic-based strategies include pseudonutrients, cationic antibodies and chimeric peptides.

Pseudo-nutrients

These are polar small molecules with a molecular structure mimicking nutrients that normally undergo carrier-mediated transport through the BBB. For example hexoses, monocarboxylic acids, basic acids, amines, nucleosides, neutral amino acid drugs, such L-dopa or a-methyl-dopa are effective neuro-pharmaceuticals because these drugs are transported into brain via the BBB through a neutral amino acid carrier (Pardridge and Bodo, 1993; Zlokovic et al., 1993).

Cationic Antibodies

Cationic antibodies undergo absorption mediated transcytosis through the BBB owing to the positive charge. When used in a homologous system, cationic antibodies have no descriminable tissue toxicity and have displayed minimal immunogenicity (Pardridge et al., 1995).

Chemeric Peptides

The brain capillary endothelial cell plasma membrane is endowed with peptide-specific receptor system and some of these receptors function as BBB transport system. The circulating peptides such as insulin or transferrin undergo transcytosis through the BBB mediated by BBB insulin and transferrin receptors, respectively. Absorptive-mediated transport systems on BBB are also available for lectins, e.g. wheat germ agglutinin or cationic proteins, such as cationic albumin. Other receptors associated with BBB could mediate only the endocytosis of ligand. The scavenger receptor present on the BBB, is identified to mediate the endocytosis of acetylated low density lipoprotein. The evidence suggesting the presence of peptide receptors on the BBB and as well as about receptors which mediate peptide transcytosis through the BBB led to the concept of chimeric peptide hypothesis (Pardridge, 1995; Bickel et al., 1994).

The approach negotiate drug delivery to the brain by anchoring drug to a peptide or protein 'vector', which is transported through BBB following absorptive or receptor mediated transcytosis. The conjugate of the vector and the non-transportable drug is referred to as a chimeric peptide system (Fig. 13-6). The vectors which has been used to date include cationic proteins, e.g. cationized albumin, or monoclonal antibodies specific to receptors on the

BBB (transferrin or insulin receptor). The murine OX26 monoclonal antibody to the red transferrin receptor is an efficacious brain transport vector. The antibody recognizes an extracellularly projected epitope of the transferrin receptor. The transferrin is excessively expressed on BBB. The ability of the OX26 antibody to engage the BBB transferrin receptor and to transcytoes through BBB explains the relatively high BBB permeability-surface area (PS) product obtained for this protein.

There are two principles concerns in using natural peptides as drug transport vectors. First, the vector itself will have biologic activity, for example, the side effects of using insulin as a drug transport vector could include hypoglycemia. The use of transferrin may alter iron homeostasis, and the use of IGF-2 as a drug transport vector is complicated by the avid binding of this peptide by specific binding proteins in plasma (Duffy et al., 1988). Second, the interaction of peptide ligands with receptor binding sites is generally highly specific, and the addition of a nontransportable pharmaceutical onto an insulin or transferring vector may result in markedly reduced rates of affinity of the modified insulin or transferrin for its native receptor. However, these two concerns are addressed with the use of polycationic proteins as BBB drug transport vectors. It has been known for many years that the cationization of proteins, in general, enhances the cellular uptake of these macromolecules. This property was demonstrated for BBB transport processes when it was shown that cationized albumin is transported across the BBB *in vivo* (Kumagai et al., 1987). Cationized albumin is prepared by converting surface carboxyl groups on the albumin molecule to extended primary amino groups using such derivatives as hexa-methylenediamine. This raises the isoelectric point of the protein from approximately four to nine and causes the modified albumin to undergo rapid absorptive-mediated transcytosis through the BBB. Native cationic proteins, such as histone, have been shown to undergo absorptive-mediated transcytosis through the BBB and to have saturable binding sites on brain capillaries (Pardridge et al., 1989) similar to cationized albumin or native peptides. However, histone has been shown to be toxic to the BBB and to cause changes in BBB permeability at relatively low doses. This property has not been observed following the infusion of cationized albumin (Triguero et al., 1989). Nevertheless, two concerns with regard to using cationized albumin as a drug transport vector are the potential toxicity of this

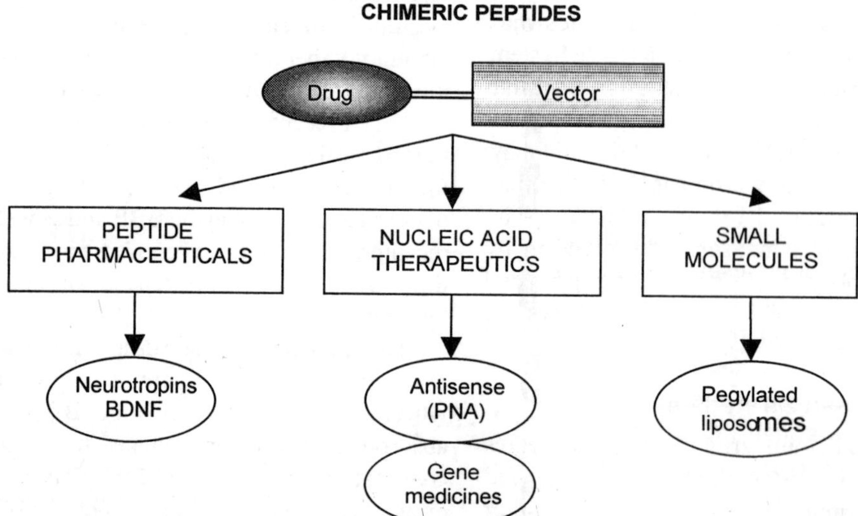

Fig. 13-6. Schematic Representation Different Therapeutic Area of Applications for Chemeric Pepdide Delivery

polycationic protein and the immunogenicity of the cationized form of the native protein. The use of cationized homologous proteins has not been found to generate a significant immune response. On the basis of these other studies, cationized rat albumin is believed to be a suitable vector for the delivery of peptides across the BBB in a physiologic setting and to provide a model for pharmacologic paradigms involving repetitive drug administration (Pardridge et al., 1992; Pardridge, 1992, Bickel and Pardridge, 1992).

β-Endorphin Chimeric Peptides

A β-endorphin-cationized albumin chimeric peptide was prepared using the disulfide-based cross-linking reagent N-succinimidyl-3-(2- pyridyldithio)-propionate (SPDP) (Carisson et al., 1978). Disulfide-based crosslinkers were chosen because previous studies have shown that disulfide bonds are relatively stable in plasma but are labile in cells (Letvin et al. 1986), which is the necessary criterion that must be established for a drug delivery vehicle. The β-endorphin was coupled via N-terminal and lysine s-amino groups on the opioid peptide to extended primary amino groups on the cationized albumin as follows (Kumagai et al., 1987):

Cationized albumin -CONH$(CH_2)_6$NHCO$(CH_2)_2$-S-S-$(CH_2)_2$CONH-β-endorphin

The transport of chimeric peptides through the BBB is viewed within the context of four individual steps that are depicted in Figure 13-7.

The first step is absorptive-mediated endocytosis at the blood side of the BBB. The absorptive-mediated endocytosis of the cationized albumin-ß-endorphin chimeric peptide was demonstrated with isolated brain capillaries using a mild acid wash technique (Kumagai et al., 1987).

The second step in the overall process is absorptive-mediated exocytosis at the brain side of the BBB, which completes the transcytosis of the chimeric peptide through the BBB, allowing for distribution of the chimeric peptide into brain interstitial fluid (Pardridge et al., 1990). Absorptive-mediated transport is triggered by the electrostatic interaction between cationic groups on the drug transport vector and anionic groups on the surface of the microvascular endothelium.

The third step in the overall chimeric peptide strategy is the cleavage of the disulfide bond joining the drug transport vector and the peptide pharmaceutical (Figure 13-7). Moreover, it is necessary that the rate of cleavage of this disulfide bond is substantially faster than the rate of degradation of the pharmaceutical peptide while it is still attached to the drug transport vector. In the setting of slow cleavage of the disulfide bond by brain, there would be little free pharmacologically active peptide generated to interact with the respective eptide receptor on brain nerve endings. However, recent studies have shown that brain is endowed with high activities of the disulfide reductase enzymatic activity that cleaves the endorphin-cationized albumin chimeric peptide (Pardridge et al., 1990).

The fourth and final step of the chimeric peptide strategy depicted in Figure 13-7 is the interaction of free pharmacologically active peptide with its respective receptor on brain nerve endings. However, significant care must be taken in choosing coupling strategies that allow for the generation of a pharmacologically active peptide subsequent to the cleavage of the peptide from its drug transport vector. For example, the principal mode of attachment of a pharmaceutical peptide through the cationized albumin vector is via free amino groups on the pharmacologically active peptide. Subsequent to the cleavage of the chimeric peptide, there is a mercaptopropionate group remaining on the amino group that participated in the coupling reaction:

HS$(CH_2)_2$CONH-β-endorphin

Therefore, the construct for opioid peptide drug design must consider the structural requirements that are necessary for preservation of opioid peptide biologic activity following cleavage from the drug transport vector.

Pharmacologic Strategies

Pharmacologic based strategies include drug inclusion in liposome or nanoparticles, a lipidization of drug or chemical delivery using redox system or synthesis of small molecular size pharmaco-dynamically active vectors of drug (Kabanov et al., 1989; Cheknonin et al., 1991).

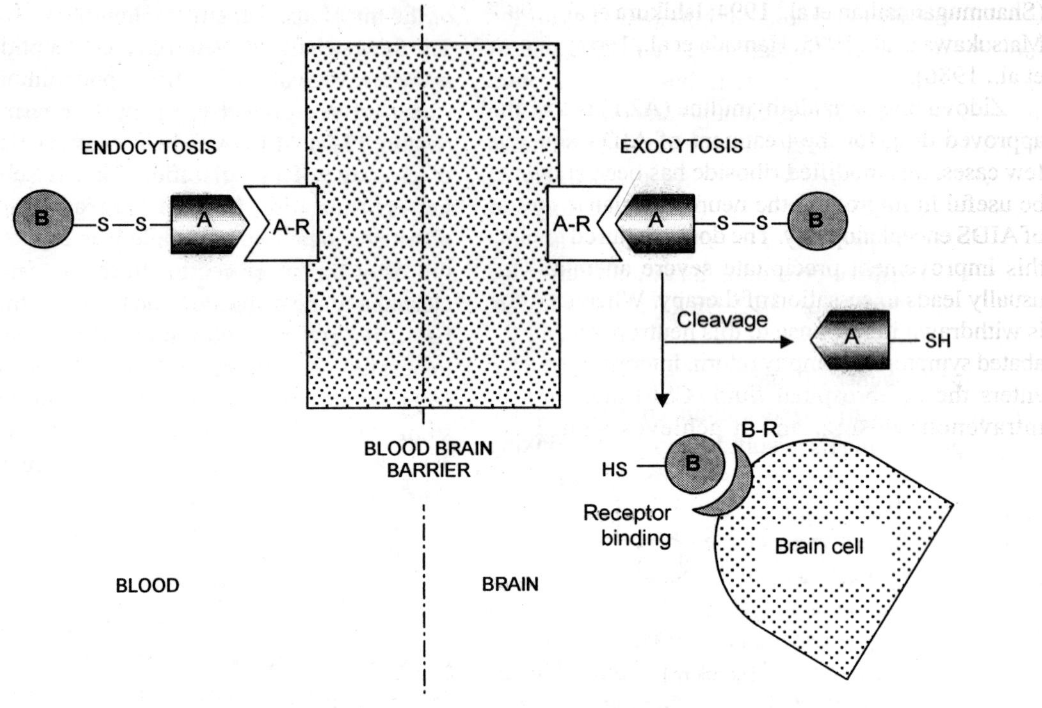

Fig. 13-7. Chimeric Peptide Drug Delivery Strategy

Chemical Delivery System

One approach for enhancing delivery of compounds to the brain is to modify them chemically so that their lipid solubility is enhanced. An elegant extension of this approach involves the chemical modification of drugs by its conjugation with methyl-dihydropyridine. The chemically modified drug is better permeable across brain capillaries, where it is immediately converted to an impermeable analogue by enzymatic reaction within the brain tissue. The dihydropyridine-pyridinium salt represent a typical redox delivery system which can be used for specific drug delivery to the brain.

The dihydropyridine-pyridinium salt redox delivery system has successfully evaluated for brain specific delivery of dopamine. *In vivo* administration of the catechol-protected dopamine coupled with 1,4-dihydrotrigonelline as a carrier resulted in brain specific, high and sustained concentrations of the 1-methyl - 3 [N {b - (3,4-dihydroxyphenyl) ethyl} carbamoyl] pyridinium salt, the direct dopamine precursor, locked in the brain for hours, while systemic concentration decrease fast, with clearece half life less than 30 minutes (Bodor and Farag, 1983).

The technical limitation of the concept, is it the facile oxidation of the dihydropyridine-modified prodrugs by oxygen in open air as well as in solution this reduces even its intravenous formulation difficult. In order to improve the stability of prodrugs; the conversion of cis-2-formylamino ethyl thio derivatives of corresponding quaternary thiazolium can be applied as an alternative drug delivery system to brain. Thiamine disulfide (TDS) is one of the most familiar representatives of the cis-2-formylamino ethyl thio derivatives and has been clinically used as fat-soluble precursor of thiamine (B_1) possessing quaternary thiazolium moiety in its structure. The conversion reaction, which proceeds mainly via gluthion and haemoglobin is similar to that of Bodar's CDS, however, the reactions of CDS within thiamine and Bodar's CDS are typically redox type. Fig. 13-8 illustrates the schematic of a redox ring-closure system designed for selective delivery to brain

(Shanmugannathan et al., 1994; Ishikura et al., 1995; Matsukawa et al., 1995; Hamada et al., 1967; Utsumi et al., 1986).

Zidovudine or azidothymidine (AZT) is the first approved drug for the treatment of AIDS and in a few cases, this modified riboside has been shown to be useful in improving the neuropsychiatric course of AIDS encephalopathy. The doses required to elicit this improvement precipitate severe anemia. This usually leads to cessation of therapy. When the drug is withdrawn in response to this neutropenia, all the abated symptoms promptly return. Interestingly, AZT enters the cerebrospinal fluid (CSF) after oral or intravenous dosing, and it achieves signtficant concentrations. Unfortunately, these CSF levels appear to greatly overestimate brain parenchymal and neuronal levels as AZT poorly penetrates the BBB. In an effort to ameliorate the prognosis of AIDS encephalopathy, the CDS approach was applied to AZT (Brewster and Bodor, 1992). This antiviral agent has primary alcohol functionality in the 5'-position, which was considered for carrier attachment. As shown in Figure 13-9, AZT was treated with nicotinic anhydride in pyridine to yield the 5'-nicotinate. This ester was subsequently quaternized with alkyl halide to yield the 5'-trigonellinate (1-methylnicotinate) and reduced in basic aqueous sodium dithionite to give the 5'-(1,4-

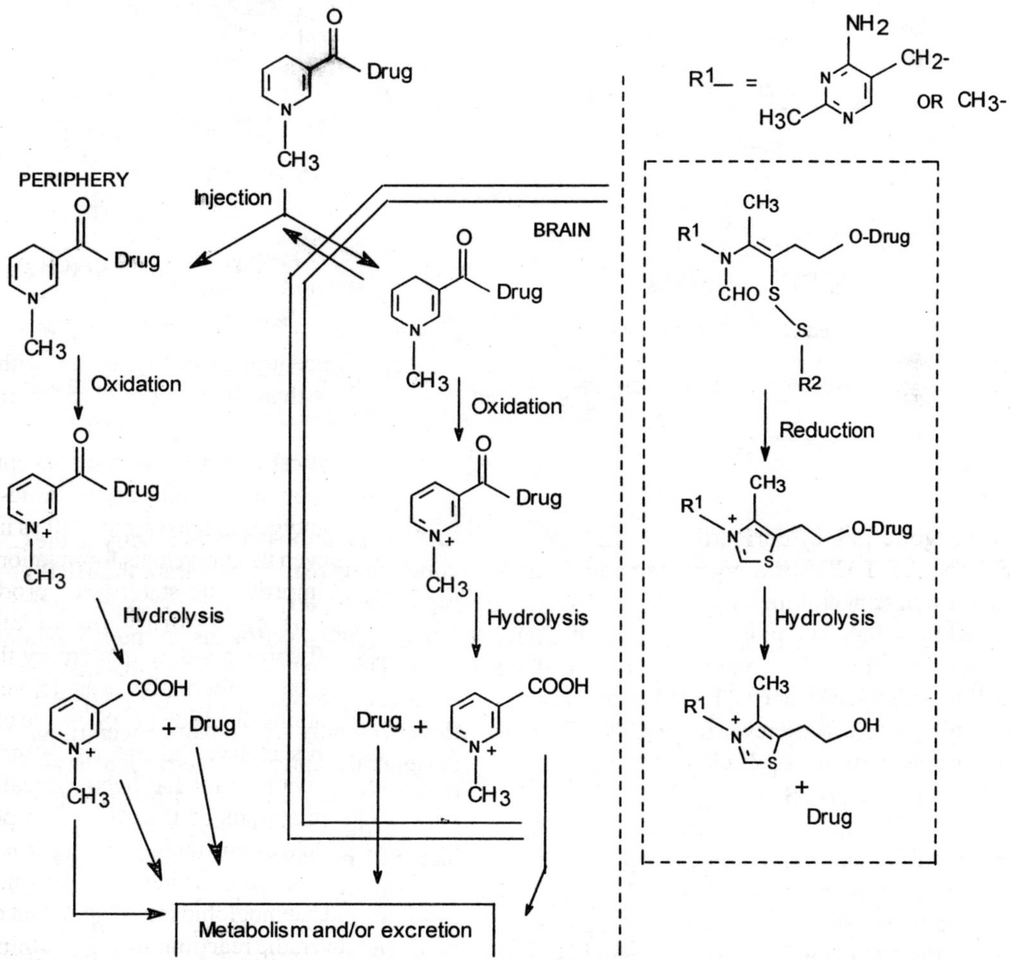

Fig. 13-8. Sequential Metabolism of a Redox Chemical Delivery System based on Ring Closure Reaction to Thiazolium (within the dashed area) in Comparison with Bodor's Dihydropyridine/Pyridinium System.

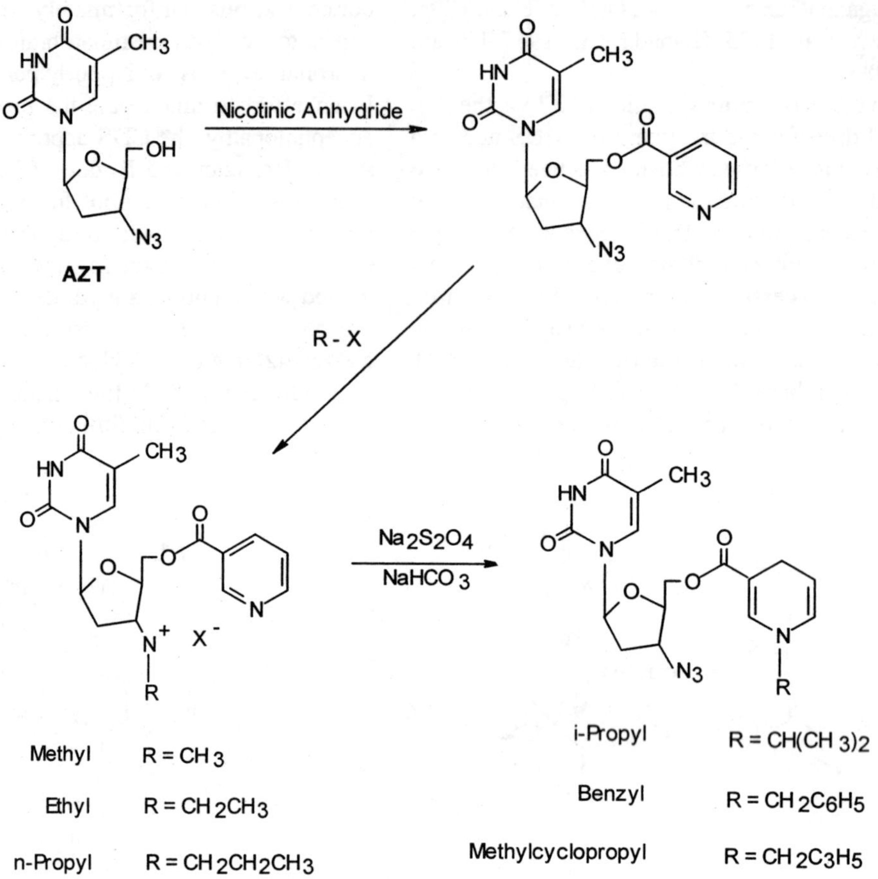

Fig. 13-9. Preparation of an Azidothymidine-CDS

dihydrotrigonellinate) derivative of AZT (AZT-CDS). The AZ-T-CDS is a crystalline solid that is stable at room temperature for several months when protected from light and moisture. The lipophilicity of the AZT-CDS and its metabolites (AZT and the AZT-5'-trigonellinate salt (AZT-Q+) is important in determining the efficiency of the CDS. The n-octanol:water partition coefficient (log P) of AZT, AZT-Q+, and AZT-CDS is 0.06, -2.00, and 1.5 for, respectively. This indicates that the CDS is 34-fold more lipophilic than the parent riboside and more than 3,900-fold more lipophilic than the AZT-Q+. These parameters should correlate with rapid brain uptake of the CDS (log P> 1.0) and rapid systemic elimination of theAZT-Q+ (Greig, 1987, Brewster and Bodor, 1992). Estrogens are lipophilic steroids that are not impeded in their entry to the CNS. These compounds readily penetrate the BBB and achieve high central levels after peripheral administration. Unfortunately, estrogens are poorly retained by the brain. This circumstance requires that frequent doses of these steroids be administered to maintain therapeutically significant concentrations. Constant peripheral exposure of estrogen has been related, however, to several pathological conditions, including cancer, hypertension, and altered metabolism. As the CNS is the target site for many of the actions of estrogens, a brain-targeted delivery form of these compounds may provide for safer and more effective estrogens. A CDS for 17β-oestradiol was generated by treatment of estradiol with nicotinoyl chloride hydrochloride to give the 3,17-

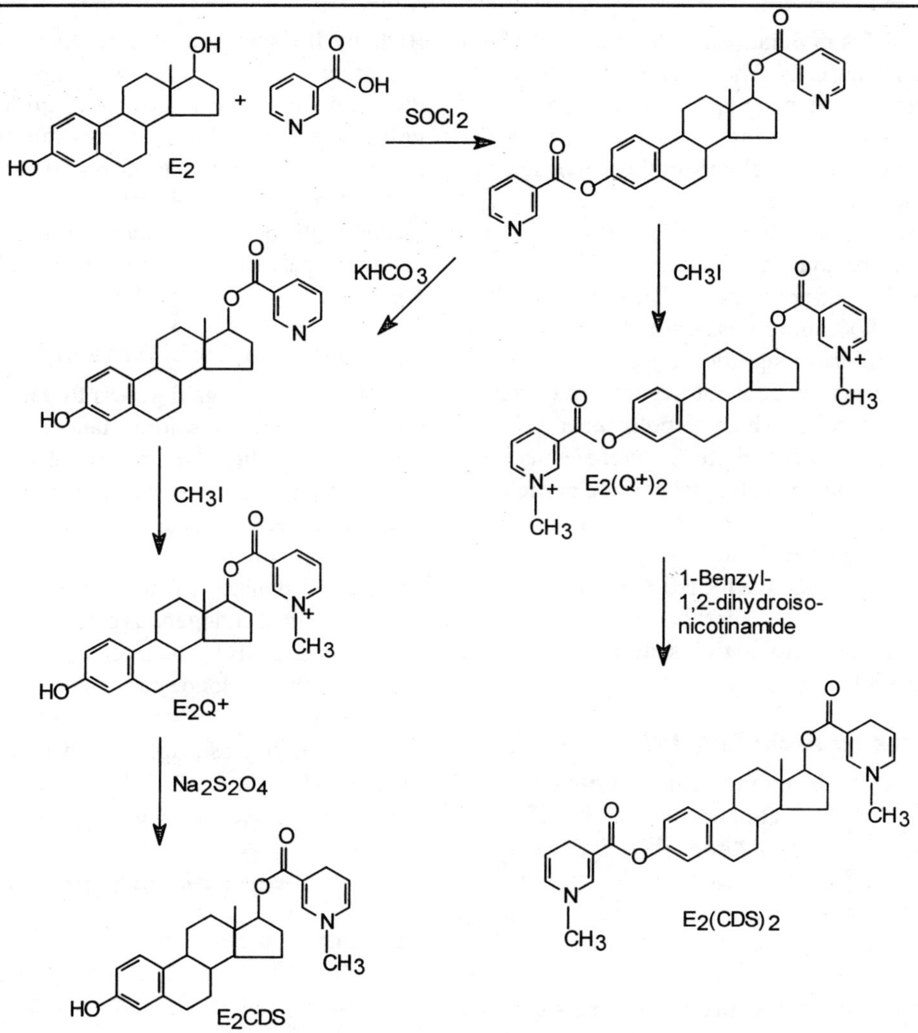

Fig. 13-10 Estrogen-CDS Synthesis

bis nicotinate (Figure 13-10). Treatment of this ester with methanol potassium bicarbonate resulted in selective cleavage of the phenolic nicotinate. The obtained secondary nicotinate was then quaternized and reduced to provide the 17-(1,4-dihydro-trigonellinate) ester of β-oestradiol or E_2CDS (Brewster and Bodor, 1992).

SMALL COLLOIDAL PARTICLES FOR BRAIN TARGETING

Small colloidal particles such as liposomes, microspheres, and nanoparticles have been suggested as possible carriers for selective delivery of drugs to tissue sites.

Nanoparticles for Brain Targeting

The coating of nanoparticles with surfactants (polysorbate 80 and 20, poloxamers 188, 338, 407 and 184, polyoxyethylene, 23-laural ether and poloxamine 908) offers the possibility to alter the body distribution of this carrier system after intravenous injection. Coating with polysorbate 80 not only can lead to higher brain concentration after intravenous injection but also can increase the uptake of nanoparticles into cultivated bovine brain blood vessel endothelial cells. The coating with polysorbate 80 may induce endocytic uptake of the particles by the endothelial cells lining the blood vessels in the brain, followed by the delivery of the active agent to brain tissues (Kreuter et al., 1997).

Among the surface modifier that led to a significantly prolonged blood circulation time are poloxamer 338 and poloxamine 908. Poloxamer 338, poloxamine 908 and polysorbate 80 (in order of decreasing efficacy) significantly increased whole brain concentrations after intravenous injection of empty nanoparticles, where as poloxamer 118 and 407 as well as polysorbate 80 were especially effective in enhancing cell uptake of the particles in bovine brain endothelial cells cultures. Schroeder et al., 1998 has reported the transport of dalargin (peptide-analgesic) across the BBB. The peptide was adsorbed onto the surface of poly(butyl-cyanoacrylate) nanoparticles and coated with polysorbate 80.

Liposomes for Brain Targeting

Liposomes are biocompatible, nontoxic, biodegradable carrier constructs which offer the possibility of carrying hydrophobic, hydrophilic or amphiphilic molecules. Despite these numerous attributes, liposomes have not gained wide spread use as drug delivery systems, due to their instability in-vivo.

Classical liposome preparations, sterically stabilized liposomes and immunoliposomes are all susceptable to clearance by immune system. The use of conventional liposomes for drug delivery across the brain capillary recently was reviewed. Briefly, even liposomes with a diameter as small as 100 nm are too large to undergo free diffusion through the BBB. However, it is possible that small unilamellar vesicles (SUVs) coupled to brain drug transport vectors may be transported through the BBB by receptor-mediated or absorptive-mediated transcytosis. Similarly, cationic liposomes recently were developed, and these structures may undergo absorptive mediated endocytosis into cells. Whether cationic liposomes successfully undergo absorptive mediated transcytosis through the BBB has not yet been determined. The transport of substances through BBB by liposomes, was extensively studied. The important finding issuing form their studies is that the addition of sulphatide (a sulphate ester of galactocerebroside) to liposome composition increases their ability to cross BBB (Rose et al., 1991). Wang et al., 1995 reported that the liposome coated with mannose reaches brain tissue and the mannose coat assists transport of loaded drug through the BBB.

Monocytes for Brain Targeting

A difficult goal to gain access to particular macrophage subpopulations, for instance, across the BBB. The unusual ability of the monocyte to cross the BBB makes it possible to consider using this cell as a 'Trojan Horse' to transport agents into the CNS. Furthermore infected brain locuses have augmented population density of monocytes, which can be utilized as ideal endogenous carriers for transporting drugs across BBB to the infected sites after loading drugs over them. Monocytes express certain receptors on their membrane, which are involved in receptor-mediated endocytosis upon interaction with suitable ligands (Molema et al., 1990). Figure 13-11 is the schematic representation of this strategy.

FUTURE PROSPECTS

Undoubtedly, the most difficult organ to be delivered with physiologically active drugs/peptides is the brain, because of its strong defense system imparted by anatomically and physiologically BBB. By chemical modification of physiologically active peptides/drugs that are very unstable and that have limited BBB transport (i.e. increasing enzymatic stability and transport activity through the BBB), it may be possible to develop several systemically effective neuropharmaceuticls that will be effective after systemic administration. Recent studies have clearly indicated that if a given peptide/protein has a transport system at the luminal side of BBB, and/or could be modified to use the existing transport mechanism, its levels in the brain and/or cerebral microvessels could be manipulated by arterial infusion and/or by intravenous administration. The eagerness for strategies such as peptide lipidization and/or enhanced passive diffusion due to increased

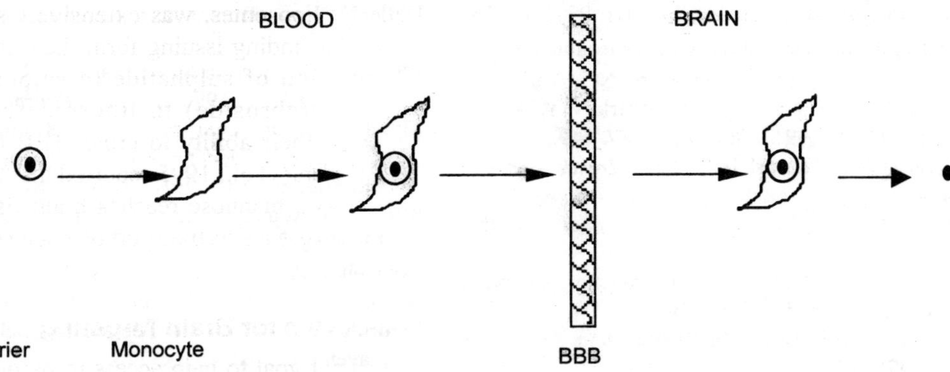

Fig. 13-11. Schematic Representation of Brain Targeting via Monocytes

lipophilicity, have been declined in recent years. New strategies based primarily on utilization of specific transport systems at the BBB are being designed and developed. The progress for delivering drug/peptide across BBB requires the integration of antibody engineering, organic chemistry, pharmacokinetics, and peptide-or receptor-based drug design. The development of a successful BBB drug delivery system seems achievable. Given the difficulties in developing successful brain drug delivery approaches, and given that most nerurophamaceuticals do not cross the BBB, it is surprising that essentially all existing CNS drug development programs are devoted solely to CNS drug discovery, with little attention paid to CNS drug delivery. Ideally, CNS drug discovery and CNS drug delivery should be integrated at the earliest possible stage as overall brain drug development program.

REFERENCES

Baba T., Black K. I., Ikezaki K., Chen K. and Becker D. P. (1991) *J. Cerebral. blood flow Metab.* **11**, 683.

Balin B.J. and Broadwell R. D. (1988) *J. Neurocytol.* **17**, 809.

Banks W. A., Kastein A. J. and Barrera C. M. (1991) *Pharm. Res.* **8**, 1345.

Baranczyk-Kuzma A., and Audus K. L. (1987) *J. Cereb. Blood Flow Metab.* **7**, 801.

Bardbury M. W. B. (1979) In: The concept of a blood brain barrier, Wiley, Chichester, 29.

Bennett G., Kan F. W. K. and O'Shaughnessy D. (1981) *J. Cell. Biol.* **88**, 16.

Betz A.L. (1992) In: Bioavailability of drugs to the brain and the blood brain barrier, Frankelhein J. and Brown R.M. (Eds.) Research Monograph, 120, U. S. Department Health and Human Services, Rockville, MD, 54.

Betz A. L. (1986) *Fed. Proc.* **45**, 2050.

Betz A. L. and Goldstein G.W. (1978) *Science* 202, 225.

Betz A.L. (1983) *J. Neurochem.* **41**, 1158.

Betz A.L. (1985) *Fed. Proc.* **44**, 2614.

Bickel U. and Pardridge W. M. (1992) In: Bioavailability of drugs to the brain and the blood brain barrier, Frankelhein J. and Brown R.M. (Eds.) Research Monograph, 120, U. S. Department Health and Human Services, Rockville, MD, 28.

Bickel Y. S., Kang S., Yoshikawa T. and Pardridge W. M. (1994) *J. Histochem. Cytochem.* **42**, 1493.

Bito L.Z., Davson H. and Hollingsworth J. (1976) *J. Physiol.* **256**, 273.

Boardwell R. D. (1992) In: Bioavailability of drugs to the brain and the blood brain barrier, Frankelhein J. and Brown R.M. (Eds.) Research Monograph, 120, U. S. Department Health and Human Services, Rockville, MD, 230.

Bodor N. and Farag H. H. (1983) *J. Med. Chem.* **26**, 528.

Bradbury M. W. B. and Stulcova B. (1970) *J. Physiol.* **208**, 415.

Brewster M. E. and Bodor N. (1992) In: Bioavailability of drugs to the brain and the blood brain barrier, Frankelhein J. and Brown R.M. (Eds.) Research Monograph, 120, U. S. Department Health and Human Services, Rockville, MD, 169.

Brightman M. W. (1977) *Exp Eye Res* **25**, 1.

Broadwell R. D. (1989) *Acta. Neuropathol. (Berl)* **79**, 117.

Broadwell, R. D., Balin B. J. and Salcman M. (1988) *Proc. Natl. Acad. Sci. USA.* **85**, 632.

Cancilla P. A., Bready J. and Berliner J. (1993) In: The blood brain barrier cellular and molecular biology, Pardridge W. M. (Ed.), Raven Press, New-York, 25.

Cheknonin V. P., Kabanov A. V., Zhirkov Y. A. and Marozov G. V. (1991) *FEBS Lett.* **287**, 149.

Dautry-Varsat A. and Lodish H. F. (1983) *Trends Neurosci.* **6**, 484.

Dautry-Varsat A. and Lodish H. F. (1984) *Sci. Am.* **250**, 52.

Davson H. (1972) In: The structure and function of nervous tissue, Academic press, NewYork, 32.

Doczi T., Joo F. and Bodosi M. (1990) *Acta. Neurochir. Suppl.* **47**, 122.

Duffy K. R., Pardridge W. M. and Resenfeid R. G. (1988) Metabolism, **37**, 136.

Frank H. J. L. and Pardridge W. M. (1981) *Diabetes* **30**, 757.

Gimbrone M. A., Jr. Majeau, G.R., Atkinson W.J., Sadler W. and Cruise S.A.

Greig N. H. (1987) *Cancer Treat. Rev.* **14**, 1.

Greig N. H., Genka S. and Rapoports I. (1990) *J. Controll. Rel.* **11**, 61.

Hamada M., Hayakawa T., Yamaguchi T. and Koike M. (1967) *Vitamins(Jap)* **35**, 474.

Hardebo J. E. and Owman C. (1980) *Ann. Neural.* 8, 1.

Harik S.I. (1986) *Proc. Natl. Acad. Sci. USA.* **83**, 4067.

Herman I. M. (1993) In: The blood brain barrier cellular and molecular biology, Pardridge W. M. (Ed.) Raven Press, NewYork, 127.

Ibaragi, M. A., Niwa M. and Ozaki M. (1989) *J. Neurochem.* **53**, 1802.

Ishikura T., Senou T., Ishikura H., Kato T. and Ito T. (1995) *International J. Pharmaceutics* **116**, 51.

Kabanov A. V., Cheknonin V. P., Alakhov V. Y., Batrakova E. V. and Lebedev A. S. (1989) *FEBS Lett.* **258**, 343.

Kalaria R.N., Stockmeier C. A. and Harik S.I. (1989) *Neurosci. Lett.* **97**, 203.

Keller B. T. and Borchardt R. T. (1987) *Fed. Proc.* **46**, 416.

Kreuter J., Petrov V. E., Kharkevich D. A. and Alautdin, R. N. (1997) *J. Controll. Rel.* **49**, 81.

Kumargai A. K., Eisenberg J. and Pardridge W. M. (1987) *J. Biol. Chem.* **262**, 15214.

Letvin N.L., Goldmacher V.S., Ritz J., Yetz J.M., Schlossman SF. and Lambert J. M. (1986) *J. C/in. Invest.* **77**, 977.

Life Sci. 25, 1075.

Matsukawa T. and Yurugi S., Yakugaku Z. (1952) **72**, 1616.

McComb J. G. and Ziokovic B. V. (1994) In: Paediatric Neurosurgery, Cheek W. R., Martin A. E., McLone D. G., Reigel D. H., W.B. Saunders Co., Philadelphia, 167.

Miller D. W. and Borchardt R. T. (1991) *J. Cell. Biol.* **115**, 261a.

Molema G., Ganessen R. W., Pauwels R., Clerca E. and Meijer D. K. F. (1990) *Biochem. Pharmacol.* **47**, 2603.

Mrsulja B. B. and Djuricic B. M. (1981) In: *Advances in Experimental Medicine and Biology* Eisenberg, H.M., and Suddith, R.L., (Eds.) Plenum, New York, 29.

Murphy V. A. and Johanson C. E. (1989) *J. Neurochem.* **52**, 1058.

Neuwelt, F. A. and Rapoport S. (1984) *Fed. Proc.* **43**, 214.

Newman E. A. (1985) *J. Neurosci.* **5**, 2225.

Pardridge W. M. (1991) In: Peptide drug delivery to brain, Raven press, NewYork, 276.

Pardridge W. M. (1992) In: Bioavailability of drugs to the brain and the blood brain barrier, Frankelhein J. and Brown R.M. (Eds.) Research Monograph, 120, U. S. Department Health and Human Services, Rockville, MD, 153.

Pardridge W. M. (1993) *Drug Delivery* **1**, 83.

Pardridge W. M. (1995) *Adv. Drug Del. Rev.* **15**, 109.

Pardridge W. M. (1996) *J. Control. Rel.* **39**, 281.

Pardridge W. M. and Boado T. J. (1991) *FEBS Lett.* **288**, 30.

Pardridge W. M. and Bodo R. J. (1993) In: The blood brain barrier cellular and molecular biology, Pardridge W. M. (Ed.), Raven Press, NewYork, 395.

Pardridge W. M., Buciak J. L. and Yoshikawa T. (1992) *J. Pharmacol. Exp. Ther.* **261**, 1175.

Pardridge W. M., Eisenberg J. and Yang J. (1987) *Metabolism* **38**, 892.

Pardridge W. M., Triguero D. and Buciak J. L. (1989) *J. Pharmacol. Exp. Ther.* **251**, 821.

Pardridge W. M., Yang J., Buciak J. and Kang Y. S. (1995) Soc. Neurosci. Abstr. **21**, 1751.

Pardridge W.M., Triguero D. and Buciak J. L. (1990) *Endocrinology* **126**, 977.

Rapoport S. I. (1970) *Am. J. Physiol.* **219**, 270.

Rapoport S. I. (1976) In: Blood brain barrier in physiology, Raven press, NewYork, 22.

Rapoport S. I.(1992) In: Bioavailability of drugs to the brain and the blood brain barrier, Frankelhein J. and Brown R.M. (Eds.) Research Monograph, 120, U. S. Department Health and Human Services, Rockville, MD, 121.

Rapoport S.I., Hori M. and Klatzo I. (1972) *Am. J. Physiol.* **223**, 323.

Rose J. K., Buoncore L. and Whitt M. A. (1991) *Biotechniques* **10**, 520.

Schroeder U., Sommerfeld P. & Sabel, B. A. (1998) *Peptides* **19**, 777.

Shanmuganathan K., Koudriakova, T., Nampalli S., Du

J., Gallo J. M., Schinazi R. F. and Chu C. K. (1994) *J. Med. Chem.* **37**, 821.

Tayarani I., Chaudiere J., Lefauconnier J. M. and Bourre J. M. (1987a) *J. Neurochem.* **48**, 1399.

Tayarani I., Lefauconnier J. M., Roux F. and Bourre J.M. (1987b) *J. Cereb. Blood. Flow Metab.* **7**, 585.

Thiebaut F., Tsuruo T., Hamada H., Gottesman M.M. Pastan I. and Willingham M.C. (1989) *J. Histochem. Cytochem.* **37**, 159.

Tresco, P. A. (1994) *J. Controll. Rel.* **28**, 253.

Triguero D., Buciak J. L., Yang J. and Pardridge W. M. (1989) *Proc. Natl. Acad. Sci. USA* **86**, 4761.

Utsumi I., Kohno K., Kakie Y. and Mizobe M. (1986) *Vitamins(Jap)* **37**, 264.

Vigne P., Champigny G., Marsault R., Barbry P., Frelin C., and Lazdunski, M. (1989) *J. Biol. Chem.* **264**, 7663.

Wang J. Y., Xu Y. R., Huang K. and Sun L. Y. (1995) *J. Pharm. Pharmacol.* **47**, 1053.

Warnke P. C., Blasberg R. G. and Groothus F. (1987) *Ann. Neurol.* **22**, 300.

Zlokovic B. V., Mackic J. B., Wang L., McComb J. G. and McDonough A. A. (1993) *J. Biol. Chem.* **268**, 8019.

CHAPTER 14

Drug Delivery to Tumour

The therapeutics of tumour is largely confined to directly encountering the tumour cells. The current cytostatic agents mainly interfere with processes involved in cell growth while the aim in immunotherapy is to make immune effector cells to selectively attack the tumour cells. A recent approach to fight tumour is to impede and interfere with its blood supply, i.e., turning off angiogenesis or neovascularization.

To lower cytotoxicity and increase therapeutic effects, targeted drug delivery systems for anti-tumour drugs have been developed over last few years. These drug delivery systems including polymeric carriers and colloidal carriers like liposomes, immunoliposomes, microspheres, are often directed against epitopes present on tumour cells and/or receptors expressed on tumour cells and carry drugs which interfere with tumour growth. In all cases, the bioactive has to cross the tumour blood vessel wall consisting of endothelial cells and basement membrane. Especially in drug delivery strategies in which polymeric, macromolecular or particulate carriers are used to increase treatment selectively, the endothelial barriers form a major obstacle. The focus of research shifts from the manipulation in barrier function or designing of carrier systems that can cross the tumour vasculature, to identification of recognition elements on tumour cells, which could be targeted using suitable ligands anchored on these carrier systems. The vasculature endothelium, basement membrane and tumour stroma may contain potential tumour specific targets. Strategies directed to these potential targets are aimed at interfering with blood vessel permeability, angiogenesis or tumour blood supply, or at manipulating endothelial cell mediated immune effector cell movement into the tumour tissue.

Tumour Vasculature vs Normal Vasculature

The tumour vasculature is different from the normal vasculature in the following respects (Molema et al., 1997):

- Permselectivity of the tumour vessels is less than that of normal vessels presumably due to the large pores in the vessel wall. This could be accounted for the absence of basement membrane adjacent to endothelial cells.

- Hampered and altered expression of adhesion molecules by tumour vasculature endothelium.
- Turnover time of normal endothelial cells is estimated in the range of 1000 days or more, whereas tumour endothelial cells grow with a turnover time of only 4-5 days.
- Heterogeneity in angiogenic peptide expression resulting in a heterogenic endothelial cell population.
- Altered vascular permeability across the tumour mass, the centre being more dense and poorly vascularized compared to peripheral region.

How Tumour Develops

Tumour seems to arise from the effects of two different kinds of carcinogens. One of these categories comprises agents that damage genes involved in controlling cell proliferation and migration. Cell adhesion is a prerequisite for cell survival in the normal condition and is thought to occur via anchoring of cells within themselves or with extracellular matrix (AREA CODES on ECM) and allow cells to survive and proliferate. Tumour cells however, survive without adhesion to extracellular matrix (Fig. 14-1). Tumour arises when a single cell accumulates a number of these mutations, usually over many years, and finally escapes from most restraints on proliferation (Bishop, 1995; Weinberg, 1996). The mutations allow the cell and its descendants to develop additional alterations and to accumulate in increasingly large numbers, forming a tumour that consists mostly of these abnormal cells. Another category includes agents that do not damage genes but instead selectively enhance the growth of tumour cells or their precursors. The primary danger of malignancies is that they can metastasize, allowing some of their cells to migrate and thus carry the disease to other parts of the body. Finally, the illness can reach and disrupt one of the body's vital organs. Development of a malignant tumour in epithelial tissue is illustrated schematically in Figure 14-2 (adopted from Weinberg, 1996). Epithelial tumours (carcinomas) are the most common malignancies. The tumour mass emerges as a result of mutations in genes and genetically altered cells.

Two gene classes (Table 14-1), namely oncogenes and tumour suppressor genes, which together constitute only a small proportion of the full genetic set, play major roles in triggering tumour (Gibbs and Oliff, 1994; Hinds and Weinberg, 1994).

In their normal configuration, they choreograph the life cycle of the cell, i.e., the intricate sequence of events by which a cell enlarges and divides. Proto-oncogenes encourage such growth, whereas tumour

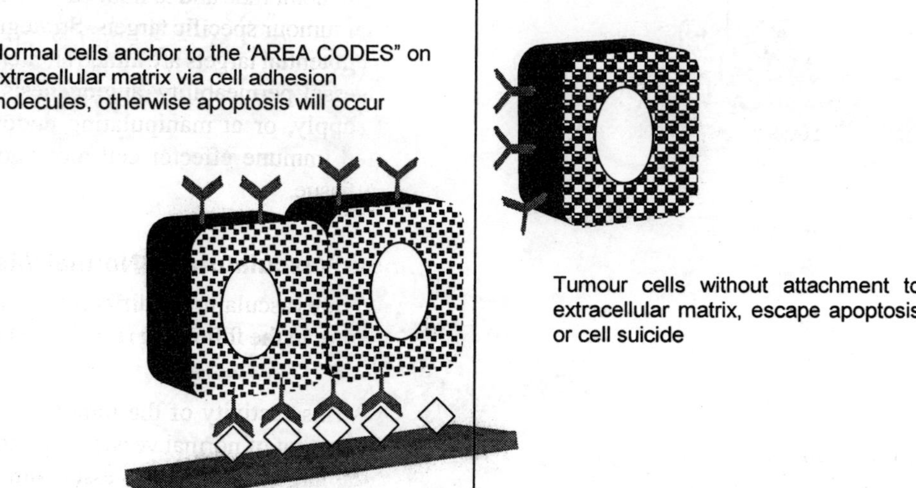

Fig. 14-1. Cellular Adhesion in Normal and Tumour Cells. Normal cells bind to area codes on ECM, whereas tumour cells do not require anchorage to ECM

suppressor genes inhibit it. Collectively these two gene classes account for much of the uncontrolled cell proliferation seen in human cancers. When mutated, proto-oncogenes can become carcinogenic oncogenes that drive excessive multiplication. The mutations may cause the proto-oncogene to yield too much of its encoded growth-stimulatory protein or an overly active form of it. Tumour suppressor genes, in contrast, contribute to tumour when they are inactivated by mutations. The resulting loss of functional suppressor proteins deprives the cell of crucial brakes that prevent inappropriate growth.

Thus proto-oncogenes code for proteins that stimulate cell division; mutated forms called oncogenes, can cause the stimulatory proteins to be overactive, with the result that tumour cells proliferate excessively (Gibbs and Oliff, 1994). Tumour suppressor genes code for proteins that inhibit cell division and these inhibitory messages are generally inactivated or lost during tumour development (Hinds and Weinberg, 1994). However, studies are aimed at introducing intact tumour suppressor genes into tumour cells to restore the normalcy to the cells (Oliff et al., 1996). Various stages of tumour development (Fig. 14-2) can be explained as follows (Vogelstein and Kinzler, 1993; Varmus and Weinstein 1993; Bishop, 1995):

1. Tumour evolution commences when a cell (or some of likes) within a normal population sustains a genetic mutation that expands its tendency to proliferate when it would normally rest.
2. Genetically altered cell and its offspring continue to appear normal, but they reproduce excessively and lead to a condition termed as hyperplasia. After some time (months or years) one in a million of these cells sustain additional mutation with subsequent loss of control on cell growth.
3. The offspring of this cell not only proliferate

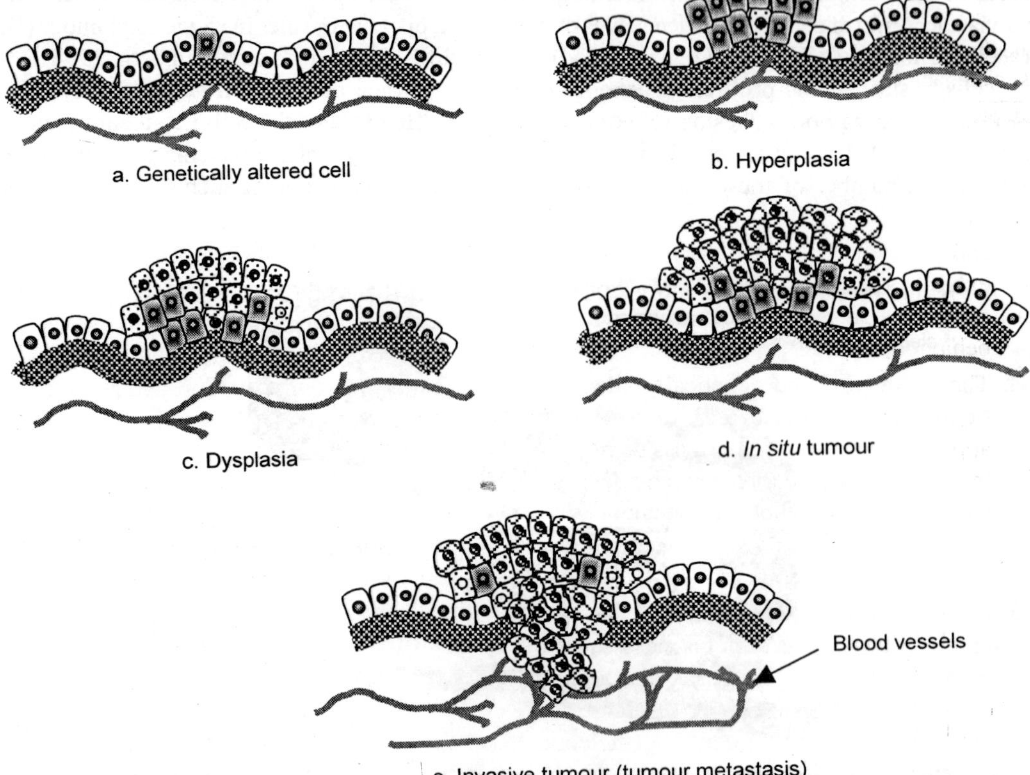

Fig. 14-2. Mechanisms and Stages of Tumour Development of Epithelial Origin

Table 14-1. Genes Involved in Human Tumours are Classified as Oncogenes and Tumour Suppressor Genes

Oncogenes	
Genes for growth factors or their receptors	PDGF codes for platelet-derived growth factor (involved in glioma, a brain cancer); erb-B codes for epidermal growth factor receptor (involved in glioblastoma and breast cancer); erb-B2 or HER-2 or neu codes for growth factor receptor (Involved in breast, salivary gland and ovarian cancers)
Genes for cytoplasmic relays in stimulatory signaling pathways	Ki-ras involved in lung, ovarian, colon and pancreatic cancers; N-ras involved in leukaemias
Genes for transcription factors that activate growth-promoting genes	c-myc Involved in leukaemias and breast, stomach and lung cancers; N-myc Involved in neuroblastoma (a nerve cell cancer) and glioblastoma; L-myc Involved in lung cancer
Genes for other kinds of molecules	Bcl-2 codes for protein that blocks cell suicide (involved in follicular B cell lymphoma); MDM2 codes for an antagonist of the p53 tumour suppressor protein (involved in sarcomas, a connective tissue cancer)
Tumour suppressor genes	
Genes for proteins in the cytoplasm	APC involved in colon and stomach cancers; DPC4 codes for a relay molecule in signaling pathway that inhibits cell division (involved in pancreatic cancer); NF-1 codes for a protein that inhibits a stimulatory (Ras) protein (involved in cancers of the peripheral nervous system)
Genes for proteins in the nucleus	RB codes for the pRB protein, a master brake of the cell cycle (involved in bone, bladder, small cell lung and breast cancer); p53 codes for the p53 protein, which can halt cell division (involved in a wide range of cancers)
Genes for proteins with unknown habitant	BRCA1 and BRCA2 involved in breast and ovarian cancers; VHL involved in renal cell cancer

Adopted from Weinberg, 1996

excessively but also appear abnormal in shape and in orientation. The tissue is now said to exhibit a condition referred as dysplasia. After some time, a further mutation that alters cell behaviour results.

4. The influenced and genetically altered cells become more abnormal in growth and appearance. If the tumour mass do not invade through any boundaries between tissues, it is termed as *in situ* tumour. This tumour may stay contained indefinitely or some cells may acquire additional mutations.
5. A malignant tumour results if the genetic changes allow the tumour mass to initiate invasion of underlying tissue and to cast off cells into the blood or lymph. The defector cells may install new tumour loci (metastases) throughout the body.

Vascularization and Localization of Drug Carriers in Tumours

Overall, the tumour vasculature within tumour tissue is highly disordered with numerous vascular shunts. Vascular haemodynamics and microvessel permeability are of utmost importance in determining the uptake of circulating drug-carrier complexes by tumours. The density of the functional vessels is lower and vascular diameters are irregular and slightly higher compared to normal tissues. Total blood flow, rates of perfusion and vessel permeability may vary significantly in different regions of the same tumours and in tumours of different types, like, spontaneous (Fig. 14-3A), transplanted (Fig. 14-3B) and metastases (Fig. 14-3C) (Peterson, 1979).

The vascular supply in tumours, transplanted subcutaneously or intramuscularly may differ significantly from that evolved through metastases. For example, implantation of a large bolus dose of tumour cells into host tissues (as occurs during animal model studies) disrupts the local micro-vasculature and surrounding tissue and enhances vasculature permeability at the injection site which persists until vasculature repair is achieved with 2-3 days time. Access of intravenous injected material is facilitated at such sites during this period and delivery of drug or drug-carrier construct within 24-48 hours of tumour implantation can result in remarkably high concentrations of drug within the tumour (Poste and Kirsh, 1983). The blood supply of transplanted tumours is established by migration of new capillary sprout (budding) from surrounding host vessels. These newly formed outgrowths are highly permeable and allow extensive movement of materials, including erythrocytes, into the extravascular tissue. Penetration of delivery systems like liposomes and immunotherapy with antibiotics or other circulating materials into transplanted tumours may thus be artificially high and will not provide an appropriate insight for the disposition of these drug-carrier constructs in the vascular bed of human tumours or spontaneous animal tumours. In latter, the vascular supply will evolve in an entirely different fashion in accordance with progressive enlargement of the tumour cell population.

In transplanted tumours new vessels grow in the peripheral region of the implant. However, in newly formed spontaneous tumours, which contain far fewer cells, the topographic relationship of tumour cells to blood capillaries will be completely different. Similarly, in formation of haematogenous metastases, a single tumour cell, or at most a few cells, extravasate and grow as pericapillary colonies before the angiogenic responses needed to support additional cell mass. These events suggest that localization of blood borne materials in the newly transplanted tumours is more likely to occur in the periphery but in spontaneous tumours and haematogenous metastases it will be central or uniform throughout the lesion.

In contrast to antibodies and macromolecules, where initial distribution is uniform throughout the capillary circulation, the disposition of particulate carriers like liposomes and microspheres is non-uniform and is influenced by particle size, surface charge, composition and vascular anatomy (Poste et al., 1984). The particulates are taken up by macrophages of RES in liver, spleen and bone marrow in size ranging from 0.1 to 5.0 μ. However, rapid clearance by RES is the major obstacle in targeting carriers to sites other than liver, spleen and bone marrow. The efforts are also being made to construct long-circulatory carriers for the targeting of extravascular tumours.

Barrier(s) Offered by Tumour Vasculature

The anatomy of the microcirculation in different tissues and organs can reasonably be expected to be of prime importance in determining whether drug carriers or antibodies conjugates can escape into the surrounding extravascular tissue. Like extravasation of circulating blood cells, extravasation of delivery systems can presumably be expected to be restricted to capillaries and small diameters post-capillary venules.

Blood capillaries are classified according to the architecture of the lining endothelium and the underlying subendothelial basement membrane (basal lamina). The three groups of capillaries have been identified (a) continuous (b) fenestrated and (c) discontinuous or sinusoidal (Fig. 14-4). In the continuous type, the endothelial cells are connected via tight junctions to form a continuous monolayer or an uninterrupted basement membrane. In the fenestrated capillaries the endothelium is interrupted by fenestrae of diameter 30-80 nm. The basal membrane in the fenestrated capillaries is continuous. The sinusoidal capillaries are found predominantly in the liver, spleen and bone marrow. They have a discontinuous endothelium and large fenestrae with a mean diameter of about 100 nm. Diagrammatic representation and the details are shown in Figure 14-4.

The natural distribution of small particulate delivery systems to RES limits the possibilities of delivering these drug carriers to other sites within the circulation. Hence, it was inferred on the basis of anatomical considerations discussed above that the extravascular compartmentalization of colloidal drug delivery systems can be achieved in the lungs, liver, spleen and bone marrow by manipulation of their

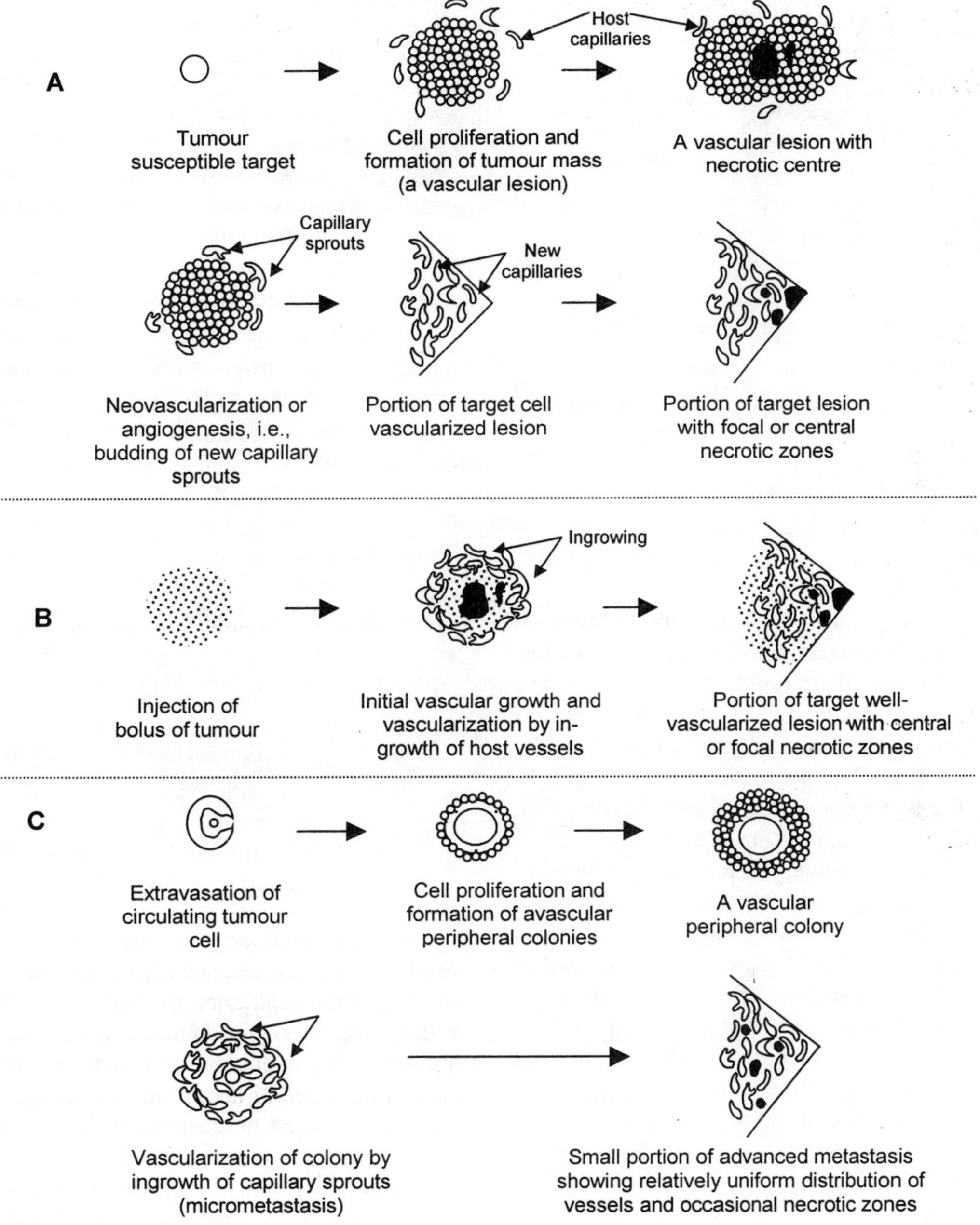

Fig. 14-3. Vascularization of Spontaneous Tumours (A), Transplanted Tumours (B) and Haematogenous Metastases (C) (Adopted from Poste, 1984 with modifications)

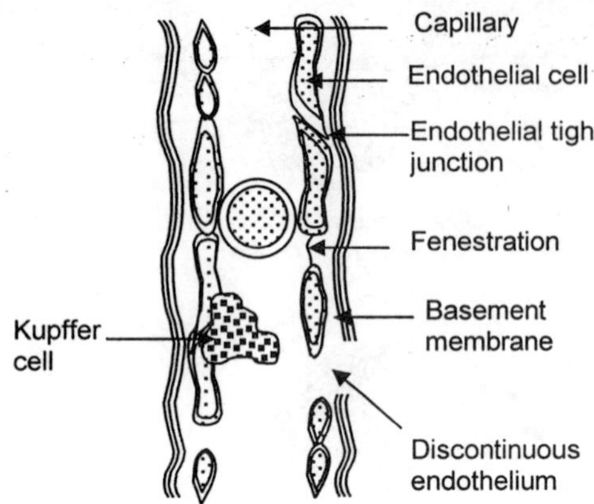

Fig. 14-4. The Capillary Endothelial Barrier

particle size. The localization of colloidal particles in the body after parenteral administration can be summarized (Illum et al., 1982; Illum et al., 1986; Illum et al., 1989) as follows:

- First, intravenous (i.v.) injection of particles of approximately 0.3-7.0 um in diameter, results into their rapid clearance from the systemic circulation via RES interception leading to their localization in the Kupffer cells of the liver. Particles of diameter between 100-300 nm pass through the fenestrations and then become localized in the hepatocytes.
- Second, i.v. delivery of particles greater than 7-13 μm in diameter leads to their mechanical filtration by the lung capillaries whereas particles of 1-8 μm diameter get localized in the liver and spleen. This has been utilized to target various macrophages activating agents to the lungs to improve the treatment of experimental lung metastases.
- Third, intraarterial administration of particles of size greater than about 13 μm leads to their retention in the first vasculature encountered.
- Fourth, alteration of the surface character of the particles allows them to avoid the RES scavenging, which leads to the possibility of directing them to other sites in the body.

Various reviews describe the barriers imposed to drug delivery to solid tumours and metastasis (Jain, 1994; Molema, 1997; Vyas et al., 2001). The major barrier posed by the tumour vasculature is the basal lamina (basement membrane) on which the endothelium rests and the endothelium itself. Permeability of the tumour blood vessels for transport of small molecules and macromolecular drug-carrier constructs is only sufficient in the blood vessels at the tumour host interface.

Down-regulation of the expression of adhesion molecules, which serve for recruitment of leukocyte molecules during inflammatory processes, subsequently facilitating the immune cell recruitment, by the tumour vasculature endothelium results in the escape of the tumour from host defense (Bates, 1995). In tumour therapy drugs or drug-carrier constructs have to cross the endothelial linings of the tumour blood vessels to reach the interstitial fluid. This is followed by travelling of constructs through the extracellular matrix towards the tumour cells. In addition to physical barrier posed by the endothelial cells, basement membrane and ECM, high interstitial pressure and low microvasculature pressure may additionally interfere with extravasation of molecules and cells into tumour tissues (Jain, 1994). Angiogenesis related factors influence both vascular permeability and immune cell recruitment. Permeability of tumour blood vessels is higher than vessels in normal tissue. There is, however, a large variation within different tumour.

MOLECULAR TARGETS FOR TUMOUR THERAPY

The drug-targeting concept was thought to be redefined as it has been severely invalidated in case of some pathological manifestations. For example, if endocytosis is required for cellular delivery, virus/tumour infected cells may be much less active in endocytosis due to the depletion of energy-rich metabolites or decreased expression of cell surface receptors. Success would seem to necessitate for some tumour cell associated receptors that are not found or expressed at extremely lower density level on the non-tumour cells. The molecular targets on the surface membrane of malignant cells may conveniently be divided in to following categories and could be targeted using the counter ligand or specially designed antibodies (Vyas et al., 2001):

- Altered expression of cell adhesion molecules and their ligands

- Altered expression of certain receptors otherwise expressed by all eukaryotic cells, like insulin receptors and MHC class-I associated compound receptors.
- Exquisite expression of receptors during certain stages of cellular differentiation, like transferrin receptor (TfR), folate receptors, apo-lipoprotein receptor, c-kit receptors, haemopexin receptor and MHC class-II associated compound receptors.
- Altered expression of certain growth factors (epidermal growth factor receptor, EGFr) and certain vasoactive and angiogenic peptides.
- Expression of tumour vasculature epitopes, either of the endothelial cells or of the basement membrane supporting the endothelial cells or tumour stroma components (30.5 kD antigen; CD19, CD34; endosialin; endoglin; F19 cell surface glycoprotein; fibronectin; fibrin; myosin and histone).
- Expression of surface determinants on malignant cells, like Ia antigens and tumour associated antigens (TAA).

Surface Determinants on the Tumour Sites

Targeting at the cellular level is particularly desirable in tumour chemotherapy where therapeutic indices are insignificant with conventional therapy. Success seems to rely on some tumour cell associated receptors that are either expressed at extremely lower density level or not expressed at all on the non-tumour cells.

There is a new search of glycoprotein and glycolipid tumour markers and/or tumour specific carbohydrate antigens (as surface determinants). The heterogeneity in the tumour population, however, raises a note of caution in the quest of cellular targeting regimen based on highly specific tumour markers. Tumour cell epitopes exploited in the cellular targeting are mainly based upon either tumour cell surface receptors or TAA (tumour associated antigens) and glyco-conjugate markers. Expression of the malignancy stigmata (i.e., tumourogenicity and metastatic activity) of the proliferating cell lines is a function of the interaction between cell membrane located receptors and epitopes in the cellular microenvironment. Tumour progression may lead to activation and expression of a number of normal genes, including those for growth factors and ligand-specific receptors, which are otherwise not expressed on normal cell lineage. The molecular receptors on the surface membrane of malignant cells may conveniently be divided in to three categories (Poste, 1984):

- Receptors expressed on virtually all the eukaryotic cells like insulin receptors and MHC class-I associated compound receptors. The MHC molecules may associate with membrane components to function as receptor sub-unit of hormone receptors (in particular insulin receptor).
- Receptors expressed during certain stages of cellular differentiation, like transferrin receptor (TfR), folate receptors, epidermal growth factor receptor (EGFR), apo-lipoprotein receptor, c-kit receptors, haemopexin receptor and MHC class-II associated compound receptors, are specifically over-expressed on proliferating tumour cell surfaces.
- Surface determinants expressed exclusively on malignant cells, like Ia antigens and tumour associated antigens (TAA). Carbohydrate epitopes and markers determine the tumour associated antigens and can be exploited to characterize and target a specific epitope of malignant cells. Carcinoembryonic antigen (CEA) and deleted in colon carcinoma (DCC) are the Ig family receptors over-expressed and down-regulated respectively in the colonic epithelial malignancies.

Folate, Transferrin, Fucose and Lipoproteins as Over-expressed Tumour Receptors

Receptor expression on the tumour cells has been considered one of the important consideration for the delivery of suitable bioactives to these sites. The receptors can be either over-expressed or down regulated in the malignant target sites. Depending upon the over-expression (folate, transferrin, fucose and lipoprotein) or down regulation (asialo-glycoprotein receptor, mannose receptor), effective cellular targeting approaches could be engineered.

Epitopes on Tumour Vascular Endothelium for Selective Drug Delivery

Tumour endothelial cells are suitable targets for targeted drug delivery and immunotherapy as they are accessible through the blood. The epitopes present on the tumour endothelial vasculature in the form of angiogenic peptides and adhesion molecules that interplay between cells, soluble factors and extracellular matrix components could be exploited to negotiate targeting and are summarized in Table 14-2. At least 20 angiogenic peptides have been found on tumour vasculature that influence the endothelial cells directly (e.g., EGF and VEGF) or indirectly by inducing host cells to produce endothelial cell growth factors (e.g., TNF and TGF).

Angiogenesis as a Target

The large number of cells within a non-operable solid tumour could only exist by virtue of formation of new capillaries, a process called as angiogenesis. It was observed that during the avascular phase of tumour growth, the size of the experimental tumour is limited. After an undefined period of time, new capillaries start to form and tumour mass increases (Folkman, 1995). Angiogenesis (or neovascularization) involves interplay between cells, soluble factors and extracellular matrix components (adhesion molecules).

Table 14-2. Potential Target Epitopes on Tumour Vascular Endothelium

Target epitope	Location of the target epitope
30.5 kD antigen	Proliferating tissue
CD34	Tips of vascular sprouts
Endosialin	Vascular endothelial cells of malignant tumours
VEGF/VEGF-R complex	VEGF-R overexpressed by endothelial cells in many tumours
Endoglin	Endothelial cells in miscellaneous human tumours
F19 cell surface glycoprotein	Stromal fibroblasts in stroma of more than 90% of epithelial tumours
Fibronectin	Basement membrane component
Fibrin	Stroma component

The knowledge of the involvement of angiogenesis in the growth of solid tumours led to new concepts in the targeted chemotherapy. New therapeutic approaches for the treatment of solid tumours are aimed at vasculature, either at the endothelial cells or at the basement membrane supporting the endothelial cells or tumour stroma components. Angiogenesis inhibitors like thrombospondin and angiostatin can selectively block angiogenesis (Folkman, 1996). These agents not only inhibit new blood vessel formation and thereby limit tumour tissue perfusion, but probably also interfere with the paracrine production of endothelial growth factors that stimulate tumour growth.

Angiogenic peptide like epidermal growth factor interacts with biological cell through their specific receptor that induces cell differentiation and proliferation upon activation through the binding of ligands and trigger tyrosine kinase mediated bioevents. It has been implicated in the development of tumour with co- or over-expression of ligand/receptor and EGFr mutations (Xu et al., 1984). The tumour necrosis factor families of cytokines are type II transmembrane proteins that are important regulators of homeostasis and have been implicated as mediators of tumour metastasis (Tsujimoto et al., 1986). These molecules serve as ligands for a family of cell surface receptors termed as tumour necrosis factor/nerve growth factor (TNF/NGF) receptor family. The receptors are type I trans-membrane proteins capable of mediating a wide range of responses *in vitro* and *in vivo*. Signal transduction is mediated by several newly discovered cytoplasmic proteins (and could be used as targeting ligand) that couple these receptors to downstream signaling events. Vascular endothelial cell growth factor (VEGF) has a central role in the regulation of angiogenesis by binding to its cognate receptor type II (VEGFr-II) (Wagner et al., 1992). VEGFr-II is an endothelial cell-specific trans-membrane tyrosine-kinase important for vascular endothelial cell development and differentiation during normal process of embryogenesis and angiogenesis under aetiological conditions (Jain, 1994).

IMMUNOTHERAPY OF TUMOUR

Immunotherapy of tumour, i.e., strategies aimed to attack disease with defense mechanism of the body, has been recognized widely and effective involvement of various immunocomponents of the body, i.e., tumour antigens (vaccine), antibodies, monoclonal antibodies, cytokines and immunotoxins may be considered as possible strategies in tumour therapeutics.

Antibodies as Targeting Tools

Antibodies bind to antigens on the surface of tumour cells, and in the process, make these cells susceptible to destruction by immunocomponents of the host defense mechanism or otherwise direct them for self-destruction (Mach, 1995). Antibodies can similarly target and attack the blood vessels feeding a tumour or the connective tissues (or stroma) supporting it. Antibodies can also block or neutralize the action of growth factors-chemicals that a tumour needs to grow. In addition, antibodies are used as guided missiles to deliver an array of therapeutic compounds to tumour sites as mentioned below (Old, 1996):

1. Enzymes that can convert prodrugs into cell killers will form an innocuous environment at or around tumours when attached to a tumour through tumour-specific antibody.
2. Chemotherapeutic agents when attached with antibodies are specifically delivered to tumour sites thus curtailing the dose and hence associated side and toxic effects.
3. Toxins, which inhibit protein synthesis and impede tumour growth, are toxic otherwise but in conjugation with antibodies they offer a great immuno-therapeutic modality.
4. Cytokines and inflammatory molecules, which include tumour necrosis factor and other messenger molecules of the immune system, can lead to tumour cell destruction owing to localized strong inflammatory responses.
5. Immune cells, guided by antibodies, such as genetically engineered T cells, can prompt tumour cell dissolution or lysis.
6. Genetic drugs, like antisense oligonucleotides may block the production of proteins needed by tumour cells, can be linked to antibodies directly, or packaged into viral particles equipped with targeting antibody on their surface.
7. Radioactive isotopes, such as ^{131}I or ^{99}Y, kill tumour cells by damaging their DNA.

Recombinant Antibodies

Immunoglobulin clustered on the surface of the target cell exposes its tail region (Fc) to be recognized by the Fc receptors (FcR) present on the surface of the macrophages and neutrophils (Garagiola et al., 1979; Cline and Sumner, 1972). Largely by means of such Fc receptors, the phagocytic cells of MPS negotiate tumour cell killing with the help of ligand-associated anti-receptor or chimeric antibodies developed against the tumour surface antigen determinants. Instead of using complete IgG or IgM, fragments with antigen binding sites (Fab) could be exploited as ligands for the FcR. F(ab') are univalent fragments with one antigen binding site, whereas F(ab')2 are bivalent with covalently linked F(ab') fragments. Receptors for the Fc portion of the Ig molecules are present on the all-developmental stages of mononuclear phagocytes but the number of the FcR increases as the cells differentiate from progenitors into monocytes and macrophages.

FcR dependent tumour cell killing of antibody coated tumour cells *in vitro* proceeds either via receptor mediated phagocytosis or by extracellular mechanisms, which operate probably through a reactive oxygen intermediate (ROI)-mediated mechanism. Monoclonal antibodies (Mabs) are now available for all the Fc receptors.

A new trend in the development of antibody-antigen (epitope) based targeting is the use of antibody fragment instead of whole immunoglobulin molecule (Unkless et al., 1981; Cho et al., 1997). The molecular size decreases from 150kD for an IgG via 50kD for a Fab' fragment to 27 kD for a single chain Fv protein (ScFv).

Recombinant antibody fragments are becoming well-sought strategy for the development of anti-tumour strategies (Fig. 14-5). The most common fragments produced in bacterial expression systems (phage display system) include Fab fragments, and single chain Fv fragments (SvFv) (Bird et al., 1988; Clackson et al., 1991; Cho et al., 1997; Neri and

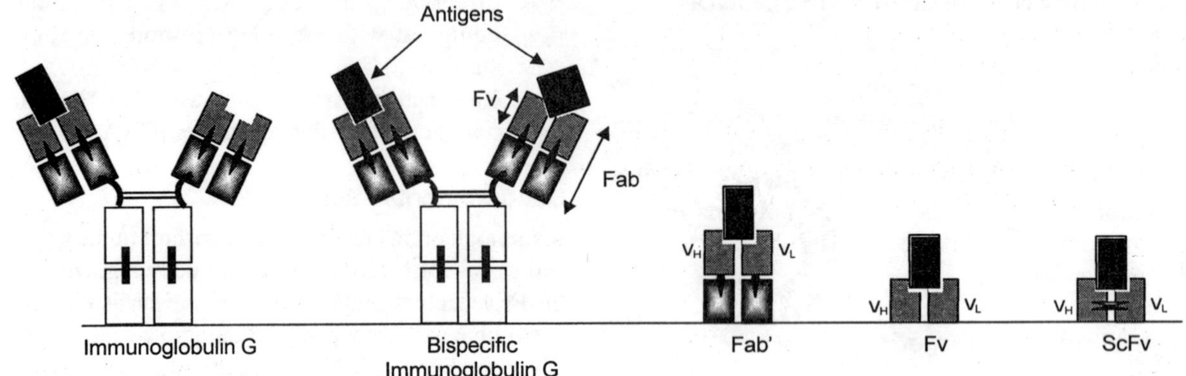

Fig. 14-5. Various Immunoglobulin Molecules and Their Fragments

Zardi, 1998). Antibodies in ScFv format consist of a single chain, comprising an antibody heavy chain variable domain (V_H) linked by a flexible polypeptide linker to a light chain variable domain (V_L). For practical applications, ScFv are generally preferred to Fv fragments. This has been suggested due to the fact that the polypeptide linker prevents the V_H and V_L domains from falling apart. ScFv and Fv fragments are the smallest antibody fragments that conserve the same binding affinity of the parent antibody. However, they may not demonstrate the same avidity.

The greatest potential of ScFv in antibody mediated ligand-targeting lies in the fact that they can be readily incorporated into fusion proteins with therapeutic entities. It was recently shown that anti-CEA ScFv located on all known tumour deposits in patients with CEA-producing tumours are exploited in tumour imaging studies.

Tumour site accumulation was slightly reduced compared to IgG and anti-CEA antibody (Begnet et al., 1996). This was proposed to be due to the monovalent antigenic nature of ScFv which, allowed for their rapid removal from circulation and tumour accumulation. In mouse tumour model, antibodies against the basement membrane component fibronectin could deliver vasoactive agents to tumour tissue.

Antibody Enzyme Conjugates

A novel strategy for the delivery of cytotoxic and antiviral agents to specific cell types is the prodrug activation by antibody-enzyme conjugates. Such antibody-coupled enzyme can be specifically delivered to the cell types that express antigenic determinant (Senter et al. 1990). Infact, the need for antibody internalization, which is one of the problems associated with immunoconjugates, is addressed in this strategy known as ADEPT (antibody directed enzyme prodrug therapy). The formation of active derivatives in the close proximity of the target cells could lead to higher cellular and lower systemic concentration of the active drug. Haisma and co-workers, 1992 described a Mab-β -glucuronidase conjugate as an activator of the prodrug epirubicin for the specific treatment of tumour.

An interesting strategy was developed towards selective and specific chemotherapeutics, namely enzymosomes. Enzymosomes are liposomal constructs engineered to provide a mini bioenvironment. Enzymes are covalently immobilized or coupled to the surface of liposomes, therefore, when a nontoxic prodrug is administered simultaneously, it is converted by the immobilized enzyme to a potent antitumour agent in the vicinity of tumour cell lines. The specificity of enzyme reaction provides the means to limit prodrug activation at the tumour site, through prior enzyme targeting by using liposomes, or via enzyme expressing gene delivery into the tumour cells (GDEPT). Figure 14-6 provides the concept of targeted delivery of antitumour prodrug activating enzymes with immunoliposomes (ADEPT based liposomal system), also known as immunoenzymosomes (Vingerhoeds et al., 1993). The enzyme bearing immunoliposomes are first targeted to tumour

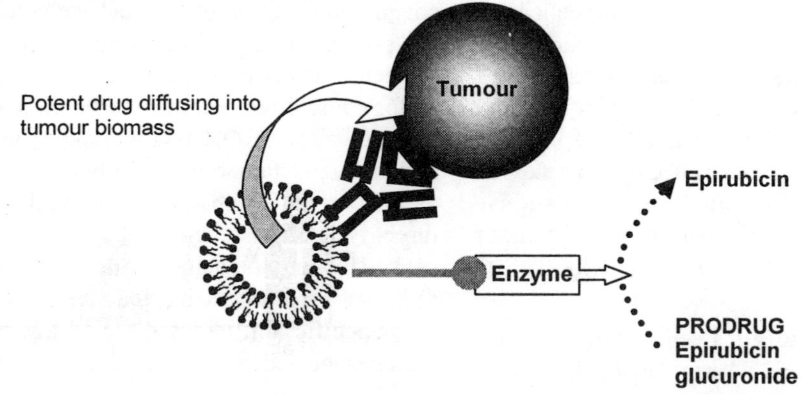

Fig. 14-6. Antibody Directed Enzyme Prodrug Therapy (ADEPT)

cell lines with the help of appropriate Mabs. After binding of the immuno-enzymes to target, a prodrug is administered, which is activated by cell bound immunoenzymes in the close proximity of the tumour cells. Vingerboeds and co-workers in 1993 reported the coupling of the enzyme β-glucuronidase, capable of activating the prodrug epirubicin-glucouronide, to epirubicin. It was found that pretreatment with enzymosomes (bearing no specific antitumour antibodies) or immunoliposomes (bearing no enzymes) were ineffective, but preincubation with immunozymes (enzymosomes) resulted into an enhanced antitumour activity of the prodrug.

It is the flexibility provided by the choice of enzymes for ADEPT/GDEPT (Antibody/Gene directed enzyme prodrug therapy) and the range of tumour antigen-targets that make these enzyme/prodrug/carrier seemingly a complex concept exploitable in tumour chemotherapy and gene therapy in the near future. There is a wide spectrum of antigen specific targets available, which provide opportunities of targeting a range of tumours with Mab-enzyme conjugates (ADEPT) and a range of antigen markers is also available which might be used for selective expression of prodrug activating enzymes coded by genes in GDEPT.

Sherwood, 1996 reported several enzyme-prodrug systems and proposed carboxypeptidase G2 enzyme and a nitrogen mustard prodrug based enzymosomes for further clinical trials. *Herpes simplex* virus-thymidine kinase (HSV-tk) has been a leading candidate conceivably suitable for VDEPT (virus directed EPT), based on large differential insensitivity to GCV (Gancyclovir) between cells expressing HSV-tk and parental cells.

Reddy and Low, 1998 has suggested the ADEPT approach that uses folic acid in place of monoclonal antibody. In their studies, penicillin-V-amidase, a fungal enzyme known to hydrolyse the prodrug, doxorubicin-N-p-hydroxy-phenoxy-acetamide (DPO) to free doxorubicin, was conjugated to folic acid and tested for *in vitro* cytotoxicity.

These workers suggested the use of folate targeted enzyme prodrug therapy *in vivo*, where factors such as tumour selectivity and immunogenic behaviour can be more accurately assessed and monitored.

Bispecific Antibodies

Bispecific antibodies is an attractive strategy for target specific drug delivery. The approach has basically been suggested in immunotherapy for circumventing the lack of MHC restricted recognition by immune effector cells (Staerz et al., 1985). Fanger et al., 1992, reported a chimeric combination of an anti-tumour antibody with an anti-lymphocyte antibody as a bi-specific protein that could redirect T-lymphocytes to lyse tumour cells. A similar approach was suggested for cytotoxic T-lymphocytes killing of HIV infected cell.

In this case, bispecific antibodies were produced that direct cytotoxic T-lymphocyte to cells expressing gp120 of HIV (Burg et al., 1991), thus specifically targeting the infected cell lines. By cross-linking effector cells (CTLs) and tumour cells, the CTLs were found to be capable of lysing the tumour cells in *in vitro* and *in vivo* (Krosen et al., 1995). In carcinoma patients, the combination treatment of interleukin-2 (subcutaneous) and BIS-1 F $(ab')_2$ (intravenous) bispecific antibody directed against epithelial glycoprotein-2 (EGP-2) and TcR/CD3 complex on T-lymphocytes elicited an immune response measured by elevated plasma levels of tumour necrosis factor-∝ and interferon-γ (Krosen et al., 1995).

Through cross-linking of T cell receptor and CD3 complex on the cytotoxic T-lymphocytes (CTLs) and epithelial glycoprotein-2 (EGP-2) on the target cell, the lymphocyte tends to be capable of actively lysing the target cells (Fig. 14-7). However, these studies indicated that the accumulation levels of bispecific antibody loaded CTLs were not sufficient for an absolute therapeutic effects at the tumour sites.

Further, to improve tumour site targeting, strategies are directed to selectively deliver CTLs against tumour endothelium, followed by site activation or site specific coagulation. Interference with tumour blood flow can inhibit tumour growth. This was achieved either by damaging the endothelial lining resulting in the formation of thrombi or by directly manipulating anti-coagulant activity (Burrow et al., 1995).

Bispecific antibodies directed against tumour endo-thelium on one hand and tissue factor (the initiator of the extrinsic pathway of blood coagulation) on the other hand were combined for the synergistic effects. *In vivo* application of the bivalent antibody plus a truncated form of tissue factor could directly induce thrombotic obstruction (Burrow et al., 1995) of the tumour blood vessels and facilitated targeting by antibody conjugates. Yet another option for obstructive blood flow is through direct lysis of endothelial cells by immune effector cells. This may be achieved using cross-linking of CTLs and tumour vascular endothelium with the help of bispecific antibodies directed against specific epitopes located on both cell types.

Bioconjugates of Immunotoxins/ Chimeric Proteins

Toxins are molecules that inactivate viral cytosolic components of the protein synthesis machinery in a catalytic manner. A major requirement of the toxins, therefore is to reach the cytosol of the target cells. Immuno-toxins (ITs) are conjugates of antibodies (Mab) or Fab' fragments and toxins (ricin) in which the cell binding moieties of the toxins are replaced by the binding specific chain of Ab (Fig. 14-8).

The complexation typically includes a disulphide bond between the antibody portion and the cytotoxic component of the conjugate to allow the release of the toxin intracellularly. Once endowed with specificity, toxin molecules inactivate vital cytosolic components of the protein synthesis machinery of viral infections in a specific and catalytic manner.

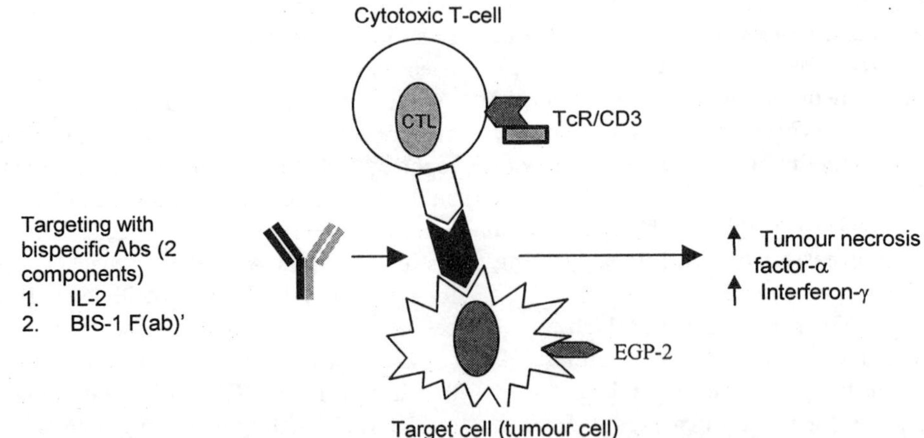

Fig. 14-7. Schematic Representation of Bispecific Antibody Mediated Lysis of Target Cells

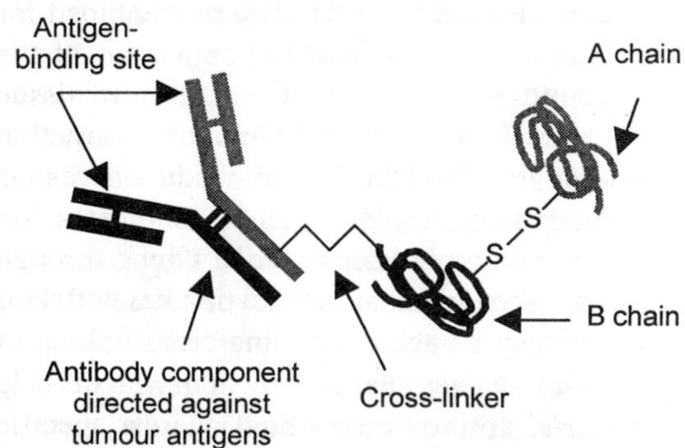

Fig. 14-8. The design of an immunotoxin conjugate consists of an antibody-targeting component cross-linked to a toxin molecule

The $F(ab)_2$ handled immuno-toxins may be anchored on the surface of carrier systems, which provide better projection to them and effectively present and place them to recognition sites, leading to receptor mediated endocytosis, eventually killing of cells which express Fc receptors. Liposomes equipped with immuno-toxins were developed for their possible use in the treatment of various tumours, the concept is well documented for antiviral therapy (Vitteta, 1990). Diphtheria toxin (DPT) is a potent cytotoxic, however, its selective and effective delivery has been a stigma. Liposomes have been appreciated to be a vector for DPT to deter them from immunoglobulin pool.

DPT inactivates vital cytosolic comp-onents of the protein synthesis machinery and can be effectively used in selective killing of target cell lines (Fig. 14-9). However, due to DPT anti-Mab pool (generated through immunization) encountered *in vivo*, DPTs are sequestered and thus obstructed for their access to the cytosol of the target cell lines (Nassander et al., 1992). The immobilization of liposomal DPT could deter them from anti-DTP-Mab and present them safely to tumour cell lines, and these engineered diphtheriosomes may be utilized as potential future strategy in 'pick and hit therapy'.

Problems of Delivery of Monoclonal Antibodies

Monoclonal antibodies to tumour-associated antigens have great theoretical potential for the specific targeting of radioactivity and anti-neoplastic agents to tumours. The clinical success of monoclonal antibody-based tumour diagnosis and therapy depends on solving a number of pharmacokinetic delivery problems (Oldham, 1983). These include: (i) slow elimination of monoclonal antibodies from the blood and poor vascular permeability; (ii) low and heterogenous tumour uptake; (iii) cross-reactivity with normal tissues; (iv) metabolism of monoclonal

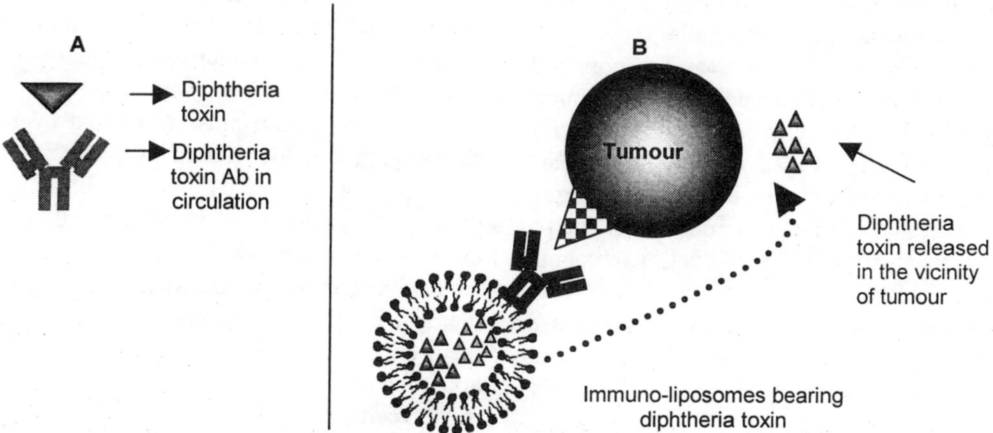

Fig. 14-9. Diphtheria toxin antibody pool encountered *in vivo* sequesters diphtheria toxin A (DTA) *en route* to cytosol of target cell (A). On the other hand, immobilization of DTA in immuno-liposome presents them safely to the tumour cell lines to affect cytosolic delivery (B)

antibody conjugates; and (v) immunogenicity of murine forms in humans. However, several potential solutions to these delivery problems have been identified and suggested. Blood concentrations of antibody conjugates may be reduced through regional administration, the use of antibody fragments (Fab', ScFv etc.), interventional strategies and various pre-targeting techniques (Unkeless et al., 1981; Cho et al., 1997).

Tumour uptake may be increased through administration of higher doses, or the use of agents to increase tumour vascular permeability. Tumour retention of antibody conjugates may be improved by inhibition of metabolism, by using more stable linkage chemistry. Alternatively, normal tissue retention may be decreased through the use of metabolisable chemical linkages inserted between the antibody and conjugated moiety. Very small antigen-binding fragments and peptides that exhibit improved tumour penetration and more rapid elimination from the blood and normal tissues have been prepared by genetic engineering techniques.

Tumour Antigens and Vaccines

In the antibody-guided immunotherapy, the immune molecules are provided to the patients (passive immunotherapy), a vaccine, on the other hand represents an active immunotherapy, as it prompts an immune response in the individual by activating their own immune system (Old, 1996). Some of the categories of tumour vaccines include:

1. Whole tumour cells: Inactivated tumour cells and their extracts can activate the immune system. Tumour cells engineered to secrete cytokines, such as IL-2 or GM-CSF, similarly augment antitumour immunity. Cells designed to express co-stimulatory molecules, such as B-7, enhance the ability of T cells to recognize tumour cells.
2. Peptides: Tumour peptides, fragments of tumour proteins recognized by T cells, are injected alone or with immune boosting adjuvants.
3. Proteins: Antigen presenting cells take up injected tumour proteins and break them down in to a range of peptidic fragments recognized by T cells.
4. Dendritic cells: These antigen presenting cells are isolated from the blood, exposed to tumour peptides or engineered to produce tumour proteins and then reinjected.
5. Gangliosides: Humans can produce antibodies to these molecules, such as GM2, found on the surface of tumour cells. Clinical studies have shown that melanoma patients with GM2 antibodies have a better diagnosis.
6. Heat-shock proteins: These cellular constituents ordinarily bind peptides, injecting heat shock proteins isolated from tumours provokes antitumour immunity in mice.
7. Viral and bacterial vectors: Genes coding for tumour antigens are incorporated into viral or bacterial genomes. When injected, these altered infectious agents trigger immunity against themselves and the encoded antigens.
8. Nucleic acid: DNA and RNA coding for tumour antigens prompt normal cells express these antigens and immunity against them.

Tumour vaccines are intended to induce T cells or other components of the immune system to recognize and vigorously attack malignant tissues. Whole tumour vaccines, whether genetically engineered or not, are giving ways to the vaccines that contain defined tumour antigens. Moreover, because peptide vaccines are easy to synthesize, they are taking the centrestage in clinical trials. Among the most promising targets for vaccines are abnormal proteins that are made when genetic mutations turn normal genes into tumour-related genes-known as oncogenes and tumour suppressor genes.

Similarly, human tumours caused by bacteria, such as gastric tumour caused by *Helicobacter pylori* infection, or caused by virus, such as cervical tumours, are prime targets for vaccine based therapies (Vyas and Sihorkar, 1999).

A recent approach, known as adoptive immunotherapy, involves stimulating T cells by exposing them to tumour cells or antigens in the laboratory and then injecting expanded populations of the treated cells into patients. However, it is not useful due to inter patient variability and thus rejection. The approach has its greatest value in treating viral tumours in patients whose immune system have been weakened by disease and therapy.

Opportunities being explored include const-ructing vaccines that combine a variety of antigens (called polyvalent vaccines); testing how well antibody- and antigen-based approach work together; and combining non-specific and specific immuno-therapies or even chemotherapy and/or drug delivery approaches.

Cytokines

Interleukin and interferon constitute a family of bio-ligands, which have their specific recognition site on the various cell types in the body and participate in the activation of the immune system and/or in the anti-viral modalities. Endogenous antiviral protein ligands like interferons (α and β) play an important regulatory role in the antiviral effect. On the other hand, γ-interferon activates neutrophils and may participate in the immune responses or may lead to macrophage activation (Tortora et al., 1998). Even γ-interferon enhances expression of cellular receptors for other regulatory molecules like tumour necrosis factor. Incubation of several human tumour cell lines with human interferon-γ (IFN-γ) increased the specific binding of subsequently added ^{125}I-labeled recombinant human tumour necrosis factor (TNF) (Depraetere and Joniau, 1995). Interferon has been investigated largely for their controlled delivery rather than site-specific delivery. However, some reports of the active targeting are documented where the conjugated recognition ligand like asialofetuin (specific for galactose specific receptors of hepatocytes), monoclonal antibody (against glioma associated antigen), and pullulan (non-specific affinity towards hepatic receptors) fortified the receptor specificity and avidity of the interferon (Ishihara et al., 1990; Mizuno et al., 1990; Xi et al., 1996; Yang and Cleland, 1997; Foldvari et al., 1999).

Interleukins constitute a family of potent lymphokines/cytokines that activate cells of the immune system (Kuby, 1994). Interleukin-2 (IL-2) is secreted by T-lymphocytes and upon activation by antigens becomes circulatory serum component. Similarly, other cytokines and non-specific mitogen equivocally stimulate the T-lymphocytes, which in turn secrete IL-2. IL-2 has been recognized as a possible therapeutic and adjuvant agent in the treatment of several diseases, including tumours, immuno-deficiency infections and for vaccination. These studies were the basis for the designing of different target oriented delivery systems, which help understand the regulation of IL-2 receptor expression and their clearance from the surface of the target (tumour) or activated cells.

Interleukins

Despite their pleiotropic properties, immuno-therapy with the respective cytokine ligands is restricted because these cytokines are rapidly cleared from the circulation and require high doses at which they induce toxic side effects (Nakamura et al., 1994; Okada et al., 1997). There have been various attempts to resolve the problems associated with the delivery of cytokines. Interleukin is gaining extensive research attention not only for its inherent therapeutic roles but also as a bio-ligand for site-specific targeting of conjugated or anchored bioactives (Table 14-3).

Recombinant cytokines are developed to circumvent unfavourable effects associated with endogenous IL-2. Sato and co-workers, 1993 investigated biological properties of an immune complex of recombinant interleukin-2 (rIL-2) and a monoclonal antibody against rIL-2 in mice for induction of killer cells and for anti-tumour activity. The results demonstrated that immune complex exerted a higher killer cell activity against YAC-1 cells and significant anti-tumour activity in a dose-dependent manner in Meth-A fibrosarcoma mice. In another development, polymer-conjugated cytokines (hybrid-cytokines), for instance PEG-modified IL-2 (Katre et al., 1987) and PEG-modified IL-6 (Tsunoda et al., 1998) were able to increase selectivity in their function but could not curtail the unfavourable functions. Targeted drug delivery using conjugates of cytokines with a variety of delivery systems including liposomes, micro-spheres, microcapsules, supramolecular biovectors, ceramics and chimeric proteins stabilizes the cytokines and potentiates only the selective functions *in vivo*. To further control the pharmacokinetics and pharmacodynamics *in vivo*, drug delivery systems using hybrid cytokines are devised with increased stability and selectivity (Anderson et al., 1992; Tsunoda et al., 1998). Though the cytokines are investigated mainly in the encapsulated/entrapped forms yet they maintain their

Table 14-3. Conjugates of Cytokine Molecules*

Target cell/ site	Delivery system	Activity
YAC-1 tumour cells/Meth A fibrosarcoma	Recombinant IL-2 immuno-complexed with Mab against rIL-2	Induction of killer cells for anti-tumour activity
Murine CTLL-2 T cell line / human mitogen activated PBLs	Interleukin-2 chemically coupled to liposomes	Receptor mediated immunotherapy
Human tumour xenograft/ Severe combined immuno-deficiency (SCID) mouse	IL-2 loaded poly(lactic acid) microsphere	Suppression of implanted tumour
IL-2 receptor bearing T cells (*in vitro*)	IL-2 in sterically stabilized liposomes	Anti-tumour activity in mice
Metastatic liver tumour	IL-2 in galactose containing liposomes	Enhancement of anti-tumour activity of lymphocytes
Hepatic sinusoidal lymphocytes/ hepatic metastasis in C3H/Me mice	IL-2 in galactose containing liposomes (Gal-lip-IL-2)	Activation of hepatic sinusoidal lymphocytes and local anti-tumour activity in liver
IL-6 transgenic mice	Alginate-poly(L)lysine-alginate membrane microencapsulating SK2 hybridoma cells	Suppression of IgG1 plasmacytosis in the IL-6 transgenic mice
Liver sites in BALB/c mice	Recombinant human interferon-pullulan conjugates	Enhancement of IFN-induced enzyme (2-5A) activity

*Adopted from Vyas and Sihorkar, 2000

ligand specificity and bind selectively to their specific receptor portals. The IL-2 bearing immunoliposomes present a new class of cell-specific systems whose entry into the cytoplasm is regulated by cell surface receptor and associated cellular events. In order to increase the targetability of the liposome encapsulate IL-2, a galactose receptor specific ligand was appended to facilitate the selective uptake by liver parenchymal cells bearing galactose-specific receptors (Okuno et al., 1998). These Gal-Lip-IL-2 liposomes were administered to C3H/He mice and *in vitro* anti-tumour activity of hepatic sinusoidal lymphocytes and *in vivo* hepatic metastases measurements were made. The results confirmed earlier reports of Nakamura and co-workers, 1994 in which they demonstrated highest accumulation and localization effects on the anti-tumour activity of the lymphocytes at the liver sites. The system with enhanced IL-2 presentation activated the hepatic sinusoidal lymphocytes and increased the local anti-tumour activity in the liver. Interleukin is also exploited as bioligand for better antigen presentation of complexed or conjugated antigen/determinants.

MOLECULAR APPROACHES IN TUMOUR THERAPY

Treating tumour at the molecular level includes repairing faulty DNA, shutting down key growth proteins, making use of cell adhesion molecules for ferrying of ligands to the tumour sites and increasing tumour cell's sensitivity towards conventional therapy, such as radiation.

Vasoactive and Angiogenic Peptides

Tumour endothelial cells constitute a suitable target for targeted drug delivery and immunotherapy, as they are accessible through the blood. The epitopes present on the tumour endothelial vasculature in the form of angiogenic peptides and adhesion molecules that interplay between cells, soluble factors and extra-cellular matrix components could be exploited for targeting. At least 20 angiogenic peptides have been found on tumour vasculature that influence the endothelial cells directly (e.g., EGF and VEGF) or indirectly by inducing host cells to produce endothelial cell growth factors (e.g., TNF and TGF) (Table 14-4).

The epidermal growth factor receptor (EGFr) is over-expressed in a variety of human tumours (Xu et al., 1984) and is reportedly involved in transduction of cell growth signals. Rosenberg et al., 1989 targeted liposomes using a sandwich strategy to the cultured rat pheochromocytoma and human melanoma cells expressing receptors for nerve growth factor (NGFr). In their study these investigators incubated cells with biotinylated NGF and treated them with liposome-coupled streptividin. Vascular endothelial growth factor mRNA antisense has shown to block expression of VEGFr and thereby suppresses the transforming phenotype of human carcinoma cell lines, KB cells (Wagner et al., 1992). However, the delivery of VEGFr anti-sense oligonucleotides (ODNs) within liposomes that are further conjugated to folate via polyethylene glycol has recorded nine times higher uptake of ODNs than the uptake resulted in the case of plain liposomes and 16 times higher than soluble or non-encapsulated ODNs. Endoglin, an essential component of the tumour growth factor receptor (TGFr) complex of human endothelial cells used as a proliferating marker that is upregulated on endothelial cells in cases of miscellaneous human solid tumours (Burrow et al., 1995).

The most of small cell lung tumours (SCLCs) ectopically express high levels of the c-kit receptors (Nishida et al., 1997). These receptors have been exploited for the selective targeting of a chimeric toxin (mSCF-PE40) composed of murine stem cell factor (SCF) genetically fused to the N-terminus of a modified form of *Pseudomonas* exotoxin (PE) lacking its cell-recognition domain. Selective cytotoxicity was recorded for human c-kit receptor-negative cells. Mabs and anti-idiotype (or, anti-anti-idiotype) Mabs directed to tumour determinants define specific epitopes along a polypeptide chain of integral membrane proteins. One such target epitope is the F19 cell surface glycoprotein of reactive stromal fibroblasts present in the basement membrane of more than 90% of common epithelial tumours. Stroma component fibrin has been identified as a tumour epitope and antibody was developed against it, on the basis of the observations that especially in tumour tissues fibrin deposition is a pre-requisite for stroma deposition and extracellular matrix formation (Molema et al., 1997).

The tumour target epitopes are not presented as homogenous target populations and are hampered most of the time by lack of basement membrane or hampered expression of adhesion molecules that can facilitate drug/carrier/immune cell adhesion and trans-endothelial migration to the tumour site.

Fas receptor-Fas ligand systems

The progress has been made in using Fas (CD95, Apo-1) ligand gene for the treatment of tumours. Fas ligand (FasL) is a member of the tumour necrosis

Table 14-4. The Use of Vasoactive and Angiogenic Peptides as Targeting Ligand*

Target cell/ site	Delivery system	Receptor
Tumour cells	Anti-EGF receptor antibody (B4G7) conjugated to poly(L-lysine)	EGFr
Human carcinoma cell lines (KB cells)	VEGFr antisense oligonucleotides in PEG-grafted liposomes	VEGFr
Human melanoma cells	'Sandwich' of biotinylated NGF and liposome coupled streptividin	NGFr
Human brain tumour	Radiolabeled EGF-Ox 26 MoAb conjugate	Transferrin receptor
Blood brain barrier	Radiolabeled NGF-Ox 26 MoAb conjugate	Transferrin receptor
Tumour cell line	EGF peptides and anti-receptor antibody	EGFr
Tumour cells	Tumour necrosis factor conjugated with dextran based on metal chelation	TNFr
Tumour cells	Amylopectin hydrogel immobilized growth factor	EGFr
Tumour cells	TNF-interferon conjugates	TNfr

*Adopted from Vyas and Sihorkar, 2000

factor family that can induce both apoptosis and activation of immune cells. While Fas ligand gene transfer eliminates tumour cells and inflammatory cells through apoptosis, it also kills normal cells and initiates inflammation in certain tissues (Fig. 14-10). Thus, new strategies that can modify the apoptotic or pro-inflammatory activities of the FasL will help to fully realize the potential of the FasL gene therapy. TNF ligand family members include TNF-α, LT-α, Fas L, CD 40L, CD 30L, CD27L and TRAILL/APO2L among others. Fas apoptosis induced systems (Fas-FasL system) has emerged as a major effector of cytotoxic T-lymphocytes (CTL)-mediated cell death along with the perforin pathway. Cell surface expression of FasL on CTLs or NK cells is used to kill target cells through the Fas receptors. In contrast with the perforin pathway the effector mechanism of Fas induced apoptosis is Ca^{++} independent. By the induction of programmed cell death of target cells, intracellular pathogens can be eradicated.

For example, hepatocytes express high levels of Fas receptors, and are thought that this may be the primary pathway used for infiltrating CTLs to target infected cells to remove viral hepatitis. Another role for the Fas-FasL system is in the maintenance of the immuno-privilege status of certain tissue. High levels of FasL are constitutively expressed in the eye epithelium and testicular Sertoli cells. Insult or injury that would normally lead to infiltration of mononuclear cells and tissue destruction by the local inflammatory response is prevented. This is due to the reason that the infiltrating cells express Fas receptors and are induced to undergo apoptotic cell death by tissue derived FasL. This mechanism has been implicated and co-opted by melanoma and hepatoma cells. These cells express FasL and are capable of killing Fas receptor-positive cells *in vitro*. This may be one of the several mechanisms by which tumours evade immuno-surveillance. Similar implications arise in graft-versus host disease (GVHD) where FasL expressing lymphocytes in transplanted tissue serve to damage host Fas-receptor bearing cells. In all these cases a potential exists for the Fas receptor-ligand antagonists to reverse these processes and provide site specific delivery and targeting to the Fas expressing systems. Equilibrium in certain factors like that of death receptors (Fas) and antiapoptotic protein (Bcl-x_L) has been suggested for the modulation of cell death signaling pathways. Anti-apoptotic protein (Bcl-x_L) promotes ADP/ATP exchange across the mitochondrial membrane and suggested that this prevents the change in the polarity of the mitochondrial membrane caused by the growth factor withdrawal that normally leads to mitochondrial swelling , cytochrome C release, and apoptotic cell death (Fig. 14-11) however, this needs to be further investigated.

Cell Adhesion Molecules

Cell adhesion molecules are glycoproteins expressed on the cell membrane and are involved in homotypic and heterotypic cell interactions through their

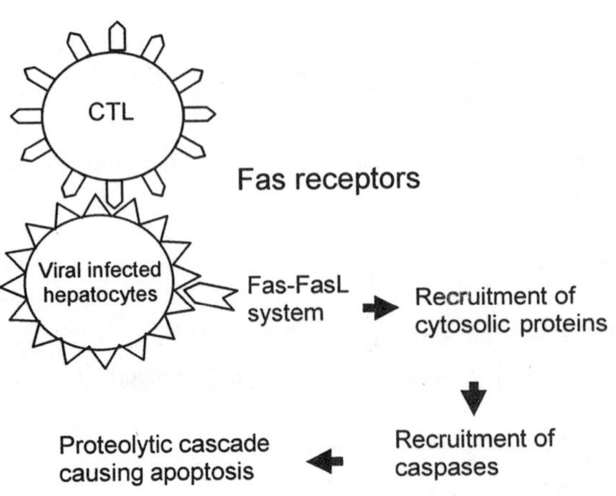

Fas-FasL SYSTEM

- Major effector of cytotoxic T-lymphocytes mediated cell death
- In infiltrating CTL to eradicate intracellular pathogenesis
- Maintenance of immunoprivilage status of certain tissues
- Maintenance of immunosurveillance of the tumour cells
- Graft versus host disease

Fig. 14-10. Mechanisms Operating for Fas-FasL System for the Apoptotic Gene Therapy

respective receptors (Frenette and Wagner 1996a, 1996b). Since cell-cell interactions are crucial in patho-physiological events, adhesion molecules play instrumental roles in processes like wound healing, tumour metastasis, lymphocyte homing and granulocyte extravasation and expression of leukocyte receptors for ligands (Berg et al., 1991) (Fig. 14-12). These include members of cadherin and immunoglobulin super family (CAM), selectins and integrins and membrane associated proteoglycans.

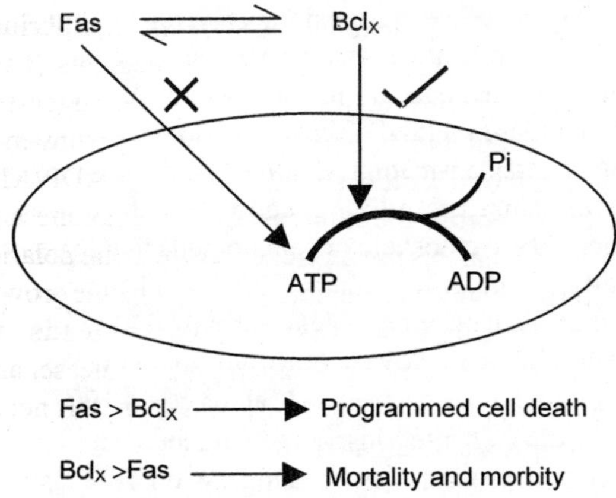

Fig. 14-11 Equilibrium Between Fas and Bclv for the Modulation of Cell Death Signaling Pathway

Cell Adhesion Molecule (CAM): Immunoglobulin Super Family and Cadherins

Induction and/or increased expression of certain cell adhesion molecules associated receptors at inflammatory and tumour loci or in various diseases, offer opportunities for the development of new targeting strategies. Monoclonal antibodies against adhesion molecules have been used to inhibit leukocyte recruitment in the areas of inflammation and metastasis. Another opportunity for therapeutic intervention is to couple these monoclonal antibodies to the liposomes for the purpose of drug targeting. CAMs include ICAM, VCAM, NCAM and PECAM (standing for intracellular, vascular, neural cell and platelet/endothelial cell adhesion molecules respectively). Strategic development of target modules using these cell adhesion molecules is hampered due to heterotypic and homotypic interactions of these adhesion molecules with their ligands *in vivo*. In contrast to NCAM and PECAM, which are homotypic calcium-independent adhesion receptor, all other IG family receptors are heterotypic in their interaction.

Bloemen and co-workers, 1995 have reported the first strategic development for the specific delivery of bioactives to the target sites, which excessively express adhesion molecules. Increased levels of VCAM-1 and ICAM-1 have been observed in tumour patients. The anti-ICAM monoclonal antibody F10.2 was conjugated to liposomes to target them to the cells expressing the cell adhesion molecule ICAM-1. The degree of ICAM-1 expression was reported

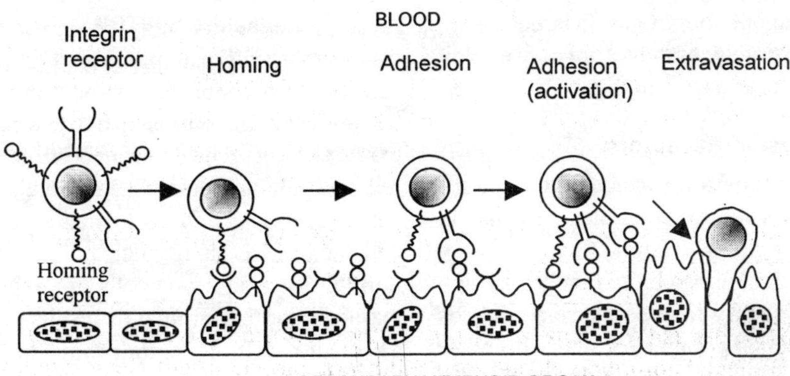

Fig. 14-12. Role of Cell-cell Adhesion Process in Leukocyte Migration to Secondary Organs

to be the limiting factor in quantitative immunoliposome binding to the target cells. Various malignant tumour cells are known to express these cell adhesion molecules on their surfaces and could be exploited as targeting ligands in the management of inflammation, metastasis and differentiation. PECAM-1 loaded liposomes associate with cell expressing human PECAM-1 receptors, however, the homotypic association may lead to aggregation and may therefore, hamper their possible utilization as ligand (Sun et al., 1996).

The cadherin receptors constitute a family of calcium-dependent adhesion receptor that are usually engaged in the cell-cell adhesion and differentiation (Frenette and Wagner, 1996a; 1996b). Three types of cadherins have been identified in mammalian tissues namely, N (neural and muscle cells)-, E (epithelium and sensory neurons)-, and P (placenta and mesothelium)-cadherins. Decreased expression of cadherins in carcinomas is associated with a malignant phenotype.

The restoration of cadherin expression by gene transfer can render the transformed cells less invasive. Thus adherin receptors in general are identified to affect tumour suppressor genes, most notably in colon carcinoma. No targeting strategy using cadherins as targeting ligands has been reported so far. Furthermore, the homotypic association (as observed with PECAM-1) may hamper its utility as a targeting ligand.

Nevertheless, the HAV (his-ala-val) tri-peptide sequence has been identified as a ligand for the N- and E-cadherins and is under investigation for its possible role in tumour metastasis (Mareel et al., 1996). A targeting strategy of the future may exploit this peptide sequence as a sensing ligand.

Integrin- cell Adhesion Receptors

Integrins are a family of cell surface glycoproteins that act as receptors for extracellular cell matrix (ECM) proteins (e.g., the β-1 family), serum components (α-v family), immunoglobulin family adhesion molecules (the β-2 family) and cell surface ligands or for membrane bound counter receptors on other cells (Lafrenie and Yamada, 1996). ECM molecules include collagen, vitronectin, fibronectin, laminin, fibrinogen and elastin, which play key roles in cell migration, differentiation and tissue structuring. Integrins can bind more than one type of ligand and latter in turn, can be recognized by different integrins. Signals can be transmitted to and from the cells through the integrins. The interaction of integrins with their ligands or counter receptors was initially considered to be a one-way process in those cells, which actively regulate the interaction of integrins with their ligands ("inside-out signaling"). In contrast, it is also obvious that cells receive a signal from outside via integrin heterodimers following ligand binding ('outside-in signaling').

Cells can modify the conformation of their integrins, controlling affinity for their ligands. The acquisition of cell adhesion, differentiation and expression by integrins may be a consequence of conformational changes in these receptors that result in an increased ligand affinity. In addition, cells can control integrin-mediated adhesion through other mechanisms, including receptor clustering and association to cytoskeleton, phenomena that regulate avidity of integrin receptors for ligand molecules without altering monovalent activity. These phenomena have collectively been designated as 'post-receptor occupancy events'(Mateos et al., 1996).

Binding of integrins to their ligands can signal either cell proliferation or suppression (Ruoslahti, 1996) and depending upon other cell signals, binding loss may induce apoptosis (Bates et al., 1995). Integrin family includes lymphocytes fusion associated antigen (LFA1) and very late antigens (VLA) that have laminin, collagen and fibronectin as ligands. Quantitative changes in integrin expression levels occur which may be specific to particular tumour type, for example loss of expression of avb1 "fibronectin receptor" in both transformed and tumour cells. In contrast to avb1, loss of cell surface expression of avb3 "vitronectin receptor" leads to reduced tumourogenicity (Bates et al., 1995). Integrin signaling has been found to mediate the programmed cell death (PCD) in normal and transformed cells. In normal or transformed cells binding of integrins to extracellular matrix ligands results in the generation of an intracellular signal that contributes to the suppression of programmed cell death. When normal cells are detached from the ECM, the un-liganded (free) integrins deliver an intracellular signal that promotes PCD. In transformed cells the loss of certain endogenous integrins may lead to tumours development by ablating the normal signals that trigger PCD, while the presence of an ectopically expressed and unliganded integrin may restore the signal that triggers PCD.

Monoclonal antibodies directed against receptor subunits, or synthetic proteins (peptide) that contain the recognizable peptide sequences, may halt integrin receptor-ligand (mainly ECM) binding. This inhibition of cell adhesion has important influence on molecular basis of ligand-integrin interactions and on malignant cell growth and metastasis. The $\alpha v\beta 3$ integrin is normally found over-expressed on endothelial cells during neovascularization (Varner et al., 1995) and is associated with diseases as diverse as metastatic tumour and macular degeneration (Filardo et al., 1995).

Barbas and co-workers, 1993 demonstrated the use of semi-synthetic human antibodies that bind integrins $\alpha v\beta 3$ and $IIb\beta 3$ with high affinity. The selected antibodies mimic natural ligands of integrins as demonstrated by their ability to compete with these ligands and RGD (arg-gly-asp)-containing peptides for binding to the integrins. Semi-synthetic or synthetic monoclonal antibodies that target integrin receptors are potential therapeutic ligands for a number of diseases including thrombosis and metastasis.

Drake and co-workers, 1995 have demonstrated that antibody (LM609) to $\alpha v\beta 3$ can block normal endothelial development causing vascular malformation during vasculogenesis (Drake et al., 1995). Sipikins et al., 1996, recently used antibodies to the $\alpha v\beta 3$ integrin to target liposomes to sites of tumour associated angiogenesis. These workers coupled approximately 50 biotinylated antibodies to each avidin-coated liposomes producing high avidity multivalent vesicles. The further exploitation of these liposomes loaded with a paramagnetic marker for MRI imaging of rabbit V2 carcinoma revealed their capability of selective targeting of chemotherapeutic agents to tumour-associated vasculature *in vivo*. Interestingly, the integrin receptors recognize small peptidic sequences in ECM molecules or on their synthetic ligands to which they bind, a tripeptide RGD (D'Souza et al., 1991).

Synthetic peptides with sequences specific for fibronectin (RGD) or laminin (YIGSR, tyrosine-isoleucine-glycine-serine-arginine) have been found to have anti-metastatic effects (Foxall et al., 1992; Gold, 1995).

When coadministered, these ECM-related peptidic fractions have been shown to bind tumour cells inhibiting their metastatic potential. Figure 14-13 explains the possible future strategy for the inhibition of metastasis of the tumour using RGD peptide. RGD tripeptide, being a fragment of fibronectin, discourages melanoma cells from spreading (metastasis), presumably RGD molecules block receptors that a wandering tumour cell needs for binding to fibronectin and hence in the extracellular matrix of the tissue.

Nishiya and Sloan, 1996 prepared DMPG/DMPC liposomes incorporating RGD-PE and demonstrated that RGD ligand could increase platelet uptake of liposomes by four to five-fold over unmodified vesicles. Zalipsky et al., 1995, coupled approximately 200-500 YIGSR molecules to liposomes through PEG chains. A slight decrease (23h vs 28 h for underivatized PEG liposomes) in mean residence time (MRT) was recorded that could be attributed to faster clearance rates for liposomes with greater amounts of surface bound peptides. Some of the targeting strategies are summarized in Table 14-5.

Selectin-cell adhesion receptors

The selectins are comprised of a recently discovered family of calcium dependent carbohydrate binding lectin like receptors. The selectins are a family of three proteins that mediate interactions between

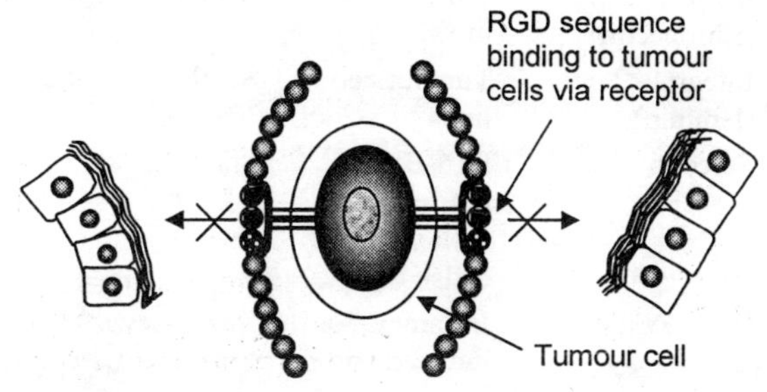

Fig. 14-13. Inhibition of Metastasis and Extracellular Adhesion of Tumour Cell by RGD Peptide

leukocytes and endothelium and between leukocytes and platelets in the blood vascular compartments (Frenette and Wagner, 1996a; 1996b).

Selectin family includes LECAM, ELCAM and PECAM adhesion factors (respectively leukocytes/endothelial, endothelial/leukocytes and platelet/endothelial adhesion molecules (CD62) that have the carbohydrate sialyl Lewis^x and heparin as counter receptors) known as L-selectin, E-selectin and P-selectin respectively (Bevilacqua and Nelson, 1993; Bevilacqua et al., 1994).

The selectins mediate cell adhesion by recognition of cell-specific carbohydrate ligands. Each membrane contains an amino-terminated C-type lectin domain or carbohydrate recognition domain followed by an epidermal growth factor (EGF)-like motif, short consensus repeats (SCRs) similar to those found in complement-regulatory proteins, a transmembrane domain, and a cytoplasmic tail. Great attention has been paid to these proteins because of their involvement in the recruitment of leukocytes to the inflammatory tissue sites and their resultant regulation profile (Springer, 1994; Lasky, 1995). Further impetus to this field derives from the fact that selectins function as lectin-like receptors by virtue of the C-type domains at their amino termini.

Unlike, other cell adhesion molecules that bind proteins, the selectins bind (with different avidities, depending upon ligand and selectin combinations) to carbohydrate ligands including the tetrasaccharide glycolipids sialyl-Lewis X (sLe^x) and sialyl-LewisA (sLe^a) (Fig. 14-14). Thus all selectins can bind to sialylated, fucosylated lactosamonoglycans, particularly sialyl Lewis X motif; such motifs can appear on glycolipids as well as glycoproteins (Rosen and Bertozzi, 1994).

Table 14-5. CAM Receptors and Ligands

Receptor	Target cell/site	Ligand
Integrin $\alpha v\beta 3$ (vitronectin)	Tumour cell	Antibodies to $\alpha v\beta 3$ (LM 609)
Integrin $\alpha 5\beta 1$ (fibronectin)	Tumour cell lines	Synthetic peptide RGD
Integrin (laminin)	Tumour cell lines	Synthetic peptide YIGSR
Selectin	B16-BL6 murine melanoma cells	Sialyl Lewis^X (sLe^X)
E-Selectin	Inflammation induced mice	Sialyl Lewis^X-Carboxy-methyl pullulan conjugates

*Adopted from Vyas and Sihorkar, 2000

Recently, mucin like glycoprotein ligands for L-selectin and P-selectins have been cloned, indicating that glycoproteins rather than glycolipids are the most significant targets of selectin. Given evidences that selectins play an important role in inflammation, reperfusion injuries and neoplastic metastases, several groups have explored the therapeutic potential of small molecular derivatives of sLe^x (Lefer et al., 1994; Albelda et al., 1995). As monomers, sLe^X ligands have low affinities, require relative large doses, and display limited selectivity for specific selectins (Foxall et al., 1992).

Liposome presentation however, can ensure higher avidities providing co-operative binding, which sLe^x and small peptidic molecules would be unable to achieve as monomers.

Saiki and co-workers, 1996 compared liposomal formulations equipped with either RGD peptide or synthetic sLe^x analogues as ligands for selectin and integrin binding respectively for the management of neoplastic metastases. These ligand appended liposomal formulations were challenged with circulating B16-BL6 murine melanoma cells, and it was demonstrated that a significantly higher tumour inhibition and cell arrest was recorded in case of liposomal sLe^x, over RGD liposomes. Liposomal sLe^x was also able to inhibit formation of lung metastases (suppressing 57% of control values). However, RGD liposomes, in contrast inhibited formation of lung tumour colonies and further suppressed formation of tumour colonies from spontaneous metastases. Ligand appended liposomes in both the cases provided co-operative binding with higher avidity and affinity via surfacial immobilization and better presentation of associated ligands as compared against free ligands.

Various strategies are adopted to target tumour site associated angiogenesis or other inflammatory environments with liposome immobilized ligands,

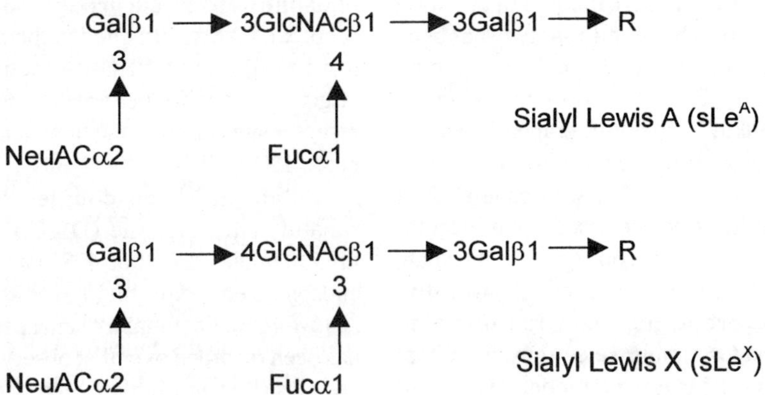

Fig. 14-14. The Binding Epitopes of the Oligosaccharide Ligands of the LEC Cell Adhesion Molecules

where adhesion receptors (or ligands) serve as molecular targets (Fig. 14-15).

Targeting can be achieved using RGD or YIGSR immobilized on liposome surface and allowing their interaction with integrin receptors on normal or malignant cells. Targeting can be achieved using synthetic antibodies anchored on the liposomes to bind to integrins and other CAM molecules by mimicking their natural ligands. Targeting can be achieved by immobilizing specific carbohydrate ligands (sLe^x and sLe^a) on liposomes, which show specific interaction with selectin. These strategies are directed either to block the normal recruitment of leukocytes during vasculogenesis or for selective targeting of chemotherapeutic agents to tumour-associated vasculature (Vyas and Sihorkar, 2000).

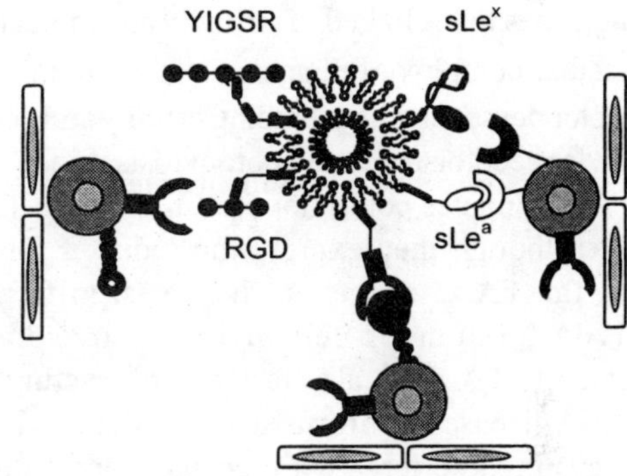

Fig. 14-15. Liposome Immobilized Ligands to Target the Cell Adhesion Molecules on Tumour Vasculature and Extracellular Matrix

Altered/Over Expression of Cell Specific Receptors

It is appropriate with the ligand-receptor mediated targeting approaches to consider the receptors, which are either over-expressed or down regulated in the malignant target sites. Depending upon the over-expression (folate, transferrin, fucose and lipoprotein) or down regulation (asialoglycoprotein receptor, mannose receptor), effective cellular targeting approaches could be engineered (Table 14-6).

Targeted Drug Delivery via the Folate Receptor

The folate receptor is a highly selective tumour marker over-expressed in greater than 90% of ovarian carcinomas and epithelial tumours and has been used as a targeting ligand (Campbell et al., 1991). Two general strategies have been developed for the targeted delivery of drugs to folate receptor-positive tumour cells: by coupling to a monoclonal antibody against the receptor and by coupling to a high affinity ligand, folic acid (FA). First, antibodies against the folate receptor, including their fragments and derivatives, have been evaluated for tumour imaging and immunotherapy clinically and have shown significant targeting efficacy in ovarian tumour patients.

Folic acid, a high affinity ligand of the folate receptor, retains its receptor binding properties when derivatized via its γ-carboxyl. Folate conjugation, therefore, presents an alternative method of targeting through folate receptor. This second strategy has been successfully applied *in vitro* for the receptor-specific delivery of protein toxins, anti-T-cell receptor antibodies, interleukin-2, chemo-therapeutic agents, γ-emitting radio-pharmaceuticals, magnetic resonance imaging contrast agents, liposomal drug carriers, and gene transfer vectors. Low molecular weight radiopharmaceuticals conjugated with folate ligand showed much more favourable pharmacokinetic properties than radiolabeled antibodies and greater tumour selectivity in animal tumour models expressing tumour models. The small size, convenient availability, simple conjugation chemistry, and presumed lack of immunogenicity of folic acid make it an ideal ligand for targeted delivery to tumours.

Conjugates to FA linked to virtually any molecule or molecular complex of diameter <150 nm bind to the receptor possessing high binding affinity and enter the cell via receptor-mediated potocytosis. Since the same FA conjugates could not bind to FR negative cells even though they express the reduced folate carrier, the FA conjugates display significant selectivity for tumour cell *in vivo*. Liposomes conjugated to FA were also tested for targeting to neoplastic diseases. Unfortunately, poly(ethylene glycol) coating interfered with receptor recognition when the folate was directly linked to a PEG-linked phospholipid head group. To circumvent this problem, FA was attached to the distal ends of a few lipid conjugated PEG-molecules, allowing the targeting ligand for better exposition and to reach the receptor sites far from the liposomal surface (Gabizon et al., 1999).

Folate has been coupled to distearoylphosphatidylethanolamine (DSPE) using a PEG2000 linker (folate-PEG2000-DSPE) to deliver liposome encapsulated doxorubicin to epithelial tumour cells. A 45-fold higher uptake of encapsulated doxorubicin has been recorded over that observed for non-targeted vesicles (Lee and Low, 1994a, 1994b).

Lectin Receptors Exploited in Tumour Targeting

An interesting observation of the receptor up-or down-regulation in normal and malignant cells could be seen in the case of lectin membrane receptors. Seymour, 1994 has suggested that asialo-glycoprotein receptor on the cell surface is depleted in normal hepatocytes of cirrhotic or tumour bearing livers, possibly due to a cellular redistribution and hence lower level of targeting was anticipated in patients with liver malignancies. On the other hand, the presence of fucose specific receptors for endogenous fucose-terminated ligands was identified on the surface of murine leukaemia L1210 (Monsigny et al., 1988; 1994). These over-expressed receptors were targeted by using polymers of N-(2-hydroxypropyl)

Table 14-6. Over-expressed Receptors as Molecular Ports

Target Receptors	Expression	Delivery strategies
Up-regulation		
Folate	Ovarian carcinomas and epithelial tumours	Folic acid-Cys[287] (Pseudomonas exotoxin) conjugate, Folic acid-maytansinoid (DM1) conjugate
Fucose	Leukaemia	N-(2-hydroxypropyl)methacrylamide co-polymer conjugates bearing N-linked fucosylamine and daunomycin
Transferrin	T-cell leukaemia, haematopoietic/tumour cells	Tf-methotrexate, Tf-adriamycin conjugate; Tf-polycation (poly-L-lysine/protamine) conjugate, Biotinylated Tf-DNA conjugate
Lipoprotein	Certain tumours	Porphyrin loaded lipoprotein (Photodynamic therapy)
Down-regulation		
Asialoglycoprotein (ASGP)	Cirrhotic or tumour bearing livers	-
Mannose	Certain tumours	-

*Adopted from Vyas et al., 2001

methacrylamide bearing sacrolysin (an alkylating agent) and additionally linked N-fucosylamine (Seymour, 1994). It was demonstrated that conjugates containing fucosylamine were more cytotoxic than fucose free material against L1210 leukaemia cells. Similarly, N-(2-hydroxypropyl)-methacrylamide co-polymer conjugates bearing N-linked fucosylamine as well as the anthracycline daunomycin were targeted to leukaemia cell lines (Seymour, 1994). The latter was conjugated via a lysosomally degradable tetrapeptide (Gly-Phe-Leu-Gly) to the skeleton of the ligand-appended polymer. A 8-fold higher cytotoxic effect was recorded against L1210 cells cultured *in vitro* as compared to control, fucosylamine free conjugates. However, these ligand-based conjugates showed no differential cytotoxic activity to CCRF leukaemia cells *in vitro* as compared against fucose free control. It clearly indicates that the over expression of fucose binding lectins on the surface of certain tumour cell (L1210) turns them susceptible to receptor-mediated targeting.

Lipoprotein Receptors for Tumour Targeting

Some tumour cells also express affinity receptors for low-density lipoprotein (LDL), which may serve as a means for ligand driven targeting of cytotoxic/ bioactives to these cell lines. The number of receptors on normal cells is regulated by metabolic factors that regulated as a function of intracellular amount of cholesterol and the rate of intracellular cholesterol synthesis. However, tumour cells lack many of the regulatory bio-events of normal cells, and in some tumour cells the regulation of the LDL-receptor is even lost. Such tumour cells over-express LDL receptors under conditions where receptors in normal tissues are down-regulated. Not only cyto-toxic drugs, but also photo-sensitizers porphyrins that incorporate well into lipoprotein carriers, may be delivered to tumour cells in this manner (Bijsterbosch and van Berkel, 1990). In the so-called photodynamic therapy, the tumour is localized with the help of porphyrin loaded lipoprotein using receptor mediated bio-events. This porphyrin-loaded tumour is subsequently exposed to irradiation or visible light. The porphyrin released at the target site act as photo-sensitizer and converts light energy to chemical energy, which results in severe biological damage of the target tissue (Fig. 14-16). However, solid tumours are poorly perfused and therefore not readily accessible for LDL, and this was the reason that these workers proposed drug-loaded or porphyrin-loaded LDL carriers for the eradication of the residual tumour cells.

Transferrin Receptors for Tumour Targeting

Transferrin receptors are also expressed on some tumour cells and this could be exploited in designing the carrier constructs to target these tumour cells. Liposomes appended with an anti-transferrin receptor antibody were more efficiently internalized by a number of human T-cell leukaemic cell lines than liposomes carrying antibodies against other surface antigens of these cells (Fig. 14-17). In an interesting study, Hege et al., 1989, reported a comparison of liposome immobilized Anti-Tac (a monoclonal antibody directed against the IL-2 receptor) and Anti-TfR (a monoclonal antibody against transferrin receptor) for specific binding, internalization and intracellular drug delivery to adult T-cell leukaemia. They reported better growth inhibition potential of Anti-TfR coupled liposomes over Anti-Tac coupled liposomes when methotrexate-γ-aspartate was used as an entrapped cytotoxic drug. Receptor targeted lipid formulations appended with transferrin as a targeting ligand find their applications in gene therapy of haematopoietic/tumour cells (Wagner et al., 1994).

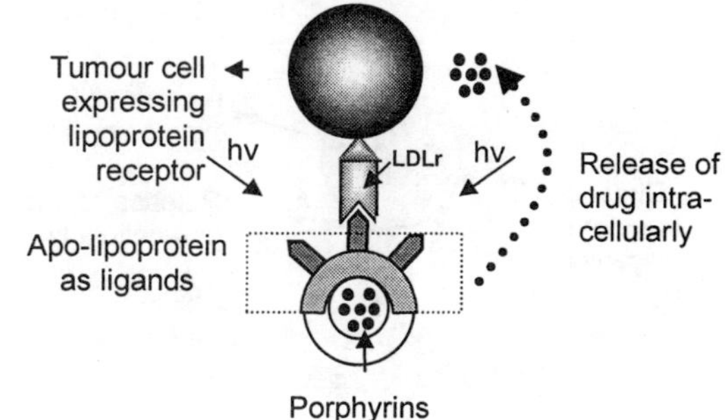

Fig. 14-16. Porphyrin Loaded Lipoproteins Bind to the Tumour Site through Specific LDL Receptors Expressed on the Surface. The Tumour Loaded with Porphyrin-lipoprotein Complex when Irradiated with Visible Light, Results in Severe Biological Damage of Target Cell

Sarti and co-workers, 1996 developed a liposomal carrier system able to interact specifically with HL60 leukaemia cell lines. The small unilamellar vesicles made up of pure phospholipids were chemically cross-linked to human transferrin. The modified liposomes interacted specifically with the cells and subsequently internalized via active-receptor-mediated endocytosis, as demonstrated by the full inhibition of internalization by circulatory free ligand. Ishida and Maruyama, 1998 further conjugated transferrin to the PEG-grafted liposomes at the distal ends of PEG chains. The biodistribution and intracellular uptake studies revealed the localization of the Tf-PEG liposomes at the tumour cell surface, coated pits and endosomes. These results suggested the endocytic pathway as internalization route for Tf-PEG liposomes, which were found to retain specificity for the tumour site mediated by transferrin receptor driven bio-events.

Tanaka and co-workers, 1996 in a study have synthesized and characterized transferrin-Mitomycin C conjugates as a target-oriented system. This tumour specific drug carrier (Tf-G-MMC) was bound specifically to the Tf receptors over-expressed on Sarcoma 180 cell lines. A recent review summarizes the role of transferrin as a targeting ligand for liposomes and antitumour drugs. Transferrin-methotrexate and transferrin-adriamycin complexes both in the conjugated form or on the liposomal surfaces were compared and found superior to anti-transferrin receptor antibody (7D-3) linked to MTX liposomes (Singh, 1999). Munns and co-workers, 1998 on the other hand, assessed the ability of transferrin-adriamycin complex to target transferrin receptor positive tumour cells and reported that Tf-ADR conjugates failed as cytotoxic delivery system as it neither prevent toxicity to the Tf-R negative cells nor did it overcame the resistance of the adriamycin-resistant cells.

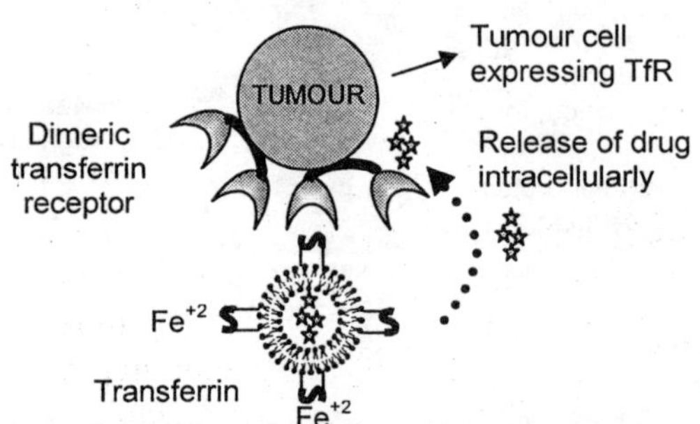

Fig. 14-17. Transferrin Appended onto the Liposomal Surface Negotiates Delivery of Entrapped Drug/ bioactive to the Proliferating Neoplastic Cells Expressing the Transferrin Specific Receptors

Role of anti-transferrin-receptor antibody (OX-26) has been well documented for the brain delivery of bioactives. On the same lines, Watanabe and his colleague, 1998 developed a simple method to conjugate biotinylated double strand DNA to biotinylated transferrin via streptavidin and demonstrated successful transduction of the conjugate into the TfR-positive human tumour cells.

GENE THERAPY

Gene therapy by definition aims at modifying the genetic program of a cell towards a therapeutic or prophylactic goal (Oliff et al., 1996). Several gene therapy strategies (Table 14-7) for tumour are currently under evaluation and some of them include: 1) modification of the function of oncogenes and tumour suppressor genes; 2) modification of the host immune response towards the tumour; 3) disruption of the tumour neovascularization; 4) lysis of tumour cells with replication-competent viruses, and 5) "suicide" gene therapy where an inactive prodrug is converted into a cytotoxic drug by gene expressed enzymes. Both viral and non-viral gene vectors have been investigated and well documented (Ledley, 1995). However, the inefficiency of current gene vectors in infecting targeted cells and their inability to selectively access the diseased cells distributed systemically are two major impediments that have to be overcome for further successful clinical applications. Various approaches are put forward for the gene therapy of tumours :

1. First approach is to locate single gene defect such as retinoblastoma, familial adenomatous polyposis or new gene mutation, i.e., leukaemia and lymphoma. Most studies attempt to enhance the quantity and specific cytotoxicity of lymphocytes that react and kill tumour cells. One of the possibilities could be to mark

Table 14-7. Gene and Molecular Delivery Approaches for Tumour

- Use of antisense oligonucleotides for inhibiting oncogenes, Targeting antisense oligonucleotides to cell signaling, Antisense oligonucleotides targeted to growth factors, Antisense oligonucleotides targeted to matrix metalloproteinase, Inhibition of fusion genes by antisense oligonucleotides, Combination of antisense and chemotherapy, Oligonucleotides that are antisense to p-glycoprotein, Antisense approaches to induce apoptosis in tumour, Antisense chimeric molecule, Antisense bcl-2 therapy
- Nucleic acid tumour vaccines, DNA tumour vaccines, DNA inoculation technology, self-replicating RNA vaccine for tumour therapy, tumour-targeted bacteria as novel antitumour vectors, naked DNA prostate tumour vaccine
- Direct gene delivery to the tumour, Particle-mediated *in vivo* gene therapy for tumour, Direct injection of adenoviral vectors, Direct injection of a plasmid DNA-liposome complex, Electroporation technology for gene transfer, Haematopoietic gene transfer, Tumour-infiltrating lymphocyte gene marking and therapy, Genetic modification of human haematopoietic stem cells and progenitor cells
- Cytokine gene therapy, use of the interleukin-2 gene, interleukin-7, interleukin-12, interleukin-13, γ-interferon gene transfer, granulocyte-macrophage colony-stimulating factor, chemokines
- Immunogene therapy, Monoclonal antibody gene transfer, Transfer and expression of intracellular adhesion-1 molecules, Other techniques of immunotherapy of tumour relevant to gene therapy, Fas/APO-1, Direct intratumoural injection of MHC gene HLA-B7, Genetically modified lymphocytes as a new class of killer cells, Major histocompatibility complex class I, Insulin-like growth factor, p53 and p21

tumour-infiltrating lymphocytes (TIL) to follow progress of malignant melanoma. TIL cells are trapped and removed in liver, spleen and lung, however, uncontrolled production of TNF in normal tissue has toxic side effects.

2. Second approach is to increase the immunogenicity of the tumour cells by gene therapy. Cytokines (e.g. IL2, IL4, TNF, GMCSF) and cell adhesion molecules are transducted to preselected portion of the tumour and reimplanted into the patient.
3. Third method is the transfer of protective or killing genes, e.g. transfer of multiple drug resistance to normal haemopoietic cells, which would allow higher tolerance to chemotherapy, killer genes like diphtheria toxin and TNF to kill tumour cells.

However, to achieve above mentioned goals various methods have been used and put forward, which include:

1. *In vivo* / *ex vivo* delivery followed by autologous return of cells to patient
2. *Ex vivo* : gene transfer into bone marrow stem cells
3. *In vivo* : direct gene delivery by using viral vectors, gene transfer by ligand-mediated DNA conjugates and fusogenic lipid vesicles (liposomes), simple direct injection or even pneumatically delivered DNA-coated gold particles (the "gene gun")
4. Viral vectors are rendered replication-defective by deletion of essential genes. Therapeutic genes and their regulatory elements are inserted into the engineered virus. Virus are then propagated in packaging (helper) cell line that complement the deleted essential gene in the virus and used to infect the target tissue

Molecular Targets (Defective Genes) for Tumour Therapy

The molecular defects that transform normal cells into the malignant consist of mutations in key classes of genes that are responsible in some ways for the reproduction, or growth of cells. These mutations alter the quantity or behaviour of the proteins encoded by growth regulating genes and, in so doing, disrupt functions that control cell division. Knowledge of mutant genes is enabling pharmaceutical researchers to design new drugs and delivery systems that will specifically act upon disrupted genes or their proteins (Table 14-8).

The defects targeted by molecular therapy are found in three major classes and some minor classes of genes (Gibbs and Oliff, 1994; Hinds and Weinberg, 1994) (Table 14-8).

The oncogenes stimulate cell progression through the cell cycle, i.e., the sequence of events in which a cell gets larger, replicates its DNA and divides, passing a complete set of genes to each daughter cell. The most common tumour causing mutation of this kind occurs in the *ras*-gene. The protein encoded by the *ras* gene (the *ras* protein) ordinarily behaves as relay switch within the signaling pathway that tells the cells to divide in response to stimuli transmitted to it from outside of the cell, it activates the rest of the signaling pathway. In the absence of outside prompt, the *ras* protein would normally remain in the "off" state. The mutated (tumourous) *ras* protein however, behaves like a switch struck in the "on" position. Members of the second class, i.e., tumour suppressor genes restrict such growth. The two primary tumour suppressor proteins are the pRB and the p53 protein. pRB protein helps to regulate the cell cycle and mutations in the RB gene render its protein inactive and as a result the cells divide non-stop. p53 protein, which is often called "guardian of the genome" prevents replication of damaged DNA in normal cells and prompts suicide or apoptosis, of cells with abnormal DNA.

Faulty or mutated p53 gene allows cell carrying damaged DNA to survive and to mutate and in most human tumours the p53 gene appears defective. Genes in the third group governs the replication and repair of DNA. Most tumours possess mutations in one or more of these defective gene categories (Oliff et al., 1996).

The means of targeting tumour at the molecular level include repairing faulty DNA, shutting down key growth factors and increasing sensitivity of tumour cells to conventional therapies like radiation. Signaling pathway in a mammalian cell includes many components that, when altered in quantity or structure, can lead to tumourous growth. Among these components are growth factor receptor, *ras* protein (oncogene) and kinase enzymes that aid their function, such as abl and src. Perturbation of prb and p53 (tumour suppressor gene) can promote tumour development as well. Figure 14-18 explains various genetic defects and therapeutic strategies developed or under development.

Non-viral Gene Delivery for p53

Abnormality in the tumour suppressor gene p53 is one of the most common occurrences associated with human neoplasia. Consequently, restoration of wild-type p53 function is seen as a promising approach for tumour gene therapy. In recent years, considerable research effort has centred upon developing and improving non-viral delivery systems as alternatives

Table 14-8. Molecular Approaches in Tumour Therapy

Tumour feature	Molecular targets	Therapeutics
Oncogene	Ras proteins	Farnesyl transferase inhibitors
Activation leading to excessive Ras protein or kinase activity	Abl, EGF receptor, Erb-B2 and Src kinase	Tyrosine kinase inhibitors: tryphostins, lavendustins, quinazolines and antisense
	PKC-α, Raf and cyclin-dependent kinases	Serine/threonine kinase inhibitors: olomoucine, staurosporine and antisense
Loss of tumour suppressor gene	APC, AT, DCC, RB and P53 genes	Gene therapy to restore normal suprresor gene function; antisense agents to block E2F synthesis
Abnormal DNA repair mechanisms	DNA mismatch repair enzymes	Gene therapy to restore normal enzyme activity
Lack of cell aging (senescence) in tumour cells	Telomerase	Telomerase inhibitors
Angiogenesis	FGF, VEGF-growth factors	TNP-470, suramin
	Integrin receptors	$\alpha_v\beta_3$, $\alpha_v\beta_3$ antagonists
Metastases	Metalloproteases ollagenases	Proteases inhibitors
		Collagenases inhibitors

to viral vectors for gene delivery. These methods include the use of lipoplexes and polyplexes, and even delivery of naked DNA. Optimally effective tumour gene therapy requires treatment of metastatic as well as local disease, and to achieve this end, systemic delivery systems for therapeutic genes will be required. Thus to improve targeting, transfection efficiency and stability for systemic, non-viral p53 gene therapy holds promise.

Targeted, Non-viral Gene Delivery for Tumour Gene Therapy

The ability to mediate target specific delivery of therapeutics to tumour cells remains one of the most important unmet goal in effective tumour therapy. This aspect also remains as one of the greatest limitations of gene therapy. Targeted vectors based on DNA-binding agents attached to cell specific ligands or "molecular conjugates" were developed to overcome this hurdle. Various ligands have been utilized as molecular conjugates for targeting the resulting protein/DNA polyplex to cells efficiently *in vitro* while mediating limited delivery *in vivo*. This limited delivery is due to many reasons such as the need to identify non-viral agents that can help in escaping endosome entrapment as well as decreasing the complexity that evolves during the creation of these "synthetic viruses".

Cationic lipid-DNA complexes are being evaluated for local or systemic therapeutic gene transfer. These positively charged liposomes fuse with negatively charged cell membranes and deliver enclosed plasmid and its encoded gene to the target tissues. This system has relevance for delivering genes to both normal and damaged or malignant tissues including phagocytes, tumour cells, endothelium and possibly parenchymal cells. Among the approaches being actively persuaded is the delivery of immuno-stimulatory cytokine genes (such as IL-2, IFN alpha or IL-12) into tumours. It is hypothesized that the local cytokine release will attract or induce antitumour immune responses. Valentis, (formerly Gene-Medicine), has developed a plasmid encoding human IL-2 complexed with the liposomal preparation of DOTMA and cholesterol.

Suicide Gene Therapy

Suicide gene therapy is one of several gene thera-peutic approaches being evaluated to treat tumour. A suicide gene is a gene that encodes a protein,

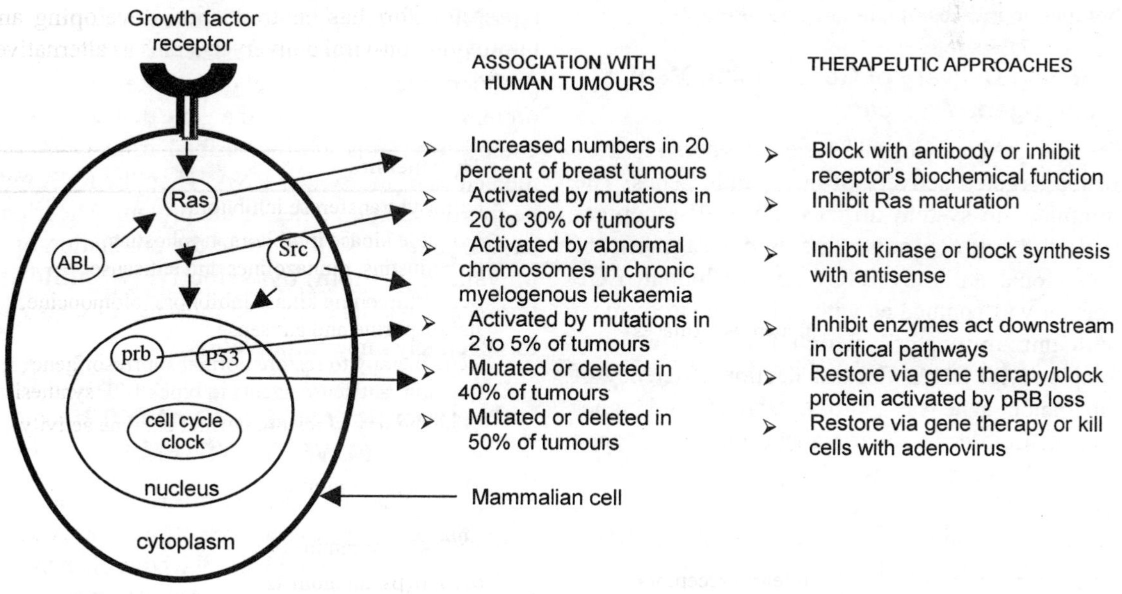

Fig. 14-18. Molecular Approaches in Tumour Targeting (Adopted from Jain, 1994)

frequently an enzyme, that in itself is nontoxic to the genetically modified cell. However, when a tumour cell is exposed to a specific nontoxic prodrug, the latter is selectively converted into toxic metabolites by the gene encoding the enzyme. The suicide gene most commonly employed, both in experimental and clinical settings, is herpes simplex thymidine kinase (HSVtk). Some suicide gene products also induce a so-called 'bystander effect', i.e. a toxic effect on adjacent nongene modified tumour cells and sometimes also on more distant tumour cells. The bystander effect is most evident in tumour cells that have a high number of gap junctions, cellular channels build up by proteins called connexins. Many tumours, mainly haematological in origin, have a low number of gap junctions. Therefore, it is important to develop gap junction independent drug delivery systems. Suicide gene technology may also be used for the *ex vivo* purging of tumour cells in bone marrow or peripheral blood stem cell autografts or for inactivation of effector cells, such as antitumour T donor lymphocytes in allogeneic transplantation to prevent severe graft versus host reactions. New constructs, e.g. combining suicide genes and immune response enhancing genes or suicide genes and connexin inducing genes may further improve the therapeutic indices of suicide gene therapy.

Targeting Delivery of Genes using Mab; Immunogene Approach

Recently an "immunogene" system has been reported for the targeted delivery of therapeutic genes. The immunogene system utilizes the EGF receptor-mediated endocytosis. The Fab' fragment of monoclonal antibody B4G7 against human EGF receptor was conjugated with polylysine to form an "Fab immunoporter", which forms an affinity complex with DNA. The transfection efficiency of Fab immunogene was approximately 10-fold higher than the Lipofectin. Gene transfer of HSV-tk gene into A431 tumour cells with Fab' immunoporter was successful and the subsequent treatment with ganciclovir induced remarkable suicide effects conferring 1000-fold higher drug sensitivity. The immunogene system promises to be useful as a gene transfer vehicle targeting the EGF receptor-hyperproducing tumour cells.

Antisense Oligonucleotides as Genetic Medicines

Antisense oligonucleotides are the first of new genetic medicines to have reached clinical trials. Following the arrival of triplex and antisense strategies, researchers are attempting to design drug or delivery systems that will bind to the selective sites on the nucleic acids (DNA or RNA) responsible for (if not targeted) the synthesis of disease related proteins. The concept of exploiting antisense or triplex strategy is based upon the fact that the unique gene that specifies the composition of a specific protein must be expressed. Thus the gene must be transcribed, or copied from double stranded DNA into individual molecules of single-stranded messenger RNA. Then the RNA molecules must be translated into the specific proteins. Novel research is based upon the attachment of a novel drug delivery device to chosen segments of DNA (in the triplex approach) or messenger RNA (in the antisense approach). The construct so formed will impede transcription or translation of selected genes (or mutated genes thus selectively and specifically disrupting their function) (Fig. 14-19). There are three mechanisms, namely, triplex helix formation, translation arrest via antisense-mRNA hybrid formation and RNase H based destruction of mRNA translation. Two innovative strategies are tested for inhibiting the production of disease-related proteins. For any protein to be synthesized, the gene that specifies its composition must be transcribed from DNA into molecules of messenger RNA. Then the RNA must be translated into copies of the protein. The triplex strategy aims to stall or route the production of an unwanted protein by selectively inhibiting transcription of its gene. The antisense strategy aims to selectively impede translation.

TUMOUR TARGETING AND DRUG DELIVERY SYSTEMS

A wide variety of cellular, macromolecular and particulate carriers have been investigated as potential drug delivery systems with the objective of improving tumour chemotherapy. These include erythrocytes, antibodies, nucleic acids, heat or chemically denaturated plasma proteins, cytokines and a diverse

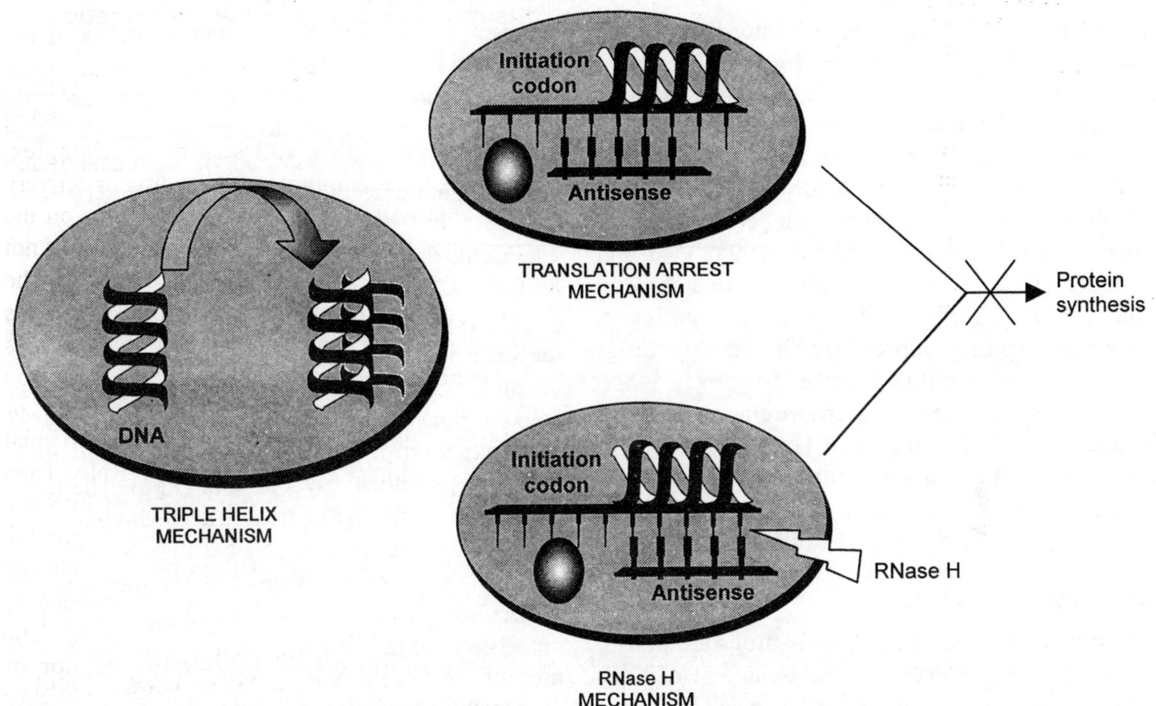

Fig. 14-19. Antisense Oligonucleotide Therapy

range of particulate carriers of different sizes and composed of diverse range of biodegradable and/or biocompatible materials like polymers, dextran, gelatin, albumin, cyclodextrin (micro/nanoparticles), lipoproteins and phospholipids (liposomes) (Table 14-9).

Site Specific Drug Delivery

Site specific drug delivery requires completion of several sequential but independent events. These include the localization of drug and carrier within the desired target organ; recognition and interaction of the carrier with specific target cell(s) and delivery of therapeutic concentration of drug to the target cell(s) with little or no uptake by non-target (normal) cells (Vyas and Dixit, 1999). Site specific drug delivery can be classified according to the level of specificity achieved in the delivery process:

1. Delivery to individual organs or tissues (organ targeting);
2. Targeting to a specific cell type(s) within a tissue (cellular targeting); and
3. Delivery to different intracellular compartments in target cells by engineering the internalization of drug and drug-carrier construct via specific transport pathways (intracellular targeting).

However, the role of carrier systems in providing site specificity can be evident from the terms like "passive" and "active" targeting approaches (Lazo and Hacker, 1986; Karajgi et al., 1993; Vyas and Sakthivel, 1994; Vyas et al., 2000). "Passive targeting" involves therapeutic exploitation of the natural (intrinsic/inherent) distribution pattern of a drug-carrier construct *in vivo*. For example the role of the reticuloendothelial system (RES) in clearing foreign particulate materials from the blood permits drug encapsulated in particulate carriers like liposomes and microspheres to be passively targeted to macrophages. In contrary, "active targeting" is aimed at altering the natural distribution pattern of a drug-carrier construct either away from RES (long circulatory) or to the specific cells, tissues or organs (ligand intervention).

Ligand mediated targeting is the major focus of the current research that involves ligands developed against cell receptors or antigenic determinants expressed on tumour cells or vasculature. These include ligands like antibodies, glycolipids, glycoproteins, polysaccharides, proteins, and immuno-regulatory molecules (Meijer et al., 1992; Jones, 1994; Molema and Meijer, 1994; Vyas and Sihorkar, 2000; Vyas et al., 2001). Another strategy that could be exploited for tumour targeting is "physical targeting" approach, which employs drug-carrier constructs that release drug only when exposed to specific micro-environments such as changes in pH (Connor and Huang, 1985) and temperature (Hayashi et al., 1998), irradiation to UV light (Lamparsk et al., 1992) or subjecting to the external magnetic fields (Scheffold et al., 1995).

Multidrug Resistance

Although nearly 50 antineoplastic drugs are in use, only a few are effective in the treatment of each specific tumour type because of intrinsic or primary drug resistance. The initial and subsequent chemotherapy allows a tumour to develop acquired or secondary resistance because malignant cells that survive the drug are, of course, resistant to that drug. Ultimately, by a variety of mechanisms, a multidrug-resistant tumour evolves. At this point, additional chemotherapy only induces toxic effects in the patient without reducing the tumour. For example, Paclitaxel is strongly cytotoxic against drug-sensitive breast tumour cells (IC_{50} = 2.5nM; IC_{50} is the concentration of a compound necessary to inhibit the cell growth by 50%), but it exhibits only very weak activity against the drug-resistant breast tumour cells (IC_{50} = 860 nM).

The broad-spectrum resistance to structurally and mechanistically diverse antitumour agents constitutes the multidrug resistance (MDR) phenotype. Tumour cells carrying this phenotype are characterized by the over-expression of an energy-dependent drug transport protein, P-glycoprotein (Pgp). The over-expression results in a decreased accumulation of the drug within the tumour cell because the cell can efficiently pump out the hydrophobic antitumour drug molecules. Located across the cell membrane, Pgp detects and expels the drug as it enters the plasma membrane much like a hydrophobic "vacuum cleaner". Often, tumour cells develop a natural defense mechanism against cytotoxic agents, and any effective chemotherapy must find a way to disable or circumvent that defense. Fortunately, specific drugs are able to inhibit the MDR mechanism in tumour cells, clearing the path for effective delivery of the

Table 14-9. Drug Delivery Systems for Tumour

- Liposomes for antitumour drugs, immunoliposomes, stealth liposomes, tumour-selective targeted drug delivery via folate-PEG liposomes, hyperthermia and liposomal drug delivery, liposome-mediated oligonucleotide delivery, lipid-coated microbubbles as a delivery vehicle for Taxol, use of thermosensitive liposomes and localized hyperthermia, photodynamic therapy for chemosensitization
- Microspheres as drug delivery systems in tumour therapy, subcutaneous injection of microspheres carrying antitumour drugs, magnetic targeted microparticle technology, nanoparticles for delivery of antitumour drugs, chemoembolization, antitumour drugs bound to carbon particles, nanoerythrosomes, albumin-based drug carriers
- Monoclonal antibodies, bispecific antibody fusion protein, radio-immunoconjugates, drug immunoconjugates, immunotoxins, combined use of Mabs and cytokines, humanized Mabs, two-step targeting using a bispecific antibody, single-chain antibody-binding protein technology
- Ultrasonic activated drug carrying micelles, tumour-activated pro-drug therapy, site-specific delivery and light-activation of antitumour proteins
- Targeting antitumour drugs to tumour blood vessels, peptides targeted against integrin cell adhesion proteins, drugs to induce clotting in tumour vessels, vascular targeting agents, cytoporter
- Antineoplastic drug implants into tumours, PEG technology, pressure-induced filtration of drugs across vessels to the tumour, use of vitamins as carriers for antitumour agents, delivery across the blood-brain barrier, chemotherapeutic agents incorporated in biodegradable polymer wafers, boron neutron capture therapy, tumour necrosis therapy (TNT), iontophoretic delivery into subcutaneous tumours

antitumour agent. By binding preferentially to Pgp, these inhibitors block the efflux channel, allowing the antitumour agent to slip into the tumour cell unnoticed and then kill cell (Fig. 14-20). These inhibitors are called MDR reversal agents.

Role of Drug Carriers in Overcoming Multidrug Resistance

Multidrug resistance is the main cause of the failure of chemotherapy. This can severely affect the effectiveness of chemotherapeutic agents. It is often associated with the over-expression of some drug efflux pumps, known as P-glycoprotein pump (Pgp) and multidrug resistance associated protein pump (MRP) (Kartner et al., 1985). However, Pgp is the best-characterized efflux pump responsible for multidrug resistance. Pgp is a cell membrane glycoprotein of 170 Kda molecular weight and is a membrane spanning ATPase located in the plasma membrane. This multidrug resistance transporter could act as an efflux pump and reject positively charged amphipathic drugs (mostly antitumour drugs) from the cells as shown for bacterial transport proteins. Over-expression of P-glycoprotein in tumour cells can lead to a marked decrease in sensitivity to drugs. Thus multidrug resistance is associated with a low intracellular accumulation of drugs. This is more pronounced with drugs which enter the cell by passive diffusion through the lipid bilayer, for example, doxorubicin (an antitumour drug) (Endicott

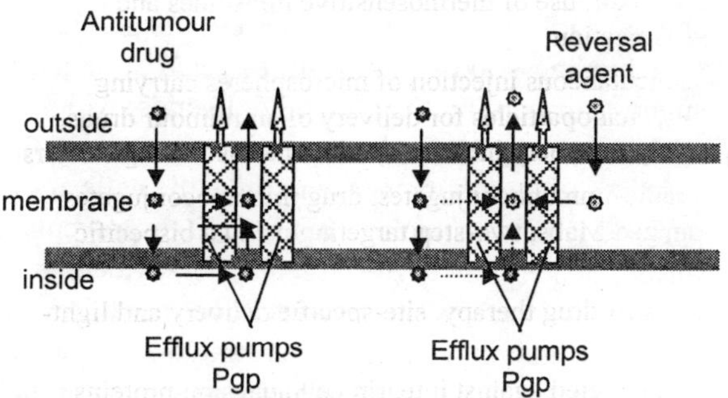

Fig. 14-20. Reversal Agents Block the Efflux of Antitumour Drugs. Pgp pumps the antitumour drug out of the cell before it can affect antimitotic activity (Left). The reversal agent blocks this mechanism, making the cell sensitive to the antitumour drug (Right).

and Ling, 1989). Upon entering the cell, these drugs bind to P-glycoprotein, which forms transmembrane channels and uses the energy of ATP hydrolysis to pump these compounds out of the cell.

Various delivery systems including liposomes and nanoparticles/microspheres have reported effective therapeutic indices in a number of chemotherapy refractory tumours both in animal models and in the clinic and these results are well documented with antitumour drugs such as doxorubicin (Vaage et al., 1994; Muggia et al., 1997). Several mechanisms are proposed through which liposomes and microparticulates avoid multi-drug resistance of encapsulated drugs:

1. Negatively charged phospholipids (phosphatidylserine or cardiolipin) used in the liposomal formulations may directly regulate the P-glycoprotein transporter.
2. Liposomes may provide sustained high levels of drug to the resistant cells over long period of time.
3. After endocytosis of drug loaded liposomes, the lysosomal localization of the drug protects it from the action of the P-glycoprotein, thus avoiding immediate contact with P-glycoprotein transporter located at the plasma membrane.
4. Along with cell sensitization, liposomal drug delivery may help overcome a broader range of drug resistance due to favourable pharmacokinetics.

Nanoparticle loaded drugs demonstrated effective treatment of a number of chemotherapy refractory tumours in animal models (Kubiak et al., 1989; Cuvier et al., 1992). The lysosomal localization of the particulate system protects the loaded drug from the action of the P-glycoprotein, thus avoiding immediate contact with P-glycoprotein transporter located at the plasma membrane (Fig. 14-21). Along with cell sensitization, nanoparticulate drug delivery may help overcome a broader range of drug resistance due to favourable pharmacokinetics.

Irrespective of the mechanism(s) operating for MDR the probability of the complete reversal of multidrug resistance is low than what is required at clinical levels. Thus, to treat patients resistant to a particular type of chemotherapy, it is important to combine liposome encapsulated drug with other presently used chemotherapeutic agents or to develop additional liposomal chemotherapeutic agents with non-overlapping mechanisms of drug resistance.

Problems Associated with Tumour Targeted Delivery Systems

Several problems have been identified (Allen, 1997) which impede and partially or fully disable the targeting strategies particularly, *in vivo*. These include:

Rapid Clearance of Targeted Systems Specially Antibody Targeted Carriers

Conventional liposomes, i.e., liposomes lacking surface sterically stabilizing molecules (such as PEG), are rapidly removed from circulation via recognition of the Fc portion of the antibodies by cells of MPS when antibodies are anchored to the liposomal surface. Therefore, it would be necessary to increase the circulation half-life of the immunoliposomes over conventional liposomes.

Immune Reactions against Intravenously Administered Systems

Immunogenic nature of the ligand mediated delivery systems in particular for antibody anchored drug carriers is quite common. However, the problem can be reduced by using fragments like Fab' and $F(ab)_2$ instead of taking whole immunoglobulin molecule. Another solution to the problem may be the use of humanized or chimerized antibodies or fragments for clinical applications. Alternatively, the use of antibodies can be avoided by using receptor specific ligands. The receptor however, should be either over-expressed or uniquely expressed on target cells, i.e., folate, asialofetuin, peptides recognizing adhesion molecules, transferrin and cytokines.

Targeı ı issue Heterogeneity

The majority of target cells exhibit a varied degree of heterogeneity in their expression of target epitopes. The question of heterogeneity is even profound with tumour cells. However, by using a pool of monoclonal (or polyclonal) antibodies or ligands, which can recognize all of the cells of a heterogenous population, a "Bystander release pattern" could be

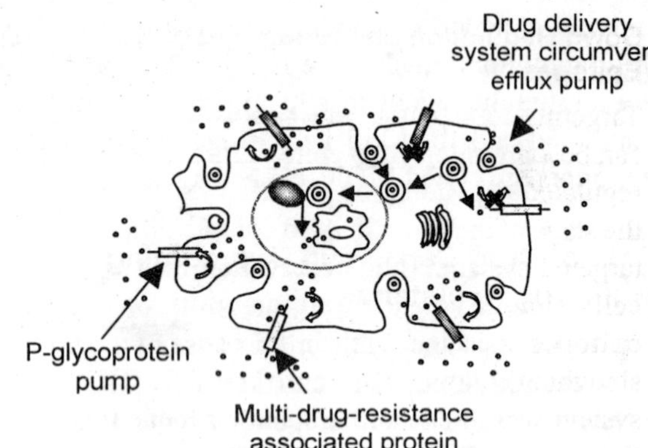

Fig. 14-21. Schematic diagram of possible trafficking of free drug associated in a carrier into multi-drug resistant cell

achieved using passively targeted system.

Bystander Effect and Binding Site Barrier Concept

Problems of insufficient localization of targeted systems into tumour cells can be a problem in designing targeted drug therapy. "Bystander release pattern" achieved using passively targeted system indicate that non-targeted systems are better than actively targeted systems in tumour localization. This release pattern indicates localization and diffusion of the passively vectorized systems throughout the tumours and gradual leaking of their contents into the interstitial fluid where they diffuse, reaching many tumour cells, which otherwise are remote from the actual locale of the delivery system. The "binding site barrier" concept further rules out the possibility of achieving good results with targeted systems. It suggests that antibodies (and other ligands) will bind to the first target cell they encounter, which in the case of solid tumours will tend to be the cells at the periphery of the tumour. This retards or prevents a further penetration of the targeted therapy deep into the tumour interior. This however does not follow in the case of micrometastases where angiogenic factors predominate, as passively targeted systems can not take advantage of this extravasation mechanism to localize in tumours. Here antibody- or ligand-mediated systems may have an edge since the "binding site barrier" concept should not exist for micrometastases, which consisted of only a few cells.

Down Regulation and Sloughing of Surface Epitopes

Targeting to specific cells against surface epitopes can be a problem when epitopes are "up" or "down" regulated depending on the life cycle of the cell or the stage of the growth. Also complicating the use of targeted system is the observation that some target cells slough considerable amounts of the target epitopes into the blood. The presence of these sloughing epitopes may cause binding of the targeted system with these and this may impede the system from reaching the target cell. A possible solution would be to inject free antibody or ligand to clear the antigen from blood prior to injecting the targeted system.

Diffusion and Redistribution of Released Drug

Diffusion and redistribution of the drug from the target device due to turbulent environment allow diffusion of drug away from the target site and may decrease the level of targetability.

Liposomes in Tumour Therapy

Most of the medical applications of liposomes that have reached the pre-clinical and clinical stages are in the tumour treatments. Several clinical studies did not support the use of conventional liposomes in tumour treatment. Although it is still not clear whether such liposomes (especially the ones remote loaded with anthracyclines) can be beneficial in tumour therapy. It has been demonstrated that small and stable liposomes can passively target several different tumours because they can (owing to their biological stability) circulate for prolonged times and extravasate (owing to their small size, 50-150 nm) in tissues with enhanced vascular permeability (Gabijon and Papahadjopoulos, 1988). However, recent trends in research predominately opt for the specially engineered long-circulatory liposomes (Stealth™ liposomes) to ensure the long circulation times and increased probability for extravasation to the tumour vascular endothelium (Woodle and Lasic, 1992; Allen, 1994; Gabizon et al., 1999).

Tumour Vasculature and Targets for Anti-neoplastic Drugs Loaded Liposomes

In tumour therapy drugs or drug-carrier constructs (liposomes) have to cross the endothelial linings of the tumour blood vessels into the interstitial fluid, followed by their movement through extracellular matrix towards the tumour cells. In addition to the physical barrier posed by the endothelial cells, basement membrane and ECM, high interstitial pressure and low microvascular pressure may also interfere with extravasation of molecules and cells into tumour tissues. New therapeutic approaches for the treatment of solid tumours are aimed at vasculature, either at the endothelial cells or at the basement membrane supporting the endothelial cells or tumour stroma components. Targeting to these components require extravasation of the delivery system at sites with a leaky vasculature.

Tumour targeting strategies using liposomes can be designed in different ways:

- Natural targeting (lysosomotropism) of conventional liposomes (passive vectorization)
- Use of long-circulatory (Stealth liposomes):
- Use of ligand mediated targeting (active targeting).
- The use of anti-receptor antibodies or antibodies developed against specific surface antigens on the tumour vascular endothelium (immunoliposomes).
- The use of angiogenic peptides and adhesion molecules as ligands against receptors expressed on tumour vascular endothelium.

Mechanistic rationale of tumour accumulation of various liposomes

The accumulation of liposomes or large macromolecules in tumours is a result of a "leaky" microvasculature and an impaired lymphatic supporting the tumour area (also known as "enhanced permeability and retention effect"). Various liposomes like passively vectorized slow release/rapid release, triggered release and actively targeted liposomes have different mechanisms operating for their tumour accumulation. Figure 14-22 demonstrates various passive and active targeting approaches with liposome accumulation in tumour. A indicates slow release passively targeted liposomes, able to carry some of the drug in circulation; B signifies rapid release liposomes that leak their drug to a greater extent in circulation, which (drug) then takes the normal pharmacokinetic profile as the free drug; C

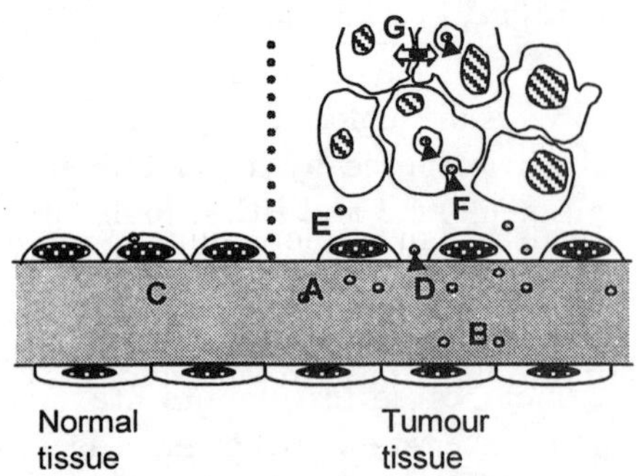

Fig. 14-22. Various Passive and Active Targeting Approaches with Liposome Accumulation in Tumour

demonstrates normal vasculature that prevents leakage of liposomes through these tissues; D shows extravasation of liposomes from leaky tumour vasculature (~100-780 nm), where non-targeted liposomes accumulate in the tumour interstitium and leak their drug (E), or otherwise targeted liposomes also accumulate in the tumour and subsequently endocytosed by tumour cells, undergoing lysosomotropism in the tumour cell (F). A strategy may be combined where hyperthermia in combination with targeted or stealth liposomes may result in enhanced distribution in the tumour interstitium and hence enhanced lysosomotropism (G).

The principle pathway for the movement of liposomes into the tumour interstitium is via extravasation through the discontinuous endothelium of the tumour microvasculature. Even the size of the liposomes in passive targeting approach determines the degree or extent of extravasation from the normal vasculature (Fig. 14-23). Once in the tumours, non-targeted liposomes are localized in the interstitium surrounding the tumour cells. However, a limited distribution of liposomes within the tumour interstitium results from a typically high interstitial pressure (which though helps in trapping the liposomes within the tumour area but prevents the access of drug into the necrotic zone) and a large interstitial space compared with normal tissue.

Moreover, the literature is abound concerning antibody anchored liposomes (immunoliposomes), i.e., liposomes with enhanced and more uniform access to the tumours after the addition of an internalizing anti-target Ab (Fab') fragment (Wright and Huang, 1989). The approach of combining local hyperthermia with immunoliposomes, thermo-sensitive liposomes and magnoresponsive liposomes is also under clinical investigation.

Passive Targeting of Drug Carriers to Tumours of RES Macrophages

The localization of liposomes and other particulate drug carriers within fixed macrophages of the RES and circulating blood monocytes after intravenous injection offers an efficient method for targeting biological response modifiers and immuno-modulators (that can selectively enhance macrophage mediated tumouricidal activity *in vivo*) to tumour cells (Gregoriadis and Florence, 1993). Systemic administration of liposomes containing immuno-modulators like muramyldipeptide (MDP) that activate macrophages to render them cytotoxic for tumour cells and significantly enhances host resistance to tumour metastases and augments macrophage-mediated destruction of tumour cells. Not only biological response modifiers but also chemotherapeutic drugs can be localized passively to tumours of RES origin. Passive localization of systemically administered particulate drug carriers in mononuclear phagocytes offers opportunities for delivering cytotoxic drugs to destroy malignancies arising in these cells such as histiocytes medullary reticulosis, monocytic leukaemia, hairy cell

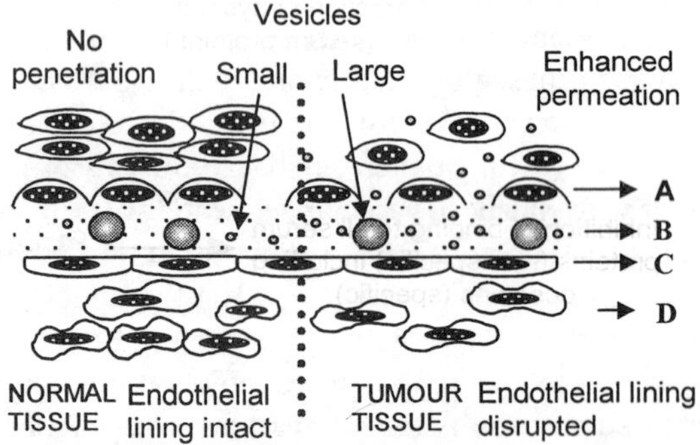

Fig. 14-23. Accumulation of Liposomes (size dependency) within Solid Tumours-Right-Liposome Extravasation from the Disorganized Structure and Left-Liposomes in Normal Tissue. A=Endothelial cells, B=Blood vessels, C=Basal membrane, and D= Perivascular tissue

leukaemia and certain forms of Hodgkin's diseases.

Sterically Stabilized (Stealth) Liposomes (SSL)

The dream of site specific drug targeting requires properly designed and intelligent delivery systems which can avoid scavenging through receptor mediated uptake by mononuclear phagocytic cells of RES-rich organs. Moreover, several targeting strategies require the system to be placed either into tumour cells or their extravasation into non-RES cellular lineage. As a matter of fact, recently described approaches to avoid RES-uptake of the drug-carrier composites, lead to the concept of long-circulatory ligand-appended system, which resist opsonization and serum protein binding to the surface (Fig. 14-24). Sterically stabilized liposomes thus avoid their recognition from RES uptake and this "stealthing" behaviour makes them long circulatory in nature (Woodle and Lasic, 1992; Allen, 1994; Gabizon et al., 1997; Lasic, 1997 and 1998).

Major aims of SSL are as follows:

- Generating more stable liposomal systems against various bio-environmental conditions
- Creating the long circulatory (i.e., less recognizable to serum proteins specially opsonins and hence less recognizable to phagocytic cells of RES) version
- Providing them targetability along with long circulatory behaviour by anchoring site-specific ligands
- Making them more sensitive towards external stimuli and signals like pH, substrates and temperatures
- Rendering them more suitable for tumour targeting

Tumour Targeting through Determinants on Tumour Cells

Ligand-directed targeting of drug carriers to determinants expressed on surface of vascular endothelial cells (under a normal and/or aetiological conditions) is most promising approach for drug targeting to tumour. The antigens and anti-target or anti-receptor antibodies developed against them can be conjugated to drug carriers like liposomes (immunoliposomes). Similarly, the emergence of various vasoactive and angiogenic peptides may serve as ligands to *en route* drug-carrier constructs to the tumour sites specifically (Vyas et al., 2001).

Stealth and Non-Stealth Immunoliposomes

Immunoglobulin fragments Fab' and F(ab')$_2$ or chimera IgG developed against surface antigens or antigenic determinants is a well exploitable strategy to negotiate Fc receptor mediated drug/gene therapy. Liposomes coated with heat aggregated isologous

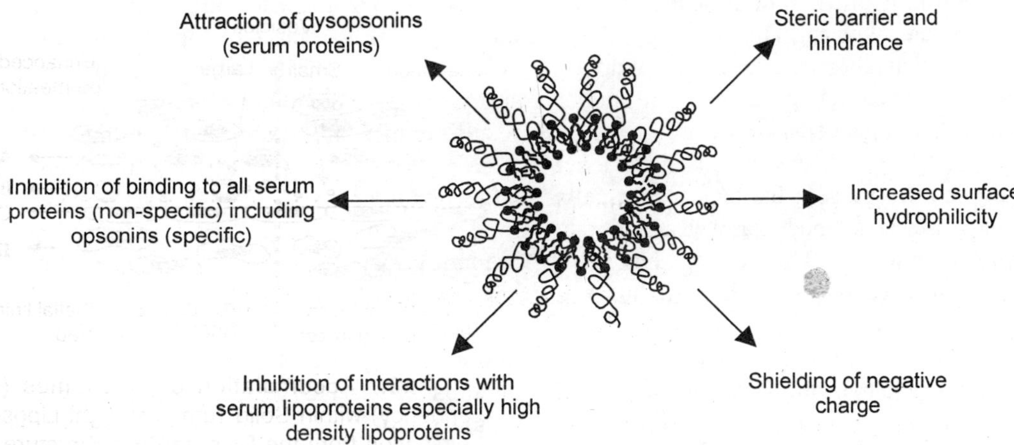

Fig. 14-24. Various Mechanisms Proposed for the Stealth or Long Circulatory Behaviour of Polymer Grafted or Glycolipid Anchored Liposomes

IgM have been efficiently taken up by lysosomes of peroxidase deficient phagocytes for the delivery of encapsulated horse-raddish peroxidase (HRP) (Weissmann et al., 1975). Owing to the instability of liposomes coupled with aggregated immunoglobulin, Gregoriadis, 1990 has reported the use of liposomes coated with polyclonal antibodies against a variety of tumour cell lines for better activity. Recent developments in liposome technology make it possible to explore therapeutic applications involving site specific delivery of Mabs. Antitarget mono-clonal antibody anchored on liposomes (immunolipo-somes) with specific avidity directed to carbohydrate containing antigens have been investigated to deliver the drugs like iodoxyuridine or acyclovir in the treatment of Herpes simplex virus (HSV) infected cell lines (Norley et al., 1986). Instead of using complete IgG portion or immunologically active fragments [$F(ab)_2$ and Fab'] have been used with improved access to the receptor bearing cells (Roer-dink et al., 1983).

The haptenated liposomes are based on biological target sensor and pilot module. The vesicular constructs were developed using PE lipids, containing the hapten linked to the liposome surface via carbon spacers of various lengths, in the presence of specific antibody. It can be exploited for the fixation to target cells that express surface immunoglobulin with specified affinity for the hapten. Hapten-bearing liposomes were pioneered by Kinsky et al., 1972. PE was modified by dinitrophenyl hapten (DNP) and incubated with anti-DNP antibody. These workers reported that rabbit antinitrophenyl antibody interacts with DNP bearing liposomes in the similar way as murine myeloma cells, which are known to express surface IgG that interacts with nitrophenyl hapten. Liposomes present haptens to the cells equipped with surfacial antibodies as well as antibody sequestering receptor(s). The concept has been effectively exploited to direct hapten bearing liposomes to Fc receptor bearing tumour and/or normal cells. The DNP bearing liposomes, opsonized by rabbit anti-nitrophenyl antibodies, bind to cells of the murine macrophage (tumour cell lines) that express Fc receptor for IgG. No binding was evident to the cells lacking the macrophage Fc receptor or when liposomes were opsonized by $F(ab)_2$ or IgA antibodies, confirming their specificity to the Fc portion of IgG. Lewis et al., 1980 reported haptenated liposomes where PE modified with a nitroxide spin-labeled hapten was used and studied the interaction of liposomes with Fc receptor bearing cells in the presence of antibody to hapten.

Recently designed immunoliposomes have been ameliorated by coating the outermost surface of large oligolamellar vesicles of egg PC with the poly-saccharide pullulan, to carry both cholesterol as the hydrophobic anchor and the monoclonal antibodies fragment (anti-sialosyl Lewis x : IgMs) as a site directing sensory device. The system showed better *in vivo* targetability. The concept of bivalent anti-bodies immobilized on the liposomal surface has been exploited in immuno-diagnostic assays and could be constructed for specific cellular targeting.

Antibody-associated liposomes containing antisense oligomer provide dual specificity: the antibody mediated selection of the particular cell lines along with the selectivity of the chosen mRNA sequence which is complementary to the liposome delivered oligomer (Leonetti et al., 1990). Zelphati and co-workers, 1996 reported immunoliposome as a carrier for intracellular delivery of antisense oligonucleotides.

The hydrophilic, opsonin repelling and sterically stabilized surface of SSL modified using GM1 gangliosides or PEG polymers (protein PEGylation), i.e. polymer-grafted immuno-liposomes make them long circulatory and hence suitable for extravascular tumour targeting. The development of new tech-nologies for an efficient attachment of Mab at the surface of PEG containing liposomes permits the resulting sterically stabilized immunoliposomes (SSIL) not only to exhibit greater recognition and target binding but also allow them to remain longer in circulation time relative to conventional immunoliposomes. SSL mediated targeting of antitumour drug doxorubicin has been reported in the treatment of murine solid tumours, human solid tumour xenografts and human haematological tumours. The surface immobilized Mabs directed to tumour associated antigens for immuno-specific binding produce better therapeutic effect and reduce the level of non-specific binding to nontarget cells (Allen, 1994; Emanuel et al., 1996).

Liposome Targeting to Tumours using Vitamin and Growth Factor Receptors

Liposome-encapsulated antitumour drugs reveal their potential for increased therapeutic efficacy and decreased nonspecific toxicities due to their ability to enhance the delivery of chemotherapeutic agents selectively to solid tumours. Advances in liposome technology have resulted in the development of ligand-targeted liposomes capable of selectively increasing the efficacy of carried agents against receptor bearing tumour cells. Receptors for vitamins and growth factors have become attractive targets for ligand-directed liposomal therapies due to their high expression levels on various forms of tumour and their ability to internalize after binding to the liposomes conjugated to receptors' natural ligands (vitamins) or synthetic agonists (receptor-specific antibodies and synthetic peptides).

Targeted Vs Non-targeted Liposomes in Tumour Targeting

In an exhaustive study, Allen, 1997 reported problems associated with targeting using monoclonal antibodies against surface epitopes on tumour cells. In his study solid tumours were implanted either subcutaneously or administered intravenously in pseudo-metastatic animal models. Figure 14-25 explains the interaction of non-targeted and ligand-mediated liposomes with tumour cells within the vasculature. Non-targeted liposomes have very limited inter-actions with single cells and released drug rapidly diffuses and redistributes to other tissues throughout the body. Targeted liposomes can interact either through non-internalizing or internalizing surface epitopes. Diffusion and redistribution of drug occur when interaction is mediated via non-internalizing receptors however, internalizing receptors deliver drug into the cellular interior. The author explained "bystander effect" for non-targeted liposomes and targeted liposomes equipped with non-internalizing epitopes for the fact that drug diffuses in the vicinity and into the interstitial fluid of a solid tumour. On the other hand, in the case of targeted liposomes equipped with internalizing epitope, the system gets ingested to cellular interiors well before a significant amount of drug is released outside the cells by diffusion (bystander effect) to take place.

Coupled with the bystander effect, the "binding site barrier" hypothesis (Weinstein and van Osdol, 1992) suggested that non-targeted (passively targeted) liposomes had greater penetrability into solid tumours with leaky vasculature compared to targeted liposomes.

However, this may or may not lead to increased cytotoxicity relative to targeted systems. Nevertheless, in the cases where extravasation mechanism has a critical interplay, for example in micrometastases prior to angiogenesis and haematological tumours, targeted liposomes are preferred over non-targeted liposomes. Further, the problems related to epitope mediated tumour targeting in terms of down regulation or sloughing of surface epitopes, the non-availability of appropriate ligands or antibodies against internalizing tumour epitopes and the lack of developing a true metastatic model for the otherwise available epitopes, have been explored.

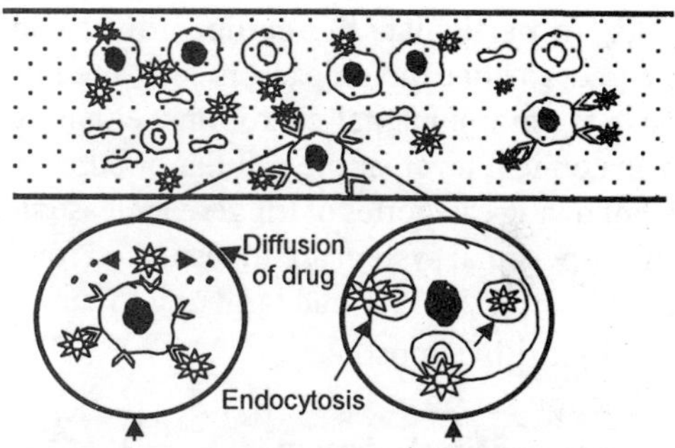

Fig. 14-25. The Interaction of Targeted Liposomes with Tumour cells within Vasculature. Non-targeted liposomes rapidly diffuse and redistribute the encapsulated contents with the interstitial fluid to tumour site and other sites in the body. Targeted liposomes show the same effect if the appended ligand is a non-internalizing epitope (Adopted from Allen, 1997)

Physicochemical Approaches (Triggered Release) of Liposomes in Tumour Therapy

An ideal system may involve some time-dependent or other specific inducible changes in the liposome membrane or its coating to produce "intelligent" liposomes that will change their properties (e.g. leakage rate, fusogenic activity and interaction with particular cells) upon getting specific stimulus following their application. Liposomes that are sensitive towards applied signal or environmental stimuli are being investigated as a tool for the targeted tumour therapy. The triggering of the release with the help of physical modulation or manipulation of the internal or external environment of the lipid constructs has been discussed under various titles, viz. signal sensitive, stimuli sensitive or physical targeting approaches. Signal sensitive liposomes belong to a class of ligand appended liposomal constructs which are responsive to biosignals and environmentally modulated by physical means to program and monitor selective release of entrapped contents. In particular, the compositions can be engineered so that the release is site specific in response to environmental conditions, either at the gross anatomical level, at the cellular or subcellular level. Following categories of triggered release signal sensitive liposomal system are investigated for their potential in drug delivery and targeting to tumour:

- pH sensitive liposomes
- Thermo sensitive liposomes
- Target sensitive liposomes
- Magneto-liposomes
- Photoactivated liposomes

Mechanisms operate for targeting at each of these levels are confined to pH and temperature sensitive liposomes.

The use of thermosensitive liposomes as drug delivery system was suggested by the observations that a dramatic increase in permeability of liposomes occurred at a temperature (above physiologic temperature) where molecules start arranging from one stable state to a second stable state and in the process destabilizing the structure. The fluctuations in temperature *in situ* similar to the fluctuations in pathological states like tumours, metastasis and inflammed tissues could trigger the release of the contents delivering them at the cellular level. In addition, the temperature of the desired site can be artificially manipulated by applying local heating (local hyperthermia, HT) that could increase the temperature of the desired site and hence concomitant release of the contents. The use of pH sensitive liposomes as drug delivery system was suggested by the observations that pathological tissues (tumours, metastases, inflammation and infection) have an ambient pH that is considerably lower than the normal tissue. Incorporation of the anti-target Mabs on pH sensitive liposome surface allows selective delivery to the respective target cells (Connor and Huang, 1985; Collins et al., 1990). These pH sensitive immunoliposomes possesses the ability to specifically deliver entrapped dye (calcein) and cytotoxic drugs (Ara-C and methotrexate) (Connor and Huang, 1985) to the cytoplasm of cell *in vitro*.

Temperature sensitive immunoliposomes (Sullivan and Huang, 1985; 1986) are designed to release their contents at the cell surface (target) upon heating to their intrinsic transition temperature. The anchored antibody confers recognition and specificity towards the target cell and once attached to the target cells the change in internal (or intrinsic) or external temperature modulates the release of the contents. Rapid release of entrapped carboxyfluorescein from immunoliposomes bound to target cells at 4°C was achieved upon brief exposure of (less than 3 min) at 41 °C (Sullivan and Huang, 1985).

Immunoliposomes composed of DPPC with entrapped uridine showed a heat-induced release of uridine at the target cell surface followed by transport and phosphorylation of uridine by the target cells (Sullivan and Huang, 1986). Khoobehi et al., 1988, proposed the design of temperature sensitive immunoliposomes containing calcein. The liposome could be activated through photo-excitation or thermal relaxation and irradiation after they arrive at the target tissue, offering a second degree of targeting. Aicher and co-workers, 1994 on the other hand reported photodynamic therapy of human bladder carcinoma cells *in vitro* with pH sensitive liposomes loaded with phototoxic drug 9-acetoxy-tetra-n-propylporphyrine.

Engineering vesicular constructs that destabilize upon binding of one of the lipid constituent with the target cells, offers enormous opportunity for intracellular and cytoplasmic delivery (target sensitive liposomes). Similarly, using magno-responsive or photosensitive lipid physically triggered release of the encapsulated contents constructs can be induced. Such systems respond to external/physical sources and get destabilized. Liposomal system can be customized as being thermosensitive and at the same time magno-responsive too. The system offers opportunities of active targeting under the guidance of external magnetic field of appropriate strength, and utilizes physical means for auto-destruction of liposomes in the target vicinity in response to local hyperthermia, negotiating a triggered delivery of the liposomal contents.

Magnoresponsive thermosensitive liposomes have been demonstrated in tumour treatment for their magnetically modulated localization followed by drug release in response to hyperthermia (Fig. 14-26). Positively charged liposomes with encapsulated paramagnetic materials, named as magneto-cationic liposomes (MCLs) were reported as potentially effective tools for hyperthermic treatment of solid tumours, because in addition to killing of the tumour cells by heat (Yanase et al., 1997) a host immune response was also induced (Yanase et al., 1998). Furthermore, immuno-cytochemical assay revealed that the host immune response induced by the hyperthermia treatment was mediated by both CD8+ and CD4+ T cells with a marked augmentation of tumour-selective cytotoxic T lymphocyte activity.

The use of photosensitizing drugs associated with different types of delivery vehicle has received distinctive interest within the field of the photodynamic therapy of tumours. Lipid-based delivery vehicles, such as liposomes and oil emulsions, allow the administration of water-insoluble photo-sensitizers, widening the choice of photo-sensitizers potentially useful for treating tumours. In some cases, these delivery vehicles increase the selectivity of tumour targeting by favouring photosensitizer uptake in tumour tissue. However, a higher selectivity of tumour targeting could be designed through association of photo-sensitizers with delivery vehicles, which can interact preferentially or specifically with tumour cells. With this aim in mind, low-density lipoproteins (LDLs) and monoclonal antibodies, in particular, are regarded as the most promising delivery systems for antitumour drugs. Some pharmacokinetic studies with LDL-associated photo-sensitizers have demonstrated a higher tumour uptake compared to the same photo-sensitizers delivered with other formulations. Monoclonal antibody-coupled photo-sensitizers have been tested mainly *in vitro*, and have shown a high selectivity towards cells expressing specific antigens. However, liposomal systems appear to be most promising for photo-sensitizers in the photodynamic therapy of tumours. Specific targeting of phototoxic haptenated liposomes to a hapten specific B cell lymphoma upon irradiation has been reported (Avirilions and Boggs, 1996). The photosensitizer eosin was coupled to a phospholipid and incorporated into trinitrophenol (TNP)-bearing SUVs of egg PC in order to target the photosensitizer to B lymphoma cells (A20-HL) that expressed TNP-specific membrane IgM receptors *in vitro*. These liposomes were consisted of TNP-DPPE:eosin-DPPE:EPC :Chol at a molar ratio of 2:5:48:45, respectively. Upon irradiation the production of singlet oxygen by TNP-targeted eosin containing liposomes cause elimination of B lymphoma cells (which otherwise have low internalization property or do not express sufficient membrane antigen (i.e. TNP) specific Ig receptors (Fig. 14-27).

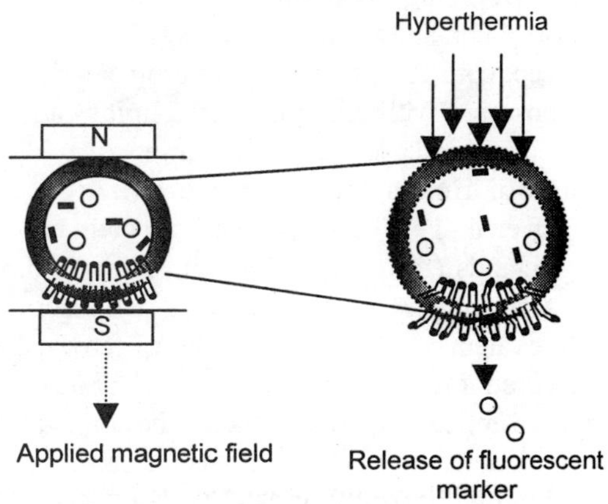

Fig. 14-26. Magnoresponsive Thermosensitive System for Tumour Targeting

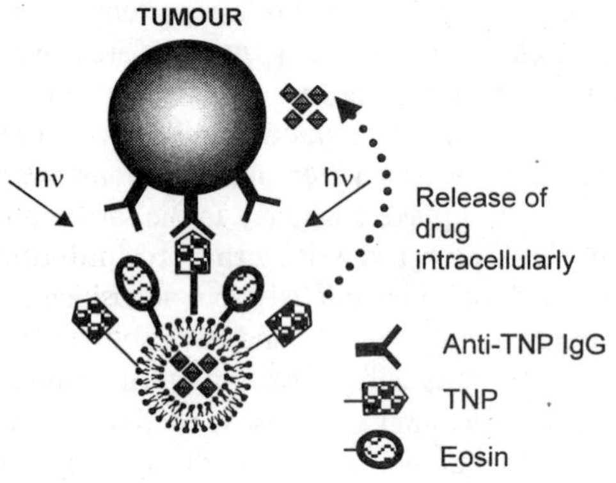

TUMOUR
hν
hν
Release of drug intracellularly
Anti-TNP IgG
TNP
Eosin

Fig. 14-27. Haptenated (TNP)-liposomes with Phototoxic Eosin Released upon Irradiation following Specific Interaction of TNP with Anti-TNP IgG of the Tumour Cell

Two step Targeting Approach: Biotin-avidin Conjugates with Anti-tumour Drugs

One of the most promising methods of tumour targeting is to make use of natural strong binding of avidin or streptavidin to small molecule biotin (Longman et al., 1995a). Biotinylated molecules can be targeted in complex mixtures by using appropriate avidin or streptavidin conjugates. If the biotinylated component has affinity for binding to a particular antigen or receptor of tumour, then the same can be located by the use of an avidin/streptavidin conjugate containing a detecting molecule. A series of avidin or streptavidin-biotin interactions can be built upon each other-utilizing the multivalent nature of each tetrameric avidin/streptavidin molecule (Fig. 14-28). The concept could be exploited with drug carriers as well. Liposomes with biotin modified lipids can be easily prepared and used to attach a variety of avidin/ streptavidin linked targeting proteins/ligands (Longman et al., 1995b). Non-specific protein based binding ligands (for example, avidin, streptavidin, protein A or protein G) can be attached to liposomes through covalent conjugation methods. Moreover, the site directed targeting ligands, an antibody or biotinylated antibody, can subsequently be conjugated to the liposomes non-covalently using some non-specific binding ligands (Fig. 14-28). This however, restricts the use of only anti-target immunoglobulin molecules as site-directing ligands.

Micro/Nanoparticles in Chemotherapy

The most promising application of micro/ nanoparticles is their possible use as carriers for antitumour agents (Convreur and Vauthier, 1991; Kreuter, 1991). Enhanced endocytic activity and leaky vasculature of the tumour, favours accumulation of intravenously administered nanoparticles. In addition, targeting to tumour tissues could be facilitated and optimized using stealth version of microparticulates for better extravasation. Stealth nanoparticles are prepared by coating them with soluble polyoxyethylene, or by using dialykyl polyoxyethylene and phospholipids. Sometimes the accumulation of non-stealth (conventional) nano-particles in RES may be exploited for organ localized tumour chemotherapy.

Chemoembolization- Intraarterial Infusion Chemotherapy

In order to improve targeting and retention of antitumour agents in the tumour area, drug delivery systems involving the haemodynamics of the tumour area are being designed and developed. These include balloon-occluded arterial infusion therapy, administration with vasoconstrictive agents such as noradrenaline or angiotensin II. Intraarterial

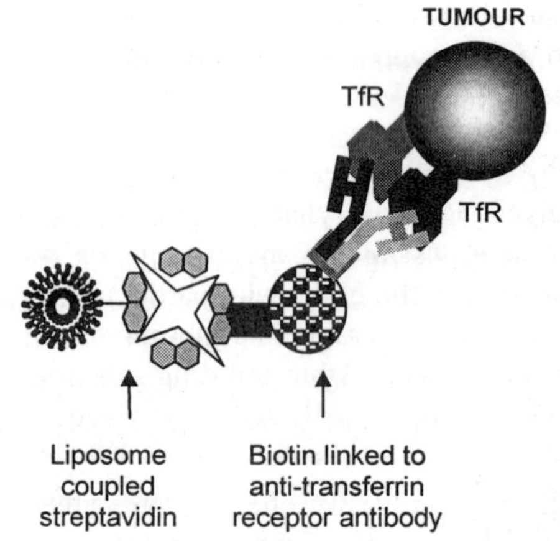

Fig. 14-28. Biotin-avidin/streptavidin Conjugated Carriers, where Avidin/Streptividin Links the Delivery Systems and Biotinylated Targeting Ligand. This sandwich-targeting carrier then can target receptor (or antigen) against which the targeting ligand (antibody) has been linked.

administration of anti-tumour drugs with various drug carriers, i.e., microcapsules, lipiodol, albumin microspheres, degradable starch microspheres and liposomes have been proposed and clinically evaluated with various tumours. Furthermore, development of totally implantable equipment for intraarterial use for continuous infusion or one-shot injection of antitumour agents, could treat the patients longer and more frequently with less trouble. One of the approaches, defined as, chemoembolization, makes use of the biodegradable particles administration to the liver tumours using a catheter that passes directly into an artery leading to the tumour (Fig. 14-29). The accumulation of mitomycin-C bearing microparticles within the Kupffer cells (liver) has been explored and used to target hepatic neoplasm indirectly (Natsume et al., 1990). A depot of drug for killing nearby neoplastic tissues was used *in vivo*, as the particles (non-stealth) are not actually taken up by the neoplastic tissue. Similar targeting strategies using trans-catheter chemoembolization have been reported for cisplatin (Li et al., 1994), doxorubicin (Cay et al., 1996), taxol (Wang et al., 1996), rifampicin (Kassab et al., 1997) and 5-fluorouracil (Denkbas et al., 1999). Several studies report prolonged drug retention in tumours, reduction in tumour growth, and prolonged survival of tumour bearing animals following administration of nanoparticle loaded antitumour agents compared to free drug treatment.

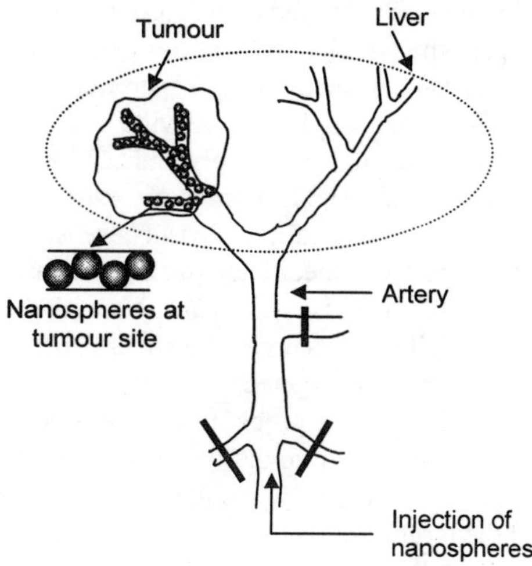

Fig. 14-29. Infusion of Albumin Particles for Chemo-embolization into the Liver

Delivery of Antitumour Drugs

The polyalkylcyanoacrylate nanoparticles have been studied as a possible means of targeting drugs to specific sites in the body, with particular emphasis on tumour chemotherapy. The sub-micron colloidal carriers are biodegradable and drug substances can be incorporated normally by a process of surface adsorption. Some of the antitumour drugs that are reported either entrapped or adsorbed onto nano-particles are:

- Doxorubicin in polyisohexylcyanoacrylate nanoparticles (Chiannilkulchai et al., 1989)
- Mitoxantrone in polybutylcyanoacrylate nano-particles (Beck et al., 1993)
- Aclacinomycin A in polyisobutylcyano-acrylate nanoparticle
- Granulocyte-colony stimulating factor (G-CSF) in polyalkylcyanoacrylate nanoparticles (Gibaud et al., 1998),
- Acyclovir in polybutylcyanoacrylate nanoparticles (Zhang et al., 1995), and
- Doxorubicin-loaded polyalkylcyanoacrylate nanoparticles (Soma et al., 2000).

However, other biodegradable polymers like poly(lactide-co-glycolide) and polyvinyl-pyrrolidone have also been investigated for drug delivery in tumour therapy. These include dexamethasone in poly(lactide-co-glycolide) nanoparticle (Guzman et al., 1996) and Taxol in polyvinylpyrrolidone nanoparticles (Sharma et al., 1996).

Nanoparticles Coated with Antibodies

The anchoring of target specific antibodies to the nanoparticle surface may further facilitate their delivery to the specific sites. Selectivity in drug targeting can, in theory, be achieved by the attachment of monoclonal antibody as a site-directing device. Work *in vitro* and *in vivo*, where nanoparticles have been coated with monoclonal antibodies, is described (Douglas et al., 1987). Monoclonal antibodies can be fixed on nanoparticles by direct adsorption or via a spacer molecule (protein A) or by covalent linkage (e.g., carbodiimide, cyanogen bromide and glutaraldehyde reaction) (Illum et al., 1989). In this way, antibodies are anchored to the particles through their Fc part thus projecting the antigen specific binding sites (Fab') for the target specificity. This technique has been applied to a wide variety of nanoparticles including PACA, polymethacrylate and albumin (Illum et al., 1982; Illum et al., 1986; Illum et al., 1989; Breton et al., 1996). These studies however, suggest the specificity of these immuno-nanoparticles to tumour cells *in vitro*. Nevertheless, such systems failed to record a significant accumulation of the carriers in targeted tumours *in vivo*. This could be attributed to a probable competitive displacement of the blood components or secondary coating of opsonin components and/or insufficient access to the target site.

Ramsen and co-workers, 1996 reported that tumour-specific monoclonal antibodies conjugated to super-paramagnetic monocrystalline iron oxide nanoparticles (MION) could be used to yield specific diagnoses with the use of MR imaging. Tiefenauer and co-workers, 1996 evaluated magnetic nanoparticles as a tumour contrast agent in MRI. Magnetite nanoparticles, coated by three different artificial polypeptides, were conjugated to an antibody specific to the carcinoembryonic antigen (CEA). To protect the particles from fast blood elimination, the surfaces were modified using various macromolecules, i.e., polyethylene-glycol, albumin, and sialoprotein, respectively. The protective effect was determined by using a specific *in vitro* test and by analyzing the biodistribution of the nanoparticles in nude mice grafted with CEA-tumours. The tumour accumulation was slightly improved in the case of the nanoparticles coated with sialoprotein glycophorin B.

However, coating long circulatory and sterically stabilized nanoparticles with site-specific antibodies or lectins remain to be explored for better biomedical applications.

FUTURE PERSPECTIVES

Vascular Targeting with Phage Peptide Libraries

Recent research is being focused on developing *in vivo* selection system in which phages capable of selective homing to different tissues are recovered from phage display peptide libraries following intravenous administration. Using this strategy, several organ and tumour-homing peptides have been separated. Each of these peptides binds to different receptors that are selectively expressed on the vasculature of the target tissue. The tumour-homing peptides bind to receptors that are upregulated in tumour angiogenic vasculature. Targeted delivery of doxorubicin to angiogenic vasculature using these peptides in animal models decreased toxicity and increased the therapeutic efficacy of the drug. Vascular targeting may facilitate the development of other treatment strategies that rely on inhibition of angiogenesis and lead to advances in tumour treatment.

Application of Peptide Nucleic Acid in Tumour Therapy

Peptide nucleic acid (PNA) is a DNA mimic with a pseudopeptide backbone composed of aminoethyl glycine units. Several features of PNA, such as superior hybridization affinities to RNA and DNA, high biological stability, and convenient solid-phase synthesis, make it a promising candidate for use as a gene targeting and potential as an anti-tumour drug.

Polyethylene Glycol Modifications in Tumour Targeting

Soluble polymer (macromolecule) conjugates have only recently been introduced into clinical practice. They can be subdivided into two main categories: polymer-protein conjugates, so far the most widely studied; and polymer-drug conjugates, particularly those containing conventional antitumour agents.

Of all the polymers applied to molecule altering structural chemistry, polyethylene glycol (PEG) modification has numerous benefits for tumour targeting. PEG is now increasingly being applied in tumour targeting, both in the context of the passive targeting of PEG-liposomes and in active targeting strategies using PEGylated anti-tumour antibodies. PEG can also serve as a useful linker molecule between targeting moieties and other agents, including cytotoxic or imaging agents and target-oriented liposomes. Despite established benefits of PEGylation, relatively little considerations have been given to optimize their implementation. First issue is the extent to which the coupling method has an impact on both the functionality of the PEG-adduct and the acquisition of beneficial properties. Another issue focuses on the effect of PEGylation on complex biodistribution, thus any attempt to optimize a PEG-peptide or PEG-liposome for a particular task must involve a critical examination of all the individual facets of the effects relating to PEGylation.

Local Delivery of Anti-neoplastic Agents using Biodegradable Polymers

Controlled delivery of chemotherapeutic agents by biodegradable polymers is a new strategy that has been added to the therapeutic arsenal available for the treatment of malignant neoplasms. This approach is particularly suitable for the management of brain tumours because of the constraints imposed by the blood brain barrier (BBB). The use of polymers for local drug delivery minimizes systemic toxicity, while achieving prolonged elevation of intratumoural drug concentrations that results in improved efficacy.

Others

The innovation in the field of research on the targeted drug delivery in the coming years would be a shift from "receptor to nucleus" reflecting a desire to construct defined pathway linking the end points of different regulatory cellular events. However, for basic and technical reasons, research efforts have been focused overwhelmingly on receptor/ligand or transcription factor/DNA interactions. The task confronting molecular targeting is to link up these two extremes. It is clear that signal transduction involves many intermediate cellular events from membrane to nucleus. One of the simplest types of signal transduction pathway involves the generation of second messenger and cascade of events thereafter. A second type of signal transduction pathway is the kinase cascade, which is activated in response to events occurring at the cell surface. In each of these, the target transcription factors appear related to the nucleus under most circumstances giving an insight of the communication of the signals across the nuclear membranes. Whiteside and Goodbourn, 1993 have reviewed a number of studies in which the transcription factors themselves are actually located in the cytoplasm prior to activation and become relocated in the nucleus as a consequence of response to appropriate signals/ligands.

In the future, targeted drug-delivery systems may also prove particularly valuable to enable the use of a drug that seems to be ineffective or toxic, if delivered systemically [e.g., neural growth factor (which need to cross blood-brain barrier) or vaccines (which need to be taken up by antigen presenting cells)]. At the current pace of gene cloning and recombinant-protein production within the bio-pharmaceutical industry, many more site-specific drug-delivery products will be clinically investigated and implemented in near future.

REFERENCES

Aicher A., Miller K., Reich E. and Hautmann R. (1994) *Urol. Res.* **22**, 25.

Albelda S. M., Smith C. W. and Ward P. A. (1995) *FASEB J.* **8**, 504.

Allen T. M. (1997) *J. Liposome Res.* **7**, 315.

Allen T. M. (1994) Trends Pharmacol. Sci. **15**, 215.

Anderson P., Hasz D., Dickrell L. and Sencer S. (1992) *Drug Deliv. Res.* **27**, 15.

Avrilionis K. and Boggs J. M. (1996) *Cell. Immunol.* **168**, 13.

Barbas C. F., Languino L. R. and Smith J. W. (1993) *Proc. Natl. Acad. Sci. USA* **90**, 10003.

Bates R. C., Lincz L. F. and Burns G. F. (1995) *Cancer Metastasis Rev.* **14**, 191.

Beck P., Kreuter J., Reszka R. and Fichtner I. (1993) *J. Microencap.* **10**, 101.

Begnet R. H. J., Verhaar M. J., Chester K. A., Casey J. L., Green A. J., Napier M. P., Hope-Stone L. D., Cushen N., Keep P. A. and Johnson C. J. (1996) *Nature Med.* **2**, 979.

Berg E. L., Goldstein L. A., Picker L. J., Streeter P. R., Jutilla M. A., Bergatze R. F., Zhou D. F. H. and Butcher E. C. (1991) In: Glycobiology, Welplay J. K. and Jaworski E. (Eds.) New York, Wiley-Liss, 91.

Bevilacqua M. P. and Nelson R. M. (1993) *J. Clin. Invest.* **91**, 379.

Bevilacqua M. P., Nelson R. M., Mannori G. and Cecconi O. (1994) *Annu. Rev. Med.* **45**, 361.

Bigsterbosch M. K. and Van Berkel Th. J. C. (1990) *Adv. Drug Deliv. Rev.* **5**, 231.

Bird R. E., Hardman K. D., Jacobson J. W., Johnson S., Kaufman B. M., Lee S. M., Lee T., Pope S. H., Riordan

G. S., Whitelow M. (1988) *Science* **242**, 423.

Bishop J. M. (1995) *Genes and Development* **9**, 1309.

Bloemen P. G. M., Henricks P. A. J., van Bloois L., van den Tweel M. C., Blqem A. C., Nijkamp F. P., Crommelin D. J. A. and Storm G. (1995) *FEBS Lett.* **357**, 140.

Breton P. (1996) *Eur. J. Pharm. Biopharm.* **43**, 95.

Burg J., Lotscher E., Steimer K. S., Capon D. J., Baenziger J., Jick H. M. and Wabl M. (1991) *Proc. Natl. Acad. Sci. USA* **88**, 4723.

Burrow F. J., Tazzari P., Amlot P., Gajdar A. F., Derbyshire E. J., King S. W., Vitetta E. S. and Thorpe P. E. (1995) *Clinical Cancer Res.* **1**, 1623.

Campbell I. G., Jones T. A., Foulkes W. D. and Trowsdale J. (1991) *Cancer Res.* **51**, 5329.

Cay O., Kruskal J., Thomas P. and Clouse (1996) *J. Vasc. Interv. Radiol.* **7**, 409.

Chiannilkulchai N., Driouich Z., Benoit J. P., Parodi A. L. and Couvreur P. (1989) *Sel. Cancer Ther.* **5**, 1.

Cho B. K., Roy E. J., Patrik T. A. and Kranz D. M. (1997) *Bioconjug. Chem.* **8**, 338.

Clackson T., Hoogenboom H. R., Griffiths A. D., Winter G. (1991) *Nature* **352**, 624.

Cline H. J. and Sumner H. A. (1972) *Blood* **40**, 62.

Collins D., Connor J., Ting-Beall H. P. and Huang L. (1990) *Chem. Phys. Lipid.* **55**, 339.

Connor J. and Huang L. (1985) *J. Cell Biol.* **101**, 582.

Convreur P. and Vauthier C. (1991) *J. Control. Rel.* **17**, 187.

Cuvier C., Roblot-Treupel L., Millot J. M., Lizard G., Chevillard S., Manfait M., Couvreur P. and Poupon M. F. (1992) *Biochem. Pharmacol.* **44**, 509.

D'Souza S. E., Ginsberg M. H. and Plow E. F.(1991) *Trends Biochem. Sci.* **16**, 246.

Denkbas E. B., Seyyal M. and Piskin E. (1999) *J. Microencapsul.* **16**, 741.

Depraetere S. and Joniau M. (1995) *Leuk. Res.* **19**, 803.

Dittrich E. (1994) *J. Biol. Chem.* **269**, 19014.

Douglas S. J., Davis S. S. and Illum L. (1987) *CRC Crit Rev.* **3**, 233.

Drake C. J., Cheresh D. A. and Little C. D. (1995) *J. Cell Sci.* **108**, 2655.

Emanuel N., Kedar E., Bolotin E.M., Smorodinsky N. I. and Bareholz Y. (1996) *Pharm. Res.* **13**, 861.

Endicott J. A. and Ling V. (1989) *Annu. Rev. Biochem.* **58**, 137.

Fanger M. W., Morganelli P. M. and Guyre P. M.(1992) *Crit. Rev. Immunol.* **12**, 101.

Filardo E. J., Brooks P. C., Deming S. L., Damsky C. and Cheresh D. A.(1995) *J. Cell Biol.* **130**, 441.

Foldvari M., Baca-Estrada M. E., He Z., Hu J., Attah-Poku S. and King M. (1999) *Biotechnol. Appl. Biochem.* **30**, 129.

Folkman J. (1995) In: The Molecular Basis of Cancer, Mendelsohn J., Howley P. M., Israel M. A. and Liotta L. A. (Eds.) W.B. Saunders, Philadelphia, 1.

Folkman J. (1996) *Scientific American* **9**, 150.

Foxall C., Watson S. R., Dowbenko D., Fennie C., Lasky L. A., Kiso M., Hasegawa A. and Asa D. (1992) *J. Cell Biol.* **117**, 895.

Frenette P. S. and Wagner D. D. (1996a) *New. Eng. J. Med.* **334**, 1526.

Frenette P. S. and Wagner D. D. (1996b) *New. Eng. J. Med.* **335**, 43.

Gabizon A., Horowitz A.T., Goren D. , Tzemach D., Mondelbaum-Shavit F., Qazen M. M. and Zalipsky S. (1999) *Bioconjugate Chem.* **10**, 289.

Gabizon A. and Papahadjopoulos D. (1988) *Proc. Natl. Acad. Sci. USA* **85**, 6949.

Gabizon A., Goron D., Horowitz A. T., Tzemach D., Lossos A. and Siegal T. (1997) *Adv. Drug Del. Rev.* **24**, 337.

Garagiola D. M., Huard T. K. and Lo Buglio A. F. (1979) *Blood* **54**, 84a.

Gibaud S., Rousseau C., Weingarten C., Favier R., Douay L., Andreux J. P. and Couvreur P. (1998) *J. Control. Rel.* **52**, 131.

Gibbs J. F. and Oliff A. (1994) *Cell* **79**, 193.

Gold L. (1995) *Nucleic Acid Symp. Ser.* **33**, 20.

Gregoriadis G. and Florence A. T. (1993) *Drugs* **45**, 1993.

Gregoriadis G. (1990) *Immunol. Today* **11**, 89.

Gregoriadis G. (1993) *Lancet* **2**, 241.

Guzman L., Labhasetwar V., Song C., Jang Y., Lincoff M. A., Levy R. J. and Topol E. J. (1996) *Circulation* **92**, I-292.

Haisma H. J., Boven M., Vanmuijen M., Dejong J., Vander Vijgh W. J. F. and Pinedo H. M. (1992) *Br. J. Cancer* **66**, 474.

Hayashi H., Kono K. and Takagishi T. (1998) *Bioconjug. Chem.* **9**, 382.

Hege K. M., Daleke D. L., Waldmann T. A. and Matthay K. K.(1989) *Blood* **74**, 2043.

Hinds P. W. and Weinberg R. A. (1994) *Current Opinion in Genetics and Development* **4**, 135.

Illum L., Davis S. S., Wilson C. G., Frier M., Hardy J. G. and Thomas N. W. (1982) *Int. J. Pharm.* **12**, 135.

Illum L., Thomas N. W. and Davis S. S. (1986) *J. Pharm. Sci.* **29**, 53.

Illum L., Wright J. and Davis S. S. (1989) *Int. J. Pharm.* **52**, 1989.

Ishida O. and Maruyama K. (1998) *Nippon. Rinsho.* **56**, 657.

Ishihara H., Hara T., Aramaki Y., Tsuchiya S. and Hosoi

K. (1990) *Pharm. Res.* **7**, 542.

Jain R.K. (1994) *Scientific American* **271**, 58.

Jiang X. and Liao G. (1995) *Hua. His. I. Ko. Ta. Hsueh. Hsueh. Pao.* **26**, 163.

Jones M. N. *(1994) Adv. Drug Deliv. Rev.* **13**, 215.

Karajgi J., Jain N. K. and Vyas S. P. (1993) *J. Drug Target.* **1**, 197.

Kartner N., Evernden-Porelle D., Bradley G. and Ling V. (1985) *Nature* **316**, 820.

Kassab A. C., Xu K., Denkbas E. B., Dou Y., Zhao S., Piskin E. (1997) *J. Biomater. Sci. Polym. Ed.* **8**, 947.

Katre N., Knauf M. and Laird W. (1987) *Proc. Natl. Acad. Sci. USA* **84**, 1487.

Kedar E., Rutkowski Y., Braun E., Emanuel N. and Barenholz Y. (1994) *J. Immunother. Emphasis Tumour Immunol.* **16**, 47.

Khoobehi B., Peyman G. A., Mcturnan W.G., Niesman, M. R. and Magin R. L. (1988) *Opthalmology* **95**, 950.

Kinsky S. C. (1972) *Biochim. Biophys. Acta.* **265**, 1.

Konigsberg P. J., Godtel R., Kissel T. and Richer L. L.(1998) *Biochim. Biophys. Acta.* **1370**, 243.

Kreuter J. (1991) *J. Control. Rel.* **16**, 169.

Kroesen B. J., Helfrich W., Bakker A., Wubbena A. S., Bakker H., Kal H. B., The T. H. and Dleij L (1995) *Int. J. Cancer* **61**, 812.

Kubiak C., Manil L., Clausse B. and Couvreur P. (1989) *Biomaterials* **10**, 553.

Kuby J. (1994) Immunology, IInd edition. W.H. Freman and Company, New York, 1.

Lafrenie R. M. and Yamada K. M. (1996) *J. Cell Biochem.* **61**, 543.

Lamparsk H., Liman U., Barry J. A., Frankel D. A., Ramaswami V., Brown M. F. and O'Brien D. F. (1992) *Biochemistry* **31**, 685.

Lasic D. D. (1997) Liposomes in gene therapy, CRC Press, Boca Raton, FL, 1.

Lasic D. D. (1998) *Trends in Biotechnology* **16**, 307.

Lasky L. A. (1995) *Annu. Rev. Cell Dev. Biol.* **11**, 601.

Lazo J. S. and Hacker M. P. (1986) *Fred. Proc.* **44**, 2335.

Ledley F. D. (1995) *Human Gene Therapy* **6**, 1129.

Lee R. J. and Low P. S. (1994) *J. Biol. Chem.* **269**, 3198.

Lee R. J. and Low P. S. (1994) *Biochim. Biophys. Acta* **1233**, 134.

Lefer A. M., Weyrich A. S. and Buerke M. (1994) *Cardiovasc. Res.* **28**, 289.

Leonetti J. P., Degols G. and Lebleu B. (1990) *Bioconjugate. Chem.* **1**, 149.

Lewis J. T., Hafeman D. G. and McConnell H.M. (1980) *Biochemistry* **19**, 5376.

Li C., Yang D. J., Nikiforow S., Tansey W., Kuang L. R., Wright K. C. and Wallace S. (1994) *Pharm. Res.* **11**, 1792.

Longman S. A., Cullis P. R. and Bally M. B. (1995a) *Drug Delivery* **2**, 156.

Longman S. A., Cullis P. R., Choi L., de Jong G. and Bally M. B. (1995b) *Cancer Chemother. Pharmacol.* **36**, 91.

Mach J. P. (1995) In: Oxford Textbook of Oncology, Vol. 1, Peckham J., Pinedo M. and Veronesi U. (Eds.) Oxford University Press, 25.

Mareel M., Berx F., Van Roy F. and Bracke M. (1996) *J. Cell Biochem.* **61**, 524.

Mateos S. P., Cabanas C. and Madrid S. F. (1996) *Semin. Cancer Biol.* **7**, 99.

Meijer D. K. F., Jansen R. W. and Molema G. (1992) *Antiviral Res.* **18**, 215.

Mizuno M., Yoshida J., Sugita K., Inoue I., Seo H., Hayashi Y., Koshizaka T. and Yagi K. (1990) *Cancer Res.* **50**, 7826.

Molema G. and Meijer D. K. F. (1994) *Adv. Drug Deliv. Rev.* **14**, 25.

Molema G., de Leij L. F. M. H. and Meijer K. F. (1997) *Pharm. Res.* **14**, 2.

Monsigny, M., Roche, A.C. and Midoux, P. (1988) *Ann. NY Acad. Sci.* **551**, 195.

Monsigny M., Roche A. C., Midoux P. and Mayer R. (1994) *Adv. Drug Deliv. Rev.* **14**, 1.

Muggia F. M., Hainsworth J. D., Jeffers S., Miller P., Groshen S., Tan M., Roman L., Uziely B., Muderspach L., Garcia A., Burnett A. and Greco F. A. (1997) *J. Clin. Oncol.* **15**, 987.

Munns J., Yaxley J., Coomer J., Lavin M. F., Gardinger R. A. and Watters D. (1998) *Br. J. Urol.* **82**, 284.

Nakamura K., Okuno K., Hirohata T., Shigeoka H., Jinnai H. and Yasutomi M. (1994) *Gan To Kagaku Ryoho* **21**, 2105.

Nassander U. K., Steerenberg P. A., Poppe H., Storm G., Jap P. H. K., Poels L. G., de Jong W. H. and Cromellin D. J. A. (1992) *Cancer Res.* **52**, 646.

Natsume H., Sugibayashi K., Juni K., Morimoto Y., Shibata T. and Fujimoto S. (1990) *Int. J. Pharm.* **58**, 79.

Neri D. and Zardi L. (1998) *Adv. Drug Deliv. Rev.* **31**, 43.

Nishida K., Seto M., Takahashi T., Oshima Y., Asano S. and Ueda R. (1997) *Cancer Lett.* **113**, 153.

Nishiya T. and Sloan S. (1996) *Biochim. Biophys. Res. Commun.* **224**, 242 .

Norley S. G., Huang L. and Rouse B.T. (1986) *J. Immunol.* **136**, 681.

Okada N., Miyamoto H., Yoshioka T., Katsume A., Saito

H., Yorozu K., Ueda O., Itoh N., Mizuguchi H., Nakagawa S., Ohsugi Y. and Mayumi T. (1997) *Biochim. Biophys. Acta.* **1360**, 53.

Okuno K., Nakamura K., Tanaka A., Yachi K. and Yasutomi M. (1998) *Surg Today* **28**, 64.

Old J. L. (1996) *Scientific American* **9**, 136.

Oldham R. E. (1983) *Clin. Immunol. News* **4**, 131.

Oliff A., Gibbs J. B. and McCormick F. (1996) *Scientific American* **9**, 144.

Peterson, H.I. (1979) In;Tumour Blood Circulation: Angiogenesis, Vascular Morphology and Blood flow of Experimental and Human Tumours, CRC Press, Boca raton, 1.

Poste G. and Kirsh R. (1983) *Biotechnology* **1**, 869.

Poste G. (1984) In: Drug Targeting In Cancer Chemotherapy, In Receptor Mediated Targeting Of Drugs. Gregoriadis G., Poste G., Senior J. and Trout A. (Eds.) Plenum Press, New-York, 1.

Reddy J. A. and Low P. S. (1998) *Crit. Rev. Ther. Drug Carrier Syst.* **15**, 587.

Roerdink F., Wassef N. M., Richardson E. C. and Alving C. R. (1983) *Biochim. Biophys. Acta.* **734**, 33.

Rosen S. D. and Bertozzi C. R. (1994) *Curr. Opin. Cell Biol.* **6**, 663.

Rosenberg M. B., Breakfield X. O. and Hawrot E. (1989) *J. Neurochem.* **48**, 865.

Ruoslahti E. (1996) *Annu. Rev. Cell Dev. Biol.* **12**, 697.

Saiki I., Koike C., Obata A., Fuji H., Murata J., Kiso M., Hasegawa A., Komazawa H. (1996) *Int. J. Cancer* **65**, 833.

Sarti P., Ginobbi P., D'Agostino I., Arancia G., Lendaro E., Molinari A., Ippoliti R. and Citro G. (1996) *Biotechnol. Appl. Biochem.* **24**, 269.

Sato J., Hamaguchi N., Doken K., Gotoh K., Ootsu K., Iwasa S., Ogawa Y. and Toguchi H. (1993) *Biotherapy* **6**, 225.

Scheffold A., Miltenyi S. and Radbrunch A. (1995) *Immunotechnology* **1**, 127.

Senter P. D. (1990) *FASEB J.* **4**, 188.

Seymour L. W. (1994) *Adv. Drug Deliv. Rev.* **14**, 89.

Sharma D., Chelvi T. P., Kaur J., Chakravorty K., De T. K., Maitra A. and Ralhan R. (1996) *Oncol. Res.* **8**, 281.

Sherwood R. F. (1996) *Adv. Drug Deliv. Rev.* **22**, 269.

Singh M. (1999) *Curr Pharm. Des.* **5**, 443.

Sipkins D. A., Brooks P. C., Cheresh D. A., Li K. P. C. and Bednarski M. D. (1996) *Proc. Am. Assoc. Cancer Res.*, Washington DC.

Soma C. E., Dubernet C., Bentolia D., Benita S. and Couvreur P. (2000) *Biomaterials* **21**, 1.

Springer T. A. (1994) *Cell* **76**, 301.

Staerz U. D., Kanagawa O. and Bevan M. J. (1985) *Nature* **314**, 628.

Sullivan S. M. and Huang L. (1985) *Biochem. Biophy. Acta* **812**, 116.

Sullivan S. M. and Huang L. (1986) *Proc. Natl. Acad. Sci. USA.* **83**, 6117.

Sun Q. H., De Lisser H. M., Zukowski M. M., Paddock C., Albelda S. M. and Newman P. J. (1996) *J. Biol. Chem.* **271**, 11090.

Tanaka T., Kaneo Y., Miyashita M. (1996) *Biol. Pharm. Bull.* **19**, 774.

Tortora G. J., Funke B. R. and Case C. L. (1998) In: Microbiology: An introduction. 6th edition. Addison Wesley Longman, California. 456.

Tsujimoto M., Yip Y. K. and Vilcek J. (1986) *J Immunol.* **136**, 441.

Tsunoda S., Tsutsumi Y. and Mayumi T. (1998) *Nippon Rinsho.* **56**, 573.

Unkeless J. C., Fleit H. B. and Mellman I. S. (1981) *Adv. Immunol.* **31**, 247.

Vaage J., Donavan D., Loftus T., Abra R., Working P. and Hunag A. (1994) *Cancer* **73**, 2366.

Varner J. A., Brooks P. C. and Cheresh D. A. (1995) *Cell Adhes. Commun.* **3**, 367.

Vingerhoeds M. H., Haisma H. J., Van Muijen M., Van de R., Cromellin D. J. A. and Storm G. (1993) *FEBS Lett.* **336**, 485.

Vitetta E. S. (1990) *J. Clin. Immunol.* **10**, 515.

Vogelstein B. and Kinzler K. W. (1993) *Trends in genetics* **9**, 138.

Vyas S. P. and Dixit V. K. (1999) In: Pharmaceutical Biotechnology, CBS Publishers, New Delhi.

Vyas S. P. and Sakthivel T. (1994) *J. Microencap.* **11**, 373.

Vyas S. P. and Sihorkar V. (1999) *J. Clin. Pharm. Ther.* **24**, 259.

Vyas S. P. and Sihorkar V. (2000) *Adv. Drug Deliv. Rev.* **43**, 101.

Vyas S. P., Katare Y. K. Mishra V. and Sihorkar V. (2000) *Int. J. Pharm.* **210**, 1.

Vyas S. P., Singh A. and Sihorkar V. (2001) *Crit Rev. Ther. Drug Carr. Syst.* **18**, 1.

Wagner E., Curiel D. and Cotton M. (1994) *Adv. Drug Deliv. Rev.* **14**, 113.

Wagner E., Zatloukal K., Cotton M., Kirlappos H., Mechtler K. and Curiel D. T. (1992) *Proc. Natl. Acad. Sci. USA.* **89**, 6099.

Wang S., Lee R. J., Mathias C. J., Green M. and Low P. S. (1996) *Bioconjug. Chem.* **7**, 56.

Watanabe N., Sato Y., Yamauchi N. and Nitsu Y. (1998) *Nippon Rinsho.* **56**, 724.

Weinberg R. A. (1996) *Scientific American.* **9**, 62.

Weinstein J. N. and Van Osdol W. (1992) 52, 2747.

Weissmann G., Bloomgarden D., Kalpan R., Cohen C., Hoffstein S., Collins T., Gottlieb A. and Nagle D. (1975) *Proc. Natl. Acad. Sci. USA*. **72**, 88.

Whiteside S. T. and Goodbourn S. (1993) *J. Cell Biol.* **104**, 949.

Woodle M. C. and Lasic D. D. (1992) *Biochim. Biophys. Acta* **1113**, 171.

Wright S. and Huang L. (1989) *Adv. Drug Deliv. Rev.* **3**, 343.

Xi K., Tabata Y., Uno K., Yoshimoto M., Kishida T., Sokawa Y. and Ikada Y. (1996) *Pharm. Res.* **13**, 1846.

Xu Y. H., Richert N., Ito S., Merlino G. T. and Pasten I. (1984) *Proc. Natl. Acad. Sci. USA*. **81**, 7308.

Yanase M., Shinkai M., Honda H., Wakabayashi T., Yoshida J. and Kobayashi T. (1998) *Jpn. J. Cancer Res.* **89**, 775.

Yanase M., Shinkai M., Honda H., Wakabayashi T., Yoshida J. and Kobayashi T. (1997 *Jpn. J. Cancer Res.* **88**, 630.

Yang J. and Cleland J. L. (1997) *J. Pharm. Sci.* **86**, 908.

Zalipsky S., Puntambekar B., Boulikas P., Engbers C. M. and Woodle M. C. (1995) *Bioconj. Chem.* **6**, 705.

Zelphati O., Francis C. and Szoka Jr. F. C. (1996) *J. Control. Rel.* **41**, 99.

Zhang Q., Liao G. and Yin H. (1995) *Hua. His. I. Ko. Ta. Hsueh. Hsueh. Pao.* **26**, 172.

CHAPTER 15

Drug Delivery to Bone Marrow

The bone marrow is basically a connective spongy tissue found inside bones. There are two types of bone marrows in the human body, yellow marrow and red marrow. Yellow marrow consists mostly of adipose tissue, and red marrow consists of haematopoietic or blood forming tissue that produces red and white blood cells. The yellow marrow is normally located in the shafts of long bones and the red marrow is found at the ends of long bones and short, flat and irregularly shaped bones.

The bone marrow in the breast, bone, skull, hips, ribs and spine contains stem cells also know as "mother" cells as mature blood cells evolve from these stem cells. The most primitive of these stem cells is the pluripotent stem cell that is believed to be the origin of all blood cells. In contrast to a unipotent cell, which differentiate into a single cell type, a haematopoietic stem cell is pluripotent. It is able to differentiate following number of pathways and thereby generate erythrocytes, granulocytes, monocytes, mast cells, lymphocytes and megakaryocytes (Yoffey and Tavassol, 1983). Pluripotent stem cells differ from other blood cells in that they are capable both of unlimited self-renewal and differentiation. Self-renewal is the ability of the cell to reproduce another cell identical to itself, thus maintaining a steady number of these types of cells in the body. Differentiation is the process of generating one or more subsets of more mature cells that eventually evolve into components of blood either as erythrocytes, neutrophils, eosinophils, basophils, lymphocytes, monocytes or platelets.

STEM CELLS AND PROGENITOR CELLS OF BONE MARROW

The bone marrow is a fundamental haematopoietic organ and assist in the production of blood cells. The production begins with the cells and progenitor cells located in the extravascular compartment of the adult bone marrow. Stem cells are defined by their capability to self-renewal with subsequent production of restricted cells, the progenitor cells, which are believed to have less capacity for self-renewal. Finally, progenitor cells give rise to blood cells of different lineage such as erythrocytes, granulocyte and platelets to assist in functioning of events like oxygenation; immunity and coagulation, respectively (Wichramasinghe, 1975). Thus every functionally specialized mature blood cell is derived from a common stem cell.

Pluripotent stem cells produce other stem cells like the lymphoid stem cell and the myeloid stem cell from which the various types of mature blood cells evolve. Like pluripotent stem cells, the myeloid and lymphoid stem cells can self-renewable as well as produce colonies of offspring that eventually evolve into mature cells. However, their ability to self-renew is believed to be more limited than that of pluripotent stem cells and they are capable of producing fewer different types of offspring. Progenitor cells since do not have the capacity to self renovate themselves, and thus are committed to a given cell lineage. The lymphoid stem cells generate T and B progenitor lymphocytes. The myeloid stem cell generates progenitor stem cells for erythrocytes, granulocytes, monocytes, mast cells and platelets. The myeloid and Iymphoid stem cells produce colonies of "committed progenitor" cells. Unlike stem cells, committed progenitors are only capable of developing into one specific type of mature cell. Cells passing through the final stages of maturation are called precursor cells (Fig. 15-1).

In healthy human beings, the number of each type of stem cell and their offspring is contained within very narrow limits. Certain proteins, such as interleukins and colony-stimulating factors, play a key role in determining whether a stem cell will replicate itself or produce offspring that evolve into mature cells, do both or do neither at any given time. These proteins also regulate the maturation of precursor cells. If this regulatory mechanism breaks down, too many or too few stem cells will be present in the bone marrow and/or certain progenitor or precursor cells will proliferate and fail to properly mature. In patients with leukaemia, for example, one or more types of blood cells (usually white blood cells) fail to properly mature. They stall at one stage of development and self-replicate uncontrollably.

ANATOMY AND PHYSIOLOGY OF BONE MARROW

The bone marrow is a highly organized organ composed of haemopoietic cells, fat cells and vascular structures, surrounded by bony tissue. Within the marrow, haemopoietic progenitor cells at various stages of development continually replenish the peripheral blood cell populations. Haemopoietic tissue is traversed by an extensive network of vascular sinusoids that communicate with the peripheral circulation. Mature haemopoietic cells must egress from the extravascular space of the bone marrow across the marrow/blood barrier to enter the vascular sinusoids and the peripheral blood. The medullary sinusoidal system of the bone marrow is formed from an uninterrupted layer of spindle shaped endothelial cells, an outer discontinuous layer of adventitial cells which covers a variable proportion of the abluminal surface of the endothelium (to provide support for developing haematopoietic cells and for the sinus endothelial cells) and a discontinuous basal lamina.

The bone marrow is divided into wedge-shaped haematopoietic compartments filled with proliferating and differentiating blood cells in connective tissue matrices bordered by venous sinuses. Radial venous sinuses that merge with a central longitudinal vein are major components of mouse bone marrow structure. Blood cells complete maturation immediately adjacent to the dilated vascular channels into which they subsequently emigrate. The microenvironment of the bone marrow is produced by a unique endothelium and connective tissue stroma combined with locally deposited cytokines that regulate compartmentalization, proliferation and differentiation of haematopoietic stem cells (Heller, 1992). Adventitial cells lining the interstitial side of venous sinuses extend cytoplasmic processes into the haematopoietic compartment, making contact with numerous cells. Stromal cells are essential for regulation of haematopoietic cell development. *In situ* hybridization with probes for allotypic markers proved that stromal cells are capable of transferring the haematopoietic microenviroment of the donor after allogeneic bone

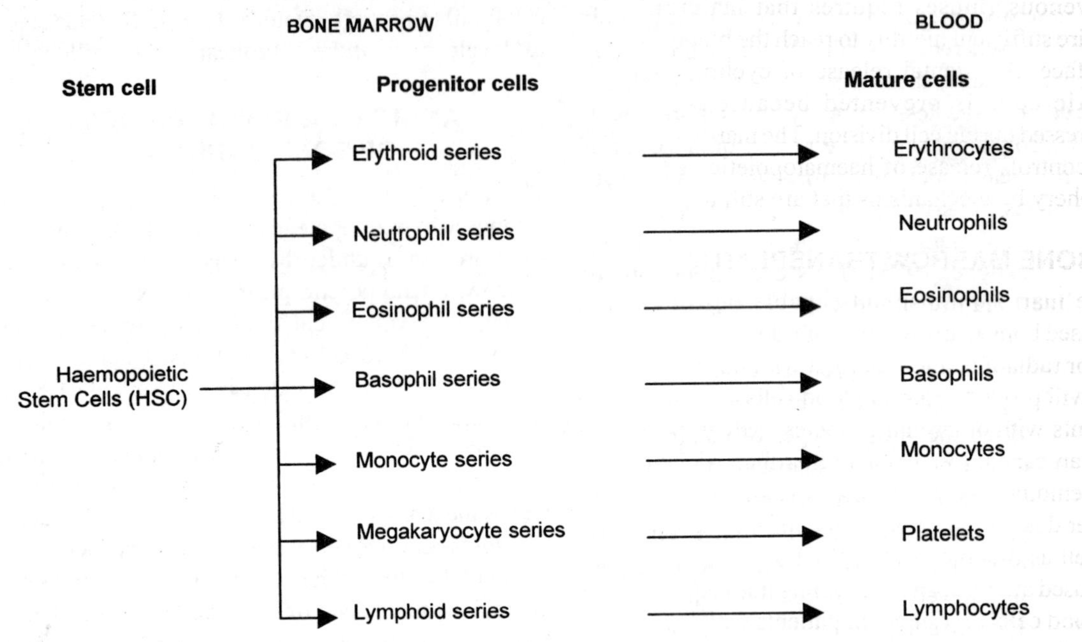

Fig. 15-1. Diagrammatic Representation of the Relationship Between Progenitor Cells and Mature Blood Cells of the Haemopoietic System

marrow transplantation. One way marrow stroma assists haematopoiesis through the glycosaminoglycan-rich extracellular matrix that binds and distributes growth factors such as granulocyte-myelocyte colony stimulating factor (GM-CSF). It is in the sinusoids that the essential functions of the bone marrow are released from the marrow into the blood. Release of these cells into the blood stream is regulated by the requirement of the body (e.g. low O_2 → production of erythropoietin → stimulate stem cells in bone marrow → produce RBC). This in the long run regulates the production rate. The walls of marrow veins are extremely thin but the veins of the marrow are disproportionately large. The vein wall consists of a single layer of endothelium, like the sinusoids. Because of the thinness of the marrow veins, they are easily compressible. When a blood cell is ready to exit the marrow, it is discharged into thin walled blood vessels called blood sinuses, which is found throughout the bone marrow. Generally, the cellular passage across the endothelium is transendothelial rather than interendothelial. Cellular passage proceeds through newly formed pores. Each passing cell opens a new pore, which is immediately closed after the passage is completed. A cell entering the sinus must press against the abluminal membrane of the endothelium bringing it into an ultimate contact with the luminal membrane. The two membranes then fuse in one direction perpendicular to the first. This opens a pore through which the cell enters the lumen. Immediately after the passage is complete, a fusion-fission in a reverse direction leads to the closure of the pore. Not all blood cells formed in the bone marrow are released into the blood stream after maturation (Yoffey and Tavassol, 1983). Megakaryocytes remain in the bone marrow when mature. They lie close beside the blood sinuses, as do many developing cells, and extend processes through holes in the endothelial lining of these vessels. Platelets pinch off from the processes and are swept away into the blood (Fig. 15-2).

The vascular system of the marrow is anatomically closed with little leakage. Mature cells are transported from interstitium to venous sinus through cytoplasmic apertures in the endothelium. Location of immature cells at sites far removed from the venous sinuses requires that maturing cells acquire sufficient motility to reach the blood vascular interface. Accidental release of cycling haematopoietic cells is prevented because motility is suppressed during cell division. The marrow monitors and controls release of haematopoietic cells to the periphery by mechanisms that are still unknown.

BONE MARROW TRANSPLANTATION

Bone marrow transplants enable destruction of diseased bone marrow with high-dose chemotherapy and/or radiation, and replace it with healthy marrow that will produce normal blood cells. It also enables patients with other malignancies such as breast and ovarian cancer to receive higher than normal doses of chemotherapy to treat their disease. Although the higher doses of chemotherapy destroy bone marrow as well as the tumour, healthy bone marrow can be reinfused after treâtment, enabling normal production of blood cells to resume. In patients with leukaemia, aplastic anemia, and some immune deficiency diseases, the stem cells in the bone marrow malfunction, producing an excessive number of defective or immature blood cells (in the case of leukaemia) or low blood cell counts (in the case of aplastic anemia). The immature or defective blood cells interfere with the production of normal blood cells, accumulate in the bloodstream and may invade other tissues (Hassan et al., 1998).

Large doses of chemotherapy and/or radiation are required to destroy the abnormal stem cells and abnormal blood cells. These therapies, however, not only kill the abnormal cells but can destroy normal cells found in the bone marrow as well. Similarly, aggressive chemotherapy used to treat some lymphomas and other cancers can destroy healthy bone marrow. A bone marrow transplant enables to treat these diseases with aggressive chemotherapy and/or radiation by allowing replacement of the diseased or damaged bone marrow after the chemotherapy/radiation treatment. While bone marrow transplants do not provide an absolute assurance that the disease will not recur, a transplant can increase the probability of a cure or at least prolong the period of disease-free survival for many patients.

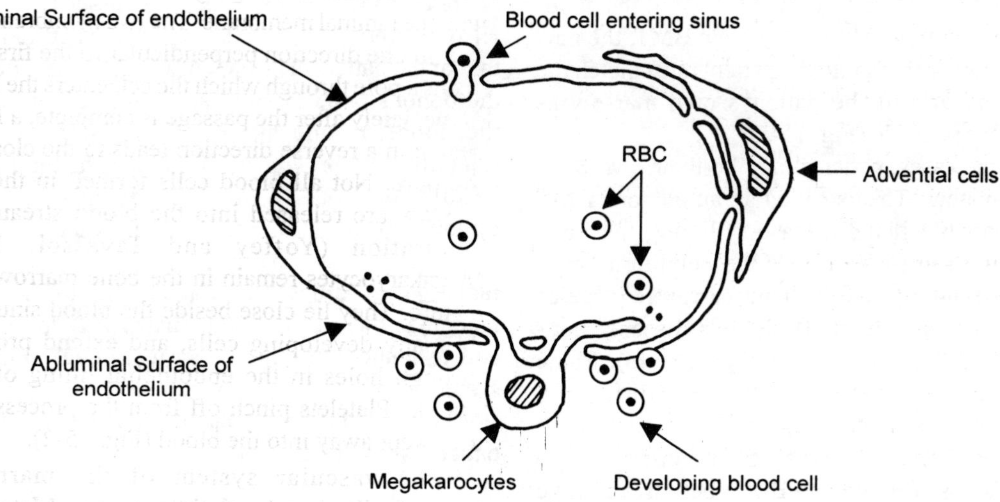

Fig. 15-2. Schematic Diagram Depicting Various Cell Types in Bone Marrow and Release of Cells into the Venous Sinus

The bone marrow and specially the stem cells are harvested for use in a transplant. Stem cells resemble medium sized white blood cells. It has been estimated that less than 1% in 100,000 cells in the bone marrow are stem cells. When stem cells are infused into a patient's bloodstream, they will migrate to the interior of certain bones, set up housekeeping or "colonize" and begin producing immature cells called "committed progenitors." These committed progenitors produce colonies of cells that eventually mature into red blood cells, white blood cells, or platelets. Although the largest concentration of stem cells in the body is found in the bone marrow, stem cells also can be found in the bloodstream or "peripheral blood." The concentration of stem cells in the bloodstream is normally 1/100 of that in bone marrow. Extracting stem cells from the peripheral blood is referred to as "peripheral stem cell harvest" or PSCH (Hassan et al., 2000).

Types of Transplants

In a bone marrow transplant, the patient's diseased bone marrow is destroyed and healthy marrow is infused into the patient's blood-stream. In a successful transplant, the new bone marrow migrates to the cavities of the large bones, engrafts and begins producing normal blood cells. If bone marrow from a donor is used, the transplant is called an "allogeneic" BMT, or "syngeneic" BMT if the donor is an identical twin. In an allogeneic BMT, the new bone marrow infused into the patient must match the genetic makeup of the patient's own marrow as perfectly as possible (Fig. 15-3).

In some cases, patients may be their own bone marrow donors. This is called an autologous BMT and is possible if the disease afflicting the bone marrow is in remission or if the condition being treated does not involve the bone marrow (e.g. breast cancer, ovarian cancer, Hodgkin's disease, non-Hodgkin's lymphoma, and brain tumours). Some complications associated with allogeneic BMTs such as graft-versus-host defense are avoided with autologous BMTs. The risk of infection is also somewhat less in autologous BMTs because the large doses of immunosuppressive medications given to patients in allogeneic BMTs to prevent graft versus host disease (GVHD) are not needed. Recently, introduced peripheral stem cell (PSC) transplants differ from autologous BMTs only in the method of collecting "stem cells," the cells that are reinfused into the patient during the transplant. Diseases treated with PSC transplants include Acute Leukemias, Brain Tumours, Breast Cancer, Hodgkin's Disease, Multiple Myeloma, Neuroblastoma, Non-Hodgkin's Lymphomas, Ovarian Cancer, Sarcoma and Testicular Cancer.

T-cells are special white blood cells that recognize foreign matter in the body. T-cells orchestrate attacks on bacteria, viruses and other substances foreign to the body. They can also distinguish "self" from "non-self" (human cells that belong in one person's body and those that do not). On the surface of many human cells is an inherited set of genetic markers called "human leukocyte antigens" (HLA). Like a fingerprint, no two person's set of HLA markers are exactly alike (except for identical twins). The T-cells use these HLA markers to distinguish "self" from "non-self." If a "non-self" human cell is encountered in the body, the T- cells quickly activate the immune system to destroy it. The greater the disparity between the body's HLA markers or "tissue type" and that of the foreign human cell, the swifter and more vigorous the attack. The ability of the immune system's T-cells to distinguish "self" from "non-self" can create a serious problem after allogeneic BMTs. Unless the donor is an identical twin, his or her tissue type (those HLA markers or genetic fingerprints) will differ from that of the patient. The patient's T-cells may identify the donor's bone marrow as "non-self" and attack the donated bone marrow. This is called graft rejection. To prevent graft rejection, total body irradiation (TBI) and/or drugs such as cyclophosphamide are used to kill the cancerous cells and to suppress a patient's immune system. The radiation and drugs disrupt the ability of T-cells to recognize the donated bone marrow as "non- self" and to launch an immune system attack. Immune system suppression is not required in autologous BMTs since the bone marrow transfused into the patient is his or her own.

BONE MARROW TARGETING

The clinical advantages that would arise from a system with bone marrow homing specificity are

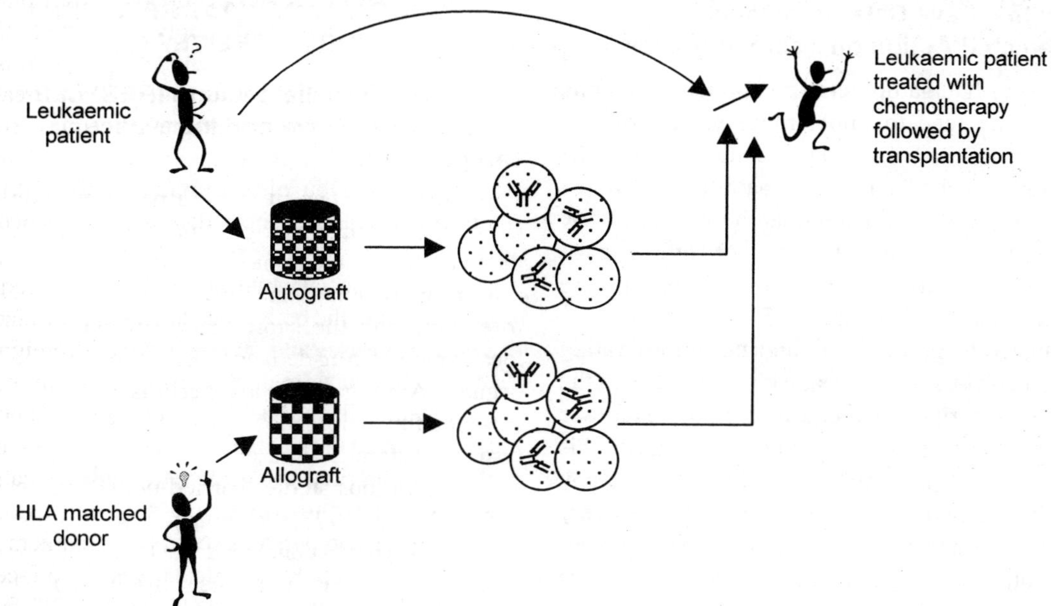

Fig. 15-3. Treatment of Leukaemia after Superlethal X-irradiation or Chemotherapy with Bone Marrow Transplantation

quite obvious as explained for the under mentioned reasons. Therapeutic approaches might include gene therapy, selective delivery and local release of antimicrobials, as well agents that could induce self-renewal, proliferation and maturation of stem and progenitor cells.

Reduction in the Haemopoietic Damage During Chemo or Radio-therapy

Encapsulation of antigens or antigenic peptides which are able to protect an organism from some viral infections has been reported to provide stimulation of nonspecific immunity, haemopoiesis and protection of mice against radiation injury. Thus the system could be therapeutically beneficial to moderate the haemopoietic damage (undesirable effect of radiotherapy or chemotherapy) and induce the non-specific immunity to support the antimicrobial treatment of immuno-compromised patients.

Hereditary and Congenital Disorders

Hereditary disorders of the bone marrow which represent a large diverse group affecting either the stem cell or committed lineage and subsequently the numbers and function of the end cells they produce, also require bone marrow localization. Selective trapping of the circulatory pool of haematopoietic stem cells by marrow sinus endothelium has provided an effective form of correction of congenital marrow disorders and new approaches for gene therapy.

Bone Marrow Related Diseases

There are numerous diseases associated with the bone marrow transplantation. If the donor's bone marrow is not a good genetic match, it will perceive the patient's body as foreign material to be attacked and destroyed. This condition is known as graft-versus-host disease (GVHD) and can be therapeutically unacceptable. Diseases frequently treated with allogeneic BMTs are : Aplastic Anemia, Hodgkin's Disease, Leukaemia, Myelodysplasia, Non-Hodgkin's Lymphoma, Multiple Myeloma, Osteopetrosis, Severe Combined Immune Deficiency Syndrome (SCIDS), Thalassemia, Wiskott-Aldrich Syndrome and Peripheral Stem Cell Transplants. Alternatively, the patient's immune system may destroy the new bone marrow and this is known to as graft rejection.

Drugs that have Catastrophic and Unpredicted Action on Haematopoiesis

Damage to haematopoietic components of bone marrow can lead to undesirable effects on the physiology of the body and associated diseases like invasion of bone marrow by pathogenic micro-organisms resulting in the quantitative leukocyte alterations, anaemia and the continuation of disseminated intravascular coagulation in the peripheral blood (Van Furth, 1981).

Damage to proliferating and non-proliferating cells in bone marrow stroma, which may lead to the absence of peripheral blood and tissue leukocyte necessary for host defense against infection and this is the most common side effect of chemotherapy (cytotoxic agents) or radiation therapy. Drug delivery systems present therapeutic concentrations of chemo-therapeutic agents to the diseased bone marrow cells avoiding interaction with normal marrow and thus provide targeted delivery.

Distinct Physiological Functions of the Components of the Bone Marrow

Some approaches are adopted for distinct physiological functions of the components of the bone marrow like sinuses. Sinuses are relatively large blood vessels (5-30 μm in mice and somewhat larger in humans) forming a barrier, referred to as marrow-blood barrier (MBB), between the haematopoietic compartments and the circulation. The MBB serves to control cellular traffic in and out of the marrow. On the other hand, the circulatory pool of haemato-poietic stem cells (administered or transplanted) is selectively trapped by marrow sinus endothelium, permitting them to enter the haematopoietic area. This selective trapping is evident during bone marrow transplantation, when a relatively high concentration of stem cells is introduced in the circulation.

Certain genetic diseases can be treated by transplantation of either normal allogeneic bone marrow or potentially autologous bone marrow into which the normal gene has been inserted *in vitro*. Introduction of foreign genes into stem cells can constitute a possible approach to the treatment of non-genetic diseases and to complement the effect of conventional therapies.

BONE MARROW TARGETS FOR DRUG DELIVERY

Reticuloendothelial System (RES) of Bone Marrow for Passive and Intravascular Targeting

The rapid clearance of foreign particles from the circulation by macrophages lining the sinusoids in the liver, spleen and bone marrow is one of the most important mechanisms in host defense against infections and the same has been exploited for localization of drug delivery systems in the RES-rich organs. Among these are serious parasitic and systemic fungal infections as well as RES-localized lysosomal storage diseases.

From various studies carried out (Biozzi et al., 1953; Griffin, 1977; Van Furth, 1981; Illum and Davis, 1987) it was concluded that (a) major function of the macrophages, lining the sinusoids in the liver, spleen and bone marrow, is to remove foreign particles from the circulation; and (b) the clearance of the particles from the circulation is dependent on the opsonins (serum components which mediate phagocytic clearance via macrophages) and the dose of the particles given. Figure 15-4 represents various sites for the reticuloendothelial clearance of particles from the circulation. The RES of the bone marrow

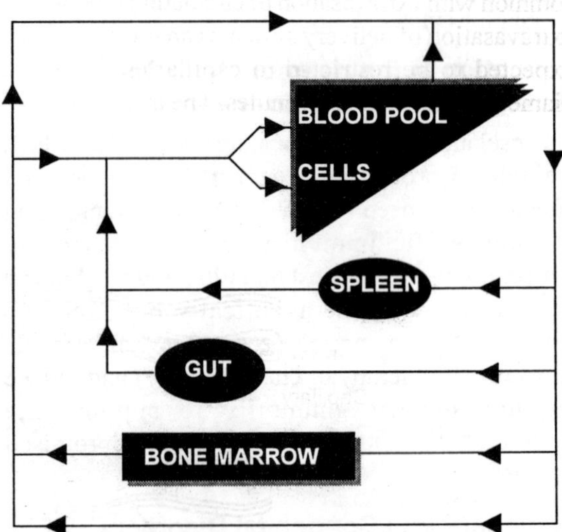

Fig. 15-4. Sites of Reticuloendothelial Mediated Blood Clearance

has been well exploited in diagnostic imaging where colloidal radionucleotides have traditionally provided a non-invasive method for the evaluation of a number of clinical situations.

Sinusoidal Capillaries for Extravascular Targeting

Traffic across the MBB is not limited to cellular elements; the endothelium of bone marrow sinusoids is unique among post-capillary venules in that it removes particulate materials from the blood. The endothelium is not only capable of phagocytic uptake and storage of particles (thus functioning as part of body's reticuloendothelial system) but also provides for transmural passage of particulate material to the extravascular space where the particles are then phagocytosed by central macrophages or by other cells. The successful delivery of particulates to the RES-rich organs focused interest on the possible delivery to other sites in the body, such as various extravascular tissues. This is not only a consequence of the rapid clearance of particulates by the RES but also of natural anatomical barriers in the blood vessels. The anatomy of the microcirculation in different tissues and organs can reasonably be expected to be of prime importance in determining whether drug carriers or antibodies conjugates can escape into the surrounding extravascular tissue. In common with extravasation of circulating blood cells, extravasation of delivery systems can presumably be expected to be restricted to capillaries and small diameters postcapillary venules. The anatomy of the microcirculation in different tissues and organs can reasonably be expected to be of prime importance in determining whether drug carriers or antibodies conjugates can escape into the surrounding extravascular tissue. In common with extravasation of circulating blood cells, extravasation of delivery systems can presumably be expected to be restricted to capillaries and small diameters postcapillary venules.

Based upon the architecture of the lining endothelium and the underlying sub-endothelial basement membrane (basal lamina), three groups of capillaries are described (Fig. 15-5).

- Continuous
- Fenestrated and
- Discontinuous or sinusoidal

Continuous Capillaries

The endothelial cells are connected via tight junctions to form a continuous monolayer or an uninterrupted basement membrane.

Fenestrated Capillaries

The endothelium is interrupted by fenestrae of diameter 30-80 nm. The basal membrane in the fenestrated capillaries is continuous.

Sinusoidal Capillaries

These are found predominantly in the liver, spleen and bone marrow. They have a discontinuous endothelium and large fenestrae with a mean diameter of about 100 nm.

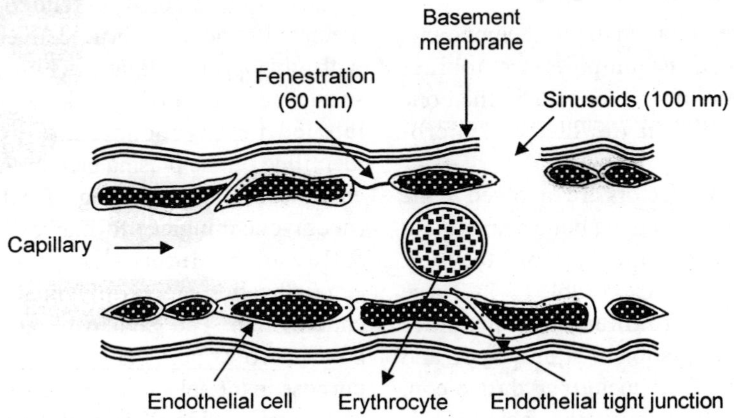

Fig. 15-5. The Capillary Endothelial Barrier

Drug loaded particulates localize intrinsically to RES-rich organs and this concept has been exploited to deliver drugs and bioactives to macrophages of liver, spleen and bone marrow. Several workers (Kanke et al., 1980; Illum et al., 1982; Tomlinson et al., 1984; Fidler, 1980) investigated the role of localization of colloidal particles in the body after parenteral administration and their conclusions are summarized as follows :

- Particulates of approximately 10-30 nm in diameter after intravenous (i.v.) administration localize in bone marrow however, even with these systems a high proportion still reaches to liver and spleen.
- Particulates (0.3-7.0 μm) clear rapidly from circulation via macrophags however smaller particles (100-300 nm) escape through fenestrae and localize in hepatocytes.
- Particulates greater in size (7-13 μm) on i.v. administration are mechanically filtered by alveolar macrophages.
- Intra arterial administration of particles of size greater than 15 microns leads to their retention in first vasculature encountered.

Alteration of the surface character of the particles allows them to avoid the RES scavenging, which leads to the possibility of directing them to bone marrow macrophages (polaxamer 407 coating) or other sites in the body (coating with other PEG and PEO polymers) (Illum and Davis, 1987).

HAEMOPOIETIC CYTOKINES AS HOMING MOLECULES

Proliferation and differentiation in the haemopoietic system is regulated by haemopoietic cytokines produced by a network of stromal cells in the bone marrow and other cells in the marrow micro-environment.

Haemopoietic growth factors are involved in the production of blood cells from the bone marrow and are useful in reducing bone marrow toxicity associated with anticancer agents (Table 15-1). These growth factors are cytokines that promote proliferation and differentiation of granulocytes and monocyte/macrophages. They include erythropoietin, granulocyte-macrophage stimulating factor (GM-CSF) and granulocyte stimulating factor (G-CSF). GM-CSF and G-CSF increase the neutrophil count in peripheral blood after high dose chemotherapy followed by bone-marrow transplantation, thus resulting in lesser chances of infections. Erythropoietin can help to replenish red blood cells in aplastic anaemia and after cancer chemotherapy. Recently, thrombopoietin has been described; this agent may alleviate thrombocytopaenia due to inadequate marrow production.

Carbohydrate Determinants as Possible Homing Ligands

Various studies conducted on rat bone marrow suggested that the luminal surface of bone marrow sinus endothelium possesses both exposed sialic acid moieties (mostly made from sialoglycoproteins) and some unidentified and poorly characterized non-neuraminidase-sensitive anionic material with a pKa higher than sialic acid. These later anionic sites on the abluminal surface are throughout to capture circulating particulate materials for endocytosis across the sinus endothelium of bone marrow.

The presence of lectin receptors on the bone marrow sinusoidal endothelium specially the luminal plasalemma (and not by abluminal plasmalemma) of rat has been confirmed by ultrastructural localization studies. These cells were found to express glycoproteins including mannosyl, N-acetyl-gluosaminyl, galactosyl and N-acetylgalactosaminyl residues. These glycoproteins may act as receptors for selective uptake of a variety of circulating substances, e.g., erythropoietin and viruses and the concept may also be extended for the receptor mediated removal of drug delivery systems grafted with glycoprotein ligands (Fig. 15-6). Lectin-like substances recognizing galactosyl residues of gold-labeled neoglycoconjugate probes have been identified on the plasma membrane of marrow sinus endothelium. The binding of galactosyl-BSA-gold (neoglycoconjugate) to marrow endothelium was followed by internalization and subsequent externalization on the abluminal side of the marrow endothelium. The galactosyl recognition system of bone marrow sinus endothelium may serve a biologic purpose in the selective uptake of certain cell-bound or circulating glyco-conjugates terminating in correct orientation of galactosyl residues.

Table 15-1. Major Haemopoietic Growth Factors

Growth factors	Sources	Cell types produced
IL-3	T-cells	Neutrophils, monocytes, eosinophils, basophils, megakaryocytes, erythrocytes
GM-CSF	T-cells, monocytes, fibroblasts	Neutrophils, monocytes, eosinophils, dendritic cells
G-CSF	Monocytes, fibroblasts, endothelial cells	Neutrophils
M-CSF	Monocytes, fibroblasts, endothelial cells	Monocytes
IL-5	T-cells	Eosinophils
EPO	Kidney	Erythrocytes, megakaryocytes
TPO	Liver, kidney	Megakaryocytes (platelets)

Abbreviations: IL-3: interleukin-3; GM-CSF: granulocyte-macrophage colony-stimulating factor; G-CSF: granulocyte colony-stimulating factor; M-CSF: macrophage colony-stimulating factor; IL-5: interleukin-5; EPO: erythropoietin; TPO: thrombopoietin

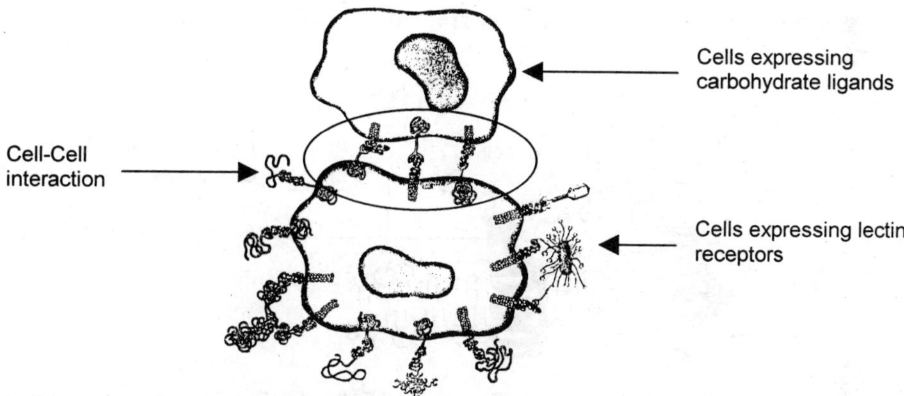

Fig. 15-6. Lectin Receptors and Carbohydrate Ligands Exploited for the Homing of Viruses, Erythropoietin and Other Particulates to the Bone Marrow Endothelium

Adhesion Molecules as Possible Homing Ligands

The regulation of expression of specific adhesion molecules by bone marrow endothelium or mature myeloid or erythroid elements may allow for selective exit of these cells out of the marrow parenchyma. Adhesion molecules like CD34, PECAM and thrombospondin have been identified by bone marrow microvascular endothelial cells monolayers. However, in majority they function as a trans-migratory bridge permitting the exit of mature cells out of the bone marrow. The selective homing of transplanted progenitor cells to the bone marrow is also likely to involve expression of specific adhesion molecules. The expression of CD34 on haematopoietic progenitor cells has been demonstrated. Because mucin can bear lineage-specific carbohydrate determinants, CD34 can act as skeleton for the attachment of lineage-specific glycans, allowing progenitor cells to bind to lectins expressed by bone marrow components.

Adhesion molecules may also be responsible for selective attachment of prostatic, breast, and follicular carcinoma to bone marrow microvascular endothelium (Fig. 15-7). Such homing molecules may be envisaged as new tools for selective targeting of drug carriers to the bone marrow.

COLLOIDAL CARRIERS FOR BONE MARROW TARGETING

The ability of the bone marrow to remove particulate matters from the circulation, opens up perhaps an opportunity for the delivery of therapeutic agents by means of colloidal drug carrier systems such as liposomes, emulsions, nanoparticles, etc. for the treatment of diseases and disorders of this multifunctional organ of the body (Fig. 15-8).

Colloidal Particles

Certain colloidal particulates have been investigated for site specific imaging of bone marrow. Some of the colloidal carriers used are radiolabeled albumin microspheres and micro-aggregates (10-30 μm) and fine (1-13 μm) poly vinyl pyrrolidone particles. However, with all these systems a high proportions of the dose still reaches the liver and spleen within a few minutes after intravenous administration. Since intravenously administered colloidal particles are normally removed efficiently by the reticulo-endothelial cells of the liver and spleen, only a small fraction of these particles reaches the bone marrow (Illum and Davis, 1987). By coating particulates with certain polymers it has been possible effectively to by pass the liver/spleen uptake and obtain a deposition of the microspheres primarily in the bone marrow. Such carrier systems are used in radiodiagnosis and in the treatment of various diseases of bone marrow. The body distribution of the particles after intra-venous injection was shown to be mainly depending upon surface properties of the particles. After injection of these particles into the blood stream, certain blood components (opsonins) are rapidly adsorbed. This adsorption of opsonins leads to a rapid phagocytic or endocytic uptake into cells of the

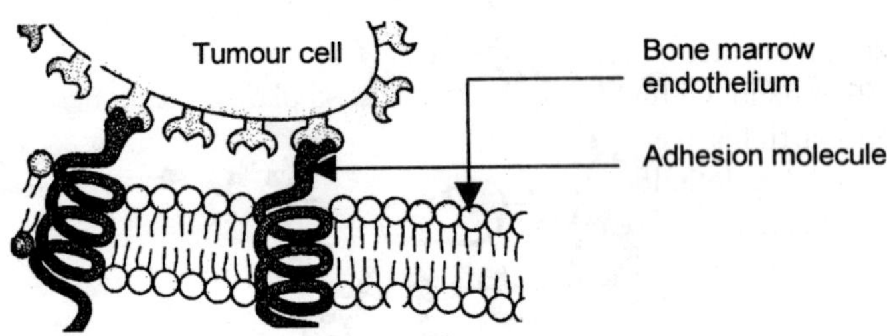

Fig. 15-7. Selective Attachment of Prostatic, Breast, and Follicular Carcinoma Cells Expressing Ligands for Adhesion Molecules on Bone Marrow Microvascular Endothelium

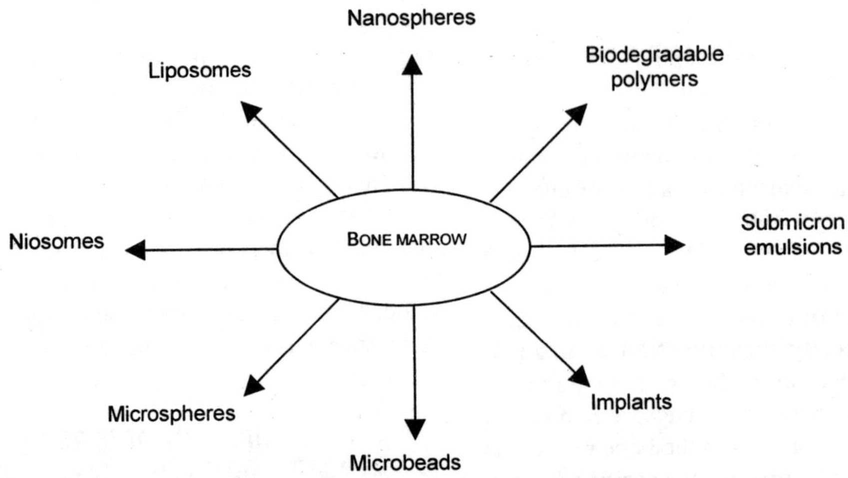

Fig. 15-8. Various Colloidal Carrier Systems Used for Bone Marrow Targeting

reticuloendothelial system (RES), especially into the liver (60 - 90 %), spleen (2 - 20 %), bone marrow (0.1 - 1 %), and a varying amount into the lungs (Fig. 15-9). Certain synthetic substances have been shown to exhibit "bone marrow homing" activity. One such substance is polaxamer 407, a non-ionic block copolymer containing a central block of hydrophobic polyoxypropylene (POP) flanked by blocks of hydrophilic polyoxyethylene (POE).

This material can adhere firmly to the surface of polystyrene microspheres via its central POP block which leaves the POE chains in mobile states as they extend outwards from the surface of the particles. Following i.v. administration into rabbits, polaxamer 407 coated particles (150 μm in diameter or below) displayed two distinct behaviours in their mode of clearance from the blood. On the one hand, the polaxamer coating dramatically hampered particle recognition by Kupffer cells and concomitantly increased the blood circulation half-life of microspheres. On the other hand, within a few hours of administration, nanoparticles were selectively recognized by the sinusoidal endothelial cells of the bone marrow where they eventually become localized internally in groups of 5-20 particles in large vesicles (Porter et al., 1992). While sinusoidal endothelium was vigorously active in the uptake process, the endothelium of marrow vessels remained indifferent to the presence of intravascular polaxamer 407 coated particles (Fig. 15-9).

These observations are interesting since the polaxamer 407 makes microspheres both anti-adhesive (by virtue of its extended POE configuration on the particle surface which acts as a steric barrier) and pro-adhesive (by virtue of recognition by bone marrow sinusoidal endothelial cells), a process analogues to the anti-adhesive and pro-adhesive behaviour of mucin.

Bone marrow homing of polaxamer 407 coated particles is apparently specific to rabbit model as demonstrated by the percent activity associated with Femar (represent activity associated with bone marrow) and Carcass (represent activity associated with bones including marrow, muscles and skin). In addition, homing of nanospheres to the rabbit bone marrow could not be demonstrated with other polymers of similar structure and molecular weight to that of polaxamer 407 (termed as Polymer A) exhibiting a molecular mass of 13310 Da and contains 84.6 mol % ethylene oxide (Porter et al., 1992). Other Polaxamer 407 polymers exhibiting a molecular mass of 10400 and 11540 Da with 76.2 and 80.8 mol % ethylene oxide (termed as Polymer B and C respectively) failed to offer significant bone marrow targetability however, they remained in the circulation for a longer period of time (Fig. 15-10).

Another report also suggested the ability of polaxamer 338 to redirect a significant portion of intravenously (i.v.) administered nanospheres to the rabbit bone marrow (Bradfield, 1984; Illum and Davis, 1987). The mechanism responsible for selective recognition of polaxamer 407 coated particles by sinusoidal endothelial cells of rabbit bone marrow still remains unknown but may be related to the density and conformation of the polymer on the nanosphere surface. It can also be assumed that the surface of the polymer-coated particles adsorbs a critical plasma component, which exhibits specificity for certain micro-domains on the bone marrow sinusoidal endothelial cell plasma membrane (Fig. 15-11). The application of the site-specific targeting of drug carriers to bone marrow and the prevention of the adherence of metastases of tumours, which selectively colonize the bone marrow endothelium can be addressed.

Studies were performed using particulate systems to provide successful bone marrow allografts by pre-saturation and blockade of reticuloendothelial system. Kadowaki and co-workers, 1993 reported poly(L-lactic acid) particles for the suppression of genetic resistance to bone marrow allografts by reticulo-endothelial system-blockade.

Controlled release of transforming growth factor-beta1 (TGF-beta1) to a bone defect may be beneficial for the induction of a bone regeneration cascade. Lu and co-workers, 2001 assessed the feasibility of using biodegradable polymer microparticles as carriers for controlled TGF-beta1 delivery and the effects of released TGF-beta1 on the marrow stromal cell proliferation and osteoblastic differentiation of marrow stromal cells *in vitro*. Gibaud and co-workers, 1996 addressed that the affinity of nanoparticles for haematopoietic organs could be valuable for the targeting of certain stimulating factors to bone

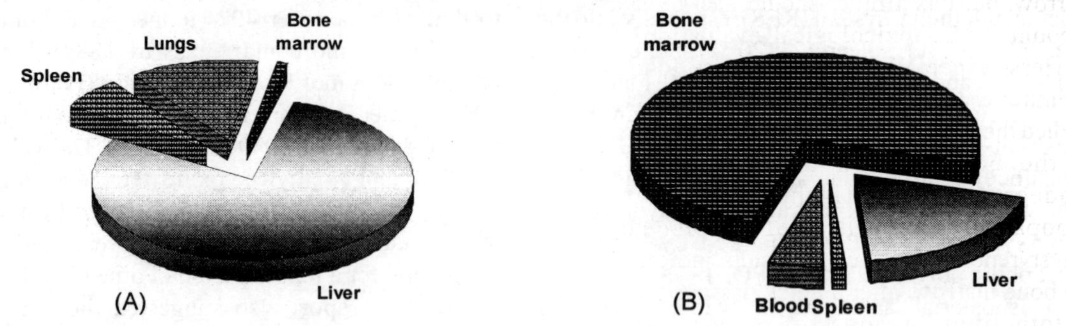

Fig. 15-9. Uptake of Particles to Various RES-rich Organs after Intravenous Administration Before (A), and After (B) Polaxamer 407 Coating

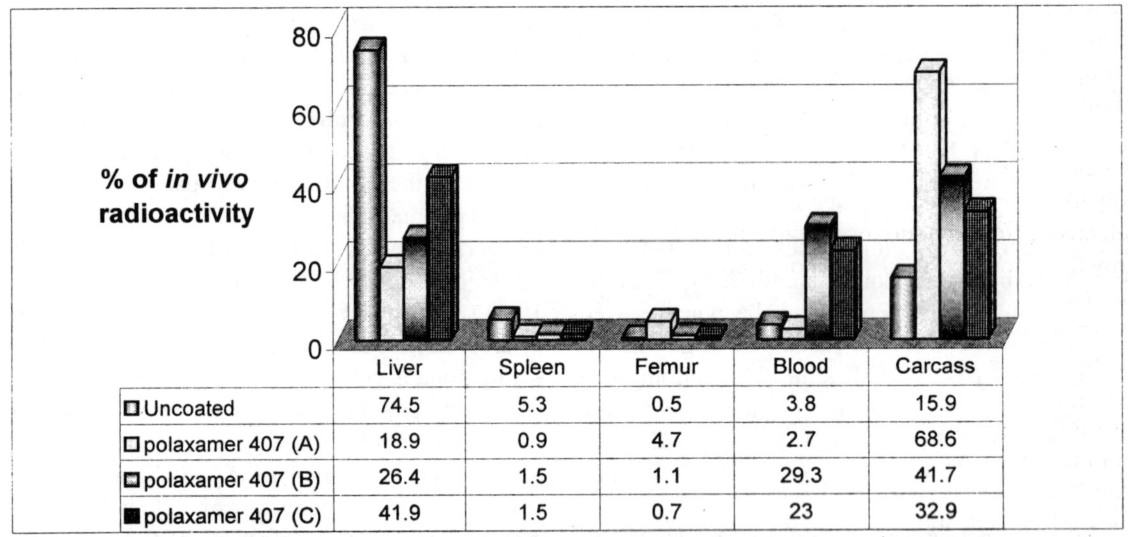

	Liver	Spleen	Femur	Blood	Carcass
Uncoated	74.5	5.3	0.5	3.8	15.9
polaxamer 407 (A)	18.9	0.9	4.7	2.7	68.6
polaxamer 407 (B)	26.4	1.5	1.1	29.3	41.7
polaxamer 407 (C)	41.9	1.5	0.7	23	32.9

Fig. 15-10. Biodistribution of Uncoated and Polymer Coated Microspheres 24 h Following intravenous Administration into Rabbit (produced from data of Porter et al., 1992)

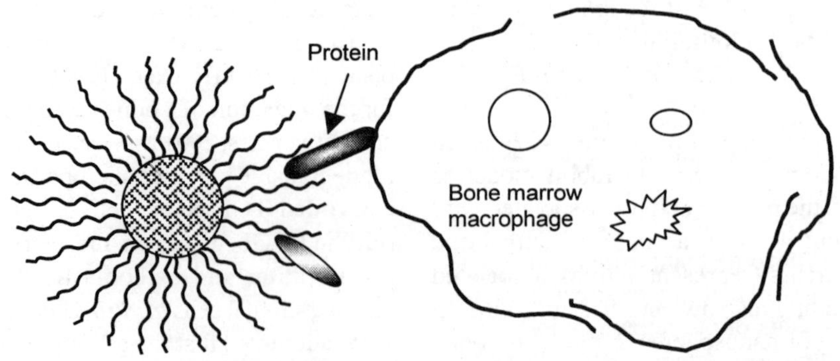

Fig. 15-11. Adsorption of Certain Plasma Proteins over Polaxamer 407 Coated Nanoparticles, which in turn Demonstrate Affinity for BMs

marrow, but this affinity should also be taken into account in the toxicological evaluation of those carriers, especially when they are loaded with antimitotic compounds such as doxorubicin. They studied the capture, the localization, and the retention in the bone marrow and in the spleen of biodegradable poly(isohexyl cyanoacrylate) nanoparticles as well as of nonbiodegradable polystyrene nanoparticles. Results indicate that, in the bone marrow, after a quick passage through the endothelium, nanoparticles were dispersed throughout in the tissue and captured by all types of phagocytic cells. In the spleen, nanoparticles were mainly localized in large angular capturing cells in the marginal zone of the lymphoid follicles. Gibaud et al., 1998 also reported polyalkylcyanoacrylate nanoparticles as carriers for granulocyte-colony stimulating factor (G-CSF).

Gibaud et al., 1999 in a recent study reported the targeting of bone marrow with the help of polyalkylcyanoacrylate nanoparticles. These workers selected cytotoxic (doxorubicin) and stimulating growth factor (rhG-CSF) as model compounds for entrapment in polyalkylcyanoacrylate nanoparticles. Histological studies showed rapid capture of nanoparticles by bone marrow macrophages and granulocytes as soon as 15 minutes after injection into the blood stream. Doxorubicin nanoparticles, administered at a dose of 11 mg/kg were more toxic than free doxorubicin on all blood and marrow cell lines. Moreover, the nature of the polymer had an influence on toxicity: Doxorubicin polyisohexylcyanoacrylate nanoparticles were more toxic than polyisobutylcyanoacrylate particles. The bone marrow concentrations suggested for a high level of targeting towards the bone marrow. Nevertheless, rhG-CSF nanoparticles did not show better efficacy than free rhG-CSF. Table 15-2 summarizes various studies carried out for bone marrow localization and targeting with their significant outcomes.

Liposomes

A wide range of liposome compositions have been examined *in vivo* for their ability to affect the uptake of liposomes into cells of the reticuloendothelial of bone marrow (Allen and Chonn, 1987; Allen et al., 1989). Similar to successful studies of coating polystyrene microspheres with polaxamer 407 to achieve bone marrow targeting, attempts were made to study the effect of Polaxamer 407 on liposome stability and targeting to bone marrow by Moghimi and co-workers, 1990. However, in contrast to Polaxamer 407 effect on polystyrene microspheres, no apparent difference on biodistribution of Polaxamer pre-incubated liposomes and hence on bone marrow targeting was recorded (Fig. 15-12).

Liposomes (150 nm in diameter and below) composed of equimolar amounts of cholesterol and either saturated phospholipids or sphingomyelin exhibit low tendency for accumulation in Kupffer cells following intravenous administration. In contrast, their uptake from blood to spleen and bone marrow remains relatively high. For example, 25% of the injected dose of vesicles, formed from equimolar amount of cholesterol and disteroyl phosphatidylcholine, were localized in to the rat bone marrow 72 h post intravenous administration. Not much is known regarding the mechanism of liposome uptake and their deposition within the bone marrow. Opsonization mechanisms are believed to regulate vesicles recognition by marrow endothelium and persinial macrophages (Moghimi et al., 1990). Moghimi and Patel, 1992 studied the role of liver, spleen and bone marrow specific opsonin factors and complement components for the uptake of cholesterol rich and cholesterol poor liposomes. However, it remained an unexplored fact whether same or different opsonin factors are responsible on the uptake of different types and sized liposomes by RES-rich organs (liver spleen and bone marrow). Other small-sized liposomes (150 nm or below in diameter) with long-circulatory half-life, such as PEG-PE containing vesicles do not substantially accumulate in bone marrow following i.v. administration into experimental animals (Fig. 15-13) (Allen et al., 1989).

Recently, Mercadal and co-workers, 2000 reported that immunoliposomes bearing poly-(ethylene glycol)-coupled monoclonal antibody linked via a cleavable disulfide bond can be used for *ex vivo* applications as sorting of haematopoietic stem cells.

Liposomal formulations of anthracyclines have been developed to increase their delivery to solid tumours while reducing toxicity in normal tissues.

Table 15-2. Various Studies of Bone Marrow Localization and Targeting Using Particulate Sytems

System investigated	Drug(s)	Inferences	Reference
Polystyrene microspheres coated with polyoxyethylene/ polyoxy-propylene block copolymer poloxamer-407	-	Selective delivery of intravenously injected microspheres to sinusoidal endothelial cells of rabbit bone marrow.	Porter et al., 1992
Biodegradable poly(phosphazene) nanoparticles surface modified with poly(phosphazene)-poly(ethylene oxide) copolymer	Model compound	Prolonged systemic circulation lifetime and reduced liver uptake, and targeting to bone marrow	Vandorpe et al., 1997
Polyalkylcyanoacrylate nanoparticles	Doxorubicin; G-CSF	Rapid capture of nanoparticles by bone marrow macrophages and granulocytes	Gibaud et al., 1998; 1999
Polymethyl methacrylate nanoparticles	^{14}C lebeled	After peroral administration highest radio-activity was recorded in bone marrow, fatty renal tissue, stomach, liver, and lymph nodes	Nefzger et al., 1984
Microparticles of blends of poly(DL-lactic-co-glycolic acid) (PLGA) and poly(ethylene glycol) (PEG)	Recombinant human TGF-beta1	Effective carriers for controlled delivery of transforming growth factor and proliferation and differentiation of marrow stromal cells *in vitro*	Lu et al., 2001
Blends of biodegradable polymers, poly(caprolactone) and poly(D, L-lactic-co-glycolic acid)	-	Novel polymer/ceramic composites as scaffold in bone tissue engineering applications	Marra et al., 1999
Plaster of Paris implants coated with polylactide-co-glycolide polymer	Vancomycin	Sustained release delivery system of antibiotics for the treatment of bone and joint infections	Beniot et al., 1997a
PF-PEO(5000)-coated poly(organo phosphazene) nanoparticles	-	Prolonged systemic circulation and reduced liver uptake and increased uptake to the bone marrow	Vandrope et al., 1997
HIV-Tat peptide derivatized superparamagnetic nanoparticles	-	Internalized into hematopoietic and neural progenitor cells and allow *in vivo* tracking and recovery of progenitor cells	Lewin et al., 2000
Polybutylcyanoacrylate nanoparticles (PBCN)	Mitomycin C; Farmorubicin	Genotoxic activity of antitumor drugs diminished or even abolished after their incorporation in PBCN	Blagoeva et al., 1992

DaunoXome (DNX, NeXstar) is a liposomal-encapsulated preparation of daunorubicin registered for treatment of Kaposi's sarcoma that during prior *in vitro* studies showed a toxicity to leukaemic cells at least comparable to that of free daunorubicin. Liposomal formulation may allow a reduction of daunorubicin captation in normal tissues. thus minimizing toxicity of the parent drug, and guarantee an unimpeded access to leukaemic cells in the bloodstream and bone marrow, thus theoretically improved efficacy (Pea et al., 2000). Oussoren and co-workers, 1999 reported that liposomes may serve as carriers of the antiretroviral agent dideoxycytidine-5'-triphosphate to bone marrow, To overcome problems associated with the administration of free nucleosides and to improve targeting to bone marrow mononuclear phagocyte system (MPS), dideoxy-cytidine-5'-triphosphate (ddCTP) was encapsulated

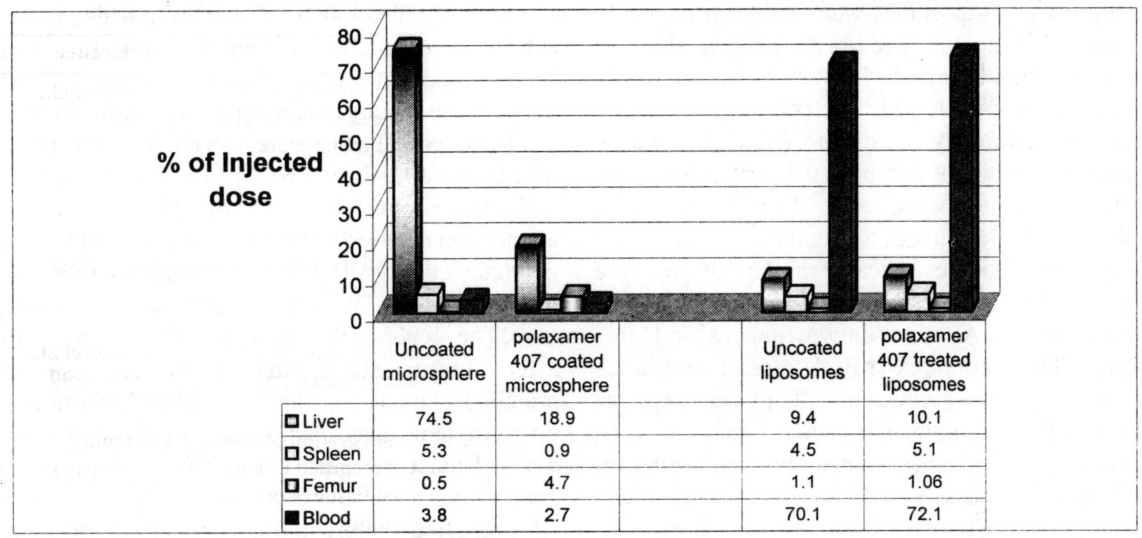

	Uncoated microsphere	polaxamer 407 coated microsphere		Uncoated liposomes	polaxamer 407 treated liposomes
Liver	74.5	18.9		9.4	10.1
Spleen	5.3	0.9		4.5	5.1
Femur	0.5	4.7		1.1	1.06
Blood	3.8	2.7		70.1	72.1

Fig. 15-12. Biodistribution of Control and Polaxamer-Treated Liposomes versus Control and Polaxamer-Coated Microspheres After 1 h Following Intravenous Administration into Rats

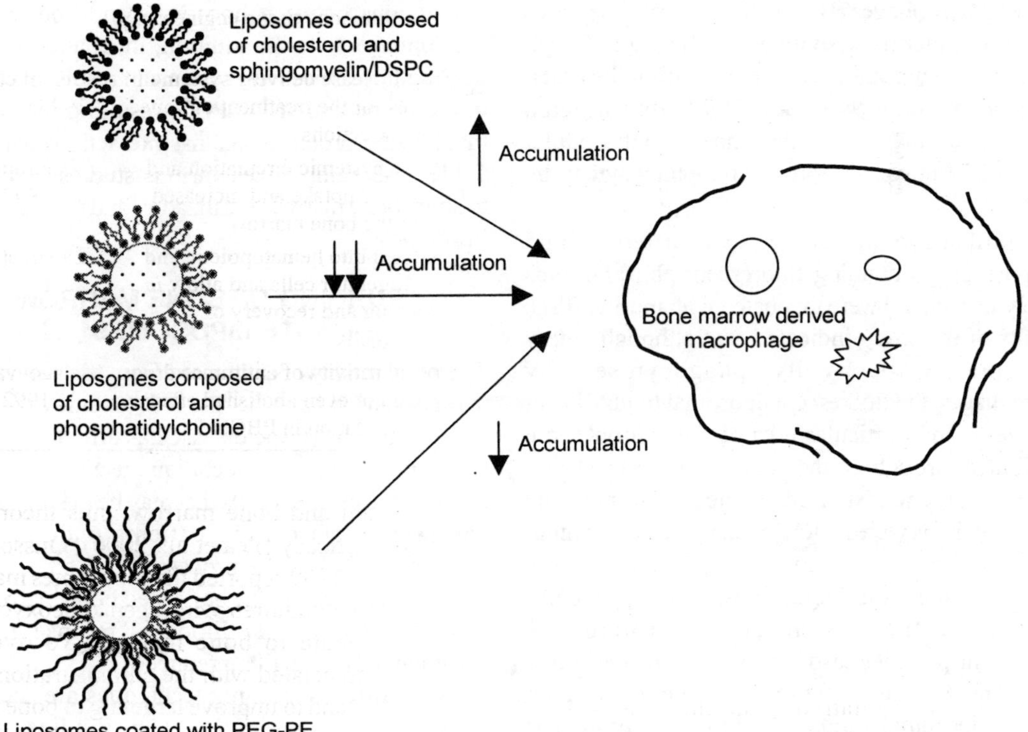

Fig. 15-13. Role of Type and Nature of Lipids in Preferential Accumulatrion to Bone Marrow

in liposomes. Liposomes were stable in regard to retention of the entrapped drug, particle size and chemical stability of ddCTP. Results obtained with liposome encapsulated ddCTP in the murine acquired immunodeficiency syndrome (MAIDS) model indicate that ddCTP encapsulated in liposomes can reduce proviral DNA in cells of the MPS in both spleen and bone marrow. Rao and co-workers, 1999 in a series of studies revealed the fate of liposome protein after being uptaken by bone marrow derived macrophages. As it is known that major histocompatibility complex (MHC) class I molecules found on antigen-presenting cells present peptides derived from cytoplasmic proteins to T cells. In contrast, peptides from exogenous proteins are mostly presented by class II molecules. It has been well established that liposomes can serve as an efficient delivery system for entry of exogenous protein antigens into the MHC class I pathway. Rao et al., 1999 utilized fluorophore-labeled proteins encapsulated in liposomes and demonstrated that after phagocytosis of the liposomes by bone marrow-derived macrophages (BMs), the processed peptides were subsequently visualized in the trans-Golgi, while free conalbumin was excluded from the trans-Golgi area. Same workers, 1997, investigated whether liposomal lipids follow the same intracellular route as the liposomal proteins after phagocytosis by BMs.

Multilamellar liposomes with different lipid compositions containing fluorescent phospholipids (empty liposomes) were incubated with murine BMs. Results of the study indicated that although empty liposomes were avidly phagocytosed by macrophages, the fluorescent liposomal lipids did not localize to any particular area of the cell but were distributed throughout the cell. In contrast, when a protein was encapsulated in the liposomes, the liposomal lipids were no longer dispersed throughout the cell, but were concentrated and localized in the trans-Golgi area. Furthermore, when the liposomes contained a fluorescent-labeled protein, the fluorescent peptides also localized in to the trans-Golgi. These results demonstrate that the combination of both liposomal lipids and liposomal protein is required for Golgi-specific targeting of liposomal antigens. Transport of both liposomal lipids and liposomal proteins to the Golgi complex, a major subcellular organelle in the passage of MHC class I molecules, might explain why antigens encapsulated in liposomes readily induce cytotoxic T lymphocytes.

The effect of serum protein on binding and uptake of phosphatidylglycerol, phosphatidylserine, cardiolipin, and N,N-dioleyl-N,N-dimethylammonium chloride (DODAC) containing as well as poly(ethylene glycol) (PEG) containing liposomes by mouse bone marrow macrophages were studied *in vitro*. They reported that serum proteins which adsorb after administration (surface-associated serum proteins) inhibit the uptake of phosphatidylserine and poly(ethylene glycol) liposomes by bone marrow derived macrophages. These reports were quite contrast to earlier reports by Hume and Nayer, 1989 who reported preferential accumulation and bone marrow internalization of vesicles composed of both PE and PS or succinylated PE. In the case of phosphatidylserine liposomes, the bound serum protein can provide a non-specific surface-shielding property that reduces the charge-mediated interactions between liposomes and bone marrow macrophage cells. In addition, incubation of PEG-bearing liposomes with serum can result in a change in the properties of the PEG, resulting in a surface that is better protected against interactions with cells. Table 15-3 summarizes various studies carried out to study bone marrow localization and targeting using liposomes.

PURGING OF BONE MARROW WITH LIPOSOMES

The bone marrow is extracted from the patient prior to transplant and may be "purged" to remove lingering malignant cells (if the disease has afflicted the bone marrow). Purging is a technique used to reduce the number of cancerous cells that may be in bone marrow harvested from certain patients undergoing an autologous BMT. The process reduces the number of cancerous cells in the harvested bone marrow and subsequently the likelihood of relapse after an autologous BMT will be reduced.

Two different purging techniques are used. The first involves "monoclonal antibodies"special proteins that distinguish malignant cells from normal cells and attach to the surface of the malignant cell.

Table 15-3. Various Studies of Bone Marrow Localization and Targeting using Liposomal Systems

System investigated	Inference	Reference
Stilbogluconate loaded liposomes and niosomes	Failure to reach therapeutic concentration at bone marrow in *Leishmania donovani* infected BALB/c mice	Carter et al., 1989
Cholesterol-poor and cholesterol-rich liposomes	Opsonophagocytosis of liposomes by bone marrow reticuloendothelial cells	Moghimi and Patel, 1992
Liposomes composed of macrophage activating alkyl-lysophospholipids	Liposomally activated bone marrow macrophages; subsequent interaction with L1210 leukaemic cells	Luckenbach and Layton , 1981
Stilbogluconate loaded niosomes	Improve parasite suppression in the liver, spleen and bone marrow	Williams et al., 1995
Liposome-loaded with dichloromethylene diphosphonate (Cl2MDP)	Decrease in total number of bone marrow macrophages; Serve as a model for studying the role of macrophages in erythropoiesis	Giuliani et al., 2001
Fluorophore-labeled proteins encapsulated in liposomes; fluorescent liposomal lipids	Trafficking of liposomal antigen to the trans-Golgi area of bone marrow macrophages through MHC-I pathway, requires both liposomal lipid and liposomal protein	Rao et al. , 1997, 1999
Liposome encapsulated synthetic analogs of muramyldipeptide	Stimulation of haemopoiesis (through cytokine production) and radio-protection in subsequently irradiated mouse	Turanek et al., 1997
Macrophage activator muramyl tripeptide phosphatidylethanolamine encapsulated in liposomes	Administration of MTP-PE/MLV (24 h) to mouse prior to irradiation exerted radioprotective effect and haemopoietic recovery in irradiated mouse	Fedorocko, 1994
Carboplatin loaded liposomes	Stimulation of hematopoiesis during or after the treatment with radiation or chemotherapy	Fichtner et al., 1993
γ- interferon associated with liposomes composed of phosphatidylethanolamine (PE) and phosphatidylserine (PS)	Bone marrow internalization of vesicles composed of both PE and PS or succinylated PE with subsequent improvement of the therapeutic potential of gamma interferon	Hume and Nayar, 1989

These "marked" malignant cells are then broken apart with additional proteins called "complement" or "immunotoxins". Alternatively, small magnetic beads or "microspheres" are coated with the monoclonal antibodies and mixed with the bone marrow. The marrow is then passed over electromagnets, which remove the microspheres and malignant cells to which they have become attached.

A second technique is chemical or pharmacological purging. The bone marrow is incubated with chemicals more toxic to cancerous cells than normal cells. The marrow is then transplanted into the patient. Generally purging of bone marrow harvested from patients with leukaemia is done before an autologous transplant.

Recently, though drug delivery systems have been adopted to affect purging of bone marrow during transplantation. Morgan et al., 1992 reported the use of photosensitive, antibody directed liposomes to destroy target populations of cells in bone marrow as a potential purging method for autologous bone marrow transplantation.

Liposomes containing the photosensitive dye, sulphonated aluminium phthalocyanine (AlSPc) were coupled to polyclonal sheep anti-mouse-Ig antibody and bound to cells coated with specific mouse monoclonal antibody. When illuminated with red light, the AlSPc in the liposomes was activated to produce singlet oxygen and the antibody and liposome targeted cells were destroyed. DW-BCL cells (an *Epstein barr* virus immortalized B-cell line) were targeted with an anti-B-cell antibody and killed specifically, both alone and in the presence of bone marrow mononuclear cells (BM-cells), without phototoxic effects on the untargeted bone marrow CFU-GM progenitor cells. Similar results were obtained on T-lymphocytes as target cells using anti-CD3 antibody.

MONOCLONAL ANTIBODIES AND IMMUNOCONJUGATES FOR *EX VIVO* DRUG DELIVERY

Monoclonal antibodies coupled to drugs and toxic agents (immunotoxins) or radionuclides (radio-immunoconjugates) represent new tools for immuno-therapy of haematological malignancies (Falini et al., 1997). The main problems with immunotoxin therapy remain the inability of immunotoxins to target tumour cells in the presence of a high burden of disease, the host immune response against both the antibody and the toxin moieties, which precludes repeated administration of immunotoxins, and the vascular leak syndrome.

Targeting of tumour cells with specific antibodies armed with radionuclides (usually iodine-131 or yttrium-90) appears to be an even more attractive approach. Preliminary clinical studies have clearly demonstrated the ability of radioimmuno-conjugates, especially when administered at high dose followed by bone marrow rescue, to induce durable complete remission in patients with non-Hodgkin's lymphomas refractory to conventional therapies. Radioimmuno-therapy also overcomes the antigenic heterogeneity of the tumour cell population, since antigen negative tumour cells will be irradiated by the nearby targeted antigen-positive cells. Efforts should now be focused on defining more precisely the optimal clinical setting for administration of immunotoxin and radioimmunoconjugates (e.g. minimal residual disease), to reduce the immuno-genicity of these compounds and solve the problem of vascular leak syndrome. Traditional chemotherapy for acute leukaemia often causes life-threatening toxic effects due to a lack of specificity for haematopoietic cells. Monoclonal antibodies and fusion proteins that target cell surface antigens on leukaemic blasts are being evaluated for their cytotoxic effects and as a means of delivering chemotherapeutic agents or radiation directly to malignant cells. It is hoped that this strategy might selectively ablate malignant cells without many of the toxic effects commonly associated with conventional chemotherapy. In acute myeloid leukaemia (AML), the cell surface antigens CD33 and CD45 are especially suitable targets (Sievers, 2000). Although CD33 is expressed on AML blast cells from about 90% of patients, normal haematopoietic stem cells lack this antigen, as do essentially all nonhaematopoietic tissues. For that reason, anti-CD33 antibodies have been created to target malignant myeloid and immature normal cells selectively while sparing normal stem cells. Anti-CD33 antibodies have also been used to deliver radiation or a cytotoxic agent directly to leukaemic cells. Since the vast majority of leukaemias and normal stem cells express the cell surface antigen CD45, another targeting approach allows the delivery of myeloablative radiation to bone marrow and spleen, common sites of leukaemic involvement. Consequently, ^{131}I-labeled anti-CD45 antibody has been combined with traditional preparative regimens for patients receiving bone marrow transplantation for acute leukaemia.

Finally, fusion proteins such as that combining diphtheria toxin with granulocyte-macrophage colony-stimulating factor (GM-CSF) to target the GM-CSF receptor are now being evaluated in clinical trials. Both unconjugated and conjugated antibodies have shown promise in early clinical trials, and may represent appealing therapeutic alternatives for patients with AML.

Humanized monoclonal anti-CD20 has impressive activity with radioimmunoconjugates (Longo, 1996). Monoclonal antibodies (Mabs) and radioimmunoconjugates targeting B-cell differen-tiation antigens have emerged as promising new treatments for patients with relapsed non-Hodgkin's lymphoma) (Johnson and Press, 2000).

Bone marrow transplantation is currently used to treat a variety of life-threatening diseases. Its applications could be expanded if the risks of graft-versus-host disease (GVHD), a complex pathologic disease, could be reduced. Immunotoxins may provide a means to control drug refractory GVHD (Vallera, 1996).

DIAGNOSTIC IMAGING OF BONE MARROW USING RADIOLABELLED PARTICULATES

Carrier systems like liposomes and nanoparticles containing the paramagnetic contrast agent manganese chloride were shown to selectively enhance the intensity of the proton NMR signal from the livers of experimental mice. This may be due to their rapid removal from the circulation and deposition in high concentration within the RES-rich organs (liver, spleen and bone marrow). This process is known to involve the phagocytic activity of macrophages. It may also be possible to use these carriers to selectively deliver contrast agents to tissue regions of developing pathology that are rich in macrophage activity. In recent years, scintigraphic studies with radiolabeled microparticles (RMIPs) have been declined due to increasing amount of molecular (nanoparticulate) radiopharmaceuticals. However, RMIPs are indispensable in nuclear medicine because diagnostic procedures such as lung perfusion and RES studies (liver, spleen and bone marrow imaging) can not entirely be performed with non-particulate radiopharmaceuticals. Recently, there is also great interest in biodegradable RMIPs, and liposomes and poly(lactic acid) microspheres are likely to establish themselves among other radiopharmaceuticals in nuclear medicine. Bone marrow scintigraphy is used to evaluate bone marrow infarcts, diffuse benign or malignant infiltration, focal metastases, benign and malignant haematological disorders and infection and inflammatory disorders.

Different RMIPs visualize different cellular components of normal bone marrow, i.e., erythropoietic precursor cells, granulopoietic bone marrow or reticuloendothelial system. Therefore, any disorder altering the normal bone marrow tissue can be detected by scintigraphy with a specific radiolabeled microparticulate or molecular system (Table 15-4).

Presently, the most commonly used bone marrow imaging agent is ^{99m}Tc-sulphur colloid (^{99m}Tc-SC) with varying particle sizes in the range of 100 nm-1 µm. About 5% of the injected dose is taken up by RES of bone marrow, with considerable liver and spleen accumulation. This may cause an obscure scintigraphy of thoracic and abdominal spine activities and hence shielding of liver and spleen is necessary to visualize these organs. ^{99m}Tc-nanocolloid is a colloidal serum albumin (nanoparticles, <80 nm) which reportedly accumulate in bones (1-20 %) as compared to accumulation of ^{99m}Tc-SC particles (~5%). Although accumulation of albumin nanoparticles in liver and spleen is relatively lower than that of ^{99m}Tc-SC, it is still sufficient to obscure thoracic and lumber bone marrow (Fig. 15-14).

Nanoparticulate (molecular) radiopharmaceuticals used for bone marrow imaging include ^{52}Fe-ferric chloride, ^{111}In-indium chloride. ^{111}In-WBC, ^{99m}Tc-WBC and ^{99m}Tc-NCA95-leukocytes are also used for bone marrow imaging. *In vivo* labeling by ^{99m}Tc-labeled monoclonal antibodies directed against granulocyte and recently by radio-iodinated antibodies against CD33 antigen has also been reported for bone marrow targeting. The ability to track the distribution and differentiation of progenitor and stem cells by high-resolution *in vivo* imaging techniques would have significant clinical and research implications. Lewin and co-workers, 2000 developed a cell labeling approach using short HIV-Tat peptides to derivatize superparamagnetic

Table 15-4. Different Radiopharmaceuticals Used for Bone Marrow Imaging, and Their Localization in Specific Bone Marrow Components

Radiotracer	Type	Particle size (µm)	Bone marrow component
^{99m}Tc-sulphur colloid	Particulate	0.1-1	RES
^{99m}Tc-nanocolloid	Particulate	<0.080	RES
^{52}Fe-ferric chloride	Molecular	-	Erythropoietic cells
^{111}In-indium chloride	Molecular	-	General
^{111}In-WBC	Cells	7-10	RES
^{99m}Tc-WBC	Cells	7-10	RES
^{99m}Tc-NCA95-leukocytes	Cells	7-10	Granulopoietic cells

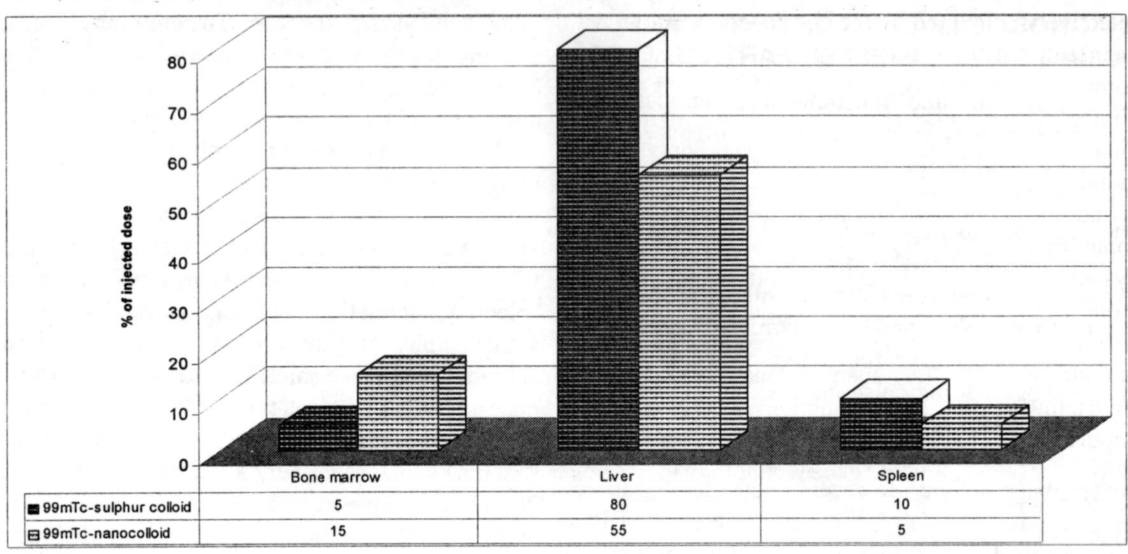

Fig. 15-14. Accumulation of ^{99m}Tc-sulphur Colloid and ^{99m}Tc-nanocolloid in Bone Marrow, Liver and Spleen

nanoparticles. The particles were efficiently internalized into haematopoietic and neural progenitor cells in quantities up to 10-30 picogram of superparamagnetic iron per cell. Iron incorporation did not affect cell viability, differentiation, or proliferation of CD34+ cells. Following intravenous injection into immunodeficient mice, 4% of magnetically CD34+ cells homed to bone marrow per gram of tissue, and single cell could be detected by magnetic resonance (MR) imaging in tissue samples. Localization and retrieval of cell populations *in vivo* enable detailed analysis of specific stem cell and organ interactions critical for advancing the therapeutic use of stem cells.

Remarkable progress has been made in the last 5 years in the use of gene therapy for the treatment of inherited diseases and acquired disorders of bone marrow with the use of genetically modified haematopoietic cells (Schmidt-Wolf and Schmidt-Wolf, 1995).

All gene therapy strategies have two essential technical requirements. These are :

1. The efficient introduction of the relevant genetic material into the target cell, and
2. The expression of the transgene at therapeutic levels.

To date, the most widely used and best understood vectors for gene transfer in haematopoietic cells are derived from retroviruses, although they suffer from several limitations. However, as gene transfer mechanisms become more efficient and long-term gene expression is enhanced, the variety of diseases that can be tackled by gene therapy will continue to expand.

Existing modes of gene therapy can restrain the replication of pathogenic microorganisms, can eliminate defective cells, and can increase the resistance of normal cells to drugs harmful to them (e.g., certain anticancer agents). For example the Multiple Drug Resistance (MDR) gene enables production of a protein that removes various foreign chemicals from cells. Introduction of the MDR gene into the bone-marrow cells of patients with advanced cancer seems safe and may protect their bone marrow from the toxic side effects of chemotherapy. It may thus make high-dose chemotherapy safer and improve recovery (Fredric and Steinberg, 1998).

Suicide gene therapy is one of several gene therapeutic approaches demonstrated to treat bone marrow derived cancer (Dilber and Gahrton, 2001). A suicide gene is a gene encoding a protein, frequently an enzyme, that in itself is nontoxic to the genetically modified cell. However, when a cell is exposed to a specific nontoxic prodrug, this is selectively converted by the gene product into toxic metabolites that kill the cell. The suicide gene most commonly employed, both in experimental and a clinical settings, is *Herpes simplex* Virus thymidine kinase (HSVtk). Some suicide gene products also induce a so-called 'bystander effect', i.e. a toxic effect on adjacent nongene modified tumour cells and sometimes also on more distant tumour cells. The bystander effect is most evident in tumour cells that have a high number of gap junctions, cellular channels build up by proteins called connexins. Many tumours, amongst them many haematological ones, have a low number of gap junctions. Therefore, it is important to develop gap junction independent drug delivery systems. Suicide gene technology may also be used for the *ex vivo* purging of tumour cells in bone marrow or peripheral blood stem cell autografts or for inactivation of effector cells, such as antitumour T donor lymphocytes in allogeneic transplantation to prevent severe graft versus host reactions. New constructs, e.g. combining suicide genes and immune response enhancing genes or suicide genes and connexin inducing genes may further improve the pharmacodynamic effects of suicide gene therapy.

BONE MARROW TRANSPLANTATION USING CYTOSTATIC DRUG LOADED CARRIERS

The main cause of failures during allogeneic bone marrow transplantation is the development of graft versus host reactions. The methods of its prevention and treatment include the use of large doses of human toxic cytostatics and immuno-suppressants aimed against donor immuno-competent cells. A way of preventing the adverse effects of cytostatics are targeted transport of long-acting cytostatic dosage forms to an organ or target cell using carriers, such as liposomes, microcapsules, microspheres and their conjugates with monoclonal antibodies.

Pan'ko and co-workers, 2000 used gelatin and gum arabic microspheres containing the immunosuppressive cytostatic adriamycin to enhance the efficiency of cytostatic depositing at the site of transplantation. The approach not only deposits the agent, but substantially increases the proportion of donor cells localization at the site of grafting as compared to the intravenous and intraosseous infusion of donor cells. The main advantage of use of carrier systems for allogenous bone marrow transplantation in combination with a long-acting cytostatic dosage form can be inhibited by using adriamycin in subtherapeutic dosages.

Busulphan is an alkylating agent currently used in conditioning regimen prior to stem cell transplantation (SCT). High dose therapy with busulphan has been shown to contribute to transplantation-related toxicities. The distributions of liposomal busulphan was higher to bone marrow and spleen, and lower to brain, lung and heart, compared with free drug, while the distribution to liver was similar. Liposomal busulphan was found suitable formulation for high dose treatment in conditioning regimen prior to stem cell transplantation (Hassan et al., 1998; Hassan et al., 2000).

ANTIGEN PRESENTATION TO BONE MARROW

Tkaczyk and co-workers, 1998 reported that specific antigen targeting to surface IgE and IgG on mouse bone marrow-derived mast cells enhances efficiency of antigen presentation. Since this was earlier known that bone marrow-derived mast cells can express major histocompatibility complex class II molecules and act as antigen-presenting cells. They evaluated when antigen is internalized through fluid-phase endocytosis or via specific uptake by using IgG and IgE antibodies. These workers concluded that tissue distribution and strategic location of mast cells at the mucosal barriers and their capacity to process the antigen through efficient fluid-phase pinocytosis as well as IgG- and IgE-dependent targeting of antigens provides mast cells with a prominent role in immune surveillance.

Krishan and co-workers, 2001 reported vesicles composed of glycerolipids of archaea (archaeosomes) with potent adjuvant activity. These workers studied the effect of archaeosomes on APCs to elucidate the mechanism(s) of adjuvant action. Exposure of bone marrow derived macrophages to archaeosomes *in vitro* resulted in up-regulation of MHC class II molecules to an extent comparable to that achieved with lipopolysaccharides.. In contrast, conventional liposomes made from ester phospholipids failed to modulate the expression of these activation markers.

APCs treated with archaeosomes exhibited increased TNF production and functional ability to stimulate allogenic T cell proliferation. More interestingly, archaeosomes enhanced APC recruitment and activation *in vivo*. The activation of APCs correlated to the ability of archaeosomes to induce strong humoral, T helper, and CTL responses to entrapped antigen. Thus, the recruitment and activation of professional APCs by archaeosomes constitutes an efficient self-adjuvanting process for induction of Antigen-specific responses to encapsulated Antigens.

Encapsulation of 1-Adamantylamide-L-alanyl-D-isoglutamine (adamantylamide dipeptide, AdDP) belongs to a group of desmuramyl muramyl peptide derivatives (which are able to protect an organism from some viral infections) has been reported to provide stimulation of nonspecific immunity, haemopoiesis and protection of mice against radiation injury. Thus the system could be therapeutically beneficial to moderate the haemopoietic damage (undesirable effect of radiotherapy or chemotherapy) and induce the non-specific immunity to support the antimicrobial treatment of immuno-compromised patients.

FUTURE TRENDS

Benoit and co-workers, 1997a,b reported vancomycin -loaded plaster of Paris implants coated with poly lactide-co-glycolide as a controlled release delivery system for the treatment of bone infections. In all bone tissues (bone marrow and cortical bone) surrounding the implanted pellets, the drug concentration exceeded MIC for the common causative organisms of bone infections (*Staphylococcus aureus*) and thus system appears to be a promising sustained release delivery system of antibiotics for the treatment of bone and joint infections.

Recently, the use of biopolymers as a culture vehicle for mesenchymal progenitor cells has been advocated. Radice et al., 2000 reported hyaluronan-based biopolymers as delivery vehicles for bone-marrow-derived mesenchymal progenitors. The proliferation patterns and extracellular matrix production of rabbit and human mesenchymal, bone-marrow-derived progenitors first were characterized *in vitro*. Subsequently, rabbit autologous cells were cultured in the hyaluronan-based scaffold and implanted in a full-thickness osteochondral lesion. *In vitro* histologic findings showed that mesenchymal progenitor cells adhered and proliferated onto the hyaluronan-derived scaffold.

Haematopoietic stem cells (HSC) are able to reconstitute the haematopoietic system in disease-related bone marrow failure and bone marrow aplasia. Nowadays, HSC can be mobilized from the bone marrow into the peripheral blood using haematopoietic cytokines, allowing a convenient harvesting of these cells for clinical transplantation (Gunsilius et al., 2001).

REFERENCES

Allen T. M. and Chonn A. (1987) *FEBS Lett.* **223**, 42.

Allen et al. (1989) *Biochim. Biophys. Acta* **981**, 27

Benoit M. A., Mousset B., Delloye C., Bouillet R., Gillard J. Vandorpe J., Schacht E., Dunn S., Hawley A., Stolnik S, Davis S. S., Garnett, M. C., Davies M. C. and Illum L. (1997a) *Biomaterials* **18**, 1147.

Benoit M. A., Mousset B., Delloye C., Bouillet R., Gillard J. (1997b) *Int. Orthop.* **21**, 403.

Biozzi G., Benacerraf B. and Halpern B. N. (1953) *Br. J. Exp. Pathol.* **34**, 441.

Blagoeva P. M., Balansky R. M., Mircheva T. J. and Simeonova M. I. (1992) *Mutat. Res.* **268**, 77.

Bradfield J. W. B. (1984) In: Microspheres and Drug Therapy Davis, S.S, et al.(Eds.) Elsevier Science, Amsterdom 25.

Carter K.C., Dolan T.F., Alexander J., Baillie A.J. and McColgan C. (1989) *J. Pharm. Pharmacol.* **41**, 87.

Dilber M. S., Gahrton G. (2001) *J. Intern. Med.* **249**, 359.

Falini B., Terenzi, A., Liso A., Flenghi L., Solinas A. and Pasqualucci L. (1997) *Cancer Surv.* **30**, 295.

Fedorocko P. (1994) *Int. J. Radiat. Biol.* **65**, 465.

Fichtner I., Reszka R., Schutt M., Rudolph M., Becker M., Lemm M., Richter J. and Berger I. (1993) *Oncol. Res.* **5**, 65.

Fidler I. J. (1980) *Science* **208**, 1469.

Fredric M. and Steinberg J. (1998) *Pharm. Pharmaceut. Sci.* **1**, 48.

Gibaud S., Demoy M., Andreux J. P., Weingarten C., Gouritin B. and Couvreur P. (1996) *J. Pharm. Sci.* **85**, 944.

Gibaud S., Rousseau C., Weingarten C., Favier R., Douay L., Andreux J.P. and Couvreur P. (1998) *J. Control. Rel.* **2**, 131.

Gibaud S., Weingarten C., Andreux J.P. and Couvreur P. (1999) *Ann. Pharm. Fr.* **57**, 324.

Giuliani A. L., Wiener E., Lee M. J., Brown, I. N., Berti G. and Wickramasinghe S. N. (2001) *Eur. J. Haematol.* **66**, 221.

Griffin F. M. Jr. (1977) Comprehensive immunology, 2, Plenum Press, New York, 85.

Gunsilius E., Gastl G. and Petzer A. L. (2001) *Biomed. Pharmacother.* **55**, 186.

Hassan Z., Ljungman P., Ringdén O., Winiarski J., Nilsson C., Aschan J. and Rosengren Whitley H., (2000) *Bone Marrow Transplant* **27**, 579.

Hassan Z., Nilsson C. and Hassan M. (1998) *Bone Marrow Transplant* **22**, 913.

Heller C. H. (1992) Life: The Science of Biology. Sinaur Associates Inc., Utah, 1.

Hume D. A. and Nayar R. (1989) *Lymphokine Res.* **8**, 415.

Illum L. and Davis S. S. (1987) *Life Sci.* **20**, 1553.

Illum L., Davis S .S., Wilson C. G., Thomas N., Frier M. and Hardy J. G. (1982) *Int. J. Pharm.* **12**, 135.

Johnson T. A. and Press O. W. (2000) *Ann. Haematol.* **79**, 175.

Kadowaki S., Sugimoto K., Tsurumaki Y., Tabata Y., Ikada Y., Fujita J. and Mori K. J. (1993) *Biomed. Pharmacother.* **47**, 385.

Kanke M., Simmons G. H., Weiss D. L., Bivins B. A. and Deluca P. P. (1980) *J. Pharm. Sci.* **69**, 755.

Krishnan L., Sad S., Patel G. B. and Sprott G. D. (2001) *J. Immunol.* **166**, 1885.

Lewin M., Carlesso N., Tung C. H., Tang X. W., Cory D., Scadden D. T. and Weissleder R. (2000) *Nat. Biotechnol.* **18**, 410.

Longo D. L. (1996) *Curr. Opin. Oncol.* **8**, 353.

Lu L., Yaszemski M. J. and Mikos A. G. (2001) *J. Bone Joint Surg. Am.* **83**, S82.

Luckenbach G. A. and Layton D. (1981) *Int. J. Cancer* **15**, 837.

Marra K. G., Szem J. W., Kumta P. N., DiMilla P. A. and Weiss L. E. (1999) *J. Biomed. Mater. Res.* **47**, 324.

Mercadal M., Domingo J. C., Petriz J., Garcia J. and de Madariaga M. A. (2000) *Biochim. Biophys. Acta* **1509**, 299.

Moghimi S. M., Illum L. and Davis S. S. (1990) *Crit. Rev. Ther. Drug Carrier Syst.* **7**, 187.

Moghimi S. M. and Patel H.M. (1992) *Biochim. Biophys. Acta* **1135**, 269.

Morgan J., MacRobert A. J., Gray A. G. and Huehns E. R. (1992) *Br. J. Cancer* **65**, 58.

Nefzger M., Kreuter J., Voges R., Liehl E. and Czok R. (1984) *J. Pharm. Sci.* **73**, 1309.

Oussoren C., Magnani M., Fraternale A., Casabianca A., Chiarantini L., Ingebrigsten R., Underberg W. J. and Storm G. (1999) *Int. J. Pharm.* **180**, 261.

Pan'ko S. V., Antipov I. G., Semenido I. N., Sosnovskaia O. I., Golovanova T. A. and Sanin A. V. (2000) *Vestn Ross Akad Med Nauk* **3**, 10.

Pea F., Russo D., Michieli M., Baraldo M., Ermacora A., Damiani D., Baccarani M. and Furlanut M. (2000) *Cancer Chemother. Pharmacol.* **46**, 279.

Porter C. J., Moghimi S. M., Illum L. and Davis S. S. (1992) *FEBS Lett.* **305**, 62.

Radice M., Brun P., Cortivo R., Scapinelli R., Battaliard C., Abatangelo G. (2000) *J. Biomed. Mater. Res.* **50**, 101.

Rao M., Rothwell S. W., Wassef N. M., Koolwal A. B, Alving C. R. (1999) *Exp. Cell Res.* **246**, 203.

Rao M., Rothwell S. W., Wassef N. M., Pagano R. E. and Alving C. R. (1997) *Immunol. Lett.* **59**, 99.

Schmidt-Wolf G. D. and Schmidt-Wolf I. G. (1995) *J. Haematother.* **4**, 551.

Sievers E. L. (2000) *Cancer Chemother. Pharmacol.* **46** Suppl, S18.

Tkaczyk C., Viguier M., Boutin Y., Frandji P., David B., Hebert J. and Mecheri S. (1998) *Immunology* **94**, 318.

Tomlinson E., Burger J. J., Mevie J. G. and Hoefnagel K. (1984) In: Recent advances in drug delivery systems, Anderson J. H. and Kim J. W. (Eds.), Plenum Press, New York, 199.

Turanek J., Zaluska D., Hofer M., Vacek A., Ledvina M. and Jezek J. (1997) *Int. J. Immunopharmacol.* **19**, 611.

Vallera D. A. *Semin. (1996) Cancer Biol.* **7**, 57.

Van Furth, R. (1981) In: Disorders of the monocyte macrophage system, Schmalzl F. (Eds.) Springer-Verlag, Dermstadt, 3.

Vandorpe J., Schacht E., Dunn S., Hawley A., Stolnik S., Davis S. S., Garnett M.C., Davies M. C. and Illum L. (1997) *Biomaterials* **18**, 1147.

Wichramasinghe S. N. (1975) Human Bone Marrow. Blackwell, Oxford, 1.

Williams D. M., Carter K. C. and Baillie A. J. (1995) *J. Drug Target.* **3**, 1.

Yoffey T. and Tavassol P. S. (1983) Bone Marrow: Structure and Function, Alan R. Liss Inc., New York, 1.

Index

C

D

E

F

G

H

I

L

M

N

O

P

R

S